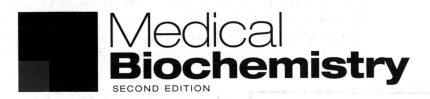

Medical
Biochemistry
SECOND EDITION

John W Baynes • Marek H Dominiczak

Medical
Biochemistry

SECOND EDITION

John W Baynes PhD
Carolina Distinguished Professor
  Department of Chemistry and Biochemistry,
  and School of Medicine
  University of South Carolina
  Columbia, South Carolina, USA

Marek H Dominiczak MD FRCPath FRCP(Glasg) FACB
Consultant Chemical Pathologist
  NHS Greater Glasgow
  Western Infirmary and Gartnavel General Hospital;
  Honorary Clinical Senior Lecturer
  University of Glasgow, UK;
  Docent in Laboratory Medicine
  University of Turku, Finland

ELSEVIER
MOSBY

Philadelphia • Edinburgh • London • New York • Oxford • St Louis • Sydney • Toronto • 2005

An imprint of Elsevier Limited

Commissioning Editor:	Alex Stibbe
Project Development Manager:	Duncan Fraser
Project Manager:	Glenys Norquay
Illustration Manager:	Mick Ruddy
Designer:	Stewart Larking
Illustrator:	Tim Loughhead and Antbits Illustration

First published 1999
Reprinted 2001, 2002, 2003
Second edition 2005
Reprinted 2005

ISBN 0 7234 3341 0

British Library Cataloguing in Publication Data
A catalogue record for this book is available from the British Library

Library of Congress Cataloging in Publication Data
A catalog record for this book is available from the Library of Congress

---

Notice

Medical knowledge is constantly changing. Standard safety precautions must be followed, but as new research and clinical experience broaden our knowledge, changes in treatment and drug therapy may become necessary r appropriate. Readers are advised to check the most current product information provided by the manufactactureer of each drug to be administered to verify the recommended dose, the method and duration of administration, and contraindications. It is the responsibility of the practitioner, relying on experience and knowledge of the patient, to determine dosages and the best treatment for each individual patient. Neither the Publisher nor the editors assume any liability for any injury and/or damage to persons or property arising from this publication.

The Publisher

ELSEVIER your source for books, journals and multimedia in the health sciences

www.elsevierhealth.com

Working together to grow libraries in developing countries

www.elsevier.com | www.bookaid.org | www.sabre.org

ELSEVIER   BOOK AID International   Sabre Foundation

Printed in China
Last digit is the print number: 9 8 7 6 5 4 3 2

The publisher's policy is to use **paper manufactured from sustainable forests**

Contents

List of Contributors xi
Preface to First Edition xiii
Preface to Second Edition xv
Dedication xvi

1. Introduction 1
J W Baynes and M H Dominiczak
The value of biochemistry 1
How this book tells the story of biochemistry 1

2. Amino Acids and Proteins 7
N Taniguchi
Introduction 7
Amino acids 7
Buffers 12
Peptides and proteins 12
Purification and characterization of proteins 16
Analysis of protein structure 21
Protein folding and folding disease 23

3. Blood: Cells and Plasma Proteins . . . 25
W D Fraser
Introduction 25
Plasma and serum 25
Formed elements of blood 25
Plasma proteins 26
The acute phase response and C-reactive protein
   (CRP) 32

4. Oxygen Transport 35
G M Helmkamp
Introduction 35
Structure of the heme prosthetic group 35
Characteristics of mammalian globin proteins 36
Recently identified vertebrate globins 43
Insights from myoglobin knockout mice 44
Interactions of hemoglobin with nitric oxide 44
Normal hemoglobin variants 45
Sickle cell disease 45
Other hemoglobinopathies 47

5. Catalytic Proteins–Enzymes 51
J Fujii
Introduction 51
Enzymatic reactions 51
Enzyme kinetics 55

Enzyme inhibition 57
Regulation of enzyme activity 59

6. Hemostasis and Thrombosis 63
G Lowe
Introduction 63
Hemostasis 63
The vessel wall 65
Platelets 66
Coagulation 69
Fibrinolysis 74

7. Membranes and Transport 77
M Maeda
Introduction 77
Membrane lipids 77
Composition of biomembranes 78
Types of transport processes 80

8. Bioenergetics and Oxidative
   Metabolism 93
L W Stillway
Introduction 93
Oxidation as a source of energy 93
Free energy 94
Conservation of energy by coupling with ATP 95
Mitochondrial synthesis of ATP from reduced
   coenzymes 96
The mitochondrial electron transport system 97
The ATP-synthetic proton gradient 102
P:O ratios and respiratory control 105
Inhibitors of oxidative metabolism 106
Regulation of oxidative phosphorylation 110

9. Function of the Gastrointestinal
   Tract 113
I Broom
Introduction 113
The mechanical and anatomical basis of digestion . . . 113
General principles of digestion 115
Digestion and absorption of carbohydrates 116
Digestion and absorption of lipids 120
The pancreas 120
Digestion and absorption of proteins 123

10. Micronutrients: Vitamins and Minerals 127
M H Dominiczak and I Broom

Introduction 127
Fat-soluble vitamins 128
Water-soluble vitamins 133
Trace elements 139

11. Anaerobic Metabolism of Glucose in the Red Blood Cell 143
J W Baynes

Introduction 143
The erythrocyte 143
Glycolysis 144
Synthesis of 2,3-bisphosphoglycerate 150
The pentose phosphate pathway 150
Concentrations of redox coenzymes in the cell 151

12. Carbohydrate Storage and Synthesis in Liver and Muscle 157
J W Baynes

Introduction 157
Structure of glycogen 157
Pathway of glycogenesis from blood glucose in liver 158
Pathway of glycogenolysis in liver 159
Hormonal regulation of hepatic glycogenolysis 160
Mechanism of action of glucagon 160
Mobilization of hepatic glycogen by epinephrine 163
Glycogenolysis in muscle 164
Regulation of glycogenesis 165
Gluconeogenesis 167

13. The Tricarboxylic Acid Cycle 175
L W Stillway

Introduction 175
Energy production in the TCA cycle 175
Biosynthesis linked to TCA cycle 175
Pyruvate carboxylase 177
The pyruvate dehydrogenase complex (PDC) 178
Enzymes and reactions of the TCA cycle 180
Energy yield from the TCA cycle 184
Regulation of the TCA cycle 184
Anaplerotic ('filling up') reactions 186

14. Oxidative Metabolism of Lipids in Liver and Muscle 189
J W Baynes

Introduction 189
Activation of fatty acids and their transport to the mitochondrion 189
Oxidation of fatty acids 190
Ketogenesis in liver 194

15. Biosynthesis and Storage of Fatty Acids in Liver and Adipose Tissue 199
I Broom

Introduction 199
Fatty acid synthesis 199
Fatty acid elongation 202
Desaturation of fatty acids 203
Essential fatty acids 203
Storage and transport of fatty acids: the synthesis of triacylglycerols 203
Regulation of total body fat stores 204

16. Biosynthesis of Cholesterol and Steroids 209
M H Dominiczak and G Beastall

Introduction 209
Cholesterol structure 209
Free and esterified cholesterol 209
Cholesterol biosynthesis 216
Bile acids 217
Cholesterol excretion 218
Steroid hormones 218
Vitamin D_3 220

17. Lipids and Lipoproteins 225
M H Dominiczak

Introduction 225
Structure and function of lipoproteins 226
Lipoprotein receptors 230
Measurement of lipoproteins 230
Metabolism of lipoproteins 231
Dyslipidemias 234
Atherogenesis 236
Cardiovascular risk and its assessment 240

18. Biosynthesis and Degradation of Amino Acids 245
A B Rawitch

Introduction 245
Metabolism of the carbon skeletons of amino acids 253
Amino acid biosynthesis 256
Inherited diseases of amino acid metabolism 256
Amino acids as precursors of signaling molecules 259

19. Muscle: Energy Metabolism and Contraction 261
J A Carson and J W Baynes

Introduction 261
Structure of muscle 261
Muscle proteins 263
Muscle energy metabolism 268
Metabolism and muscle contraction 268

20. Glucose Homeostasis, Fuel Metabolism, and Insulin 273
M H Dominiczak
Organ-fuel interactions 273
Glucose homeostasis 274
Insulin 275
Hypoglycemia 278
Metabolism after a meal and in the fasting state 279
Metabolism during stress, and the metabolic response to injury 282
Diabetes mellitus: the principal disorder of fuel metabolism 286
Treatment of diabetes 293
Assessment of fuel metabolism 294

21. Nutrition 299
M H Dominiczak
Introduction 299
Key definitions and recommendations used in nutrition science 299
Nutrition and genetics 299
The main classes of nutrients 301
The essential (limiting) nutrients 303
Water and minerals 303
Energy homeostasis 304
Regulation of food intake 305
Assessment of nutritional status 305
Malnutrition 307
Obesity 308
Diet in health and disease 309
Nutrition and chronic disease 311

22. Water and Electrolyte Balance: Kidney Function 315
M H Dominiczak and M Szczepanska-Konkel
Introduction 315
Water, sodium, and potassium metabolism . . . 315
Osmolality and volume of ECF and ICF 317
The water balance 319
The kidney 319
The importance of plasma potassium concentration . . . 325
The renin–angiotensin system 326
Water reabsorption in the distal tubule and collecting duct 328
Water metabolism and sodium metabolism are interrelated 330

23. Lung and Kidney: The Control of Acid–Base Balance 333
M H Dominiczak and M Szczepanska-Konkel
The body buffer systems 333
The lungs and the gas exchange 336
Kidneys and the handling of bicarbonate 340
Clinical disorders of the acid–base balance . . . 341

24. Calcium and Bone Metabolism 345
W D Fraser
Calcium metabolism 347
Disorders of calcium metabolism and bone . . . 352
Metabolic bone disease 356

25. Complex Carbohydrates: Glycoproteins 359
A D Elbein
Glycoproteins: structures and linkages 359
Interconversions and activation of dietary sugars 362
Other pathways of sugar nucleotide metabolism 365
Biosynthesis of oligosaccharides 366
Functions of the oligosaccharide chains of glycoproteins 369

26. Complex Lipids 375
A D Elbein
Introduction 375
Glycerophospholipids (phospholipids) 375
Sphingolipids 379

27. The Extracellular Matrix 387
G P Kaushal and A D Elbein
Introduction 387
Collagens 387
Noncollagenous proteins in the extracellular matrix . . . 390
Proteoglycans 394

28. Special Liver Function 399
A F Jones
Introduction 399
Structure of the liver 399
Participation of the liver in carbohydrate metabolism . . . 399
Liver and protein metabolism 401
Heme synthesis 403
Bilirubin metabolism 403
Drug metabolism 405
Pharmacogenomics 408
Genomics of liver disease 408
Biochemical tests of liver function 409
Classification of liver disorders 410

29. Biosynthesis and Degradation of Nucleotides 413
R Thornburg
Introduction 413
Purine metabolism 413
Pyrimidine metabolism 417
Formation of deoxynucleotides 421

30. Deoxyribonucleic Acid (DNA) 425
R Thornburg

Introduction 425
Structure of DNA 425
The cell cycle 430

31. Ribonucleic Acid (RNA) 437
G A Bannon

Molecular anatomy of RNA molecules 437
RNA polymerases 439
The process of transcription 440
Post-transcriptional processing 442

32. Protein Synthesis and Turnover 447
G A Bannon

Introduction 447
The genetic code 447
The machinery of protein synthesis 449
The process of protein synthesis 451
Protein targeting and post-translational
    modifications 455

33. Control of Gene Expression 459
D M Hunt and A Jamieson

Introduction 459
Basic mechanisms of gene expression 459
Steroid receptors 464
Alternative approaches to gene regulation in
    humans 465
Gene expression 467

34. Recombinant DNA Technology 473
W S Kistler and A Jamieson

Introduction 473
Hybridization 473
DNA amplification and cloning 480
Specific methods used in the analysis of DNA . . . 485
DNA sequencing 492

35. Oxygen and Life 497
J W Baynes

Introduction 497
The inertness of oxygen 497
Reactive oxygen species (ROS) and oxidative stress
    (OxS) 499
Reactive nitrogen species (RNS) 499
The nature of oxygen radical damage 500
Antioxidant defenses 501

36. The Immune Response 507
A Farrell

Introduction 507
The nonspecific immune response 507
The specific immune response 509
Lymphoid tissues and traffic between them 510
Lymphocytes 511
Molecules involved in antigen recognition 511
The reaction with, the response to, and the
    elimination of, antigens 514
Major histocompatibility complex (MHC) 516
MHC expression patterns and MHC restricted
    stimulation 517
Humoral specific immune response 518
The cellular and molecular elements of the
    integrated immune response 519
Immunologic dysfunction 521

37. Biochemical Endocrinology 523
F F Bolander Jr

Introduction 523
Hormones 523
The hypothalamo–pituitary regulatory system . . . 525
The hypothalamo–pituitary–thyroid axis 526
The hypothalamo–pituitary–adrenal axis 529
The hypothalamo–pituitary–gonadal axis 531
The growth hormone axis 536
The prolactin axis 539

38. Membrane Receptors and Signal
Transduction 541
M M Harnett and H S Goodridge

Introduction 541
Hormone receptors 541
Receptor coupling to intracellular signal
    transduction 542
Second messengers 546

39. Neurochemistry 559
E J Thompson

Introduction 559
Brain and peripheral nerve 559
Cells of the nervous system 560
Synaptic transmission 563
The mechanism of vision 566

40. Neurotransmitters 569
S Heales

Introduction 569
Definitions of a neurotransmitter 569
Classification of neurotransmitters 569
Neurotransmission 570
Various classes of neurotransmitters 573

41. Cell Growth, Differentiation, and Cancer . . . 583
M M Harnett and H S Goodridge

Introduction . . . 583
The cell cycle . . . 583
Growth factors . . . 584
Regulation of the cell cycle . . . 589
Apoptosis . . . 590
Cancer . . . 594

42. Aging . . . 599
J W Baynes

Introduction . . . 599
Theories of aging . . . 601
Aging of muscle – damage to mitochondrial DNA . . . 606
Interventions to delay aging – what works and what doesn't . . . 606
Genetic models of aging . . . 607

Appendix: Reference values and clinical decision limits for laboratory tests . . . 609
M H Dominiczak

Selected serum proteins . . . 609
Blood gases . . . 609
Calcium and phosphate . . . 609

Cerebrospinal fluid . . . 610
Coagulation . . . 610
Electrolytes . . . 610
Endocrine tests . . . 610
Full blood count . . . 610
Glucose and glycated hemoglobin . . . 610
Lipids . . . 611
Liver function . . . 611
Key metabolites . . . 611
Diagnosis of myocardial infarction . . . 611
Neurotransmitters . . . 611
Marker of pancreatitis . . . 611
Trace metals and metal-binding proteins . . . 611
Vitamins . . . 612

Self-assessment

Multiple-choice questions (MCQs) . . . 613
Patient-oriented problems (POPs) . . . 635
Short-answer questions (SAQs) . . . 643
MCQ answers . . . 649
POP answers . . . 651
SAQ answers . . . 655
Abbreviations . . . 665
Index . . . 671

List of Contributors

Gary A Bannon, PhD
Team Leader, Protein Analytics
Regulatory Division
Monsanto
St. Louis, MO, USA

Graham Beastall, PhD FRCPath
Consultant Clinical Scientist
NHS Greater Glasgow
Department of Clinical Biochemistry
Royal Infirmary
Glasgow, UK

Franklyn F Bolander Jr, MD PhD
Associate Professor in Biological
Sciences
Department of Biological Sciences
University of South Carolina
Columbia, SC, USA

**Iain Broom, MBChB MIBiol FRCPath
FRCP**
Research Professor and Consultant in
Clinical Biochemistry and Metabolic
Medicine
The Robert Gordon University
School of Life Sciences
Aberdeen, UK

James A Carson, PhD
Associate Professor
Department of Exercise Science
University of South Carolina
Columbia, SC, USA

Alan D Elbein, PhD
Professor and Chair
Department of Biochemistry and
Molecular Biology
University of Arkansas for Medical
Sciences
Little Rock, AR, USA

Alex Farrell, FRCPath
Consultant Immunologist and Head of
Department of Clinical Immunology,
Immunopathology, Histocompatibility
and Immunogenetics
NHS Greater Glasgow
Western Infirmary;
Honorary Clinical Senior Lecturer
University of Glasgow
Glasgow, UK

**William D Fraser, BSc MD MRCP
FRCPath**
Professor of Clinical Chemistry and
Honorary Consultant
Department of Clinical Chemistry and
Metabolic Medicine
Royal Liverpool University Hospital
Liverpool, UK

Junichi Fujii, PhD
Professor
Department of Biomolecular Function
Graduate School of Medical Science
Yamagata University
Yamagata, Japan

**Peter J Galloway, DCH FRCP (Edin)
MRCPath**
Consultant Chemical Pathologist
NHS Greater Glasgow
Yorkhill Hospital for Sick Children
Glasgow, UK

Helen S Goodridge, BSc PhD
Division of Immunology, Infection and
Inflammation
Western Infirmary
University of Glasgow
Glasgow, UK

Margaret M Harnett, BSc PhD
Professor of Immune Signalling
Division of Immunology, Infection and
Inflammation
Western Infirmary
University of Glasgow
Glasgow, UK

Simon Heales, PhD FRCPath
Consultant Clinical Scientist
Neurometabolic Unit
National Hospital
London, UK

George M Helmkamp Jr, PhD
Professor of Biochemistry
Department of Biochemistry and
Molecular Biology
University of Kansas School of Medicine
Kansas City, KS, USA

Diana M Hunt, BA PhD
Associate Professor
Department of Pathology and
Microbiology
University of South Carolina School of
Medicine
Columbia, SC, USA

**Andrew Jamieson, MBChB (Hons) PhD
FRCP (Glas)**
Consultant Physician
Department of Medicine
Hairmyres Hospital
East Kilbride, UK

Alan F Jones, DPhil FRCP FRCPath
Consultant Physician and Chemical
Pathologist
Department of Clinical Biochemistry
and Immunology
Birmingham Heartlands and Solihull
NHS Trust
Birmingham, UK

Gur P Kaushal, PhD
Associate Professor of Medicine
Department of Medicine
University of Arkansas for Medical
Sciences
Little Rock, AR, USA

W Stephen Kistler, PhD
Professor of Biochemistry
Department of Chemistry
University of South Carolina
Columbia, SC, USA

Gordon Lowe, MD FRCP
Professor of Vascular Medicine
University of Glasgow
University Department of Medicine
Royal Infirmary
Glasgow, UK

Masatomo Maeda, PhD
Professor of Pharmaceutical Sciences
Laboratory of Biochemistry and
Molecular Biology
Graduate School of Pharmaceutical
Sciences
Osaka University
Osaka, Japan

Allen B Rawitch, PhD
Professor of Biochemistry and
Molecular Biology
Department of Biochemistry and
Molecular Biology
University of Kansas Medical Center
Kansas City, KS, USA

Peter F Semple, MD FRCP
Senior Lecturer and Consultant
Physician
Department of Medicine and
Therapeutics
University of Glasgow
Western Infirmary
Glasgow, UK

L William Stillway, PhD
Professor of Biochemistry and
Molecular Biology
Department of Biochemistry and
Molecular Biology
Medical University of South Carolina
Charleston, SC, USA

Mirosława Szczepanska-Konkel, PhD
Professor of Clinical Biochemistry
Laboratory of Pharmacogenetics and
Therapy Monitoring
Medical University of Gdansk
Gdansk, Poland

Naoyuki Taniguchi, MD PhD
Professor and Chair
Department of Biochemistry
Osaka University Medical School
Osaka, Japan

Edward J Thompson, PhD MD DSc
FRCPath FRCP
Professor of Neurochemistry
Department of Neuroimmunology
Institute of Neurology
London, UK

Robert Thornburg, PhD
Professor of Biochemistry
Department of Biochemistry, Biophysics
and Molecular Biology
Iowa State University
Ames, IA, USA

Preface to First Edition

One of the physician's most important skills is the ability to apply basic science in a clinical setting. To help develop this skill, *Medical Biochemistry* combines the chemical, physiologic and pathologic perspectives on human biochemistry.

Anyone involved in medical education has grumbled at some point that, despite the enormous amount of knowledge taught during the preclinical years, students are often unable to recall relevant information or apply it clinically. This is now being addressed in the new medical curricula, which focus on understanding principles rather than ingesting fact after fact.

In the early stages of planning this book, we decided *Medical Biochemistry* would provide students with the biochemistry they need to know when they practice medicine. We have been particular about maintaining scientific rigor and, at the same time, have made conscious decisions to reduce the number of facts irrelevant to clinical practice including the molecular weights of enzyme molecules, thermodynamic parameters of reactions, and the numerous intermediates in some metabolic pathways.

In each chapter core knowledge is enriched by Advanced Concepts which point the reader to new developments or more specialist topics. The information is presented in a clinical context: the core is illustrated by clinical examples to simulate a ward-round environment. Special effort has been made to select cases that illustrate important concepts in metabolism, but also to provide down-to-earth examples of clinical situations that the future physician will confront on a daily basis. For such cases, a problem-solving approach has been taken and clinical laboratory data are given for interpretation. This combination of the metabolic aspects of biochemistry with its application to the diagnosis and monitoring of disease is critical in providing a context for learning biochemistry.

Another issue in medical education is the need to integrate knowledge from separate basic science disciplines. This integration involving molecular, anatomical and physiologic information is essential for developing a perspective on the function of the human body in health and disease. We have avoided presenting biochemistry as a collection of metabolic pathways, which operate in isolated systems. Instead, the reader will find chapters dedicated to the function of the lungs, kidneys and liver, to the regulation of acid-base and electrolyte balance, and to biochemical endocrinology.

All in all, we hope that *Medical Biochemistry* will help students to develop an understanding of biochemistry as an everyday science, a science that is as useful in the laboratory as in the hospital ward or the physician's office.

John W Baynes
Marek H Dominiczak

1999

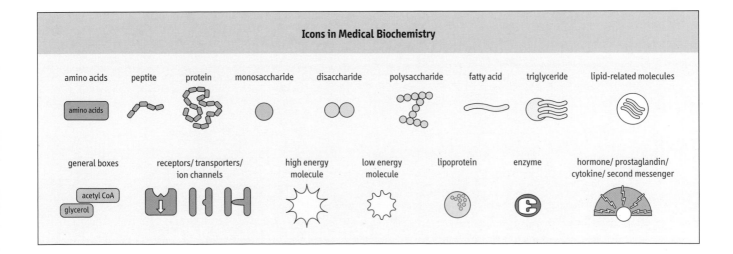

Preface to Second Edition

Biochemistry marches on! Within the five years, since the last edition of *Medical Biochemistry* we have witnessed a massive explosion of knowledge in the biomedical sciences: the sequencing of the human genome; great leaps in technology leading to new fields such as genomics, proteomics, metabolomics and bioinformatics; and development of more powerful diagnostic tools for diagnosis and treatment of disease. The quantity of material to be mastered by the medical student had been a major concern when we worked on the first edition of this book. Now, five years later, our principal challenge remains: to limit the mass of information while including new data important to future doctors. We have made a number of adjustments without changing the philosophy of the book, which is to emphasize a core of biochemical knowledge relevant to the work of a clinician.

The chapters have been thoroughly updated, particularly in the areas of regulatory biology and recombinant DNA; each chapter now contains a set of *Learning Objectives*, which lists the tasks the student should be able to carry out after mastering the material. We have also added information related to laboratory medicine, and included more clinical vignettes designed to develop the habit of applying biochemical data in day-to-day medical practice. Each chapter also now has an *Active Learning* section to facilitate independent study. This is supplemented by updated references and a listing of relevant websites (typically links to educational, organizational and governmental resources). We have also worked with the team at Elsevier to upgrade the content and usefulness online material for both medical students and faculty, and we will continue to improve the web support for this book.

We have added three brand new chapters. One of these focuses on nutrition, an increasingly important issue in a world that, depending on one's economic and geopolitical environment, is either under- or over-nourished. A second new chapter deals with oxidative stress, a pro-inflammatory process now recognized as a ubiquitous factor in the pathogenesis of chronic and age-related diseases, such as diabetes, atherosclerosis, neurodegenerative diseases and arthritis; as populations receive better medical care and grow older, the prevention and treatment of these diseases are becoming even more important in medical practice. The final new chapter, the last in the book, deals with aging itself, the set of chemical and biochemical mechanisms that gradually degrade the performance of the human body – why are there limits and how can they be challenged? With all this, we hope that by presenting the journey from protein chemistry through metabolic pathways, regulatory mechanisms and organ function, to medical genetics, and recombinant DNA technology, we have conveyed the excitement of a dynamic and evolving science that biochemistry is and have made its clinical relevance clearly evident.

Over the last five years – through five printings in English, and translations into Chinese, Greek, Italian and Portuguese – we have learned much from our readers. We are indebted to many students and faculty who have given us feedback, not only in the form of corrections, but also as creative and constructive suggestions. We also thank all the contributing authors, experts in their respective fields – those who contributed to the first edition, the many who remained on board for this new edition, and those who have joined us for the first time. We appreciate their guidance in improving the presentation of existing material and in updating rapidly advancing areas.

As for the others who contributed in many ways, the limits of space do not allow us to mention everyone by name. However, we would like to express our particular gratitude to Dr Peter Semple, consultant physician at the Western Infirmary in Glasgow for scrutinizing all the patient cases from the point of view of their relevance to everyday clinical work, and to Dr Peter Galloway, consultant chemical pathologist at the Yorkhill Hospital in Glasgow who provided many of the pediatric case histories. We are obliged to Dr Mike Wallace for providing the picture of the steroid separation by GC-MS, and to the members of the Dietetic Department at the Western Infirmary in Glasgow, Ms Laurie McFarlane, Mrs Samina Ahmed and Ms Jane Wilson, for many helpful comments on the new nutrition chapter. We are very grateful to Dr J Newman and Dr A Bannerjee from the Birmingham Solihull Hospital for letting us use the images in chapter 28 and to Mr D Galloway, consultant surgeon in Glasgow for allowing us to present the results of his work. We also thank Dr Jeanne Stewart in Columbia for redrawing and standardizing chemical structures, and Ms Jacky Gardiner in Glasgow for her excellent secretarial assistance.

Finally, we greatly appreciate the work of the Elsevier editorial team, particularly Alex Stibbe, Duncan Fraser and Glenys Norquay, whose organizational skills and publishing expertise guided us throughout the preparation of this edition.

John W Baynes
Marek H Dominiczak   2004

Dedication

To my parents John and Marie Baynes, my mentors William J Ruppenthal, Ed Heath and Finn Wold, and my wife Susan Thorpe.
– John W Baynes

To my teachers, H Gemmell Morgan and Stefan Angielski, who showed me how exciting laboratory medicine can be. To Anna, my parents, and to Peter Jacob.
– Marek H Dominiczak

1. Introduction

J W Baynes and M H Dominiczak

THE VALUE OF BIOCHEMISTRY

The study of human biochemistry will open your eyes to how the body works as a chemical system. From a physician's point of view, biochemistry not only describes how the system works, but also provides a foundation for understanding how to improve its operation (e.g. by appropriate nutrition and exercise), how to diagnose problems and, where possible, how to remedy them. Knowing biochemistry helps to understand current therapies, which include recombinant proteins, such as human insulin or erythropoietin synthesized by bacteria. It helps to understand the action of new drugs, such as thiazolidinediones used in type 2 diabetes, which act through cell signaling systems. In the future, therapies will possibly involve gene rather than organ transplants. Pharmacogenomics and nutritional genomics will create a basis for designer treatments, customized to an individual's genetic makeup.

To understand all this it is essential to know something not only about the 'nuts and bolts', but to appreciate functional interactions between metabolic pathways, organs, and tissues. This, in a broad sense, is the realm of physiologic biochemistry, and the scope of this text.

The living organism communicates with its environment

It is useful to consider the human organism from two points of view: as a tightly controlled, internally integrated metabolic system, and as a flexible, open system that communicates with its environment. Interactions between these two are essential for the maintenance of our internal, homeostatic environment. We regularly consume fuel (food) and water, and we constantly take up oxygen from inspired air and transport it to tissues for oxidative metabolism. We use the energy from metabolism of foods to perform work and to maintain body temperature – respiration is in fact a controlled, low-temperature combustion reaction. We exhale or excrete the primary metabolic products, carbon dioxide, and water. Water represents approximately 50% of our total body mass; we control its loss, its electrolyte and metabolite concentrations, and use it as the common medium for biochemical reactions. Carbon dioxide, before elimination, is used for buffering the pH of body fluids.

The amount and composition of food we consume is immensely important for our health, and forms a background for a wide range of treatments and preventive actions. To understand links between nutrients, metabolism, and health and disease, is one of the most important reasons to study biochemistry.

Metabolic processes occur in a variety of spaces within cells

Most metabolism occurs within the complex ecosystem of the cell, in subcellular organelles such as the nucleus, cell membrane, rough and smooth endoplasmic reticulum, Golgi apparatus, mitochondrion, lysosomes, or peroxisomes. Such compartmentalization of metabolic processes is important for several reasons: to protect the organism from autodigestion, to concentrate pathways and metabolites in space, and to enable different pathways, such as synthesis and degradation of proteins, to operate at the same time.

HOW THIS BOOK TELLS THE STORY OF BIOCHEMISTRY

The main pathways of carbohydrate and lipid metabolism are routes of access to other processes in biochemistry

Therefore we start with an introduction to the structure and function of proteins, lipids, and biological membranes. Figure 1.1 is a simplified flow chart giving an overview of human biochemistry. Proteins are the building-blocks and catalysts of biochemical systems: as structural units, they form the architectural framework of our tissues; as enzymes, together with helper molecules known as coenzymes and cofactors, they catalyze and control biochemical reactions. We describe the elements of the homeostatic environment in which human metabolism takes place, such as pH, oxygen tension, inorganic ion and buffer concentrations. This is important to understand, because treatments which aim to maintain the stability of this environment are a significant part of clinical medicine. The chapter on blood is particularly important, because plasma is an accessible 'window' on metabolism and serves as a source of clinical information for the diagnosis and management of disease. On the other hand, the enzymatic reactions involved in blood coagulation, and the complexity of the immune system, illustrate the sophistication of our defenses against disturbances in this environment.

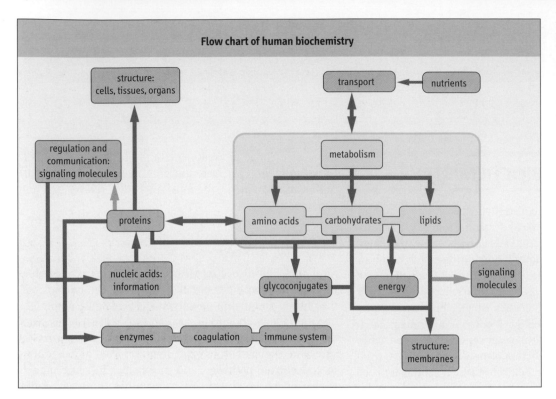

Fig. 1.1 **Flow chart of human biochemistry.** Throughout this book we will be discussing interrelationships between nutrients, energy metabolism and structure of cells and organs. We will highlight the role of catalytic and regulatory molecules and the control of cell cycle and metabolism by the information encrypted in the nucleic acids.

Biological membranes compartmentalize metabolic processes and process signals which control them

Biological membranes perform important roles in the compartmentalization of metabolites and metabolic pathways. Linked with this role is their fundamental function in metabolite transport, and also their role in receiving signals from other cells and organs. We discuss the structure of membranes both in the separation of different subcellular spaces and in the transport of ions, metabolites and larger biomolecules. Note that most of the body's energy is consumed in the maintenance of ion charge and metabolite gradients across biological membranes.

Energy released from nutrients is distributed throughout the cell in the form of adenosine triphosphate

We introduce bioenergetics, the science of energy recovery and utilization in biological systems, through the function of mitochondrial membranes in oxidative phosphorylation. This is the process involving oxygen consumption, or respiration, by which we capture the energy of fuels, produce a hydrogen ion gradient, and convert this energy to adenosine triphosphate (ATP). The molecules of ATP are the 'common currency of metabolism' for exchange of metabolic energy: they transduce the energy from fuel metabolism for use in work, transport, and biosynthesis.

Glucose is a key molecule in fuel metabolism

We introduce fuel metabolism by describing the digestion and absorption of nutrients in the gut, followed by discussion of our nutritional requirements for both main nutrients (proteins, carbohydrates, fats, and minerals) and the micronutrients – vitamins and trace elements. We also discuss the role of diet in health and disease.

The metabolism of fuels is introduced through glycolysis, an ancient, universal anaerobic metabolic pathway for glucose metabolism and energy production. Glycolysis proceeds through identical steps both in our brain cells and in the anaerobic bacteria in our intestines; it transforms glucose to pyruvate, setting the stage for oxidative metabolism in the mitochondrion. This pathway provides an opportunity to introduce the mechanisms of regulation of metabolic pathways by small-molecule allosteric effectors, by reversible chemical modification of key enzymes, and by control of gene expression.

Glucose is not only our major carbohydrate fuel, but also a stringently regulated circulating form of carbohydrate in blood. The maintenance of a normal concentration of blood glucose, only one-fifth of a teaspoon of sugar in a liter of blood (100 mg/dL; 1 g/L; 5 mmol/L) is essential for our survival. When blood glucose decreases to less than 45 mg/dL (2.5 mmol/L), we may fall into a hypoglycemic coma; when it remains consistently greater than 125 mg/dL (7 mmol/L), we are diabetic and are at risk for renal, vascular, and eye disease. Several chapters in this book explain different aspects of glucose metabolism. We also discuss the metabolism of glycogen, the storage form of glucose in liver and muscle. While talking about glycogen, we introduce the role of hormones in the regulation of metabolic pathways, and describe how organs use hormones to communicate with one another, and how hormones activate, inactivate, and coordinate metabolic activities within and among cells and organs.

Oxygen is essential for metabolism but the body needs to protect itself against its excess

Although oxygen is not required for conversion of glucose to lactate during glycolysis, it is needed for oxidative metabolism of pyruvate to carbon dioxide and water – a process that is essential for maximal extraction of the energy available from glucose. However, oxygen can also be toxic, causing oxidative stress and widespread tissue damage. We discuss both the advantageous and disadvantageous features of oxygen, emphasizing how we harness it usefully and, at the same time, protect ourselves from its more damaging effects through antioxidant defenses.

In aerobically-operating cells, pyruvate is transformed into another key metabolite, acetyl coenzyme A (acetyl-CoA), which is the common intermediate in the energy metabolism of carbohydrates, lipids, and amino acids. Acetyl-CoA enters the central metabolic engine of the cell, the tricarboxylic acid cycle (TCA cycle, also known as citric acid cycle or Krebs cycle) in the mitochondrial matrix. The TCA cycle oxidizes acetyl CoA to carbon dioxide and reduces the important coenzymes, nicotinamide adenine dinucleotide (NAD^+) and flavin adenine dinucleotide (FAD). These reduced nucleotides capture the energy from fuel oxidation and are the substrates for the final pathway: oxidative phosphorylation in the mitochondrion. Their oxidation provides the energy for synthesis of ATP.

Eating and fasting shift body metabolism between the anabolic and catabolic states

The fed and fasting states represent two entirely different patterns of metabolism – anabolism and catabolism. As you work your way through energy metabolism, a complex web of interactions between biochemical pathways will become evident. The process of glycolysis, in addition to its role in setting the stage for energy metabolism, produces metabolites that are the starting point for synthesis of amino acids, proteins, lipids, and nucleic acids.

An important principle that evolves is the partial reversibility of the main pathways of carbohydrate and lipid metabolism – catabolism versus anabolism, in response to food intake. The direction of metabolism is constantly shifting during the feed–fast cycle. In the fed state, the active pathways are glycolysis, glycogen synthesis, lipogenesis, and protein synthesis, rejuvenating tissues and storing the excess of metabolic fuel. In the fasting state, which begins only a few

hours after our last meal, the direction of metabolism is reversed: glycogen and lipid stores are degraded, protein is converted into glucose by the pathway of gluconeogenesis, and other biosynthetic processes are slowed down. We placed particular emphasis on explaining the mechanisms for adaptation to the changes in energy status induced by feeding, fasting, changing diets and starvation. We also consider the integration of fuel metabolism within and among tissues, storage of fuel in tissues and its transport in plasma, fuel preferences of individual tissues, and the derangements in fuel metabolism that occur in diabetes and atherosclerosis.

Tissues perform specialized metabolic functions

To illustrate the diversity of biochemistry in specialized tissues, we describe the mechanism of muscle contraction, the roles of the lung and kidneys in acid-base and electrolyte balance, that of the liver in biosynthesis and detoxification, and the processes of bone metabolism and biological mineralization. We then focus on the role of specialized microstructures, such as glycoconjugates (glycoproteins, glycolipids, and proteoglycans) and their role in cell-cell interactions and in the extracellular matrix.

The genome and cellular signaling underlie it all

We then turn your attention to the structure of the genome, the mechanism of conservation and transfer of genetic information, the control of protein synthesis, and the regulation of gene expression. These pathways are complex – protein synthesis is controlled by information encoded in deoxyribonucleic acid (DNA) and transcribed into ribonucleic acid (RNA), which is then translated into peptides that fold into functional protein molecules. Not only is the spectrum of expressed proteins important, but also the control of their temporal expression during development, adaptation, and aging. Information presented in these chapters offers many opportunities for understanding the therapies and strategies for fighting bacterial and viral infections. This is followed by a discussion of applications of recombinant DNA and polymerase chain reaction (PCR) technology in the clinical laboratories and in molecular medicine. The remaining chapters of the book deal with integrated topics, such as the function of the immune system, biochemical endocrinology, and the specialized biochemistry of nerve tissue. In separate chapters we deal with the issues of cell growth, the decline of biochemical systems during aging, the failure of biochemical controls in cancer, and the fascinating field of cell signaling systems.

Integrating the knowledge of metabolism with clinical medicine

Biochemistry is often perceived by students as excessively complicated – but then, we are the most complicated machine

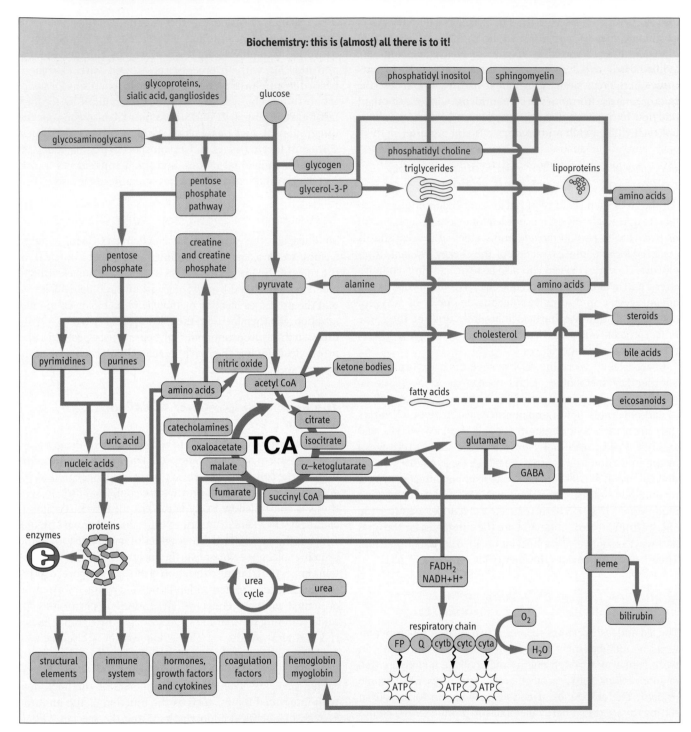

Fig. 1.2 Biochemistry: all in one. Interrelationships between biochemical pathways. This figure has been designed to give you a bird's-eye view of the field. It may help to structure your study, or revision.

on Earth – and much more! We believe that you will find biochemistry more comprehensible once you gain a mental picture of how the different parts of metabolism interact. For this purpose, we have included a general (and necessarily much simplified) scheme (Fig. 1.2) that looks not unlike the drawing of the London Underground! It is designed to help

you to place a particular aspect/pathway/class of substances in the context of the whole system, as you proceed through the various chapters in the text.

In many places around the world, cutting-edge medical curricula emphasize integration of basic and clinical disciplines and introduce clinical contact at an early stage. Following this way of thinking, our important goal was that the study of biochemistry should, at its every stage, help you understand aspects of clinical practice. Therefore, throughout this book, we strive to link the basic science you learn with clinical practice, in as relevant way as possible. Our clinical examples have been carefully scrutinized by experienced practicing clinicians and laboratorians, and most of them illustrate problems that hospital residents encounter in their daily work. This should make the biochemistry you learn easier to apply and, hopefully, will turn the journey through the metabolic pathways into a relevant, enjoyable, and rewarding experience.

Further reading

Dominiczak MH. Teaching and training laboratory professionals for the 21st century. *Clin Chem Lab Med* 1998;**36**:133–36.

Jolly B, Rees L, eds. *Medical education in the millenium*. Oxford: Oxford University Press; 1998;1–268.

2. Amino Acids and Proteins

N Taniguchi

LEARNING OBJECTIVES

After reading this chapter you should be able to:

- Classify the amino acids based on their chemical structure and charge.
- Explain the meaning of the terms, pK_a and pI, as they apply to amino acids and proteins.
- Describe the elements of the primary, secondary, tertiary, and quaternary structure of proteins.
- Describe the principles of ion exchange and gel filtration chromatography, and electrophoresis and isoelectric focusing, and describe their application in protein isolation and characterization.
- Explain the principle of MALDI and electrospray mass spectrometry and its application to proteomics.

INTRODUCTION

Proteins are the primary structural and functional polymers in living systems. They have a broad range of activities, including catalysis of metabolic reactions and transport of vitamins, minerals, oxygen, and fuels. Some proteins make up the structure of tissues, while others function in nerve transmission, muscle contraction, and cell motility, and still others in blood clotting and immunologic defenses, and as hormones and regulatory molecules. Proteins are synthesized as a sequence of amino acids linked together in a linear polyamide (polypeptide) structure, but they assume complex three-dimensional shapes in performing their function. There are approximately 300 amino acids present in various animal, plant and microbial systems, but only 20 amino acids are coded by DNA to appear in proteins. Many proteins also contain modified amino acids and accessory components, termed prosthetic groups. A range of chemical techniques is used to isolate and characterize proteins by a variety of criteria, including mass, charge, and three-dimensional structure. Proteomics is an emerging field which studies the full range of expression of protein in a cell or organism, and changes in protein expression in response to growth, hormones, stress, and aging.

AMINO ACIDS

Stereochemistry: configuration at the α-carbon, D- and L-isomers

Each amino acid has a central carbon, called the α-carbon, to which four different groups are attached (Fig. 2.1):

- a basic amino group (—NH$_2$)
- an acidic carboxyl group (—COOH)
- a hydrogen atom (—H)
- a distinctive side chain (—R).

One of the 20 amino acids, proline, is not an α-amino acid but an α-imino acid (see below). Except for glycine, all amino acids contain at least one asymmetric carbon atom (the α-carbon atom), giving two isomers that are optically active, i.e. can rotate plane-polarized light. These isomers, referred to as enantiomers, are said to be chiral, a word derived from the Greek word for hand. Such isomers are non-superimposable mirror images and are analogous to left and right hands, as shown in Figure 2.2. The two amino acid configurations are called D (for dextro or right) and L (for laevo or left). All amino acids in proteins are of the L-configuration, because proteins are biosynthesized by enzymes that insert only L-amino acids into the peptide chains.

Classification of amino acids based on chemical structure

The properties of each amino acid are dependent on its side chain (—R); the side chains are the functional groups that are the major determinants of the structure and function of proteins, as well as the electrical charge of the molecule. Knowledge of the properties of these side chains is important for understanding methods of analysis, purification, and identification of proteins. Amino acids with charged, polar, or hydrophilic side chains are usually exposed on the surface of proteins. The nonpolar hydrophobic residues are usually buried in the hydrophobic interior or core of a protein and are out of contact with water. The 20 amino acids in proteins encoded by DNA are listed in Table 2.1 and are classified according to their side-chain functional groups.

Structure of an amino acid

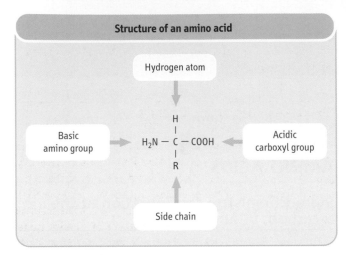

Fig. 2.1 **Structure of an amino acid.** Except for glycine, four different groups are attached to the α-carbon of an amino acid. Table 2.1 on this page lists the structures of the R moiety.

Enantiomers

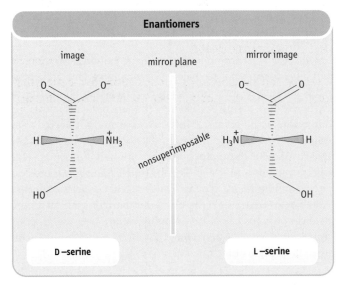

Fig. 2.2 **Enantiomers.** The mirror-image pair of amino acids. Each amino acid represents nonsuperimposable mirror images. The mirror-image stereoisomers are called enantiomers.

 NONPROTEIN AMINO ACIDS

Some amino acids occur in free or combined states, but not in proteins. Measurement of abnormal amino acids in urine (aminoaciduria) is useful for clinical diagnosis (see Chapter 18). In plasma, free amino acids are usually found in the order of 10 to 100 μmol/L, including many that are not found in protein. Citrulline, for example, is an important metabolite of L-arginine and a product of nitric oxide synthase, an enzyme that produces nitric oxide, an important vasoactive signaling molecule. Urinary amino acid concentration is usually expressed as μmol/g creatinine. Creatinine is an amino acid derived from muscle, and is excreted in relatively constant amounts per unit body mass per day. Thus, the creatinine concentration in urine, normally about 1 mg/mL, can be used to correct for urine dilution. The most abundant amino acid in urine is glycine, which is present as 400–2000 μg/g creatinine.

The 20α-amino acids specified by the genetic code

Amino acids	Structure of R moiety
Aliphatic amino acids	
glycine (Gly, **G**)	—H
alanine (Ala, **A**)	—CH$_3$
valine (Val, **V**)	—CH(CH$_3$)CH$_3$
leucine (Leu, **L**)	—CH$_2$—CH(CH$_3$)CH$_3$
isoleucine (Ile, **I**)	—CH(CH$_3$)—CH$_2$—CH$_3$
Sulfur-containing amino acids	
cysteine (Cys, **C**)	—CH$_2$—SH
methionine (Met, **M**)	—CH$_2$—CH$_2$—S—CH$_3$
Aromatic amino acids	
phenylalanine (Phe, **F**)	—CH$_2$—(ring)
tyrosine (Tyr, **Y**)	—CH$_2$—(ring)—OH
tryptophan (Trp, **W**)	—CH$_2$—(indole ring)
Imino acid	
proline (Pro, **P**)	(pyrrolidine ring)—COOH (Whole structure)
Neutral amino acids	
serine (Ser, **S**)	—CH$_2$—OH
threonine (Thr, **T**)	—CH(OH)—CH$_3$
asparagine (Asn, **N**)	—CH$_2$—C(=O)—NH$_2$
glutamine (Gln, **Q**)	—CH$_2$—CH$_2$—C(=O)—NH$_2$
Acidic amino acids	
aspartic acid (Asp, **D**)	—CH$_2$—COOH
glutamic acid (Glu, **E**)	—CH$_2$—CH$_2$—COOH
Basic amino acids	
histidine (His, **H**)	—CH$_2$—(imidazole ring)
lysine (Lys, **K**)	—CH$_2$—CH$_2$—CH$_2$—CH$_2$—NH$_2$
arginine (Arg, **R**)	—CH$_2$—CH$_2$—CH$_2$—NH—C(=NH)—NH$_2$

Table 2.1 **The 20 amino acids found in proteins.** The three-letter and single-letter abbreviations in common use are given in parentheses.

Aliphatic amino acids

Alanine, valine, leucine, and isoleucine, referred to as aliphatic amino acids, have saturated hydrocarbons as side chains. Glycine, which has only a hydrogen side chain, is also included in this group. Alanine has a relatively simple structure, a side chain methyl group, while leucine and isoleucine have *sec-* and *iso-*butyl groups. All of these amino acids are hydrophobic in nature.

Aromatic amino acids

Phenylalanine, tyrosine, and tryptophan have aromatic side chains. The nonpolar aliphatic and aromatic amino acids are normally buried in the protein core and are involved in hydrophobic interactions of the protein core. Tyrosine has a weakly acidic hydroxyl group and may be located on the surface of proteins. Reversible phosphorylation of the hydroxyl group of tyrosine in some enzymes is important in the regulation of metabolic pathways. The aromatic amino acids are responsible for the ultraviolet absorption of most proteins, which have absorption maxima ~280 nm. Tryptophan has a greater absorption in this region than the other two aromatic amino acids. The molar absorption coefficient of a protein is useful in determining the concentration of a protein in solution, based on spectrophotometry. Typical absorption spectra of aromatic amino acids and a protein are shown in Figure 2.3.

Neutral polar amino acids

Neutral polar amino acids contain hydroxyl or amide side-chain groups. Serine and threonine contain hydroxyl groups. These amino acids are sometimes found at the active sites of catalytic proteins, enzymes (Chapter 5). Reversible phosphorylation of peripheral serine and threonine residues of enzymes is also involved in regulation of energy metabolism and fuel storage in the body (Chapter 12). Asparagine and glutamine have amide-bearing side chains. These are polar, but uncharged under physiological conditions. Serine, threonine and asparagine are the primary sites of linkage of sugars to proteins, forming glycoproteins (Chapter 25).

Acidic amino acids

Aspartic and glutamic acids contain carboxylic acids on their side chains and are ionized at pH 7.0, and, as a result, carry

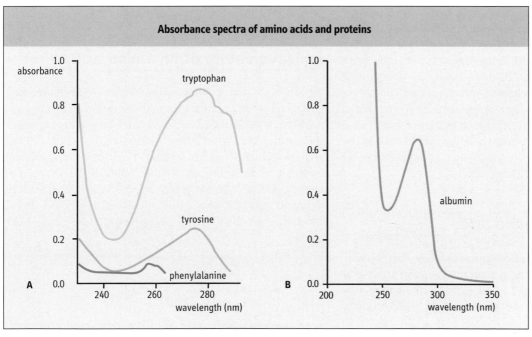

Fig. 2.3 **Ultraviolet absorption spectra of the aromatic amino acids and bovine serum albumin.**
(A) Aromatic amino acids such as tryptophan, tyrosine, and phenylalanine have absorbance maxima at ~280 nm. Each purified protein has a distinct molecular absorption coefficient at around 280 nm, depending on its content of aromatic amino acids.
(B) A bovine serum albumin solution (1 mg dissolved in 1 ml of water) has an absorbance of 0.67 at 280 nm using a 1 cm cuvette. The absorption coefficient of proteins is often expressed as $E^{1\%}$ (10 mg/ml solution). For albumin, $E1\%_{280\,mm} = 6.7$. Although proteins vary in their Trp, Tyr, and Phe content, measurements of absorbance at 280 nm are useful for estimating protein concentration in solutions.

negative charges on their β- and γ-carboxyl groups, respectively. In the ionized state, these amino acids are referred to as aspartate and glutamate, respectively.

Basic amino acids

The side chains of lysine and arginine are fully protonated at neutral pH and, therefore, positively charged. Lysine contains a primary amino group (NH_2) attached to the terminal ε-carbon of the side chain. The ε-amino group of lysine has a $pK_a \approx 11$. Arginine is the most basic amino acid ($pK_a \approx 13$), and its guanidine group exists as a protonated guanidinium ion at pH 7.0.

Histidine ($pK_a \approx 6$) has an imidazole ring as the side chain and functions as a general acid–base catalyst in many enzymes. The protonated form of imidazole is called an imidazolium ion.

Sulfur-containing amino acids

Cysteine and its oxidized form, cystine, are sulfur-containing amino acids characterized by low polarity. Cysteine plays an important role in stabilization of protein structure, since it can participate in formation of a disulfide bond with other cysteine residues to form cystine residues, crosslinking protein chains and stabilizing protein structure. Two regions of a single polypeptide chain, remote from each other in the sequence, may be covalently linked through a disulfide bond (intrachain disulfide bond). Disulfide bonds are also formed between two polypeptide chains (interchain disulfide bond), forming covalent protein dimers. These bonds can be reduced by enzymes, or by reducing agents such as 2-mercaptoethanol or dithiothreitol to form cysteine residues. Methionine is the third sulfur-containing amino acid and contains a nonpolar methyl thioether group in its side chain.

Proline, a cyclic amino acid

Proline is different from other amino acids in that its side-chain pyrrolidine ring includes both the α-amino group and the α-carbon. This structure forces a 'bend' in a polypeptide chain, sometimes causing abrupt changes in the direction of the chain.

Classification of amino acids based on the polarity of the amino acid side chains

Table 2.2 depicts the functional groups of amino acids and their polarity (hydrophilicity). Polar side chains can be

Summary of the functional groups of amino acids and their polarity			
Amino acids	**Functional group**	**Hydrophilic (polar) or hydrophobic (apolar)**	**Examples**
acidic	carboxyl, —COOH	polar	Asp, Glu
basic	amine, —NH₂	polar	Lys
	imidazole	polar	His
	guanidino	polar	Arg
neutral	glycine, —H	nonpolar	Gly
	amides, —CONH₂	polar	Asn, Gln
	hydroxyl, —OH	polar	Ser, Thr,
	sulfhydryl, —SH	nonpolar	Cys
aliphatic	hydrocarbon	nonpolar	Ala, Val, Leu, Ile, Met, Pro
aromatic	C-rings	nonpolar	Phe, Trp, Tyr

Table 2.2 **Summary of the functional groups of amino acids and their polarity.**

involved in hydrogen bonding to water and to other polar groups. The hydrophobic nature of side chains contributes to protein folding by hydrophobic interactions.

Ionization state of an amino acid

Amino acids are amphoteric molecules – they have both basic and acidic groups. Monoamino and monocarboxylic acids are ionized in different ways in solution, depending on the solution pH. At pH 7, the 'zwitterion' $^+H_3N—CH_2—COO^-$ is the dominant species of glycine in solution, and the overall molecule is therefore electrically neutral. On titration to acidic pH, the α-amino group is protonated and positively charged, yielding the cation $^+H_3N—CH_2—COOH$, while titration with alkali yields the anionic $H_2N—CH_2—COO^-$ species.

$$^+H_3N—CH_2—COOH \underset{\longleftarrow}{\overset{H^+}{\longrightarrow}} {}^+H_3N—CH_2—COO^- \underset{\longleftarrow}{\overset{OH^-}{\longrightarrow}} H_2N—CH_2—COO^-$$

pK_a values for the α-amino and α-carboxyl groups and side chains of acidic and basic amino acids are shown in Table 2.3. The overall charge on a protein depends on the contribution from basic (positive charge) and acidic (negative charge) amino acids, but the actual charge on the protein varies with the pH of the solution. To understand how the side chains affect the charge on proteins, it is worth recalling the Henderson–Hasselbalch equation.

pK values and ionized groups in proteins

Group	Acid (protonated form) (conjugate acid)	H⁺+ Base (unprotonated form) (conjugate base)	pKa
terminal carboxyl residue (α-carboxyl)	—COOH (carboxylic acid)	—COO⁻ + H⁺ (carboxylate)	3.0–5.5
aspartic acid (β-carboxyl)	—COOH	—COO⁻ + H⁺	3.9
glutamic acid (γ-carboxyl)	—COOH	—COO⁻ + H⁺	4.3
histidine (imidazole)	(imidazolium)	(imidazole)	6.0
terminal amino (α-amino)	—NH₃⁺ (amino)	—NH₂ + H⁺ (amine)	8.0
cysteine (sulfhydryl)	—SH (thiol)	—S⁻ + H⁺ (thiolate)	8.3
tyrosine (phenolic hydroxyl)	(phenol)	(phenolate)	10.1
lysine (ε-amino)	—NH₃⁺ (ε-amino)	—NH₂ + H⁺ (ε-amine)	10.5
arginine (guanidino)	(guanidinium)	(guanidino)	12.5

Table 2.3 **pK values and ionized groups in proteins.** pK_a indicates the approximate value, because it depends on temperature, buffer, etc.

Henderson–Hasselbalch equation and pK_a

The general dissociation of a weak acid, such as a carboxylic acid, is given by the equation:

$$HA \rightleftharpoons H^+ + A^- \qquad (1)$$

where HA is the protonated form (conjugate acid or associated form) and A⁻ is the unprotonated form (conjugate base, or dissociated form).

The dissociation constant (K_a) of a weak acid is defined as the equilibrium constant for the dissociation reaction (1) of the acid:

$$K_a = \frac{[H^+][A^-]}{[HA]} \qquad (2)$$

The hydrogen ion concentration [H⁺] of a solution of a weak acid can then be calculated as follows. Equation (2) can be rearranged to give:

$$[H^+] = K_a \times \frac{[HA]}{[A^-]} \qquad (3)$$

Equation (3) can be expressed in terms of a negative logarithm:

$$-\log[H^+] = -\log K_a - \log \frac{[HA]}{[A^-]} \qquad (4)$$

Since pH is the negative logarithm of [H⁺], i.e. −log[H⁺] and pK_a equals the negative logarithm of the dissociation constant for a weak acid, i.e. −log K_a, the Henderson–Hasselbalch equation (5) can be developed and used for analysis of acid-base equilibrium systems:

$$pH = pK_a + \log \frac{[A^-]}{[HA]} \qquad (5)$$

For a weak base, such as an amine, the dissociation reaction can be written as:

$$RNH_3^+ \rightleftharpoons H^+ + RNH_2 \qquad (6)$$

and the Henderson–Hasselbalch equation becomes:

$$pH = pK_a + \log \frac{[RNH_2]}{[RNH_3^+]} \qquad (7)$$

From equations (5) and (7), it is apparent that the extent of protonation of acidic and basic functional groups, and therefore the net charge will vary with the pK_a of the functional group and the pH of the solution. For alanine, which has two functional groups with pK_a = 2.4 and 9.8, respectively (Fig.

2.4), the net charge varies with pH, from +1 to −1. At a point intermediate between pK_{a1} and pK_{a2}, alanine has a net zero charge. This pH is called its isoelectric point, pI (Fig. 2.4).

BUFFERS

Buffers are solutions that minimize a change in [H⁺], i.e. pH, on addition of acid or base. A buffer solution, containing a weak acid or weak base and a counter-ion, has maximal buffering capacity at its pK_a when the acidic and basic forms are present at equal concentrations. The acidic, protonated form reacts with added base, and the basic unprotonated form neutralizes added acid, as shown below for an amino compound:

$$RNH_3^+ + OH^- \rightleftharpoons RNH_2 + H_2O$$
$$RNH_2 + H^+ \rightleftharpoons RNH_3^+$$

An alanine solution (Fig. 2.4) has maximal buffering capacity at pH 2.4 and 9.8, i.e. at the pK_a of the —COO⁻ and NH₂ groups, respectively. When dissolved in water, alanine exists as a dipolar ion, or zwitterion, in which the carboxyl group is unprotonated (—COO⁻) and the amino group is protonated (—NH₃⁺). The pH of the solution is 6.1, the pI, halfway between the pK_a of the amino and carboxyl groups. The titration curve of alanine by NaOH (Fig. 2.4) illustrates that alanine has minimal buffering capacity at its pI, and maximal buffering capacity at a pH equal to the pK_{a1} or pK_{a2}.

PEPTIDES AND PROTEINS

Primary structure of proteins

The primary structure of the protein is the linear sequence of amino acids

In proteins, the primary amino group of one amino acid is linked to the carboxyl group of the next amino acid, forming

 GLUTATHIONE

Glutathione (GSH) is a tripeptide with the sequence L-γ-glutamyl-L-cysteinylglycine (Fig. 2.6). If the thiol group of the cysteine is oxidized, the disulfide GSSG is formed. GSH is the major peptide present in the cell. In the liver, the concentration of GSH is ~5 mmol/L. GSH plays a major role in the maintenance of proteins in their reduced forms and in antioxidant defenses (Chapter 35). The enzyme γ-glutamyl transpeptidase is involved in the metabolism of glutathione and is a marker for some liver diseases, including hepatocellular carcinoma and alcoholic liver disease.

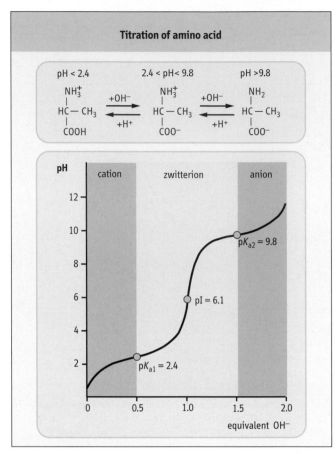

Fig. 2.4 **Titration of amino acid.** The curve shows the number of equivalents of NaOH consumed by alanine while titrating the solution from pH 0 to pH 12. Alanine contains two ionizable groups: an α-carboxyl group and an α-amino group. As NaOH is added, these two groups are titrated. The pK_a of the α–COOH group is 2.4, whereas that of the α-NH₃⁺ group is 9.8. At very low pH, the predominant ion species of alanine is the fully protonated form:

$$^+H_3N - \underset{\underset{CH_3}{|}}{CH} - COOH$$

At the mid-point in the first stage of the titration (pH 2.4), equimolar concentrations of proton-donor and proton-acceptor species are present, providing good buffering power.

$$^+H_3N - \underset{\underset{CH_3}{|}}{CH} - COOH \quad H_2N - \underset{\underset{CH_3}{|}}{CH} - COO^-$$

The second stage of the titration corresponds to the removal of a proton from the –NH₃⁺ group of alanine. The pH at the mid-point of this stage is 9.8, equal to the pK_a for the –NH₃⁺ group. The titration is complete at a pH of about 12, at which point the predominant form of alanine is:

$$H_2N - \underset{\underset{CH_3}{|}}{CH} - COO^-$$

The pH at which a molecule has no net charge is known as its isoelectric point, pI. For alanine, it is calculated as:

$$pI = \left[\frac{pKa1 + pKa2}{2}\right] = \left[\frac{2.4 + 9.8}{2}\right] = \frac{12.2}{2} = 6.1$$

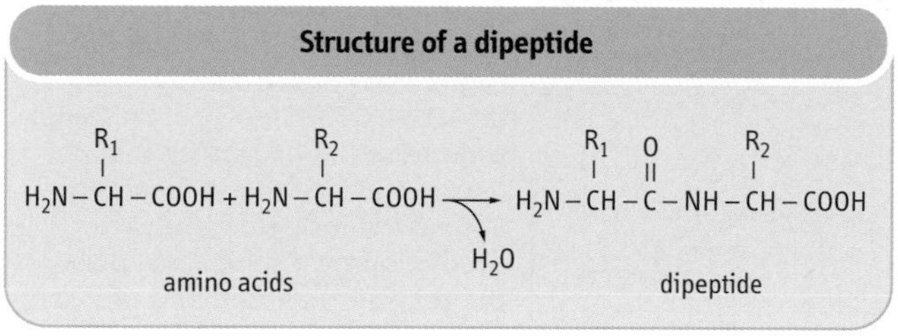

Structure of a dipeptide

$$H_2N-\underset{\underset{R_1}{|}}{C}H-COOH + H_2N-\underset{\underset{R_2}{|}}{C}H-COOH \longrightarrow H_2N-\underset{\underset{R_1}{|}}{C}H-\underset{\underset{O}{\|}}{C}-NH-\underset{\underset{R_2}{|}}{C}H-COOH$$

amino acids $\quad\quad$ H_2O $\quad\quad\quad$ dipeptide

Fig. 2.5 **Structure of a peptide bond.**

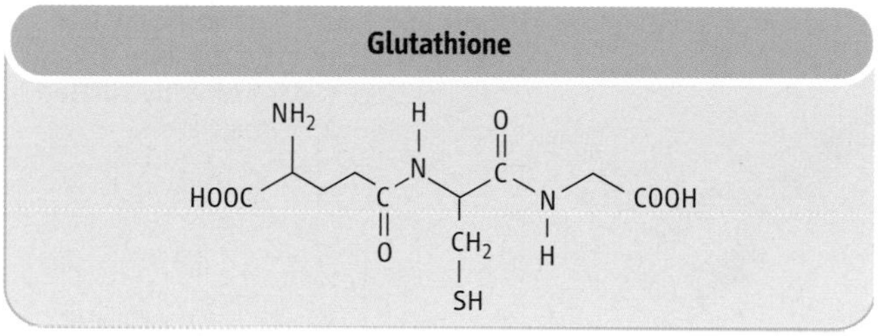

Glutathione

(structure of glutathione showing: NH_2, HOOC, C, O, N, H, CH₂, SH, COOH)

Fig 2.6 **Structure of glutathione.**

---

an amide (peptide) bond (Fig. 2.4). During the formation of a peptide bond, a molecule of water is eliminated, as shown in Figure 2.5. The amino acid units on a peptide chain are referred to as amino acid residues. A peptide chain consisting of three amino acid residues is called a tripeptide, e.g. glutathione in Figure 2.6. By convention, the amino terminus (N-terminus) is taken as the first residue, and the sequence of amino acids is written from left to right. When writing the peptide sequence, one uses either the three-letter or the one-letter abbreviations of amino acids, such as Asp-Arg-Val-Tyr-Ile-His-Pro-Phe-His-Leu or D-R-V-Y-I-H-P-F-H-L (see Table 2.1). This peptide is angiotensin, a peptide hormone that affects blood pressure. The amino acid residue having a free amino group at one end of the peptide, Asp, is called the N-terminal amino acid (amino terminus), whereas the residue having a free carboxyl group at the other end, Leu, is called the C-terminal amino acid (carboxyl terminus). Proteins contain between 50 and 2000 amino acid residues. The mean molecular mass of an amino acid residue is about 110 dalton units (Da). Therefore the molecular mass of most proteins is between 5500 and 220 000 Da. Human carbonic anhydrase I, an enzyme that plays a major role in acid–base balance in blood (see Chapter 23), is a protein with a molecular mass of 29 000 Da (29 kDa).

The charge and polarity characteristics of a peptide chain

The amino acid composition of a peptide chain has a profound effect on its physical and chemical properties. Proteins

---

MASS SPECTROMETRY AND MALDI–TOF MS

Mass spectrometry is used to measure the molecular weight of proteins and to detect posttranslational modification of proteins and peptides and in proteome research (see below). Matrix Assisted Laser Desorption Ionization Time-of-Flight Mass Spectrometry (MALDI–TOF MS) is a particularly sensitive and powerful technique for the characterization of proteins, peptides, and various biomolecules as shown in Figure 2.7. Another powerful method, electrospray ionization mass spectrometry (ESI MS), permits the measurement of the molecular weight of a protein directly from an aqueous solution of a protein. Two researchers, Drs Koichi Tanaka and John B Fenn were awarded the 2002 Nobel Prize in chemistry for their contribution to the development of the soft desorption ionisation methods for mass spectrometry.

---

rich in aliphatic or aromatic amino groups are relatively insoluble in water and more soluble in cell membranes. Proteins rich in polar amino acids are more water-soluble. Amides are neutral compounds so that the amide backbone of a protein, including the α-amino and α-carboxyl groups from which it is formed, does not contribute to the charge of the protein. Instead, the charge on the protein is dependent on the functional side chain groups of amino acids. Amino acids with side-chain acidic (Glu, Asp) or basic (Lys, His, Arg) groups will confer charge and buffering capacity to a protein. The balance between acidic and basic side chains in a protein determines its isoelectric point (pI) and net charge in solution. Proteins rich in lysine and arginine are basic in solution and have a positive charge at neutral pH, while acidic proteins, rich in aspartate and glutamate residues, are acidic and have a negative charge. Because of their side-chain functional groups, all proteins become more positively charged at acidic pH and more negatively charged at basic pH. Proteins are an important part of the buffering capacity of blood cells and biological fluids.

Secondary structure is determined by hydrogen bonding interactions of carbonyl and amide residues in the peptide backbone

The secondary structure of a protein refers to the local structure of the polypeptide chain. This structure is determined by hydrogen bond interactions between the carbonyl oxygen group of one peptide bond and the amide hydrogen of another nearby peptide bond. There are two types of secondary structure, the α-helix and the β-pleated sheet.

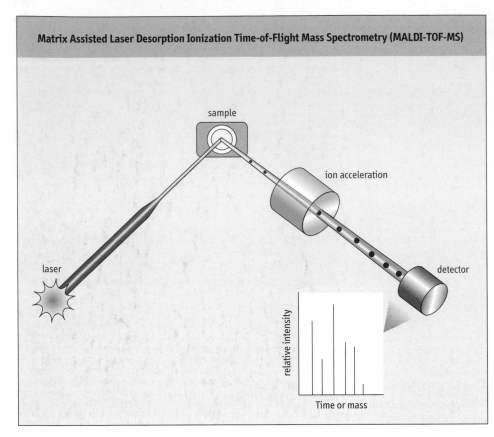

Matrix Assisted Laser Desorption Ionization Time-of-Flight Mass Spectrometry (MALDI-TOF-MS)

Fig. 2.7 **Matrix Assisted Laser Desorption Ionization Time-of-Flight Mass Spectrometry (MALDI–TOF MS).** A protein sample is dispersed in a large excess of matrix material that will strongly absorb the incident light. After irradiation by a short laser pulse, the protein is ionised and desorbed from the matrix. The ionized protein molecules are exposed to a voltage gradient in a vacuum and accelerate at a rate that is dependent on their mass to charge ratio. Each molecule reaches the detector after a time (time-of-flight) that can be directly related to its molecular mass.

The α-helix

The α-helix is a rod-like structure with the peptide chain tightly coiled and the side chains of amino acid residues extending outward from the axis of the spiral. Each amide carbonyl group is hydrogen-bonded to the amide hydrogen of a peptide bond that is four residues away along the same chain. There are on average 3.6 amino acid residues per turn of the helix, and the helix winds in a right-handed (clockwise) manner in almost all natural proteins (Fig. 2.8A).

The β-pleated sheet

If the H-bonds are formed between peptide bonds in different chains, the chains become arrayed parallel or antiparallel to one another in what is commonly called a β-pleated sheet. The β-pleated sheet is an extended structure as opposed to the coiled α-helix. It is pleated because the carbon–carbon (C—C) bonds are tetrahedral and cannot exist in a planar configuration. If the polypeptide chain runs in the same direction, it forms a parallel β-sheet (Fig. 2.8B), but in the opposite direction, it forms an antiparallel structure. The β-turn or β-bend refers to the segment in which the polypeptide abruptly reverses direction. Glycine (Gly) and proline

COLLAGEN

Human genetic defects involving collagen illustrate the close relationship between amino acid sequence and three-dimensional structure. Collagens are the most abundant protein family in the mammalian body, representing about a third of body proteins. Collagens are a major component of connective tissue such as cartilage, tendons, the organic matrix of bones, and the cornea of the eye.

Comment. Collagen contains 35% Gly, 11% Ala, and 21% Pro plus Hyp (hydroxyproline). The amino acid sequence in collagen is generally a repeating tripeptide unit, Gly-Xaa-Pro or Gly-Xaa-Hyp, where Xaa can be any amino acid; Hyp = hydroxyproline. This repeating sequence adopts a left-handed helical structure with three residues per turn. Three of these helices wrap around one another with a right-handed twist. The resulting three-stranded molecule is referred to as tropocollagen. Tropocollagen molecules self-assemble into collagen fibrils and are packed together to form collagen fibers. There are metabolic and genetic disorders which result from collagen abnormalities. Scurvy, osteogenesis imperfecta (Chapter 27) and Ehlers-Danlos syndrome result from defects in collagen synthesis and/or crosslinking.

Protein secondary structural motifs

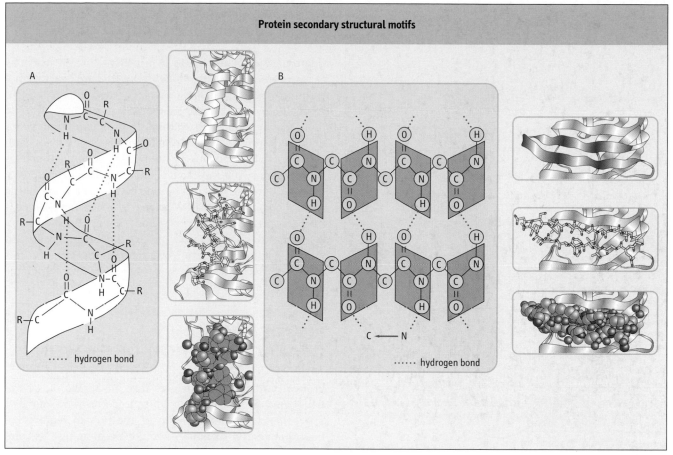

Fig. 2.8 **Protein secondary structural motifs.** (A) An α-helical secondary structure. Hydrogen bonds between 'backbone' amide NH and C=O groups stabilize the α-helix. Hydrogen atoms of OH, NH or SH group (hydrogen donors) interact with free electrons of the acceptor atoms such as O, N or S. Even though the bonding energy is lower than that of covalent bonds, they play a pivotal role in the stabilization of protein molecules. R: side chain of amino acids which extend outward from the helix. Ribbon, stick and space-filling models are shown. (B) The parallel β-sheet secondary structure. In the β-conformation, the backbone of the polypeptide chain is extended into a zigzag structure. When the zigzag polypeptide chains are arranged side by side, they form a structure resembling a series of pleats. Ribbon, stick and space-filling models are also shown.

(Pro) residues often occur in β-turns on the surface of globular proteins.

Tertiary structure results from folding of the peptide chain

The three-dimensional, folded and biologically active conformation of a protein is referred to as its tertiary structure. This structure reflects the overall shape of the molecule. The tertiary structures of over 1000 proteins have been determined by X-ray crystallography and nuclear magnetic resonance spectroscopy. The folded conformation of proteins that contain more than 200 residues consists of several smaller folded units termed domains.

The three-dimensional tertiary structure of a protein is stabilized by interactions between side-chain functional groups, covalent disulfide bonds, hydrogen bonds, salt bridges, and hydrophobic interactions (Fig. 2.8). The side chains of tryptophan and arginine serve as hydrogen donors, whereas asparagine, glutamine, serine, and threonine can serve as both hydrogen donors and acceptors. Lysine, aspartic acid, glutamic acid, tyrosine, and histidine also can serve as both donors and acceptors in the formation of ion pairs (salt bridges). Two opposite-charged amino acids, such as glutamate with a γ-carboxyl group and lysine with an ε-amino group, may form a salt bridge, primarily on the surface of proteins (Fig. 2.9).

Compounds such as urea and guanidine hydrochloride frequently cause denaturation or loss of tertiary structure when

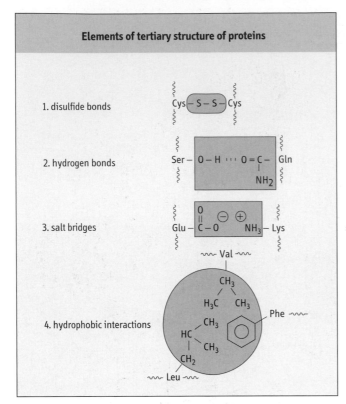

Fig. 2.9 **Elements of tertiary structure of proteins.** Examples of amino acid side-chain interactions contributing to tertiary structure.

LENS DISLOCATION IN HOMOCYSTINURIA (INCIDENCE 1 IN 350 000)

The most common ocular manifestation of homocystinuria is lens dislocation occurring around age 10 years.
Fibrillin, found in the fibres that support the lens, is rich in cysteine residues. Disulphide bonds between these residues are required for the cross-linking and stabilization of protein and lens structure. Homocysteine, a homolog of cysteine, can disrupt these bonds by homocysteine-dependent disulphide exchange.
Another equally rare sulfur amino acid disorder – sulfite oxidase deficiency – is also associated with lens dislocation by a similar mechanism (usually presenting at birth with early refractory convulsions). Marfan's syndrome, also associated with lens dislocation, is associated with mutations in the fibrillin gene.

present at high concentrations such as, for example, 8 mol/L urea. These reagents are called denaturants or chaotropic agents.

Quaternary structure is formed by interactions between peptide chains

Quaternary structure refers to a complex or an assembly of two or more separate peptide chains that are held together by noncovalent or, in some cases, covalent interactions. In general, most proteins larger than 50 kDa consist of more than one chain and are referred to as dimeric, trimeric, or multimeric proteins. Many multisubunit proteins are composed of different kinds of functional subunits, such as the regulatory and catalytic subunits. Hemoglobin is a tetrameric protein (Chapter 4), and beef heart mitochondrial ATPase has 10 protomers (Chapter 8). The smallest unit is referred to as a monomer or subunit. Figure 2.10 indicates the structure of the dimeric protein Cu,Zn-superoxide dismutase. Figure 2.11 is an overview of the primary, secondary, tertiary, and quaternary structures of a tetrameric protein.

PURIFICATION AND CHARACTERIZATION OF PROTEINS

Protein purification procedures take advantage of separations based on charge, size, binding properties, and solubility. The complete characterization of the protein requires an understanding of its amino acid composition, and its complete primary, secondary, and tertiary structure and, for multimeric proteins, its quaternary structure.

In order to characterize a protein, it is first necessary to purify the protein by separating it from other components in complex biological mixtures. The source of the proteins is commonly blood or tissues, or microbial cells such as bacteria and yeast. First, the cells or tissues are disrupted by grinding or homogenization in buffered isotonic solutions, commonly at physiologic pH and at 4°C to minimize protein denaturation during purification. The 'crude extract' containing organelles such as nuclei, mitochondria, lysosomes,

POST-TRANSLATIONAL MODIFICATIONS OF PROTEINS

Most proteins undergo some form of enzymatic modification after the synthesis of the peptide chain. The 'post-translational' modifications are performed by processing enzymes in the endoplasmic reticulum, Golgi apparatus, secretory granules, and extracellular space. The modifications include proteolytic cleavage, glycosylation, lipation and phosphorylation. Mass spectrometry is a powerful tool for detecting such modifications, based on differences in molecular mass.

Three-dimensional structure of a dimeric protein

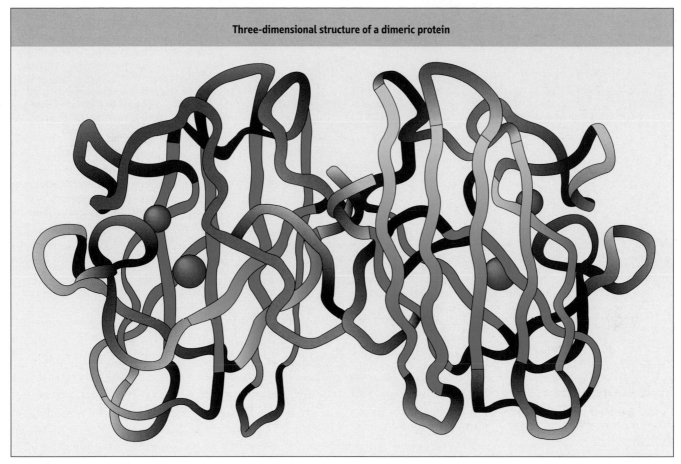

Fig. 2.10 **Three-dimensional structure of a dimeric protein.** Quaternary structure of Cu,Zn-superoxide dismutase from spinach. Cu,Zn-superoxide dismutase has a dimeric structure, with a monomer molecular mass of 16 000 Da. Each subunit consists of eight antiparallel β-sheets called a β-barrel structure, in analogy with geometric motifs found on native American and Greek weaving and pottery. Courtesy of Dr Y Kitagawa.

microsomes, and cytosolic fractions can then be fractionated by high-speed centrifugation or ultracentrifugation. Proteins that are tightly bound to the other biomolecules or membranes may be solubilized using organic solvent or detergent.

Salting-out (ammonium sulfate fractionation)

The solubility of a protein is dependent on the concentration of dissolved salts, and the solubility may be increased by the addition of salt at a low concentration (salting-in) or decreased by high salt concentration (salting-out). When ammonium sulfate, one of the most soluble salts, is added to a solution of a protein, some proteins precipitate at a given salt concentration while others do not. Human serum immunoglobulins are precipitable by 33–40% saturated

$(NH_4)_2SO_4$, while albumin remains soluble. Saturated ammonium sulfate is about 4.1 mol/L. Most proteins will precipitate from an 80% saturated $(NH_4)_2SO_4$ solution.

Separation on the basis of size

Dialysis and ultrafiltration

Small molecules, such as salts, can be removed from protein solutions by dialysis or ultrafiltration. Dialysis is performed by adding the protein-salt solution to a semipermeable membrane tube (commonly a nitrocellulose or collodion membrane). When the tube is immersed in a dilute buffer solution, small molecules will pass through and large protein molecules will be retained in the tube, depending on the pore size of the dialysis membrane. This procedure is particularly useful for removal of $(NH_4)_2SO_4$ or other salts during protein purification, since the salts will

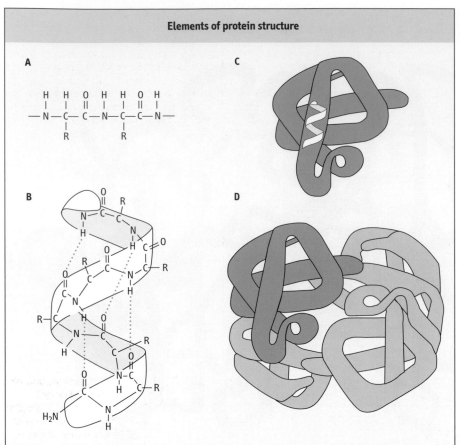

Elements of protein structure

Fig. 2.11 **Primary, secondary, tertiary, and quaternary structures.** (A) The primary structure is composed of a linear sequence of amino acid residues of proteins. (B) The secondary structure indicates the local spatial arrangement of polypeptide backbone yielding an extended α-helical or β-pleated sheet structure as depicted by the ribbon. Hydrogen bonds between the 'backbone' amide –NH– and –CO– groups stabilize the helix. (C) The tertiary structure illustrates the three-dimensional conformation of a subunit of the protein; while the quaternary structure (D) indicates the assembly of multiple polypeptide chains into an intact, tetrameric protein.

interfere with the purification of proteins by ion-exchange chromatography (below). Figure 2.12 illustrates the dialysis of proteins.

Gel filtration (molecular sieving)

Gel filtration, or gel-permeation, chromatography uses a column of insoluble but highly hydrated polymers such as dextrans, agarose, or polyacrylamide. Gel-filtration chromatography depends on the differential migration of dissolved solutes through gels that have pores of defined sizes. This technique is frequently used for protein purification and for desalting protein solutions. Figure 2.13 describes the principle of gel filtration. There are commercially available gels made from carbohydrate polymer beads designated as dextran (Sephadex series), polyacrylamide (Bio–Gel P series), and agarose (Sepharose series), respectively. The gels vary in pore size, and one can chose the gel filtration materials according to the molecular weight fractionation range desired.

Separation on the basis of charge: ion-exchange chromatography

When a charged ion or molecule with one or more positive charges exchanges with another positively charged component bound to a negatively charged immobilized phase, the process is called cation exchange. The inverse process is called anion exchange. The cation exchanger, carboxymethyl-cellulose ($-O-CH_2-COO^-$), and anion exchanger, diethyl-aminoethyl (DEAE) cellulose ($-O-C_2H_4-NH^+[C_2H_5]_2$, are frequently used for the purification of proteins. Consider purifying a protein mixture containing albumin and immunoglobulin. At pH 7.5, albumin, with a pI of 4.8, is negatively charged; immunoglobulin with a pI ~8 is positively charged. If the mixture is applied to a DEAE column, the albumin sticks to the positive-charged DEAE column whereas the immunoglobulin passes through the column. Figure 2.14 illustrates the principle of ion-exchange chromatography. As with gel permeation chromatography, proteins can be separated from one another, based on small differences in their pI.

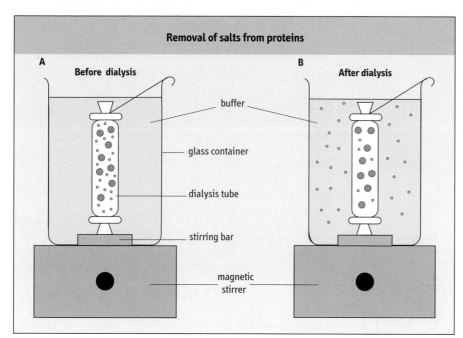

Fig. 2.12 **Dialysis of proteins.** Protein and low-molecular-mass compounds are separated by dialysis on the basis of size. (A) A protein solution with salts is placed in a dialysis tube in a beaker and dialyzed with stirring against an appropriate buffer. (B) The protein is retained in the tube whereas salts will pass through the membrane.

Removal of salts from proteins

A **Before dialysis**   B **After dialysis**

buffer

glass container

dialysis tube

stirring bar

magnetic stirrer

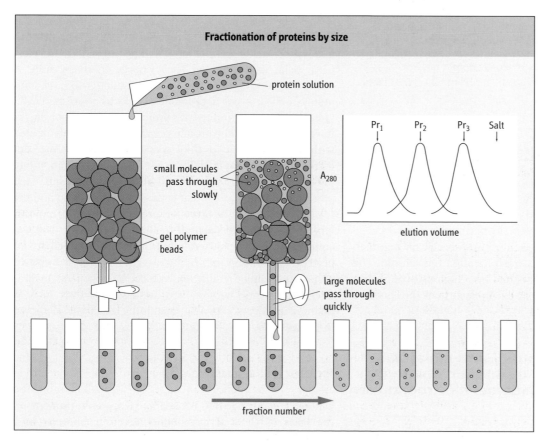

Fractionation of proteins by size

protein solution

small molecules pass through slowly

gel polymer beads

A_{280}

Pr$_1$ Pr$_2$ Pr$_3$ Salt

elution volume

large molecules pass through quickly

fraction number

Fig. 2.13 **Fractionation of proteins by size: gel filtration chromatography of proteins.** Proteins with different molecular sizes are separated by gel filtration based on their relative size. The smaller the protein, the more readily it exchanges into polymer beads, whereas larger proteins may be completely excluded. Larger molecules flow more rapidly through this column, leading to fractionation on the basis of molecular size. The chromatogram on the right shows a theoretical fractionation of three proteins, Pr$_1$–Pr$_3$ of decreasing molecular weight.

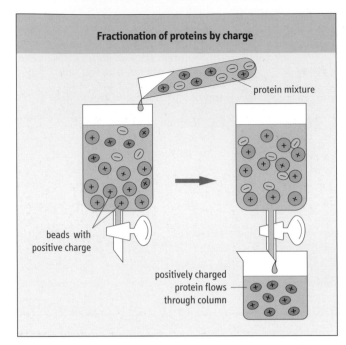

Fractionation of proteins by charge

protein mixture

beads with positive charge

positively charged protein flows through column

Fig. 2.14 **Fractionation of proteins by charge: ion-exchange chromatography.** Mixtures of proteins can be separated by ion-exchange chromatography according to their net charges. Beads that have positive-charge groups attached are called anion exchangers, whereas those having negative-charge groups are cation exchangers. This figure depicts an anion-exchange column. Negatively charged protein binds to positively charged beads, and positively charged protein flows through the column.

Affinity chromatography

Affinity chromatography is a convenient and specific method for purification of proteins. A porous chromatography column matrix is derivatized with a ligand that interacts with, or binds to, a specific protein in a complex mixture. The protein of interest will be selectively and specifically bound to the ligand while the others wash through the column. The bound protein can then be eluted by a high salt concentration, mild denaturation, or by a soluble form of the ligand or ligand analogs (see Chapter 5).

Determination of purity and molecular weight of proteins by sodium dodecyl sulfate-polyacrylamide gel electrophoresis (SDS–PAGE)

Electrophoresis can be used for the separation of a wide variety of charged molecules, including amino acids, polypeptides, proteins, and DNA. When a current is applied to molecules in dilute buffers, those with a net negative charge at the selected pH migrate toward the anode

HIGH PERFORMANCE LIQUID CHROMATOGRAPHY (HPLC)

HPLC is a powerful chromatographic technique for high-resolution separation of proteins, peptides, and amino acids. The principle of the separation may be based on the charge, size, or hydrophobicity of proteins. The narrow columns are packed with a noncompressible matrix of fine beads coated with a thin layer of a stationary phase. A protein mixture is applied to the column, and then the components are eluted by either isocratic or gradient chromatography. The eluates are monitored by ultraviolet absorption, refractive index, or fluorescence. This technique gives high-resolution separation with high specificity and high sensitivity and is the most common technique for purification of proteins and peptides.

and those with a net positive charge toward the cathode. A porous support, such as paper, cellulose acetate, or polymeric gel, is commonly used to minimize diffusion and convection.

Like chromatography, electrophoresis may be used for preparative fractionation of proteins at physiologic pH. Different soluble proteins will move at different rates in the electrical field, depending on their charge to mass ratio. A denaturing detergent, sodium dodecylsulfate (SDS), is commonly used in a polyacrylamide gel electrophoresis (PAGE) system to separate and resolve protein subunits according to molecular weight. The protein preparation is usually treated with both SDS and a thiol reagent, such as β-mercaptoethanol, to reduce disulfide bonds. Because the binding of SDS is proportional to the length of the peptide chain, each protein molecule has the same mass-to-charge ratio and the relative mobility of the protein is proportional to the molecular mass of the polypeptide chain. Varying the state of crosslinking of the polyacrylamide gel provides selectivity for proteins of different molecular weights. A purified protein preparation can be readily analyzed for homogeneity on SDS-PAGE by staining with sensitive and specific dyes such as Coomassie Blue, or with a Silver staining technique, as shown in Figure 2.15.

Isoelectric focusing (IEF)

Isoelectric focusing (IEF) is used for to separate proteins on the basis of their pI by conducting electrophoresis in a microchannel or gel containing a pH gradient. A protein applied to the system will be either positively or negatively charged, depending on its amino acid composition and the ambient pH. Upon application of a current, the protein will move towards either the anode or cathode until it encounters

Polyacrylamide gel electrophoresis

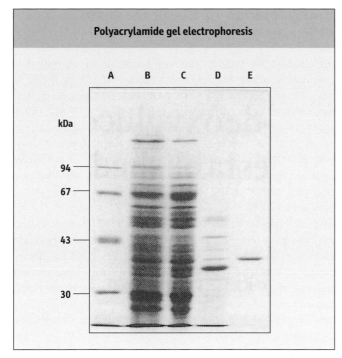

Fig. 2.15 **SDS–PAGE.** Sodium dodecylsulfate-polyacrylamide gel electrophoresis is used to separate proteins on the basis of their molecular weights. Larger molecules are retarded in the gel matrix, whereas the smaller ones move more rapidly. Lane A contains standard proteins with known molecular masses (indicated in kDa on the left). Lanes B, C, D, and E show results of SDS–PAGE analysis of a protein at various stages in purification: B = total protein isolate; C = ammonium sulfate precipitate; D = fraction from gel permeation chromatography; E = purified protein from ion exchange chromatography.

that part of the system that corresponds to its pI, where the protein has no charge and will cease to migrate. IEF is used in conjunction with SDS–PAGE for two-dimensional gel electrophoresis (Figure 2.16). This technique is particularly useful for the fractionation of complex mixtures of proteins for proteomic analysis (below).

ANALYSIS OF PROTEIN STRUCTURE

The typical steps in the purification of a protein are summarized in Figure 2.17. Once purified, for the determination of its amino acid composition, a protein is subjected to hydrolysis, commonly in 6 mol/L HCl at 110°C in a sealed and evacuated tube for 24–48 h. Under these conditions, tryptophan, cysteine, and most of the cystine are destroyed, and glutamine and asparagine are quantitatively deaminated to give glutamate and aspartate, respectively. Recovery of serine and threonine is incomplete and decreases with increasing time of hydrolysis. Alternative hydrolysis procedures may be used for measurement of tryptophan, while cysteine and

 ## THE PROTEOME

A proteome is defined as the full complement of proteins produced by a particular genome. Proteomics is an important field of study of protein properties and is defined as the qualitative and quantitative comparison of proteomes under different conditions with the goal of further unraveling biological process. To analyze the proteome of a cell, proteins from a cell are extracted and subjected to 2-dimensional gel electrophoresis. Individual protein spots are extracted and digested with proteases. Small peptides from such a gel are sequenced by mass spectrometry, permitting the identification of the protein. A typical analysis of a rat liver extract is shown in Fig. 2.16.

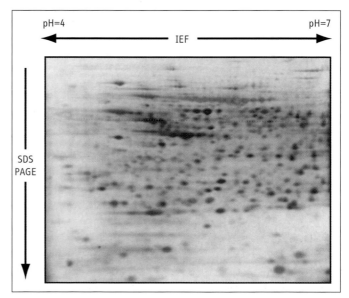

Figure 2.16 **Two-dimensional gel electrophoresis.** A crude rat liver extract was first subjected to isoelectric focusing (IEF) in cylindrical gel within the pH range 4–7. The gel was then laid horizontally on a second slab gel and separated by SDS–PAGE according to molecular mass. The gel was then stained with Coomassie Blue.

cystine may be converted to an acid-stable cysteic acid prior to hydrolysis. Following hydrolysis, the free amino acids are separated on an automated amino acid analyzer using an ion-exchange column, or by reversed-phase high-performance liquid chromatography (HPLC). The amino acids are reacted with chromogenic or fluorogenic reagents, such as ninhydrin or dansyl chloride, Edman's reagent (see below), or *o*-phthalaldehyde. These techniques allow the measurement of as little as 1 pmol of each amino acid. A typical elution pattern of amino acids in a purified protein is shown in Figure 2.18.

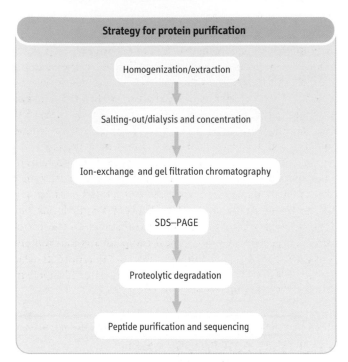

Strategy for protein purification

Homogenization/extraction

↓

Salting-out/dialysis and concentration

↓

Ion-exchange and gel filtration chromatography

↓

SDS–PAGE

↓

Proteolytic degradation

↓

Peptide purification and sequencing

Fig. 2.17 **Strategy for protein purification.** Purification of a protein involves a sequence of steps in which contaminating proteins are removed, based on difference in size, charge and hydrophobicity. Purification is monitored by SDS–PAGE. The primary sequence of the protein is determined by automated Edman degradation of peptides. The three-dimensional structure of the protein may be determined by X-ray crystallography.

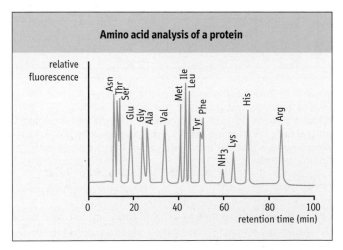

Amino acid analysis of a protein

relative fluorescence

0   20   40   60   80   100
retention time (min)

Fig. 2.18 **Typical chromatogram from an amino acid analysis by cation–exchange chromatography.** A protein hydrolysate is applied to the cation exchange column in a dilute buffer at acidic pH (~3.0), at which all amino acids are positively charged. The amino acids are then eluted by a gradient of increasing pH and salt concentrations. The most anionic (acidic) amino acids elute first, followed by the neutral and basic amino acids. Amino acids are derived by post-column reaction with a fluorogenic compound, such as o-phthalaldehyde.

Determination of the primary structure of proteins

Information on protein primary sequence of a protein is essential for understanding its functional properties, the identification of the family to which the protein belongs, as well as characterization of mutant proteins that cause disease. A protein may be cleaved first by digestion by specific endoproteases, such as trypsin (see Chapter 5), V8 protease, or lysyl endopeptidase, to obtain peptide fragments. Trypsin cleaves peptide bonds on the C-terminal side of arginine and lysine residues, provided the next residue is not proline. Lysyl endopeptidase is also frequently used to cleave at the C-terminal side of lysine. Cleavage by chemical reagents such as cyanogen bromide is also useful. Cyanogen bromide cleaves on the C-terminal side of methionine residues. Before cleavage, proteins with cysteine and cystine residues are reduced by 2-mercaptoethanol (MeSH) and then treated with iodoacetate to form carboxymethylcysteine residues. This avoids spontaneous formation of inter- or intra-molecular disulfides during analyses.

$$R_1 - S - S - R_2 + 2MeSH$$
$$\downarrow$$
$$R_1SH + R_2SH + MeSSMe$$
$$\downarrow$$
$$ICH_2COOH$$
$$\downarrow$$
$$R_{1(2)}S - CH_2COO^-$$

The cleaved peptides are then subjected to reversed-phase HPLC to purify the peptide fragments, and then sequenced on an automated protein sequencer, using the Edman degradation technique (Fig. 2.19). The sequence of overlapping peptides is then used to obtain the primary structure of the protein. Mass spectrometry may also be used to obtain both the molecular mass and sequence of polypeptides simultaneously (see below). Both techniques can be applied directly to proteins or peptides recovered from SDS–PAGE or two-dimensional electrophoresis (IEF plus SDS–PAGE). Once the partial amino acid sequence is obtained, one can determine the nucleotide sequence of the DNA that encodes this polypeptide segment. After chemically synthesizing this DNA, it can be used to identify and isolate the gene containing its nucleotide sequence (Chapter 34).

Determination of the three-dimensional structure of proteins

X-ray crystallography and NMR spectroscopy are usually used for the determination of the three-dimensional structure of proteins.

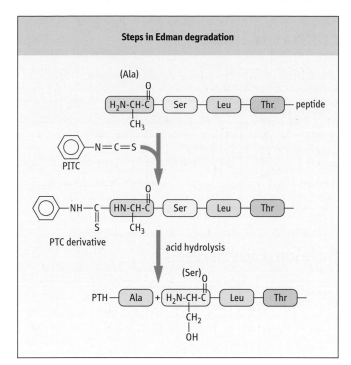

Steps in Edman degradation

Fig. 2.19 **Steps in Edman degradation.** The Edman degradation method sequentially removes one residue at a time from the amino end of a peptide. Phenyl isothiocyanate (PITC) converts the N-terminal amino group of the immobilized peptide to a phenylthiocarbamyl derivative (PTC amino acid) in alkaline solution. Acid treatment removes the first amino acid as the phenylthiohydantoin (PTH) derivative, which is identified by HPLC.

X-ray crystallography involves the diffraction of X-rays by the electrons of the atoms constituting the molecule. However, since the X-ray diffraction caused by an individual molecule is immeasurably weak, the protein must exist in the form of a well-ordered crystal, in which each molecule has the same conformation in a specific position and orientation on a three dimensional lattice. Based on diffraction of a collimated beam of electrons, the distribution of the electron density, and thus the location of atoms, in the crystal can be calculated to determine the structure of the protein. For protein crystallization, the most frequently used method is the hanging drop method which involves the use of a simple apparatus that permits a small portion of a protein solution (typically 10 μl droplet containing 0.5–1 mg/protein) to evaporate gradually to reach the saturating point at which the protein begins to crystallize. NMR spectroscopy is usually used for structural analysis of small organic compounds, but high-field NMR is also useful for determination of the structure of a protein in solution and complements information obtained by X-ray crystallography. Kurt Wuthrich was awarded the 2002 Nobel Prize in chemistry for his applications of NMR to macromolecules in solution.

PROTEIN FOLDING AND FOLDING DISEASE

For proteins to function properly, they must fold into the correct shape. Proteins have evolved so that one fold is more favourable than all others, the native state. Numerous proteins assist other proteins in the folding process. These proteins, termed chaperones, include 'heat shock' proteins, HSP 60 and HSP 70, and protein disulfide isomerase. A protein folding disease is a disease that is associated with abnormal conformation of a protein. This occurs in chronic, age-related diseases, such as Alzheimer disease, amyotrophic lateral sclerosis, and Parkinson's disease.

CREUTZFELDT–JACOB DISEASE

A 56-year-old male cattle rancher presented with epileptic cramp and dementia and was diagnosed as having Creutzfeldt–Jacob disease, a human prion disease. The prion diseases, also known as transmissible spongiform encephalopathies, are neurodegenerative diseases that affect both humans and animals. This disease in sheep and goats is designated as scrapie, and in cows as spongiform encephalopathy (mad cow disease). The diseases are characterized by the accumulation of an abnormal isoform of a host-encoded protein, prion protein-cellular form (PrPC), in affected brains.

Comment. Prions appear to be composed only of PrPSc (Scrapie form) molecules, which are abnormal conformers of the normal, host-encoded protein. PrPC has a high α-helical content and is devoid of β-pleated sheets, whereas PrPSc has a high β-pleated sheet content. The conversion of PrPC into PrPSc involves a profound conformational change. The progression of infectious prion diseases appears to involve an interaction between PrPC and PrPSc, which induces a conformational change of the α-helix-rich PrPC to the β-pleated sheet-rich conformer of PrPSc. PrPSc-derived prion disease may be genetic or infectious. The amino acid sequences of different mammalian PrPCs are similar, and the conformation of the protein is virtually the same in all mammalian species. The central protein of the transmissible agent, or prion, was discovered by Stanley B Prusiner, the Nobel Prize winner in physiology in 1997.

Summary

There are thousands of different proteins in cells, and each protein has a different structure and function. The higher order structure of a protein is the product of its primary, secondary, tertiary, and quaternary structure. Purification and characterization of proteins is essential for elucidating their structure and function. By taking advantage of differences in their size, solubility, charge and ligand binding properties, proteins can be purified to homogeneity using various chromatographic and electrophoretic techniques. The molecular mass and purity of a protein, and its subunit composition, can be determined by SDS–PAGE. The primary structure can be determined by hydrolysis of a protein and automated Edman degradation. Deciphering the primary and three-dimensional structures of a protein by X-ray analysis or NMR spectroscopy leads to an understanding of structure-function relationships in proteins. Mass spectrometry has become a powerful technique for elucidating protein structure, chemical modification, function and homology.

ACTIVE LEARNING

1. Mass spectrometry analysis of blood, urine and tissues is now being applied for clinical diagnosis. Discuss the merits of this technique with respect to specificity, sensitivity, through-put and breadth of analysis, including proteomic analysis for diagnostic purposes.
2. Study the role of chaperone proteins in the folding and transport of newly synthesized proteins in the cell.
3. Review the importance of protein misfolding and deposition in tissues in age-related chronic diseases.

Further reading

Collinge J. Prion diseases of humans and animals: their cause of molecular basis. *Annu Rev Neurosci* 2001;**2**:519–550.

Frydman J. Folding of newly translated proteins *in vivo*: the chaperones. *Annu Rev Biochem* 2001;**70**:603–647.

Imai J, Yashiroda H, Maruya M, Yahara I, Tanaka K. Proteasomes and molecular chaperones: cellular machinery responsible for folding and destruction of unfolded proteins. *Cell Cycle* 2003;**2**:585–590.

Petricoin EF, Liotta LA. Clinical applications of proteomics. *J Nutr* 2003;**133**: 2476S–2484S.

Valentine JS, Hart PJ. Misfolded CuZnSOD and amyotrophic lateral sclerosis. *Proc Natl Acad Sci USA* 2003;**100**:3617–3622.

Zhu H, Bilgin M, Snyder M. Proteomics. *Annu Rev Biochem* 2003;**72**:783–812.

Relevant websites

SWISS-PROT http://www.expasy.ch/sprot
Protein Data Bank http://www.rcsb.org/pdb
Protein structure: http://kinemage.biochem.duke.edu/

3. Blood: Cells and Plasma Proteins

W D Fraser

LEARNING OBJECTIVES

After reading this chapter you should be able to:

- Describe the major components of blood.
- Explain the difference between plasma and serum.
- Define the roles of plasma proteins and their broad classification.
- Identify diseases associated with deficiency of specific proteins.
- Discuss the structure and function of the immunoglobulins.
- Appreciate the pathological significance of monoclonal gammopathy.
- Define the acute phase response and the change it induces in the concentrations of circulating plasma proteins.

INTRODUCTION

Blood functions as a transport and distribution system for the body, delivering essential nutrients to tissues and at the same time removing waste products. It is composed of an aqueous solution containing molecules of varying sizes and a number of cellular elements. Some of the components of blood perform important roles in the body's defense against external insult and in the repair of damaged tissues.

PLASMA AND SERUM

Plasma is the natural environment of blood cells but most chemical measurements are done in serum

The formed elements of blood are suspended in an aqueous solution that is termed plasma. Plasma is the supernatant obtained by centrifuging a blood sample that has been treated with an anticoagulant to prevent clotting of red cells. Serum is the supernatant obtained if a blood sample is allowed to clot (usually requires 30–45 minutes) and then centrifuged. In laboratory practice, the most common anticoagulants are lithium heparinate and ethylenediamine tetraacetic acid (EDTA). Heparinate prevents clotting by binding to thrombin. EDTA and citrate bind Ca^{++} and Mg^{++} thus interfering with the action of calcium/magnesium-dependent enzymes (prothrombin-converting complex, thromboplastin and thrombin) involved in the clotting cascade. When blood is collected for transfusion, citrate is used as an anticoagulant, as this preserves procoagulants and its effects are readily reversible by calcium. During clotting, fibrinogen is converted to fibrin as a result of proteolytic cleavage by thrombin, and so a major difference between plasma and serum is the absence of fibrinogen in serum.

FORMED ELEMENTS OF BLOOD

There are three major cellular components circulating in the bloodstream:

Erythrocytes

Erythrocytes are not true cells, as they do not possess nuclei and intracellular organelles. They are cellular remnants, containing specific proteins and ions, which can be present in high concentrations. Erythrocytes are the end-product of erythropoiesis in the bone marrow, which is under the control of erythropoietin produced by the kidney (Fig. 3.1). Hemoglobin is synthesized in the erythrocyte precursor cells – erythroblasts and reticulocytes – under a tight control dictated by the concentration of heme, the synthesis of which involves the chelation of reduced ferrous iron (Fe^{2+}) by 4 nitrogen atoms in the centre of a porphyrin ring (see Chapter 28). The main functions of erythrocytes are the transport of oxygen and the removal of carbon dioxide and hydrogen ion; as they lack cellular organelles, they are not capable of protein synthesis and repair. As a result, erythrocytes have a finite life span of 60–120 days before being trapped and broken down in the spleen.

Leukocytes

Leukocytes are cells, the main function of which is to protect the body from infection.

Most leukocytes are produced in the bone marrow, some are produced in the thymus, and others mature within several tissues (Fig. 3.2) (see Chapter 36). Leukocytes can

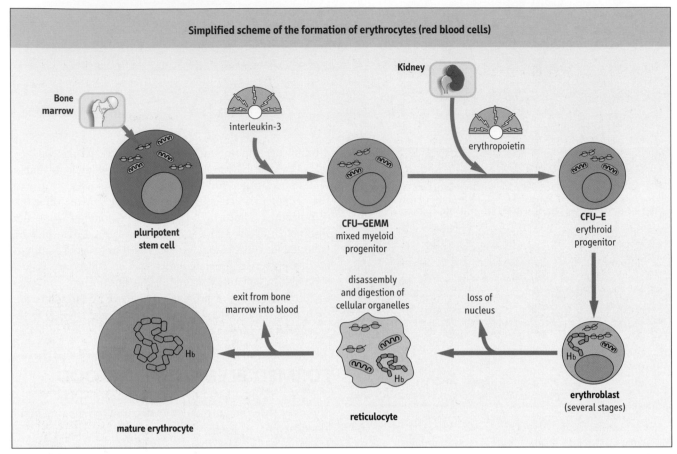

Simplified scheme of the formation of erythrocytes (red blood cells)

Fig. 3.1 **Simplified scheme of the formation of erythrocytes.** In an average day, 10^{11} erythrocytes are formed. Hemoglobin is synthesized in the erythrocyte and reticulocyte before the loss of ribosomes and mitochondria. CFU, colony-forming unit. GEMM: granulocyte, erythroid, monocyte, megakaryocyte. CFU-E, colony-forming unit erythroid.

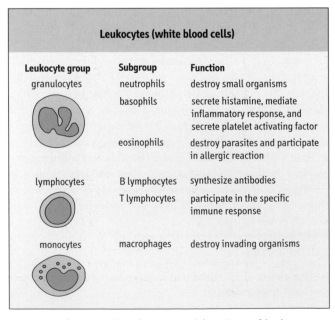

Leukocytes (white blood cells)

Leukocyte group	Subgroup	Function
granulocytes	neutrophils	destroy small organisms
	basophils	secrete histamine, mediate inflammatory response, and secrete platelet activating factor
	eosinophils	destroy parasites and participate in allergic reaction
lymphocytes	B lymphocytes	synthesize antibodies
	T lymphocytes	participate in the specific immune response
monocytes	macrophages	destroy invading organisms

Fig. 3.2 **Leukocytes.** Classification and functions of leukocytes.

control their own synthesis by secreting into the blood signal peptides that subsequently act on the bone marrow stem cells. In order to function correctly, leukocytes have the ability to migrate out of the bloodstream into surrounding tissues.

Thrombocytes (platelets)

Thrombocytes (platelets) are not true cells, but are membrane-bound fragments derived from megakaryocytes residing in the bone marrow. They have a key role in the process of blood clotting (see Chapter 6).

PLASMA PROTEINS

Plasma proteins can be broadly classified into two groups: those, including albumin, that are synthesized by the liver, and the immunoglobulins, which are produced by plasma cells of the bone marrow, usually as part of the immune response.

A number of plasma proteins have the ability to bind certain ligands with a high affinity and specificity. These

PLASMA AND SERUM

The role of the clinical laboratory

The clinical laboratory performs a large number of biochemical analyses on body fluids, which can give answers to specific clinical questions about an individual patient. Such analyses are usually requested to aid in the diagnosis or treatment of specific conditions. The majority of specimens received by the laboratory are blood and urine samples . Whereas some measurements are performed on whole blood, serum or plasma are preferred for most analyses of molecules and ions. In general, the time devoted to the analysis of each sample is relatively short, but the entire process from a request for analysis to receipt of a result involves many steps and can take several hours. Throughout the process, constant checking, attention to detail, and quality assurance are performed to ensure that the produced results are analytically and clinically valid. An outline of the laboratory workflow is shown in Figure 3.3.

NEPHROTIC SYNDROME 24

A 44-year-old woman was admitted to hospital because of weakness, anorexia, recurrent infections, bilateral leg edema, and breathlessness. Her plasma albumin concentration was 19 g/L (normal range 35–45 g/L) and her urinary protein excretion 10 g/24 h (normal value <0.15 g/24 h). There was microscopic haematuria. Renal biopsy confirmed the diagnosis as membranoproliferative glomerulonephritis.

Comment. This woman had the classic triad of the nephrotic syndrome: hypoalbuminemia, proteinuria, and edema. The nephritis has resulted in damage to the glomerular basement membrane, with resultant leak of albumin. Continued loss of albumin exceeds the synthetic capacity of the liver, and results in hypoalbuminemia; consequently, the capillary osmotic pressure is significantly reduced. This leads to both peripheral (leg) edema and pulmonary edema (breathlessness). With increasing glomerular damage, proteins of larger molecular mass, such as immunoglobulins and complement (Chapter 36) are lost.

proteins can then act as a reservoir for the ligand and help control its distribution and availability by transporting it to tissues throughout the body. Binding to a protein can also render a toxic substance less harmful to the tissues. Major binding proteins and their ligands are shown in Table 3.1.

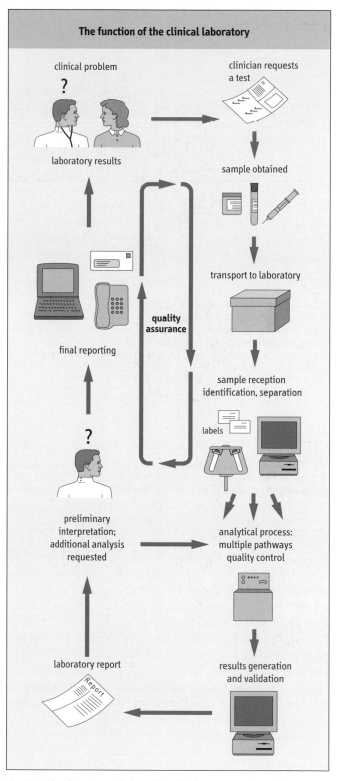

Fig. 3.3 **The function of the clinical laboratory.** Flow diagram indicating the steps involved in the generation of results from the clinical laboratory.

Transport proteins and their ligands

Proteins	Ligands
Cation binding	
Albumin	divalent and trivalent cations, e.g. Cu^{2+}, Fe^{3+}
Ceruloplasmin	Cu^{2+}
Transferrin	Fe^{3+}
Hormone binding	
Thyroid-binding globulin (TBG)	Thyroxine (T_4), Tri-iodothyronine (T_3)
Cortisol-binding globulin (CBG)	Cortisol
Sex hormone-binding globulin (SHBG)	Androgens (testosterone), estrogens (estradiol)
Hemoglobin/protoporphyrin binding	
Albumin	Heme, bilirubin, biliverdin
Haptoglobin	Hemoglobin dimers
Fatty acid binding	
Albumin	Non-esterified fatty acids, steroids

Table 3.1 **Transport proteins and their ligands.** Almost all plasma proteins bind ligands, and this is a major function of many proteins. Albumin can bind many molecules weakly and nonspecifically, but other proteins bind tightly to specific molecules – for example, transferrin is specific for ferric iron (Fe^{3+}).

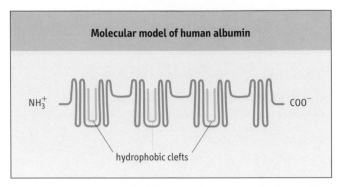

Fig. 3.4 **Molecular model of human albumin.** The hydrophobic clefts are globular segments of albumin that are able to bind fatty acids with high affinity.

Albumin

Albumin, in addition to its functions as a protein reserve in nutritional depletion and as an osmotic regulator, is a major transport protein

Albumin, the predominant plasma protein having no known enzymatic or hormonal activity, accounts for approximately 50% of the protein found in human plasma, and is present normally at a concentration of 35–45 g/L. It is easy to isolate, and has been extensively studied. With a molecular weight of about 66 kDa, albumin is one of the smallest plasma proteins and, given its highly polar nature, dissolves easily in water. At pH 7.4, it is an anion with 20 negative charges per molecule; this gives it a vast capacity for non-selective binding of many ligands. The presence of large amounts of albumin in the body (4–5 g/kg body weight), with at least 38% being present intravascularly, also helps to explain the critical role that it has in exerting colloid osmotic pressure.

The rate of synthesis of albumin (14–15 g daily) is critically dependent on nutritional status, especially the extent of amino acid deficiencies. The half-life of albumin is about 20 days, and degradation appears to occur by pinocytosis in all tissues.

Albumin is the primary plasma protein responsible for the transport of hydrophobic fatty acids, bilirubin, and drugs

Albumin demonstrates a unique ability to solubilize, in aqueous phase, a heterogeneous range of substances that include the long-chain fatty acids, sterols, and several synthetic compounds. The transport of long-chain fatty acids underpins much of the body's distribution of energy-rich substrates. Through binding, consequently solubilizing, and ultimately transporting fatty acids such as stearic acid, oleic acid, and palmitic acid, albumin enables the transport of these hydrophobic molecules in the predominantly hydrophilic milieu of the plasma. Associative studies have demonstrated the presence of numerous fatty acid binding sites on the albumin molecule, with variable affinities. The highest-affinity sites are believed to lie in the globular segments within specialized clefts of the albumin molecule (Fig. 3.4).

In addition to binding fatty acids, albumin has an important role in binding unconjugated bilirubin, thereby rendering it, not only water soluble and transportable from the reticuloendothelial system to the liver, but also temporarily nontoxic. In the presence of excessively high concentrations of unconjugated bilirubin the binding capacity of albumin is exceeded and in children this can contribute to the development of kernicterus (see Chapter 28).

The presence of sites within the albumin molecule that are capable of binding a variety of drugs, including salicylates, barbiturates, sulfonamides, penicillin, and warfarin, is of great pharmacologic relevance. Chiefly, such interactions are weak and the ligands become easily displaced by competitors for the binding site. Given such binding, not only does albumin play a part in drug solubilization, but it may also determine the proportion of free, and thus pharmacologically active, drug available in the plasma.

Albumin is not essential for human survival and rare congenital defects have been described where there is hypoalbuminaemia or complete absence of albumin (analbuminaemia).

HEMOLYSIS AND FREE HEMOGLOBIN

Handling of free hemoglobin

When erythrocytes are prematurely hemolyzed, they release hemoglobin into the plasma, where it dissociates into dimers that bind to haptoglobin. The hemoglobin-haptoglobin complex is metabolized more rapidly than haptoglobin alone, in the cells of the liver and reticuloendothelial system, producing an iron-globulin complex and bilirubin. This prevents the loss of iron in the urine. When excessive hemolysis occurs, the plasma haptoglobin concentration can become very low. If hemoglobin breaks down into heme and globin, the free heme is bound by hemopexin; unlike haptoglobin, which is an acute phase protein, hemopexin is not affected by acute phase response. The heme-hemopexin complex is taken up by liver cells, where iron binds to ferritin. A third complex, called methemalbumin, can form between oxidized heme and albumin. These mechanisms have evolved to allow the body not only to scavenge iron and prevent major losses, but also to complex free heme, which is toxic to many tissues.

Proteins that transport metal ions

The ability of proteins to bind and transport metal ions is of major importance

Iron is an essential element for many metabolic processes, and is an important component of the heme proteins, myoglobin, hemoglobin, and cytochromes. Within the plasma, iron is transported bound to transferrin as ferric ions (Fe^{3+}) and is released from the protein into tissues after it has bound to specific cell receptors and the resulting complex has been internalized. The iron is then deposited in storage sites as ferritin or hemosiderin, or is used in synthesis of heme proteins. The binding of ferric ions to transferrin protects against the toxic effects of these ions. In inflammatory reactions, the iron-transferrin complex is degraded by the reticuloendothelial system without a corresponding increase in the synthesis of either of its components; this results in low plasma concentrations of transferrin and iron.

■ Ferritin is the major iron storage protein found in almost all cells of the body. It acts as the reserve of iron in the liver and bone marrow. The concentration of ferritin in plasma is proportional to the amount of stored iron, and so measurement of plasma ferritin is one of the best indicators of iron deficiency;

■ Hemosiderin is a derivative of ferritin and is found in the liver, spleen, and bone marrow. It is insoluble in aqueous solutions, and forms aggregates that slowly release iron when deficiency exists;

■ Ceruloplasmin is the major transport protein for copper, an essential trace element. Ceruloplasmin helps export copper from the liver to peripheral tissues, and is essential for the regulation of the oxidation-reduction reactions, transport, and utilization of iron (Fig. 3.5). Increased concentrations of ceruloplasmin occur in active liver disease and in tissue damage.

Low concentrations of ceruloplasmin and total copper are observed in Wilson's disease, the autosomal recessive disorder of copper transport. The genetic defect is on chromosome 13 resulting in a mutation in copper-transporting P-type adenosine triphosphatase (ATP7B) which is responsible for transport of copper into ceruloplasmin and elimination of copper through bile. Mutation of ATP7B results in the accumulation of copper in the liver, brain and kidney. These mutations are readily identified by haplotype and mutational analysis and so genetic screening of patients and their families for Wilson's disease is possible.

WILSON'S DISEASE

A 14-year-old girl was admitted as an emergency. She was jaundiced with abdominal pain and had an enlarged, tender liver with drowsiness and asterixis (flapping tremor) due to acute liver failure. Previous history revealed behavior disturbance, difficulty with movement in the recent past, and truancy from school. Her ceruloplasmin concentration was 50 mmol/L (normal range 200–450 mmol/L [20–45 mg/dL]), serum copper was 8 mmol/L (normal range 13–19 µmol/L [80–120 µg/dL]), urinary excretion of copper was 2.2 mmol/24 h (normal range 2–3.9 µmol/24 h [13–25 µg/dL]), and a liver biopsy established the diagnosis of Wilson's disease.

Comment. This case highlights the importance of measurement of ceruloplasmin. In Wilson's disease, a deficiency of ceruloplasmin results in low plasma concentrations of copper. The metabolic defect is in the excretion of copper in bile and its reabsorption in the kidney; copper is deposited in liver, brain, and kidney. Liver symptoms are present in patients of younger age, and cirrhosis and neuropsychiatric problems are manifest in those who are older. Detection of low plasma concentrations of ceruloplasmin and copper, increased urinary excretion of copper, and markedly increased concentrations of copper in the liver confirms the diagnosis.

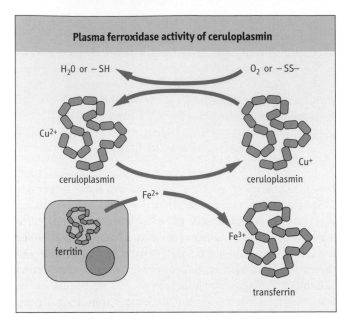

Plasma ferroxidase activity of ceruloplasmin

Fig. 3.5 **Plasma ferroxidase activity of ceruloplasmin.** Oxidation of Fe^{2+} by ceruloplasmin permits the binding and transport of iron by plasma transferrin. The cuprous ion (Cu^{2+}) bound to ceruloplasmin is regenerated by reaction with oxygen or with oxidized thiol groups.

Immunoglobulins

Immunoglobulins are proteins produced in response to foreign substances (antigens) (see also Chapter 36)

The immune system may be conceptualized as two independent entities, served by separate lymphoid cells: thymically derived T lymphocytes oversee immunoregulation and cell-based immune function, and B lymphocytes that synthesize and secrete antibodies (immunoglobulins) (see Chapter 36). These antibodies are proteins, produced by the immune system, which have a defined specificity for a foreign particle (immunogen) that stimulated their synthesis. Not all foreign substances entering the body can elicit this response, however; those that do are called immunogens, whereas any agent that can be bound by an antibody is termed an antigen.

The immunoglobulins are a uniquely diverse group of molecules, recognizing and reacting with a wide range of specific antigenic structures (epitopes) and giving rise to a series of effects that result in the eventual elimination of the presenting antigen. Some immunoglobulins have additional effector functions: for example, IgG is involved in complement activation.

Structure of immunoglobulins

Immunoglobulins share a common Y-shaped structure of two heavy and two light chains

The basic immunoglobulin is a Y-shaped molecule containing two identical units termed heavy (H) chains, and two identical, but smaller, units termed light (L) chains. Several H chains exist, and the nature of the H chain determines the class of immunoglobulin: IgG, IgA, IgM, IgD, and IgE are characterized by γ, α, μ, δ, and ε heavy chains, respectively. L chains are of only two types κ and λ, and both types may be found in any one class of immunoglobulin, although obviously not within the same molecule. Each polypeptide chain within the immunoglobulin is characterized by a series of globular regions, which have considerable sequence homology and, in evolutionary terms, are probably derived from protogene duplication.

The N-terminal domains of both H and L chains contain a region of variable amino acid sequence (the V region); together, these determine antigenic specificity. Both H and L chains are required for full antibody activity, as the physically apposed V regions in the L and H chains form a functional pocket into which the epitope fits; this is termed the antibody recognition (Fab_2) region. The domain immediately adjacent to the V region is much less variable, in both H and L chains. The remainder of the H chain consists of a further constant region (Fc region) consisting of a hinge region and two additional domains. This constant region is responsible for immunoglobulin functions other than epitope recognition, such as complement activation (Chapter 36). This basic structure of immunoglobulins is depicted in Figure 3.6. When antigen binds to the immunoglobulin, conformational changes are transmitted through the hinge region of the antibody, to the Fc region, which is then said to have become activated.

Major immunoglobulins

IgG is the most common immunoglobulin, protecting tissue spaces and freely crossing the placenta

IgG 'with an overall molecular mass of 160 kDa' consists of the basic 2H2L immunoglobulin subunit joined by a variable number of disulfide bonds. The γ H chains have several antigenic and structural differences, allowing classification of IgG into a number of subclasses according to the type of H chain present; however, functional differences between the subclasses are minor.

IgG circulates in high concentrations in the plasma, accounting for 75% of immunoglobulin present in adults, and has a half-life of 22 days. It is present in all extracellular fluids, and appears to eliminate small, soluble antigenic proteins through aggregation and enhanced phagocytosis by the

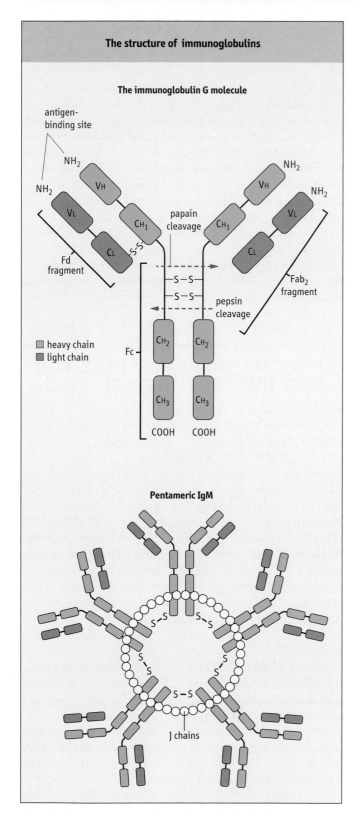

The structure of immunoglobulins

The immunoglobulin G molecule

Pentameric IgM

Fig. 3.6 **The structure of immunoglobulins.** Diagrammatic representation of the basic structure of a monomeric immunoglobulin and that of pentameric immunoglobulin (IgM). V, variable region; C, constant region; H, heavy chain; L, light chain; J chain, joining chain; Fab$_2$, fragment generated by pepsin cleavage of the molecule; Fc, Fd, fragments generated by papain proteolysis (See also Chapter 36).

reticuloendothelial system. From weeks 18–20 of pregnancy, IgG is actively transported across the placenta and provides humoral immunity for the fetus and neonate before maturation of the immune system.

IgA is found widely in secretions and presents an antiseptic barrier, which protects mucosal surfaces

IgA has an H chain similar to the γ chain of IgG, and α chains possess an extra 18 amino acids at the C-terminus. The extra peptide sequence enables the binding of a 'joining' or J chain. This short (129-residue) acidic glycopeptide, synthesized by plasma cells, allows dimerization of secretory IgA. IgA is often found in noncovalent association with the so-called secretory component, a highly glycosylated 71kDa polypeptide, synthesized by mucosal cells and capable of protecting IgA against proteolytic digestion.

IgA represents 7–15% of plasma immunoglobulins and has a half-life of 6 days. It is found, in particular in the dimerized form, in parotid, bronchial, and intestinal secretions. It is a major component of colostrum. IgA appears to function as the primary immunologic barrier against pathogenic invasion of mucous membranes. It can promote phagocytosis, cause eosinophilic degranulation, and activate complement via the so-called alternate pathway.

IgM is confined to the intravascular space and helps eliminate circulating antigens and micro-organisms

Immunoglobulins belonging to this final major class are polyvalent, with a high molecular mass. IgM has a basic form similar to that of IgA, having the extra H chain domain that allows for J chain binding, and is thus capable of polymerization. IgM normally circulates as a pentamer (with a molecular mass of 971 kDa) linked by disulfide bonds and the J chain (see Fig. 3.6).

IgM accounts for 5–10% of plasma immunoglobulins and has a half-life of 5 days. With its polymeric nature and high molecular mass, most IgM is found confined to the intravascular space, although lesser amounts may be found in secretions, usually in association with secretory component. It is the first antibody to be synthesized after an antigenic challenge.

Minor immunoglobulins

IgD is the surface receptor for antigen in B lymphocytes

IgD differs from the standard immunoglobulin structure chiefly by its high carbohydrate content of numerous oligosaccharide units, resulting in an increased molecular mass of 190 kDa. δ chains are characterized by having only a single interconnecting disulfide bridge, and an elongated hinge region that is particularly susceptible to proteolysis.

Accounting for less than 0.5% of circulating plasma immunoglobulin mass, IgD has a role that remains elusive, although, as a surface component of the mature B cell, it probably has some role in response to antigens. Rare cases of isolated IgD deficiency seem to be associated with no obvious pathology.

IgE is present only in trace amounts and acts to bind antigen and promote a release of vasoactive amines from mast cells

Similar to IgM in its unit structure, IgE has ε heavy chains that consist of five, rather than four, domains, but J chain binding and polymers do not occur. The extended H chain helps to explain the high molecular mass of IgE which is approximately 200 kDa.

IgE has a high affinity for binding sites on mast cells and basophils. Antigenic binding at the Fab_2 region induces crosslinking of the high-affinity receptor, granulation of the cell, and release of vasoactive amines. By this mechanism, IgE plays a major part in allergy/atopy and mediates antiparasitic immunity.

MULTIPLE MYELOMA

A 65-year-old man presented with a sudden onset of low back pain. Radiography revealed a crush fracture of the second lumbar vertebra, and discrete and so-called 'punched out' lesions in the skull. Serum electrophoresis demonstrated the presence of a monoclonal immunoglobulin. This proved to be an IgG immunoglobulin and, on electrophoresis, excess free κ chains (Bence-Jones protein) were found in the patient's urine.

Comment. Multiple myeloma affects men and women with equal incidence and presents mostly after the age of 50 years. The clinical features are due to both the malignant proliferation of monoclonal plasma cells and the synthesis and secretion of antibody by these cells. Bone lesions affect the skull, vertebrae, ribs, and pelvis. There may be generalized osteoporosis and pathologic fractures. In up to 20% of cases, no plasma protein is detected, although Bence–Jones proteins are present in urine. Such cases are commonly associated with suppression of production of other immunoglobulins (immunoparesis). The presence of excess light chains may cause renal failure as a result of the deposition of Bence–Jones proteins in the renal tubules or amyloidosis. Other common findings in myelomatosis include anemia and hypercalcemia.

Monoclonal immunoglobulins

Monoclonal immunoglobulins are the product of a single B cell, and arise from benign or malignant transformations of B cells

Monoclonal immunoglobulins result from the proliferation of a single B cell clone, which thus produces identical antibodies. Usually, these are structurally normal molecules, but sometimes they may be in some way fragmented or truncated. The absolute physical identity of the monoclonal immunoglobulins leads to a single band in gel electrophoresis, revealed by protein staining as a single, dense band in the gamma region (the paraprotein band) (Fig. 3.7).

Monoclonal immunoglobulins are associated with diverse malignant pathologies such as myeloma and Waldenström's macroglobulinemia, and also from more benign transformations that are usually termed monoclonal gammopathies of uncertain significance (MGUS).

THE ACUTE PHASE RESPONSE AND C-REACTIVE PROTEIN (CRP)

The acute phase response is a nonspecific response to tissue injury or infection; it affects several organs and tissues

During the acute phase response, there is a characteristic pattern of change in certain proteins–in particular, a marked increase in the synthesis of some proteins (predominantly in the liver), along with a decrease in the plasma concentration of some others (Fig. 3.8). An increase in the synthesis of proteins such as proteinase inhibitors (α_1-antitrypsin), coagulation proteins (fibrinogen, prothrombin), complement proteins, and CRP is of obvious clinical benefit (Fig. 3.9). The synthesis of albumin, transthyretin (prealbumin), and transferrin decreases during the acute phase response, and they are thus termed the 'negative acute phase reactants'.

CRP is a major component of the acute phase response and a marker of bacterial infection. It is synthesized in the liver and is constructed of five polypeptide subunits, having a molecular weight of around 130 kDa. It is present in only minute quantities (<1 mg/L in normal serum) and is believed to mediate binding of foreign polysaccharides, phospholipids, and complex polyanions, and also activating complement via the classical pathway (see Chapter 36).

Using assay for CRP, which is approximately a hundred times more sensitive than the conventional CRP measurement method, one may detect minimal fluctuations in the concentration of this protein. Interestingly, very small increases in CRP concentration, much smaller than those seen in an acute infection, seem to indicate a state of

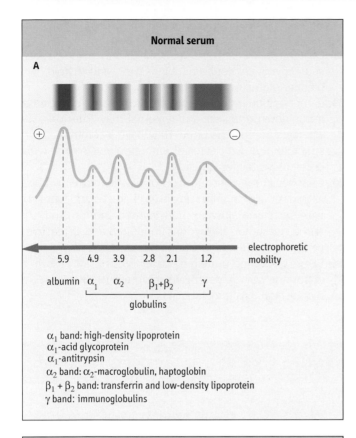

Normal serum

A

$\oplus$ $\ominus$

electrophoretic mobility

5.9   4.9   3.9   2.8   2.1   1.2

albumin α_1 α_2 $\beta_1+\beta_2$ γ

globulins

α_1 band: high-density lipoprotein
α_1-acid glycoprotein
α_1-antitrypsin
α_2 band: α_2-macroglobulin, haptoglobin
$\beta_1 + \beta_2$ band: transferrin and low-density lipoprotein
γ band: immunoglobulins

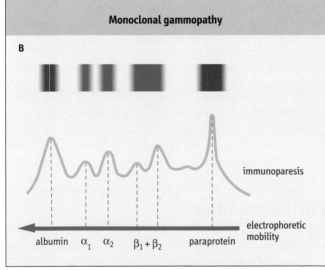

Monoclonal gammopathy

B

immunoparesis

electrophoretic mobility

albumin α_1 α_2 $\beta_1 + \beta_2$ paraprotein

Fig. 3.7 **Comparison of gel electrophoretic appearance of normal serum and that containing monoclonal immunoglobulins.** The scanning pattern peaks (solid line) represent the relative concentrations of the separated proteins. (A) Normal serum. (B) Monoclonal gammopathy: a strongly stained band is present in the γ-globulin region on electrophoresis, and there is an associated reduction of staining in the remainder of the γ-region (immunoparesis).

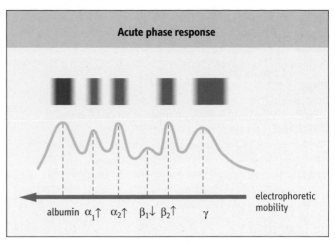

Acute phase response

electrophoretic mobility

albumin $\alpha_1\uparrow$ $\alpha_2\uparrow$ $\beta_1\downarrow$ $\beta_2\uparrow$ γ

Fig. 3.8 **Acute phase response.** Gel electrophoretic pattern observed in serum during the acute phase response. Albumin is decreased, the sum of α_1- and α_2-globulins is increased, β_1-globulins are decreased, β_2-globulins are increased and there is a mild increase in γ-globulins.

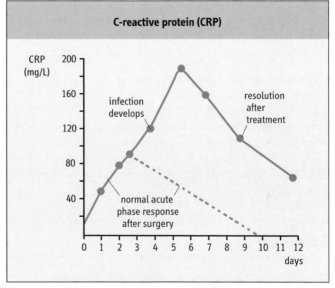

C-reactive protein (CRP)

CRP (mg/L)

200

160

infection develops

resolution after treatment

120

80

40

normal acute phase response after surgery

0   1   2   3   4   5   6   7   8   9   10   11   12

days

Fig. 3.9 **C-reactive protein (CRP) and the post-operative acute phase reaction.** The concentration of CRP increases as part of the acute phase response to surgical trauma, and a further increase may be observed if recovery is complicated by infection. (The dotted line represents response to uncomplicated surgery).

ACUTE PHASE RESPONSE

A 45-year-old woman suffered severe lower limb injuries in a road traffic accident. After her admission to hospital, biochemical profiling revealed slightly decreased concentrations of total serum protein (58 g/L) (normal 63–86 g/L) and serum albumin (35 g/L) (normal 35–45 g/L). Serum electrophoresis revealed an increase in the α_1 and α_2 protein fractions. Four days after her operation, the patient's condition deteriorated, and she developed an increased temperature, sweating, and confusion. An acute infection was diagnosed and treatment with appropriate antibiotics was commenced. CRP concentrations peaked 5 days after the operation (Fig. 3.9).

Comment. Increased concentrations of α_1 and α_2 proteins (which include α_1-antitrypsin, α_1-acid glycoprotein, and haptoglobin), together with a decrease in serum albumin concentration, suggest an acute phase response. This response is also associated with an increase in CRP, the erythrocyte sedimentation rate (ESR), and increased plasma viscosity. A therapeutic response to treatment of infection can be assessed by a decrease in plasma CRP concentration.

chronic-low-grade inflammation which is associated, for instance, with an increased risk of heart disease (see Chapter 42). Other inflammatory conditions such as inflammatory bowel disorders, type 2 diabetes and the metabolic syndrome (see Chapter 20). Abdominal aortic aneurysm and premature rupture of membranes during pregnancy have also been associated with these minute increases in serum CRP concentration.

Summary

- The formed elements of blood are erythrocytes, leukocytes and platelets. They are suspended in an aqueous solution (plasma) and have several specialized functions such as transport of oxygen, destruction of external agents, and clotting of blood. Plasma which is allowed to clot yields serum. Most biochemical tests are done on serum. To obtain plasma, blood must be taken into a test tube containing an anticoagulant.
- Plasma contains many proteins broadly classified into albumin and globulins (predominantly immunoglobulins). Albumin functions as a major

transport protein for several ligands – trace metals, hormones, bilirubin, and free fatty acids.

- Other proteins are more specialized: they bind specific ligands, e.g. ceruloplasmin binds Cu^{2+}, and thyroid binding globulin (TBG) binds thyroid hormones.
- Immunoglobulins are unique molecules that participate in the defense against antigens that may enter or attempt to enter the body. They have a common structure and five classes of immunoglobulin exist with different protective functions.
- Changes in the concentration of plasma proteins give important clinical information. A characteristic pattern with decreased albumin, transthyretin and transferrin and increased α_1-antitrypsin, fibrinogen and C-reactive protein indicates the acute phase response.
- Serum and urine protein electrophoresis is an important way of identifying the presence of monoclonal immunoglobulins.

ACTIVE LEARNING

1. Compare and contrast plasma and serum and discuss the different types of blood samples taken for laboratory tests.
2. Discuss the transport role of serum albumin.
3. Describe the core structure of immunoglobulins and different roles played in immunity by different classes of immunoglobulins.
4. How does acute phase reaction affect the results of blood tests?
5. Characterize Wilson's disease.
6. How is hemoglobin handled if erythrocytes become disrupted?

Further reading

Anderson KC, Shaughnessy JD, Barlogie B, Harousseau JL, Roodman GD. Multiple Myeloma. *Hematology.* American Society of Hematology Education Program Book 2002;214–240. (Full text available at *www.asheducationbook.org*)

El-Youssef M. Wilson's Disease. *Mayo Clin Proc* 2003;**78**:1126–1136.

Hayashi T, Hideshima T, Anderson KC. Novel therapies for multiple myeloma. *Br J Haematol* 2003;**120**:10–17.

Lewis SM, Bain B, Bates I, eds. *Practical Haematology* 9th Ed. London: Churchill Livingston; 2001.

Pepys MB, Hirschfield GM. C-reactive protein: a critical update. *J Clin Invest* 2003;**111**:1805–1812. (full text available at www.jci.org)

4. Oxygen Transport

G M Helmkamp

LEARNING OBJECTIVES

After reading this chapter you should be able to:

- Describe the mechanism of oxygen binding to myoglobin and hemoglobin.
- Describe conformational differences between deoxygenated and oxygenated hemoglobins.
- Define the concept of cooperativity in oxygen binding to hemoglobin.
- Describe the Bohr effect and its role in modulating the binding of oxygen to hemoglobin.
- Explain how 2,3-bisphosphoglycerate interacts with hemoglobin and influences oxygen binding.
- Summarize the processes by which carbon dioxide is transported from peripheral tissues to the lungs.
- Describe the major classifications of hemoglobinopathies.
- Describe the molecular basis of sickle cell disease.

INTRODUCTION

Humans are aerobic organisms. Our lungs extract oxygen (O_2) from air and deliver carbon dioxide (CO_2) in exhaled gases. The inspired O_2 leads to a more efficient utilization of metabolic fuels, such as glucose and fatty acids, and expired CO_2 is a major product of cellular metabolism. Living systems contain proteins that interact with O_2 and, consequently, increase its solubility in water and sequester it for transport. In mammals, these proteins are myoglobin (Mb) and hemoglobin (Hb). Mb, found primarily in skeletal and striated muscle, serves to store O_2 in the cytoplasm and deliver it on demand to the mitochondrion. Hb, restricted to the erythrocytes, is responsible for the transport of O_2 from the lungs to peripheral tissues. This chapter presents the molecular features of heme, the biochemical and physiologic relationships between the structures of Mb and Hb and their interaction with O_2, and the pathologic aspects of selected Hb mutations.

Properties of O_2

In mixtures of gases each component makes a specific contribution, known as its partial pressure that is directly proportional to its concentration. It is customary to use the partial pressure of a gas as a measure of its concentration in physiologic fluids. For atmospheric O_2 at a barometric pressure of 760 mmHg (760 torr, 101.3 kPascal (kPa), the partial pressure of oxygen, pO_2, is 150–160 mmHg, i.e. air contains about 20% oxygen. The amount of O_2 in solution is, in turn, directly proportional to its partial pressure. Thus, in arterial blood the pO_2 is ~100 mmHg (13.3 kPa), which produces a concentration of dissolved O_2 of 0.13 mmol/L (4.2 mg/L).

The major fraction of O_2 in blood is transported in blood and stored in muscle in complexes with the proteins Hb and Mb, respectively. Hb is a tetrameric protein with four O_2-binding sites. In arterial blood with an Hb concentration of 150 g/L (2.3 mmol/L), the contribution of Hb-bound O_2 is about 275 mg/L (8.6 mmol/L). The overall effect is a dramatic 60-fold increase in the O_2 content of this physiologic fluid, yielding almost 200 mL dissolved O_2/L of blood.

STRUCTURE OF THE HEME PROSTHETIC GROUP

Heme is the O_2-binding molecule common to Mb and Hb; it is a porphyrin molecule to which an iron atom (Fe^{2+}) is coordinated (Fig. 4.1). The Fe-porphyrin prosthetic group is, with the exception of two propionate groups, hydrophobic, and planar. Heme becomes an integral component of the globin proteins during polypeptide synthesis; it is heme that gives globin proteins their characteristic purple-red color. Globins increase the aqueous solubility of the otherwise poorly soluble, hydrophobic heme prosthetic group. Once sequestered inside a hydrophobic pocket created by the folded globin polypeptide, heme encounters a protective environment that minimizes the oxidation (rusting) of Fe^{2+} to Fe^{3+} in the presence of O_2. Such an environment is also essential for globins to bind and release O_2. Should the iron atom become oxidized to Fe^{3+}, generating the proteins metmyoglobin or methemoglobin, heme can no longer interact reversibly with O_2. Ultimately, O_2 storage and transport become compromised.

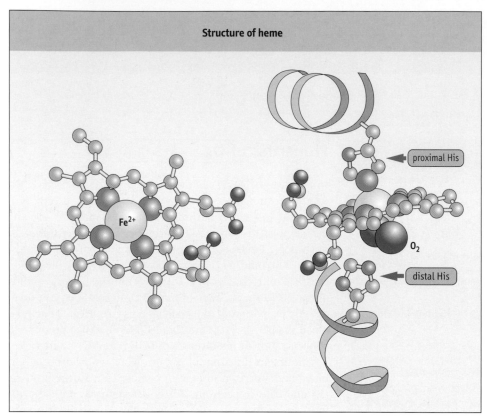

Structure of heme

Fe²⁺

proximal His

O₂

distal His

Fig. 4.1 **Structure of heme.** Heme is a complex of porphyrin and iron. Left (top view): The carbon framework of protoporphyrin IX, a conjugated tetrapyrrole ring, is depicted in gray; O_2 molecules are red. Iron (yellow sphere) prefers six ligands in an octahedral coordination geometry; pyrrole nitrogen atoms (blue spheres) provide four of these. Right (side view): In the globin structure, the planar heme is positioned between the proximal and distal histidines (His); only the former has an imidazole nitrogen (blue sphere) close enough to bond with iron. The α-helices that contain these histidines are shown in pink. In deoxygenated globins, the sixth position remains vacant, leaving a pentacoordinated iron. For globins in the oxygenated state, O_2 occupies the sixth position.

CHARACTERISTICS OF MAMMALIAN GLOBIN PROTEINS

Globins constitute an ancient family of soluble metalloproteins whose structure and function have been preserved for several million years among leguminous plants, certain invertebrates, and vertebrates. These proteins most likely evolved to convert heme from an electron carrier to an oxygen carrier. Mb and Hb are examples of globins found in all mammals. Mb consists of a single globin polypeptide and a heme prosthetic group (Fig. 4.2). Hb is a tetrameric assembly of closely related globin subunits. The globin polypeptide is a single chain of approximately 150 amino acids. Each globin molecule contains one noncovalently bound heme prosthetic group. The most significant aspect of the secondary structure of globins is the high proportion of α-helix: over 75% of the amino acids are associated with eight helical segments containing as few as six and as many as 28 residues. These α-helices are organized into a tightly packed, nearly spherical, globular tertiary structure (Fig. 4.2).

Polar amino acids are located almost exclusively on the exterior surface of globin polypeptides and contribute to the remarkably high solubility of these proteins (for example, 5.2 mmol/L [335 g/L] Hb in the erythrocyte, or >30% protein). Amino acids that are both polar and hydrophobic,

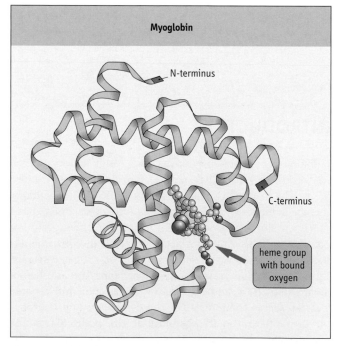

Myoglobin

N-terminus

C-terminus

heme group with bound oxygen

Fig. 4.2 **Model of myoglobin.** Myoglobin is a compact globular protein. In this depiction of mammalian Mb only the globin polypeptide backbone is shown, with emphasis on the high proportion of secondary structure (exclusively α-helix). The N-terminus is blue; the C-terminus is red. The heme group, with bound O_2, is illustrated as a 'ball-and-stick' structure.

HYPERBARIC O₂ THERAPY IN TREATMENT OF ACUTE CO POISONING

A 22-year-old pregnant female, carrying a fetus of 31 weeks gestational age, was transported to the maternity clinic of a hospital for suspected CO poisoning. The patient was experiencing headache, nausea, and visual abnormalities. She stated that her workplace had been undergoing repairs to the heating and ventilation systems during the past 2 weeks, and on the day of her hospital visit the fire department had evacuated the building after detecting a high level of CO (200 ppm). Vital signs were blood pressure of 116/68 mm Hg, pulse rate of 100, and respiratory rate of 24. Noteworthy in the patient's evaluation was a carboxyhemoglobin component of 15% of total Hb at time of admission (normal <3%, but may exceed 10% in heavy smokers). External fetal monitoring indicated a fetal heart rate of 135, with occasional, moderate irregularities. Uterine contractions were occurring every 3–5 min. The patient was treated in the hospital's hyperbaric O₂ chamber: 30 min at 250 kPa (2.5 atmospheres), then 60 min at 200 kPa. She also received magnesium sulfate intravenously to resolve the premature contractions. The patient was discharged 2 days later. She delivered a healthy female infant at 38 weeks of gestational age who, on examination at birth and at 6 weeks of age, exhibited no apparent sequelae to her *in utero* exposure to CO.

Comment. Like O₂, CO binds to heme prosthetic groups. Because the affinity of globin-bound heme for CO is more than 10^4 times that of O₂, prolonged exposure of hemoglobin (Hb) to CO would be virtually irreversible ($t_{1/2}$ = 4–5 h) and lead to highly toxic levels of carboxyhemoglobin. Hyperbaric O₂ is the treatment of choice for severe or complicated CO poisoning. The administration of 100% O₂ at 200–300 kPa creates arterial and tissue pO₂ values of 2000 mmHg and 400 mmHg respectively (~20 times normal). The immediate result is a reduction in the $t_{1/2}$ of carboxyhemoglobin to less than 20 min. Hyperbaric O₂ is also used in the treatment of decompression sickness, arterial gas embolism, radiation-induced or ischemic tissue injury, and severe hemorrhage.

such as threonine, tyrosine, and tryptophan, are oriented with their polar functions toward the protein's exterior. Hydrophobic residues are buried within the interior, where they stabilize the folding of the polypeptide and form a pocket that accommodates the heme prosthetic group. Notable exceptions to this general distribution of amino acid residues in globins are the two histidines that play indispensable roles in the heme pocket. The side chains of these histidines are oriented perpendicular to and on either side of the planar heme prosthetic group. One histidine has an imidazole nitrogen that is close enough to bond directly to the Fe²⁺ atom: this is the proximal histidine. On the opposite side of the heme plane

is the other histidine: this is the distal histidine. The distal histidine is too far from the heme iron for direct bonding; rather, it confers important geometrical constraints on the sixth coordination site and makes a hydrogen bond with the bound O₂. The alignment of heme and the distal histidine permits O₂ to bind favorably to the Fe²⁺ atom.

Myoglobin: an O₂-storage protein

Located in the cytosol of muscle cells, Mb binds O₂ that has been released by Hb in the tissue capillaries and has subsequently diffused across cellular membranes. This stored O₂ is readily available to organelles, particularly the mitochondrion, that carry out oxidative metabolism. With its single ligand-binding site, the reversible reaction of Mb with O₂

$$Mb + O_2 \rightleftharpoons Mb \bullet O_2$$

may be described by the following equations,

$$K_a = \frac{[Mb \bullet O_2]}{[Mb][O_2]}$$

$$Y = \frac{[Mb \bullet O_2]}{[Mb \bullet O_2] + [Mb]}$$

in which K_a is an affinity or equilibrium constant and Y is the fractional O₂ saturation. Combining these two equations, expressing the concentration of O₂ in terms of its partial pressure pO₂, and substituting the term P_{50} for $1/K_a$ yields the equation for the O₂ saturation curve of Mb:

$$Y = \frac{pO_2}{(pO_2 + P_{50})}$$

By definition, the constant P_{50} is the value of pO₂ at which $Y = 0.5$ or half the ligand sites are occupied (saturated by O₂). In a plot of Y versus pO₂, the equation for ligand binding by Mb describes a hyperbola (Fig. 4.3) with $P_{50} \approx 4$ mm Hg. The low value of P_{50} reflects a high affinity for O₂. In the capillary beds of muscle tissues, pO₂ values are in the range of 20–40 mm Hg. Predictably, working muscles exhibit lower pO₂ values than muscles at rest. With its high affinity for O₂, myocyte Mb readily becomes saturated with O₂ that has entered from the blood. As O₂ is consumed during aerobic metabolism, O₂ dissociates from Mb and diffuses into mitochondria, the power plants of the muscle cell.

Hemoglobin: an O₂-transport protein

Hb, the principal O₂-transporting protein in blood, is localized in the erythrocytes. As a delivery vehicle, Hb must be able to bind O₂ efficiently as it enters the lung alveoli during

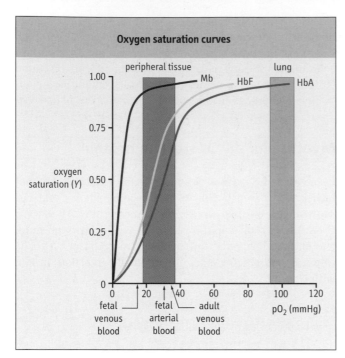

Oxygen saturation curves

Fig. 4.3 **Oxygen saturation curves of myoglobin and hemoglobin.** Mb and Hb have different O_2 saturation curves. The fractional saturation (Y) of O_2-binding sites is plotted against the concentration of O_2 [pO_2 (mm Hg)]. Curves are shown for Mb, fetal Hb (HbF), and adult Hb (HbA). Also indicated, by arrows and shading, are the normal levels of O_2 measured in various adult and fetal blood samples.

respiration and to release O_2 to the extracellular environment with similar efficiency as erythrocytes circulate through tissue capillaries. This remarkable duality of function is achieved by cooperative interactions among the globin subunits of Hb.

Quaternary structure of human hemoglobin

Human Hb is a tetramer of two α-globin and two β-globin subunits: $\alpha_2\beta_2$. These subunits are organized in a tetrahedral array, a geometry that predicts several types of subunit-subunit interactions (Fig. 4.4). Experimental analysis of the quaternary structure indicates multiple noncovalent interactions (hydrogen and electrostatic bonds) between each pair of dissimilar subunits, i.e. at the α–β interfaces. In contrast, there are fewer interactions between identical subunits, at the α–α or β–β interfaces. Thus, Hb is more appropriately considered a dimer of heterodimers: $(\alpha–\beta)_2$. The actual number and nature of contacts differ in the presence or absence of O_2 and allosteric effectors. Strong associations within the α–β heterodimer and at the interface between the two heterodimers (Fig. 4.4) are now recognized as major factors determining O_2 binding and release.

Interactions of hemoglobin with O_2

Hb can bind up to four molecules of O_2. With its multiple ligand-binding sites, the binding affinity and the fractional saturation of Hb are more complex functions than those of Mb. Consequently, the equation for the fractional O_2 saturation curve is modified to

$$Y = \frac{pO_2^n}{pO_2^n + P_{50}^n}$$

where n is the Hill coefficient. In a plot of Y versus pO_2 when $n > 1$, the equation for ligand binding describes a sigmoid (S-shaped) curve (Fig. 4.3).

The Hill coefficient, determined experimentally, is a measure of cooperativity among ligand-binding sites, i.e., the extent to which the binding of O_2 with one subunit influences the affinity of O_2 with other subunits. For fully cooperative binding, n is equal to the number of sites, an indication that binding at one site maximally enhances binding at other sites in the same molecule. In the absence of cooperativity, even with multiple sites, the Hill coefficient would be 1, i.e. binding of one molecule of O_2 does not influence the binding of the

 ARTIFICIAL HEMOGLOBINS

Red cell substitutes are allogeneic transfusion alternatives; they are potentially useful during major surgical procedures and in hemorrhagic shock emergencies. The supply-and-demand curves of whole blood and packed red cell availability and use point to an impending crisis and the need to develop alternatives. Three classes of products have been investigated: Hb-based oxygen carriers (HBOC), liposome-encapsulated Hb, and perfluorocarbon emulsions. HBOCs are polymerized forms of hemoglobin; otherwise, the hemoglobin dissociates into monomers (MW ~16 000 kDa) in plasma and is excreted in urine. Retention of hemoglobin in the kidney may also cause renal failure. Advantages of HBOCs include ease of purification, long-term stability, and minimal immunogenicity. Glutaraldehyde-polymerized bovine Hb (Hemopure®) and diaspirin cross-linked human Hb exhibit increased O_2 affinity (P_{50} = 32–35 mm Hg), diminished cooperativity (n = 1.3–2.1), and decreased sensitivity to allosteric effectors, compared to normal Hb. Both also are more susceptible to autooxidation, a process that leads to significant, although sub-clinical increases in methemoglobin levels. These and other HBOCs have been investigated in clinical trials. In single- and multidose administration, polymerized bovine Hb appears to be well-tolerated in surgical and anemic patients; it has recently been approved for use in some countries. On the other hand, increased mortality with the use of diaspirin cross-linked human Hb has forced the termination of its clinical evaluation.

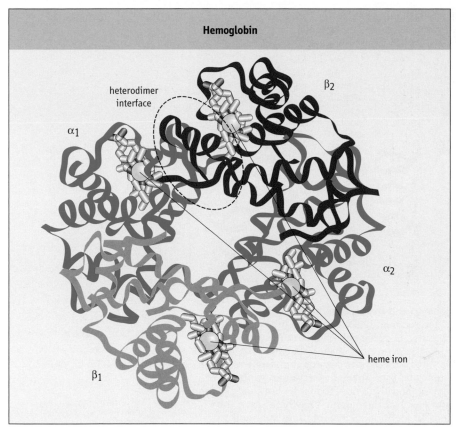

Hemoglobin

heterodimer
interface

α_1

β_2

α_2

β_1

heme iron

Fig. 4.4 **Model of hemoglobin.** Hemoglobin is a tetramer of four globin subunits. Hb is a tetrahedral complex of two identical α-globins (α_1 and α_2, greens) and two identical β-globins (β_1 and β_2, purples). With this geometry each globin molecule contacts the other three, creating the subunit interfaces and interactions that define cooperativity.

next. This is observed for Hb mutants that have lost functional subunit-subunit contacts.

In practice, a Hill coefficient between 1 and n, the theoretical maximum, is commonly observed. The normal value for adult Hb ($n = 2.7$) is an indication of strongly cooperative ligand binding. Hb has a P_{50} of 27 ± 2 mmHg, significantly greater than that of Mb. The steepest slope of the saturation curve for Hb lies in a range of pO_2 that is found in most tissues (Fig. 4.3). Thus, relatively small changes in pO_2 will result in considerably larger changes in the interaction of Hb with O_2. Accordingly, slight shifts of the curve in either direction will also dramatically influence O_2 affinity.

Transition between deoxygenated and oxygenated hemoglobin

As deoxygenated Hb becomes oxygenated, significant structural changes extend throughout the protein molecule. In the heme pocket, as a consequence of O_2 coordination to iron and a new orientation of atoms in the heme structure, the proximal histidine and the helix to which it belongs shift their positions (see Fig. 4.1). This subtle conformational change triggers major structural realignments elsewhere within each subunit. In turn, these tertiary structural changes are trans-

mitted, even amplified, in the overall quaternary structure such that one αβ heterodimer rotates ~15° and slides ~0.10 nm relative to the other. Because of the inherent asymmetry of the Hb tetramer, these combined motions result in quite dramatic changes within and, more importantly, between the αβ heterodimers.

Contact between the two heterodimers (Fig. 4.4) is stabilized by a mixture of hydrogen and electrostatic bonds. Approximately 30 amino acids participate in the noncovalent interactions that characterize the deoxygenated and oxygenated Hb conformations. The two quaternary conformations are known as the T- and R-states, respectively (see Fig. 5.10). In the T-state (tense), interactions between the heterodimers are stronger; in the R-state (relaxed), these noncovalent bonds are, in summation, weaker. O_2 affinity is lower for the T-state and higher for the R-state. The transition between these structures is accompanied by the dissolution of existing noncovalent bonds and formation of new ones at the heterodimer interfaces (Fig. 4.5).

Several models have been developed to describe the transition between the T- and R-states of hemoglobin. At one extreme is a model in which each hemoglobin subunit sequentially responds to O_2 binding with a conformational change, thereby permitting hybrid intermediates of the T- and R-states. At the opposite extreme is a model in which all four subunits

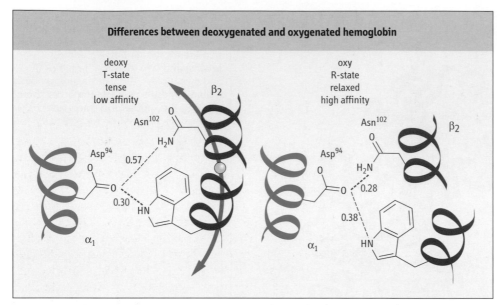

Fig. 4.5 **Noncovalent bonds differ in deoxygenated and oxygenated hemoglobin.** In the middle of the interface between the two $\alpha\beta$ heterodimers are the residues Asp[94] α_1 on one heterodimer and Trp[37] β_2 and Asn[102] β_2 on the other. Each has side-chain atoms capable of non-covalent interactions. Left: In the deoxygenated T-structure the distance between the Asp and Trp residues favors a hydrogen bond, whereas the distance between Asp and Asn is too great. Right: As a result of the conformational changes that accompany the transition to the oxygenated R-structure, the distance between Asp and Trp is now too large, but that between Asp and Asn is compatible with formation of a new hydrogen bond. Elsewhere along this interface, other bonds are created and broken. An identical alignment of residues and noncovalent interactions is found between the α_2 and β_1 monomers (Fig. 4.4). Distances are shown in nm. Hydrogen bonds are commonly 0.27–0.31 nm in length.

switch concertedly; hybrid states are forbidden, and O_2 binding shifts the equilibrium between T- and R- states. The molecular structures of deoxygenated and partially and fully liganded Hb have been studied extensively. Despite a wealth of thermodynamic and kinetic data and recent elegant investigations of ligand interactions with Hb crystals and silica-encapsulated Hb, progress toward reconciling inconsistencies with both models has been slow. Much evidence appears to support an allosteric mechanism with features of both models, in part because fundamental questions still remain unanswered. Do the α- and β-subunits differ in ligand affinity? Which subunit binds the first (or releases the last) molecule of O_2?

Interactions with allosteric effectors

Allosteric proteins and effectors

Hb is one of the best-studied examples of an allosteric protein, a protein that exhibits changes in ligand (or substrate) affinity under the influence of small molecules. These small

 PULSE OXIMETRY

Pulse oximetry ('pulse-ox') is a non-invasive method of estimating the oxygen saturation of arterial Hb. Two physical principles are involved: first, the visible (650–660 nm) and infrared (850–940 nm) spectral characteristics of oxy- and deoxy-Hb are different; second, arterial blood flow has a pulsatile component that results from volume changes with each heart beat. Therefore, transmission or reflectance measurements are made in a translucent tissue site with reasonable blood flow, commonly a finger, toe, or ear of adults and children, or a foot or hand of infants. The pulse oximeter's photodetector and microprocessor calculate an oxygen saturation (SpO$_2$) that typically correlates within 4–6% of the value found by arterial blood gas analysis. Pulse oximetry is used to monitor the cardiopulmonary status during local and general anesthesia, in intensive care and neonatal units, and during patient transport. Body movement, radiated ambient light, elevated bilirubin, artificial or painted fingernails can interfere with pulse oximetry.

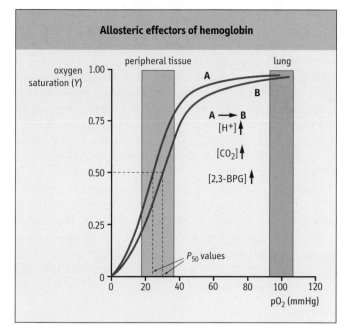

Allosteric effectors of hemoglobin

Fig. 4.6 **Allosteric effectors decrease the oxygen affinity of hemoglobin.** O_2 interaction with hemoglobin is regulated by allosteric effectors. Under physiologic conditions HbA exhibits a highly cooperative O_2 saturation curve. With an increase in the erythrocyte concentration of any of three allosteric effectors, H^+, CO_2, or 2,3-bisphosphoglycerate (2,3-BPG), the curve shifts to the right (position B), indicating a decreased affinity for O_2 (increase in the P_{50} value). Actions of the effectors that modulate O_2 affinity appear to be additive. Conversely, a decrease in any of the allosteric effectors shifts the curve to the left (position A). Increasing temperature will also shift the curve to the right. The sensitivity of O_2 saturation to [H^+] is known as the Bohr effect. Normal ranges of O_2 measured in pulmonary and peripheral tissue capillaries are indicated by shaded areas.

molecules, called allosteric (meaning other place or site) effectors, bind to proteins at sites that are spatially distinct from the ligand-binding sites. Through long-range conformational effects, they alter the ligand or substrate binding affinity of the protein. Allosteric proteins are typically multisubunit proteins. An allosteric effector may exert either a positive influence on ligand interaction (increased affinity) or a negative influence (decreased affinity). The O_2 binding affinity of hemoglobin is affected positively by O_2 (above), and also also by a number of chemically different allosteric effectors, including H^+, CO_2, and 2,3-bisphosphoglycerate (2,3-BPG) (Fig. 4.6). When an allosteric effector affects its own binding to the protein (at other sites), the process is termed homotropic, e.g. the effect of binding of O_2 at one site on hemoglobin enhances the affinity for binding of O_2 to other sites on hemoglobin. When the allosteric effector is different from the ligand whose binding is altered, the process is termed

heterotropic, e.g. the effect of H^+ on the P_{50} for oxygen binding to hemoglobin.

Bohr effect

The O_2 affinity of Hb is exquisitely sensitive to pH, a phenomenon called the Bohr effect. It is most readily described as a right shift in the O_2 saturation curve with decreasing pH. Thus, an increased concentration of H^+ (decreased pH) favors an increased P_{50} (lower affinity) for O_2 binding to hemoglobin. To understand the Bohr effect at the level of protein structure and to appreciate the role of H^+ as an allosteric effector, it is important to recall that Hb is a highly charged molecule. Experimental evidence suggests that the residues that participate in the Bohr effect are the N-terminal amino group of the α-chains and the side chains of His[122] α and His[143] β. The pK values of these residues differ sufficiently between the deoxygenated and oxygenated forms of Hb to cause the uptake of about two H^+ by the T-structure (deoxygenated Hb). These interactions, in turn, are linked directly to the decrease in O_2 affinity of the T-state of Hb.

When Hb binds O_2, protons dissociate from the weak acid functions. Conversely, in acidic media, protonation of the conjugate bases inhibits O_2 binding. During their circulation between pulmonary alveoli and peripheral tissue capillaries, erythrocytes encounter markedly different conditions of pO_2 and pH. The high pO_2 in the lungs promotes ligand saturation, yet it also forces protons from the Hb molecule to stabilize the R-state. In the capillary bed, particularly in metabolically active tissues, the pH is slightly lower, due to the production of acidic metabolites, such as lactate. Oxygenated Hb, upon entering this environment, will acquire some 'excess' protons and shift toward the T-state, promoting release of O_2 for uptake in tissues for aerobic metabolism (Chapter 23).

Effects of CO_2 and temperature

Closely related to the Bohr effect is the ability of CO_2 to alter the O_2 affinity of Hb. Like the negative allosteric effect of H^+, the increase in pCO_2 in venous capillaries decreases the affinity of hemoglobin for O_2. Accordingly, a right shift in the ligand saturation curve occurs as pCO_2 increases. It should be emphasized that the allosteric effector is, in fact, CO_2, not HCO_3^-. CO_2 reacts reversibly with the unprotonated N-terminal amino groups of the globin polypeptides to form carbamino–Hb:

$$Hb - NH_2 + CO_2 \rightleftharpoons Hb - NH - COO^- + H^+$$

This transient chemical modification of Hb is not only a specialized example of allosteric control, resulting in a stabilization of deoxygenated Hb; it also represents one form of transport of CO_2 to the lungs for clearance from the body.

❋ ACUTE MOUNTAIN SICKNESS (TOO HIGH TOO FAST)

Acute mountain sickness (AMS) develops in 20–25% of individuals who ascend rapidly to altitudes above 2500–4000 m and in the majority of those who climb even higher. Symptoms include shortness of breath, rapid heart rate, headache, nausea, anorexia, and sleep disturbance. AMS is usually benign; it occurs with greater frequency in the young. The most severe form is high-altitude cerebral edema (HACE), a potentially life-threatening condition that is characterized by ataxia and other neuromuscular and neurological problems. HACE has been proposed to be a hypoxia-induced, vasogenic edema whose pathophysiology involves altered permeability of the blood-brain barrier and imbalance among fluid compartments in the central nervous system.

At 4000 m the barometric pressure is 460 torr, leading to an ambient partial pressure of O_2 of 96 torr (sea level, 159). Physiological calculations yield values of tracheal pO_2 = 86 torr (sea level, 149), alveolar pO_2 = 50 torr (sea level, 105), and arterial pO_2 = 45 torr (sea level, 100). At this arterial partial pressure of O_2, hemoglobin saturation is only 81% (see Fig. 4.3). Consequently, the O_2 content of arterial blood decreases to ~16.0 mL/L (sea level, 19.5), based on an Hb concentration of 150 g/L. Decreased tissue O_2 can potentially disrupt cellular metabolism. Humans adapt to high altitude (acclimatization) by several mechanisms. Hyperventilation is a critical short-term response that serves to decrease alveolar pCO_2 and, in turn, increase alveolar pO_2. Arterial pH is also increased during hyperventilation, leading to a higher affinity of Hb for O_2. A gradual increase in 2,3-bisphosphoglycerate also occurs in response to chronic hypoxia. Another important adaptive mechanism is polycythemia, an increase in erythrocyte concentration that results from erythropoietin stimulation of bone marrow cells. Within 1 week of acclimatization the Hb concentration can increase by as much as 20% (30 g/L) to provide near-normal arterial O_2 content.

There is a strong physiologic correlation between pCO_2 and O_2 affinity. CO_2 is a major product of mitochondrial oxidation and, like H^+, will be particularly abundant in metabolically active tissues. Upon diffusing into the blood, a small portion of CO_2 reacts with oxygenated Hb, shifts the equilibrium toward the T-state, and thereby promotes the dissociation of bound O_2 (Fig. 4.6). The vast majority of peripheral-tissue CO_2, however, is hydrated in the presence of erythrocyte carbonic anhydrase to carbonic acid (H_2CO_3), a weak acid that dissociates partially to H^+ and HCO_3^- (see Chapter 23):

$$CO_2 + H_2O \rightleftharpoons H_2CO_3 \quad \text{enzyme-catalyzed reaction}$$

$$H_2CO_3 \rightleftharpoons H^+ + HCO_3^- \quad \text{acid-conjugate base reaction}$$

Interestingly, from both the carbamination reaction and hydration/dissociation reactions involving CO_2, an additional pool of protons is generated, protons that become available to participate in the Bohr effect and facilitate O_2–CO_2 exchange. During its return to the lungs, blood transports two forms of CO_2: carbamino-Hb and the H_2CO_3/HCO_3^- acid-conjugate base pair. Blood and Hb are now exposed to a low pCO_2, and through mass action the carbamination reaction is reversed and binding of O_2 is again favored. Similarly, in the pulmonary capillaries, erythrocyte carbonic anhydrase converts H_2CO_3 into CO_2 and H_2O, products whose gaseous forms are expelled into the atmosphere, as discussed in Chapter 23.

Working muscles not only produce the allosteric effectors H^+ and CO_2 as byproducts of aerobic metabolism, but they liberate heat as well. Because the binding of O_2 to heme is an exothermic process, the O_2 affinity of Hb decreases with increasing temperature. Thus, the microenvironment of an exercising muscle favors a more efficient release of Hb-bound O_2 to the surrounding tissue.

Effect of 2,3-bisphosphoglycerate

An organic phosphate compound, 2,3-bisphosphoglycerate, is another important modulator of the O_2 affinity of hemoglobin. A side product in the glycolytic pathway (Chapter 11), this molecule is synthesized in human erythrocytes. Like H^+ and CO_2, it is an indispensable negative allosteric effector that, when bound to Hb, causes a marked increase in P_{50}. Indeed, if it were not for the high erythrocyte concentration of 2,3-BPG (~4.1 mmol/L [1.1 g/L], nearly equal to that of Hb), the O_2 saturation curve of Hb would approach that of Mb!

At one end of the two-fold symmetry axis within the quaternary structure of Hb there is a shallow cleft defined by cationic amino acids of the juxtaposed β subunits (Fig. 4.7). One molecule of 2,3-BPG binds to this site. A critical consequence of the conformational differences between the T- and R-states is that only deoxygenated Hb interacts with the negatively charged 2,3-BPG. Electrostatic interactions stabilize the complex between the effector and Hb. The cleft is too narrow in oxygenated Hb to accommodate 2,3-BPG.

The importance of 2,3-BPG as an allosteric effector is underscored by observations that its concentration in the erythrocyte changes in response to various physiologic and pathologic conditions. During chronic hypoxia (decreased pO_2) because of pulmonary disease, anemia or shock, the level of 2,3-BPG increases. Such compensatory increases have also been described in cigarette smokers and on adaptation to high altitudes. The net result is a greater stabilization of the deoxygenated, low-affinity T-state and a further shift of the saturation curve to the right, thereby facilitating release of more O_2 to the hypoxic tissues. Under most circumstances, the rightward shift has an insignificant effect on the O_2 saturation of Hb in the lungs.

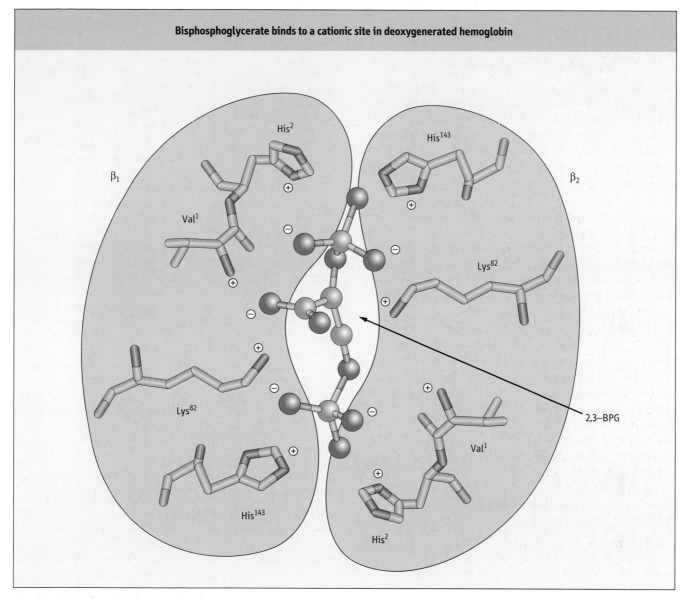

Bisphosphoglycerate binds to a cationic site in deoxygenated hemoglobin

Fig. 4.7 **2,3-Bisphosphoglycerate binding to deoxygenated hemoglobin.** On the surface of the deoxygenated Hb tetramer where the two β-globin (purple) interact, there is a cleft formed by the N-terminal amino acid residue (Val[1] β) and the side chains of His[2] β, Lys[82] β, and His[143] β (stick models). This site consists of eight cationic groups, sufficient to bind with high affinity one molecule of 2,3-BPG (ball-and-stick model; phosphorus, orange), a molecule with five anionic groups at physiological pH. This array of positive charges does not exist in oxygenated Hb. In fetal Hb (HbF) His[143] β is replaced by a Ser residue.

RECENTLY IDENTIFIED VERTEBRATE GLOBINS

In addition to Mb and Hb, two new cytosolic members of the vertebrate globin family have been identified since 2000. Neuroglobin is expressed primarily in brain and other nerve tissues; cytoglobin (or histoglobin) is ubiquitously expressed. Both human proteins share only about 25% sequence identity with Mb and Hb. Yet all key elements of the globin domain are present, including the proximal and distal His residues and a hydrophobic pocket in which heme is inserted. The O_2 affinities of the monomeric neuroglobin and cytoglobin are similar to that of Mb. Recent evidence suggests an Mb-like role in O_2 storage and diffusion in tissues such as the retina, adrenal cortex, and pituitary. Other possible functions include scavenging reactive oxygen species and sensing cellular O_2 concentration.

INSIGHTS FROM MYOGLOBIN KNOCKOUT MICE

Access to embryonic stem cells and complementary DNA fragments permits selected gene disruption in whole animals. With deletion of exon 2 in the gene encoding mouse Mb, three genotypes could be compared: wild-type, heterozygous, and homozygous null (or knockout). Quite unexpectedly, mice lacking Mb exhibited no obvious phenotypic abnormalities under normal conditions or even during exercise or hypoxia. Thus, Mb does not appear to be essential for normal cardio-vascular, musculoskeletal, and reproductive function. How-ever, this 'normal' phenotype was the result of numerous compensatory mechanisms, all of which contributed to a steeper pO_2 gradient between the capillary and the mito-chondrion. Some of the adaptations were increased capillary density, more rapid coronary flow, transition to fast-twitch myofibers, and elevated Hb concentration.

These findings have prompted a reappraisal of the function of Mb in muscle tissues. In the knockout animals the devel-opment of broad compensatory measures strongly suggests that Mb is normally important in facilitating O_2 diffusion and maintaining mitochondrial electron transport, particularly in muscles that produce slow, repetitive, and forceful activity. In the fast-twitch muscles of Mb-deficient mice, however, there is a significant increase in nitric oxide (NO), a potent vasodilator and an inhibitor of electron transport. This has led to the intriguing idea that Mb, with a recognized capacity to convert NO to nitrate, may be a key mediator of O_2 delivery and a regulator of O_2 utilization.

HYPERVENTILATION, NUMBNESS, AND DIZZINESS

A college student with severe muscle spasms in her arms, numbness in her extremities, some dizziness, and respiratory difficulty was brought to the student health center. The patient had been vigorously exercising in an attempt to relieve the stress of forthcoming examinations when she suddenly began to experience forced, rapid breathing. Suspecting hyperventilation, a health care worker began to reassure the student and helped her recover by getting her to breathe into a paper bag. After 20 minutes the spasms ceased, feeling returned to her fingers, and the lightheadedness resolved.

Comment. Alveolar hyperventilation is an abnormally rapid, deep, and prolonged breathing pattern that leads to respiratory alkalosis, i.e. a profound decrease in pCO_2 and an increase in blood pH that can be attributed to the increased loss of CO_2 from the body. With decreased $[CO_2]$ and $[H^+]$, two allosteric effectors of O_2 binding and release, the affinity of Hb for O_2 increases sufficiently to reduce the efficiency of delivery of O_2 to peripheral tissues, including the central nervous system. Another characteristic of alkalosis is a decreased level of ionized calcium in plasma, a situation that contributes to muscle spasms and cramps. In general, hyperventilation may be triggered by hypoxemia, pulmonary and cardiac diseases, metabolic disorders, pharmacologic agents, and anxiety.

INTERACTIONS OF HEMOGLOBIN WITH NITRIC OXIDE

Notwithstanding its well-established role as an important mediator of vascular signal transduction (see Chapter 6), NO (nitric oxide) is a highly reactive, gaseous free radical that can

ACQUIRED (TOXIC) METHEMOGLOBINEMIA

In a rural region of the state, a 4-month-old infant was seen at the local emergency room for episodes of seizures, breathing difficulty, and vomiting. The infant's skin and mucous membranes were bluish, indicating cyanosis. Analysis of arterial blood revealed a chocolate brown color, a normal pO_2, an O_2 saturation of 60%, and a ferric-heme methemoglobin level of 35%. The tentative cause of the acute toxic methemoglobinemia was found to be well water contaminated by a nitrate/nitrite concentration of 34 mg/L. The infant was treated successfully by intravenous administration of methylene blue (1–2 mg/kg), a potent reducing agent.

Comment: Methylene blue reduces ferric hemoglobin (methemoglobin) to normal (ferrous) hemoglobin. Methemoglobin is an oxidation product of Hb; it is produced spontaneously at a low rate and more rapidly in the presence of certain drugs, nitrites, and aniline dyes. Mutation of either the proximal or distal His to Tyr also makes heme iron more susceptible to oxidation (Table 4.1). Erythrocytes contain an NADH-cytochrome b_5 reductase that catalyzes the reduction of methemoglobin to Hb. Infants are particularly vulnerable to methemoglobinemia. Not only do they have a diminished activity of the reductase, but their HbF is more sensitive to oxidants compared to HbA.

modify biological macromolecules. NO has been shown to react reversibly with Hb in two rather different ways: binding to heme Fe^{2+}, a process comparable to the binding of O_2, and forming an adduct with surface-exposed Cys^{93} β side chains. The physiological significance of either nitrosyl-Hb or S-nitroso-Hb remains controversial. Some investigators favor a hypothesis that the interaction of Hb with NO is sensitive to pO_2 and the T-state/R-state conformational transition and that Hb has a role in transport and delivery of a third gas, NO. Others argue that the level of S-nitroso-Hb in blood is too low (~5 nM) and unchanged between the arterial and venous compartments to participate in an allosterically mediated release of NO (see also p 235).

NORMAL HB VARIANTS

Over 95% of the Hb found in adult humans is HbA, with the $α_2β_2$ globin chain composition. HbA_2 accounts for 2–3% of the total and has an $α_2δ_2$ polypeptide composition. HbA_2 is elevated in β-thalassemia, a disease characterized by a deficiency in β-globin biosynthesis. Functionally, these two adult Hbs are indistinguishable. Not surprisingly, mutations of the gene encoding δ-globin are without clinical consequence.

Another minor Hb is fetal Hb, HbF; its subunits are α-globin and γ-globin. While it accounts for no more than 1% of adult Hb, HbF predominates in the fetus during the second and third trimesters of gestation and in the neonate. Gene switching on chromosome 11 causes HbF to decrease shortly after birth. The most striking functional difference between HbF and HbA is its decreased sensitivity to 2,3-BPG. Comparison of the primary structures of the β- and γ- polypeptides reveals a replacement of His^{143} β by serine in γ-globin (Fig. 4.7). Consequently, two of the cationic groups that participate in the binding of the anionic allosteric effector are no longer present. Predictably, the interaction of 2,3-BPG with HbF is weaker, resulting in an increased affinity for O_2 (P_{50} = 19 mm Hg for HbF versus 27 mm Hg for HbA) and a greater stabilization of the oxygenated R-state. The direct benefit of this structural and functional change in the HbF isoform is a more efficient transfer of O_2 from maternal HbA to fetal HbF (Fig. 4.3). The HbF variant, barely detectable in most adults, often increases up to 15–20% in individuals with mutant adult Hbs, such as sickle cell disease. This is an example of the body's compensatory response to a pathologic abnormality. Evaluation of many Hb variants is performed by electrophoretic and chromatographic analysis (Fig. 4.8).

SICKLE CELL DISEASE

Sickle cell disease is caused by an inherited structural abnormality in the β-globin polypeptide. Clinically, an

ERYTHROPOIETIN TREATMENT FOR ANEMIA

Anemia, defined clinically as a decrease in hematocrit (<37%) or Hb concentration (<120 g/L), may be caused by blood loss, excessive hemolysis, and/or deficient erythropoiesis. One therapeutic strategy in the treatment of some anemias is the production of new erythrocytes, a bone marrow stem cell proliferation and differentiation process that requires the hormone erythropoietin (EPO). In the 1980s and 1990s clinical trials of recombinant human EPO (rHuEPO, Epogen®, Procrit®) showed that exogenous hormone was particularly effective in increasing Hb levels in patients with anemias associated with chronic renal failure, chemotherapy for nonmyeloid malignancies, and treatment of HIV infections.
EPO is secreted by renal peritubular endothelial cells in response to localized tissue hypoxia. Upon binding to receptors that belong to the cytokine superfamily, EPO initiates multiple signaling pathways in erythroid progenitor cells. The glycoprotein EPO contains both N-linked and O-linked oligosaccharides. Because the oligosaccharide groups exhibit microheterogeneity in sugar content and structure, particularly in the number of N-acetylneuraminic (sialic) acid residues, a family of isoforms is always observed by isoelectric focusing polyacrylamide electrophoresis. Additional heterogeneity is seen between natural EPO and rHuEPO that is produced commercially in Chinese hamster ovary cells. Darbopoetin alfa (Aranesp®), a second-generation rHuEPO, has been 'glycoengineered' to contain additional N-linked oligosaccharides, structural features that significantly enhance its stability and bioactivity.

individual with sickle cell disease presents with intermittent episodes of hemolytic and painful vaso-occlusive crises, the latter leading to severe pain in bones, chest, and abdomen. Common side effects include impaired growth, increased susceptibility to infections, and multiple organ damage. Sickle cell disease has a prevalence of 40% in some regions of equatorial Africa; among black Americans, heterozygotic carriers number 8%, yielding about 0.2% frequency of the disease in the African American population. The Hb molecule in sickle cell disease (HbS) has been studied biochemically and biophysically for over 50 years, and sickle cell disease has become the paradigm of a molecular disease.

HbA remains a true solute at rather high concentrations, largely as a result of a polar exterior surface that is compatible with and nonreactive with nearby Hb molecules. In contrast, HbS, when deoxygenated, is less soluble. It forms long, filamentous polymers that readily precipitate, distorting erythrocyte morphology to the characteristic sickle shape. The mutation is Glu^6 β→Val: a surface-localized charged amino

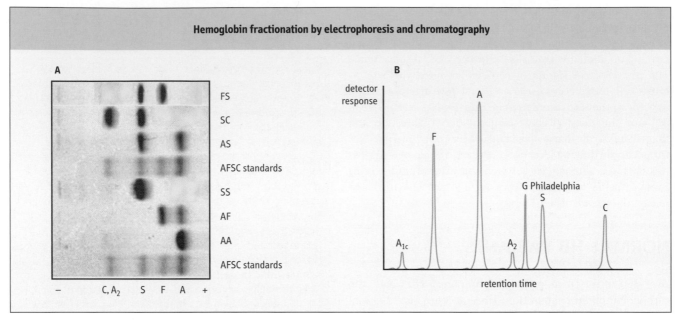

Fig. 4.8 **Normal and abnormal hemoglobins can be separated by electrophoretic and chromatographic methods.** (A) This panel shows cellulose acetate electrophoresis (pH 8.4) of blood samples obtained for neonatal screening. This rapid technique will tentatively identify HbS and HbC, two common mutant hemoglobins in the African American population. Additional tests are required for a definitive diagnosis. FS, newborn with sickle cell disease; SC, double heterozygote child with sickle cell-like disease; AS, child with sickle cell trait; AF, normal neonate. (B) This trace illustrates high-pressure liquid chromatography (HPLC) with a cation-exchanger solid phase, a technique capable of separating and quantifying more than 40 hemoglobins. HPLC may also be used to measure HbA_{1c}, a glycated protein that provides information on the progression and treatment of diabetes mellitus (Chapter 20). Also shown is the elution profile of Hb G Philadelphia ($Asn^{68}\alpha \rightarrow Lys$), a common but benign variant that co-migrates with HbS on electrophoresis.

 ## SEPARATION OF HEMOGLOBIN VARIANTS AND MUTANTS AND THE DIAGNOSIS OF HEMOGLOBINOPATHIES

The mobility of a protein during electrophoresis or chromatography is determined by its charge and interaction with the matrix. Three commonly used techniques provide sufficient resolution to separate hemoglobin variants differing in a single charge from HbA: electrophoresis, isoelectric focusing, and ion exchange chromatography. Electrophoretic and chromatographic separations of Hb are illustrated in Figure 4.8. The volume of hemolysate required (<100 µL) makes these techniques suitable for neonate and adult blood samples. Quantification is performed by scanning densitometry or absorption spectrometry. Indications of abnormalities in screening tests are followed by complete blood count (see Table 4.2), additional protein analysis, and DNA analysis to identify specific mutations to the globin genes.

 ## ANALGESIC TREATMENT OF SICKLE CELL VASO-OCCLUSIVE CRISES

Vaso-occlusive pain is the most common problem reported by individuals with sickle cell disease. It is also the most frequent reason for emergency-room treatment and hospital admission of individuals with sickle cell disease. Episodes of vaso-occlusive pain are unpredictable and are often excruciating and incapacitating. The origin of this progressive pain involves altered rheologic and hematologic properties of erythrocytes attributable to HbS polymerization and aggregation, coupled with an inflammatory leukocytosis and elevation of plasma acute-phase proteins (Chapter 3). The pain lasts an average of 4–10 days. To provide relief to the patient, nonnarcotic, narcotic, and adjuvant analgesics are used alone or in combination. Obviously, the severity and duration of the pain dictate the most appropriate analgesic regimen. Several recent studies suggest additional options for the patient and physician: continuous intravenous infusion of a nonsteroidal anti-inflammatory drug (ketoralac) reduced the requirement for opioid analgesic (meperidine); and continuous epidural administration of local anesthetic (lidocaine) and opioid analgesic (fentanyl) effectively decreased pain that was unresponsive to conventional measures.

A PATIENT WITH MUTANT HEMOGLOBIN

During a complete physical examination related to diabetes mellitus and cataracts, a 66-year-old male presented with cyanosis of the lips. The patient was found to have mild hypertension, left ventricular hypertrophy, and other electrocardiographic abnormalities. Since childhood, he has followed a restricted exercise program because of suspected heart disease. Laboratory findings indicated increases in hematocrit (HCT), erythrocyte count, and Hb concentration (see Table 4.2). Platelet and leucocyte counts were normal, as was pulmonary function. The P_{50} of the patient's whole blood was 58 mmHg (normal = 27 ± 2); the Hill coefficient was 1.6 (normal = 2.7 ± 0.2). The possibility of an abnormal Hb was considered. Biochemical analysis of his Hb revealed a mutant β-globin polypeptide in which Asn^{102} β was replaced by Thr. Electrophoretic analysis indicated that the patient was heterozygous for Hb Kansas.

Comment. Not only does this mutant Hb exhibit a dramatically reduced affinity for O_2 (increased P_{50}), but subunit cooperativity is also markedly disrupted (decreased n). Examination of the tertiary structures of deoxygenated and oxygenated Hb provides an explanation: Asp^{94}α hydrogen bonds to Asn^{102}β in the heterodimer interface, a bond that only exists in the R-state (Fig. 4.5). These residues are too far apart in the T-state to create a noncovalent interaction. In Hb Kansas the absence of this critical oxygenated Hb-stabilizing bond shifts the equilibrium between the T- and R-states toward deoxygenation, less communication among the four ligand-binding sites, and a decrease in subunit cooperativity. Although Hb Kansas is very rarely seen in a clinical setting, the phenotypes of this and other rare hemoglobinopathies continue to provide valuable insight into protein structure-function relationships.

acid is replaced by a hydrophobic residue. Valine on the mutant β-globin subunit fits into a complementary pocket (sometimes called a 'sticky patch') formed on the β-globin subunit of another Hb molecule, a pocket that becomes exposed only upon the release of bound O_2 in tissue capillaries. In the homozygous individual with sickle cell disease (HbS/HbS), the complex process of nucleation and polymerization occurs rapidly, producing about 10% of circulating erythrocytes that are sickled. In the heterozygous individual (HbA/HbS, sickle cell trait), the kinetics of sickling are decreased by at least a factor of 10^3, thereby accounting for the asymptomatic nature of this genotype. In dilute solution, HbS has interactions with O_2 (P_{50} value, Hill coefficient) that are similar to those for HbA. However, the Bohr effect on concentrated HbS is more pronounced, leading to greater release of O_2 in the capillaries and increased propensity for polymer growth.

Sickled erythrocytes exhibit less deformability; they no longer move freely through the microvasculature and often block blood flow, especially in the spleen and joints. Moreover, these cells lose water, become fragile, and have a considerably shorter life span, leading to hemolysis and anemia. Except during extreme physical exertion, the heterozygous individual appears normal. For reasons that remain to be elucidated, heterozygosity is associated with an increased resistance to malaria, specifically growth of the infectious agent *Plasmod-*

ium falciparum in the erythrocyte. This observation represents an example of a selective advantage that the HbA/HbS heterozygote exhibits over either the HbA/HbA normal or the HbS/HbS homozygote and probably explains the persistence of HbS in the gene pool.

OTHER HEMOGLOBINOPATHIES

More than 600 mutations in the genes encoding the α- and β-globin polypeptides have been documented. As with most mutational events, the majority of these lead to few, if any, clinical problems. There are, however, several hundred mutations that give rise to abnormal Hb and pathologic phenotypes. Hb mutants or hemoglobinopathies are usually named after the location (hospital, city, or geographical region) in which the abnormal protein was first identified. They are classified according to the type of structural change and altered function and the resulting clinical characteristics (Table 4.1 and 4.2). While many of these mutants have predictable phenotypes, there are others that are surprisingly pleiotropic in their impact on multiple properties of the Hb molecule. With few exceptions, Hb variants are inherited as autosomal recessive traits. Occasionally, double heterozygotes are identified, e.g., HbSC (see Fig. 4.8).

Classification and examples of hemoglobinopathies

Classification	Common name mutation		Biochemical change	Clinical consequences
abnormal solubility	HbC (common)	$Glu^6 \beta \rightarrow Lys$	cellular crystallization of oxygenated protein; increased fragility	mild anemia; splenomegaly (enlarged spleen)
decreased O_2 affinity	Hb Titusville (rare)	$Asp^{94} \alpha \rightarrow Asn$	heterodimer interface altered to stabilize T-state	mild cyanosis (blue-purple skin coloration from deoxygenated blood)
increased O_2 affinity	Hb Helsinki (rare)	$Lys^{82} \beta \rightarrow Met$	reduced binding of 2,3-BPG in T-state	mild polycythemia (increased erythrocyte count)
ferric heme (methemoglobin)	HbM Boston (rare)	$His^{58} \alpha \rightarrow Tyr$	altered heme pocket (loss of distal His) and decreased Bohr effect	cyanosis of skin and mucous membranes
unstable protein	Hb Gun Hill (rare)	$\Delta \beta 91{-}95$	misfolding caused by loss of Leu in heme pocket and shorter helix	formation of Heinz bodies (inclusions of denatured Hb); jaundice (yellow coloration of integument and sclera); pigmented urine
abnormal synthesis	Hb Constant Spring (rare)	$ter^{142} \alpha \rightarrow Gln$	loss of termination codon; decreased mRNA stability	α-thalassemia (hemolytic anemia, splenomegaly, and jaundice)

Table 4.1 **Classification and examples of hemoglobinopathies.** Hemoglobinopathies are usually classified according to the most prominent change to the protein's structure, function, or regulation. Initial identification of a mutation often involves electrophoretic or chromatographic analysis, as shown in Figure 4.8 for HbSC, a double heterozygous genotype associated with a sickle cell disease-like phenotype.

Complete blood count (CBC)

Parameter	Sample	Normal value*
white blood cell count, WBC	$6.82 \times 10^3/mm^3$	$4.5{-}11.0 \times 10^3$
red cell count, RBC	$4.78 \times 10^6/mm^3$	$4.1{-}5.1 \times 10^3$ (F)
		$4.5{-}5.3 \times 10^3$ (M)
hemoglobin, Hb	9.9 g/dL	12.0–16.0 (F)
		13.0–18.0 (M)
hematocrit, HCT	33.4%	36–46 (F)
		37–49 (M)
mean corpuscular volume, MCV	71.9 fL	78–100
mean corpuscular hemoglobin, MCH	21.3 pg/cell	25–35
mean corpuscular hemoglobin concentration, MCHC	29.6 g/dL	31–37
red cell distribution width, RDW	17.7%	11.5–14.5
platelet count, PLT	$274 \times 10^3/mm^3$	$150{-}400 \times 10^3$
mean platelet volume, MPV	8.6 fL	6.4–11.0

*A Kratz and KB Lewandrowski (1998) Normal reference laboratory values. *New Engl J Med* 339:1063–1072

Table 4.2 **Complete blood count.** Automated laboratory evaluation of blood provides invaluable information for the diagnosis and monitoring of health problems. The complete blood count (CBC) includes cell counts of erythrocytes, white cells, and platelets and quantitative indices of the red cells (MCV, MCH, MCHC, and RDW). The results describe the hematopoietic status of the bone marrow and the presence of anemia and its possible cause. Data presented are characteristic of an individual with iron deficiency anemia: low HGB, low MCV (microcytosis), and low MCH (hypochromia). $mm^3 = \mu L$.

COMPLETE BLOOD COUNT

A complete blood count (CBC) provides information on blood cell populations and their characteristics. Data are obtained from whole blood samples by automated hematology analysis. Some instruments also provide leukocyte differentials, reticulocyte count, and red cell morphology. A typical printout of the results for one individual and the range for normals is shown in Table 4.2.

Summary

This chapter describes two important proteins that reversibly interact with O_2 – myoglobin (Mb), a tissue oxygen storage molecule, and hemoglobin (Hb), a blood oxygen transport molecule. Both use an ancient heme-containing polypeptide domain motif to sequester O_2 and increase its solubility. These proteins must function efficiently in rather different biochemical environments to sustain aerobic metabolism. As a tetramer of globins, Hb is one of the best-characterized examples of cooperativity in ligand interactions. With its wide variety of effector molecules, Hb is also a prototype of an allosteric protein. Conformational changes in both the tertiary and quaternary structures characterize the transition between deoxygenated and oxygenated states. Mutations to globin genes lead to a spectrum of structural and functional variants, among which are fetal Hb and sickle cell disease.

ACTIVE LEARNING

1. Discuss why some genetic mutations to α-globin or β-globin result in a pathological phenotype while the majority remain silent or benign. Which kind are the most difficult to detect?
2. Speculate on the mechanisms by which an adult with sickle cell disease would benefits from a fetal hemoglobin (HbF) level of 20%.
3. Many Hb-based oxygen carriers have a decreased sensitivity to pH and an increased susceptibility to oxidation. Discuss the consequences of a reduced Bohr effect to oxygen delivery to the periphery, tissue acid-base balance, and CO_2 transport to the lungs.
4. Discuss the requirement for supplemental iron during rHuEPO treatment. Comment on the use of rHuEPO by athletes as a performance-enhancing drug. Design a laboratory test that could potentially differentiate endogenous EPO from rHuEPO in human urine.

Further reading

Kendall RG. Erythropoietin. *Clin Lab Haem* 2001;**23**:71–80.

Klein HG. The prospects for red-cell substitutes. *New Engl J Med* 2000;**342**:1666–8.

Ou CN, Rognerud CL. Diagnosis of hemoglobinopathies: electrophoresis vs. HPLC. *Clin Chim Acta* 2001;**313**:187–94.

Perutz MF. Molecular anatomy and physiology of hemoglobin. In: Steinberg MH, Forget BG, Higgs DR, Nagel RL, eds *Disorders of Hemoglobin: Genetics, Pathophysiology, and Clinical Management.* Cambridge: Cambridge University Press; 2001:174–96.

Pesce A, Bolognesi M, Bocedi A, Ascenzi P, Dewilde S, Moens L, Hankeln T, Burmester T. Neuroglobin and cytoglobin. Fresh blood for the vertebrate globin family. *EMBO Reports* 2002;**3**:1146–51.

Roach RC, Hackett PH. Frontiers of hypoxia research: acute mountain sickness. *J Exp Biol* 2001;**204**:3161–70.

Wittenberg JB, Wittenberg BA. Myoglobin function reassessed. *J Exp Biol* 2003;**206**:2011–20.

Relevant websites

Globin Gene Server (links to sites describing human hemoglobinopathies and thalassemias): globin.cse.psu.edu/globin/html/

The Red Cell and Anemia (a 5-part presentation by pathologist E Uthman): web2.iadfw.net/uthman/blood_cells.html

Sickle Cell Information Center (comprehensive site for both patients and professionals): www.scinfo.org/

Modified hemoglobins: www.1uphealth.com/health/hemoglobin_derivatives_info.html

5. Catalytic Proteins–Enzymes

J Fujii

LEARNING OBJECTIVES

After reading this chapter you should be able to:

- Describe the characteristics of enzymatic reactions from the viewpoint of free energy, equilibrium, kinetics and direction of the reactions in comparison with simple chemical reactions.
- Discuss the structure and composition of enzymes, including cofactors, and conditions that affect enzymatic reactions.
- Describe enzyme kinetics based on the Michaelis–Menten equation and the significance of the Michaelis constant (Km).
- Describe the elements of enzyme structure that explain their substrate specificity and catalytic activity.
- Describe regulatory mechanisms affecting enzymatic reactions, including regulation by allosteric effectors and covalent modification.
- Differentiate among the three types of enzyme inhibition from the viewpoint of enzyme kinetics.
- Discuss the therapeutic use of enzyme inhibitors and the diagnostic utility of clinical enzyme assays.

INTRODUCTION

Almost all biological functions are supported by chemical reactions catalyzed by biological catalysts, enzymes. Efficient metabolism is controlled by orderly, sequential, and branching metabolic pathways. Enzymes accelerate chemical reactions under physiologic conditions, 37 °C and neutral pH. However, an enzyme cannot alter the equilibrium of a reaction, but can only accelerate the reaction rate, by decreasing the activation energy of the reaction (Fig. 5.1). Regulation of enzymatic activities allows metabolism to adapt to rapidly changing conditions. Nearly all enzymes are proteins, although some ribonucleic acid molecules, termed ribozymes, also have catalytic activity (Chapter 31). Based on analysis of the human genome, it is estimated that about a quarter of human genes encode for enzymes that catalyze metabolic reactions.

ENZYMATIC REACTIONS

Factors affecting enzymatic reactions

Effect of temperature

In the case of an inorganic catalyst, the reaction rate generally increases with the temperature of the system. Enzymes function as catalysts at body temperature, but display a temperature optimum *in vitro*. Because the three-dimensional structure of a protein involves weak bonding interactions,

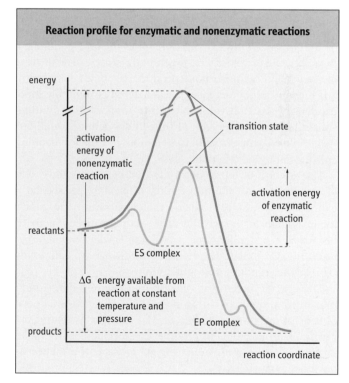

Reaction profile for enzymatic and nonenzymatic reactions

Fig. 5.1 **Reaction profile for enzymatic and nonenzymatic reactions.** The basic principles of an enzyme-catalyzed reaction are the same as any chemical reaction. When a chemical reaction proceeds, the substrate must gain activation energy to reach a point called the transition state of the reaction, at which the energy level is maximum. Since the transition state of the enzyme-catalyzed reaction has a lower energy than that of the uncatalyzed reaction, the reaction can proceed faster. ES complex, enzyme-substrate complex; EP complex, enzyme-product complex.

such as hydrogen and hydrophobic bonds, it can be disrupted by protein denaturation at high temperature.

Effect of pH

Every enzyme has a pH optimum, because ionizable amino acids, such as histidine, glutamate, and cysteine, participate in the catalytic reactions. Since the extremes of pH in our body are 6.9 and 7.7, many enzymes function optimally in this range. However, there are important exceptions. Pepsin, which is secreted by gastric cells and functions in gastric juice, has a pH optimum of 1.5–2.0; trypsin and chymotrypsin have alkaline pH optima, consistent with their digestive activity in pancreatic juice; lysosomal enzymes typically have acidic pH optima. Changes in pH affect the ionic charge of amino acid side chains of enzymes, and can have a dramatic effect on enzymatic activity. In addition, various molecules, including substrates, products, intermediates, and regulatory molecules, also affect the rate of enzymatic reactions.

Definition of enzyme activity

The activity of an enzyme is obtained by determining the rate of an enzyme-catalyzed reaction under defined conditions. Reaction rate or velocity (*v*) is generally expressed as the rate of conversion of substrate to product per min, i.e. mol/min. Since the catalytic activity of an enzyme is normally independent of reaction volume, i.e. it is unaffected by dilution, substrate turnover per unit of time under defined conditions (pH, buffer, temperature) is commonly used for defining enzyme-catalyzed reactions.

The amount of enzyme activity that catalyzes conversion of 1 mole of substrate into 1 mole of product per second is expressed as the katal (1 kat = 1 mol/s). However, the katal is inconvenient for expressing the actual enzyme activity, because it is generally a very small number. The much larger international unit (1 IU = 1 µmol/min) is more commonly used as the standard unit of activity.

The specific activity of an enzyme, expressed as µmol/min/mg of protein, or IU/mg of protein, indicates the amount of enzyme in a protein sample, and is useful for estimating the purity of an enzyme. The higher the specific activity of an enzyme, i.e. the more units/mg of protein, the higher its purity or homogeneity.

Reaction specificity and substrate specificity are determined by the active site structure

Most enzymes are highly specific for both the type of reaction catalyzed and the nature of the substrate(s). Reaction speci-ficity, i.e. the reaction that the enzyme catalyzes, is determined chemically by the amino acid residues in the catalytic center of the enzyme. In general, the active site of the enzyme is composed of the substrate binding site and the catalytic site. Substrate specificity is determined by the size, structure, charges, polarity, and hydrophobicity of the substrate binding site. This is because the substrate must bind in the active site as the first step in the reaction, setting the stage for catalysis. Highly specific enzymes such as catalase and urease, which degrade H_2O_2 and urea, respectively, catalyze only one type of reaction, but some enzymes have broader substrate specificity. The serine proteases are a typical example of such a group of enzymes. These are a family of closely related enzymes, such as the pancreatic enzymes, chymotrypsin, trypsin, and elastase, which contain a reactive serine residue in the catalytic site. They catalyze the hydrolysis of peptide bonds on the carboxyl side of a limited range of amino acids in protein. Although they have similar structures and catalytic mechanisms, their substrate specificities are quite different because of structural features of the substrate binding site (Fig. 5.2).

Isozymes are enzymes that catalyze the same reaction, but differ in their primary structure and/or subunit composition. Levels of some tissue-specific enzymes and isozymes are measured in serum for diagnostic purposes (Fig. 5.3 and Table 5.1).

Some enzymes used for clinical diagnosis of disease		
Enzyme	**Tissue source(s)**	**Diagnostic use**
AST	heart, skeletal muscle, liver, brain	liver disease
ALT	liver	liver disease, e.g. hepatitis (ALT > AST)
amylase	pancreas, salivary gland	acute pancreatitis, biliary obstruction
CK	skeletal muscle, heart, brain	muscular dystrophy, myocardial infarction
GGT	liver	hepatitis, alcohol excess
LDH	heart, liver erythrocytes	lymphoma, hepatitis
lipase	pancreas	acute pancreatitis, biliary obstruction
alkaline phosphatase	osteoblast	bone disease, bone tumors
acid phosphatase	prostate	prostate cancer

Table 5.1 **Some enzymes used for clinical diagnosis of disease.** AST = aspartate amino transferase; ALT = alanine amino transferase; CK = creatine phosphokinase; GGT = gamma glutamyl transferase; LDH = lactate dehydrogenase.

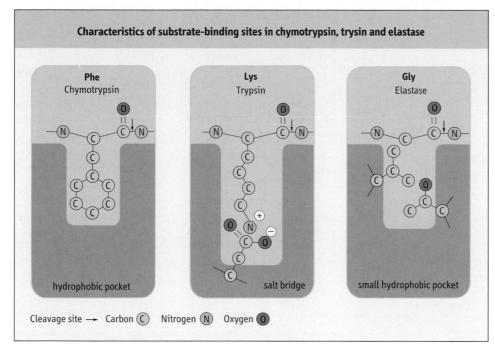

Characteristics of substrate-binding sites in chymotrypsin, trysin and elastase

| Phe Chymotrypsin | Lys Trypsin | Gly Elastase |

hydrophobic pocket   salt bridge   small hydrophobic pocket

Cleavage site → Carbon Ⓒ Nitrogen Ⓝ Oxygen Ⓞ

Fig. 5.2 **Characteristics of the substrate-binding sites in the serine proteases chymotrypsin, trypsin, and elastase.** In chymotrypsin a hydrophobic pocket binds aromatic amino acid residues such as phenylalanine (Phe). In trypsin, the negative charge of the aspartate residue in the substrate binding site promotes cleavage to the carboxyl side of positively charged lysine (Lys) and arginine (Arg) residues. In elastase, side chains of valine and threonine block the substrate binding site and permit binding of amino acids with small or no side chains, such as glycine (Gly).

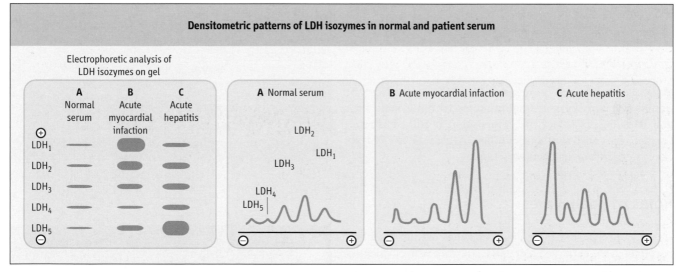

Densitometric patterns of LDH isozymes in normal and patient serum

Fig. 5.3 **Densitometric patterns of the LDH isozymes in serum of patients diagnosed with myocardial infarction or acute hepatitis.** Isozymes, differing slightly in charge, are separated by electrophoresis on cellulose acetate, visualized using a chromogenic substrate, and quantified by densitometry. Total serum LDH activity is also increased in these patients. Since hemolysis releases LDH from red blood cells and affects diagnosis, blood samples should be treated with care. The LDH measurements for the diagnosis of myocardial infarction have now been superseded by plasma troponin levels.

Nomenclature of enzymes

A systematic classification is required to organize the different enzymes that catalyze the many thousands of reactions that take place in our body. All enzymes are assigned a four-digit enzyme classification (EC) number. The first digit indicates membership of one of the six major classes of enzymes shown in Table 5.2. The next two digits indicate sub-strate subclasses and sub-subclasses. For example, the transfer of reducing equivalents from one redox system to another is catalyzed by the oxidoreductases (Class 1). The transfer of other functional groups from one substrate to another is catalyzed by the transferases (Class 2). The hydrolases (Class 3) catalyze group transfer, but the acceptor molecule is exclusively a water molecule. Reactions involving the addition or removal of H_2O, NH_3, or CO_2 are catalyzed by lyases (Class 4),

TISSUE SPECIFICITY OF LDH ISOZYMES

A 56-year-old female was admitted to an intensive care unit. The patient had suffered from a slight fever for 1 week, and had some chest pain, and difficulty breathing for the past 24 h. No abnormality was found on chest X-ray or by electrocardiography. However, a blood test showed white blood cells 12 100/mm^3 (normal: 4000 – 9000/mm^3), red blood cells 240 × 10^4/mm^3 (normal: 380 – 500 × 10^4/mm^3), hemoglobin 8.6 g/dL (normal: 11.8 – 16.0 g/dL), lactate dehydrogenase (LDH) 1400 IU/L (normal: 200 – 400 IU/L). Levels of other enzymes were normal. Based on the blood tests, the LDH isozyme profile and other data, the patient was eventually diagnosed with malignant lymphoma.

Comment. LDH is a tetrameric enzyme composed of two different 35 kDa subunits. The heart contains mainly the H type, and skeletal muscle and the liver the M type subunit, which are encoded by different genes. Five types of tetrameric isozymes can be formed from these subunits: H$_4$ (LDH$_1$), H$_3$M$_1$ (LDH$_2$), H$_2$M$_2$ (LDH$_3$), H$_1$M$_3$ (LDH$_4$), and M$_4$ (LDH$_5$). Since isozyme distributions differ among tissues, it is possible to diagnose tissue damage by assaying total LDH activity and then by isozyme profiling (Fig 5.3).
For hematological reference values, see Table 4.2.

Enzyme classification		
Class	**Reaction**	**Enzymes**
1. Oxidoreductases	$A_{red} + B_{ox} \rightarrow A_{ox} + B_{red}$	dehydrogenase, peroxidase
2. Transferases	$A—B + C \rightarrow A + B—C$	hexokinase, transaminase
3. Hydrolases	$A—B + H_2O \rightarrow$ $A—H + B—OH$	alkaline phosphatase, trypsin
4. Lyases (synthases)	$A(XH)—B \rightarrow$ $A—X + B—H$	carbonic anhydrase, dehydratases
5. Isomerases	$A \rightleftharpoons Iso—A$	triose phosphate isomerase, phosphoglucomutase
6. Ligases (synthetases)	$A + B + ATP \rightarrow$ $A—B + ADP + Pi$	pyruvate carboxylase, DNA ligase

Table 5.2 **Enzyme classification.** Major classes of enzymes.

also called synthases. Isomerases (Class 5) catalyze isomerization reactions by rearranging atoms within a molecule, and thus do not affect the composition of the substrate. Ligases, also called synthetases (Class 6), use ATP to catalyze energy-dependent synthetic reactions.

PROPORTION OF ENZYME GENES IN WHOLE HUMAN GENOME

Original data (Venter *et al.*, *Science* **291**:1335, 2001) are quoted here, and so classification does not exactly match nomenclature in Table 5.2. About a quarter of genes encodes enzymes. Names of enzyme groups with number and proportion (percentage in parenthesis) in a total of 26 383 human genes were as follows: transferase, 610 (2.0); synthase and synthetase, 313 (1.0); oxidoreductase, 656 (2.1); lyase, 117 (0.4); ligase, 56 (0.2); isomerase, 163 (0.5); hydrolase, 1227 (4.0); kinase, 868 (2.8); nucleic acid enzyme, 2308 (7.5).

Roles of coenzymes

Helper molecules referred to as coenzymes play an essential part in enzyme-catalyzed reactions. Enzymes with covalently or noncovalently bound coenzymes are referred to as holoenzymes. A holoenzyme without a coenzyme is termed an apoenzyme. Coenzymes are divided into two categories. Soluble coenzymes bind to the protein moiety of the enzyme, undergo a chemical change, and are ultimately released. Prosthetic groups are tightly bound to and remain associated with the enzyme during the entire catalytic cycle. Most coenzymes are vitamin derivatives. Derivatives of the B vitamins, niacin and riboflavin, act as coenzymes and are involved in oxidoreductase reactions. The structure and function of coenzymes will be described in later chapters. Some enzymes require inorganic (metal) ions, frequently termed cofactors, for their activity, e.g. blood-clotting enzymes that require Ca^{2+} and oxidoreductases, which use iron, copper, and manganese.

ISOZYMES

Isozyme profiles are often performed in the clinical laboratory for diagnostic purposes (see Fig. 5.3). The definition of isozymes is often operational, i.e. based on simple and reproducible assay methods that sometimes do not require precise analysis of enzyme structure. The term isozyme is commonly used to refer to: (1) genetic variants of an enzyme; (2) genetically independent proteins with little homology; (3) heteropolymers of two or more noncovalently bound polypeptide chains; (4) unrelated enzymes that catalyze similar reactions, *e.g.* enzymes conjugated with different prosthetic groups or requiring different coenzymes or cofactors; (5) different forms of a single polypeptide chain, *e.g.* varying in carbohydrate composition, deamination of amino acids, or proteolytic modification.

ENZYME KINETICS

The Michaelis–Menten equation: a simple model of an enzymatic reaction

Enzyme reactions are multistep in nature and comprise several partial reactions. In 1913, long before the structure of proteins was known, Michaelis and Menten developed a simple model for examining the kinetics of enzyme-catalyzed reactions (Fig. 5.4). The Michaelis–Menten model assumes that the substrate S binds to the enzyme E, forming an essential intermediate, the enzyme-substrate complex (ES), which then undergoes reaction on the enzyme surface and decomposes to E + product (P). The model assumes that E, S, and ES are all in rapid equilibrium with one another, so that a steady concentration of ES is rapidly achieved, and that decomposition of the ES complex to E + P is the rate-limiting step in catalysis.

The catalytic constant, k_{cat}, also known as the turnover number, is defined as the number of substrate molecules that can be converted per enzyme molecule per unit time. The proportion of ES, in relation to the total number of enzyme

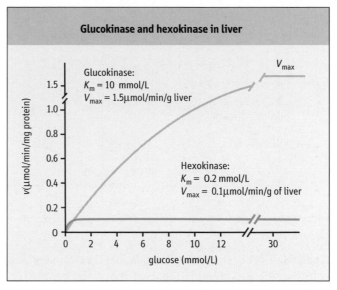

Fig. 5.4 **Properties of glucokinase and hexokinase.** Glucokinase and hexokinase catalyze the same reaction, phosphorylation of glucose to glucose 6-phosphate (Glc-6-P). They exhibit different kinetic properties and have different tissue distribution and physiologic function.

ISOZYMES: GLUCOKINASE AND HEXOKINASE

Hexokinase catalyzes the first step in glucose metabolism in all cells, namely the phosphorylation reaction of glucose by adenosine triphosphate (ATP) to form glucose 6-phosphate (Glc-6-P):

glucose + ATP → glucose 6-phosphate + ADP

This enzyme has a low K_m for glucose (0.2 mmol/L) and is inhibited allosterically by its product, Glc-6-P. Since normal glucose levels in blood are about 5 mmol/L and intracellular levels are 0.2–2 mmol/L, hexokinase efficiently catalyzes this reaction under normal conditions, e.g. in muscle. Hepatocytes, which store glucose as glycogen, and pancreatic β-cells, which regulate glucose consumption in tissues and its storage in liver by secreting insulin, contain an isozyme called glucokinase. Glucokinase catalyzes the same reaction as hexokinase, but has a higher K_m for glucose (10 mmol/L) and is not inhibited by the product, Glc-6-P. Since glucokinase has a much higher K_m than hexokinase, glucokinase phosphorylates glucose with increasing efficiency as blood glucose levels increase following a meal (see Fig. 5.4). One of the physiologic roles of glucokinase in the liver is to provide Glc-6-P for the synthesis of glycogen, a storage form of glucose. In the pancreatic beta cell, glucokinase functions as the glucose sensor, determining the threshold for insulin secretion. Mice lacking glucokinase in the pancreatic β-cell die within 3 days of birth of profound hyperglycemia, because of failure to secrete insulin.

molecules $[E]_t$, i.e. the ratio $[ES]/[E]_t$, limits the velocity of an enzyme (v) so that:

$$v = k_{cat} [ES]$$

Since E, S, and ES are all in chemical equilibrium, the enzyme achieves maximal velocity, V_{max}, at very high (saturating) substrate concentrations [S], when $[ES] \approx [E]_t$.

For the dissociation of the ES complex, the law of mass action yields

$$K_d = \frac{[E][S]}{[ES]}$$

Given that

$$[E]_t = [E] + [ES].$$

it can be shown that

$$\frac{[ES]}{[E]_t} = \frac{[S]}{(K_m + [S])}, \text{where } K_m \approx K_d$$

Consequently, v is given by

$$v = \frac{(k_{cat}[E]_t[S])}{(k_m + [S])}$$

Since $k_{cat} [E]_t$ corresponds to the maximum velocity, V_{max}, that is attained at high (saturating) substrate concentrations, we obtain the Michaelis–Menten equation:

$$v = \frac{(V_{max}[S])}{(K_m + [S])}$$

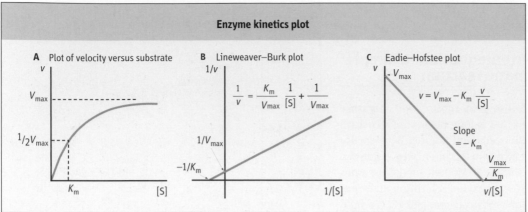

Enzyme kinetics plot

A Plot of velocity versus substrate

B Lineweaver–Burk plot

$$\frac{1}{v} = \frac{K_m}{V_{max}} \frac{1}{[S]} + \frac{1}{V_{max}}$$

C Eadie–Hofstee plot

$$v = V_{max} - K_m \frac{v}{[S]}$$

Slope $= -K_m$

Fig. 5.5 **Enzyme kinetics plot.** Kinetic representations of the properties of enzymes. (A) Michaelis–Menten plot of velocity (*v*) versus substrate concentration ([S]); (B) Lineweaver–Burk plot; and (C) Eadie–Hofstee plot.

Analysis of the above equations indicates that the Michaelis constant, K_m, is expressed in units of concentration and corresponds to the substrate concentration at which v is 50% of the maximum velocity, i.e. $[ES] = \frac{1}{2}[E]_t$ and $v = V_{max}/2$.

The Michaelis–Menten model is based on the assumptions that:

- E, S, and ES are in rapid equilibrium
- there are no forms of the enzyme present other than E and ES
- the conversion of ES into E + P is a rate-limiting, irreversible step.

Similar types of kinetic models have been developed for describing the kinetics of multisubstrate, multiproduct enzymes.

Use of the Lineweaver–Burk and Eadie–Hofstee plots for estimating K_m and V_{max}

In a plot of reaction rate versus substrate concentration, the rate of the reaction approaches the maximum velocity (V_{max}) asymptotically (Fig. 5.5A), so that it is difficult to obtain accurate values for V_{max}, and, as a result, K_m (substrate concentration required for half-maximal activity), by simple extrapolation. To solve this problem, several linear transformations of the Michaelis–Menten equation have been developed.

Lineweaver–Burk plot

The Lineweaver–Burk, or double reciprocal, plot is obtained by taking the reciprocal of the steady-state Michaelis–Menten equation (Fig. 5.5B). By rearranging the equation, we obtain:

$$\frac{1}{v} = \left(\frac{1}{V_{max}}\right) + \left\{\left(\frac{k_m}{V_{max}}\right)\left(\frac{1}{[S]}\right)\right\}$$

This equation yields a straight line ($y = mx + b$), with $y = 1/v$, $x = 1/[S]$, m = slope, b = y intercept. Therefore, a graph of $1/v$ versus $1/[S]$ (Fig. 5.5B) has a slope of K_m/V_{max}, a $1/v$ intercept of $1/V_{max}$, and a $1/[S]$ intercept of $-1/K_m$. Although

MEASUREMENT OF ENZYME ACTIVITY IN CLINICAL SAMPLES

In clinical laboratories, enzyme activity is measured in the presence of saturating substrate(s) and coenzyme concentrations. Initial kinetics are normally recorded to minimize reverse reactions, i.e. conversion of product to substrate in reversible reactions. Under these conditions ($v \approx V_{max}$), enzyme activity is directly proportional to enzyme concentration. Enzyme activity is expressed in IU/mL of plasma, serum, cerebrospinal fluid, etc. For interlaboratory comparisons, the conditions for the enzyme assay must be standardized, e.g. the substrate and coenzyme concentrations used, the buffer, buffer concentration, ionic species and ionic strength, pH and temperature. Most clinical samples are collected under fasting conditions; this assures consistency in measurement of analytes whose concentration may vary diurnally or others, such as glucose or lipids, that vary in response to food intake. Lipemic samples are cloudy and may yield unreliable data by spectrophotometric or fluorometric methods. To avoid such problems, clinical samples must be delipidated, commonly by extraction with organic solvent.

the Lineweaver–Burk plot is widely used for kinetic analysis of enzyme reactions, because reciprocals of the data are calculated, a small experimental error, especially at low substrate concentration, can result in a large error in the graphically determined values of K_m and V_{max}. An additional disadvantage is that important data obtained at high substrate concentrations are concentrated into a narrow region near the $1/v$ axis.

Eadie–Hofstee plot

A second, widely used linear form of the Michaelis–Menten equation is the Eadie–Hofstee plot (Fig. 5.5C). This is described by the equation:

$$v = V_{max} - \left(K_m \times \frac{v}{[S]}\right)$$

TREATMENT WITH AN INHIBITOR OF ANGIOTENSIN-CONVERTING ENZYME (ACE)

A 50-year-old man was admitted to hospital suffering from general fatigue, a stiff shoulder, and headache. The patient was 1.8 m tall and weighed 84 kg. His blood pressure was 196/98 mmHg (normal below 140/90 mmHg; optimal below 120/80 mmHg) and his pulse was 74. He was diagnosed as hypertensive. The patient was given captopril, an angiotensin converting enzyme (ACE) inhibitor. After 5 days' treatment, his blood pressure returned to near-normal levels.

Comment. Renin in the kidney converts angiotensinogen into angiotensin I, which is then proteolytically cleaved to angiotensin II by ACE. Angiotensin II increases renal fluid and electrolyte retention, contributing to hypertension. Inhibition of ACE activity is therefore an important target for hypertension treatment. Captopril inhibits ACE competitively, decreasing blood pressure. (See also Chapter 22.)

In this case, a plot of v versus $v/[S]$ has a y axis (v-intercept) of V_{max}, an x axis ($v/[S]$) intercept of V_{max}/K_m, and a slope of $-K_m$. The Eadie–Hofstee plot involves only one reciprocal and does not compress the data at high substrate concentrations.

ENZYME INHIBITION

Enzymes are inhibited in different ways

Among numerous substances affecting metabolic processes, enzyme inhibitors are particularly important. Many drugs, either naturally occurring or synthetic, act as enzyme inhibitors. Metabolites of these compounds may also inhibit enzyme activity. Most enzyme inhibitors act reversibly, but there are also irreversible inhibitors that permanently modify the target enzyme. Using Lineweaver–Burk plots, it is possible to distinguish three forms of reversible inhibition: competitive, uncompetitive, and noncompetitive inhibition.

Competitive inhibitors cause an apparent increase in K_m, without changing V_{max}

An enzyme can be inhibited competitively by substances that are similar in chemical structure to the substrate (Fig. 5.6). These compounds compete with substrate for the active site of the enzyme causing an apparent increase in K_m, but no change in V_{max}. The inhibition is not the result of an effect on enzyme activity, but on substrate access to the active site. The kinetic scheme for competitive inhibition, is:

METHANOL POISONING CAN BE TREATED BY ETHANOL ADMINISTRATION

A 46-year-old male presented to the emergency room 7 h after consuming a large quantity of bootleg alcohol. He could not see clearly and complained of abdominal and back pain. Laboratory results indicated severe metabolic acidosis, a serum osmolality of 465 mmol/kg (reference range 285–295 mmol/kg), and serum methanol level of 4.93 g/L. By aggressive treatment, including an ethanol drip, bicarbonate, and hemodialysis, he survived and regained his eyesight.

Comment. Methanol poisoning is uncommon but extremely hazardous. Ethylene glycol poisoning is more common and exhibits similar clinical characteristics. The most important initial symptom of methanol poisoning is visual disturbance. Laboratory evidence of methanol poisoning includes severe metabolic acidosis and increased plasma solute concentration. Methanol is slowly metabolized to formaldehyde, which is then rapidly metabolized to formate by alcohol dehydrogenase. Formate accumulates during methanol intoxication and is responsible for the metabolic acidosis in the early stage of intoxication. In later stages lactate may also accumulate as a result of formate inhibition of respiration. Ethanol is metabolized by alcohol dehydrogenase, which binds ethanol with much higher affinity than either methanol or ethylene glycol. Ethanol is therefore a useful agent to inhibit competitively the metabolism of methanol and ethylene glycol to toxic metabolites. Early treatment with ethanol, together with alkali to combat acidosis and hemodialysis to remove methanol and its toxic metabolites, yields a good prognosis.

$$\begin{array}{c} S \rightleftharpoons ES \rightarrow E + P \\ E\ \substack{+ \\ \\ +} \\ I \rightleftharpoons EI \end{array}$$

The inhibition constant (K_i) is the dissociation constant of the enzyme-inhibitor complex (EI). The lower the K_i, the more efficient the inhibition of enzyme activity.

Both K_m and V_{max} decrease in uncompetitive inhibition

An uncompetitive inhibitor binds only to the enzyme-substrate complex and not to the free enzyme. The equation shows the kinetic scheme for uncompetitive inhibition. In this case, the K_i is the dissociation constant for the enzyme-substrate-inhibitor complex (ESI).

$$\begin{array}{c} I \rightleftharpoons ESI \\ E + S \rightleftharpoons ES\ \substack{+ \\ \\ \searrow} \\ E + P \end{array}$$

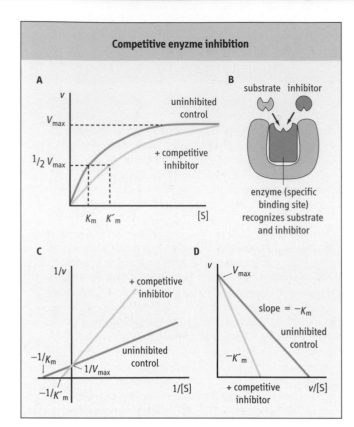

Fig. 5.6 **Competitive enzyme inhibition.** (A) Plot of velocity versus substrate concentration; (B) mechanism of competitive inhibition; (C) Lineweaver–Burk plot in the presence of a competitive inhibitor; and (D) Eadie–Hofstee plot in the presence of a competitive inhibitor. K'_m is the apparent K_m in presence of inhibitor.

ENZYME INHIBITION: TRANSITION-STATE INHIBITION AND SUICIDE SUBSTRATE

Enzymes catalyze reactions by inducing the transition state of the reaction. It should therefore be possible to construct molecules that bind very tightly to the enzyme by mimicking the transition state of the substrate. Transition states themselves cannot be isolated, because they are not a stable arrangement of atoms, and some bonds are only partially formed or broken. But for some enzymes, analogues can be synthesized that are stable, but still have some of the structural features of the transition state.

Penicillin (Fig. 5.7) is a good example of a transition state analog. It inhibits the transpeptidase that crosslinks bacterial cell-wall peptidoglycan strands, the last step in cell-wall synthesis in bacteria. It has a strained 4-membered lactam ring that mimics the transition state of the normal substrate. When penicillin binds to the active site of the enzyme, its lactam ring opens, forming a covalent bond with a serine residue at the active site. Penicillin is a potent irreversible inhibitor of bacterial cell-wall synthesis, making the bacteria osmotically fragile and unable to survive in the body.

The inhibitor causes a decrease in V_{max} because a fraction of the enzyme-substrate complex is diverted by the inhibitor to the inactive ESI complex. Bound inhibitor also affects the dissociation of substrate, causing an apparent decrease in K_m, i.e. an apparent increase in substrate affinity.

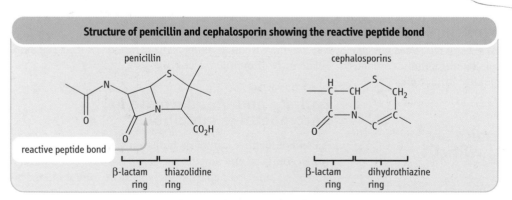

Fig. 5.7 **Structure of penicillin showing the reactive peptide bond in the β-lactam ring and core structure of cephalosporins.** Penicillins contain β-lactam ring in conjunction with thiazolidine ring. Cephalosporins are another class of compounds containing the β-lactam ring fused to a six-membered dihydrothiazine ring. Because of their effectiveness and lack of toxicity, β-lactam compounds are widely used antibiotics. Bacteria with β-lactamase, which breaks the β-lactam ring, are resistant to these antibiotics.

V_{max} decreases in noncompetitive inhibition

A noncompetitive inhibitor can bind either to the free enzyme or to the enzyme-substrate complex. Thus, noncompetitive inhibition is more complex than other types of inhibition. The next equation shows the kinetic pattern observed for noncompetitive inhibition.

$$E + S \rightleftharpoons ES \rightarrow E + P$$

$$
\begin{array}{ccc}
+ & & + \\
I & & I \\
\Updownarrow & & \Updownarrow \\
EI & & ESI
\end{array}
$$

Many drugs and poisons irreversibly inhibit enzymes

Prostaglandins are key inflammatory mediators. Their synthesis is initiated by cyclooxygenase-mediated oxidation and cyclization of arachidonate under inflammatory conditions (Chapter 38). Compounds that suppress cyclooxygenase have anti-inflammatory activity. Aspirin (acetylsalicylic acid), one of the most popular drugs, inhibits cyclooxygenase activity by acetylating Ser[530], which blocks access of arachidonate to the active site of the enzyme. Other nonsteroidal anti-inflammatory drugs (NSAIDs), such as indomethacin, inhibit cyclooxygenase activity by reversibly blocking the channel for arachidonate in the enzyme.

Disulfiram (Antabuse®) is a drug used for the treatment of alcoholism. Alcohol is metabolized in two steps to acetic acid. The first enzyme, alcohol dehydrogenase, yields acetaldehyde, which is then converted into acetic acid by aldehyde dehydrogenase. The latter enzyme has an active site cysteine residue that is irreversibly modified by disulfiram, resulting in accumulation of alcohol and acetaldehyde in the blood. People who take disulfiram become sick because of the accumulation of acetaldehyde in blood and tissues, leading to alcohol avoidance.

Alkylating reagents, such as iodoacetamide ($ICH_2 - CONH_2$), irreversibly inhibit the catalytic activity of some enzymes by modifying essential cysteine residue. Heavy metals, such as mercury and lead salts, also inhibit sulfhydryl enzymes. The mercury adducts are often reversible by thiol compounds. Eggs or egg-white are sometimes administered as an antidote for accidental ingestion of heavy metals; the egg white protein, ovalbumin, is rich in sulfhydryl groups, traps the free metal ions and prevents their absorption from the gastrointestinal tract.

In many cases, irreversible inhibitors are used to identify active-site residues involved in enzyme catalysis and to gain insight into the mechanism of enzyme action. By sequencing the protein, it is possible to identify the specific amino acid residue modified by the inhibitor and involved in catalysis.

CATALYTIC MECHANISM OF SERINE PROTEASE

In enzyme reactions, ionizable amino acids, such as histidine and cysteine, participate in the enzyme-catalyzed reaction. In the serine protease family, a specific serine residue forms the catalytic center, with aid from other amino acids. Ser[195], His[57], and Asp[102] form a 'catalytic triad' in chymotrypsin (Fig. 5.8). When the proton of the hydroxyl group of Ser[195] is hydrogen bonded to His[57], the more nucleophilic oxygen atom of Ser[195] is able to attack the carbonyl carbon atom of the peptide bond in the substrate. The role of the carboxylate group of Asp[102] is to stabilize the positively charged form of His[57] in the transition state.

Trypsin and elastase, two other digestive enzymes, are similar to chymotrypsin, in many respects. About 40% of the amino acid sequences of these three enzymes are identical, and their three-dimensional structures are very similar. All three enzymes contain a serine-histidine-aspartate-catalytic triad, and are inactivated by the binding of fluorophosphates such as diisopropylfluorophosphate to the serine residue in this triad.

A schematic model of a catalytic triad of a serine protease

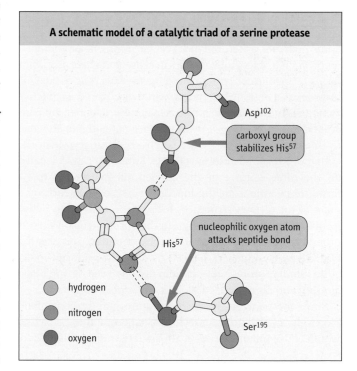

Fig. 5.8 **A schematic model of a catalytic triad of serine protease.**

REGULATION OF ENZYME ACTIVITY

In multistep metabolic pathways, the slowest step limits the overall rate of the reaction. It is therefore most efficient to regulate the metabolic pathway by controlling key enzymes that are involved in this 'rate-limiting' step. Generally, five independent mechanisms are involved in these processes:

- The expression of the enzyme protein from the corresponding gene changes in response to the cell's changing environment or metabolic demands.
- Enzymes may be irreversibly activated or inactivated by proteolytic enzymes.
- Enzymes may be reversibly activated or inactivated by covalent modification, such as phosphorylation.
- Allosteric regulation modulates the activity of key enzymes through reversible binding of small molecules at sites distinct from the active site in a process that is relatively rapid and, hence, the first response of cells to changing conditions.
- The degradation of enzymes by intracellular proteases in the lysosome or by proteasomes in the cytosol also determines the lifetimes of the enzymes and consequently enzyme activity over a much longer period of time.

Proteolytic activation of digestive enzymes

Some enzymes are stored in a specific organelle or compartment, such as exocytotic vesicles in cells, in inactive precursor forms termed proenzymes or zymogens. This type of enzyme includes the digestive enzymes, which are stored as inactive zymogens in the pancreas. The zymogens are secreted in pancreatic juice following a meal and are activated in the gastrointestinal tract; trypsinogen is converted into trypsin by the action of intestinal enteropeptidase. Enteropeptidase, located on the inner surface of the duodenum, hydrolyzes an N-terminal peptide from the inactive trypsinogen. Rearrangement of the tertiary structure yields the proteolytically active form of trypsin. The active trypsin then proteolytically digests other zymogens, such as procarboxypeptidase, proelastase and chymotrypsinogen, as well as other trypsinogen molecules. Similar proteolytic cascades are observed during blood clotting and fibrinolysis (dissolution of clots) (Chapter 6).

Since the pancreas is an important organ for controlling blood glucose, the unregulated activation of these enzymes would cause inflammation of the pancreas (pancreatitis).

Allosteric regulation of rate-limiting enzymes in metabolic pathways

The substrate saturation curve for an 'isosteric' (single shape) enzyme is hyperbolic (see Fig. 5.5A). On the other hand, allosteric enzymes often show sigmoidal plots of reaction velocity versus substrate concentration [S] (Fig. 5.9). An allosteric effector molecule binds to the enzyme at a site that is distinct and physically separate from the substrate-binding site, but which affects the overall substrate binding and/or

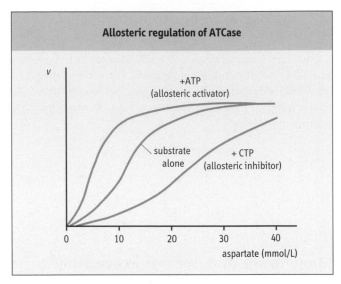

Fig. 5.9 **Allosteric regulation of ATCase.** Plot of velocity (*v*) versus substrate concentration in the presence of an allosteric activator or allosteric inhibitor. Aspartate transcarbamoylase (ATCase) is an example of an allosteric enzyme. Aspartate (substrate) homotropically regulates ATCase activity, providing sigmoidal kinetics. CTP, an end product, heterotropically inhibits, but ATP, a precursor, heterotropically activates ATCase. This enzyme is described in more detail in Chapter 29.

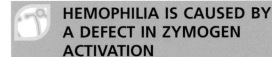

HEMOPHILIA IS CAUSED BY A DEFECT IN ZYMOGEN ACTIVATION

A child was admitted to hospital with muscle bleeding affecting the femoral nerve. Laboratory findings indicated a blood-clotting disorder, hemophilia A, resulting from deficiency of Factor VIII. Factor VIII was administered to the patient to restore blood-clotting activity.

Comment. Formation of a blood clot results from a cascade of zymogen-activation reactions. Over a dozen different proteins, known as blood-clotting factors, are involved. In the final step, the blood clot is formed by conversion of a soluble protein, fibrinogen (Factor I), into an insoluble, fibrous product, fibrin, which forms the matrix of the clot. This last step is catalyzed by the serine protease, thrombin (Factor IIa). Hemophilia is a disorder of blood clotting caused by a defect in one of the sequence of clotting factors. Hemophilia A, the major (85%) form of hemophilia, is caused by a defect of clotting Factor VIII (See Chapter 6).

reaction velocity. In some cases, the substrate exerts allosteric effects; this is referred to as a homotropic effect. If the allosteric effector is different from the substrate, it is referred to as a heterotropic effect. Homotropic effects are observed when the reaction of one substrate molecule with a multimeric enzyme affects the binding of a second substrate molecule at a different active site on the enzyme. The interaction

NUCLEOSIDE ANALOGS AS ANTI-VIRAL AGENTS

Nucleoside analogs such as acyclovir and ganciclovir have been used for treatment of herpes simplex virus (HSV), varicella-zoster (VZV), and cytomegalovirus (CMV). They are pro-drugs that are activated by phosphorylation and terminate viral DNA synthesis by inhibiting the viral DNA polymerase reaction. The thymidine kinase (TK), more properly a nucleoside kinase, of the viruses phosphorylate these compounds to their monophosphate form. Cellular kinases next add phosphates to form the active triphosphate compounds, which are competitive inhibitors of the viral DNA polymerase during DNA replication (Chapter 29). While viral TK has low substrate specificity and efficiently phosphorylates nucleoside analogs, cellular nucleoside kinases have high substrate specificity and barely phosphorylate the nucleoside analogs. Thus, virus-infected cells are prone to be arrested at specific cell cycle stage, G_2-M checkpoint (Chapter 41), but uninfected cells are resistant to the nucleoside analogs.

between subunits makes the binding of substrate cooperative and results in a sigmoidal curve in the plot of v versus [S]. The effect is essentially identical with that described for the binding of O_2 to hemoglobin (Chapter 4), except that in the case of enzymes, substrate binding leads to an enzyme-catalyzed reaction.

Positive and negative cooperativity

Positive cooperativity indicates that the reaction of a substrate with one active site makes it easier for another substrate to react at another active site. Negative cooperativity means that the reaction of a substrate with one active site makes it more difficult for a substrate to react at the other active site. Since the affinity of the enzyme changes with substrate concentration, it cannot be described by simple Michaelis–Menten kinetics. Instead, it is characterized by substrate concentration giving a half-maximal rate, $[S]_{0.5}$, and the Hill coefficient (H). The H-values are larger than 1 for enzymes with positive cooperativity and less than 1 for those with negative cooperativity. For most allosteric enzymes, intracellular substrate concentrations are poised near the $[S]_{0.5}$, so that the enzyme's activity responds to slight changes in substrate concentration.

The model most often invoked to rationalize allosteric behavior was established by Monod, Wyman, and Changeaux, the so-called concerted model (Fig. 5.10). As with O_2 binding to Hb, in the absence of substrate, the enzyme has a low affinity for substrate, and is in the T-state (tense state). The other conformation of the enzyme is the R-state (relaxed state). Binding of allosteric effector molecules shifts the fraction of enzyme from one state to the other. While enzymes are shifted to the R-state by the binding of positive allosteric effector molecules, they are stabilized in the T-form by negative allosteric effector molecules. In this model, all the

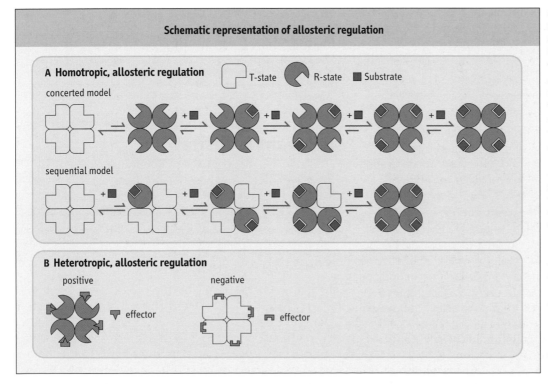

Schematic representation of allosteric regulation

A Homotropic, allosteric regulation   T-state   R-state   ■ Substrate

concerted model

sequential model

B Heterotropic, allosteric regulation

positive   negative

effector   effector

Fig. 5.10 **Schematic representation of allosteric regulation.** (A) In homotropic regulation, the substrate acts as an allosteric effector. Two models are presented. In the concerted model, all of the subunits convert from the T (tense; low affinity for substrate) – into the R (relaxed; high affinity for substrate) – state at the same time; in the sequential model, they change one by one, with each substrate-binding reaction. (B) In heterotropic regulation, the effector is distinct from the substrate, and binds at a structurally different site on the enzyme. Positive and negative effectors stabilize the enzyme in R- and T-state, respectively.

INSECTICIDE POISONING

A 55-year-old man was spraying an insecticide containing organic fluorophosphates in a rice field. He suddenly developed a frontal headache, eye pain, and tightness in his chest, typical signs of over-exposure to toxic organic fluorophosphates. He was taken to hospital and treated with an intravenous injection of 2 mg of atropine sulfate, and gradually recovered.

Comment. Organic fluorophosphates form covalent phosphoryl-enzyme complexes with acetylcholinesterase and irreversibly inhibit the enzyme. Acetylcholinesterase terminates the action of acetylcholine during neuromuscular activity (Chapter 39) by hydrolyzing the acetylcholine to acetate and choline. Inhibition of this enzyme prolongs the action of acetylcholine, leading to constant neuromuscular stimulation. Atropine competitively blocks acetylcholine binding at the neuromuscular junction.

ACTIVE LEARNING

1. In a multi-step sequence of enzymatic reactions, where is the most effective site for controlling the flux of substrate through the pathway. What effect will an inhibitor of a rate-limiting enzyme have on the concentration of substrates in a multi-step pathway?
2. Most drugs are designed to inhibit specific enzymes in biological systems. The drug, Prozac, has had a profound effect on the medical treatment of depression. Review the history of development of Prozac, illustrating the importance of specificity in the mechanism of drug action.
3. Discuss some examples of reversible and irreversible enzyme inhibitors used in medical practice.
4. Knock-out mice are mice that lack a specific gene. Discuss the impact of KO-mice on the direction of drug development in the pharmaceutical industry.

active sites in the R-state are the same and all have higher substrate affinity than in the T-state. Because the transition between the T- and R-states occurs at the same time for all subunits, this is called the concerted (two-state) model. An alternative model, the so-called sequential (multi-state) model, has also been proposed by Koshland, Nèmethy, and Filmer. It postulates that each subunit changes independently to a different conformation and that different subunits may have different affinities for substrate. It is now recognized that both models are applicable to different enzymes.

Summary

Most metabolism is catalyzed by biological catalysts – enzymes. Their catalytic activities are apparent at body temperature, and they are strictly regulated by several mechanisms. Both covalent and noncovalent modifications are involved in this regulation and allow for efficient metabolic control. Enzyme activity can be inhibited (or activated) by synthetic compounds (drugs), exogenous compounds (toxins), as well as endogenous compounds (allosteric effectors). Kinetic analyses of enzymatic reaction are beneficial for evaluating the biological role of enzymes and for elucidating their reaction mechanisms. In addition, assays of enzymes in blood are useful for diagnosis of some diseases. Uncontrolled enzymatic activity, however, sometimes causes serious diseases. In such cases, appropriate inhibitors are quite useful for therapeutic purposes.

Further reading

Hammes GG. Multiple conformational changes in enzyme catalysis. *Biochem* 2002;**41**:8221–8.

Andersson I, van Scheltinga AC, Valegard K. Towards new beta-lactam antibiotics. *Cell Mol Life Sci* 2001;**58**:1897–906.

Christen P, Mehta PK. From cofactor to enzymes. The molecular evolution of pyridoxal-5'-phosphate-dependent enzymes. *Chem Re.* 2001;**1**:436–447.

Piliero PJ. Atazanavir: a novel HIV-1 protease inhibitor. *Expert Opin Investig Drugs* 2002;**11**:1295–1301.

Matschinsky FM. Regulation of pancreatic beta-cell glucokinase: from basics to therapeutics. *Diabetes* 2002;**51**(Suppl 3):S394–S404.

Michaelis ML. Drugs targeting Alzheimer's disease: some things old and some things new. J *Pharmacol Exp Ther* 2003;**304**:897–904.

Malasky BR, Alpert JS. Diagnosis of myocardial injury by biochemical markers: problems and promises. *Cardiol Rev* 2002;**10**:306–317.

Relevant websites

Case Studies, many employing clinical enzyme analysis: http://path.upmc.edu/cases/index.html

Clinical Enzymology: http://www.qub.ac.uk/cm/cb/text/studgide; http://www.labtestsonline.org/

Enzyme Kinetics: http://www.indstate.edu/thcme/mwking/enzyme-kinetics.html; http://www-biol.paisley.ac.uk/kinetics/contents.html

International Federation of Clinical Chemistry and Laboratory Medicine: http://www.ifcc.org/ifcc.asp

6. Hemostasis and Thrombosis

G Lowe

LEARNING OBJECTIVES

After reading this chapter you should be able to:

- Outline the sequential mechanisms involved in normal hemostasis.
- Summarize the processes through which the vessel wall regulates hemostasis and thrombosis.
- Describe the role of platelets in hemostasis and thrombosis.
- Outline pathways through which antiplatelet drugs act.
- Describe the pathways of blood coagulation, and how these are tested in the clinical hemostasis laboratory to identify coagulation disorders.
- Describe the physiological inhibitors of blood coagulation.
- Outline pathways through which anticoagulant drugs act.
- Describe the main components of the fibrinolytic system.
- Describe how thrombolytic (fibrinolytic) drugs act.

INTRODUCTION

Circulation of the blood within the cardiovascular system is essential for transportation of gases, nutrients, minerals, metabolic products, and hormones between different organs. It is also essential that blood should not leak excessively from blood vessels when they are injured by the traumas of daily life. Animal evolution has therefore resulted in the development of an efficient, but complex, series of hemodynamic, cellular, and biochemical mechanisms that limit such blood loss by forming platelet-fibrin plugs at sites of vessel injury (hemostasis). Genetic disorders that result in loss of individual protein functions, and therefore in excessive bleeding (e.g. hemophilia), have played an important part in the identification of many of the biochemical mechanisms in hemostasis.

It is essential also that these hemostatic mechanisms are appropriately controlled by inhibitory mechanisms, otherwise an exaggerated platelet-fibrin plug may produce local occlusion of a major blood vessel (artery or vein) at its site of origin (thrombosis), or may break off and block a blood vessel downstream (embolism). Arterial thrombosis is the major cause of heart attacks, stroke, and the need for limb amputations in developed countries, but venous thrombosis and embolism are also major causes of death and disability.

Clinical use of antithrombotic drugs (antiplatelet, anticoagulant, and thrombolytic agents) is now widespread in developed countries, and requires an understanding of how they interfere with hemostatic mechanisms to exert their antithrombotic effects.

HEMOSTASIS

Hemostasis means 'the arrest of bleeding'

After tissue injury that ruptures smaller vessels (including everyday trauma, injections, surgical incisions, and tooth extractions), a series of interactions between the vessel wall and the circulating blood normally occur, resulting in cessation of blood loss from injured vessels within a few minutes (hemostasis). Hemostasis results from effective sealing of the ruptured vessels by a hemostatic plug composed of blood platelets and fibrin. Fibrin is derived from circulating fibrinogen, whereas platelets are small cell fragments that circulate in the blood and have an important role in the initiation of hemostasis.

Hemostasis requires the effective, coordinated function of blood vessels, platelets, coagulation factors and the fibrinolytic system

Figure 6.1 provides an overview of hemostatic mechanisms, and illustrates some of the interactions between blood vessels, platelets, and the coagulation system in hemostasis; each of these components of hemostasis also interacts with the fibrinolytic system. The initial response of small blood vessels to injury is arteriolar vasoconstriction, which temporarily reduces local blood flow. Flow reduction transiently reduces blood loss, and may also promote formation of the platelet-fibrin plug. Activation of blood platelets is followed by their adhesion to the vessel wall at the site of injury, and their subsequent aggregation to each other, building up an occlusive platelet mass that forms the initial (primary) hemostatic plug. This platelet plug is friable and, unless subsequently stabilized by fibrin, will be washed away by local blood pressure when vasoconstriction reverses.

Vascular injury also activates coagulation factors, which interact sequentially to form thrombin, which converts circulating soluble plasma fibrinogen to insoluble, crosslinked fibrin. This forms the subsequent (secondary) hemostatic plug, which is relatively resistant to dispersal by blood flow

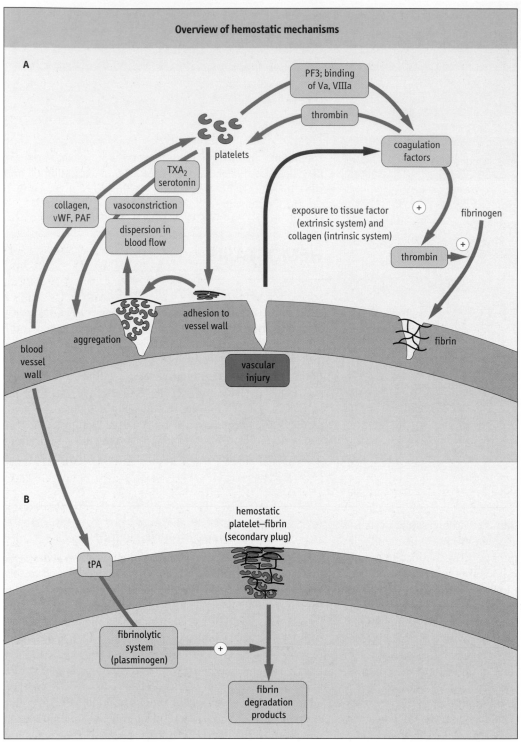

Fig. 6.1 **Overview of hemostatic mechanisms.** (A) Vascular injury sets in motion a series of events that culminate in formation of a primary plug of platelets. This can be dispersed by blood flowing through the vessel unless the plug is stabilized. (B) The primary plug is stabilized by a network of fibrin (formed from crosslinked fibrinogen). The secondary plug is stable and is degraded only when the fibrinolytic system has been activated. PAF, platelet activating factor; PF3, platelet factor 3; tPA, tissue-type plasminogen activator; TXA_2, thromboxane A_2; Va, activated coagulation factor V; VIIIa, activated coagulation factor VIII; vWF, von Willebrand factor.

or fibrinolysis. There are two pathways of the activation of coagulation factors: the extrinsic pathway which is initiated by the exposure of the flowing blood to tissue factor, released from subendothelial tissue; and the intrinsic pathway which has an important amplification role in generating thrombin and fibrin.

The lysis of fibrin is equally important to health as is its formation

Hemostasis is a continuous process throughout life, and would result in excessive fibrin formation and vascular occlusion if unchecked. Evolution has therefore produced a fibrinolytic system; this is activated by local fibrin formation, resulting in local generation of plasmin, an enzyme which digests fibrin plugs (in parallel with tissue repair processes), thus maintaining vascular patency. Digestion of fibrin results in generation of circulating fibrin degradation products (FDP). These are detectable in plasma of healthy individuals at low concentration, which illustrates that fibrin formation and lysis are continuing processes in health.

Excessive bleeding may result from defects in each of the components of hemostasis, which may be caused by disease (congenital or acquired) or by antithrombotic drugs (Table 6.1).

The vascular, platelet, coagulation and fibrinolytic components of hemostasis will now be discussed in turn.

THE VESSEL WALL

Vascular injury has a key role in initiating local formation of the platelet-fibrin plug and in its subsequent removal by the fibrinolytic system

All blood vessels are lined by a flat sheet of endothelial cells, which have important roles in the interchange of chemicals, cells, and microbes between the blood and the body tissues. Endothelial cells in the smallest blood vessels (capillaries) are supported by a thin layer of connective tissue, rich in collagen fibers, called the intima. In veins, a thin layer (the media) of contractile smooth muscle cells allows some venoconstriction: for example, superficial veins under the skin constrict in response to surface cooling. In arteries and arterioles, a well-developed muscle layer allows powerful vasoconstriction, including the vasoconstriction after local injury that forms part of the hemostatic response. Larger vessels also have a supportive connective tissue outer layer (the adventitia). Figure 6.2 illustrates the structure of the vessel wall.

Normal endothelium has an antithrombotic surface

Intact normal endothelium does not initiate or support platelet adhesion or blood coagulation. Its surface is antithrombotic. This thrombo-resistance is partly due to endothelial production of two potent vasodilators and inhibitors of platelet function: prostacyclin (prostaglandin I_2, PG_{I2}) and nitric oxide, otherwise known as endothelium-derived relaxing factor (EDRF) (see box on p. 66).

The vasoconstriction that occurs after vascular injury is partly mediated by two platelet activation products: serotonin (5-hydroxytryptamine), and thromboxane A2 (TXA2; see Fig. 6.1), a product of platelet prostaglandin metabolism. In

Causes of excessive bleeding

	Congenital	Acquired
vessel wall	disorders of collagen synthesis (Ehlers–Danlos syndrome)	vitamin C deficiency (scurvy) corticosteroid excess
platelets	vWF deficiency (von Willebrand disease) platelet GPIb-IX deficiency (Bernard–Soulier syndrome) platelet GPIIb-IIIa deficiency (Glanzmann's thrombasthenia)	antiplatelet drugs (e.g. aspirin) defective formation of platelets excessive destruction of platelets
coagulation	coagulation factor deficiencies (hemophilias)-factor VIII factor IX factor XI fibrinogen etc.	vitamin K deficiency (factors II, VII, IX, X) oral anticoagulants (vitamin K antagonists, e.g. warfarin) liver disease disseminated intravascular coagulation (DIC)
fibrinolysis	antiplasmin deficiency PAI-1 deficiency	fibrinolytic drugs (e.g. tPA, urokinase, streptokinase)

Table 6.1 **Congenital and acquired causes of excessive bleeding**. GPIb-IX, GPIIb-IIIa, glycoprotein receptors Ib-IX and IIb-IIIa; PAI-1, plasminogen activator inhibitor type 1.

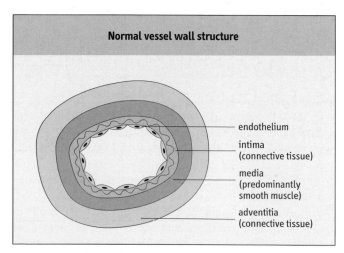

Normal vessel wall structure

- endothelium
- intima (connective tissue)
- media (predominantly smooth muscle)
- adventitia (connective tissue)

Fig. 6.2 **Normal vessel wall structure.**

PROSTACYCLIN AND NITRIC OXIDE ARE GENERATED IN THE VESSEL WALL

Biochemical mediators of vasoconstriction and vasodilatation

The diameters of arteries and arterioles throughout the body continuously alter to regulate blood flow according to local and general metabolic and cardiovascular requirements. Control mechanisms include neurogenic (sympathetic/adrenergic; see Chapter 39) and myogenic pathways, and local biochemical mediators, including prostacyclin (PGI_2) and nitric oxide.

Prostacyclin is the major arachidonic acid metabolite formed by vascular cells. It is a potent vasodilator, and also a potent inhibitor of platelet aggregation. It has a short half-life in plasma (3 minutes).

Nitric oxide is also a potent vasodilator formed by vascular endothelial cells, also with a short half-life. It was initially termed endothelium-derived relaxing factor (EDRF). In common with that of prostacyclin, its generation by endothelial cells is enhanced by many compounds, and also by blood flow and shear stress. In the normal circulation, nitric oxide appears to have a key role in flow-mediated vasodilatation. It is synthesized by two distinct forms of endothelial nitric oxide synthase (eNOS): constitutive and inducible. Constitutive eNOS rapidly provides relatively small amounts of nitric oxide for short periods, related to vascular flow regulation. The beneficial effects of nitrate drugs in hypertension and angina may partly reflect their effects on this pathway (see Chapter 17). Inducible eNOS is stimulated by cytokines in inflammatory reactions, and releases large amounts of nitric oxide for long periods. Its suppression by glucocorticoids may partly account for their anti-inflammatory effects.

Both prostacyclin and nitric oxide appear to exert their vasodilator actions by diffusing locally from endothelial cells to vascular smooth muscle cells (see Fig. 6.2), where they stimulate guanylate cyclase, resulting in increased formation of cyclic guanosine 3′,5′-monophosphate (cGMP) and relaxation of vascular smooth muscle, probably via alteration of the intracellular calcium concentration (see Chapter 38).

PLATELETS PRODUCE THROMBOXANE A_2

Thromboxane A_2 and aspirin

It has already been noted that PGI_2, the major arachidonic acid metabolite formed by vascular cells is a potent vasodilator and inhibitor of platelet aggregation. In contrast, the major arachidonic acid metabolite formed by platelets is TXA_2, which is a potent vasoconstrictor and stimulates platelet aggregation. In common with prostacyclin, TXA_2 has a short half-life. In the late 1970s, Salvador Moncada and John Vane contrasted the effects of PGI_2 and TXA_2 on blood vessels and platelets, and hypothesized that a balance between these two compounds was important in the regulation of hemostasis and thrombosis.

Congenital deficiencies of cyclo-oxygenase or thromboxane synthase (the enzymes involved in TXA_2 synthesis) result in a mild bleeding tendency. Ingestion of even low doses of acetylsalicylic acid (aspirin) irreversibly acetylates cyclo-oxygenase and suppresses TXA_2 synthesis and platelet aggregation for several days, resulting in an antithrombotic effect and a mild bleeding tendency. Bleeding is especially likely from the stomach, as a result of the formation of stomach ulcers secondary to the inhibition of cytoprotective gastric mucosal prostaglandins by aspirin. Although in persons at high risk of arterial thrombosis (e.g. previous myocardial infarction or stroke) this bleeding tendency is outweighed by a reduction in risk of thrombosis, aspirin is contraindicated in individuals with a history of bleeding disorders, or existing stomach or duodenal ulcers.

membrane glycoprotein receptor, GPIb-IX). Platelet activating factor (PAF) from the vessel wall may also activate platelets in hemostasis (see Fig. 6.1).

Collagen has a key role in the structure and the hemostatic function of small blood vessels

Because collagen has a key role in the structure and the hemostatic function of small blood vessels, vascular causes of excessive bleeding include congenital or acquired deficiencies of collagen synthesis (see Table 6.1). Congenital disorders include the rare Ehlers–Danlos syndrome. Acquired disorders include the relatively common vitamin C deficiency, scurvy (see Chapter 10), and excessive exogenous or endogenous corticosteroids.

PLATELETS

Blood platelets form the initial hemostatic plug in small vessels, and the initial thrombus in arteries and veins.

Platelets are circulating, anuclear microcells of mean diameter 2–3 mm. They are fragments of bone marrow

addition, after a vascular injury that disrupts the endothelial cell lining, flowing blood is exposed to subendothelial collagen, which activates the intrinsic pathway of blood coagulation. The endothelial cell damage also exposes flowing blood to subendothelial tissue factor, which activates the extrinsic pathway of blood coagulation (see Fig. 6.1).

Exposure of flowing blood to collagen as a result of endothelial damage also stimulates platelet activation. Platelets bind to collagen via von Willebrand factor (vWF), which is released from the endothelial cells. vWF in turn binds both to collagen fibers and to platelets (via a platelet

PLATELET ACTIVATION EXPOSES GLYCOPROTEIN RECEPTORS

Platelet membrane receptors and their ligands, vWF and fibrinogen

Platelets have a key role in hemostasis and thrombosis, through adhesion to the vessel wall and subsequent aggregation to form a platelet-rich hemostatic plug or thrombus. These processes involve exposure of specific membrane glycoprotein receptors after platelet activation by several compounds (see Fig. 6.3).

Platelet receptor GPIb-IX plays a key part in the adhesion of platelets to subendothelium. It binds vWF, which also interacts with specific subendothelial receptors, including those on subendothelial collagen. Congenital deficiencies of GPIb-IX (Bernard-Soulier syndrome) or, more commonly, of vWF, result in a bleeding tendency. In contrast, high plasma concentrations of vWF are associated with increased risk of thrombosis. For patients at high risk of thrombosis, therapeutic strategies directed against vWF (for example anti-vWF antibodies) are currently being developed, to reduce the thrombotic risk.

Another receptor, GPIIb-IIIa has a key role in platelet aggregation. After platelet activation, hundreds of thousands of GPIIb-IIIa receptors can be exposed in a single platelet. These receptors interact with fibrinogen or vWF, which bind platelets together, forming a hemostatic or thrombotic plug. Congenital deficiency of GPIIb-IIIa (the rare Glanzmann's thrombasthenia) causes a severe bleeding disorder; in contrast, deficiencies of either fibrinogen or vWF cause a milder bleeding disorder, because these two ligands can substitute for each other. High plasma concentrations of fibrinogen are associated with increased risk of thrombosis, partly because of its platelet-binding activity. For patients at high risk of thrombosis, inhibitors of the GPIIb-IIIa receptor (such as antireceptor antibodies) are being developed and are proving to be clinically effective.

megakaryocytes, and circulate for about 10 days in the blood. The concentration of platelets in normal blood is 150–400×10^9/L (150–400×10^3/mm^3).

Platelets can be activated by several chemical agents, including adenosine diphosphate (ADP, released by platelets, erythrocytes, and endothelial cells), epinephrine, collagen, thrombin, and PAF; by immune complexes (generated during infections); and by high physical shear stresses (shear stress is the tangential force applied to the cells by the flow of blood). Most of the chemical agents appear to act by binding to specific receptors on the platelet surface membrane (see Fig. 6.3). After receptor stimulation, several pathways of platelet activation can be initiated, resulting in several phenomena:

- **change in platelet shape** from a disc to a sphere with extended pseudopodia – which facilitates aggregation and coagulant activity;

- **release of several compounds involved in hemostasis** from intracellular granules – for example ADP, serotonin, TXA2, and vWF;
- **aggregation**, via exposure of GPIb-IX membrane receptor and linking by vWF (under high shear conditions), and via exposure of another membrane glycoprotein receptor, GPIIa-IIIb and linking by fibrinogen (under low shear conditions);
- **adhesion to the vessel wall** via exposure of the GPIb-IX membrane receptor, through which vWF binds platelets to subendothelial collagen.

Finally, stimulation of the platelet membrane receptor triggers the activation of platelet membrane phospholipases, which hydrolyze membrane phospholipids, releasing arachidonic acid. Arachidonic acid is metabolized by cyclo-oxygenase and thromboxane synthase to TXA$_2$, a potent but labile (half-life 30 seconds) mediator of platelet activation and vasoconstriction.

Platelet-related bleeding disorders

Congenital defects in platelet adhesion/aggregation can cause lifelong excessive bleeding

A simple screening test – measurement of the skin bleeding time (normal range, 2–10 minutes) – is sufficient to detect congenital defects of platelet adhesion/aggregation, in which the time is characteristically prolonged. The most common such defect is von Willebrand disease (see Table 6.1), a group of autosomal dominant disorders that result in low plasma concentrations of vWF multimers. These multimers are composed of subunits (molecular weight 250 kDa) that are released from endothelial cells (and platelet granules) and circulate in plasma at a concentration of 1 mg/dL. Not only does vWF have an important role in platelet hemostatic function but it also transports coagulation factor VIII (antihemophilic factor) in the circulation and delivers it to sites of vascular injury. Hence, plasma concentrations of factor VIII may also be low in von Willebrand disease. Treatment of this disease is to increase the low plasma vWF activity, usually by means of desmopressin (a synthetic analogue of vasopressin (see Chapter 23) which releases vWF from endothelial cells into plasma). Sometimes this is done using human plasma concentrates.

Less common congenital bleeding disorders include GPIb-IX deficiency (Bernard–Soulier syndrome), GPIIb-IIIa deficiency (Glanzmann's thrombasthenia), and fibrinogen deficiency (because fibrinogen bridges GPIIb-IIIa receptors of adjacent platelets).

Acquired disorders of platelets include a low platelet count (thrombocytopenia), which may be the result either of defective formation of platelets by bone marrow megakaryocytes

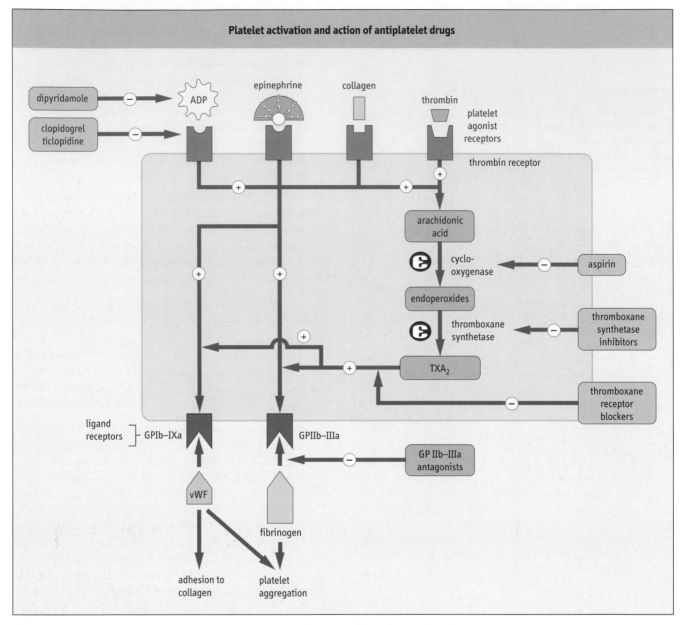

Platelet activation and action of antiplatelet drugs

Fig. 6.3 **Pathways of platelet activation and mechanisms of action of antiplatelet drugs.** Stimulation of platelet agonist receptors results in exposure of platelet ligand receptors, partly through the platelet prostaglandin (cyclo-oxygenase) pathway. Ligand receptors bind vWF and fibrinogen in platelet adhesion/aggregation.

(as in marrow neoplasia, or aplasia), or of excessive destruction of platelets (e.g. by antiplatelet antibodies, or in splenomegaly or disseminated intravascular coagulation, DIC).

Antiplatelet drugs

Antiplatelet drugs are used in the prevention or treatment of arterial thrombosis; their sites of action are illustrated in Figure 6.3. As described above, aspirin inhibits cyclo-oxygenase and hence reduces the formation of TXA_2. Because it also has the effect of reducing the formation of PGI_2, which itself has antiplatelet activity, agents acting more specifically as thromboxane synthase inhibitors or thromboxane receptor antagonists have also been investigated as potential antiplatelet agents, but do not appear to be more effective than aspirin. Dipyridamole acts by reducing the availability of ADP, and ticlopidine and clopidogrel inhibit the ADP receptor (Fig. 6.3). These drugs have antithrombotic effects similar to those of aspirin, but cause less gastric bleeding because they do not interfere with synthesis of prostaglandins in the stomach. Recently, GPIIb-IIIa antagonists have been used in acute coronary thrombosis. Each of these newer antiplatelet drugs adds to the antithrombotic efficacy of aspirin; but also increases the risk of bleeding when used in combination.

PATIENT SELF-MONITORING OF ORAL ANTICOAGULANT THERAPY

Oral anticoagulant therapy (e.g. with warfarin) is given long-term to patients at risk of thrombosis within the chambers of the heart (e.g. patients with atrial fibrillation, or heart valve prostheses), which may embolize to the brain causing a stroke. Monitoring of the prothrombin time every few weeks is essential to minimize not only risk of thromboembolism, but also of excessive bleeding. Up to 1 per cent of the adult population in developed countries now receive long-term oral anticoagulants, hence traditional monitoring by doctors and nurses (taking blood samples, sending them to the laboratory, getting results, and giving dosage instructions to patients) has become a huge workload. In recent years, portable prothrombin time measuring devices have been developed which selected patients can use for self-monitoring. A 'finger-stick' capillary sample is drawn into the machine, and the result displayed to the patient (similar to blood glucose self-monitoring by persons with diabetes). Computer algorithms have also been developed which track the patient's prothrombin time results and oral anticoagulant doses, and can recommend appropriate changes in dose not only to their supervising doctor or nurse, but also directly to the patient.

COAGULATION

Blood coagulation factors interact to form the secondary, fibrin-rich, hemostatic plug in small vessels, and the secondary fibrin thrombus in arteries and veins

Plasma coagulation factors are identified by roman numerals; they are listed in Table 6.2, together with some of their properties. Tissue factor was formerly known as factor III, calcium ion as factor IV; factor VI does not exist. Congenital deficiencies of other coagulation factors (I–XIII) result in excessive bleeding, which illustrates their physiologic importance in hemostasis. The exception is factor XII deficiency, which does not increase the bleeding tendency, despite prolonging blood clotting times *in vitro*; the same is true for its cofactors, prekallikrein or high-molecular-weight kininogen (HMWK). A possible explanation for this is given below.

Figure 6.4 illustrates the currently accepted scheme of blood coagulation. Since the early 1960s, this has been accepted as a 'waterfall' or 'cascade' sequence of interactive pro-enzyme to enzyme conversions, each enzyme activating the next pro-enzyme in the sequence(s). Activated factor enzymes are designated by the letter 'a' – for example, factor XIa. Traditionally, the scheme has been divided into three parts:

- the intrinsic pathway,
- the extrinsic pathway,
- the final common pathway.

Coagulation factors and their properties

Factor	Synonyms	Molecular weight (Da)	Plasma concentration (mg/dL)
I	Fibrinogen	340 000	200–400
II	Prothrombin	70 000	10
III	Tissue factor (thromboplastin)	44 000	0
IV	*Calcium ion	40	9–10
V	Proaccelerin, labile factor	330 000	1
VII	Serum prothrombin conversion accelerator (SPCA), stable factor	48 000	0.05
VIII	Antihemophilic factor (AHF)	330 000	0.01
(vWF)		(250 000)n	1
IX	Christmas factor	55 000	0.3
X	Stuart–Prower factor	59 000	1
XI	Plasma thromboplastin antecedent (PTA)	160 000	0.5
XII	Hageman factor	80 000	3
XIII	Fibrin-stabilizing factor (FSF)	320 000	1–2
Prekallikrein	Fletcher factor	85 000	5
High-molecular-weight kininogen (HMWK)	Fitzgerald, Flaujeac; or Williams factor, contact activation cofactor	120 000	6

*To convert calcium ion to mmol/L multiply by 0.2495

Table 6.2 **Coagulation factors and some of their properties.** n indicates number of subunits.

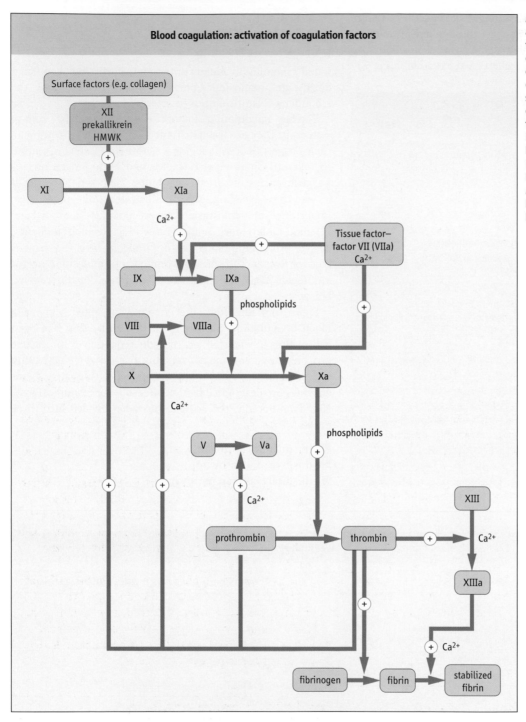

Blood coagulation: activation of coagulation factors

Fig. 6.4 **Blood coagulation: activation of coagulation factors.** After the initiation of blood coagulation, the coagulation factor pro-enzymes are activated sequentially: activated factor enzymes are designated by the letter 'a'. The purple box indicates contact factors that have no apparent function in *in vivo* hemostasis. Phospholipids are supplied *in vivo* by platelets. HMWK, high-molecular-weight kininogen.

These are described below. They are distinguished on the basis of the nature of the initiating factor and its corresponding test in the clinical hemostasis laboratory; hence, three tests of coagulation are performed in clinical laboratories on citrated, platelet-poor plasma:

- activated partial thromboplastin time (APTT),
- prothrombin time,
- thrombin time.

Platelet-poor plasma is used in these tests because the platelet count influences clotting time results. To obtain the platelet-poor plasma, citrate anticoagulant is added to blood to sequester calcium ions reversibly, and the blood is centrifuged at 2000 g for 15 minutes. The coagulation time tests are initiated by adding calcium and appropriate initiating agents.

The intrinsic pathway

The term 'intrinsic' implies that no extrinsic factor such as tissue factor or thrombin is added to the blood, other than a contact with nonendothelial 'surface'. The clinical test of this pathway is the activated partial thromboplastin time (APTT), also known as the kaolin-cephalin clotting time (KCCT) because kaolin (microparticulated clay) is added as a standard 'surface' and cephalin (brain phospholipid extract) as a substitute for platelet phospholipid. The normal range of the APTT is about 30–50 seconds; prolongations are observed in deficiencies of factors XII (or its cofactors, prekallikrein or HMWK), XI, IX (or its cofactor, factor VIII), X (or its cofactor, factor V), prothrombin (factor II), or fibrinogen (factor I) (see Table 6.1). The test is used to exclude the common congenital hemophilias (deficiencies of factors VIII, IX, or XI; see Table 6.2), and to monitor heparin treatment (see box). Hemophilias caused by factor VIII or IX deficiency occur in about 1 in 10 000 males; inheritance is X-linked recessive, transmitted by carrier females. Treatment is usually with factor VIII or IX concentrates.

The extrinsic pathway

The term 'extrinsic' refers to the effect of tissue factor, which (after combining with coagulation factor VII) greatly accelerates coagulation, by activating both factor IX and factor X (Fig. 6.4). Tissue factor is a polypeptide that is expressed in all cells other than endothelial cells. The clinical test of this pathway is the prothrombin time (PT), in which tissue factor is added to plasma. The normal range is about 10–15 seconds; prolongations are observed in deficiencies of factors VII, X, V, II, or I. In clinical practice, the test is used to diagnose both the rare congenital defects of these factors and,

HEPARIN TREATMENT IS INEFFECTIVE IN ANTITHROMBIN DEFICIENCY

A 40-year-old man was admitted from the Emergency Room of his local hospital because of acute pain and swelling of his left leg 10 days after recent major surgery. Ultrasound imaging of the leg confirmed occlusion of the left femoral vein by thrombus. He was prescribed anticoagulant therapy with low molecular weight heparin at standard doses. The patient volunteered a strong family history of 'clots in the legs' at a young age. A thrombophilia screening test was performed, and showed a low plasma antithrombin level.

Comment. The patient was treated with intravenous antithrombin concentrate, which increased his plasma antithrombin levels to within the normal range. This allows heparin to be effective. The clinical response was satisfactory, and the patient's medication was subsequently changed from heparin to oral warfarin.

much more commonly, to diagnose acquired bleeding disorders, resulting from:

- **vitamin K deficiency** (e.g. malabsorption, obstructive jaundice; see Chapters 10 and 28), which reduces hepatic synthesis of factors II, VII, IX, and X. Treatment is by injections of vitamin K;
- **oral anticoagulants** (e.g. warfarin) which are vitamin K antagonists, reducing hepatic synthesis of these factors. Excessive bleeding in patients taking warfarin can be treated by stopping the drug, giving vitamin K, or replacing factors II, VII, IX, and X with fresh frozen plasma or concentrates;
- **liver disease**, which reduces hepatic synthesis of these factors. For example, the prothrombin time is a prognostic marker of liver failure after acetaminophen (paracetamol) overdose (see Chapter 28). Treatment is by replacing factors II, VII, IX, and X with fresh frozen plasma or concentrates.

The final common pathway

The third part of coagulation is tested clinically by the thrombin time, in which exogenous thrombin is added to plasma. The normal range of values is about 10–15 seconds; prolongations are observed in fibrinogen deficiency. This may be congenital, or due to acquired consumption of fibrinogen in disseminated intravascular coagulation (DIC), or may occur after administration of fibrinolytic drugs (see below). Treatment is with fresh frozen plasma or fibrinogen concentrates.

CLASSICAL HEMOPHILIA: CONGENITAL FACTOR VIII DEFICIENCY

A 3-year-old boy was admitted from the Emergency Room of his local hospital because of extensive bruising after a fall down a few stairs (see Fig. 6.5). A routine coagulation screen test showed a greatly prolonged APTT of more than 150 seconds (normal range, 30–50 seconds). Assay of coagulation factor VIII showed a very low level; the vWF level was normal. His mother recollected a family history of excessive bleeding which had affected her brother and father.

Comment. Because of this typical history of an X-linked recessive bleeding disorder, a low coagulation factor VIII level, and a normal vWF level, a diagnosis of classical hemophilia (congenital factor VIII deficiency) was made. The family were referred to the local Hemophilia Center and counseled about the risks of further affected sons and carrier daughters. The child was treated with intravenous factor VIII concentrate for the presenting bleed, and for future bleeds, injuries, or surgery.

Thrombin

Thrombin converts circulating fibrinogen to fibrin and activates factor XIII which crosslinks the fibrin forming a clot. It is currently believed that activation of blood coagulation is usually initiated by vascular injury, causing exposure of flowing blood to tissue factor, which results in activation of factors VII and IX. Subsequently, activation of factors X and II (prothrombin) occurs preferentially at sites of vascular injury, and upon activated platelets, which provide procoagulant activity (platelet factor 3, PF3) as a result of exposure of negatively-charged platelet surface membrane phospholipids, such as phosphatidylserine. This is accompanied by the exposure, on activated platelets, of high-affinity binding sites for several activated coagulation factors (especially factors Va and VIIIa), and provision of platelet phospholipid, which further catalyzes coagulation activation. As a result of these biochemical interactions (see Figs 6.1 and 6.6), thrombin and fibrin formation are efficiently localized at sites of vascular injury.

Thrombin has a central role in hemostasis

Not only does thrombin convert circulating fibrinogen to fibrin at sites of vascular injury (producing the secondary, fibrin-rich, hemostatic plug); it also activates factor XIII (transglutaminase), which crosslinks such fibrin, rendering it resistant to dispersion by local blood pressure or by fibrinolysis (see Figs 6.1 and 6.4). Furthermore, thrombin stimulates its own generation in a positive feedback cycle in two ways:

- **it catalyzes activation of factor XI**; this may explain why congenital deficiencies of factor XII, prekallikrein, or HMWK are not associated with excessive bleeding (Fig. 6.6);
- **it catalyzes activation of factors VIII and V.**

Thrombin also activates platelets (see Fig. 6.3).

Now that the central role of thrombin in hemostasis and thrombosis has been recognized, there is current interest in the development of direct antithrombins as antithrombotic drugs; these include examples such as hirudin (originally obtained from the medicinal leech, *Hirudo medicinalis*) and its synthetic derivatives.

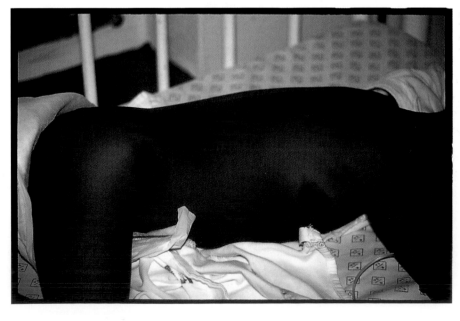

Fig. 6.5 **Severe bruising that resulted from a minor fall in a 3-year-old child with classic hemophilia.** (Courtesy of Dr S Taylor.)

Inhibitors of blood coagulation

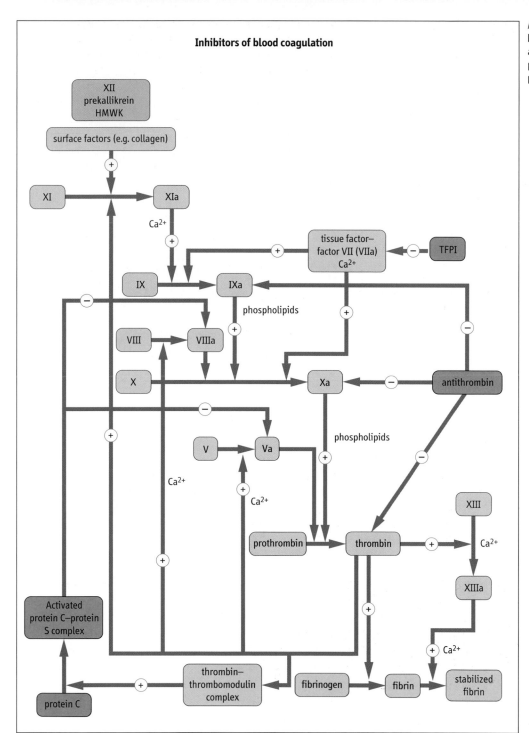

Fig. 6.6 **Sites of action of blood coagulation inhibitors:** antithrombin, protein C and protein S, and tissue factor pathway inhibitor (TFPI).

Properties of coagulation inhibitors		
Inhibitor (synonym)	Molecular weight	Plasma concentration (mg/dL)
Anthithrombin (antithrombin III)	65 000	18–30
Protein C	56 000	0.4
Protein S	69 000	2.5
Tissue factor pathway inhibitor, TFPI (lipoprotein-associated coagulation inhibitor, LACI)	32 000	0.1

Table 6.3 **Properties of coagulation inhibitors.**

Coagulation inhibitors are essential to prevent excessive thrombin formation and thrombosis

Three systems of coagulation inhibitors have been identified (see Figs 6.6 and Table 6.3):

- **antithrombin**: this is a protein synthesized in the liver. Its activity is catalyzed by the antithrombotic drug, heparin, and by heparin-like endogenous glycosaminoglycans (GAGs) that are present on the surface of vascular endothelial cells. It inactivates not only thrombin, but also factors IXa and Xa (see Fig. 6.6). Congenital antithrombin deficiency results in increased risk of venous thromboembolism. Heparin injections are given in the treatment of acute venous or arterial thrombosis; they are usually replaced by oral anticoagulants such as warfarin for longer-term anticoagulation.
- **protein C and its cofactor, protein S**: these are vitamin-K-dependent proteins, synthesized in the liver. When thrombin is generated, it binds to thrombomodulin (molecular weight 74 kDa), which is present on the surface of vascular endothelial cells. The thrombin-thrombomodulin complex activates protein C, which forms a complex with its cofactor, protein S. This complex selectively degrades factors Va and VIIIa by limited proteolysis (Fig. 6.6). Hence, this pathway forms a negative feedback upon thrombin generation. Congenital deficiencies of protein C or protein S result in increased risk of venous thromboembolism; a further cause of increased risk of venous thromboembolism is a mutation in coagulation factor V (factor V Leiden), which confers resistance to its inactivation by activated protein C. This mutation is common, occurring in about 3% of the population in Western countries.
- **tissue factor pathway inhibitor (TFPI)**: this protein is synthesized in endothelium and the liver; it circulates bound to lipoproteins. It inhibits the tissue factor-VIIa complex (Fig. 6.6), which may explain the severe bleeding in hemophilia caused by deficiency in factor VIII or IX (failure to sustain thrombin and fibrin

MEASUREMENT OF FIBRIN D-DIMER IN DIAGNOSIS OF SUSPECTED DEEP VEIN THROMBOSIS

Fibrin D-dimer (a degradation product of cross-linked fibrin and a marker of fibrin turnover) is normally present in blood at concentrations less than 0.25g/L. In deep vein thrombosis of the leg (DVT), deposition of a large mass of cross-linked fibrin within the leg veins, followed by partial lysis by the body's fibrinolytic system, increases fibrin turnover and blood D-dimer levels are elevated. Many patients attend accident and emergency departments with a swollen and/or painful leg, which may be due to DVT. Rapid immunoassays for blood D-dimer can be performed in the emergency department, and are now widely used as a adjunct to clinical diagnosis. About one-third of patients with clinically-suspected DVT have normal D-dimer levels, which usually excludes the diagnosis and allows early discharge of such patients without the need for further investigation or treatment. In patients with raised D-dimer levels, heparin treatment is started and imaging of the leg performed (usually by ultrasound) to confirm the presence and extent of DVT.

formation). Conversely, deficiency of TFPI does not appear to increase the risk of thrombosis.

FIBRINOLYSIS

The fibrinolytic system also limits excessive fibrin formation

The coagulation system acts to form fibrin; the fibrinolytic system acts to limit excessive formation of fibrin (both intra- and extravascular) through plasmin-mediated fibrinolysis. Circulating plasminogen binds to fibrin via lysine-binding sites; it is converted to active plasmin by plasminogen activators. Tissue-type plasminogen activator (tPA) is synthesized by endothelial cells; it normally circulates in plasma in low basal concentrations (5 ng/mL), but is released into plasma by stimuli that include venous occlusion, exercise, and epinephrine. Together with plasminogen, it binds strongly to fibrin, which stimulates its activity (the K_m for plasminogen decreases from 65 to 0.15 μmol/L in the presence of fibrin), thereby localizing plasmin activity to fibrin deposits. Excessive tPA activity in plasma is normally prevented by an excess of its major inhibitor, plasminogen activator inhibitor type 1 (PAI-1), which is synthesized by both endothelial cells and hepatocytes. Urinary-type plasminogen activator (uPA) circulates in plasma both as an active single-chain precursor form, uPA (scuPA, pro-urokinase) and as a more active two-chain form (tcuPA, urokinase). One activator of scuPA is surface-activated coagulation factor XII, which therefore links the coagulation and fibrinolytic systems. The major components of the fibrinolytic system are illustrated in Table 6.4 and Figure 6.7.

Excessive formation of plasmin is normally prevented by:

- binding of 50% of plasminogen to histidine-rich glycoprotein (HRG);
- rapid inactivation of free plasmin by its major inhibitor, α_2-antiplasmin.

The physiologic importance of PAI-1 and α_2-antiplasmin is illustrated by the increased bleeding tendency that is associated with the rare cases of their congenital deficiencies (see Table 6.1); the excessive plasma plasmin activity which results from the deficiencies has the effect of lysing hemostatic plugs.

THROMBOLYTIC TREATMENT IN MYOCARDIAL INFARCTION

Occlusion of a coronary artery by thrombus causes death of that part of the heart muscle which is supplied by the artery (myocardial infarction). In acute myocardial infarction, the patient typically experiences severe, substantial chest pain. Many such patients are candidates for thrombolytic treatment with a plasminogen activator drug, given intravenously (there are some exceptions). Prompt thrombolysis dissolves the coronary artery thrombus, reduces the size of the infarct, and reduces the risk of complications, including death and heart failure. Aspirin is also given routinely in acute myocardial infarction, to inhibit the platelet component of the developing coronary artery thrombus.

Comment. Thrombolytic drugs include tissue-type and urinary-type plasminogen activators (tPA and uPA) (Fig. 6.7), produced by recombinant gene technology, or their synthetic variants. Worldwide, the most commonly used thrombolytic drug is streptokinase (a plasminogen activator produced by streptococci), because of its lower cost. All thrombolytic drugs can cause bleeding (see Table 6.1), as a result of lysis of hemostatic plugs in addition to the target thrombi.

Properties of fibrinolytic system components

Component (synonym)	Molecular weight	Plasma concentration (mg/dL)
Plasminogen	92 000	0.2
Tissue-type plasminogen activator, tPA	65 000	5 (basal)
Urinary-type plasminogen activator type 1, uPA	54 000	20
Plasminogen activator inhibitor type 1, PAI-1	48 000	200
Antiplasmin (α_2 antiplasmin)	70 000	700

Table 6.4 **Properties of fibrinolytic system components.**

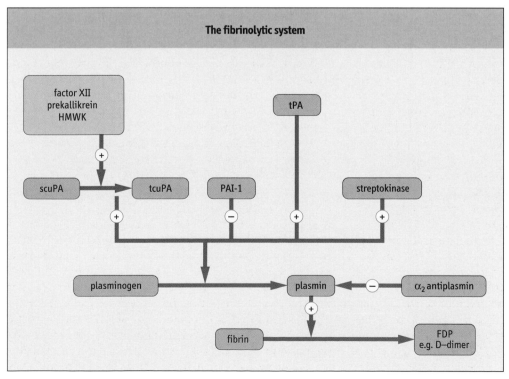

Fig. 6.7 **The fibrinolytic system.** Plasminogen can be activated to plasmin by uPA (urokinase), tPA, or streptokinase. uPA and tPA are inhibited by plasminogen activator inhibitor type 1 (PAI-1). Plasmin is inhibited by antiplasmin. Plasmin degrades fibrin to fibrin degradation products (FDP). HMWK, high-molecular-weight kininogen; scuPA, pro-urokinase; tcuPA, urokinase; tPA, tissue-type plasminogen activator.

Summary

- Hemostasis constitutes a number of processes which guard the body against blood loss.
- Injury to the blood vessel wall sets in motion complex phenomena which involve blood platelets (activation, adhesion, aggregation), and a cascade of coagulation factors, classified into intrinsic, extrinsic and final common pathways.
- The integrity of these three systems may be tested by simple laboratory tests.
- Deficiencies of factors participating in the coagulation cascade, and/or disordered platelet function, result in bleeding disorders.
- Eventually, blood clots are degraded by the fibrinolytic system. The process of fibrinolysis prevents thrombotic phenomena and there is normally a balance between hemostasis and thrombosis.
- Aspirin, and clot dissolution using intravenous infusion of enzymes such as streptokinase, are now established treatments for acute myocardial infarction.
- Aspirin (or other antiplatelet agents) are also used to reduce risk of recurrent myocardial infarction and stroke.
- Anticoagulant drugs (heparin then warfarin) are used in treatment of acute venous thrombosis or embolism.
- Anticoagulant drugs (warfarin) are used long-term to prevent thromboembolism from the heart (atrial fibrillation, heart valve prostheses).

ACTIVE LEARNING

Test your knowledge:

1. When a patient presents with excessive bleeding from multiple sites, what laboratory tests should be done to identify the likely cause of their hemostatic defect?
2. When a patient presents with a painful swollen leg, possibly due to acute deep venous thrombosis (DVT), what laboratory tests can be performed to help the clinician:
   - to establish or exclude this diagnosis?
   - to monitor anticoagulant treatment, after the diagnosis has been confirmed?
3. When a patient presents with acute coronary artery thrombosis (evolving to myocardial infarction), what antithrombotic drugs should be urgently considered to reduce the risk of complications?

Further reading

Lowe GDO, ed. State of the Art 2003. *J Thromb Haemostas* 2003;**1**:1335–1670 (available on http://www.blackwellpublishing.com/jth).

Membranes and Transport

M Maeda

LEARNING OBJECTIVES

After reading this chapter you should be able to:

■ Describe the major types of lipids and proteins in biological membranes.

■ Explain how lipids and protein interact to form the membrane, according to the fluid mosaic model of membrane structure.

■ Describe differences between passive and active carrier-mediated transport systems, with emphasis of the kinetic similarities between transport processes and enzyme catalysis.

■ Describe the basic features of membrane channels and pores.

■ Give several specific examples of ion and substrate transport systems and coupled transport systems.

■ Describe how defects in membrane transport are associated with various diseases.

INTRODUCTION

Cells are surrounded by membranes, thin films about 50 Å in width, composed of proteins and lipids, including both glycoproteins and glycolipids. Intracellular organelles are also compartmentalized by membranes. Biomembranes are not rigid or impermeable but highly mobile and dynamic structures. The plasma membrane is the gatekeeper of the cell. It controls not only the access of inorganic ions, vitamins and nutrients, but also the entry of drugs and the exit of waste products. Integral transmembrane proteins have important roles in transporting these molecules through the membrane and often maintain concentration gradients across the membranes. K^+, Na^+, and Ca^{2+} concentrations in the cytoplasm are maintained at ~140, 10, and 10^{-4} mmol/L (546, 23, and 0.0007 mg/dL), respectively, by the transporter proteins, whereas those outside (in the blood) are ~5, 145, and 1–2 mmol/L (20, 333, and 7–14 mg/dL), respectively. The driving force for transport of ions and maintenance of ion gradients is directly or indirectly provided by ATP. We will begin this chapter with a description of the composition, structure and properties of lipids, and then explain how lipids and proteins interact to form biomembranes. The transport properties of membranes will be illustrated by several important examples.

MEMBRANE LIPIDS

Structure and properties of membrane lipids

Lipids are nonpolar biomolecules that can be extracted into organic solvents. They are the major component of fat in adipose tissue and of membranes in all cells. Fatty acids (Table 7.1) are common components of both triglycerides, the storage form of fats, and phospholipids (Fig. 7.1), the major lipids in cell membranes. Fatty acids in biological systems normally contain an even number of carbon atoms – a property that stems from their synthesis in two-carbon units. Long-chain, linear aliphatic C-16 and C-18 fatty acids are the most common components of phospholipids, and nearly 50% of the fatty acids in membrane phospholipids are unsaturated, containing one or more carbon-carbon double bonds. The double bonds in unsaturated fatty acids are all in the *cis* configuration. This places a 'kink' in their structure and interferes with their molecular packing, so that lipids enriched in unsaturated fatty acids have lower melting points.

The storage form of lipids is a triacylglycerol (triglyceride) molecule, with fatty acids esterified to all three of the hydroxyl groups of glycerol. Both vegetable oils and animal fats are triglycerides, but triolein (glycerol trioleate, found in olive oil) is a liquid, whereas tristearin (glycerol tristearate, found in lard) is a solid at room temperature.

Membrane phospholipids are mostly glycerophospholipids, composed of an L-glycerol backbone with the fatty acids attached at the C-1 and C-2 positions in ester linkage. In general, saturated fatty acids are attached at the C-1 position, and unsaturated fatty acids at the C-2 position of the glycerol in phospholipids. Phosphoric acid is linked as an ester to position C-3, and a polar head group is further linked to the phosphate moiety forming a phosphate diester (Fig. 7.1). Variations in the size and degree of unsaturation of the fatty acid components in phospholipids affect the fluidity of biomembranes – shorter chain and unsaturated fatty acids decrease the freezing point of phospholipids, making the membrane more fluid at body temperature.

Naturally occurring fatty acids				
Carbon atoms	Chemical formula	Systematic name	Common name	Melting point (°C)
Saturated fatty acids				
12 12:0	$CH_3(CH_2)_{10}COOH$	n-dodecanoic	lauric	44
14 14:0	$CH_3(CH_2)_{12}COOH$	n-tetradecanoic	myristic	54
16 16:0	$CH_3(CH_2)_{14}COOH$	n-hexadecanoic	palmitic	63
18 18:0	$CH_3(CH_2)_{16}COOH$	n-octadecanoic	stearic	70
20 20:0	$CH_3(CH_2)_{18}COOH$	n-eicosanoic	arachidic	77
Unsaturated fatty acids				
16 16:1; ω-6, Δ^9	$CH_3(CH_2)_5CH = CH(CH_2)_7COOH$		palmitoleic	−0.5
18 18:1; ω-9, Δ^9	$CH_3(CH_2)_7CH = CH(CH_2)_7COOH$		oleic	13
18 18:2; ω-6, $\Delta^{9,12}$	$CH_3(CH_2)_4CH = CHCH_2CH = CH(CH_2)_7COOH$		linoleic	−5
18 18:3; ω-3, $\Delta^{9,12,15}$	$CH_3CH_2CH = CHCH_2CH = CHCH_2CH = CH(CH_2)_7COOH$		linolenic	−11
20 20:4; ω-6, $\Delta^{5,8,11,14}$	$CH_3(CH_2)_4CH = CHCH_2CH = CHCH_2CH = CHCH_2CH = CH(CH_2)_7COOH$		arachidonic	−50

Table 7.1 **Structure and melting point of naturally occurring fatty acids.** For unsaturated fatty acids, the 'ω' designation indicates the location of the first double bond from the methyl end of the molecule; the Δ superscripts indicate the location of the double bonds from the carboxyl end of the molecule. The melting point of fatty acids, triglycerides and phospholipids increases with the chain length of the fatty acid and decreases with the number of its double bonds.

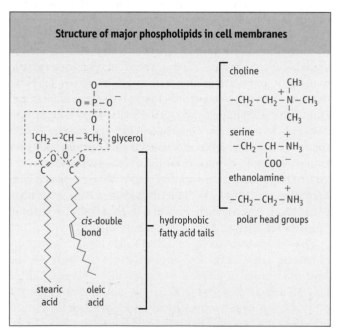

Fig. 7.1 **Structure of major phospholipids in cell membranes.** Two of the –OH groups in glycerol (at the C–1 and C–2 positions) are linked to fatty acids, while the third –OH group is phosphorylated. The phosphate is further linked to one of the variety of small polar head groups (such as choline, serine, and ethanolamine).

Phospholipids are amphipathic molecules, because they are composed of both hydrophobic fatty acids and hydrophilic or polar head groups. The characteristic head groups of membrane phospholipids are choline, serine, and ethanolamine (Fig. 7.1). When they are hydrated, phospholipids spontaneously form lamellar structures, and, under suitable conditions, they organize into extended bilayer structures – not only lamellar structures, but also closed vesicular structures termed liposomes. Liposomes having defined lipid compositions are being evaluated clinically for use as drug carrier and delivery systems.

The liposome is a model for the structure of a biological membrane, a bilayer of polar lipids with a polar face exposed to the aqueous environment and the fatty acid side chains buried in the oily, hydrophobic interior of the membrane. The liposomal surface membrane, like its component phospholipids, is a somewhat pliant, mobile and flexible structure. Biological membranes also contain another important amphipathic molecule, cholesterol, a flat, rigid hydrophobic molecule with a polar hydroxyl group. Cholesterol is found in all biomembranes and acts as a modulator of membrane fluidity. At lower temperatures it interferes with fatty acid chain associations and increases fluidity, and at higher temperatures it tend to limit disorder and decrease fluidity. Thus, cholesterol–phospholipid mixtures have properties intermediate between the gel and liquid crystalline states of the pure phospholipids; they form stable, but supple membrane structures.

COMPOSITION OF BIOMEMBRANES

Eukaryotic cells have a plasma membrane, as well as a number of intracellular membranes that define compartments with specialized functions; differences in both membrane protein and lipid composition distinguish these organelles (Table 7.2). In addition to the major phospholipids described in Figure 7.1, other important membrane lipids include phosphatidylinositol, cardiolipin, sphingolipids (sphingomyelin and glycolipids), and cholesterol, which are described in detail in later chapters.

Phospholipid composition of organelle membranes from rat liver						
	Percentage of total phospholipids in membranes from different organelles					
	Mitochondria	Microsomes	Lysosomes	Plasma membrane	Nuclear membrane	Golgi membrane
Cardiolipin	18	1	1	1	4	1
Phosphatidylethanolamine	35	22	14	23	13	20
Phosphatidylcholine	40	58	40	39	55	50
Phosphatidylinositol	5	10	5	8	10	12
Phosphatidylserine	1	2	2	9	3	6
Phosphatidic acid	–	1	1	1	2	<1
Sphingomyelin	1	1	20	16	3	8
Phospholipids (mg/mg protein)	0.175	0.374	0.156	0.672	0.500	0.825
Cholesterol (mg/mg protein)	0.003	0.014	0.038	0.128	0.038	0.078

Table 7.2 **Phospholipid composition of organelle membranes from rat liver.** This table shows the phospholipid composition (%) of various organelle membranes together with weight ratios of phospholipids and cholesterol to protein.

Cardiolipin (diphosphatidyl glycerol) is a significant component of the mitochondrial inner membrane, while sphingomyelin, phosphatidylserine and cholesterol are enriched in the plasma membrane (Table 7.2). The protein to lipid ratio also differs among various biomembranes, ranging from about 80% (dry weight) lipid in the myelin sheath that insulates nerve cells, to about 20% lipid in the inner mitochondrial membrane. Lipids affect the structure of the membrane, the activity of membrane enzymes and transport systems, and membrane function in processes such as cellular recognition and signal transduction. Each organelle membrane also has unique proteins and enzymes that may be used as markers for the purity of isolated sub-cellular fractions.

Current structural model of the membrane

The generally accepted model of biomembrane structure is the fluid mosaic model proposed by Singer & Nicolson in the early 1970s. This model represents the membrane as a fluid-like phospholipid bilayer into which other lipids and proteins are embedded (Fig. 7.2). As in liposomes, the polar head groups of the phospholipids are exposed on the external surface of the membrane, with the fatty acyl chains oriented to the inside of the membrane. Whereas membrane lipids and proteins easily move on the membrane surface (lateral diffusion), 'flip-flop' movement of lipids between the outer and inner bilayer leaflets rarely occurs without the aid of an integral membrane enzyme, flippase. Although this model is basically correct, there is also growing evidence that many membrane proteins have limited mobility and are anchored in place by attachment to cytoskeletal proteins; membrane sub-structures, described as *lipid rafts*, also demarcate regions of membranes with specialized composition and function.

Membrane proteins are classified as integral (intrinsic) membrane proteins and peripheral (extrinsic) membrane proteins. The former are embedded deeply in the lipid bilayer and some of them traverse the membrane several times (transmembrane protein), whereas peripheral membrane proteins are bound to membrane lipids and/or integral membrane proteins by noncovalent interactions (Fig. 7.2). Most of the transmembrane segments of integral membrane proteins form α-helices. They are composed primarily of amino acid residues with nonpolar side chains – about 20 amino acid residues forming six to seven α-helical turns are enough to traverse a membrane of 5 nm (50 Å) thickness. The transmembrane domains interact with one another and with the hydrophobic tails of the lipid molecules, often forming complex structures, such as channels involved in ion transport processes (Fig. 7.2).

 AMPHIPATHIC COMPOUNDS

Membrane perturbation by amphipathic compounds

Amphipathic compounds have distinct polar and nonpolar moieties. They include many anesthetics and tranquilizers. The pharmacologic activities of these compounds are dependent on their ability to interact with membranes and perturb membrane structure. A number of antibiotics and natural products, such as bile salts and fatty acids, are also amphipathic. While effective at therapeutic concentrations, some of these drugs exhibit detergent-like action in moderate to high concentrations and disrupt the bilayer structure, resulting in membrane leakage.

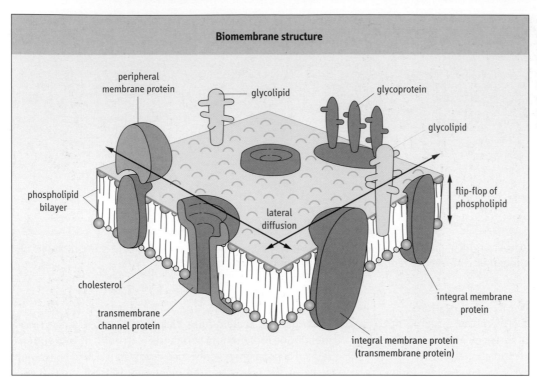

Fig. 7.2 **Fluid mosaic model of biomembranes.** In the fluid mosaic model, proteins are embedded in a fluid phospholipid bilayer. Glycolipids and glycoproteins are located mainly in the outer leaflet of the plasma membrane.

Structural and metabolic role of membranes

A major role of membranes is to maintain the structural integrity and barrier function of cells and organelles. However, membranes are not rigid or impermeable: they are fluid, and their components move around, and they are subject to metabolic turnover. The turnover of membrane components is especially important for the cellular response to information from inside and outside the cell: recognition, transfer, amplification, and signal transduction processes all occur in or on the membranes. Both small and large molecules must pass through the membrane. With few exceptions, specific membrane proteins mediate these transport processes.

Phospholipids not only provide a fluid environment, but also regulate the activities of membrane enzymes. Particular phospholipids are required for specific membrane structures, such as curved regions and junctions with adjacent membranes. The inside surface of the membrane is more suited to phosphatidylethanolamine and phosphatidylserine, in which the polar heads are small and the hydrocarbons are more spread out, because of their larger contents of polyunsaturated fatty acids. As a result of such differing requirements, phospholipids are distributed asymmetrically between outer and inner leaflets of membranes: phosphatidylcholine and sphingomyelin are more abundant in the outer leaflet, whereas phosphatidylethanolamine and phosphatidylserine are enriched in the inner leaflet. Such asymmetries are actively maintained by flippases, and cell damage often leads to loss of this membrane lipid asymmetry. Exposure of phosphatidylserine in the outer leaflet of the erythrocyte plasma membrane increases the cell's vascular adherence and is a signal for macrophage recognition and phagocytosis. Both of these processes probably contribute to the natural process of red cell turnover.

TYPES OF TRANSPORT PROCESSES

Simple diffusion through the phospholipid bilayer

Small, nonpolar molecules (such as O_2, CO_2, N_2) and uncharged polar molecules (such as urea, ethanol, and small organic acids) move through membranes by simple diffusion without the aid of membrane proteins (Table 7.3 and Fig 7.3A). The direction of net movement of these species is always 'downhill', along the concentration gradient, from high to low concentration to establish equilibrium.

The hydrophobicity of the molecules is an important requirement for simple diffusion across the membrane, as the interior of the phospholipid bilayer is hydrophobic. The rate of transport of a small molecule is, in fact, closely related to its partition coefficient between oil and water.

Although water molecules can be transported by simple diffusion, channel proteins are believed to control the movement of water across most membranes, especially in the kidney for concentration of the urine. Mutation in a water

EXTRACTION AND ANALYSIS OF MEMBRANE PHOSPHOLIPIDS

Cells (2 × 10⁷) or membranes (2 mg protein) are suspended in phosphate-buffered saline (1.6 ml) in a screw-capped glass test tube. Chloroform/methanol (1:2, v/v) (6 ml) is added into the tube and lipids are extracted by vigorous mixing. Equal volume of chloroform and the saline (2 ml each) are further added and again mixed. After centrifugation at 1,500 × g for 5 min, the lower phase (chloroform containing extracted lipids) is recovered, and the solvent is evaporated under the stream of N² gas. The lipid extract is applied to silica gel plate for two-dimensional thin-layer chromatography with chloroform/methanol/acetic acid (65:25:10, v/v) as the solvent in the first dimension, and chloroform/methanol/formic acid (65:25:10, v/v) in the second. The separated phospholipids are detectable on the plate as yellow spots by iodine vapor. Using appropriate standards, the ratio of lecithin (phosphatidylcholine) to sphingomyelin, measured in amniotic fluid, can be used to assess fetal lung maturity and risk for acute respiratory distress syndrome (ARDS, Chapter 26).

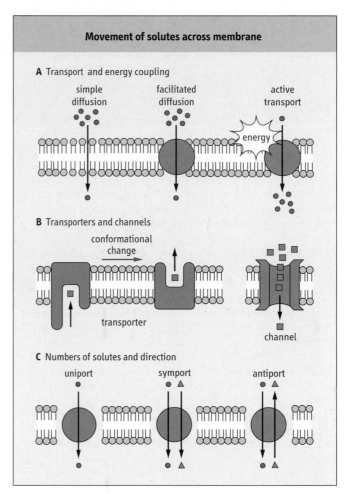

Fig. 7.3 **Various models of movement of solute across membranes.**

Transport systems of biomembranes

Type		Transport protein (example)	Energy coupling	Specificity	Saturability	Rate (molecules/transport protein/s)
Passive transport or diffusion	simple diffusion	–	–	–	–	
	facilitated diffusion	+	–	+	+	
	transporter	(GLUT-1~5)				–10²
	channel	(H₂O, Na⁺, K⁺, Ca²⁺, Cl⁻)				10⁷–10⁸
Active transport	primary	+ (see Table 7.5)	+	+	+	10²–10⁴
	secondary	+	+	+	+	10⁰–10²*
	symporter	(SGLT-1, 2, neutral amino acids)				
	antiporter	(Cl⁻/HCO₃⁻, Na⁺/Ca²⁺, Na⁺/H⁺)				
	uniporter	(Glutamate)				

Table 7.3 **Classification of transport systems of biomembranes.** Transport systems are classified according to the role of transport proteins and energy coupling. Typical substrates for various types of channels are shown in the parentheses. *The Cl⁻/HCO₃⁻ antiporter seems to be an exception to secondary active transport systems, as its transport rate is high, at 10⁵ mol/s.

MEMBRANE PATCHES

Although the fluid mosaic model is basically correct, it is recognized that there are membrane patches with unique protein and lipid compositions separated from other fluid membrane areas. Caveolae, 50–100 nm plasma membrane invaginations, and lipid rafts are plasma membrane patches (microdomains) important for signal transduction through immune and growth factor receptors. These patches are enriched in cholesterol and sphingolipids, and the interaction of the long saturated fatty acid tails of sphingolipids with cholesterol results in the stabilization of their less fluid environment. The patches are detergent-insoluble and show high buoyant density on sucrose density gradient centrifugation. While the patches are associated with specific molecules such as GPI-anchored proteins, caveolins are the principal components of caveolae. Caveolae are believed to be involved in cholesterol transport, the transport of solutes across endothelial cells, and tumor suppression. Pathogens such as viruses, parasites, bacteria and even bacterial toxins enter into the host cells through caveolae. It is interesting that the sites of γ-secretase activity and Aβ production, which are closely related to the pathology of Alzheimer's disease, are associated with membrane regions of high cholesterol content, such as lipid rafts.

Examples of patches enriched in a particular protein are the purple membrane of *Halobacterium halobium* containing bacteriorodopsin, and gap junctions containing connexin. Bacteriorodopsin is a light driven-proton pump which generates H^+-concentration gradient across the bacterial membrane. The gradient is used for ATP synthesis and nutrient uptake for bacterial growth.

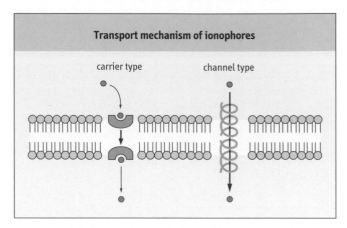

Fig. 7.4 **Mobile ion carriers and channel-forming ionophores.** Ionophores permit net movement of ions only down their electrochemical gradients.

Saturability and specificity are important characteristics of the membrane transport systems

The rate of facilitated diffusion is generally much greater than that of simple diffusion: transport proteins catalyze the transport process. In contrast to simple diffusion, in which the rate of transport is directly proportional to the substrate concentration, facilitated diffusion is a saturable process, characterized by a maximum transport rate, T_{max} (Fig. 7.5). When the concentration of extracellular molecules (transport substrates) becomes very high, the T_{max} is achieved by saturation of the transporter proteins with substrate. The kinetics of facilitated diffusion for substrates can be described by the same equations that are used for enzyme catalysis (e.g. Michaelis–Menten and Lineweaver–Burk type equations) (see Chapter 5):

$$S_{out} + transporter \underset{}{\overset{K_t}{\rightleftharpoons}} (S \cdot transporter\ complex) \rightarrow S_{in}$$

- where K_t is the dissociation constant of substrate (S) and transporter, and S_{out} is the concentration of transport substrate. Then the transport rate, t, can be calculated as:

$$t = \frac{T_{max}}{\left(1 + \dfrac{K_t}{S_{out}}\right)}$$

- where the K_t is the concentration that gives the half-maximal transport rate. The K_t for a transporter is conceptually the same as the K_m for an enzyme.

The transport process is usually highly specific: each transporter transports only a single species of molecules or structurally related compounds. The red blood cell GLUT-1 transporter has a high affinity for D-glucose, but 10–20 times lower affinity for the related sugars, D-mannose and D-galactose. The enantiomer L-glucose is not transported; its affinity is more than 1000 times less than that of the D-form.

channel protein gene (aquaporin-2) causes diuresis in some patients with nephrogenic diabetes insipidus.

Transport mediated by membrane proteins

Transport of larger, polar molecules, such as amino acids or sugars, into a cell requires the involvement of membrane proteins known as transporters, also called porters, permeases, translocases, or carrier proteins. The term 'carrier' is also applied to ionophores, which move passively across the membrane together with the bound ion (Fig. 7.4). Transporters are as specific as are enzymes for their substrates, and work by one of two mechanisms: facilitated diffusion or active transport. Facilitated diffusion catalyzes the movement of a substrate through a membrane down a concentration gradient and does not require energy. In contrast, active transport is a process in which substrates are transported uphill, against their concentration gradient. Active transport must be coupled to an energy-producing reaction (see Fig. 7.3A).

MEMBRANE PERMEABILITY

Antibiotics that induce ion permeability

Peptide antibiotics act as ionophores and increase the permeability of membranes to specific ions; bactericidal effects of ionophores are attributed to disturbance of the ion transport systems of bacterial membranes. Ionophores permit net movement of ions only down their electrochemical gradients. There are two classes of ionophores: mobile ion carriers (or caged carriers) and channel formers (Fig. 7.4). Valinomycin is a typical example of a mobile ion carrier. It is a cyclic peptide with a lipophilic exterior and ionic interior. It dissolves in the membrane and diffuses between the inner and outer surfaces. K^+ binds to the central core of valinomycin, and the complex diffuses across the membrane, releasing the K^+ and gradually dissipating the K^+ gradient. The carrier type-ionophores, nigericin and monensin, exchange H^+ for Na^+ and K^+, respectively. Ionomycin and A23187 are Ca^{2+} ionophores.

The β-helical gramicidin A molecule, a linear peptide with 15 amino acid residues, forms a pore. The head-to-head dimer of gramicidin A makes a transmembrane channel that allows movement of monovalent cations (H^+, Na^+, and K^+). Alamethicin forms volatage-gated channels developing cation conductance.

Polyene antibiotics such as amphotericin B and nystatin exert their cytotoxic action by rendering the membrane of the target cell permeable to ions and small molecules. Formation of a sterol-polyene complex is essential for the cytotoxic function of these antibiotics, as they display a selective action against organisms in which the membranes contain sterols. Thus they are active against yeasts, a wide variety of fungi, and other eucaryotic cells, but have no effect on bacteria. Because their affinity toward ergosterol, a fungal membrane component, is higher than that for cholesterol, these antibiotics have been used for the treatment of topical infections of fungal origin.

Characteristics of glucose transporters (uniporters)

Glucose transporters are essential for facilitated diffusion of glucose into cells. The glucose transporter family comprises five major species, named GLUT-1 to GLUT-5 (Table 7.4). They are transmembrane proteins similar in size, all having about 500 amino acid residues and 12 transmembrane helices. GLUT-1, in red blood cells, has a K_m of ~2 mmol/L; most of the GLUT-1 molecules are active under fasting conditions (glucose concentration of 5 mmol/L; 90 mg/dL). In contrast, pancreatic islet β-cells express GLUT-2, with a K_m of more than 10 mmol/L (180 mg/dL). In response to the intake of food and resulting increase in blood glucose concentration,

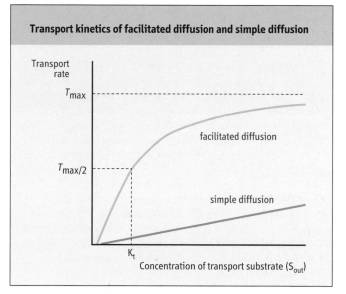

Transport kinetics of facilitated diffusion and simple diffusion

Fig. 7.5 **Comparison of the transport kinetics of facilitated diffusion and simple diffusion.** The rate of transport of substrate is plotted against the concentration of substrate in the extracellular medium. In common with enzyme catalysis, transporter-catalyzed uptake has a maximum transport rate, T_{max} (saturable). K_t is the concentration at which the rate of substrate uptake is half maximal. For simple diffusion, the transport rate is slower and directly proportional to substrate concentration.

MEMBRANE ANCHORING PROTEINS

Lateral movements of some membrane proteins are restricted by their tethering to macromolecular assemblies inside (cytoskeleton) and/or outside (extracellular matrix) the cell, and, in some cases, to membrane proteins of adjacent cells, e.g. in tight junctions between epithelial cells. Lateral diffusion of erythrocyte integral membrane proteins, band 3 ($Cl^-/HCO3^-$ antiporter) and glycophorin, is limited by indirect interaction with spectrin, a cytoskeletal protein, through ankyrin and band 4.1, respectively. Such interactions are so strong that they limit lateral diffusion of band 3. Hereditary spherocytosis and elliptocytosis are human diseases caused by genetic defects of spectrin. Ankyrin mutation causes type 4 long-QT cardiac arrhythmia and sudden cardiac death. Deficiency of ankyrin also affects the intracellular targeting of Na^+/K^+-ATPase and Na^+/Ca^{2+} antiporter in cardiac muscle cells (see Fig. 7.6), resulting in the elevation of intracellular Ca^{2+} which triggers an arrhythmia. The intracellular targeting of Na^+/K^+-ATPase in kidney is inhibited by the mutation of the γ-subunit of this ATPase. The defect is implicated in renal hypomagnesaemia.

FORMATION OF ANTIBODIES TO PHOSPHOLIPIDS

A 54-year-old woman was admitted to the hospital because of acute renal failure and thrombocytopenia. The patient had been in excellent health until 5 weeks earlier, when she began to have respiratory symptoms with fever that was unresponsive to antibiotics. Examination of the renal biopsy specimen revealed abnormalities in all components of the cortex, defining the membranoproliferative pattern of glomerular injury.

Comment. Among the conditions associated with the glomerular injury, a thrombotic angiopathy was considered, and then finally the antiphospholipid antibody syndrome was favored, since titer of anti-cardiolipin antibody was elevated. The antiphospholipid antibody syndrome was initially diagnosed on the basis of recurrent arterial and venous thrombosis leading to stroke and myocardial infarction, recurrent spontaneous abortions and fetal wastage, thrombocytopenia, and various neurologic manifestations. These antibodies are also found in systemic lupus erythematosus.

CYSTINOSIS

An 18-month-old child presented with polyuria, failure to thrive and an episode of severe dehydration. Urine dipstick testing demonstrated glucosuria and proteinuria, with other biochemical analyses showing generalized aminoaciduria and phosphaturia.

Comment. This is a classical presentation of infantile cystinosis, resulting from accumulation of cystine in lysosomes because of a defect in the lysosomal transport protein, cystinosine. Cystine is poorly soluble, and crystalline precipitates form in cells throughout the body. *In vitro* experiments with cystine loading have shown that renal proximal tubular cells become ATP-depleted, resulting in impairment of ATP-dependent ion pumps with consequent electrolyte and metabolite losses. Treatment with cysteamine increases the transport of cystine from lysosomes, delaying the decline in renal function. If untreated, renal failure occurs by 6–12 years of age. Unfortunately, there is further accumulation of cystine in the central nervous system, despite therapy, with long-term neurological damage.

GLUT-2 molecules mediate an increase in the cellular uptake of glucose, leading to insulin secretion (see Chapter 20). Cells in insulin-sensitive tissues such as muscle and adipose have GLUT-4. Insulin stimulates translocation of GLUT-4 from intracellular vesicles to the plasma membrane, facilitating glucose uptake during meals.

Transport by channels and pores

Channels are often pictured as tunnels across the membrane, in which binding sites for substrates (ions) are accessible from either side of the membrane at the same time (Fig. 7.3B). Conformational changes are not required for the translocation of substrates entering from one side of the membrane to exit on the other side. However, voltage changes and ligand binding induce conformational changes in channel structure that have the effect of opening or closing the channels – processes known as voltage or ligand 'gating'. Movement of molecules through channels is fast (10^7–10^8/s) in comparison with the rates achieved by transporters (Table 7.3).

The terms 'channel' and 'pore' are sometimes used interchangeably. However, 'pore' is used most frequently to describe more open, somewhat nonselective structures that discriminate between substrates, e.g. peptides or proteins on the basis of size. The term 'channel' is usually applied to describe more specific ion channels.

Classification of glucose transporters			
Transporter	K_t for D-glucose transport (mM)	Substrate	Major sites of expression
Facilitated diffusion (uniporter) (passive transport)			
GLUT-1	1–2	glucose, galactose, mannose	ubiquitous (erythrocyte, blood-tissue barriers)
GLUT-2	15–20	glucose, fructose	liver, intestine, kidney, pancreatic β-cells, brain
GLUT-3	1.8*	glucose	ubiquitous
GLUT-4	5	glucose	skeletal and cardiac muscles, adipose tissues
GLUT-5	6–11**	fructose	intestine
Na⁺-coupled symporter (active transport)			
SGLT-1	0.35	glucose (2Na⁺/1glucose), galactose	intestine, kidney
SGLT-2	1.6	glucose (1Na⁺/1glucose)	kidney

Table 7.4 **Classification of glucose transporters.** Km values are determined from the uptake of 2-deoxy-D-glucose (*), a non-metabolizable analog of glucose, and fructose (**).

HARTNUP DISEASE

A three-year old had been on holiday to Spain and developed pellagra-like skin changes on his face, neck, forearms and dorsal aspects of his hands and legs. His skin became scaly, rough and hyperpigmented. The child was brought to the GP complaining of headaches and weakness. Urinalysis demonstrated gross hyperaminoaciduria of neutral monoamino-monocarboxylic acids (i.e. alanine, serine, threonine, asparagine, glutamine, valine, leucine, isoleucine, phenylalanine, tyrosine, tryptophan, histidine and citrulline).

Comment. These neutral amino acids share a common transporter which is expressed only on the luminal border of epithelial cells in the renal tubules and intestinal epithelium. The pellagra-like dermatitis (see Chapter 10) and neurological involvement resemble nutritional niacin deficiency. The reduced tryptophan intake results in reduced nicotinamide production. The disease is easily treated with oral nicotinamide and sun-blocking agents to exposed areas.

Three examples of pores important for cellular physiology

The gap junction between endothelial, muscle, and neuronal cells is a cluster of small pores, in which two cylinders of six connexin subunits in plasma membranes join each other to form a pore about 1.2–2.0 nm (12–20 Å) in diameter. Molecules smaller than about 1 kDa can pass between cells through gap junctions. Such cell–cell communication is important for physiologic coupling, for example in the concerted contraction of uterine muscle during labor and delivery. These pores are usually maintained in an open state, but will close when cell membranes are damaged or when the metabolic rate is depressed. Mutations of the genes encoding connexin 26 and connexin 32 cause deafness and Charcot–Marie–Tooth disease, respectively.

Nuclear pores have a functional radius of about 9.0 nm (90 Å) through which proteins and nucleic acids enter and leave the nucleus.

A third class of pores is important for protein sorting. Mitochondrial proteins encoded by nuclear genes are transported to this organelle through pores in the outer mitochondrial membrane. Nascent polypeptide chains of secretory proteins and plasma membrane proteins also pass through pores in the endoplasmic reticulum membrane.

Active transport

ATP is a high-energy product of metabolism and is often described as the 'energy currency' of the cell. The phosphoanhydride bond of ATP releases free energy when it is hydrolyzed to produce adenosine diphosphate (ADP) and

DEFECTIVE GLUCOSE TRANSPORT ACROSS THE BLOOD-BRAIN BARRIER AS A CAUSE OF PERSISTENT HYPOGLYCORRHACHIA, SEIZURES, AND DEVELOPMENTAL DELAY

A male infant at the age of 3 months suffered from recurrent seizures. His cerebrospinal fluid (CSF) glucose concentrations were low (0.9–1.9 mmol/L; 16–34 mg/dL), and the ratio of CSF to blood glucose ranged from 0.19 to 0.33; the normal value is 0.65. The potential causes of low CSF glucose concentrations, such as bacterial meningitis, subarachnoid hemorrhage, and hypoglycemia, were not present, and high CSF lactate values would be found in all these conditions except hypoglycemia. In contrast, the CSF lactate concentrations were consistently low (0.3–0.4 mmol/L; 3–4 mg/dL) compared with the normal value (<2.2 mmol/L; <20 mg/dL). These findings suggested a defect in transport of glucose from the blood to the brain.

Comment. Assuming that the activity of GLUT-1 glucose transporter in the erythrocyte reflects that of the brain microvessels, a transport assay using his erythrocytes was carried out. The T_{max} for uptake of glucose by the patient's erythrocytes was 60% of the mean normal value. A ketogenic diet (a high-fat, low-protein, low-carbohydrate diet) was started, since the brain can use ketone bodies as oxidizable fuel sources, and the entry of ketone bodies into the brain is not dependent on the glucose-transporter system. The patient stopped having seizures within 4 days after beginning the diet.

inorganic phosphate. Such energy is used for synthesis of large and small cellular molecules, cell movement, and uphill transport of molecules against concentration gradients. Primary active transport systems use ATP directly to drive transport; secondary active transport uses an electrochemical gradient of Na^+ or H^+ ions, or a membrane potential produced by primary active transport processes. Sugars and amino acids are transported into cells by all of these transport systems.

The most important primary active transport systems are ion pumps (ion transporting ATPases or pump ATPases)

The pump ATPases are classified into four groups (Table 7.5). Coupling factor ATPases (F-ATPases) in mitochondrial, chloroplast, and bacterial membranes (see Chapter 8) hydrolyze ATP and transport hydrogen ions (H^+). This ATPase is also called H^+-ATPase (H^+-transporting ATPase). In mitochondria, the 'powerhouses' of the cell, the F-ATPase works in the backward direction, synthesizing ATP from ADP and phosphate as protons move down a concentration gradient

ION GRADIENTS

Concentration gradient and electrochemical gradient of ions

The permeability of most nonelectrolytes through membranes can be analyzed by assuming that the rate-limiting step is the diffusion within the lipid bilayer. Their permeability across a phospholipid bilayer is experimentally shown to be a function of the partition coefficient into organic solvents. The relative rate of simple diffusion of a molecule across the membrane is therefore proportional to the concentration gradient across the bilayer and to the hydrophobicity of the molecule. For charged molecules and ions, transport across the membrane must be facilitated by a transporter or channel, and is driven by the electrochemical gradient, a combination of the concentration gradient (chemical potential) and the voltage gradient across the membrane (electric potential). These forces may act in the same direction or in opposite directions. In the case of Na^+ ions, the concentration difference between outside (145 mM) and inside (12 mM) the cell is about a factor of 10, being maintained by the Na^+/K^+-ATPase. The Na^+/K^+-ATPase is an electrogenic, pumping out three Na^+ and pumping in two K^+ ions, generating an inside-negative membrane potential. K^+ leaks out through K^+ channels, down its concentration gradient (140 mM–5 mM), further increasing the electric potential. The concentration gradient of Na^+ ions and the electric potential power the import and export of other molecules with Na^+ against their concentration gradient by symporters and antiporters, respectively.

MENKES AND WILSON'S DISEASES

X-linked Menkes disease is a lethal disorder that occurs in 1 in 100,000 newborn infants and is characterized by abnormal and hypopigmented hair, a characteristic facies, cerebral degeneration, connective tissue and vascular defects, and death by the age of 3 years. A copper-transporting P-ATPase that is expressed in all tissues except liver is defective in this disease (see Table 7.5). In patients with Menkes disease, copper enters the intestinal cells, but is not transported further, resulting in severe copper deficiency. Subcutaneous administration of a copper histidine complex may be an effective treatment if started early.

The gene for Wilson's disease also encodes a copper-transporting P-ATPase and is 60% identical with that of the Menkes gene. It is expressed in liver, kidney, and placenta. Wilson's disease occurs in 1 in 35 000–100 000 newborns and is characterized by failure to incorporate copper into ceruloplasmin in the liver and failure to excrete copper from the liver into bile, resulting in toxic accumulation of copper in the liver and also in the kidney, brain, and cornea. Liver cirrhosis, progressive neurologic damage, or both, occur during childhood to early adulthood. Chelating agents such as penicillamine are used for treatment of patients with this disease. Oral zinc treatment may be useful for decreasing the absorption of dietary copper.

Comment. Copper is an essential trace metal and an integral component of many enzymes. However, it is toxic in excess, because it binds to proteins and nucleic acids, enhances the generation of free radicals, and catalyzes oxidation of lipids and proteins in membranes.

generated across the inner membrane by oxidation reactions during metabolism. The proton gradient drives the production of ATP in a process known as oxidative phosphorylation (see Chapter 8). The product, ATP, is released into the mitochondrial matrix, then transported to the outside (the cytoplasmic side) through an ATP–ADP translocase in the mitochondrial inner membrane. This translocase is an example of an antiport system shown in Figure 7.3C); it allows one molecule of ADP to enter only if one molecule of ATP exits simultaneously.

Cytoplasmic vesicles, such as lysosomes, endosomes, and secretory granules, are acidified by the V-type (vacuolar) H^+-ATPase in their membranes. Acidification by this V-ATPase is important for the activity of lysosomal enzymes that have acidic pH optima, and for the accumulation of drugs and neurotransmitters in secretory granules. The V-ATPase also acidifies the extracellular environments of osteoclasts and kidney epithelial cells. Defects in the osteoclast plasma membrane V-ATPase result in osteopetrosis (increased bone density), while mutation of the ATPase in the apical surface of α-intercalated cells of the cortical collecting duct of the distal nephron causes distal renal tubular acidosis. F- and V-type ATPases are struc-

turally similar, and seem to be derived from a common ancestor. The ATP-binding catalytic subunit and the subunit forming the H^+ pathway are conserved between these ATPases.

P-ATPases form phosphorylated intermediates that drive ion translocation: the 'P' refers to phosphorylation. These transporters have an active-site aspartate residue that is reversibly phosphorylated by ATP during the transport process. The P-type Na^+/K^+-ATPase in various tissues and the Ca^{2+}-ATPase in the sarcoplasmic reticulum have important roles in maintaining cellular ion gradients. Na^+/K^+-ATPases also create an electrochemical gradient of Na^+ that produces the driving force for uptake of nutrients (see below). The discharge of this electrochemical gradient is also fundamental to the process of nerve transmission (see Chapter 40). Mutations of P-ATPase genes cause Brody myopathy (cardiac muscle and fast twitch skeletal muscle sarcoplasmic reticulum Ca^{2+}-ATPase), familial hemiplegic migraine type 2 ($α_2$ type Na^+/K^+-ATPase), Menkes and Wilson's diseases (Cu^{2+}-ATPases), and familial intrahepatic cholestasis 1 (aminophospholipid flippase).

Various primary active transporters in eukaryotic cells				
Group	**Member**	**Location**	**Substrate(s)**	**Functions**
F-ATPase (coupling factor)	H^+-ATPase	mitochondrial inner membrane	H^+	ATP synthesis, generation of electrochemical gradient of H^+
V-ATPase (vacuolar)	H^+-ATPase	cytoplasmic vesicles (lysosome, secretory granules) plasma membranes (ruffled border of osteoclast, kidney epithelial cell)	H^+	activation of lysosomal enzymes, accumulation of neurotransmitters turnover of bone, acidification of urine
P-ATPase (phosphorylation)	Na^+/K^+-ATPase	plasma membranes (ubiquitous, but abundant in kidney and heart)	Na^+ and K^+	generation of electrochemical gradient of Na^+ and K^+
	H^+/K^+-ATPase	stomach (parietal cell in gastric gland)	H^+ and K^+	acidification of stomach lumen
	Ca^{2+}-ATPase	sarcoplasmic reticulum and endoplasmic reticulum	Ca^{2+}	Ca^{2+} sequestration into sarcoplasmic (endoplasmic) reticulum
	Ca^{2+}-ATPase	plasma membrane	Ca^{2+}	Ca^{2+} excretion to outside of the cell
	Cu^{2+}-ATPase	plasma membrane and cytoplasmic vesicles	Cu^{2+}	Cu^{2+} absorption from intestine and excretion from liver
ABC transporter (ATP binding cassette)	P-glycoprotein	plasma membrane	various drugs	excretion of harmful substances, multidrug resistance for anticancer drugs
	MRP	plasma membrane	glutathione conjugate	detoxification multidrug resistance for anticancer drugs
	CFTR*	plasma membrane	Cl^-	cAMP-dependent chloride channel, regulation of other channels
	TAP	endoplasmic reticulum	peptide	presentation of peptides for immune response

Table 7.5 **Primary active transporters in eucaryotic cells.** Various examples of primary active transporters (ATP-powered pump ATPases) are listed, together with their location. The F-ATPase is reversible, whereas others catalyze unidirectional ATP hydrolysis reactions. *Some ABC transporters function as channels or channel regulators. MRP, multidrug resistance-associated protein; CFTR, cystic fibrosis transmembrane conductance regulator; TAP, transporter associated with antigen processing.

The ATP-binding cassette (ABC) transporters comprise the fourth active transporter family. 'ABC' is the abbreviation for 'ATP-binding cassette', referring to an ATP-binding region in the transporter (Table 7.5). P-glycoprotein ('P' = permeability) and MRP (multidrug resistance-associated protein), which are thought to have a physiological role in excretion of toxic metabolites and xenobiotics, contribute to resistance of cancer cells to chemotherapy. TAP transporters, a class of ABC transporters associated with antigen presentation, are required for initiating the immune response against foreign proteins; they mediate antigen peptide transport from the cytosol into endoplasmic reticulum. Some ABC transporters are present in peroxisomal membrane where they appear to be involved in the transport of peroxisomal enzymes necessary for oxidation of very-long-chain fatty acids. Defects of ABC transporters are associated with various diseases, as shown in the clinical box.

Uniport, symport, and antiport are alternate mechanisms of facilitated transport

Transport processes may be classified into three general types: uniport (monoport), symport (cotransport), and antiport (countertransport) (see Fig. 7.3). Transport substrates move in the same direction during symport, and in opposite direc-

tions during antiport. The movement of one substrate uphill, against its concentration gradient, can be driven by movement of another substrate (usually a cation such as Na^+ or H^+) down a gradient. Uniport of charged substrates may also be electrophoretically driven by the membrane potential of the cell. The proteins participating in these transport systems are termed uniporters, symporters, and antiporters, respectively (Table 7.3). Some examples are presented below.

Examples of transport systems and their coupling

Ca^{2+} transport and mobilization in muscle

Striated muscle (skeletal and cardiac) is composed of bundles of multinucleated muscle cells (see Chapter 19). Each cell is packed with bundles of actin and myosin filaments (myofibrils) that produce contraction. During muscle contraction, nerves at the neuromuscular junction stimulate local depolarization of the membrane by opening voltage-dependent Na^+ channels. The depolarization spreads rapidly into invaginations of the plasma membrane called the transverse (T) tubules, which extend around the myofibrils (see Fig. 19.5).

ABC TRANSPORTERS AND DISEASES

Human genome data suggests that there are at least 48 genes for ABC transporters. An unusually wide range of diseases are caused by defects of ABC transporters, including Tangier disease, Stargardt disease, progressive intrahepatic cholestasis, Dubin–Johnson syndrome, pseudoxanthoma elasticum, familial persistent hyperinsulinemic hypoglycemia of infancy (PHHI), adrenoleukodystrophy, Zellweger syndrome, sitosterolemia and cystic fibrosis.

Comment. Cystic fibrosis (CF) is the most common potentially lethal autosomal recessive disease of caucasian populations, affecting 1 in 2500 newborns. CF is usually manifest as exocrine pancreatic insufficiency, an increase in the concentration of chloride ions (Cl⁻) in sweat, male infertility, and airway disease. The last of these leads to progressive lung dysfunction, which is the major cause of morbidity and mortality. CF is caused by mutations in the gene encoding a Cl⁻ channel named CFTR (cystic fibrosis transmembrane conductance regulator). ATP binding to the CFTR is required for channel opening. The lack of this channel activity in epithelia of CF patients is believed to be central to the pathogenesis of the disease.

The ATP-sensitive K⁺ channel (K_{ATP}) participates in regulation of insulin secretion in pancreatic islet β-cells. When the blood concentration of glucose increases, glucose is transported into the β-cell through a glucose transporter (GLUT-2) and metabolized, resulting in an increase in cytoplasmic ATP concentration. The ATP binds to the regulatory subunit of the K⁺ channel, K_{ATP}-β (called the sulfonylurea receptor, SUR1) causing structural change of a K_{ATP}-α subunit, which closes the K_{ATP} channel. This induces depolarization of the plasma membrane (decreased voltage gradient across the membrane) and activates voltage-dependent calcium (Ca²⁺) channels (VDCCs). The entry of Ca²⁺ stimulates exocytosis of vesicles that contain insulin. The binding of sulfonylureas such as tolubutamide and glibenclamide to K_{ATP}-β on the outside of the plasma membrane is thought to mimic the regulatory effect of intracellular ATP. Sulfonylureas stimulate insulin secretion, which decreases blood glucose concentration in diabetes. Defective K_{ATP} channels, which are unable to transport K⁺, induce low blood glucose concentration – a condition called PHHI that occurs in 1 per 50 000 persons – as a result of loss of K⁺-channel function and continuous insulin secretion.

MEASUREMENT OF GLUCOSE TRANSPORT INTO ERYTHROCYTE

Aliquots (0.2 ml) of erythrocyte suspension in phosphate-buffered saline (a hematocrit of 0.60 to 0.80) are mixed with 0.3 ml of the saline containing [^{14}C]3-O-methyl-D-glucose, and incubated at 20 °C for short period (2–15 sec). Uptake is interrupted by the rapid addition of 5 ml of ice-cold saline with 10 μM $HgCl_2$ and 100 μM phloretin to inhibit GLUT-1. The mixture is centrifuged at 2000 × g for 10 min at 4 °C. The erythrocyte pellet is washed twice with 5 ml of the same saline, and then lysed in 2.8% trichloroacetic acid (to precipitate protein). Radioactivity is measured in aliquots of the supernatant. The uptake is expressed as picomoles of 3-O-methyl-D-glucose per 10^6 erythrocyte. Nonspecific uptake is evaluated with radioactive L-glucose.

from the lumen (interior compartment) of the sarcoplasmic reticulum increases the cytoplasmic concentration of Ca²⁺ (depolarization-induced Ca²⁺ release) about 100-fold, from 10^{-4} mmol/L (0.0007 mg/L) to about 10^{-2} mmol/L (0.07 mg/dL), triggering ATP hydrolysis by myosin and muscle contraction. A Ca²⁺-ATPase in the sarcoplasmic reticulum then hydrolyses ATP to transport Ca²⁺ back out of the cell into the lumen, decreasing the cytoplasmic concentration of Ca²⁺, and the muscle relaxes (Fig. 7.6, left).

In cardiac muscle, VDCCs permit the entry of a small amount of Ca²⁺, which induces Ca²⁺ release through Ca²⁺ channel from the lumen of the sarcoplasmic reticulum (Ca²⁺-induced Ca²⁺ release). Not only the sarcoplasmic reticulum Ca²⁺-ATPase, but also an Na⁺/ Ca²⁺-antiporter and a plasma membrane Ca²⁺-ATPase are responsible for pumping out cytoplasmic Ca²⁺ from heart muscle (Fig. 7.6, right). The rapid restoration of ion gradients allows for rhythmic contraction of the heart.

Role of Na+/K+-ATPase in glucose uptake

The transport of blood glucose into cells is generally by facilitated diffusion, as the intracellular concentration of glucose is typically less than that of blood (Table 7.4). In contrast, the transport of glucose from the intestine into blood involves both facilitated diffusion and active transport processes (Fig. 7.7). Active transport is especially important for maximal recovery of sugars from the intestine when the intestinal concentration of glucose falls below that in the blood.

An Na⁺-coupled glucose symporter SGLT1, driven by an Na⁺-gradient formed by Na⁺/K⁺-ATPase, transports glucose into the intestinal epithelial cell, while GLUT-2 facilitates the

Voltage-dependent Ca²⁺ channels (VDCC) located in the T tubules of skeletal muscle change their conformation in response to membrane depolarization, and directly activate a Ca²⁺-release channel in the sarcoplasmic reticulum membrane, a network of flattened tubules that surrounds each myofibril in the muscle-cell cytoplasm. The escape of Ca²⁺

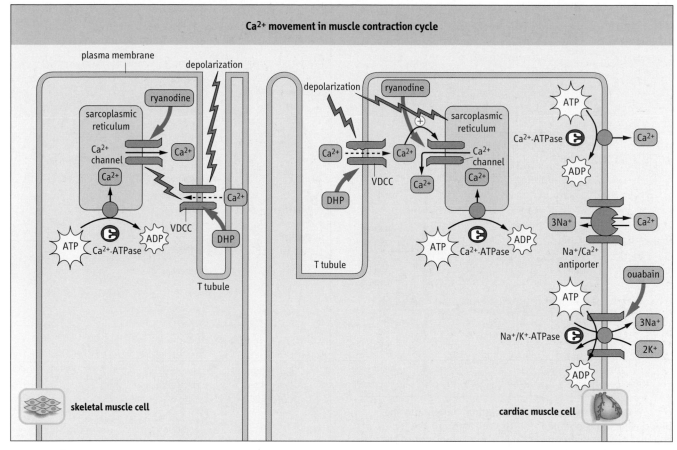

Fig. 7.6 **Ca²⁺ movement in muscle contraction cycle.** Roles of transporters in Ca^{2+} movements in skeletal (left) and cardiac (right) muscle cells during contraction. Thick arrows indicate the binding sites for inhibitors. In skeletal muscle, VDCCs (voltage-dependent calcium channels) directly activate release of Ca^{2+} from the sarcoplasmic reticulum. The increased cytoplasmic Ca^{2+} concentration triggers muscle contraction. A Ca^{2+}-ATPase in the sarcoplasmic reticulum transports Ca^{2+} back into the lumen, decreasing the cytoplasmic Ca^{2+} concentration, and the muscle relaxes. In heart muscle, VDCCs allow entry of a small amount of Ca^{2+}, which induces release of Ca^{2+} from the lumen of sarcoplasmic reticulum. Two types of Ca^{2+}-ATPases and an Na^+/Ca^{2+}-antiporter are responsible for pumping cytoplasmic Ca^{2+} out of the muscle cell. The Na^+/Ca^{2+}-antiporter uses the sodium (Na^+) gradient produced by Na^+/K^+-ATPase to antiport Ca^{2+}. DHP = dihydropyridine, nifedipine, a calcium channel blocker used for treatment of hypertension.

downhill movement of glucose into the portal circulation (Fig. 7.7).

The kidneys constitute an ultrafiltration system that filters small molecules from blood. However, glucose, amino acids, many ions, and other nutrients in the ultrafiltrate are almost completely reabsorbed in the proximal tubules, by symport processes. Glucose is reabsorbed primarily by sodium glucose transporter 2 ($SGLT_2$) (one-to-one stoichiometry), into renal proximal tubular epithelial cells. Much smaller amounts of glucose are recovered by $SGLT_1$ in a later segment of the tubule, which couples transport of one molecule of glucose to two sodium ions. The concentration of Na^+ in the filtrate is 140 mmol/L (322 mg/dL), while that inside the epithelial cells is 30 mmol/L (69 mg/dL), so that Na^+ flows 'downhill' along its gradient, dragging glucose 'uphill' against its con-

centration gradient. As in intestinal epithelial cells, the low intracellular concentration of Na^+ is maintained by an Na^+/K^+-ATPase on the opposite side of the tubular epithelial cell, which antiports three cytoplasmic sodium ions and two extracellular potassium ions, coupled with hydrolysis of a molecule of ATP. Glucose accumulated in the epithelial cell is further transported downhill across the membrane to the blood by GLUT-2 (facilitated diffusion).

Acidification of gastric juice by a proton pump in the stomach

The lumen of the stomach is highly acidic (pH ~1) because of the presence of a proton pump (H^+/K^+-ATPase; P-ATPase

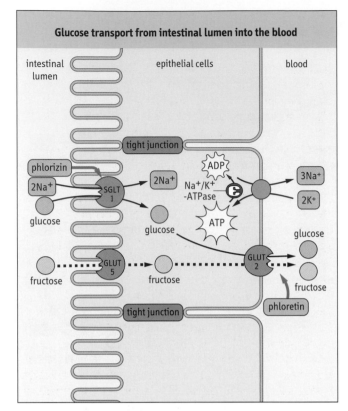

Glucose transport from intestinal lumen into the blood

Fig. 7.7 Glucose transport from intestinal lumen into the blood. Glucose is pumped into the cell through the Na^+-coupled glucose symporter (SGLT1), and passes out of the cell by facilitated diffusion mediated by the GLUT-2 uniporter. The Na^+ gradient for glucose symport is maintained by the Na^+/K^+-ATPase, which keeps the intracellular concentration of Na^+ low. SGLT1 is inhibited by phlorizin and GLUT-2 by phloretin. Phloretin-insensitive GLUT-5 catalyzes the uptake of fructose by facilitated diffusion. The fructose is then exported through GLUT-2. A defect of SGLT1 causes glucose/galactose malabsorption. Adjacent cells are connected by impermeable tight junctions, which prevent solutes from crossing the epithelium. However, leakage of salts (Na^+ and Cl^-) through tight junctions induces diarrhea as a result of inhibition of water absorption. Diarrhea is also induced by laxatives such as phenolphthalein, which is an irritant cathartic for the colon. Thick arrows indicate the binding sites for inhibitors.

in Table 7.5) that is specifically expressed in gastric parietal cells. The gastric proton pump is localized in intracellular vesicles in the resting state. Stimuli such as histamine and gastrin induce fusion of the vesicles with the plasma membrane (Fig. 7.8A). The pump antiports two cytoplasmic protons and two extracellular potassium ions, coupled with hydrolysis of a molecule of ATP, thus it is called an H^+/K^+-ATPase. The counter-ion Cl^- is secreted through a Cl^- channel, producing hydrochloric acid (HCl) (gastric acid) in the lumen (Fig. 7.8B).

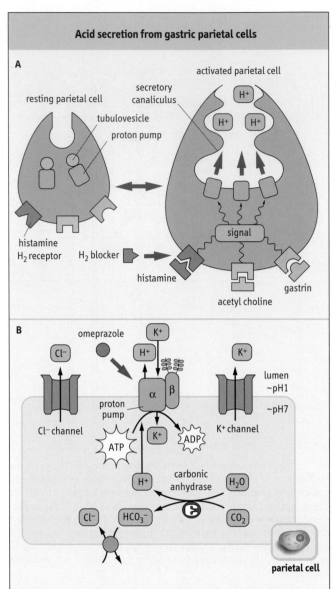

Acid secretion from gastric parietal cells

Fig. 7.8 Acid secretion from gastric parietal cells. (A) Acid secretion is stimulated by extracellular signals and accompanied by morphologic changes in parietal cells [from resting (left) to activated (right)]. The proton pump (H^+/K^+-ATPase) moves to the secretory canaliculus (plasma membrane) from cytoplasmic tubulovesicles. H_2-blockers compete with histamine at the histamine H_2-receptor. (B) Ion balance in the parietal cell. The H^+ transported by the proton pump are supplied by carbonic anhydrase. Bicarbonate, the other product of this enzyme, is antiported with Cl^- and Cl^- is secreted through a Cl^- channel. The potassium (K^+) imported by the proton pump are again excreted by a K^+ channel. The proton pump has catalytic α- and glycosylated β-subunits. The drug omeprazole covalently modifies cysteine residues located in the extracytoplasmic domain of the α-subunit and inhibits the proton pump. Thick arrows indicate the binding sites for inhibitors.

VARIOUS DRUGS INHIBIT TRANSPORTERS IN MUSCLE

Phenylalkylamine (verapamil), benzothiazepine (diltiazem), and dihydropyridine (DHP; nifedipine) are Ca^{2+}-channel blockers that inhibit VDCCs (Fig. 7.6). Ryanodine inhibits the Ca^{2+}-release channel in the sarcoplasmic reticulum. These drugs are used to inhibit both the increase in cytoplasmic Ca^{2+} concentration and the force of muscle contraction. In contrast, cardiac glycosides such as ouabain and digoxin increase heart muscle contraction and are used for treatment of congestive heart failure. They act by inhibiting the Na^+/K^+-ATPase that generates the Na^+ concentration gradient used to drive export of Ca^{2+} by the Na^+/Ca^{2+} antiporter. Snake venoms such as α-bungarotoxin, and tetrodotoxin from the puffer fish inhibit voltage-dependent Na^+ channels. Lidocaine, an Na^+-channel blocker, is used as a local anesthetic and antiarrhythmic drug. Inhibition of Na^+ channels represses transmission of the depolarization signal.

INHIBITING THE GASTRIC PROTON PUMP AND ERADICATION OF *HELICOBACTER PYLORI*

Chronic strong acid secretion by the gastric proton pump injures the stomach and the duodenum, leading to gastric and duodenal ulcers. Proton pump inhibitors such as omeprazole are delivered to parietal cells from the circulation after oral administration. Omeprazole is a prodrug: it accumulates in the acidic compartment, as it is a weak base, and is converted to the active compound under the acidic conditions in the gastric lumen. The active form covalently modifies cysteine residues located in the extracytoplasmic domain of the proton pump. H_2-blockers (receptor antagonists) such as cimetidine and ranitidine indirectly inhibit acid secretion by competing with histamine for its receptor (Fig. 7.8).

Comment. Infection of the stomach by *Helicobacter pylori* also causes ulcers and is associated with an increased risk of gastric adenocarcinoma. Recently, antibiotic treatment has been introduced to eradicate *H. pylori*. Interestingly, antibiotic treatment together with omeprazole is much more effective, possibly because of an increased stability of the antibiotic under the weakly acidic condition produced by proton pump inhibition.

Summary

Eukaryotic cells contain various organelles surrounded by membranes composed of lipids and proteins. Phospholipids are amphipathic molecules that form the bilayer structure of biomembranes. Their hydrophobic fatty acid tails are located on the interior of the membrane and their polar head groups are on the membrane surface. The unsaturated fatty acids bound to phospholipids contribute to the fluid state of the membrane. Cholesterol interacts with phospholipids and maintains the fluidity of the membrane. Peripheral membrane proteins bind to the membrane surface and integral membrane proteins are embedded in the bilayer. Transporter proteins, an example of the latter, have membrane-spanning domains. Biomembranes not only act as permeability barriers and mediators of ion and metabolite flux, but also have important roles in other cellular processes such as cellular recognition and signal transduction.

Most of the permeability properties of the membrane are determined by transport proteins. Facilitated diffusion is catalyzed by transporters that permit the movement of ions and molecules down concentration gradients, whereas uphill or active transport requires energy. Primary active transport is catalyzed by pump ATPases that use energy produced by ATP hydrolysis. Secondary active transport uses electrochemical gradients of Na^+ and H^+, or membrane potential produced by primary active transport processes. Uniport, symport, and antiport are examples of secondary active transport. Protein-mediated transport is a saturable process with high substrate specificity.

Numerous substrates such as ions, nutrients, small organic molecules including drugs and peptides, and proteins are transported by various transporters. All of these transporters are indispensable for homeostasis. The expression of unique sets of transporters is important for specific cell functions such as muscle contraction, nutrient and ion absorption by intestinal epithelial cells and resorption by kidney cells, and secretion of acid from gastric parietal cells.

ACTIVE LEARNING

1. Describe the similarities between the kinetics of enzyme action and transport processes. Compare the properties of various glucose transporters with those of hexokinase and glucokinase, both kinetically and in terms of physiological function.
2. Identify a number of transport inhibitors used in clinical medicine, e.g. Ca^{++}-channel blockers, laxatives and inhibitors of gastric acid secretion.
3. Investigate the process of glucose transport across the blood-brain barrier and explain the pathogenesis of hypoglycemic coma.
4. Study the role and specificity of ABC transporter in multidrug resistance to chemotherapeutic agents.

Further reading

Fatemi N, Sarkar B. Structural and functional insights of Wilson's disease copper-transporting ATPase. *J Bioenerg Biomemb* 2002;**34**:339–349.

Klein I, Sarkadi B, Varadi A. An inventory of the human ABC proteins. *Biochim Biophys Acta* 1999;**1461**:237–262.

Lage H. ABC-transporters: implications on drug resistance from microorganisms to human cancers. *Int J Antimicrob Agents* 2003;**22**:188–199.

Shin J-S, Abraham SN. Caveolae-Not just craters in the cellular landscape. *Science* 2001;**293**:1447–1448.

Subramanian S, Hirai T, Henderson R. From structure to mechanism: electron crystallographic studies of bacteriorhodopsin. *Philos Transact Ser A Math Phys Eng Sci* 2002;**360**:859–874.

Vereb G, *et al.* Dynamic, yet structured: The cell membrane three decades after the Singer-Nicolson model. *Proc Natl Acad Sci USA* 2003;**100**:8053–8058.

Wood IS, Trayhurn P. Glucose transporters (GLUT and SGLT): expanded families of sugar transport proteins. *Br J Nutr* 2003 Jan;**89**(1):3–9.

Relevant websites

Human ABC Transporters : http://nutrigene.4t.com/humanabc.htm

P-ATPase : http://biobase.dk/%7Eaxe/Patbase.html

Membrane Proteins of known Structure : http://www.mpibp-frankfurt.mpg.de/michel/public/memprotstruct.html

8. Bioenergetics and Oxidative Metabolism

L W Stillway

LEARNING OBJECTIVES

After reading this chapter you should be able to:

- Describe how thermodynamics is related to nutrition and obesity.
- Outline the mitochondrial electron transport system showing eight major electron carriers.
- Explain how ubiquinone, heme and the iron-sulfur complexes participate in electron transport.
- Define membrane potential and explain its role in ATP synthesis and thermogenesis.
- Explain the role of uncoupling proteins in thermogenesis.
- Describe the mechanism of ATP synthase.
- Describe the effects of inhibitors such as rotenone, antimycin A, carbon monoxide, cyanide and oligomycin on oxygen uptake by mitochondria.

INTRODUCTION

Oxidation of metabolic fuels is essential to life. In higher organisms, fuels, such as carbohydrates and lipids are metabolized to carbon dioxide and water. Most metabolic energy is provided by oxidation–reduction reactions in mitochondria. This is no small feat, because warm-blooded animals have such variable demands for energy from such processes as thermogenesis at low temperatures, stimulation of ATP synthesis during stress, degradation of excess food, efficient use of nutrients during starvation, and coupling of ATP synthesis with the rate of respiration. This chapter will provide an introduction to the concept of free energy, oxidative phosphorylation and the transduction of energy from fuels into useful work. The pathways and specific molecules through which electrons are transported to oxygen and the mechanism of generation of ATP will be described and related to the structure of the mitochondrion, the powerhouse of the cell and the major source of cellular ATP. Lastly, these biochemical processes will be applied to human health and disease.

OXIDATION AS A SOURCE OF ENERGY

Energy content of foods

Nutrition, and disorders such as obesity, diabetes, and cancer, all require an understanding of thermodynamics. Obesity, for example is a disorder in which there is an imbalance between energy expenditure and intake. It is therefore important that the energy content of foods be known; the commonly accepted energy values for the four major food categories are shown in Table 8.1; alcohol is included, because it is a significant dietary component for some people. These values are obtained by completely burning (oxidizing) samples of each food. Biologically, about 40% of food energy is conserved as ATP, and the remaining 60% is liberated as heat.

The basal metabolic rate (BMR)

The basal metabolic rate (BMR) is the total heat energy released from the body at rest

Virtually all of the reactions in the body are exothermic, and the sum of all reactions at rest is called the basal metabolic rate (BMR), which can be measured by two basic methods: direct calorimetry where the total heat liberated by an animal is measured over time and indirect calorimetry, which involves calculating BMR from the quantity of oxygen consumed, which is directly related to the BMR. Adult men (70 kg) have a BMR of about 7500 kJ (1800 kcal) and women about 5400 kJ (1300 kcal) per day. Women have a lower BMR because of an increased fat content, and the BMR typically varies by a factor of two between individuals. Heat from mitochondria accounts for the largest portion of the BMR. Elevated thyroid hormones increase the BMR.

Stages of fuel oxidation

The oxidation of fuels can be divided into two general stages: production of reduced nucleotide coenzymes during the oxidation of fuels, and ATP synthesis from the free energy provided by oxidation of the reduced coenzymes (Fig. 8.1).

The energy value of food		
Metabolic Fuel	**Energy Content**	
	kJ/g	**kcal/g**
fats	38	9
carbohydrates	17	4
proteins	17	4
alcohol	29	7

Table 8.1 **Energy content of the major classes of food.** Note that the thermodynamic term, kcal (energy required to increase the temperature of 1 kg (1 L) of water by 1 °C) is equivalent to the common nutritional Calorie (capital C), i.e. 1 Cal = 1 kcal, 1 kcal = 4.2 kJ.

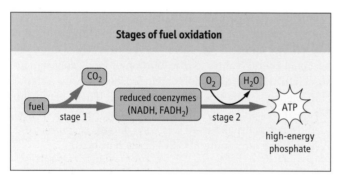

Fig. 8.1 **Stages of fuel oxidation.** NADH, reduced nicotinamide adenine dinucleotide; FADH$_2$, reduced flavin adenine dinucleotide.

FREE ENERGY

The Gibbs' free energy (ΔG) of a reaction is the maximum amount of energy that can be obtained from a reaction at constant temperature and pressure. The units of free energy are kcal/mol (kJ/mol). It is not possible to measure the absolute free energy content of a substance directly, but when reactant A reacts to form product B, the free energy change in this reaction ΔG, can be determined. For the reaction A → B:

$$\Delta G = G_B - G_A$$

where G_A and G_B are the free energy of A and B, respectively. All reactions in biologic systems are considered to be reversible reactions, so that the free energy of the reverse reaction, B → A, is numerically equivalent, but opposite in sign to that of the forward reaction.

It is clear that, if there is a greater concentration of B than of A at equilibrium, the reaction A → B is favorable – that is, it tends to move forward from a standard state in which A and

B are present at equal concentrations. In this case, the reaction is said to be a spontaneous or exergonic reaction, and the free energy of this reaction is defined as negative: that is, ΔG < 0, indicating that energy is liberated by the reaction. Conversely, if the concentration of A is greater than that of B at equilibrium, the forward reaction is termed unfavorable, nonspontaneous or endergonic, and the reaction has a positive free energy: that is, B tends to form A, rather than A to form B. In this case, energy input would be required to push the reaction A → B forward from its equilibrium position to the standard state in which A and B are present at equal concentrations. The total free energy available from a reaction depends on both its tendency to proceed forward from the standard state (ΔG) and the amount (moles) of reactant converted to product.

The free energy of metabolic reactions is related to their equilibrium constants

Thermodynamic measurements are based on standard-state conditions where reactant and product are present at 1 molar concentrations, the pressure of all gases is 1 atmosphere and the temperature is 25°C (298°K). Most commonly, the concentrations of reactants and products are then measured after equilibrium is attained. Standard free energies are represented by the symbol $\Delta G°$ and biological standard free energy change by $\Delta G°'$, with the accent symbol designating pH 7.0. The free energy available from a reaction, may be calculated from its equilibrium constant by the Gibbs equation:

$$\Delta G°' = -RT \ln K'eq$$

where T is absolute temperature (°Kelvin), lnKeq is the natural logarithm of the equilibrium constant for the reaction, and R is the gas constant:

$$R = (8.3 \text{ J K}^{-1}\text{mol}^{-1} \text{ or } \sim 2 \text{ cal K}^{-1}\text{mol}^{-1})$$

Several common metabolic intermediates that you will encounter in your studies are listed in Table 8.2, along with the equilibrium constants and free energies for their hydrolysis reactions. Those intermediates with free energy changes equal to or greater than that of ATP, the central energy transducer of the cell, are considered to be high-energy compounds, and generally have either anhydride or thioester bonds. The lower-energy compounds listed are all phosphate esters and, in comparison, do not yield as much free energy on hydrolysis. The hydrolysis reaction of glucose-6-phosphate (Glc-6-P) is written as:

$$\text{Glc-6-P} + H_2O \rightarrow \text{Glucose} + P_i$$
$$\Delta G°' = -13.8 \text{ kJ/mol} (-3.3 \text{ kcal/mol})$$

This reaction has a negative free energy and occurs spontaneously. The reverse reaction, synthesis of Glc-6-P from glucose and phosphate, would require input of energy.

Thermodynamics of hydrolysis reactions

Metabolite	K'eq	ΔG°' (kJ mol⁻¹)	(kcal mol⁻¹)
phosphoenolpyruvate	1.2×10^{11}	−61.8	−14.8
phosphocreatine	9.6×10^{8}	−50.2	−12.0
1,3-bisphosphoglycerate	6.8×10^{8}	−49.3	−11.8
pyrophosphate	9.7×10^{5}	−33.4	−8.0
acetyl coenzyme A	4.1×10^{5}	−31.3	−7.5
ATP	2.9×10^{5}	−30.5	−7.3
glucose-1-phosphate	5.5×10^{3}	−20.9	−5.0
fructose-6-phosphate	7.0×10^{2}	−15.9	−3.8
glucose-6-phosphate	3.0×10^{2}	−13.8	−3.3

Table 8.2 **Thermodynamics of hydrolysis reactions.** Equilibrium constants and free energy of hydrolysis of various metabolic intermediates at pH 7 (ΔG0')

CONSERVATION OF ENERGY BY COUPLING WITH ATP

Living systems must transfer energy from one molecule to another without losing all of it as heat. Some of the energy must be conserved in a chemical form in order to drive non-spontaneous biosynthetic reactions. In fact, nearly half of the energy obtained from the oxidation of metabolic fuels is channeled into the synthesis of ATP, a universal energy transducer in living systems. ATP is often referred to as the common currency of metabolic energy, because it is used to drive so many energy-requiring reactions. ATP consists of the purine base, adenine, the five-carbon sugar, ribose, and α, β, and γ phosphate groups (Fig. 8.2). The two anhydride linkages are said to be high-energy bonds, because their hydrolysis yields a large negative change in free energy. When ATP is used for metabolic work, these high-energy linkages are broken and it is converted to ADP or to AMP.

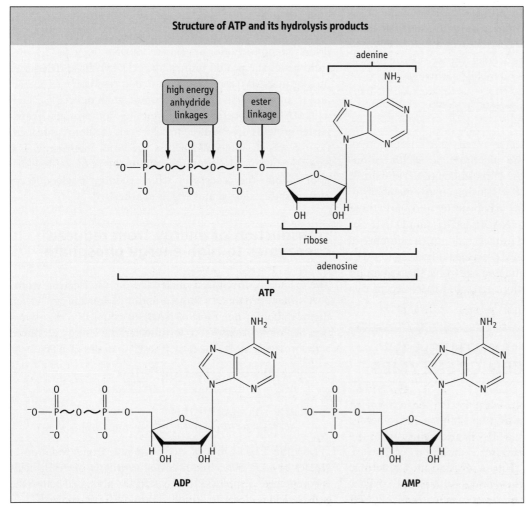

Structure of ATP and its hydrolysis products

Fig. 8.2 **Structures of high-energy phosphates.** ATP is shown, together with its hydrolysis products, adenosine diphosphate (ADP) and adenosine monophosphate (AMP).

ATP is commonly used to drive biosynthetic reactions

The free energy of a high-energy bond, such as the phosphate anhydride bonds in ATP, can be used to drive or push forward reactions that would otherwise be unfavorable. In fact, nearly all biosynthetic pathways are thermodynamically unfavorable, but are made favorable by coupling various reactions with hydrolysis of high-energy compounds. For example, the first step in the metabolism of glucose is the synthesis of Glc-6-P. As shown in Table 8.2, this is not a favorable reaction: the hydrolysis ($\Delta G^{\circ\prime} = -13.8$ kJ/mol or -3.3 kcal/mol), rather than synthesis ($\Delta G^{\circ\prime} = +13.8$ kJ/mol or $+3.3$ kcal/mol) of Glc-6-P is the favored reaction. However, as shown below, the synthesis of Glc-6-P (reaction I) can be energetically coupled to the hydrolysis of ATP (reaction II), yielding a 'net reaction' III that is favorable for synthesis of Glc-6-P:

	$\Delta G^{\circ\prime}$
I: Glc + Pi → Glc-6-P + H_2O	+3.3 kcal/mol
II: ATP + H_2O → ADP + Pi	−7.3 kcal/mol
Net: Glc + ATP → Glc-6-P + ADP	−4 kcal/mol

This is possible because of the high free energy or 'group transfer potential' of ATP. The physical transfer of the phosphate from ATP to glucose occurs in the active site of a kinase enzyme, such as glucokinase. This motif, in which ATP is used to drive biosynthetic reactions, transport processes, or muscle activity, occurs commonly in metabolic pathways.

NAD⁺, FAD, and FMN are the major redox coenzymes

The major redox coenzymes involved in transduction of energy from fuels to ATP are nicotinamide adenine dinucleotide (NAD^+), flavin adenine dinucleotide (FAD) and flavin mononucleotide (FMN) (Fig. 8.3). During energy metabolism, electrons are transferred from carbohydrates and fats to these coenzymes, reducing them to NADH, $FADH_2$ and $FMNH_2$. In each case, two electrons are transferred, but the number of protons transferred differs. NAD^+ accepts a hydride ion (H^-) that consists of one proton and two electrons; the remaining proton is released into solution. FAD and FMN accept two electrons and two protons.

MITOCHONDRIAL SYNTHESIS OF ATP FROM REDUCED COENZYMES

Metabolism of carbohydrates begins in the cytoplasm through the glycolytic pathway (see Chapter 11), whereas energy production from fatty acids occurs exclusively in the mitochondrion. Mitochondria are subcellular organelles, about the size of bacteria. They are essential for aerobic metabolism in eukaryotes. Their main function is to oxidize metabolic fuels and conserve free energy by synthesizing ATP.

EXERCISE AND MITOCHONDRIAL BIOGENESIS

It has long been known that exercise increases the oxidative capacity of skeletal muscle by inducing mitochondrial biogenesis. Continued exercise results in energy consumption, and AMP accumulates. AMP-activated protein kinase is a fuel sensor, and it plays a critical role in initiating the production of new mitochondria and electron transport components such as heme. Of course, such mechanisms are not only of importance in exercise training, but also in the regeneration of tissues after tissue injury, such as trauma, heart attacks and strokes.

Mitochondria are bounded by a dual membrane system (Fig. 8.4). The outer membrane (OMM) contains enzyme and transport proteins, and via the pore-forming protein porin (P), it is permeable to virtually all ions, small molecules (S) and proteins less than 10 000 D. Large proteins must be transported via the TOM complex (translocase in the outer mitochondrial membrane) and TIM complexes (translocases in the inner mitochondrial membrane). This is especially vital to the cell, because almost all mitochondrial proteins are nuclear encoded and must be transported into the mitochondrion. The mitochondrial genome, mtDNA, encodes 13 vital subunits of the proton pumps and ATP synthase. The inner membrane (IMM) is pleated with structures known as cristae, and is impermeable to most ions and small molecules, such as NADH, ATP, coenzymes, phosphate, and protons. Transporter proteins are required to selectively facilitate translocation of specific molecules across the inner membrane. The inner membrane also contains components of oxidative phosphorylation –the process by which reduced nucleotide coenzymes are oxidized and ATP is synthesized.

Transduction of energy from reduced coenzymes to high-energy phosphate

The oxidation of reduced nucleotides by the electron transport system produces a large amount of free energy. When the oxidation of one mole of NADH is coupled to the reduction of $\frac{1}{2}$ mole of oxygen to form water, the energy produced is theoretically sufficient to synthesize 7 moles of ATP:

$$NADH + H^+ + \tfrac{1}{2}O_2 \rightarrow NAD^+ + H_2O$$
$$\Delta G^{\circ\prime} = -220 \text{ kJ/mol } (-52.4 \text{ kcal/mol})$$

$$ADP + Pi \rightarrow ATP + H_2O$$
$$\Delta G^{\circ\prime} = -30.5 \text{kJ/mol } (-7.3 \text{ kcal/mol}) \text{ (Table 8.2)}$$

Dividing 220 kJ/mol of $\Delta G^{\circ\prime}$ available from oxidation of NADH by $\Delta G^{\circ\prime}$ 30.5 required for synthesis of ATP yields theoretically ~7 mol ATP/mol NADH. As discussed below, the actual yield is closer to 3 mol ATP/mol NADH oxidized.

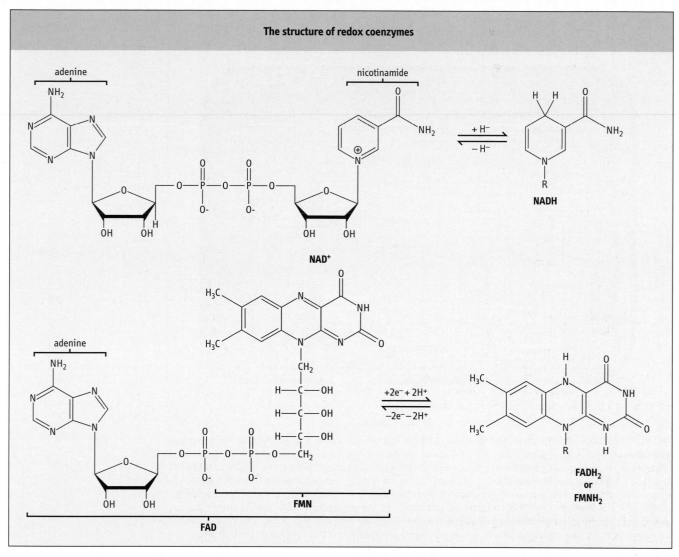

Fig. 8.3 The structure of redox coenzymes. NAD$^+$ and its reduced form, NADH (nicotinamide adenine dinucleotide), consists of adenine, two ribose units, two phosphates, and nicotinamide; FAD and its reduced form, FADH$_2$ (flavin adenine dinucleotide) consists of riboflavin, two phosphates, ribose and adenine; FMN and FMNH$_2$ consist of riboflavin phosphate. The nicotinamide and riboflavin components of these coenzymes are reversibly oxidized and reduced during electron transfer (redox) reactions. NADH and FADH$_2$ are often called reduced nucleotides or reduced coenzymes.

 ## METABOLIC FUNCTION OF ATP REQUIRES MAGNESIUM

ATP readily forms a complex with magnesium ion, and it is this complex that is required in all reactions in which ATP participates, including its synthesis. A magnesium deficiency impairs virtually all of metabolism, because ATP can neither be made nor utilized in adequate amounts.

The free energy of oxidation of NADH is used via the electron transport system to pump protons into the intermembrane space. The energy produced when these protons re-enter the mitochondrial matrix are used to synthesize ATP. This process is known as oxidative phosphorylation (Fig. 8.4).

THE MITOCHONDRIAL ELECTRON TRANSPORT SYSTEM

The entire electron transport system, also known as the electron transport chain or respiratory chain, is located in the

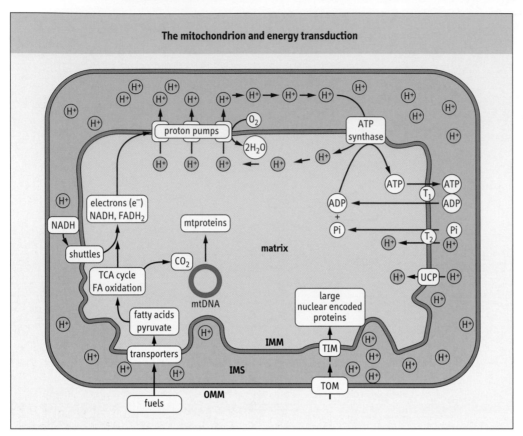

The mitochondrion and energy transduction

Fig. 8.4 **Mitochondrial structure and pathways of energy transduction: the mechanism of oxidative phosphorylation.** Major fuels, such as pyruvate and fatty acids (FA), are transported into the matrix where they are oxidized to generate CO_2 and the reduced nucleotide coenzymes NADH and $FADH_2$. Oxidation of these nucleotides via the electron transport system reduces oxygen to water and pumps protons by three proton pumps out of the matrix and into the intermembrane space (IMS), creating a pH gradient, which is the major contributor to the membrane potential. It should be noted that protons in the intermembrane space freely diffuse through the outer membrane via the protein porin, so the intermembrane space is roughly equivalent to the cytosol. Although the membrane potential is mostly comprised of the proton gradient it actually consists of several electrochemical gradients and is expressed as a voltage. Controlled influx of protons through ATP synthase powers the synthesis of ATP by ATP synthase. Mitochondrial ATP is then exchanged for cytoplasmic ADP through the ADP-ATP translocase (T_1). Phosphate (Pi), which is also required for ATP synthesis is transported by the phosphate translocase (T_2). The inner membrane also contains uncoupling proteins (UCP) that may be used to allow the controlled leakage of protons back into the matrix. OMM, outer mitochondrial membrane; IMM, inner mitochondrial membrane; mtproteins, mitochondrial proteins; mtDNA, mitochondrial DNA; TOM and TIM, protein translocase complexes in outer and inner mitochondrial membrane; TCA, tricarboxylic acid cycle.

inner mitochondrial membrane (Fig. 8.5). It consists of several large protein complexes and two small, independent components, ubiquinone and cytochrome *c*. Each step involves a redox reaction where electrons leave components with more negative reduction potentials and go to components with more positive reduction potentials. Electrons are conducted through this system in a defined sequence from reduced nucleotide coenzymes to oxygen, and the free energy changes drive the transport of protons from the matrix into the intermembrane space via the three proton pumps. After each step, the electrons are at a lower energy state.

Electrons are funneled into the electron transport chain by several flavoproteins. Of these, there are four major species, including complex I, which contains FMN, and three that contain FAD. These pathways all reduce the small, lipophilic molecule, ubiquinone (Q or coenzyme Q_{10}), at the beginning of the common electron transport pathway, consisting of Q, complex III, cytochrome c, and complex IV.

$$Flavoprotein_{(reduced)} + Q \rightarrow Flavoprotein_{(oxidized)} + QH_2$$

Protons are pumped from the matrix into the intermembrane space by complexes I, III, and IV. Oxygen (O_2) is the final

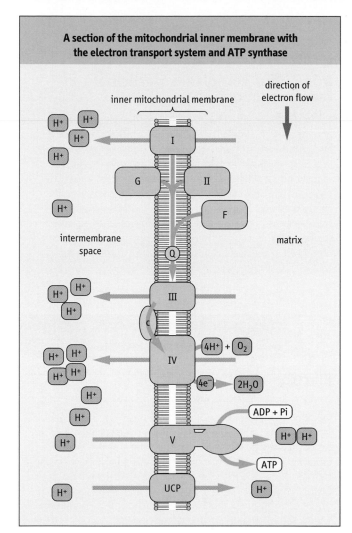

A section of the mitochondrial inner membrane with the electron transport system and ATP synthase

Fig. 8.5 **A section of the mitochondrial inner membrane with the electron transport system and ATP synthase.** I, Complex I; II, Complex II; III, Complex III; IV, Complex IV; V, Complex V or ATP synthase; G, glycerol 3-phosphate dehydrogenase; F, fatty acyl CoA dehydrogenase; Q, ubiquinone; c, cytochrome c; UCP, uncoupling protein.

 IRON DEFICIENCY LEADS TO ANAEMIA

A 45-year-old woman complains of tiredness and appears pale. She is a vegetarian and is experiencing a monthly menstrual flow that is heavy and prolonged. Her hematocrit is 0.32 (reference range 0.36–0.46) and her hemoglobin concentration 90 g/L (normal range 120–160 g/L; 12–16 g/dL).

Comment. Iron deficiency anemia is a common nutritional problem and is especially common in menstruating and pregnant women because of their increased dietary requirement for iron. Men require about 1 mg iron/day, menstruating women about 2 mg/day, and pregnant women about 3 mg/day. Iron is required to maintain normal amounts of hemoglobin, the cytochromes, and iron-sulfur complexes that are central to oxygen transport and energy metabolism. All these processes are impaired in iron deficiency. Heme iron, which is found in meats, is absorbed much more readily than inorganic iron such as that found in egg yolks, vegetables, and nuts. For hematology reference values, see Table 4.2 on p. 48.

If electron transport begins with an electron pair from NADH, approximately three moles of ATP are synthesized, whereas an electron pair from any of the other three FADH$_2$-containing flavoproteins, yields about two moles of ATP, because the proton-pumping capability of complex I is bypassed.

Flavoproteins contain FAD or FMN prosthetic groups

Complex I, also called NADH-Q reductase or NADH dehydrogenase, is a flavoprotein containing FMN. It oxidizes mitochondrial NADH, and transfers electrons through FMN and iron-sulfur (FeS) complexes to ubiquinone, providing enough energy to pump four protons from the matrix in the reaction:

$$NADH + Q + 5H^+_{matrix} \rightarrow NAD^+ QH_2 + 4H^+_{intermembrane\ space}$$

Three other flavoproteins transfer electrons from oxidizable substrates via FADH$_2$ to ubiquinone (Q) (Fig. 8.5):

- succinate – Q reductase (complex II or succinate dehydrogenase of the TCA cycle) (see Chapter 13) oxidizes succinate to fumarate and reduces FAD to FADH$_2$
- glycerol-3-phosphate – Q reductase, a part of the glycerol-3-P shuttle (see below), oxidizes cytoplasmic glycerol-3-P to dihydroxyacetone phosphate (DHAP) and reduces FAD to FADH$_2$

electron acceptor at the end of the chain, and it is reduced to two water molecules by the transfer of four electrons from complex IV.

For bookkeeping purposes in research (see P:O ratios and respiratory control, below), the efficiency of oxidative phosphorylation is measured by dividing the amount of phosphate incorporated into ADP by the amount of atomic oxygen reduced. One atom of oxygen is reduced by two electrons (one electron pair).

$$ADP + Pi + \tfrac{1}{2}O_2 + 2H^+ + 2e^- \rightarrow ATP + H_2O$$

For each pair of electrons transported through complexes I, III, or IV, a sufficient number of protons is pumped by each complex for the synthesis of approximately one mole of ATP.

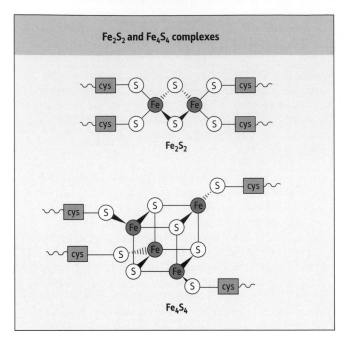

Fe₂S₂ and Fe₄S₄ complexes

Fe₂S₂

Fe₄S₄

Fig. 8.6 **Iron-sulfur complexes.** Cys, cysteine.

A RARE COENZYME Q₁₀ DEFICIENCY

A 4-year-old boy presented with seizures, progressive muscle weakness, and encephalopathy. Accumulation of lactate, a product of anaerobic metabolism of glucose, in the cerebrospinal fluid (CSF) suggested a defect in mitochondrial oxidative metabolism. Muscle mitochondria were isolated for study. The activities of the individual Complexes I, II, III, and IV were normal, but the combined activities of I + III and II + III were significantly decreased. Treatment with coenzyme Q₁₀ improved the muscle weakness, but not the encephalopathy.

Comment. Severe muscle weakness, encephalopathy, or both, may be caused in so-called mitochondrial myopathies by mitochondrial defects involving the electron transport system. The finding of increased lactate in the CSF suggests a defect in oxidative phosphorylation. The decreased activities of complexes I + III and II + III suggested a deficiency in coenzyme Q₁₀, which was confirmed by direct measurements.

■ fatty acyl CoA dehydrogenase catalyzes the first step in the mitochondrial oxidation of fatty acids and also produces FADH₂

Both FMN and FAD contain the water-soluble vitamin riboflavin. A dietary deficiency of riboflavin can severely impair the function of these and other flavoproteins.

IRON-SULFUR COMPLEXES

Iron-sulfur complexes participate in redox reactions

Iron is an important constituent of heme proteins, such as hemoglobin, myoglobin, cytochromes, and catalase, but it is also associated with iron-sulfur (FeS) complexes or nonheme iron proteins that function as electron transporters in the mitochondrial electron transport system. The Fe₂S₂ and Fe₄S₄ types are shown in Figure 8.6. In each case, the iron-sulfur center is bound to a peptide through cysteine residues. The FeS complexes undergo reversible distortion and relaxation during redox reactions. The redox energy is said to be conserved in the 'conformational energy' of the protein.

TRANSFER OF ELECTRONS FROM NADH INTO MITOCHONDRIA

Electron shuttles

NADH is produced in the cytosol during carbohydrate metabolism. Since it cannot cross the inner mitochondrial membrane, it cannot donate electrons directly to the electron transport system. Two redox shuttles that transfer the electrons from NADH into mitochondria rather than physical transfer of the NADH solve this problem. A characteristic feature of these shuttles is that they are powered by cytoplasmic and mitochondrial isoforms of the same enzyme. The glycerol-3-P shuttle is the simpler of the two (Fig. 8.7). It transfers the electrons of NADH from the cytoplasm to mitochondrion by reducing FAD to FADH₂. Cytoplasmic glycerol-3-P dehydrogenase catalyzes reduction of DHAP with NADH to glycerol-3-P. The cytoplasm-derived glycerol-3-phosphate is oxidized back to DHAP by another glycerol-3-phosphate dehydrogenase isoform of in the inner mitochondrial membrane, a flavoprotein in which FAD is reduced to FADH₂. The electrons are then transferred to the common pathway via ubiquinone. The yield of ATP from cytoplasmic NADH by this pathway is approximately 2 moles, rather than the maximum of 3 moles available from mitochondrial NADH via the NADH-Q reductase complex (Complex I).

Many cells use the glycerol 3-P shuttle, but heart and liver rely on the malate-aspartate shuttle, which yields 3 moles of ATP per mole of NADH. This shuttle is more complicated, because the substrate, malate, can cross the inner mitochondrial membrane, but the membrane is impermeable to the product, oxaloacetate – there is no oxaloacetate transporter. The exchange is therefore accomplished by interconversion between α-keto- and α-amino acids, involving cytoplasmic and mitochondrial glutamate and α-ketoglutarate, and isozymes of glutamate-oxaloacetate transaminase (aspartate aminotransferase).

Redox shuttles in the inner mitochondrial membrane

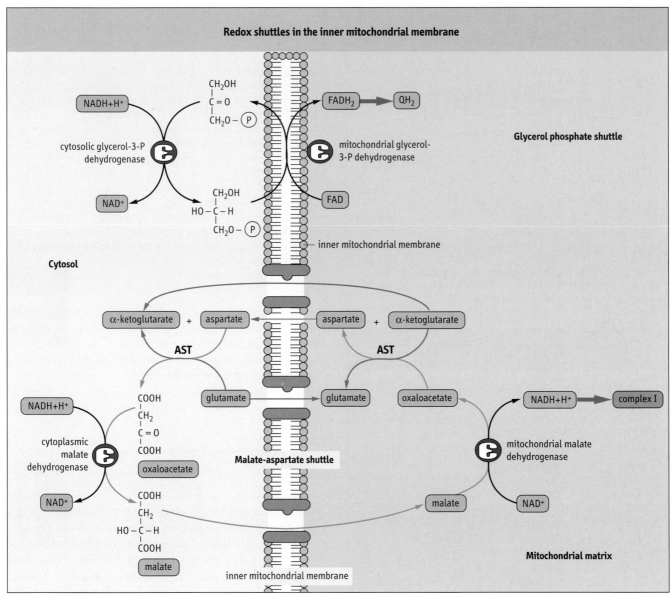

Fig. 8.7 **Redox shuttles in the inner mitochondrial membrane.** The glycerol phosphate and malate-aspartate shuttles. AST, aspartate aminotransferase.

Ubiquinone (coenzyme Q_{10}) transfers electrons to complex III

Ubiquinone is so named, because it is ubiquitous in virtually all living systems. It is a small, lipid-soluble compound found in the inner membrane of animal and plant mitochondria and in the plasma membrane of bacteria. The primary form of mammalian ubiquinone contains a side chain of 10 isoprene units and is often called CoQ_{10}. It diffuses in the inner membrane, accepts electrons from the four major mitochondrial flavoproteins, and transfers them to complex III (QH_2-cytochrome c reductase). It can carry either one or two electrons (Fig. 8.8). It is also thought to be a major source of superoxide radicals in the cell (see Chapter 35).

Complex III – Cytochrome c reductase

This enzyme complex, also known as ubiquinone-cytochrome c reductase or QH_2-cytochrome c reductase, oxidizes ubiquinone and reduces cytochrome c (Fig. 8.8). Reduced ubiquinone funnels electrons that it gathers from mitochondrial flavoproteins and transfers them to complex III. Electrons from ubiquinone are transferred through two species of cytochrome b, to an FeS center, to cytochrome c_1, and finally to cytochrome c. Transport of two electrons to cytochrome c yields sufficient free energy change and protons pumped to synthesize about one mole of ATP. The overall reaction is:

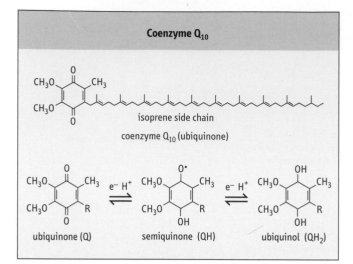

Coenzyme Q$_{10}$

isoprene side chain

coenzyme Q$_{10}$ (ubiquinone)

ubiquinone (Q)   semiquinone (QH)   ubiquinol (QH$_2$)

Fig. 8.8 **Coenzyme Q$_{10}$, or ubiquinone**, accepts one or two electrons, transferring them from flavoproteins to Complex III. The semiquinone form is a free radical.

CYTOCHROMES

Cytochromes, found in the mitochondrion and endoplasmic reticulum, are proteins that contain heme groups, but which are not involved in oxygen transport (Fig. 8.9). The core structure of heme groups is a tetrapyrrole ring similar to that of hemoglobin, differing only in the composition of the side chains. The heme group of cytochromes *b* and c$_1$ is known as iron protoporphyrin IX and is the same heme that is found in hemoglobin, myoglobin, and catalase. Cytochrome c contains heme C, covalently bound to the protein through cysteine residues. Cytochromes a and a$_3$ contain heme A, which, in common with ubiquinone, contains an isoprene side chain. In hemoglobin and myoglobin, heme must remain in the ferrous (Fe^{2+}) state; in cytochromes, the heme iron is reversibly reduced and oxidized between the Fe^{2+} and Fe^{3+} states as electrons are shuttled from one protein to another.

$$QH_2 + 2cyt\ c_{oxidized} + 2H^+_{matrix} \rightarrow$$
$$2Q + 2cyt\ c_{reduced} + 4H^+_{intermembrane\ space}$$

Four protons are pumped, two from fully reduced ubiquinone and two from the matrix.

Cytochrome *c*

Cytochrome *c*, a small heme protein that is loosely bound to the outer surface of the inner membrane, shuttles electrons from complex III to complex IV. Each cytochrome c carries only one electron, so the reduction of O$_2$ to 2 H$_2$O by complex IV requires four reduced cytochrome c molecules. The binding of cytochrome *c* to complexes III and IV is largely

COPPER DEFICIENCY IN NEONATES

Copper is required in trace amounts for optimal human nutrition. Although copper deficiency is rare in adults, premature infants have low stores of copper and may suffer from its deficiency. This may lead to anemia and cardiomyopathy, because of failure to synthesize adequate amounts of cytochrome c oxidase and other enzymes, including several cuproenzymes involved in the synthesis of heme.

Comment. Copper deficiency can impair ATP production by inhibiting the terminal reaction of the electron transport chain, leading to pathology in the heart, where energy demand is high. Dietary formulae for premature infants must contain adequate copper; cow's milk alone is unsuitable, because it is low in copper.

electrostatic, involving a number of lysine residues on the protein surface. Reduction of ferricytochrome c (Fe^{3+}) to ferrocytochrome *c* (Fe^{2+}) by cytochrome c$_1$, leads to a change in the three-dimensional structure of the protein, promoting transfer of electrons to cytochrome a in complex IV (Fig. 8.5). Under certain conditions (at low membrane potentials), cytochrome *c* leaks out of mitochondria, inducing apoptosis (cell death).

Complex IV

Complex IV, known as cytochrome *c* oxidase, or cytochrome oxidase, exists as a dimer in the IMM. It oxidizes the mobile cytochrome *c*, and conducts electrons through cytochromes a and a$_3$, finally reducing oxygen to water in a four-electron transfer reaction (Fig. 8.10). Copper is a common component of this and other oxidase enzymes. Small molecule poisons, such as azide, cyanide, and carbon monoxide, bind to the heme group of cytochrome a$_3$ in cytochrome *c* oxidase and inhibit complex IV. In common with complexes I and III, the cytochrome oxidase complex pumps protons out of mitochondria, providing for the synthesis of about one mole of ATP per pair of electrons transferred to oxygen. The actual number of protons pumped is four. In addition, another four are required in the reduction of O$_2$ to water. The overall reaction catalyzed by complex IV is:

$$4cyt\ c_{reduced} + 4H^+_{(matrix)} + O_2 \rightarrow 4cyt\ c_{oxidized} + 2H_2O$$

THE ATP-SYNTHETIC PROTON GRADIENT

According to the chemiosmotic hypothesis, mitochondria produce ATP using the free energy from the proton gradient.

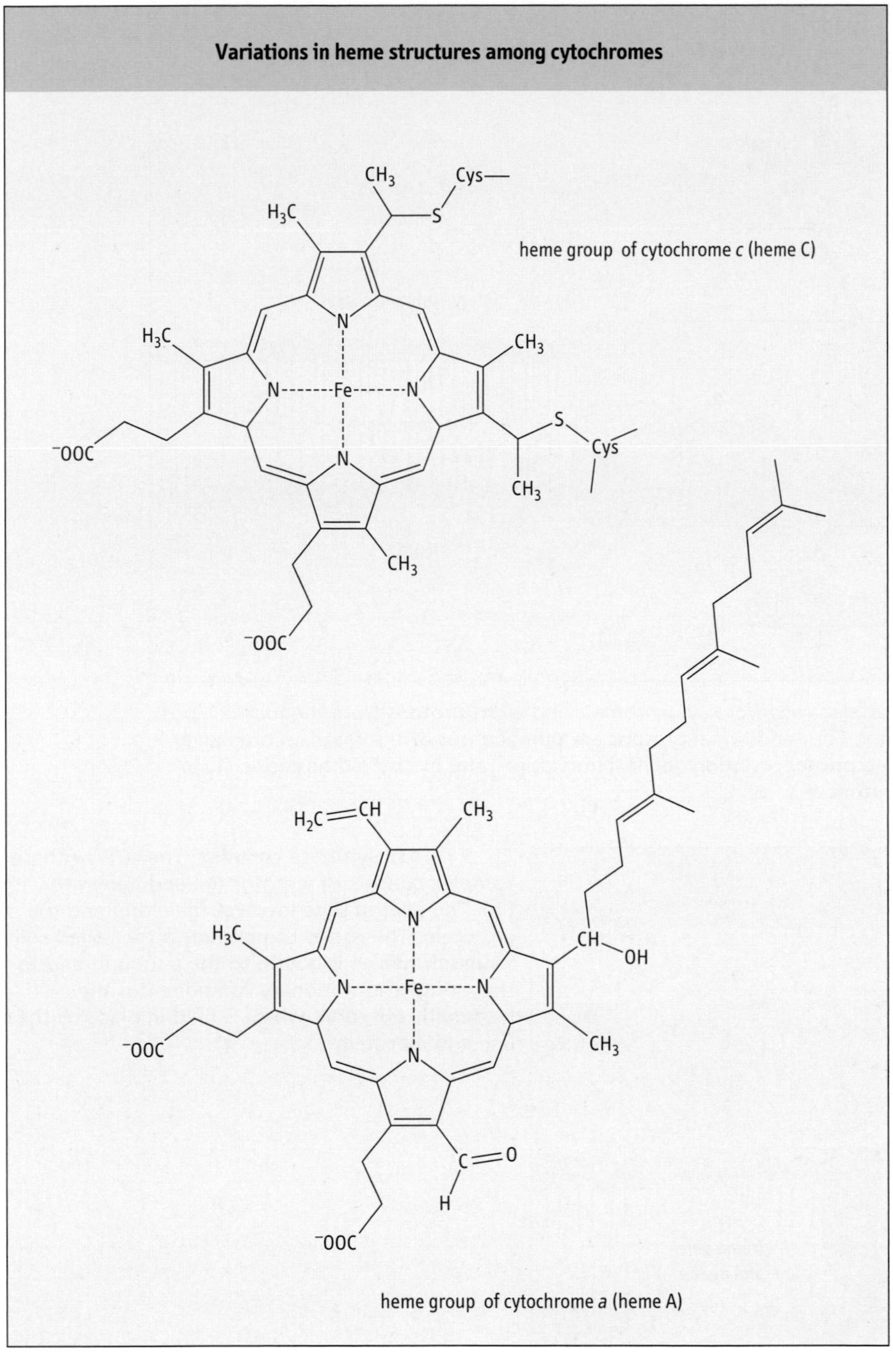

Variations in heme structures among cytochromes

heme group of cytochrome *c* (heme C)

heme group of cytochrome *a* (heme A)

Fig. 8.9 **Variations in heme structures among cytochromes.** The cytochromes are proteins that contain heme groups.

This energy is described as a proton motive force, the result of a pH gradient (concentration gradient) and a charge imbalance (electrochemical gradient) across the inner mitochondrial membrane. To operate, it requires an inner membrane system that is impermeable to protons, except through ATP synthase or other complexes in a regulated fashion. When protons are pumped out of the matrix, the intermembrane space becomes more acidic and more positively charged than the matrix, which is basic and negatively charged.

The ATP synthase complex (complex V) is an example of rotary catalysis

Lining the inner matrix face of the inner membrane of each mitochondrion are thousands of copies of the ATP synthase complex, also called complex V or F_0F_1-ATP synthase (F = coupling factor; see Inhibitors of ATP synthase). ATP synthase is also called an ATPase, because it can hydrolyze ATP. ATP synthase consists of two major complexes (Fig. 8.11). The inner membrane component, termed F_0, is the

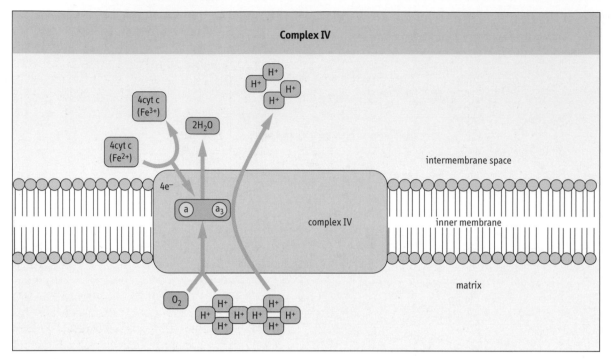

Fig. 8.10 **Complex IV.** Complex IV utilizes four electrons from cytochrome c and eight protons from the matrix. Four protons and electrons reduce oxygen to water. Four additional protons are pumped out of the matrix. Complex IV is regulated allosterically by ATP, by reversible phosphorylation/dephosphorylation, and by thyroid hormone (T_2 or diiodothyronine). a, cytochrome a; a_3, cytochrome a_3.

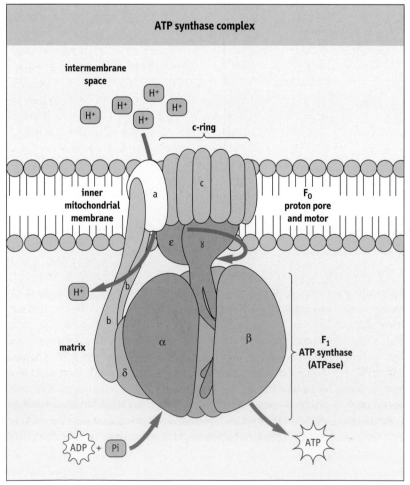

Fig. 8.11 **ATP synthase complex.** The ATP synthase complex consists of a motor (F_0) and generator (F_1). The proton pore involves the *c*-ring and the a-protein. The rotary component is the coiled-coil γ-subunit, which is bound to the ε-subunit and to the *c*-ring. The stationary component is the hexameric $\alpha_3\beta_3$ unit, which is held in place by the δ, b and a-proteins.

is in a different conformation at any given moment. This complex is a proton-driven motor, and it is an example of rotary catalysis. About three protons are required for the synthesis of each ATP. This complex acts independently of the electron transport chain; addition of a weak acid, such as acetic acid, to a suspension of isolated mitochondria is sufficient to induce the biosynthesis of ATP *in vitro*.

P:O RATIOS AND RESPIRATORY CONTROL

The P:O ratio is a measure of the number of high-energy phosphates (*i.e.* amount of ATP) synthesized per atom of oxygen ($\frac{1}{2}O_2$) consumed, or per mole of water produced. The P:O ratio can be calculated from the amount of ADP used to synthesize ATP and the amount of oxygen taken up by mitochondria. For example, if 2 mmol of ADP is converted to ATP, and 0.5 mmol of oxygen (1.0 atom of oxygen) is taken up, the P:O ratio is 2.0. As discussed earlier, the theoretical yield of ATP per mole of NADH is about 7 moles; however, by actual measurement with isolated mitochondria, the P:O ratio for oxidation of metabolites that yield NADH is about 3 and the ratio for those that yield $FADH_2$ is about 2.

'Respiratory control' is the dependence of oxygen uptake by mitochondria on the availability of ADP

Normally, oxidation and phosphorylation are tightly coupled: substrates are oxidized, electrons are transported, and oxygen is consumed only when synthesis of ATP is required (coupled respiration). Thus, resting mitochondria consume oxygen at a slow rate, which can be greatly stimulated by addition of ADP (Fig. 8.13). ADP is taken up by the mitochondria, and it stimulates ATP synthase, which lowers the proton gradient. Respiration increases, because the proton pumps are stimulated to re-establish the proton gradient. When the ADP is depleted, ATP synthesis terminates and respiration returns to the original rate. Oxygen uptake declines to the original rate when the concentration of ADP is depleted and ATP synthesis terminates.

Mitochondria can become partially uncoupled if the inner membrane loses its structural integrity. They are said to be 'leaky', because protons can diffuse through the inner membrane without involving ATP synthase. This occurs if isolated mitochondria are treated with mild detergents that disrupt the inner membrane, or if they have been stored for a period of time. Such mitochondria become uncoupled and lose respiratory control, and their P:O ratio declines.

The mechanism of respiratory control probably depends on the requirement for ADP and Pi binding to the ATP synthase complex: in the absence of ADP and Pi, protons cannot enter

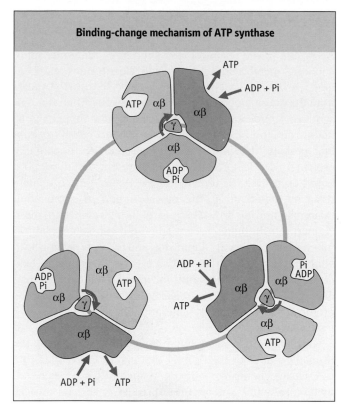

Fig. 8.12 **Binding-change mechanism of ATP synthase.** Powered by protons, the rotation of the γ-subunit of ATP synthase induces simultaneous conformational changes in all three αβ-dimers. Each 120-degree rotation results in ejection of an ATP, binding of ADP and Pi and ATP synthesis.

proton-driven motor with the stoichiometry of a, b_2 and c_{10-14}. The *c*-subunits form the *c*-ring, which rotates in a clockwise direction in response to the flow of protons through the complex. Since the γ and ε-subunits are bound to the *c*-ring, they rotate with it, inducing large conformational changes in the three-αβ dimers. The two b proteins immobilize the second complex (F_1-ATP synthase).

F_1 has a stoichiometry of $α_3$, $β_3$, γ, δ, ε. The major part of F_1 consists of three αβ dimers arranged like slices of an orange, with the catalytic activity residing on the β-subunits. Each 120-degree rotation of the γ-subunit induces conformational changes in the αβ-dimeric subunits such that the nucleotide-binding sites alternate between three states: the first binds ADP and Pi, the second synthesizes ATP, and the third releases ATP, so each complete turn produces 3 ATP. This is known as the binding-change mechanism (Fig. 8.12). Surprisingly, the proton-motive free energy used by ATP synthase is not for ATP synthesis itself, but for its release. So, when the proton gradient is too low to support ATP release, ATP remains stuck to ATP synthase and further ATP production ceases. ADP and Pi are bound to the complex as soon as ATP leaves. The αβ-dimers are asymmetrical, because each

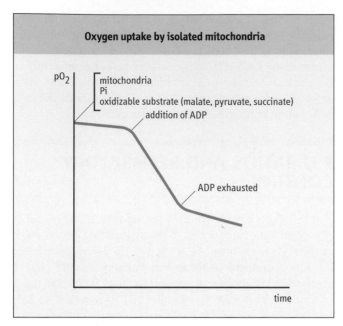

Fig. 8.13 **Effect of ADP on the uptake of oxygen by isolated mitochondria.** This may be studied in an isolated (sealed) system with an oxygen electrode and a recording device. The graph shows a typical recording of oxygen consumption (pO_2, partial pressure of oxygen) by normal mitochondria on introduction of ADP.

the mitochondrion through this complex, and oxygen consumption markedly decreases, because the proton pumps cannot transport protons against a high proton back-pressure. This happens because the free energy of the electron transport reactions is sufficient to generate a pH gradient of only 2 units across the membrane.

Uncouplers

Uncouplers of oxidative phosphorylation dissipate the proton gradient by transporting protons back into mitochondria, bypassing the ATP synthase. This stimulates respiration, because the system makes a futile attempt to restore the proton gradient by oxidizing more fuel and pumping more protons out of mitochondria. Uncouplers are typically hydrophobic compounds, either weak acids or bases, with pK_a near pH 7. The classical uncoupler, 2,4-dinitrophenol (DNP) (Fig. 8.14), accepts a proton on the outer, more acidic side of the inner mitochondrial membrane. Because of its hydrophobicity, it may then freely diffuse through the inner mitochondrial membrane. When it reaches the matrix side, it encounters a more basic pH, and the proton is released, effectively discharging the pH gradient. Other uncouplers include preservatives and antimicrobial agents, such as pentachlorophenol and *p*-cresol.

Uncoupling proteins (UCP)

According to the chemiosmotic hypothesis, the inner mitochondrial membrane is topologically closed. However, it has long been known that protons are transported into the matrix from the intermembrane space by routes other than the ATP synthase complex. Much of the BMR is now thought to be mainly due to inner membrane components called uncoupling proteins (UCP). The first discovered was uncoupling protein-1 (UCP1), formerly known as thermogenin, which is found exclusively in brown adipose tissue. Brown adipose tissue is abundant in the newborn and in some adult mammals, and it is brown because of its high content of mitochondria. In humans, brown adipose tissue is abundant in infants, but it gradually diminishes and is barely detectable in adults. The sole function of UCP1 is to provide body heat during cold stress in the young and in some adult animals and during hibernation. It accomplishes this by uncoupling the proton gradient, thereby generating heat (thermogenesis) instead of ATP.

Four additional uncoupling proteins are expressed by the human genome, UCP2, UCP3, UCP4 and UCP5. While UCP1 is exclusive to brown adipose tissue, UCP2 is expressed ubiquitously, UCP3 is mainly expressed in skeletal muscle, and UCP4 and UCP5 are expressed in the brain. Except for UCP1, the physiological functions of these proteins are not well understood, but could be of profound significance in our understanding of such health issues as diabetes, obesity, cancer, thyroid disease and aging. As uncouplers, they have been linked to a number of fundamental functions. For example, there is strong evidence that obesity induces the synthesis of UCP2 in β-cells of the pancreas. This may play a role in the β-cell dysfunction found in type 2 diabetes, because it lowers the intracellular concentration of ATP, which is required for secretion of insulin. The thyroid hormone (T_3) has been shown to stimulate thermogenesis in rats by promoting the synthesis of UCP3 in skeletal muscle. Of course, the common fever that is induced by infectious organisms is probably due to uncoupling by UCPs, but the mechanism is unknown. The UCP system may also be important in regulating the membrane potential.

INHIBITORS OF OXIDATIVE METABOLISM

Electron transport system inhibitors

Inhibitors of electron transport selectively inhibit complexes I, III, or IV, interrupting the flow of electrons through the respiratory chain. This stops proton pumping, ATP synthesis, and oxygen uptake. Several inhibitors are readily-available poisons that could be encountered in the practice of medicine.

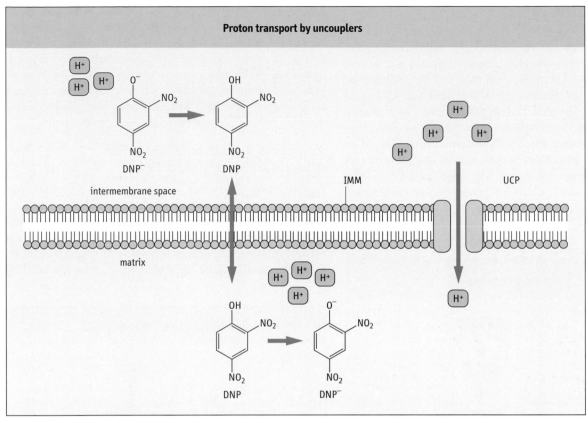

Fig. 8.14 **Proton transport by uncouplers.** Uncouplers transport protons into the mitochondrion, dissipating the proton gradient. DNP is an example of an exogenous uncoupler. The uncoupling proteins (UCP) are endogenous uncouplers in the IMM and are regulated by hormones. The gradient consisting of protons and other factors constitute the mitochondrial membrane potential (MMP), which is expressed in millivolts (mV). DNP, 2,4-dinitrophenol; IMM inner mitochondrial membrane.

 ## 2,4-DINITROPHENOL POISONING

An unresponsive 25-year-old woman is carried into the emergency room by her boyfriend, because after taking two doses of 'weight loss' pills, she complained of headache, fever, chest pain, profuse sweating, and weakness. Initial findings were: rectal temperature, 40.8 °C (105.5 °F), pulse 151 beats per minute, respiratory rate, 56 per minute, blood pressure 40/10. In 15 minutes she died and could not be resuscitated. After death, rigor mortis set in after 10 minutes and her temperature rose to 46 °C (115 °F) in 10 additional minutes. It was found that she was a body builder and that she took 'weight loss' capsules purchased from a friend, because she wanted to have a leaner body for a show. Among her personal effects, was a plastic bottle containing capsules that proved to contain 2,4-dinitrophenol.

Comment. Dinitrophenol (DNP) is an uncoupler of oxidative phosphorylation (see Fig. 8.14). It was first discovered to induce weight loss during World War I when it was noticed that French munitions workers who were exposed to dinitrophenol during the synthesis of dynamite (trinitrotoluene, TNT) rapidly lost weight. In the 1930s it was prescribed by physicians for weight loss and was also available over-the-counter, but because people suffered significant side effects, such as cataracts, blindness, kidney and liver damage and death, it was banned for medical use in United States after a congressional investigation. The case above was adapted from those hearings. Dinitrophenol is currently used industrially in the manufacture of dyes, explosives, herbicides, insecticides and lumber preservatives. DNP kills bacteria and fungi by uncoupling phosphorylation. Unfortunately, DNP has resurfaced as an illegal weight-loss product. It radically increases consumption of oxygen and metabolic fuels, and nearly all metabolic energy is wasted as heat. Cells die both because of excess temperature and lack of ATP.

Rotenone inhibits complex I (NADH-Q reductase)

Rotenone, a common insecticide, and some barbiturates (e.g. amytal) inhibits complex I. Because malate and lactate are oxidized by NAD^+, their oxidation will be inhibited by rotenone. However, substrates yielding $FADH_2$ can still be oxidized, because Complex I is bypassed and electrons are donated to ubiquinone. Addition of ADP to a suspension of mitochondria supplemented with malate and phosphate (Fig. 8.15) markedly stimulates oxygen uptake as ATP synthesis occurs. Oxygen uptake is markedly inhibited by rotenone, but, when succinate is added, ATP synthesis and oxygen consumption resume until the supply of ADP is exhausted.

Rotenone inhibition of Complex I causes reduction of all components prior to the point of inhibition, because they cannot be oxidized, whereas those after the point of inhibition become fully oxidized. This is known as a crossover point, and it can be determined spectrophotometrically, because light absorption by respiratory-chain components changes according to redox state. Such analyses were used to define the sequence of components in the respiratory chain.

Antimycin A inhibits complex III (QH₂-cytochrome c reductase)

The inhibition of Complex III by antimycin A prevents transfer of electrons from either complex I or $FADH_2$-containing flavoproteins to cytochrome *c*. In this case, components preceding complex III become fully reduced, and those after it become oxidized. The oxygen uptake curve (Fig. 8.16) shows that the stimulation of respiration by ADP is inhibited by

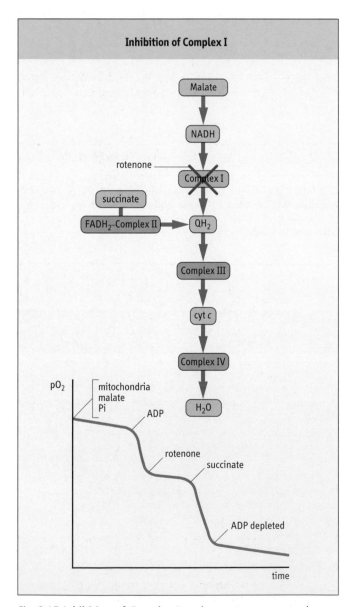

Fig. 8.15 **Inhibition of Complex I**, such as rotenone, retard oxygen uptake by mitochondria when NADH-producing substrates are being oxidized.

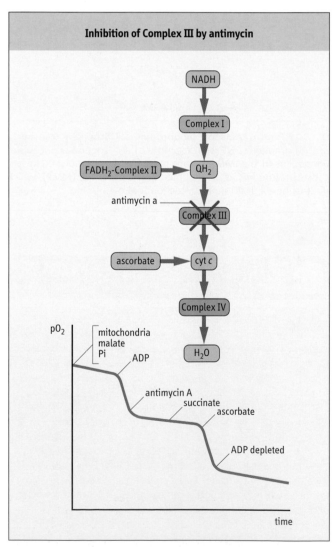

Fig. 8.16 **Inhibition of Complex III by antimycin.** Antimycin A inhibits Complex III, blocking transfer of electrons from both Complex I and flavoproteins, such as Complex II.

antimycin A, but that the addition of succinate does not relieve the inhibition. Ascorbic acid can reduce cytochrome *c*, and addition of ascorbic acid restores respiration, illustrating that complex IV is unaffected by antimycin A.

Cyanide and carbon monoxide inhibit Complex IV

Azide (N_3^-), cyanide (CN^-), and carbon monoxide (CO) inhibit Complex IV (cytochrome *c* oxidase) (Fig. 8.17). Because complex IV is the terminal electron transfer complex, its inhibition cannot be bypassed. All components preceding complex IV become reduced, oxygen cannot be reduced, none of the complexes can pump protons and ATP is not synthesized. Uncouplers such as DNP have no effect, because there is no proton gradient. Cyanide and carbon monoxide also

bind to hemoglobin, and it cannot carry oxygen (see Chapter 4). In these poisonings, both the ability to transport oxygen and to synthesize ATP are impaired. The administration of oxygen is used for the treatment of such poisonings. It is of interest that sodium azide is the nitrogen source for the inflation of air bags; it may pose an environmental problem if it is accidentally released, i.e. non-explosively.

Inhibitors of ATP synthase

Oligomycin inhibits respiration, but, in contrast to electron transport inhibitors, it is not a direct inhibitor of the electron transport system. Instead, it inhibits the proton channel of ATP synthase. It causes an accumulation of protons outside the mitochondrion, because the proton pumping system is still intact, but the proton channel is blocked. The addition of the uncoupler DNP after oxygen uptake has been inhibited by oligomycin illustrates this point: DNP dissipates the proton gradient and stimulates oxygen uptake as the electron transport system attempts to re-establish the proton gradient (Fig. 8.18).

Inhibitors of the ADP–ATP translocase

Most ATP is synthesized in the mitochondrion, but used in the cytosol for biosynthetic reactions. Newly synthesized

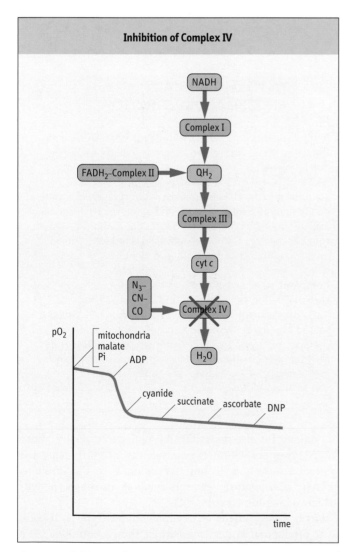

Fig. 8.17 **Inhibition of Complex IV.** The inhibition of Complex IV interrupts the transfer of electrons, in the final step of electron transport. Electrons cannot be transferred to oxygen, and the synthesis of ATP is halted.

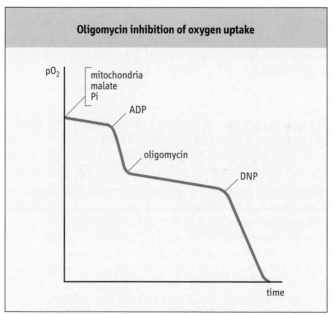

Fig. 8.18 **Oligomycin inhibition of oxygen uptake.** Oligomycin inhibits oxygen uptake in ATP-synthesizing mitochondria. Oligomycin inhibits ATP synthase and oxygen uptake in coupled mitochondria. However, DNP stimulates oxygen uptake after oligomycin inhibition, by dissipating the proton gradient.

mitochondrial ATP and spent cytosolic ADP are exchanged by a mitochondrial ADP–ATP translocase, representing about 10% of the protein in the inner mitochondrial membrane (Fig. 8.4). This translocase can be inhibited by unusual plant and mold toxins, such as bongkrekic acid and atractyloside. Their effects are similar to those of oligomycin *in vitro* – a proton gradient builds up and electron transport stops, but in this case respiration can be reactivated by uncouplers.

REGULATION OF OXIDATIVE PHOSPHORYLATION

Respiratory control and feedback regulation

The oldest and simplest known mechanism of respiratory control is accomplished by the supply of ADP. This is based on the fact that when added to isolated mitochondria, it stimulates respiration and ATP synthesis. When ADP is completely converted to ATP, respiration returns to the initial rate. Oxidative phosphorylation is tightly coupled to fundamental pathways such as glycolysis, fatty acid oxidation and the TCA cycle through feedback regulatory mechanisms. The ratios of NADH/NAD and ATP/ADP feedback on key enzymes, such as PFK-1, pyruvate dehydrogenase and isocitrate dehydrogenase. If, for example, oxidative phosphorylation is switched off because of high ATP, both NADH and ATP will negatively feedback on other energy-producing pathways. Since oxidative phosphorylation responds to the supply of $FADH_2$, NADH, ADP, and Pi as well as the ATP/ADP ratio, magnitude of the membrane potential, uncoupling and hormonal factors, its modes of regulation are clearly more complex than was once thought.

Regulation by covalent modification and allosteric effectors (ATP–ADP)

The main target for regulating oxidative phosphorylation appears to be Complex IV. It is phosphorylated in response to hormone action (Chapter 12) by cyclic-3′5′-adenosine monophosphate (*c*AMP)-dependent protein kinase (PKA) and dephosphorylated by a Ca^{2+}-stimulated protein phosphatase. Phosphorylation enables allosteric regulation by ATP (ATP/ADP ratio). A high ATP/ADP ratio inhibits, and a low ratio stimulates oxidative phosphorylation. It is thought that the complex is normally phosphorylated and inhibited by ATP, but with high Ca^{2+} levels, e.g. in muscle during exercise (Chapter 19), the enzyme is dephosphorylated, the control by ATP/ADP is abolished, and its activity greatly stimulated, increasing ATP production.

CYANIDE AND CARBON MONOXIDE ARE MITOCHONDRIAL POISONS

Both cyanide and carbon monoxide bind to hemoglobin and inhibit oxygen transport. They also inhibit electron transport and production of ATP.

Comment. Cells respond to cyanide or carbon monoxide poisoning by switching to anaerobic metabolism, resulting in lactic acidosis and ultimate death, unless immediate measures are taken. Carbon monoxide poisoning is treated with oxygen. In both cyanide and carbon monoxide poisoning, methylene blue can be administered: it alleviates the inhibition of Complex IV by accepting electrons from Complex III (cytochrome c reductase), allowing both Complex I and Complex III to pump protons, so that ATP can continue to be synthesized. Cyanide can also be converted to the relatively harmless thiocyanate ion by the administration of thiosulfate.

MITOCHONDRIAL ENCEPHALOMYOPATHY

A 16-year-old boy presented with headache, seizures and visual loss. There was a long history of inability to exercise due to muscle weakness. There have been episodes of hemianopia and mild hemiparesis lasting several days. His maternal aunt had a similar illness. Accumulation of lactate during and after exercise suggested a defect in mitochondrial oxidative metabolism. Muscle mitochondria were isolated for study. Respiratory Complex I activity was reduced. A point mutation in mitochondrial DNA was identified.

Comment. A diagnosis of mitochondrial myopathy, encephalopathy, lactic acidosis and stroke-like episodes (MELAS) was made. MELAS is one of a group of conditions caused by defects in oxidative phosphorylation and characterized by defects in the process whereby NADH drives electrons along the mitochondrial respiratory chain complex and generates ATP.

Complex I is also reversibly phosphorylated/dephosphorylated. Phosphorylation is catalyzed by a *c*AMP-dependent protein kinase and dephosphorylation by a Ca^{2+}-inhibited protein phosphatase. Phosphorylation increases activity, which is maintained at high Ca^{2+}.

Lastly, based on the observation that in type 2 diabetes, ATP production is decreased when the β-subunit of ATP-synthase is phosphorylated, it has also been proposed that this complex is also regulated by phosphorylation/dephosphorylation.

Regulation by thyroid hormones

Thyroid hormones act at two levels in mitochondria. It has been shown that in rats T_3 stimulates the synthesis of UCP2 and UCP3, which can uncouple the proton gradient. Additionally, T_2 binds to complex IV on the matrix side, inducing slip in cytochrome c oxidase. The term slip means that complex IV pumps fewer protons per electron transported through the complex, resulting in thermogenesis. The action of T_3 could explain, in part, the long-term and T_2 the short-term thermogenic effects of thyroid hormones.

Summary

The electron transport system consists of at least eight major electron carriers that are located in the inner mitochondrial membrane, each of which is isolable as a complex or as a single molecule. Electrons from four major flavoproteins feed electrons to ubiquinone, the first member of the common pathway. Energy derived from the conductance of electrons through the electron transport system is used by three of the complexes to pump protons into the intermembrane space, creating an electrochemical gradient or proton motive force. The proton gradient is used to power ATP synthase for synthesis of ATP by rotary catalysis. Numerous toxins can severely impair the electron transport system, the ATP synthase and the translocase that exchanges ATP and ADP across the inner mitochondrial membrane. The rate of ATP production by the electron transport system is regulated by modulation of the proton gradient, by allosteric modification and phosphorylation-dephosphorylation and by thyroid hormones. At least five uncoupling proteins (UCP) with specific tissue distributions occur in the inner mitochondrial membrane, and they all regulate the membrane potential and thermogenesis. Chronic diseases or conditions, such as diabetes, cancer, obesity, and aging all have metabolic links to dysregulation of oxidative phosphorylation through effects on electron transport system and ATP synthase.

ACTIVE LEARNING

Test your knowledge:

1. The glycerol-3-phosphate and malate-aspartate shuttles both transport electrons into the mitochondria from cytoplasmic NADH. Explain how the glycerol-3-phosphate shuttle is more thermogenic than the malate-aspartate shuttle. Why are there two separate transport systems?
2. Describe how increased synthesis of a UCP could decrease ATP synthesis.
3. How many 360-degree rotations of ATP synthase occur as a result of one turn of the TCA cycle if all components are fully coupled?
4. Which type of inhibitors would mimic a genetic defect in cytochrome oxidase?
5. Describe how a deficiency in riboflavin could severely impair ATP synthesis.

Further reading

Argyropoulos G, Harper ME. Uncoupling proteins and thermoregulation. *J Appl Physiol* 2002;**92**(5):2187–98.

Bender E and Kadenbach B. The allosteric ATP-inhibition of cytochrome c oxidase is reversibly switched on by cAMP-dependent phosphorylation. *FEBS Lett* 2000;**466**:130–134.

Dimauro S, Schon EA. Mitochondrial respiratory chain diseases. *N Engl J Med* 2003; **348**:2656–2668

Højlund K. *et al.* Proteome analysis reveals Phosphorylation of ATP synthase subunit in human skeletal muscle and proteins with potential roles in type 2 diabetes. *J Biol Chem* 2003;**278**(12):10436–10442.

Jezek P. Possible physiological roles of mitochondrial uncoupling proteins, *UCPn*. *Int J Biochem Cell Biol* 2002;**34**(10):1190–206.

Kadenbach B. Instrinsic and extrinsic uncoupling of phosphorylation. *Biochim Biophys Acta -Bioenergetics* 2003;**1604**(2):77–94.

McFarland R, Taylor RW, Turnbull DM. The neurology of mitochondrial DNA disease. *Lancet Neurol* 2002; **1**:343–351.

Oldfors A, Tulinius M. Mitochondrial encephalomyopathies. *J Neuropathol Exp Neurol* 2003;**62**:217–227.

S. Papa, *et al.* Minireview. The NADH: ubiquinone oxidoreductase (complex I) of the mammalian respiratory chain and the cAMP cascade. *J Bioenerg Biomembr* 2002;**34**: 1–10.

Vidal-Puig, AJ. Uncoupling expectations. *Nature Genet* 2000;**26**(4):387–388.

Zhang, CY. *et. al.* Uncoupling protein-2 negatively regulates insulin secretion and is a major link between obesity, cell dysfunction, and type 2 diabetes. *Cell* 2001;**105**:745–755.

Relevant websites

An excellent site for ATP synthase movies:
    http://www.cnr.berkeley.edu/~hongwang/Project/ATP_synthase/
Neuromuscular Disease Center:
    http://www.neuro.wustl.edu/neuromuscular/mitosyn.html
The Children's Mitochondrial Disease Network: http://www.emdn-mitonet.co.uk/
Mitochondrial diseases: http://www.umdf.org/mitodisease/;
    http://www.neuro.wustl.edu/neuromuscular/mitosyn.html

9. Function of the gastrointestinal tract

I Broom

LEARNING OBJECTIVES

After reading this chapter you should be able to:

- Describe the main stages of digestion.
- Discuss mechanisms involved in the absorption of nutrients from the gastrointestinal tract.
- Discuss the role of digestive enzymes.
- Discuss digestion of the main classes of nutrients: carbohydrates, proteins, and fats.
- Identify compounds arising from the digestion of carbohydrates, proteins, and fats that become substrates for further metabolism

INTRODUCTION

Food provides an organism with sources of energy and with materials for building up, or renewing, body structures.

The eaten food enters the gastrointestinal (GI) tract. The GI tract together with the organs functionally associated with it, the liver and the pancreas, are responsible for the process of digestion and absorption. Digestion is the degradation of nutrient molecules into components simple enough to be subsequently absorbed in the intestine. Absorption is the uptake of digested components by the intestinal cells (enterocytes). Digestion and absorption of nutrients are closely linked. Digestion is regulated by the nervous system, several hormones, and various paracrine factors. The physical presence of food particles in the GI tract also stimulates the process.

The main classes of macromolecules contained in food are carbohydrates, lipids, and proteins

Carbohydrates and lipids function primarily as sources of energy (metabolic fuels) but also have a nonfuel function in the body. Protein, on the other hand, is primarily used for nonfuel purposes but can, under certain circumstances, serve as an energy source. The composition of foods varies in the proportions of protein, carbohydrate, and fats. In addition, some ingested materials, particularly some complex carbohydrates of plant origin, are indigestible and constitute what is termed 'fiber'.

DIGESTION

The GI tract is effectively a large coiled tube with liver and pancreas connected to it by secretory ducts. Its function is to transfer the components of food from the outside to the inside the body (Fig. 9.1). The gut is organized into different anatomical areas, each having a specific function related to digestion and absorption: the stomach and duodenum dealing with the initial process of mixing ingested food and its digestion; the jejunum continuing with the digestive processes, and beginning the process of absorption; the ileum absorbing digested foodstuffs and the large bowel being involved in the absorption of fluid and electrolytes (Table 9.1). Along the lengths of the gut, various added fluids, electrolytes, and proteins aid in the mixing, hydration, and digestion of the food. The gut does more than simply pass all digested food to the other organs. It will, for example, treat the simple monosaccharide, glucose, differently when this is received from the lumen or via the mesenteric blood supply. Glucose taken up from the lumen is transferred directly to the liver unaltered, whereas glucose received via the blood supply is metabolized to lactate prior to passage to the liver. The amino acid glutamine, which is derived from the dietary protein, is used by the enterocytes as a major energy source and does not enter the portal blood supply (see below).

The mechanical and anatomical basis of digestion

There is a purely mechanical component to digestion. Mastication (chewing) and preliminary digestion of food take place in the mouth. The food is then transferred into the esophagus in a process driven by the esophageal reflex. As the ever smaller particles appear in different parts of the GI tract, such as stomach and then duodenum, they themselves trigger peristalsis, which helps mixing and stimulates the secretory function. The major stimulator of peristalsis is the parasympathetic system.

Stomach and intestine have invaginated surfaces which multiply their surface area. The small intestine contains mucosal folds, intestinal villi, and microvilli making it the main absorptive surface.

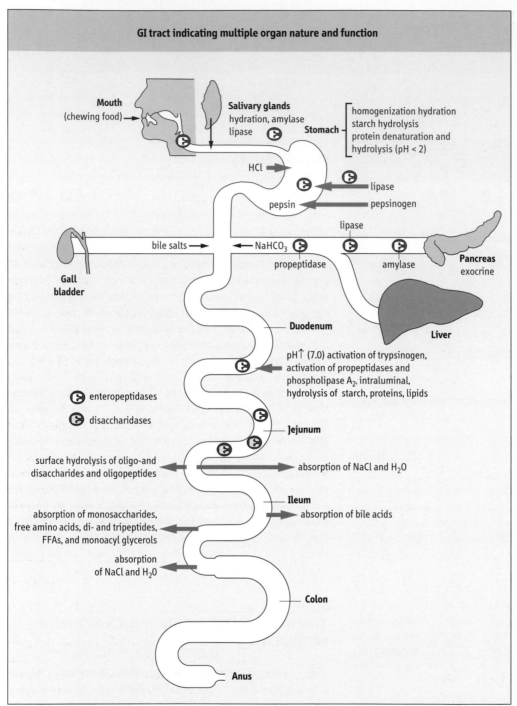

GI tract indicating multiple organ nature and function

Mouth (chewing food)

Salivary glands hydration, amylase lipase

Stomach — [homogenization hydration starch hydrolysis protein denaturation and hydrolysis (pH < 2)]

HCl

lipase

pepsin ← pepsinogen

lipase

bile salts → ← NaHCO$_3$

propeptidase

amylase

Pancreas exocrine

Gall bladder

Duodenum

Liver

pH↑ (7.0) activation of trypsinogen, activation of propeptidases and phospholipase A$_2$, intraluminal, hydrolysis of starch, proteins, lipids

enteropeptidases

disaccharidases

Jejunum

surface hydrolysis of oligo-and disaccharides and oligopeptides

absorption of NaCl and H$_2$O

Ileum

absorption of bile acids

absorption of monosaccharides, free amino acids, di- and tripeptides, FFAs, and monoacyl glycerols

absorption of NaCl and H$_2$O

Colon

Anus

Fig. 9.1 **GI tract indicating multiple organ nature and function.** The gastrointestinal (GI) tract includes several organs and functions. FFA, free fatty acids.

Volume and pH of intestinal secretions

Maintaining the appropriate pH in different parts of the GI tract is crucial for the digestive process, and also for the preservation of the underlying tissues. Thus, saliva secreted in the mouth, due to its bicarbonate content, is alkaline. The lumen of the stomach is strongly acidic, while the mucus lining its walls is again alkaline. The acidic content of the stomach is then neutralized by the strongly alkaline pancreatic juice.

Intestinal secretions reach the volume of about 7.5 liters a day. This is in addition to the average water intake of about 1.5L. In normal circumstances only about 150–250 mL of water is contained in the stool, the rest being absorbed in the GI tract.

Gastrointestinal (GI) tract organization by functional requirements

Gastrointestinal organ	Primary function in absorption of foodstuffs
salivary glands	production of fluid and digestive enzymes for homogenization, lubrication and digestion of carbohydrate (amylase) and lipid (lingual lipases)
stomach	secretion of HCl and proteases to initiate hydrolysis of proteins
pancreas	secretion of HCO_3^-, proteases and lipases to continue digestion of proteins/lipids and amylase to continue digesting starch
liver/gall bladder	secretion and storage of bile acids for release to small bowel
small bowel	final intraluminal digestion of foodstuffs, digestion of carbohydrate dimers, and specific absorptive pathways for digested material
large bowel	absorption of fluid and electrolytes and products of bacterial action in the colon

Table 9.1 **Organization of the GI tract in relation to functional requirements.**

Loss of fluid from the gastrointestinal tract may leads to disturbances of fluid, electrolyte, and acid base balance

Vomiting, i.e. the loss of primarily stomach contents, and diarrhoea, which causes the loss of intestinal contents, may lead to problems with water, electrolyte, and acid–base balance.

Prolonged vomiting causes the loss of water, potassium, and hydrogen ion. Diarrhoea might be caused by the increased intestinal secretion due to, for instance, inflammation, or may be caused by the malabsorption of nutrients. Severe diarrhoea may lead to dehydration and metabolic acidosis due to the loss of alkaline fluids. It also induces loss of sodium, potassium, and other minerals (see Chapters 10 and 22 for more details).

General principles of digestion

Digestion is a sequential, ordered process with links between each stage

The process of digestion is characterized by several specific stages, which occur in characteristic sequence, allowing the interaction of fluid, pH, emulsifying agents, and enzymes. This, in turn, requires concerted action of the liver, pancreas, gall bladder, and salivary glands. The processes that are involved are outlined in Figure 9.1 and can be summarized as follows:

- lubrication and homogenization of food with fluids secreted by glands of the GI tract, starting in the mouth;
- secretion of enzymes whose prime function is the hydrolytic breakdown of polymeric macromolecules to a mixture of oligomers, dimers and monomers;
- secretion of electrolytes, hydrogen ion and bicarbonate within different regions of the GI tract, to optimize the conditions for enzymic hydrolysis specific to a particular region of the GI tract;
- secretion of bile acids to emulsify dietary lipid, allowing appropriate enzymic hydrolysis and absorption;
- further hydrolysis of oligomers and dimers within the jejunum by membrane-bound surface enzymes;
- specific transport of digested material into enterocytes and thence to blood or lymph.

Numerous sections of the gut are involved in these processes and each area contains specialized glands and unique surface epithelial properties, as outlined in Table 9.1. Before signs and symptoms of GI maldigestion or malabsorption occur, there needs to be a considerable impairment of structural/functional relationships within the GI tract.

There is considerable functional reserve in all aspects of digestion and absorption. Minor functional loss may go unnoticed by the individual, allowing pathology to progress for some time before being diagnosed.

Each of the organs involved in digestion and absorption has the capacity to increase its activity several fold in response to specific stimulation; this adds to the gut's reserve capacity. For pancreatic disease to become manifest, 90% of the pancreatic function has to be destroyed. In addition, the gut can accommodate loss of function of one particular organ. For example, both the pancreas and the small intestine can take over after a total loss of gastric digestion, and lingual lipases can accommodate, in part, some loss of pancreatic lipase production.

Digestive enzymes and zymogens

Most digestive enzymes in the gut are secreted as inactive precursors

With the exception of amylase and lingual (tongue-associated) lipases, digestive enzymes secreted into the gut lumen are present as inactive precursors termed zymogens. The secretion of all gut enzymes is similar in the salivary glands, gastric mucosa and pancreas. These organs contain specialized cells for the synthesis, packaging, and transport of enzymes to the cell surface, and thence to the intestinal lumen. These secretions are termed exocrine, that is, 'secreting to the outside' (as opposed to the endocrine secretion of hormones).

Enzymes involved in protein digestion (proteases) and the lipase, phospholipase A_2, are synthesized as inactive zymogens and are only activated on their release to the gut lumen. In general, these enzymes, once in their active form, can activate their own precursors. Activation of their precursors can occur by either change in pH (e.g. pepsinogen in the stomach

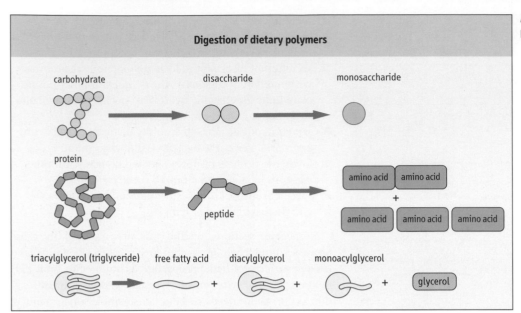

Digestion of dietary polymers

Fig. 9.2 **Digestion of dietary polymers.**

is converted at pH below 4.0 to the active enzyme, pepsin), or by the action of specific enteropeptidases bound to the mucosal membrane of the duodenum (see Fig. 9.1).

All digestive enzymes are hydrolases

All digestive enzymes hydrolyze their substrates. The products of such hydrolytic procedures are oligomers, dimers, and monomers of parent macromolecules. Thus carbohydrates are hydrolyzed to a mixture of disaccharides and monosaccharides. Proteins are broken down to a mixture of di- and tripeptides and amino acids. Lipids, however, are treated differently – they are broken down to a mixture of fatty acids (FA), glycerol, and mono-, and diacylglycerols (Fig. 9.2).

Digestion and absorption of carbohydrates

Dietary carbohydrates enter the gut as mono-, di-, and polysaccharides

Dietary carbohydrates consist of mainly plant and animal starches (polysaccharides), the disaccharides sucrose and lactose, and monosaccharides such as glucose and fructose (Fig. 9.3). Monosaccharides, glucose, fructose, and galactose, are either constituents of the diet, or are produced by digestion of di- and polysaccharides – galactose is derived mainly from dairy products. The sugar monomers require no further digestion to be absorbed from the GI tract.

 POLYSACCHARIDE DIGESTION

During the eating process and the homogenization that occurs with mastication in the mouth and the action of gastric folds, dietary polysaccharides become hydrated. Hydration of polysaccharides is essential for the appropriate action of amylase. This enzyme is specific for internal $\alpha_1 \rightarrow 4$-glycosidic linkages and is totally inert towards $\alpha_1 \rightarrow 6$ linkages. In addition amylase does not act on $\alpha_1 \rightarrow 4$ linkages of glycosyl residues serving as branching units (see Fig. 9.4). The cleaved units thus formed are the trisaccharide maltotriose, the disaccharide maltose and an oligosaccharide with one or more $\alpha_1 \rightarrow 6$ branches and containing on average eight glycosyl units termed the 'α-limit dextrin'. These compounds are then further cleaved to glucose units by oligosaccharidase and α-glucosidase, the latter removing single glucose residues from $\alpha_1 \rightarrow 4$-linked oligosaccharides (including maltose) from the nonreducing end of the oligomer. A sucrase-isomaltase complex, secreted as a single polypeptide precursor molecule and activated to two separate active polypeptide enzymes, one of which (isomaltase) is responsible for the hydrolytic cleavage of $\alpha_1 \rightarrow 6$ glycosidic linkages. This final product of digestion of starches is thus glucose, but it is generated through a complex series of enzyme reactions. The initial digestion involves amylase, which occurs free in the lumen, whereas the final processes involve α-glucosidases and isomaltase, which are attached to the mucosal membrane of the enterocyte.

Dietary carbohydrates

Carbohydrate	Food source	Structure
starch (amylose) [plant]	potatoes, rice, bread, onions	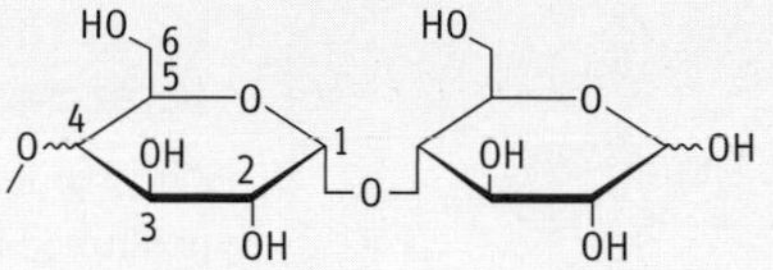
amylopectin (glycogen) [plant, animal]	potatoes, rice, bread, muscle, liver	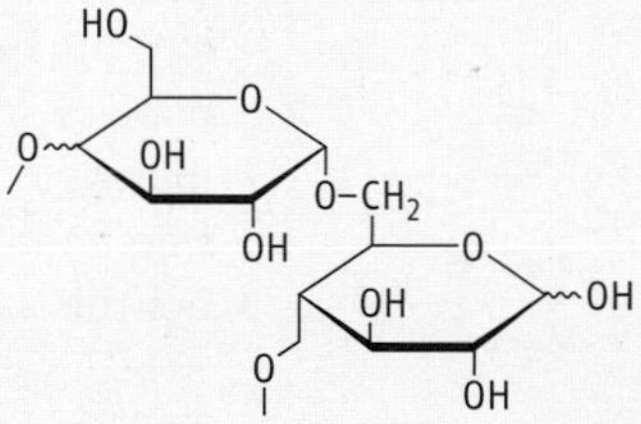
sucrose	desserts, sweets, 'sugar'	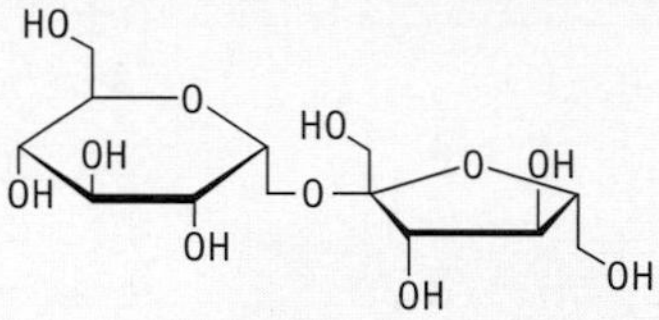
lactose	milk	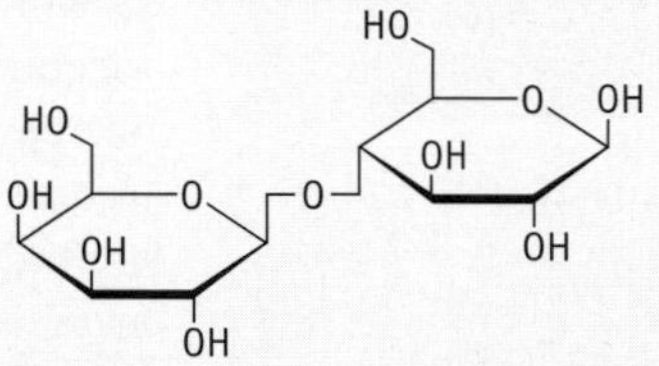
fructose	fruits, honey	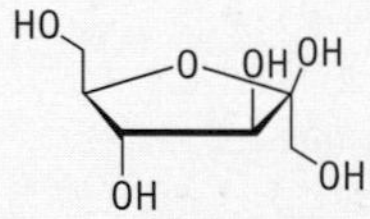
glucose	fruits, honey	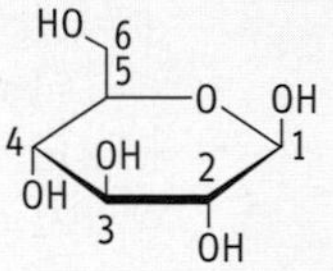

Fig. 9.3 **Structure of the main dietary carbohydrates.** The notation below the formulas of oligosaccharides and polysaccharides indicates the carbon atoms, which are involved in the linkages between the component monosaccharides. Refer to the glucose molecule for the standard numbering of carbon atoms. Monosaccharides exist in several isomeric forms. Their classification into D- and L-forms is based on the orientation of the hydrogen and hydroxyl groups at the asymmetric carbon atom adjacent to the terminal alcohol group. These isomers rotate the polarized light to the right (D) or left (L). The reference molecule for this system of classification is the simplest monosaccharide (triose), glyceraldehyde. In the ring forms of pentoses and higher sugars the carbon atom at position 1 also becomes asymmetric (anomeric). Different steric arrangements in this position result in either α or β anomers. α-Anomers have hydroxyl group pointing below the plane of the ring structure, and β anomers have hydroxyl group pointing above the plane.

Disaccharides and polysaccharides (starch and glycogen) require hydrolytic cleavage prior to absorption

Disaccharides are acted upon by membrane-bound disaccharidases on the intestinal mucosal surface. Starch and glycogen require additional hydrolytic capacity of the enzyme amylase found in the secretions of the salivary glands and pancreas (Fig. 9.4).

Starch is a plant polysaccharide and glycogen is its animal equivalent. Both contain a mixture of linear chains of glucose molecules linked by $\alpha_1 \rightarrow 4$ glycosidic bonds (amylose) and by branched glucose chains with $\alpha_1 \rightarrow 6$ linkages (amylopectin). Glycogen contains more branches than starch. The digestion of these polysaccharides is carried out by endosaccharidases and amylase produced by the salivary glands and pancreas. Amylase in the gut lumen is not bound to the mucosal membranes of enterocytes.

The products of hydrolysis of starch are the disaccharide maltose, the trisaccharide maltotriose and a branched unit, termed the α-limit dextrin. These products are then further hydrolyzed by the α-glucosidases, enzymes bound to the enterocyte mucosal membrane, to form the monosaccharide glucose (Fig. 9.5A).

Dietary disaccharides such as lactose, sucrose, and trehalose are hydrolyzed to their constituent monomeric sugars by a series of specific disaccharidases, which are attached to the small intestinal brush-border membrane.

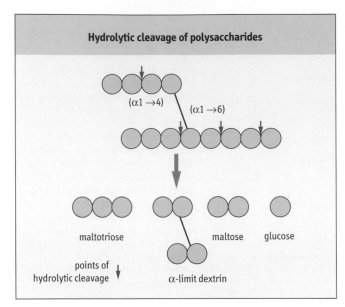

Hydrolytic cleavage of polysaccharides

$(\alpha1 \rightarrow 4)$ $(\alpha1 \rightarrow 6)$

maltotriose   maltose   glucose

points of
hydrolytic cleavage α-limit dextrin

Fig. 9.4 **Hydrolytic cleavage of polysaccharides.**

CYSTIC FIBROSIS AND PANCREATIC INSUFFICIENCY (INCIDENCE 1 IN 2000)

A three-year-old girl was brought the outpatient clinic by her parents because they felt that she was not growing and was underweight. She had good appetite but was still wearing clothes size appropriate for 12–18 month child. The parents indicated she passed stool four times a day. She had been diagnosed with asthma at 18 months and had been given oral salbutamol daily. Despite this, she had since needed four courses of antibiotics to clear chest infections.

Comment. When this child's height and weight are compared with normative data, they are both below the third centile. She thus demonstrates failure to thrive. With recurrent respiratory symptoms, a re-evaluation of the diagnosis of asthma is required. Here the measurement of chloride concentration in a sample of sweat demonstrated raised concentration (>60 mmol/L); this is diagnostic for cystic fibrosis. Also, the 3-day faecal fat collection showed grossly elevated fat content, indicating intestinal malabsorption. The increased bronchial secretions, which give rise to recurrent respiratory infections and lung damage, similarly affect other organs, particularly the pancreatic ducts where the mucus blocks the pancreatic ducts. The auto-digestion of pancreatic tissue ensues and this damages the exocrine pancreas. With time, glucose intolerance or overt diabetes may develop.
The treatment is with oral capsules containing pancreatic enzymes, which dissolve in the alkaline environment of the jejunum, releasing the content, are required. Careful assessment of fat-soluble vitamin concentration is also necessary to prevent deficiency. Malabsorption may be the presenting complaint in this common inherited disorder.

The catalytic domains of these proteins are present in the lumen to react with their substrates, while their noncatalytic, structural domain(s) are attached to the enterocyte membrane.

With the exception of lactase, all disaccharidases are inducible

The greater the amount of a disaccharide found in the diet or produced by digestion, the greater is the amount of a specific disaccharidase produced by the enterocyte. The rate-limiting step in absorption of dietary disaccharides is thus the transport of resultant monomeric sugars. Lactase is a non-inducible brush-border disaccharidase and therefore the rate-limiting factor in lactose absorption is its hydrolysis and not the transport of glucose and galactose.

There are active and passive transport systems which transport carbohydrates across the brush-border membrane

Since the process of digestion adds to the osmotic load within the gut lumen, water moves from the vascular compartment to the gut (see Chapter 22). Increased brush-border hydrolysis will thus increase the osmotic load, while increased monosaccharide transport across the enterocyte brush border will decrease it. As discussed above, for most oligo- and disaccharidases the transport of the produced monomers is rate-limiting and thus compensatory mechanisms exist to avoid accumulation of fluid in the gut. As concentrations of monomeric sugars increase in the gut lumen causing an increase in osmolality, there is a compensatory decrease in the activity of brush-border disaccharidases. This controls the osmotic load and prevents fluid shifts.

Glucose, fructose, and galactose are the primary monosaccharides produced by the digestion of dietary carbohydrate. The absorption of these sugars and other minor monosaccharides is via specific carrier-mediated mechanisms (Fig. 9.5B), all of which demonstrate substrate specificity and stereospecificity, show saturation kinetics and can be specifically inhibited. In addition, all monosaccharides can cross the brush-border membrane by a simple diffusion process, although this is extremely slow.

At least two carrier-mediated transport systems for monosaccharides exist – an Na^+-dependent co-transporter and an Na^+-independent transporter

At the brush-border membrane both glucose and galactose are transported by the Na^+-dependent glucose transporter. This membrane-linked protein binds with glucose (galactose) and Na^+ at separate sites and transports both into cytosol. The Na^+ is thus transported down its concentration gradient (a concentration in the gut lumen versus that inside of the cell), carrying glucose along against its concentration gradient. This transport mechanism is linked to Na^+-dependent

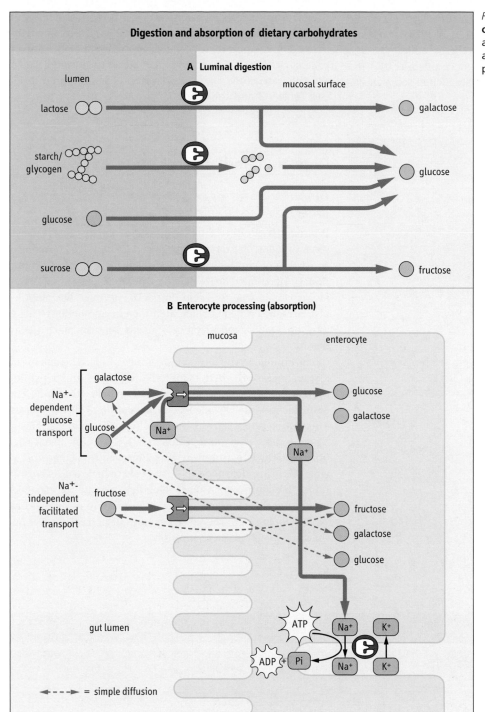

Digestion and absorption of dietary carbohydrates

A Luminal digestion

lumen

mucosal surface

lactose → galactose

starch/glycogen → glucose

glucose → glucose

sucrose → fructose

B Enterocyte processing (absorption)

mucosa

enterocyte

galactose

Na⁺-dependent glucose transport

glucose

Na⁺

glucose

galactose

Na⁺

Na⁺-independent facilitated transport

fructose

fructose

galactose

glucose

gut lumen

ATP

ADP + Pi

Na⁺ K⁺

Na⁺ K⁺

- - - → = simple diffusion

Fig. 9.5 **Digestion and absorption of dietary carbohydrates.** ADP, adenosine diphosphate; ATP, adenosine triphosphate; Pi inorganic phosphate.

ATPase, which then removes Na^+ from the cell in exchange for K^+, with the concomitant hydrolysis of ATP. The transport of glucose (galactose) is thus an indirect active process. The interesting consequence of this mechanism is that the sodium absorption in the gut is facilitated when some carbohydrates are present in the lumen.

 ## THE PANCREAS

Pancreas contains the exocrine part secreting digestive enzymes and an endocrine part, the islets of Langerhans which secrete insulin, glucagon and other hormones such as somatostatin (see Chapter 20) .Anatomically, it consists of multiple subunits called acini.

The exocrine pancreatic secretions are secreted into the pancreatic duct which then joins the common bile duct before it enters duodenum. Food particles entering the duodenum stimulate the secretion of cholecystokinin and it in turn activates pancreatic enzyme production and secretion. Also, acid secreted in the stomach stimulates the production of hormone secretin, which in turn stimulates the production of bicarbonate-rich pancreatic juice. This neutralizes the acid contained in the food entering the duodenum from the stomach.

Pancreas secretes enzymes, which digest all three main types of nutrients: proteases and peptidases are secreted as proenzymes to protect itself from autodigestion; they are activated by enzymic degradation in the small intestine. Pancreatic amylase digests carbohydrates to oligosaccharides and monosaccharides. Lipase digests triacylglycerols yielding monoglycerides and free fatty acids, and cholesteryl esterase yields free cholesterol and fatty acids.

Fructose is transported across the brush-border membrane by an Na^+-independent facilitated diffusion process involving a specific membrane-associated protein, possibly glucose transporter (GLUT-5), which is present on the luminal side of the enterocyte, and GLUT 2 present on the antiluminal side (see Table 9.2 and Table 7.5).

Digestion and absorption of lipids

Globules of fat need to be emulsified before digestion can take place

Approximately 90% of fat contained in the diet is as triacylglycerols (TAG), also termed triglycerides, with the remainder consisting of cholesterol, cholesteryl ester, phospholipid and nonesterified fatty acids (NEFA). The hydrophobic nature of fats excludes water-soluble digestive enzymes. Fat globules also present limited surface area for enzyme action. This is why an emulsification process needs to take place before digestion can begin.

The change in the physical structure of lipids begins in the stomach where the heat helps to liquefy lipids, and peristaltic movements aid in the formation of a lipid emulsion. The emulsification is also aided by the salivary and gastric lipases. The initial rate of hydrolysis is slow due to the separate aqueous and lipid phases and relatively small lipid–water interface. Once hydrolysis begins, however, the water-immiscible TAGs are degraded to fatty acids, which act as surfactants, breaking down lipid globules to smaller particles increasing their surface and facilitating more rapid hydrolysis. The lipid phase therefore becomes dispersed throughout the aqueous phase as an emulsion.

Enzymes that digest proteins				
Source	Zymogen/enzyme	Activation	Substrate	End product
stomach				
fundus	pepsinogen A	HCl	protein	peptides
pylorus	pepsinogen B	pH 1–2 autoactivation	protein	peptides
pancreas	trypsinogen	enteropeptidase, trypsin	protein, peptides	polypeptides, dipeptides
	chymotrypsinogen	trypsin	protein, peptides	as for trypsin
	proelastase	trypsin	protein, peptides	polypeptides dipeptides
	procarboxy-peptidases	trypsin	polypeptides at –COOH end	small peptides, amino acids
small intestine (no inactive precursor)	aminopeptidase	not applicable	polypeptide at –NH_2 end dipeptides	small peptides, amino acids amino acids
	dipeptidases endopeptidases		polypeptides	small peptides, dipeptides

Table 9.2 **Enzymes responsible for protein digestion.**

PANCREATITIS

The inflammatory reaction affecting pancreas (pancreatitis) is a serious disease. Acute pancreatitis is most often caused by gallstones or excessive alcohol intake. It may also be caused by some drugs and by high concentration of plasma triacylglycerols. The patients present with a severe abdominal pain, nausea, and vomiting. The most important biochemical marker is the increased serum activity of the enzyme amylase. Acute pancreatitis is also usually accompanied by hypocalcemia and by increased activity of serum lipase. Because in a proportion of patients amylase remains normal or only a little elevated, other tests such as pancreatic imaging (computed tomography (CT) or ultrasound) are used together with biochemical tests to confirm the diagnosis. Chronic inflammatory process affecting the pancreas (chronic pancreatitis) may lead to more metabolic complications such as hyperglycemia, malnutrition, and, characteristically, steatorrhoea defined as an increased excretion of fat in stools.

Other dietary components also act as surfactants. These include phospholipids, fatty acids and monoacylglycerols. They aid in the emulsification process and promote the binding of the acid-stable lipases to the interface. This in turn facilitates the hydrolysis of TAGs and the emulsification of lipids.

In the duodenum, pancreatic enzymes and bile salts act on the lipid emulsion

The lipid emulsion is ejected from the stomach into the duodenum where dietary lipid undergoes its major digestive process using enzymes secreted by the pancreas. There, solubilization is further aided by the release of bile salts from the gall bladder. The secretion of bile from the gall bladder is stimulated by the hormone cholecystokinin.

The major enzyme secreted by the pancreas is pancreatic lipase. This enzyme is, however, inactivated in the presence of bile salts normally secreted during lipid digestion into the small intestine. This inhibition is overcome by the concomitant secretion of co-lipase by the pancreas. Co-lipase binds to both the water-lipid interface and to pancreatic lipase, simultaneously anchoring and activating the enzyme. As indicated in Figure 9.6, very little dietary TAG is completely hydrolyzed to glycerol and fatty acids. The 'second' and 'third' fatty acids in TAGs are hydrolyzed with increasing difficulty; therefore the action of pancreatic lipase produces mainly 2-monoacylglycerol (2-MAG) for absorption into enterocytes.

Bile salts are essential for solubilizing lipids during the digestive process

Without bile salts acting as detergents, the digested lipid would not be in a form suitable for absorption from the gut. The structure of bile acids is demonstrated by cholic acid

(Fig. 9.7, also Chapter 28). Its molecule is planar with both a hydrophobic and hydrophilic surface. The hydrophobic region of bile acids is formed by the upper surface of the fused-ring system, while the carboxyl group and all hydroxyl groups are on the opposite surface, conveying hydrophilicity (see also Chapter 16, Fig. 16.6). Bile acids (or actually bile salts at the alkaline pH of the intestine), reversibly form aggregates at concentrations above a critical level, the so-called critical micellar concentration. Such aggregates are termed 'micelles' and their constituent bile acids are in equilibrium with free bile acids. Micelles are thus equilibrium structures of well-defined size (which is considerably smaller than lipid emulsion droplets). The size of these micelles is dependent on the bile acid concentration and the ratio of bile acid to lipids.

Thus, fat emulsion turns into micellar structures. This facilitates the transport of fat through the aqueous environment of the gut. Bile salt micelles can solubilize other lipids and these mixed micelles have disc-like shapes. During digestion of TAGs, the lipid digest changes from the fat emulsion droplets into micellar structures. The micelles mediate the transport of lipid digest through the aqueous environment of the gut lumen to the brush border of the enterocytes, where the digest is absorbed. Most fatty acids and 2-MAG are absorbed into the epithelial cells, however, water-insoluble lipids, such as cholesterol, are poorly absorbed in the small intestine.

The absorption of lipids into epithelial cells of the small intestine occurs by diffusion through the plasma membrane. Almost 100% of fatty acids and 2-MAGs is absorbed, both being slightly water-soluble. Water-insoluble lipids are poorly absorbed – only 30–40% of dietary cholesterol is absorbed. The bile salts pass on to the ileum where they themselves are absorbed and passed back to the liver via the so-called enterohepatic circulation.

The fate of fatty acids entering enterocytes dependents on their chain length

Medium- and short-chain (containing less than 10 carbon atoms) fatty acids pass directly through the cells to the hepatic portal blood supply. In contrast, fatty acids of more than 12 carbon atoms are bound to a fatty acid-binding protein and transferred to the rough endoplasmic reticulum for resynthesis into TAGs. The glycerol for this process is provided by the absorbed 2-MAGs (the MAG pathway; see Fig. 9.6), by the hydrolysis of 1-MAGs producing free glycerol, or via glycerol-3-phosphate generated during glycolysis (the phosphatidic acid pathway; see Fig. 9.6). Glycerol produced in the intestinal lumen is not reutilized in the enterocyte for TAG synthesis but passes directly to the portal system.

TAG synthesis requires activation of fatty acids

Fatty acid activation is accomplished by the formation of acyl-CoA derivatives by acyl-CoA synthase. All long-chain

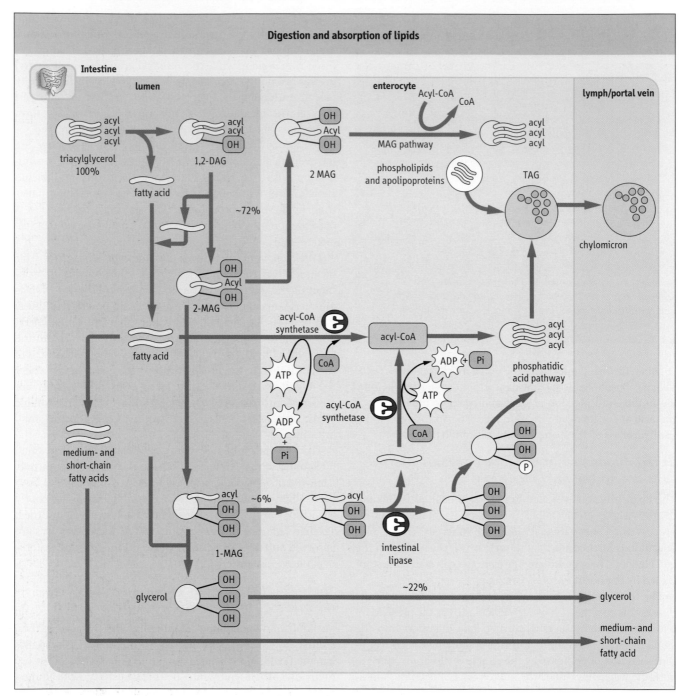

Fig. 9.6 Digestion and absorption of dietary lipids. The percentages can vary widely, but they indicate the relative importance of the three routes indicated. TAG, triacylglycerol; DAG, diacylglycerol; MAG, monoacylglycerol; CoA, coenzyme A. This diagram does not take into account the solubilization factors involved or micelle formation (see below). Note that enterocytes do not possess glycerol kinase. The formation of glycerol phosphate requires the presence of glucose.

fatty acids absorbed by the intestinal epithelial cells are neutilized to form TAG before being transferred to the lymphatic system as chylomicrons. Chylomicrons are large, lipid-rich (99% lipid, 1% protein) particles assembled within enterocytes on the rough endoplasmic reticulum. They are released into the intercellular space by exocytosis and then leave the intestine via the lymphatics. The protein component, apolipoprotein B48 is essential for the final release of chylomicrons from the enterocyte (see Chapter 17).

Bile acid – structure and stereochemistry

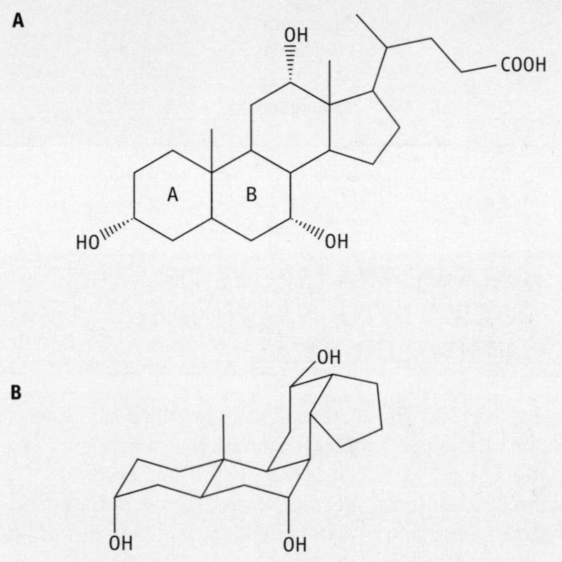

Fig. 9.7 **Bile acid structure and stereochemistry.** Cholic acid is one of the main bile acids. (A) Structure of cholic acid. (B) Stereochemical structure of cholic acid. Compare Fig. 16.6.

GASTRIC ULCER

Gastric ulcer results from the damage to the lining of the stomach of the duodenum

Its treatment is focused on neutralizing the effects of acid on the lining of the stomach and includes the use of alkali suspensions to neutralize the hydrogen ion, the proton pump inhibitors, and the drugs which block histamine H_2 receptors, inhibiting acid secretion (see Chapter 7).

Digestion and absorption of proteins

The protein load received by the gut is derived from two primary sources: 70–100 g dietary protein and 35–200 g endogenous protein, the latter being either proteins secreted and into the gut (mostly enzymes) or shed as a result of turnover of epithelial cells. Only 1–2 g nitrogen, equivalent to 6–12 g protein, are lost in the feces daily. Thus, the digestion and absorption of protein is extremely efficient.

Proteins are hydrolyzed by peptidases

Proteins are broken down by hydrolysis of peptide bonds and hence the enzymes involved are termed 'peptidases'. These enzymes can either cleave internal peptide bonds (endopeptidases) or cleave off one amino acid at a time from either the –COOH or –NH_2 terminal of the polypeptide (exopeptidases subclassified into carboxypeptidases and aminopeptidases, respectively). The endopeptidases cut the large polypeptides to smaller oligopeptides, which can be acted upon by the exopeptidases to produce the final products of protein digestion, di- and tripeptides and amino acids, which are then absorbed by the enterocytes. Depending on the source of the peptidases, protein digestion can be divided into gastric, pancreatic and intestinal phases (Fig 9.8 and Table 9.2). The specificity of peptidases is illustrated in Table 9.1.

Protein digestion begins in the stomach

In the stomach, secreted HCl reduces the pH to 1–2 with consequent denaturation of dietary proteins (Fig. 7.8).

THE STOMACH

Different cell types present in the stomach perform different digestive functions. The chief cells secrete pepsinogen, a precursor of a peptidase, pepsin. Pepsinogen is activated to pepsin in the acid environment of the stomach lumen. The parietal cells generate hydrogen ion in the stomach by the action of carbonic anhydrase (see Chapter 23). Hydrogen ion is secreted by the ATP-dependent proton pump located on the luminal membrane of these cells (see Chapter 7, Fig. 7.8). The secretion of the parietal cells is stimulated by the histamine-secreting cells, histamine acting on the H_2 receptors on the parietal cells. The G-cells in the stomach secrete the hormone gastrin. Gastrin secretion is stimulated by food entering stomach.

Stomach cells also secrete the intrinsic factor (IF) which facilitates the absorption of vitamin B_{12}. Finally stomach cells secrete mucus which is alkaline and protects the stomach lining against the effects of the acid.

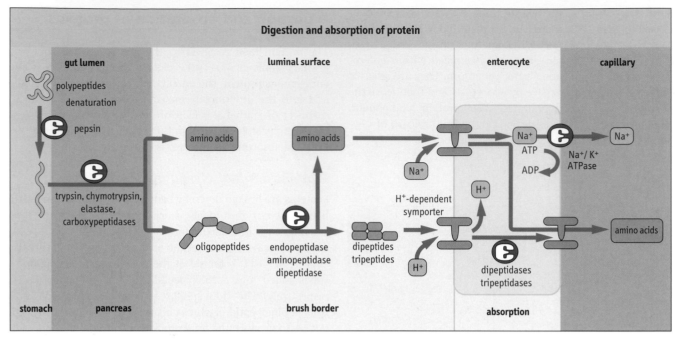

Fig. 9.8 **Digestion and absorption of proteins.**

Denaturation makes proteins more accessible to protease activity by the unfolding of the polypeptide chain. In addition, pepsins are secreted by the chief cells of the gastric mucosa. These acid proteases are released as the inactive precursors, pepsinogens A and B, and are activated by either an intramolecular reaction (autoactivation) at a pH below 5 or by active pepsin (autocatalysis). At a pH above 2, the liberated peptide remains bound to pepsin and acts as an inhibitor of pepsin activity. This inhibition is removed by either a decrease in pH below 2 or by further pepsin action. The major products of pepsin digestion of proteins are large peptide fragments and some free amino acids. The gastric protein digests in turn stimulate cholecystokinin release in the duodenum, initiating the release of the main digestive enzymes by the pancreas.

The proteolytic enzymes released from the pancreas are, similarly to the pepsins, released as inactive zymogens: the duodenal enteropeptidase converts trypsinogen to the active trypsin. This enzyme is then capable of autoactivation and and the activation of all other pancreatic zymogens, thus activating chymotrypsin, elastase, and carboxypeptidases A and B. Since the prime role of trypsin is activating other pancreatic enzymes, its activity is controlled within the pancreas and pancreatic ducts by a low molecular weight inhibitory peptide.

 ACTIVE TRANSPORT OF AMINO ACIDS INTO INTESTINAL EPITHELIAL CELLS

These mechanisms are similar to those described for glucose uptake. At the brush border membrane Na$^+$-dependent symporters (membrane transporters which transport two substances in the same direction – see Chapter 7) for amino acid uptake are linked to ATP-dependent pumping out of Na$^+$ at the contraluminal membrane. A similar H$^+$-dependent symporter is present on the brush-border surface for di- and tri-peptide active transport into the cell. Na$^+$-independent transporters are present on the contraluminal surface, thus allowing the facilitated transport of amino acids to the hepatic portal system.

From both genetic and transporter studies, at least six specific symporter systems have been identified for the uptake of L-amino acids from the intestinal lumen:

- neutral amino acid symporter for amino acids with short or polar side-chains (Ser, Thr, Ala);
- neutral amino acid symporter for aromatic or hydrophobic side-chains (Phe, Tyr, Met, Val, Leu, Ileu);
- imino acid symporter (Pro, OH-Pro);
- basic amino acid symporter (Lys, Arg, Cys);
- acidic amino acid symporter (Asp, Glu);
- β-amino acid symporter (β-Ala, Tau).

These transport systems are also present in the renal tubules and defects in their constituent protein structure can lead to disease (e.g. Hartnup disease). Pathologies of similar mechanism can thus be produced in both the kidney and intestine.

LACTOSE INTOLERANCE

A 15-year-old African-American boy came across to the UK on an exchange visit for 2 months. After 2 weeks in the UK, he complained of abdominal discomfort, a feeling of being bloated, increased passage of urine and, more recently, the development of diarrhoea. His only change in diet noted at the time was the introduction of milk into his diet. He had developed a considerable liking for milk and was consuming 1–2 large cartons per day. A lactose tolerance test was performed, whereby the young man was given 50 g lactose in an aqueous vehicle to drink. Plasma glucose levels did not rise by more than 1 mmol/L (18 mg/dL) over the next 2 hours, with sampling at 30-minute intervals. A diagnosis of lactose intolerance was made.

Comment. Lactose intolerance is a physiologic change resulting from acquired lactase deficiency. Lactase activity decreases with increasing age in children but the extent of the decline in activity genetically determined and demonstrates ethnic variation. Lactase deficiency in the adult black population varies from 45–95%. If symptoms of malabsorption occur after the introduction of milk to adult diets, the diagnosis of acquired lactase deficiency should be considered. A diagnosis is made by challenging the small bowel with lactose and monitoring the rise in plasma glucose. An increase of more than 1.7 mmol/L (30 mg/dL) is considered normal. A rise of less than 1.1 mmol/L (20 mg/dL) is diagnostic of lactase deficiency. A rise of 1.1–1.7 mmol/L (20–30 mg/dL) is inconclusive.

COELIAC DISEASE

A 22-year-old man presented with a history of weight loss, diarrhea, abdominal bloating and anemia. He described his stools as pale and bulky. Laboratory features included hemoglobin of 90 g/L (9 g/dL) (reference range 130–180 g/L; 13–18 g/dL). Biopsy of his small bowel demonstrated flattening of the mucosal surface, villous atrophy and disappearance of microvilli. A diagnosis of gluten-induced enteropathy or coeliac disease was made. All wheat products were removed from the patient's diet and the symptoms resolved.

Comment. Coeliac disease is an autoimmune condition characterized by malabsorption and specific diagnostic features exhibited by the intestinal mucosa. Since the absorptive surface is markedly reduced, the resulting indigestion/malabsorption is severe. The histologic changes are due to the interaction of gluten, the principal protein of wheat, with the epithelium. There is evidence to suggest that the deficit is located within the mucosal cells of the intestine and permits polypeptides, resulting from peptic and tryptic digestion of gluten, not only to exert local harmful effects within the intestine but also to be absorbed and to induce an antibody response. Circulating antibodies to wheat gluten and its fractions are frequently present in cases of coeliac disease. The use of sensitive and specific serological screening tests, such as endomysial antibodies of IgA subclass has shown that coeliac disease is under-diagnosed, especially in patients with unexplained anaemia.
For hematology reference values, refer to Table 4.2 on p. 48.

Pancreatic proteases have different substrate specificity with respect to peptide bond cleavage

Trypsin cleaves proteins at lysine and arginine residues, chymotrypsin at aromatic amino acids and elastase at smaller hydrophobic amino acids. The combined effect of these pancreatic enzymes is to produce an abundance of free amino acids and small molecular weight peptides of two to eight residues in length.

In association with protease secretion, the pancreas also produces copious amounts of sodium bicarbonate ($NaHCO_3$). This results in the neutralization of the acid contents of the stomach, promoting pancreatic alkaline protease activity.

Endopeptidases, dipeptidases and aminopeptidases complete the digestion of proteins

The final digestion of oligo- and dipeptides is dependent on membrane-bound small intestinal endopeptidases, dipeptidases, and aminopeptidases. The end-products of this surface enzyme activity are free amino acids, and di- and tripeptides which can then be absorbed across the enterocyte membrane by specific carrier-mediated transport. Di- and tripeptides are further hydrolyzed to their constituent amino acids inside the enterocyte. The final step is the transfer of the free amino acids across the contraluminal plasma membrane into the portal system.

Certain carbohydrates and proteins cannot be properly digested by some individuals and lead to the development of disease. The commonest of these is lactose intolerance and gluten (wheat protein) sensitivity, the latter also known as coeliac disease (see the two boxes on this page). Elimination of these foods from the diet is, in essence, the treatment for these particular pathologies.

Summary

- Absorption and digestion of foods make the metabolic fuels available to the organism.
- Carbohydrates are digested to simple sugars.
- Fats are hydrolzed to di- and monoglycerides.
- Proteins are hydrolyzed to di- and tripeptides and free amino acids.

- Digestion is a series of processes which prepare food for absorption.
- Defects in these mechanisms result in a variety of malabsorption and food intolerance syndromes.

ACTIVE LEARNING

1. Describe the process of digestion of starch.
2. Discuss the possible complications of persistent vomiting.
3. Which hormones aid digestion?
4. List the secretory products of the stomach.
5. Outline the mechanisms of sugar transport in the small intestine.
6. What is the role of micelles in the digestion of fat?

Further reading

Bronner F. Calcium absorption – a paradigm for mineral absorption. *J of Nutr* 1998;**128**:917–20.

Duerksen DR, Nehra V, Bistrian BR, Blackburn GL. Appropriate nutritional support in acute and complicated Crohn's disease. *Nutition* 1998;**14**:462–465.

Rose RC. Intestinal absorption of water soluble vitamins. *Proceedings of the Society for Experimental Biology and Medicine* 1996;**212**:191–198.

Green PHR Jabri B. Coeliac disease. *Lancet* 2003; **362**:383–91

Mowat AM. Coeliac disease – a meeting point for genetics, immunology, and protein chemistry. *Lancet* 2003;**361**:1290–92

Mitchell RMS *et al.* Pancreatitis. *Lancet* 2003;**361**:1447–55.

10. Micronutrients: Vitamins and Minerals

M H Dominiczak and I Broom

LEARNING OBJECTIVES

After reading this chapter you should be able to:

- Describe the groups of fat-soluble and water-soluble vitamins.
- Discuss the actions, sources and signs and symptoms of deficiencies of vitamins.
- List methods of measurement of vitamins relevant to clinical assessment of nutritional status.
- Describe the role of trace metals in metabolism.

INTRODUCTION

Vitamins and trace metals are an important part of nutrition and many of them are essential nutrients. Deficiencies of micronutrients lead to specific clinical syndromes. They accompany general malnutrition or become manifested during illness. They also may occur as a result of surgical procedures on the gastrointestinal tract. Importantly, multiple deficiencies of micronutrients are much more common than single deficiencies. This chapter should be read in conjunction with Chapter 21.

Vitamins are an inherent part of functional protein molecules. They act as coenzymes in the specific reactions, e.g. riboflavin in oxidoreductase reactions or biotin in carboxylation reactions. There are fat-soluble and water-soluble vitamins. Fat-soluble vitamins are vitamins A, D, E, and K, and water-soluble are vitamins B_1, B_2, B_3, B_5, B_6, B_{12}, folate, biotin and C.

Several trace metals are also essential nutrients

Many of the trace metals function as part of protein molecules or metalloenzymes. Such proteins, without their trace metal prosthetic groups, e.g. Zn, Mn, or Mg, lose their biological function. Some trace elements are cytotoxic. In addition to the essential trace elements, other trace metals (e.g. cadmium, mercury, and aluminium) find their way into the food chain and can be toxic to cells. The toxic metals also include essential trace elements when taken in large amounts, e.g. copper and manganese. The essential requirements for these metals in the prevention of disease and their association with certain pathologies only came to light when suitable analytical methods such atomic absorption spectrometry and mass spectrometry were developed.

To prevent the development of pathologies caused by vitamin or trace metal deficiencies, certain levels of intake have been recommended for healthy people. The requirement for vitamins depends, to some extent, on the macronutrient intake (Chapter 21). Although single deficiency states may occur, poor diets are often characterized by multiple nutrient deficiencies. Specific vitamin-associated pathologies are also well recognized.

Malnutrition is usually associated with multiple nutrient deficiencies

Assessment of nutrient status is fraught with difficulties since malnutrition is usually associated with multiple nutrient deficiencies, each one having functional implications, and all being interrelated. Micronutrient assessment is even more difficult in situations where subclinical deficits exist. Measurements of circulating vitamin levels are inappropriate in the case of water-soluble vitamins, because these levels relate to the recent intake and do not reflect overall vitamin status. Therefore, measurement of enzyme function associated with particular water-soluble vitamins has been suggested as the most appropriate way to assess micronutrient status. This is usually carried out as stimulation tests, i.e., enzyme activity is measured in the absence and then in the presence of the vitamin as reagent. Deficit is recognized if there is a stimulation of enzyme activity in the presence of added vitamins.

There are also potential problems with interpretation of circulating concentrations of fat-soluble vitamins. These vitamins are associated with body fat and are often stored in specific tissues with circulating concentrations kept relatively constant; for example, vitamin A is stored in the liver and transported by specific binding proteins in the plasma. Furthermore, a decrease in level of a nutrient within blood or plasma does not need to indicate a deficiency or an increased requirement: it could be simply reflecting a metabolic adjustment to stress or a change in physiologic status, such as pregnancy. Similar principles apply to trace metals, where the circulating levels bear little relation to nutrient status. For evaluation of trace element toxicity, tissues other than blood may need to be analyzed before a definite diagnosis of metal poisoning can be made.

FAT-SOLUBLE VITAMINS

Fat-soluble vitamins are stored in tissues

Fat-soluble vitamins are not as readily absorbed or extracted from the diet as water-soluble vitamins but ample reserves are stored in tissues. With the exception of vitamin K they do not act as coenzymes. Indeed, vitamins A and D behave more like hormones. Note that vitamin A and vitamin D can be toxic in excess amounts. This is not true of either vitamin E or K.

Vitamin A

'Vitamin A' is a generic term for three compounds, retinol, retinal and retinoic acid, all of which are found in animals. Vitamin A is found in animals as retinol, retinal, and retinoic acid; its provitamin, β-carotene, is found in plant food. The term 'retinoids' has been used to define these three substances as well as other synthetic compounds associated with vitamin A-like activity. Vitamin A provitamin, β-carotene, is converted to all-*trans* retinal by the action of β-carotene dioxygenase in the small bowel. Further metabolism in the enterocytes produces retinol and retinoic acid (Fig. 10.1)

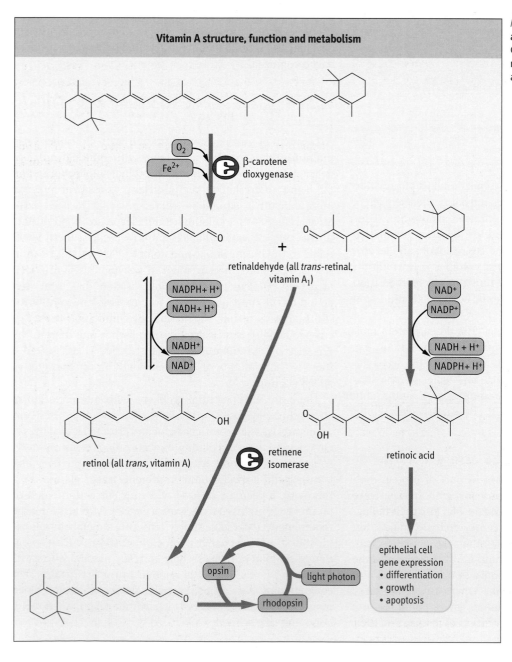

Vitamin A structure, function and metabolism

O₂
Fe²⁺
β-carotene dioxygenase

retinaldehyde (all *trans*-retinal, vitamin A₁)

+

NADPH+ H⁺
NADH+ H⁺
NADH⁺
NAD⁺

NAD⁺
NADP⁺
NADH + H⁺
NADPH+ H⁺

retinol (all *trans*, vitamin A)

retinene isomerase

retinoic acid

opsin
light photon
rhodopsin

epithelial cell gene expression
• differentiation
• growth
• apoptosis

Fig. 10.1 **Structure, metabolism and function of vitamin A.** Conversion of retinaldehyde to retinoic acid is irreversible. (See also Chapter 39.)

which are then transported to the liver where vitamin A is stored as retinol palmitate. The stores of vitamin A in the liver comprise approximately 1 year's supply. Liver, egg yolk, butter, and milk are good sources of pre-formed vitamin A. Dark-green and yellow vegetables are good sources of β-carotene. Conversion of carotenoids to vitamin A is rarely 100% efficient and the potency of foods is described in retinol equivalents (RE; 1 RE equals 1 mg of retinol or 6 mg β-carotene, or 12 mg of other carotenes).

Is vitamin A protective against cancer and cardiovascular disease?

Recently β-carotene has received attention in its role as an antioxidant. Since normal epithelial cell growth and differentiation depends on retinoids, and many human tumors (carcinomas) arise from epithelial cells, it has been proposed that vitamin A may be protective against these diseases. Indeed, some epidemiologic studies have demonstrated an inverse relationship between the vitamin A content of the diet and the risk of cancer. However, no practical conclusions regarding clinical use of vitamin A can be drawn at this time (see below).

Vitamin A is stored in the liver and needs to be transported to its sites of action

Owing to the fat-soluble nature of the vitamin, specific transport mechanisms are involved, both in the blood and at tissue sites of action. It is transported by specific proteins – serum retinal-binding protein (SRBP) and cytosolic retinal binding proteins (CRBP). In addition, retinoic acid is thought to be transported to cells either bound to albumin or to a specific retinoic acid binding protein (RABP). Other tissue proteins are also involved in the molecular trafficking of retinol to the nucleus of the cell.

Vitamin A deficiency presents as 'night blindness'

The visual pigment, rhodopsin, is found in the rod cells of the retina and is formed by the binding of 11-*cis*-retinal to the apoprotein opsin. When rhodopsin is exposed to light, it is bleached, retinal dissociates and is isomerized and reduced to all-*trans*-retinol (see Fig. 10.1). This reaction is accompanied by a conformational change and elicits a nerve impulse perceived by the brain as light (see also Chapter 39). Rod cells are responsible for vision in poor light.

Vitamin A deficiency often presents as defective night vision or 'night blindness'. Vitamin A also affects growth and differentiation of epithelial cells; thus its deficiency produces defective epithelialization and keratomalacia – corneal softening and opacity. Severe vitamin A deficiency leads to progressive keratinization of the cornea and to permanent blindness. In fact, vitamin A deficiency is the commonest cause of blindness in the world.

Subclinical vitamin A deficiency may lead to increased susceptibility to infection. Severe vitamin A deficiency occurs in the developing world. However, it is also fairly common in patients with severe liver disease or fat malabsorption.

Vitamin A is toxic in excess

Excess vitamin A administration is toxic, with symptoms including bone pain, hair loss, dermatitis, hepatosplenomegaly, nausea, vomiting, double vision, headaches and diarrhea. It is virtually impossible to develop vitamin A toxicity by ingesting normal foods; however, toxicity may result from the use of pure vitamin A supplements. Increased intake of vitamin A is also associated with teratogenicity and should be avoided during pregnancy.

Vitamin D

Vitamin D (calciol) is really a hormone; it is only under conditions of inadequate exposure to sunlight that dietary intake is required. Vitamin D is the only vitamin that is not usually required in the diet. It is, in fact, a group of closely related sterols produced by the action of ultraviolet light (wavelength 290–310 nm) on provitamins, ergosterol in plants and 7-dehydrocholesterol in animals (Fig. 10.2). The latter is synthesized in the liver and is found in the skin. The products of the photolytic reaction are ergocalciferol (vitamin D_2) and cholecalciferol (vitamin D_3), respectively. They are equipotent. Both are converted to a series of hydroxylated

VITAMIN A DEFICIENCY

A 47-year-old woman with a long history of Crohn's disease (a chronic inflammatory bowel disease) had to be fed for some months using intravenous nutrition. Initially, this treatment included intravenous fat and fat-soluble vitamins. As a result of complications in the administration of the intravenous feed, the fat component was removed and more energy supplied using a carbohydrate source. Prior to her starting intravenous feeding she had been receiving supplements of oral vitamins: these had been discontinued. Three months after the alteration of her intravenous feeding regimen she began to complain of being unable to see appropriately in dim light. Measurement of her serum vitamin A indicated a level well below the reference range.

Comment. Intravenous feeding solutions are highly purified and micronutrients must be added. The removal of fat from the prescription precluded the administration of fat-soluble vitamins intravenously. This was not noted at the time and the patient proceeded to develop symptoms of vitamin A deficiency, i.e. night blindness. This could have been avoided by providing a separate infusion of fat emulsion one or two days per week to act as a carrier for the fat-soluble vitamins.

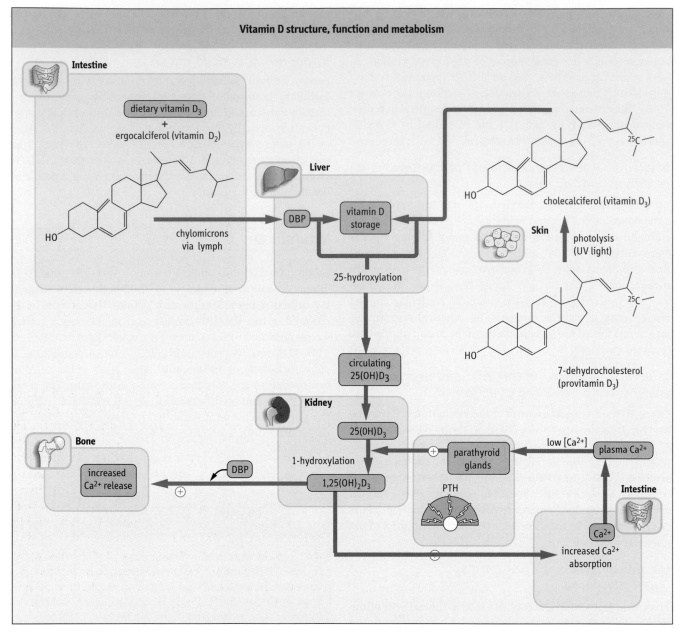

Fig. 10.2 **Structure, function and metabolism of vitamin D.** Note that excess of 25(OH)D$_3$ can mimic 1,25(OH)2D$_3$ but at greater concentrations. PTH, parathyroid hormone. DBP, vitamin D-binding protein. See also Fig. 16.9 and Fig. 23.5.

derivatives, firstly at the 25-position in the liver producing 25-hydroxycholecalciferol (25(OH)$_{D3}$; calcidiol) and at the 1-position in the kidney, producing the active compound 1α-,25-dihydroxycholecalciferol (1,25(OH)$_2$D$_3$; calcitriol)). The details of of vitamin D metabolism and action are described in Chapter 24.

Most of the vitamin intake is via milk and other fortified foodstuffs. Fish oils, egg yolks and liver are also rich in vitamin D. Insufficient sunlight and increased metabolism of vitamin D due to low calcium intake or absorption may lead to deficiency. Vitamin D requirements are greater in winter due to lower exposure to sunlight.

Deficiency of vitamin D produces rickets in children and osteomalacia in adults

Rickets is characterized by the soft pliable bones due to defective mineralization secondary to calcium deficiency. The characteristic bowing of the leg bones and the formation of the rickety rosary around costochondral junctions results. In the adult, demineralization of pre-existing bones takes place, increasing susceptibility to fractures. Vitamin D deficiency is also characterized by low circulating concentrations of calcium and an increased serum alkaline phosphatase activity (see Chapter 24).

VITAMIN D DEFICIENCY

A 42-year old devout woman of Asian origin presented to her Scottish female GP with knee and tibia pains, which had been present for 3 months. During the GP's initial screen her adjusted calcium (2.2 mmol/l) was at the low end of normal, but her alkaline phosphatase was four times the upper limit of normal, with a raised PTH of 20 pmol/l (normal range 1–6.9 pmol/l). The woman ate her normal cultural diet including curries and chapattis, and was always covered up when outside.

Comment. Osteomalacia is still common in certain groups in the UK. Painful tibia, pain in the groins and sore wrists are frequent symptoms. While vitamin D is produced by the action of ultraviolet light, the further away from the equator the shorter this light is available, such that in Scotland only sunlight between the end of April and early September is of the correct wavelength. With little skin exposure when out for religious reasons and chapattis, which bind vitamin D supplemented foods, vitamin D deficiency is common. Particular problems can occur during pregnancy, and both mother and baby should receive vitamin D supplementation.

Vitamin D is toxic in excess

Vitamin D excess leads to enhanced calcium absorption and bone reabsorption, leading to hypercalcemia and metastatic calcium deposition. There is also a tendency to develop kidney stones from the hypercalciuria secondary to hypercalcemia.

Vitamin E

Vitamin E occurs in the diet as a mixture of several closely related compounds, called tocopherols. Ninety percent of vitamin E present in human tissues is in the form of the natural isomer, α-tocopherol. Tocopherols have a substituted chromanone nucleus, with a polyisoprenoid side chain of variable length; usually three isoprene units (Fig. 10.3). The richest sources of naturally occurring vitamin E are vegetable oils and nuts. In European folklore, vitamin E has been associated with fertility and sexual activity. This is certainly true in other animal species where vitamin E plays a role in sperm production and egg implantation, but this is not the case in man.

Vitamin E is a membrane antioxidant

Vitamin E functions as an antioxidant, in particular a membrane antioxidant, and as such it is associated with the membrane lipid structure. It is the most abundant natural

Structure of vitamin E

chromanone nucleus

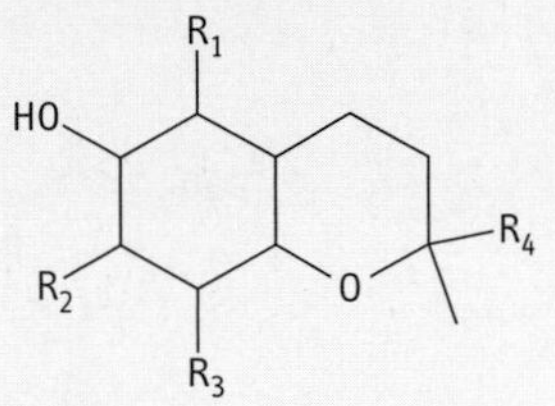

R_1–R_3	R_4
α-tocopherol R_1,R_2,R_3, Me	
β-tocopherol R_1,R_3, Me	$-CH_2(CH_2-CH_2-\overset{CH_3}{\underset{\mid}{CH}}-CH_2)_3-$
γ-tocopherol R_2,R_3, Me	
δ-tocopherol R_2,R_3, Me	

Fig. 10.3 **Structure of vitamin E family (tocopherols).** R_1–R_3 can be methylated in a variety of combinations. The polyisoprenoid side chain occurs at R_4. Me, methyl.

antioxidant and, owing to its lipid solubility, it is associated with all lipid-containing structures: membranes, lipoproteins and fat deposits. It is absorbed from the diet with other lipid components and there is no specific transport protein. In the circulation it is associated with lipoproteins. Fat malabsorption reduces the body fat content of vitamin E and, after a prolonged period, neurologic symptoms related to vitamin E deprivation have been reported. Low vitamin E intake in pregnancy and newborn infants is associated with hemolytic anemia. This is usually found only in preterm infants fed on formula milk with low vitamin E content. Deficiency of vitamin E in premature infants causes haemolytic anaemia, thrombocytosis and edema. There is little evidence in support of vitamin E toxicity.

Vitamin K

Vitamin K is necessary for blood coagulation

The name vitamin K refers to a group of related compounds, varying in the number of isoprenoid units in their side chain. Like vitamin E, the absorption of vitamin K depends on appropriate fat absorption. The structure, nomenclature and sources of the vitamin Ks are outlined in Figure 10.4. Vitamin K circulates as phylloquinone and its hepatic stores are in the form of manaquinones. It is required for the post-translational modification of several proteins (factors II, VII, IX, and X) in the coagulation cascade. All of these proteins are synthesized by the liver as inactive precursors and are activated by the carboxylation of specific glutamic acid

Structure of the different forms of vitamin K		
Source	Structure	Group
plants	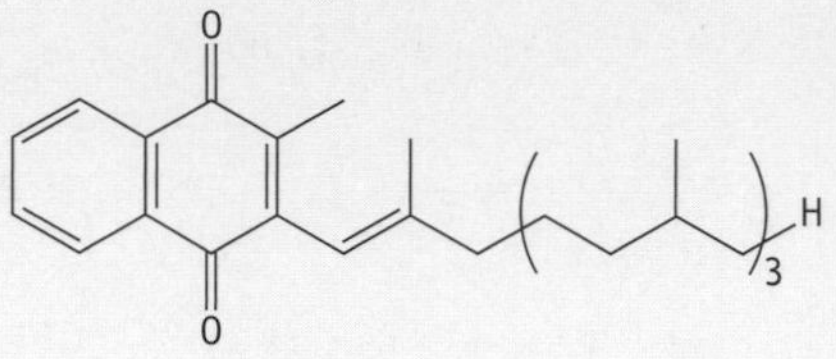	phylloquinone (vitamin K₁)
animal tissue bacteria	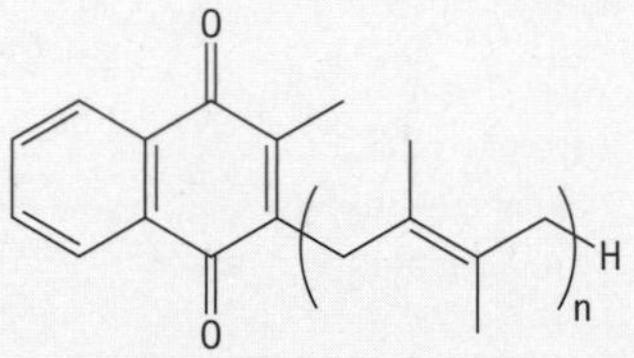	menaquinones (vitamin Kn₂)

Fig. 10.4 **The structure and nomenclature of vitamin K.**

residues by a vitamin K-dependent enzyme (Fig. 10.5). Prothrombin (factor II) contains 10 of these carboxylated residues (Gla) and all are required for this protein's specific chelation of Ca²⁺ ions during its function in coagulation. Recently, other proteins containing vitamin K-dependent Gla residues, such as osteocalcin, have been identified in tissues. Vitamin K is widely distributed in nature: its dietary sources are green leafy vegetables also fruits, dairy products, and vegetable oils, cereals, and meats; its production by the intestinal microflora virtually ensures that dietary deficiency does not occur in man.

Vitamin K deficiency causes bleeding disorders

Deficiency of vitamin K is rare but may develop in those with liver disease, fat malabsorption, or in the newborn, and it is associated with bleeding disorders. Premature infants are especially at risk and may suffer from hemorrhagic disease of the newborn. The placental transfer of maternal vitamin K to the fetus is inefficient. Immediately after birth the circulating concentration decreases, but it recovers on absorption of food; this is possibly delayed in preterm infants. In addition, the gut of the newborn is sterile, so that the intestinal microflora does not provide a source of vitamin K for several days after birth.

Inhibitors of vitamin K action are valuable antithrombotic drugs

Specific inhibitors of vitamin K-dependent carboxylation reactions are used in the treatment of thrombosis-related diseases, e.g. in patients with deep vein thrombosis and pulmonary thromboembolism, or patients with atrial fibrillation who are at risk of thrombosis. These are drugs of the dicoumarin group, e.g. warfarin, which inhibit the action of

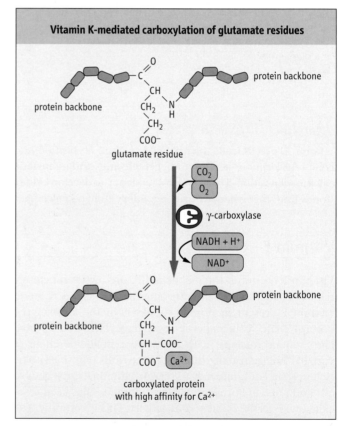

Fig. 10.5 **Vitamin K-mediated carboxylation of glutamate residues (Glu).** This reaction produces carboxylated residues, which are required for Ca²⁺ chelation. Gla-γ-carboxyglutamate.

vitamin K – probably via the mechanisms involved in the regeneration of the active hydroquinone. This drug is also used as rat poison and vitamin K is thus the antidote for human poisoning by this agent.

WATER-SOLUBLE VITAMINS

B-complex vitamins

B-complex vitamins act as coenzymes in many metabolic pathways

With the exception of vitamin B_{12} there is no storage capacity for water-soluble vitamins. As a consequence of the absence of storage, all water-soluble vitamins must be regularly supplied as constituents of the diet. Any excess of these vitamins is excreted in the urine. In contrast to the fat-soluble vitamins there is no common toxicity associated with excess of these vitamins.

B-complex vitamins are essential to the normal metabolism of all cells and are involved as coenzymes in many reactions. The B vitamins and their deficiency states are listed in Figure 10.6. Patients often present with multiple deficiencies: a deficiency of a single B vitamin is rare.

Thiamin (vitamin B₁)

Thiamin is essential for carboxylation reactions

Thiamin, in its active form as thiamin pyrophosphate, is essential for carboxylation and some reactions catalyzed by transferases, and for normal carbohydrate energy metabolism (see Chapter 8). Thiamin is required for the transketolase reaction in the hexose monophosphate pathway (see Chapter 11). Although the pathways which require thiamin are well characterized, their failure in deficiency states and the signs and symptoms of deficiency are not clearly related.

Thiamin deficiency is associated with alcoholism

Loss of appetite, constipation, and nausea are early symptoms of thiamin deficiency, progressing to depression, peripheral neuropathy, and unsteadiness, the latter related to impaired nerve cell function. Further deterioration in thiamin status results in mental confusion (loss of short-term memory), ataxia and loss of eye coordination. This combination, often seen in alcoholic patients, is termed Wernicke–Korsakoff psychosis. Severe thiamin deficiency results in beri-beri, either 'dry' (without fluid retention), or 'wet' (associated with cardiac failure with edema). Beri-beri is characterized primarily by advanced neuromuscular symptoms, and occurs in populations relying exclusively on polished rice for food. Wet beri-beri is particularly associated

with alcoholism. The signs and symptoms of deficiency may be also seen in the elderly or in low-income groups with poor diet. The measurement of erythrocyte transketolase activity is the most frequently used test to assess thiamin status. Recently is has also been measured by high-pressure liquid chromatography (HPLC).

The greater the caloric intake, the larger the requirement for B vitamins

Diseases that are associated with high caloric requirement require greater intake of thiamin and other B vitamins. Importantly, increased energy supply, in particular from carbohydrates, requires increased amounts of B vitamins as to cope with the increased enzyme activity. Therefore, beriberi might develop on a high-carbohydrate diet.

Riboflavin (vitamin B₂)

Riboflavin is associated with oxidoreductases

Riboflavin is attached to the sugar alcohol, ribitol. The molecule is colored, fluorescent, decomposes in visible light but is heat-stable. It is found in the oxidoreductases as flavin mononucleotide (FMN) and flavin adenine dinucleotide (FAD), and is required for the energy metabolism of both sugars and lipids (see Chapter 8). The activation of riboflavin is via an ATP-dependent enzyme system resulting in the production of FMN and FAD.

Lack of riboflavin in the diet causes a generally nonfatal deficiency syndrome of inflammation of the corners of the mouth (angular stomatitis), the tongue (glossitis) and scaly dermatitis. A degree of photophobia may also exist. Owing to its light sensitivity, riboflavin deficiency may occur in newborn infants with jaundice, who are treated by phototherapy. Hypothyroidism is also known to affect the conversion of riboflavin to FMN and flavin adenine FAD. The measurements of erythrocyte glutathione reductase activity are used to determine the riboflavin status.

Niacin (vitamin B₃)

Niacin is required for NAD⁺ and NADP⁺ synthesis

Niacin is a generic name for nicotinic acid or nicotinamide, either of which is an essential nutrient.

Niacin is active as part of the coenzyme nicotinamide adenine dinucleotide (NAD^+) or nicotinamide adenine dinucleotide phosphate ($NADP^+$) which participate in in oxidoreductase reactions. The active form of the vitamin required for synthesis of NAD^+ or $NADP^+$ is nicotinate, and therefore nicotinamide must be deamidated before becoming available for synthesis of these coenzymes. Niacin can be synthesized from tryptophan and hence, in the truest sense, is not a vitamin. The conversion is, however, very inefficient and

Vitamin B-complex			
Vitamin	**Structure**	**Deficiency disease**	**Food source**
Thiamin (vit B$_1$)	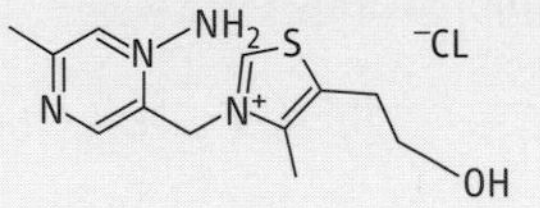	beri-beri	seeds, nuts, wheatgerms, legumes, lean meat
Riboflavin (vit B$_2$)	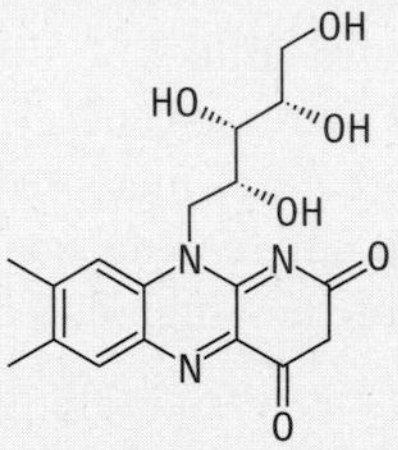	pellagra	meats, nuts, legumes
Niacin (vit B$_3$)	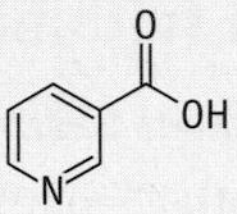	pellagra	meats, nuts, legumes
Panthothenic acid (vit B$_5$)	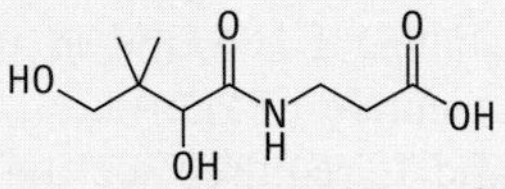		yeast, grains, egg yolk, liver
Pyridoxine (vit B$_6$)	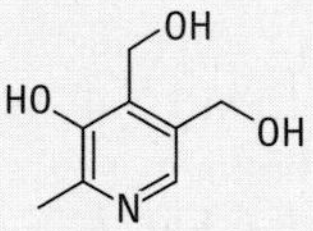	neurologic disease	yeast, liver, wheatgerm, nuts beans, bananas
Biotin	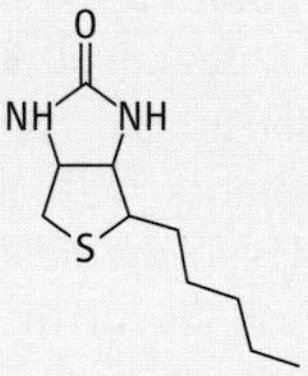	widespread injury	corn, soy, egg yolk, liver, kidney, tomatoes
Folate	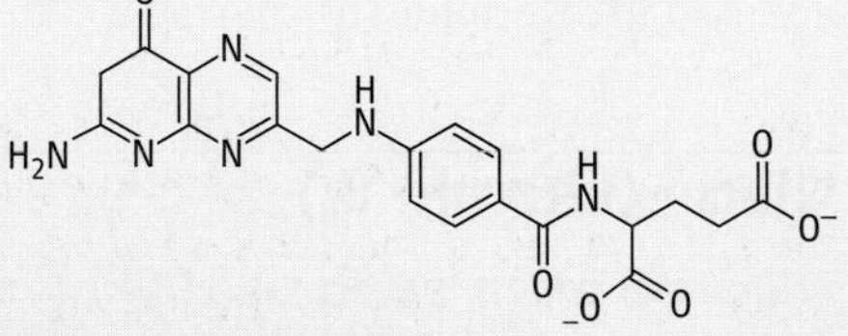	anemia	yeast, liver, leafy vegetables
Cobalamin (vit B$_{12}$)	complex	pernicious anemia	liver, kidney, egg, cheese

Fig. 10.6 **Structure, sources and deficiency diseases of B vitamins** (see also Fig. 13.6).

cannot supply sufficient amounts of niacin. In addition, the conversion requires thiamin, pyridoxine, and riboflavin, and on marginal diets such a synthesis would be problematic. The requirement for niacin is also related to energy expenditure.

Severe niacin deficiency produces dermatitis, diarrhea and dementia

Niacin deficiency initially produces a superficial glossitis but may progress to pellagra, which is characterized by dermatitis, sunburn-like skin lesions in areas of body exposed to sunlight and to pressure, diarrhea, and dementia. Untreated pellagra is fatal. Certain drugs, e.g. isoniazid, also predispose to niacin deficiency. In the modern world pellagra is a medical curiosity. Very high doses of niacin can cause hepatotoxicity which is reversible on withdrawal.

Pyridoxine (vitamin B$_6$)

Pyridoxine is important in amino acid metabolism

Vitamin B$_6$ is a mixture of pyridoxine, pyridoxal, pyridoxamine, and their 5'-phosphates. Pyridoxine is the major form of vitamin B$_6$ in the diet, and pyridoxal phosphate is the active form of the vitamin. Pyridoxal phosphate participates as a cofactor in amino acid metabolism, and also in the glycogen phosphorylase reaction.

All forms of the vitamin are absorbed from the gut, during which some hydrolysis of the phosphates occurs. Most tissues, however, contain pyridoxal kinase, thus resynthesizing the active phosphorylated forms required for the synthesis, catabolism and interconversion of amino acids (see Chapter 18). Pyridoxine is also required for synthesis of the neurotransmitters, serotonin and noradrenaline (see Chapter 40), for the synthesis of sphingosine, a component of sphingomyelin and sphingolipids (see Chapter 26), and for the synthesis of heme (see Chapter 28).

Vitamin B$_6$ requirements increase with high protein intake

Owing to the central role of vitamin B$_6$ in amino acid metabolism, requirements for this vitamin increase with protein intake. Vitamin B$_6$ deficiency causes irritability, nervousness and depression in its mild form, progressing to peripheral neuropathy, convulsions and coma in severe deficiency. Severe deficiency is also associated with a sideroblastic anemia. The antituberculosis drug, isoniazid, by binding to pyridoxine, and the oral contraceptive pill, by increasing the synthesis of enzymes requiring the vitamin, interfere strongly with pyridoxine and deficiency may occur. Peripheral neuropathy in association with isoniazid is also well recognized. The debate concerning the contraceptive pill continues but it is generally accepted that there is an increased requirement

for pyridoxine. As with other B vitamins, assessment of pyridoxine status is based on the measurement of erythrocyte enzymes, in this case, aspartate aminotransferase.

Biotin

Biotin is important for carboxylation reactions

Biotin is normally synthesized by intestinal flora. It serves as a coenzyme in multienzyme complexes involved in carboxylation reactions. It is important in lipogenesis, gluconeogenesis, and the catabolism of the branched-chain amino acids. The majority of the requirement for biotin is met from synthesis in the bowel by intestinal bacteria. Consumption of raw eggs can cause biotin deficiency because the egg-white protein, avidin, combines with biotin, preventing its absorption. Interestingly, certain inherited single or multiple carboxylase deficiencies can also lead to apparent biotin deficiency syndrome. Symptoms of biotin deficiency include depression, hallucinations, muscle pain and dermatitis. Children with multiple decarboxylase deficiency also demonstrate immunodeficiency disease.

Panthotenic acid

Panthotenic acid forms a part of the coenzyme A (CoA) molecule.

It is widely distributed in animals and plants. There is no evidence of deficiency in man, except on experimental diets. No method of its measurement is available in clinical laboratories.

Folic acid

Folic acid derivatives are important in single carbon transfer reactions

Folic acid (pteroyl glutamic acid) has a number of derivatives known collectively as folates. It participates in single carbon transfer reactions in numerous pathways including the synthesis of choline, serine, glycine, methionine and nucleic acids. Deficiency of folate contributes to hyperhomocysteinemia, which is regarded as a risk factor for cardiovascular disease (see Chapter 17).

Folic acid is physiologically inactive until reduced to dihydrofolic acid. Its main forms are tetrahydrofolate, 5-methyl tetrahydrofolate (N^{5}MeTHF) and N^{10}-formyltetrahydrofolate-polyglutamate forms based on 5MeTHF predominate in fresh food. Before polyglutamates can be absorbed, they must be hydrolyzed by glutamyl hydrolase (conjugase) in the small intestine. Main circulating form of folate is the monoglutamate N^5-THF.

Folic acid is necessary for the synthesis of DNA

Rapidly dividing cells have high requirements for this vitamin since its role is in the synthesis of purines and pyrimidine thymine required for DNA synthesis (see Chapter 30). On the basis of selective toxicity in rapidly growing cells, e.g. bacteria and cancer cells, this function of folate has also formed the basis for development of drug such as antibiotics (e.g. trimethoprim) and anticancer agents (methotrexate). Folic acid is present in liver yeast, green leafy vegetables. It is measured by HPLC methods.

Folate deficiency causes megaloblastic anemia

Failure to synthesize methionine and nucleic acids in deficiency states accounts for the signs and symptoms of megaloblastic anemia, i.e. the presence of enlarged blast cells in the bone marrow. Deficiency of folate is one of the commonest vitamin deficiencies and the hematologic abnormalities associated with this cannot be distinguished from those of vitamin B_{12} deficiency (see below). The neurologic changes are also similar. The block in synthesis slows down the production of erythrocytes, causing the appearance of macrocytic erythrocytes with fragile membranes and a tendency to hemolyze. A macrocytic anemia thus ensues in association with a megaloblastic bone marrow.

There are many causes of folate deficiency, including inadequate intake, impaired absorption, impaired metabolism, and increased demand. The most common examples of increased demand are pregnancy and lactation. Folic acid requirements increase dramatically as the blood volume and number of erythrocytes increase in pregnancy. By the third trimester of pregnancy folic acid requirements double. However, megaloblastic anemias in pregnancy, other than multiple pregnancy, are rare. The common practice is to provide folate supplements during pregnancy. Folate deficiencies are seen in the elderly as a result of poor diet and poor absorption.

Vitamin B₁₂

Vitamin B₁₂ is part of the structure of heme

Vitamin B_{12} (cobalamin) has a complex ring structure similar to the porphyrin system of heme (see Chapter 28) but is more hydrogenated. The iron of the heme system is replaced by a cobalt ion (Co^{3+}) at the center. It is the only known function of cobalt in the body. In addition, and essential for the chelation of the cobalt ion, a dimethylbenzimidazole ring is also part of the active molecule (Fig. 10.7). Vitamin B_{12} participates in the recycling of folates, and in the methionine synthesis.

Vitamin B_{12} is synthesized solely by bacteria. It is absent from all plants but is concentrated in the livers of animals in three forms: methylcobalamin, adenosylcobalamin, and

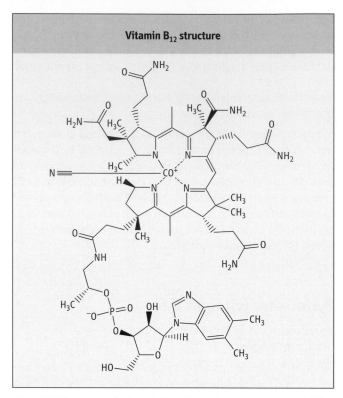

Vitamin B₁₂ structure

Fig. 10.7 **Structure of vitamin B₁₂.** There is a cyano-group (CN) attached to the cobalt: this is an artifact of extraction but it is also the most stable form of the vitamin and indeed is the commercially available product for treatment. The cyano group does require removal for conversion to the active form of the vitamin.

hydroxycobalamin. Liver is therefore a useful source of this vitamin and has been used in the treatment of deficiency states in the past.

It is impossible to consider the function of vitamin B₁₂ in isolation from folate

That the roles of vitamin B_{12} and folate are interrelated is exemplified by the fact that deficiency of either produces the same signs and symptoms of disease. The reaction involving both these vitamins is the conversion of homocysteine to methionine – a methylation reaction (Fig. 10.8).

Vitamin B_{12} is required in only one further reaction, that is the conversion of methylmalonyl-CoA to succinyl-CoA. The coenzyme form of the vitamin in this case is 5′-deoxyadenosyl cobalamin. Specific mechanisms exist for the absorption and transport of cobalamin (Fig. 10.9).

The megaloblastic anemia characteristic of vitamin B_{12} deficiency is probably due to a secondary deficiency of reduced folate and a consequence of the accumulation of N^5-methyltetrahydrofolate; therefore, the folate/B_{12}-associated syndrome. A neurologic presentation also can develop in the absence of anemia. This is known as subacute combined degeneration of the cord. This neurologic disorder is probably secondary to a relative deficiency of methionine in the cord. Since vitamin B_{12} is required in only two reactions, deficiency of this vitamin results in an accumulation of methylmalonic acid and homocysteine and consequent methylmalonic aciduria and homocystinuria.

Vitamin B_{12} deficiency causes pernicious anemia

Vitamin B_{12} deficiency can occur through several mechanisms. The one most commonly seen is known as pernicious anemia, and is due to lack of intrinsic factor (IF) in the stomach; this prevents the vitamin absorption in the terminal ileum. IF lack can also be caused by gastric surgery. A similar situation, albeit caused through different mechanism, arises upon surgical removal of the ileum, for instance in Crohn's disease (see Chapter 9). Vegans are at risk of developing a dietary deficiency of vitamin B_{12} since the vitamin is found only in foods of animal origin (the vegetable diet may contain some vitamin only if it is contaminated with microorganisms, such as yeasts). Vitamin B_{12} is secreted in the bile and there is a marked enterohepatic circulation. Disturbances of this circulation can have major effects on vitamin B_{12} status (Table 10.1).

Vitamin B_{12} must be supplemented when folate treatment is given

Importantly, giving folate alone in a case of vitamin B_{12} deficiency aggravates the neuropathy. Therefore, if supplementation is required during investigation of the cause of megaloblastic anemia, folate needs to be given together with

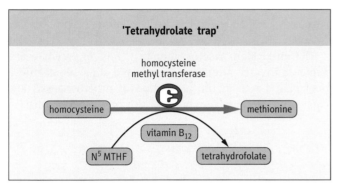

Fig. 10.8 **'Tetrahydrolate trap'.** Vitamin B_{12} and folate are involved together in the conversion of homocysteine to methionine. An absence of vitamin B_{12} inhibits the reaction and leads to the buildup of N^5 methyltetrahydrofolate (N^5MTHF), known as the 'tetrahydrafolate trap'.

Mechanisms of B_{12} deficiency	
Mechanism	Time to develop clinical deficiency (years)
vegan diet	10–12
intrinsic factor failure	1–4
ileal dysfunciton	rapid

Table 10.1 **Mechanism of development of vitamin B_{12} deficiency.**

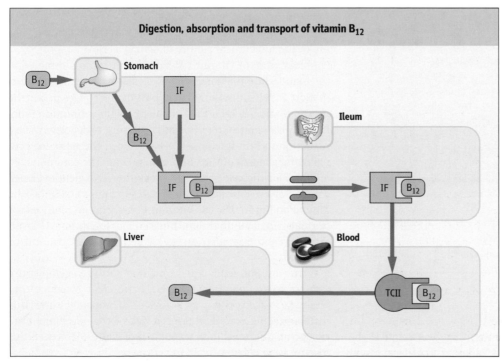

Fig. 10.9 **Digestion, absorption and transport of vitamin B_{12}.** Simple diffusion of free vitamin B_{12} across the intestinal membrane accounts for 3% of transported vitamin, and complexing with intrinsic factor (IF) accounts for 97%. Vitamin B_{12} derivatives are released from food by peptic digestion in the stomach and become attached to specific binding on IF, secreted by the parietal cells of the gastric mucosa. IF-B_{12} complex is required for absorption by specific receptor sites on the ileal mucosa. The rate-limiting factor in this process is the number of ileal receptor sites. Other transport proteins (transcobalamin I, II and III (TC I, II and III) and R-proteins) are involved in the delivery or storage of the cobalamins. The latter are secreted by the salivary glands and gastric mucosa.

VITAMIN B₁₂ TRANSPORT PROTEINS

Intrinsic factor (IF) is a highly specific glycoprotein. Other cobalamin-binding proteins, R-proteins, secreted by the salivary glands and stomach, are also glycoproteins and along with trans-cobalamin (TC)I and III are now termed cobalaphilins. The third type of cobalamic protein, also a glycoprotein, is TCII. All three classes of B₁₂-transport proteins have similar properties:

- single polypeptide chain (340–375 amino acid residues),
- single binding site for cobalamin,
- glycoproteins.

They do not, however, cross-react with each other immunologically, and are coded for by different genes. At acid pH, R-proteins bind cobalamin stronger than IF, but they are normally degraded by pancreatic proteinases in contrast to IF, which is not. Thus, in pancreatic disease where R-proteins are not degraded, there is less cobalamin available to bind to IF, with loss of absorptive capacity for this vitamin. In the final absorption process, a specific site on the IF molecule binds with the ileal receptor in the presence of Ca^{2+} and at neutral pH. As the IF-B₁₂ complex crosses the ileal mucosa, IF is released and the B₁₂ is transferred to a plasma transport protein TCII. Other cobalamin-binding proteins, e.g. TCI and possibly TCIII, exist in the plasma and liver. In the latter, these provide excellent storage forms of the vitamin, a situation that is unique for water-soluble vitamins.
Once cobalamin is bound to TCII in portal blood, it disappears from the plasma in a few hours. The major circulating form is methylcobalamin with only a trace of hydroxycobalamin. In the liver, 5'-deoxyadenosyl cobalamin accounts for 70% of the total and methylcobalamin for only 3% of the total amount.
The TCII-cobalamin complex delivers exogenous cobalamin to the tissues, where it binds to specific cell-surface receptors and enters the cell by a process of endocytosis, ultimately releasing the cobalamin as hydroxycobalamin. Conversion of hydroxycobalamin to methylcobalamin occurs in the cytosol for participation in the homocysteine-methionine conversion. 5-deoxy-adenosyl cobalamin is derived from hydroxycobalamin to allow the mitochondrial conversion of methylmalonyl CoA to succinyl CoA. TCII is also thought to be necessary for the delivery of vitamin B₁₂ to the central nervous system (CNS).

vitamin B₁₂ (after blood and bone marrow specimens have been taken to confirm the diagnosis).

Vitamin C

Vitamin C is a reducing agent

While most of the animal kingdom synthesizes vitamin C, the human species does not. Vitamin C, ascorbic acid, is an essential nutrient in human beings, the higher primates, the guinea pig and fruit-eating bats. In all other animals, a specific pathway exists for its synthesis. The synthetic pathway and structure of vitamin C are shown in Figure 10.10. Vitamin C is labile: it is easily destroyed by oxygen, metal ions, increased pH, heat and light. Vitamin C serves as a reducing agent and its active form is ascorbic acid, which is oxidized during the transfer of reducing equivalents to dehydroascorbic acid (which also can act as a source of the vitamin). Vitamin C participates in the synthesis of collagen and adrenaline, steroidogenesis, degradation of tyrosine, bile acid formation, absorption of iron and in bone mineral metabolism. The prime function of this compound is to maintain metal cofactors in their lower valence state, e.g. Fe^{2+} and Cu^{+}. This is the case in its role in the synthesis of collagen where it is required specifically for the hydroxylation of proline (see Chapter 27).

The antioxidant role of vitamin C has, in recent years, achieved greater attention. There were suggestions that it may play a role in the prevention of atherosclerosis and cancer but no conclusive proof of this has been obtained.

Vitamin C deficiency causes scurvy and compromises immune function

Scurvy is related to a defective collagen synthesis associated with vitamin C deficiency. It is characterized by subcutaneous and other hemorrhages, muscle weakness, soft, swollen, bleeding gums, osteoporosis, and poor wound healing and anemia. The osteoporosis results from the inability to maintain bone matrix in association with demineralization. This latter aspect results in the appearance of Looser's zones on radiography, especially in the hands.

Except in the elder individuals, vitamin C deficiency resulting in the full clinical picture of scurvy is rare.

Milder forms of vitamin C deficiency are more common and the manifestation of such includes easy bruising and the formation of petechiae (small, pinpoint hemorrhages under the skin) both due to increased capillary fragility. Immune function is also compromised in mild vitamin C deficiency. This reduction in immuncompetence has been the basis for providing megadoses of the vitamin to prevent the common cold and also for the role in cancer prevention. No clear evidence exists, however, to substantiate these claims first made by Linus Pauling in 1970s. Vitamin C is certainly required for normal leukocyte function, and leukocyte vitamin C levels drop precipitously after stress related to either trauma or infection.

Citrus and soft fruits and growing points of vegetables are rich sources of vitamin C. There is no clear evidence that vitamin C taken in excess is toxic. Theoretically, since it is metabolized to oxalate, there is a risk of the development of renal oxalate stones in susceptible individuals. However, this has not been substantiated in practice.

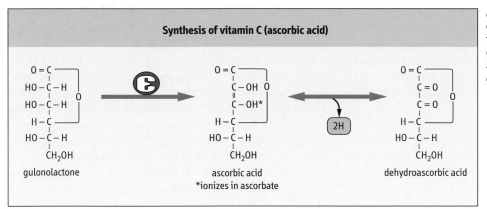

Fig. 10.10 **Structure and synthesis of vitamin C (ascorbic acid).** Note that the enzyme that converts gulonolactone to ascorbic acid is absent in man, higher primates, the guinea pig and the fruit-eating bat.

Dietary supplementation of vitamins

Supplementation of some vitamins provides clear health benefit

Areas where the benefits of vitamin supplementation are clear include supplementation of folic acid to women who are pregnant or are planning pregnancy, to prevent neural tube defects. Vitamin D provision to people living in areas of low sunlight has also been beneficial.

Benefits of vitamin supplementation in cancer and cardiovascular disease are uncertain

Because the supplementation of folic acid and vitamin B_6 and B_{12} lowers plasma homocysteine concentration, it has been suggested that it could be beneficial for the prevention of cardiovascular disease. There also were suggestions that supplementation of vitamins A, C and E is protective against cancer. Some observational studies suggested that the supplementation of vitamins C and E could also be useful in the prevention of cardiovascular disease. However, prospective studies of this yielded controversial results. The recommendations of the US Preventive Services Task Force published in 2003 (www. preventiveservices.ahrq.gov) say that 'current evidence is insufficient to recommend for or against the use of supplements of vitamins A, C, or E , multivitamins with folic acid, or antioxidant combinations for the prevention of cancer or cardiovascular disease' (note that these recommendations do not apply to people with nutritional deficiencies, pregnant and lactating women, children, elderly persons and people with chronic illnesses).

As mentioned above, high-dose vitamin supplementation may be harmful: the example is the reduction of bone mineral density, hepatotoxicity, and teratogenecity associated with high doses of vitamin A. β-carotene supplementation to smokers was also harmful, resulting in an increase in lung cancer mortality.

Fruit and vegetables are the best sources of vitamins

In the clinical studies mentioned above the vitamins were supplemented in a pure form, rather than as complete foodstuffs: and it might be that this is why the benefit of supplementation was not evident. Clearly there are benefits of eating diets rich in vegetables and fruit, which are the most important sources of vitamins. However, apart from proven instances of toxicity in excess, there is no reason to discourage people from taking vitamin supplements.

TRACE ELEMENTS

Metal ions are required as active components of several proteins.

The most obvious of these is iron, it forms part of the proteins involved in the transfer of molecular oxygen (see Chapter 4). Other metals have been found to be essential for normal biological function. These include metals previously thought to be toxic; indeed, environmental excesses of these do result in toxicity. Such elements include chromium, selenium, manganese, copper and zinc, and are termed essential trace elements.

Iron

Iron is important in the transfer of molecular oxygen and is a component of heme in hemoglobin and myoglobin. Cytochromes a,b, and c also contain iron.

Iron is present in the body in in the ferrous (2^+) form in the heme molecule and is transported and stored in the ferric (3^+) form. Altogether, there are 3–4 g of iron in the body. Seventy five percent of body iron is in hemoglobin and myoglobin, and 25% is stored in the tissues such as bone marrow, liver, and reticuloendothelial system. It is absorbed in the upper small intestine, and about 10% is absorbed from diet. Meat and ascorbic acid increase its absorption, and vegetable fibre inhibits it. It is transported in blood bound to transferrin and is stored as ferritin and hemosiderin. Transferrin is normally about 30% saturated with iron. Iron is lost through the skin and through the gastrointestinal tract. Human beings cannot excrete excess iron and free iron is toxic.

Requirement for iron increases during growth and pregnancy. Iron deficiency results in defective erythropoiesis and in normocytic or microcytic (small erythrocytes) hypochromic anemia. This is most likely to develop in infants and adolescents, in pregnant and menstruating women, and also in the elderly. Iron deficiency most often develops as a result of abnormal blood loss, and therefore persons who present with iron deficiency anemia are always investigated for causes of bleeding, particularly from the gastrointestinal tract.

Dietary sources of iron include organ meats, poultry and fish and oysters, and also egg yolks, dried beans, dried figs and dates, and some green vegetables. The assessment of iron status includes the measurements of transferrin and ferritin in plasma, the assessment of hematological variables, and the bone marrow smear.

Zinc

Zinc is an integral part of numerous enzymes associated with carbohydrate and energy metabolism, protein synthesis and degradation, nucleic acid synthesis, intercellular transport functions and protection from oxidative damage.

Its effects, however, are most obviously seen in the maintenance of skin integrity and in wound healing. It plays a role in maintaining exocrine and endocrine pancreatic function. Spermatogenesis is also a zinc-dependent process based on the metal's role in testosterone metabolism.

Absorption of zinc from the diet is an active process and shares gut transport mechanisms with copper and iron

On absorption, zinc is found bound to the protein metallothioneine, a cysteine-rich protein, which is also associated with the binding of other divalent metal ions such as copper. Its synthesis is dependent on the amount of trace metals present in the diet. Its excess may interfere with copper absorption. Zinc is probably the least toxic of the trace metals but increased oral doses of zinc interfere with copper absorption leading to deficiency of the latter.

Zinc deficiency affects growth, skin integrity and wound healing

Zinc deficiency is not uncommon: in children it is characterized by growth retardation, skin lesions, and impairment of sexual development. A specific inherited defect in the absorption of zinc from the gut was identified in the 1970s; it was termed acrodermatitis enteropathica with the clinical

appearance of severe skin lesions, diarrhea, and loss of hair (alopecia). Its deficiency also leads to impairment in taste and smell and to delayed wound healing.

Increased losses of zinc occur in patients with major burns and in those with renal damage. Zinc loss in renal disease is due to its association with plasma albumin, and it accompanies urinary protein loss. Substantial amounts of zinc may be also lost during dialysis. Increased metallothioneine synthesis is part of the metabolic response to trauma and results in a reduction of serum zinc concentration. During intravenous feeding, in situations where there is frequently an increased demand, failure to replace it may produce a symptomatic deficiency.

Measurement of serum zinc concentration is the usual method of assessing zinc status. However, many conditions and environmental factors can affect its concentration in plasma, including inflammation, stress, cancer, smoking, steroid administration and hemolysis. More recently, erythrocyte metallothioneine levels have proved more appropriate in assessing zinc status.

ZINC DEFICIENCY

A 34-year-old man who required total intravenous feeding had been receiving the same prescription for some 4 months, with no assessment of his trace metal status. During this time, he continued to have major gastrointestinal losses and intermittent pyrexia. Initially, he developed a rash across his face, head, and neck, with accompanying hair loss and, by the end of the 4-month period, was clearly zinc-deficient. He had a widespread acne-type rash and was virtually devoid of hair. His serum zinc concentration at that time was less than 1 µmol/L (range: 9–20 µmol/L; 60–130 µg/dL).

Comment. Patients with major catabolic illness and increased gastrointestinal losses have markedly increased zinc requirements. The zinc-depleted state the patient developed would aggravate his illness: (a) by preventing healing of his gastrointestinal lesions; and (b) by making him more susceptible to infection due to defects in his immune competence. Patients receiving intravenous feeding need to have their micronutrient status checked regularly and prescriptions altered if required.

Copper

Copper scavenges superoxide and other reactive oxygen species

Copper is associated with several oxygenase enzymes. These include cytochrome oxidase and superoxide dismutase, the latter also requiring zinc for activity. One of the main roles of copper, especially in superoxide dismutase, but also in association with the plasma copper-carrying protein ceruloplasmin, is the scavenging of superoxide and other reactive oxygen species. Copper is also required for the crosslinking of collagen, being an essential component of lysyl oxidase.

Absorption of copper from the gut is associated with metallothioneine. Copper availability in the diet is less affected by dietary constituents than zinc, although high fiber intake reduces availability by complexing with copper.

Rare copper deficiency produces an anemia; skin and hair may also be affected. Copper deficiency is most likely to occur from reduced intake or excess loss, e.g. during renal dialysis. Deficiency manifests itself as a microcytic hypochromic (pale erythrocytes) anemia that is resistant to iron therapy. There is also a reduction in the number of leukocytes in the blood (neutropenia) and degeneration of vascular tissue with bleeding (due to defects in elastin and collagen production). Skin depigmentation and alteration in hair structure also occur in severe deficiency.

Copper excess causes liver cirrhosis

When taken orally, copper is generally nontoxic but in large doses it accumulates in tissues and can interfere with other metal ions such as iron and zinc. Chronic excessive intake, however, results in liver cirrhosis. Acute toxicity is manifested by marked hemolysis and damage to both liver and brain cells. The latter is seen in the inherited metabolic defect of Wilson's disease, where the liver's capacity to synthesize ceruloplasmin is compromised. This results in a reduced excretion of copper and its chronic accumulation of in tissues.

Selenium

Selenium occurs in all cells as amino acids selenomethionine and selenocysteine

Selenium forms a part of glutathione peroxidase, an antioxidant enzyme. Selenium is also a part of type I iodothyronine 5-deiodinase which participates in the hepatic deiodination of thyroxine; in animals it is a component of muscle proteins selenoprotein P and selenoprotein W. Selenium is absorbed from the small intestine. It is protein bound in circulation, and is excreted in urine.

Selenium is present in diet as selenomethionine and selenocysteine. Its content in plant food depends on the content in the the soil. Its dietary sources include organ meats, fish (tuna) and shellfish, and cereals.

Increased intake of selenium might be required during lactation. There is a rare selenium-responsive cardiomyopathy (Keshan disease), which is endemic in China in areas of very low selenium intake. Deficiency of selenium can also develop during total parenteral nutrition and may result in chronic muscle pain, abnormal nail beds, and cardiomyopathy. The excess of selenium leads to liver cirrhosis, splenomegaly, gastrointestinal bleeding and depression.

Numerous other trace metals are required for normal biologic function, for example manganese, molybdenum, vanadium, nickel, and even cadmium. The latter is probably better known for its renal toxic effects and has been seen especially in shipyard workers exposed to this metal over long periods of time. No doubt, as techniques for separation and analysis develop, other metals and other functions of known essential minerals will become known. This will lead to a better understanding of the epidemiology of certain diseases which may have, at least in part, an environmental aetiology.

Summary

- Vitamins function mostly as cofactors to enzymes.
- Fat soluble vitamins can be stored in the adipose tissue but there usually is only a short-term supply of the water-soluble ones.
- Dietary micronutrient deficiencies are most likely to occur in susceptible groups with increased demand, or in people unable to maintain sufficient intake. Children, pregnant women, the elderly and low-income groups are particularly vulnerable.
- Gastrointestinal disease and gastrointestinal surgery are potential causes of micronutrient deficiencies.
- Vitamin and trace metal supplements are particularly important in patients who remain on artificial diets and on parenteral nutrition.
- While there are controversies regarding some vitamin supplementation, the intake of fruit and vegetables as sources of micronutrients is unequivocally recommended.

ACTIVE LEARNING

1. Compare and contrast the deficiencies of vitamin B_{12} and folic acid.
2. When may an increased intake of a nutrient or energy precipitate vitamin deficiencies?
3. Is vitamin A supplementation safe?
4. Describe the clinical importance of copper.
5. Which vitamins play a role in the development of hyperhomocysteinemia?

Further reading

Dietary reference values for food energy and nutrients for the United Kingdom. *Report of the Panel on Dietary reference Values of the Committee on Medical aspects of Food Policy.* London,TSO, 2003.

Colquhoun DM. Nutraceuticals: vitamins and other nutrients in coronary heart disease. *Current Opinion Lipidol* 2001;**12**:639–46.

Asplund K. Antioxidant vitamins in the prevention of cardiovascular disease: a systematic review. *J Int Med* 2002;**251**:372–92.

Fairfield, KM, Fletcher, RH. Vitamins for chronic disease prevention in adults: *Scientific review. JAMA* 2002;**287**:3116–26.

Fletcher RH. Fairfield KM. Vitamins for chronic disease prevention in adults: *Clinical applications. JAMA* 2002;**287**:3127–29.

Brown BG. Cheung MC,Lee, A C, Zhao Xue-Qiao, Chait A. Antioxidant vitamins and lipid therapy: End of a long romance? *Arteriosclerosis, Thrombosis & Vascular* Biology 2002;**22**:1535–46.

Jones, G. Eating fruit and vegetables. *BMJ* 2003;**326**:888.

Websites

US Preventive Services Task Force www. preventiveservices.ahrq.gov
National Guideline Clearinghouse www.guideline.gov)

11. Anaerobic Metabolism of Glucose in the Red Blood Cell

J W Baynes

LEARNING OBJECTIVES

After reading this chapter you should be able to:

- Outline the sequence of reactions in anaerobic glycolysis, the central pathway of carbohydrate metabolism in all cells.
- Summarize the energetics of anaerobic glycolysis, including the reactions involved in the utilization and formation of ATP, and the net yield of ATP during glycolysis.
- Identify the primary site of allosteric regulation of glycolysis and the mechanism of regulation of this enzyme by AMP.
- Identify reactions in glycolysis that illustrate the use of coupled reactions to drive thermodynamically unfavored reactions, including substrate-level phosphorylation.
- Describe the major roles of the pentose phosphate pathway in erythrocytes and nucleated cells.
- Describe the principles of the glucose oxidase/peroxidase assay and how it is used for measurement of blood glucose concentration.
- Describe the role of anaerobic glycolysis in development of dental caries and acidosis.
- Explain the metabolic origin of acidosis in chronic obstructive pulmonary disease.
- Explain why glycolysis is essential for normal red cell functions, including consequences of deficiencies in glycolytic enzymes and the role of glycolysis in adaptation to high altitude.
- Explain the origin of drug-induced hemolytic anemia in persons with G6PD deficiency.

INTRODUCTION

Glucose is the major carbohydrate on Earth, the backbone and monomer unit of cellulose and starch. It is also the only fuel that is used by all cells in our body. All of these cells, even the microbes in our intestines, begin the metabolism of glucose by a pathway termed glycolysis, i.e. carbohydrate (glyco) splitting (lysis). Glycolysis is catalyzed by soluble cytosolic enzymes and is the ubiquitous, central metabolic pathway for glucose metabolism. The erythrocyte, commonly known as the red blood cell (RBC), is unique among all cells in the body – it uses glucose and glycolysis as its sole source of energy. Thus, the RBC is a useful model for an introduction to glycolysis.

Pyruvate, a three-carbon acid, is the end product of glycolysis; 2 moles of pyruvate are formed per mole of glucose. In cells with mitochondria and oxidative metabolism, pyruvate is converted completely into CO_2 and H_2O – glycolysis in this oxidative setting is termed aerobic glycolysis. In RBCs, which lack mitochondria and oxidative metabolism, pyruvate is reduced to lactic acid, a three-carbon hydroxyacid, the product of anaerobic glycolysis. Each mole of glucose yields 2 moles of lactate, which are then excreted into blood. Two molecules of lactic acid contain exactly the same number of carbons, hydrogens, and oxygens as one molecule of glucose (Fig. 11.1); however, there is sufficient free energy available from the cleavage and rearrangement of the glucose molecule to produce 2 moles of ATP per mole of glucose converted into lactate. The RBC uses most of this ATP to maintain electrochemical and ion gradients across its plasma membrane.

In the red cell, 10–20% of the glycolytic intermediate, 1,3-bisphosphoglycerate, is diverted to the synthesis of 2,3-bisphosphoglycerate (2,3-BPG), an allosteric regulator of the O_2 affinity of Hb. The pentose phosphate pathway, a shunt from glycolysis, accounts for about 10% of glucose metabolism in the red cell. In the red cell this pathway has a special role in protection against oxidative stress, while in nucleated it also serves as a source of NADPH for biosynthetic reactions and pentoses for nucleic acid synthesis.

THE ERYTHROCYTE

The erythrocyte, or red blood cell (RBC), represents 40–45% of blood volume and over 90% of the formed elements (erythrocytes, leukocytes, and platelets) in blood. The RBC is, both structurally and metabolically, the simplest cell in the body – the end product of the maturation of bone-marrow reticulocytes. During its maturation, the RBC loses all its subcellular organelles. Without nuclei, it lacks the ability to synthesize DNA or RNA. Without ribosomes or an endoplasmic reticulum, it cannot synthesize or secrete protein. Because it cannot oxidize fats, a process requiring mitochondrial activity, the RBC relies exclusively on blood glucose as a fuel. Metabolism of glucose in the RBC is entirely anaerobic, consistent with

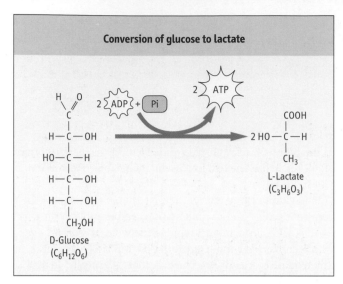

Conversion of glucose to lactate

Fig. 11.1 **Conversion of glucose to lactate during anaerobic glycolysis.** One mole of glucose is converted to 2 moles of lactate during anaerobic glycolysis. No oxygen is consumed, nor is CO_2 produced in this pathway. There is a net yield of 2 mol ATP per mol glucose converted to lactate.

the primary role of the RBC in oxygen transport and delivery, rather than its utilization.

GLYCOLYSIS

Overview

Glucose enters the RBC by facilitated diffusion, via the insulin-independent glucose transporter, GLUT-1. The glucose concentration in the RBC is not significantly different from that in plasma, and clinical laboratory measurements of glucose concentration in plasma, serum and whole blood are essentially identical.

Glycolysis proceeds through a series of phosphorylated intermediates, starting with the synthesis of glucose-6-phosphate (Glc-6-P). During this process, which involves 10 distinct enzymatically catalyzed steps, two molecules of ATP are expended (*investment* stage) to build up a nearly symmetric intermediate, fructose-1,6-bisphosphate (Fru-1,6-BP), which is then cleaved (*splitting* stage) to two three-carbon triose phosphates. These are eventually converted into lactate during the *yield* stage of glycolysis. The yield stage includes both redox and phosphorylation reactions, leading to formation of four molecules of ATP during the conversion of the two triose phosphates into lactate. Two moles of ATP are formed from each mole of triose phosphate, yielding a net 2 moles of ATP per mole of glucose converted into lactate. Glycolysis is a relatively inefficient pathway for extracting energy from glucose: the yield of 2 moles of ATP per mole of glucose is only about 5% of the 36–38 ATP that are avail-

able by complete oxidation of glucose to CO_2 and H_2O in other tissues.

One might ask why a 10-step pathway is required to convert glucose to lactate – couldn't it have been done in fewer steps? The answer, from a metabolic point of view, is that glycolysis is a central pathway and most glycolytic intermediates serve as branch points to other metabolic pathways. In this way, the metabolism of glucose intersects with the metabolism of fats, proteins and nucleic acids, as well as other pathways of carbohydrate metabolism. Some of these metabolic interactions are shown in Figure 11.2.

The investment stage of glycolysis

Glucose-6-phosphate

Glucose is taken up into the red cell via the facilitated transporter, GLUT-1 (Chapter 7); this protein accounts for approximately 5% of total red cell membrane protein, so that transport is not rate limiting for glycolysis. The first step in the commitment of glucose to glycolysis is the phosphorylation of glucose to Glc-6-P, catalyzed by the enzyme hexokinase (Fig. 11.3, top). The formation of Glc-6-P from free glucose and inorganic phosphate is energetically unfavorable, so that a molecule of ATP must be expended or invested in the phosphorylation reaction – the hydrolysis of ATP is coupled to the synthesis of Glc-6-P. The Glc-6-P is trapped in the RBC, along with other phosphorylated intermediates in glycolysis, because there are no transport systems for sugar phosphates in the plasma membranes of mammalian cells.

GLUCOSE UTILIZATION IN THE RED CELL

In a 70-kg person, there are about 5 L of blood and a little over 2 kg (2 L) of RBCs. These cells constitute about 3% of total body mass and consume about 20 g (0.1 mole) of glucose per day, representing about 10% of total body glucose metabolism. The RBC has the highest specific rate of glucose utilization of any cell in the body, approximately 10 g of glucose/kg of tissue/day, compared with ~2.5 g of glucose/kg of tissue/day for the whole body.

In the RBC, about 90% of glucose (~18 g or 0.1 mole) is metabolized via glycolysis, yielding ~0.2 mole of lactate (~18 g/day). Despite its high rate of glucose consumption, the RBC has one of the lowest rates of ATP synthesis of any cell in the body, ~0.2 mole of ATP per day, reflecting the fact that most of its glucose metabolism is carried out by anaerobic glycolysis, which produces lactate and traps only a fraction of the energy available from complete combustion of glucose to CO_2 and H_2O.

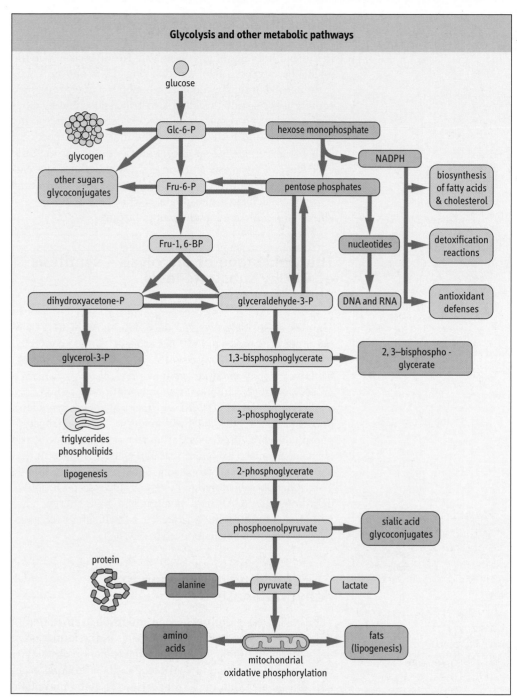

Fig. 11.2 **Interactions between glycolysis and other metabolic pathways.** The green colored boxes indicate intermediates involved in the pathway of glycolysis. Other boxes illustrate some of the metabolic interactions between glycolysis and other metabolic pathways in the cell. Not all of these pathways are active in the red cell which has limited biosynthetic capacity and lacks mitochondria. Glc-6-P, glucose-6-phosphate; Fru-6-P, fructose-6-phosphate; Fru-1,6-BP, fructose-1,6-bisphosphate.

Fructose-6-phosphate

The second step in glycolysis is the conversion of Glc-6-P into Fru-6-P by phosphoglucose isomerase (Fig. 11.3, middle). Isomerases catalyze freely reversible equilibrium reactions, in this case an aldose-ketose interconversion. The Fru-6-P can now be phosphorylated at C-1 by phosphofructokinase-1 (PFK-1) to yield the pseudosymmetric intermediate, fructose 1,6-bisphosphate (Fru-1,6-BP), which has a phosphate ester on each end of the molecule. PFK-1 requires ATP as a substrate and, like hexokinase, catalyzes an essentially irreversible reaction ($K_{eq} \approx 500$). Both hexokinase and PFK-1 are important regulatory enzymes in glycolysis, but PFK-1 is the critical step. This reaction commits glucose to glycolysis, the only pathway for metabolism of Fru-1,6-BP.

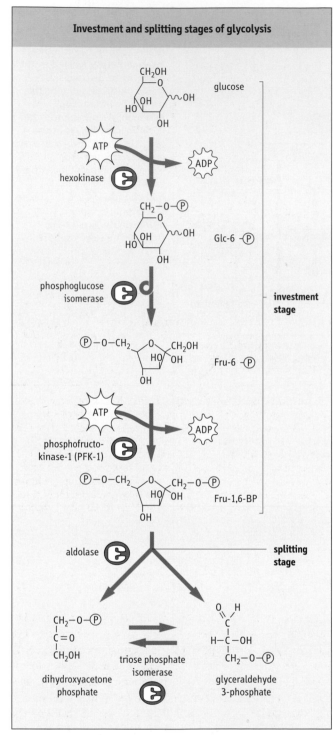

Investment and splitting stages of glycolysis

Fig. 11.3 **The investment and splitting stages of glycolysis.** Note the consumption of ATP at the hexokinase and phosphofructokinase-1 reactions.

The splitting stage of glycolysis

In the splitting stage of glycolysis, Fru-1,6-BP is cleaved in the middle by a reverse-aldol reaction (Fig. 11.3, bottom), thus the name aldolase. The aldolase reaction is a freely reversible equilibrium reaction, yielding two triose-phosphates, dihydroxyacetone phosphate and glyceraldehyde-3-phosphate, from the top and bottom half of the molecule, respectively. Only the glyceraldehyde-3-phosphate continues through the yield stage of glycolysis, but triose phosphate isomerase catalyzes the interconversion of dihydroxyacetone phosphate into glyceraldehyde 3-phosphate, so that both halves of the glucose molecule are metabolized to lactate.

The yield stage of glycolysis – synthesis of ATP by substrate-level phosphorylation

The yield stage of glycolysis produces four moles of ATP, yielding a net of 2 moles of ATP per mole of glucose converted into lactate (Fig. 11.4). The synthesis of ATP is accomplished by kinases that catalyze *substrate-level phosphorylation*, a process in which a high-energy phosphate compound transfers its phosphate to ATP. To set the stage for substrate level phosphorylation, the aldehyde group of glyceraldehyde-3-phosphate is oxidized to a carboxylic acid and the energy available from the oxidation reaction is used, in part, to trap a phosphate from the cytoplasmic pool as an acyl phosphate. This reaction is catalyzed by glyceraldehyde-3-phosphate dehydrogenase (GAPDH), yielding the high-energy compound, 1,3-bisphosphoglycerate (1,3-BPG). The coenzyme, NAD^+ is simultaneously reduced to NADH.

Glyceraldehyde-3-phosphate dehydrogenase

The GAPDH reaction provides an interesting illustration of the role of enzyme-bound intermediates in the formation of high-energy phosphates. How does the oxidation of an aldehyde and the reduction of NAD^+ lead to the formation of an acyl phosphate bond in 1,3-BPG? How does the phosphate enter the picture, and become activated to a high-energy state? The inhibition of GAPDH by reagents such as iodoacetamide, *p*-chloromecuribenzoate and N-ethylmaleimide pointed to involvement of an active-site sulfhydryl residue, leading to the proposed mechanism of action of this enzyme, described in Figure 11.5.

Substrate-level phosphorylation

Phosphoglycerate kinase catalyzes transfer of the phosphate group from the high energy acyl phosphate of 1,3-BPG to

Yield stage of glycolysis

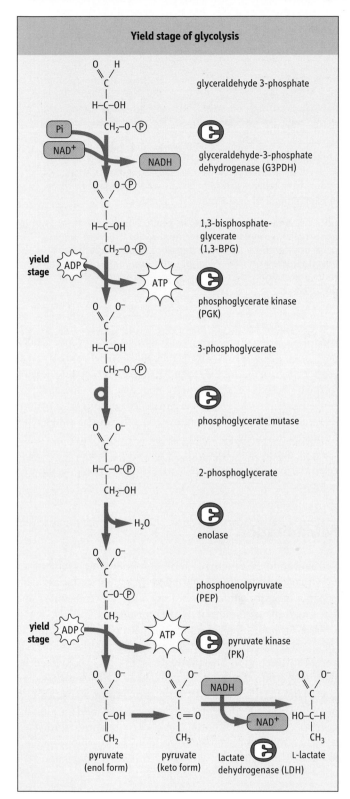

Fig. 11.4 **The yield stage of glycolysis.** Substrate-level phosphorylation reactions catalyzed by phosphoglycerate kinase and pyruvate kinase produce ATP, using the high-energy compounds, 1,3-bisphosphoglycerate and phosphoenolpyruvate, respectively. Note that the NADH produced during the glyceraldehyde-3-phosphate dehydrogenase reaction is converted back into NAD+ during the lactate dehydrogenase reaction, permitting continued glycolysis in the presence of only catalytic amounts of NAD+.

G3PDH reaction

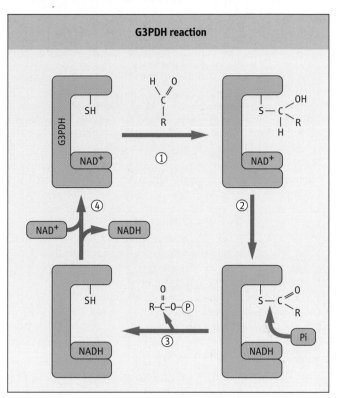

Fig. 11.5 **Mechanism of the glyceraldehyde-3-phosphate dehydrogenase (G3PDH) reaction.** In Step 1, an active-site sulfhydryl group of G3PDH forms a thiohemiacetal adduct with glyceraldehyde-3-phosphate. In Step 2, the thiohemiacetal is oxidized to a thioester by NAD+, also bound in the active site of the enzyme. In Step 3, phosphate enters the active site and, in a phosphorylase reaction, displaces the thiol group, yielding 1,3-bisphosphoglycerate and regenerating the sulfhydryl group. In Step 4, the enzyme exchanges NADH for NAD+, completing the catalytic cycle.

ADP, forming ATP. This substrate level phosphorylation reaction yields the first ATP produced in glycolysis. The remaining phosphate group in 3-phosphoglycerate is an ester phosphate and does not have enough energy to phosphorylate ADP, so a series of isomerization and dehydration reactions is enlisted to convert the ester phosphate into a high-energy enol phosphate. The first step is to move the phosphate to C-2 of glycerate, converting 3-phosphoglycerate into 2-phosphoglycerate, catalyzed by the enzyme phosphoglycerate mutase (see Fig. 11.4). Mutases catalyze the transfer of functional groups within a molecule. Phosphoglycerate mutase has an active-site histidine residue, and a phosphohistidine adduct is formed as an enzyme-bound intermediate during the phosphate transfer reaction.

2-Phosphoglycerate then undergoes a dehydration reaction, catalyzed by enolase, to yield phosphoenolpyruvate (PEP), a high-energy phosphate compound. PEP is used by pyruvate kinase to phosphorylate ADP, yielding pyruvate and the second ATP, again by substrate-level phosphorylation. It

INHIBITION OF SUBSTRATE-LEVEL PHOSPHORYLATION BY ARSENATE

Arsenic is just below phosphorus in the Periodic Chart of the Elements, and it might be expected to share some of the properties and reactivity of phosphate. In fact, arsenate has pKa values similar to those of phosphate and can actually be used by G3PDH, producing 1-arsenato-3-phosphoglycerate. However, the acyl-arsenate bond is unstable and hydrolyzes rapidly in water. Because the high-energy acyl-phosphate bond is discharged nonenzymatically, ATP is not generated by substrate-level phosphorylation. While arsenate does not inhibit any of the enzymes of glycolysis, it dissipates the redox energy available from the G3PDH reaction and prevents the formation of ATP by substrate-level phosphorylation at the phosphoglycerate kinase reaction. In effect, arsenate uncouples the energy available from oxidation of G3PDH for the phosphorylation of adenosine diphosphate (ADP). In the presence of arsenate, the net yield of ATP from anaerobic glycolysis drops to zero moles of ATP per mole of glucose converted to lactate.

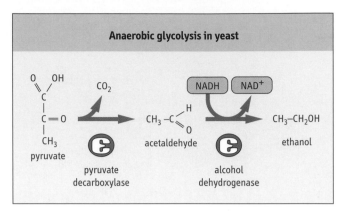

Fig. 11.6 **Anaerobic glycolysis in yeast.** Formation of ethanol by anaerobic glycolysis during fermentation. Pyruvate is decarboxylated by pyruvate decarboxylase, yielding acetaldehyde and CO_2. Alcohol dehydrogenase uses NADH to reduce acetaldehyde to ethanol, regenerating NAD^+ for glycolysis.

seems strange that the high-energy phosphate bond in PEP can be formed by a simple sequence of isomerization and dehydration reactions. However, the thermodynamic driving force for these reactions is probably derived from charge-charge repulsion between the phosphate and carboxylate groups of 2-phosphoglycerate and the isomerization of enolpyruvate to pyruvate following the phosphorylation reaction.

Lactate dehydrogenase (LDH)

Phosphoglycerate kinase and pyruvate kinase catalyze the ATP-generating reactions of glycolysis, yielding 2 moles of ATP per mole of triose phosphate, or a total of 4 moles of ATP per mole of Fru-1,6-BP. After adjustment for the ATP invested in the hexokinase and PFK-1 reactions, the net energy yield is 2 moles of ATP per mole of glucose converted into pyruvate. Two molecules of pyruvate have exactly the same number of carbons and oxygens as one molecule of glucose; however, there is a deficit of four hydrogens – each pyruvate has four hydrogens, a total of eight hydrogens for two pyruvates, compared with 12 in a molecule of glucose. The 'missing' four hydrogens remain in the form of the 2NADH and 2 H+ formed in the G3PDH reaction. Since NAD+ is present in only catalytic amounts in the cell and is an essential cofactor for glycolysis (and other reactions), there must be a mechanism for regeneration of NAD+ if glycolysis is to continue.

The oxidation of NADH is accomplished under anaerobic conditions by lactate dehydrogenase (LDH) which catalyzes reduction of pyruvate to lactate by NADH + H+, regenerating NAD+. In mammals, all cells have LDH, and lactate is the end

product of glycolysis under anaerobic conditions. Under aerobic conditions, mitochondria oxidize NADH to NAD+ and convert pyruvate to CO_2 and H_2O, so that lactate is not formed. Despite their capacity for oxidative metabolism, however, some cells may at times 'go glycolytic', forming lactate, e.g. in muscle during oxygen debt and in phagocytes in pus or in poorly perfused tissues. Under anaerobic conditions or in red cells, lactate is excreted into blood, where it is retrieved by liver for use as a substrate for gluconeogenesis (Chapter 12).

Fermentation

Fermentation is a general term for anaerobic metabolism of glucose. Some anaerobic bacteria, such as lactobacilli, produce lactate, while others have alternative mechanisms for anaerobic oxidation of NADH formed during glycolysis. During fermentation in yeast, the pathway of glycolysis is identical with that in the RBC, except that pyruvate is converted into ethanol. The pyruvate is first decarboxylated by pyruvate decarboxylase to acetaldehyde, releasing CO_2. The NADH produced in the GAPDH reaction is then re-oxidized by alcohol dehydrogenase, regenerating NAD+ and producing ethanol (Fig. 11.6). Ethanol is a toxic compound, and yeast die when the ethanol concentration in their medium reaches about 12%, which is the approximate concentration of alcohol in natural wines.

Regulation of glycolysis in erythrocytes

RBCs consume glucose at a fairly steady rate. They are not physically active like muscle, and do not require energy for

✳ INHIBITION OF ENOLASE BY FLUORIDE

Measurement of blood glucose concentration is used for the diagnosis of diabetes. Frequently these measurements are made in the clinical laboratory more than 1 h after the collection of the blood sample. Because RBCs can metabolize glucose to lactate, even in a sealed, anaerobic vial, the glucose in blood will be consumed, with concomitant production of lactate, which will lead to acidification of the blood sample. These reactions proceed in RBCs at room temperature, so that both blood glucose concentration and pH will decrease during standing. How can this be prevented? This is readily achieved by adding an inhibitor of glycolysis. Sulfhydryl reagents would work – they are inhibitors of GAPDH; however, most blood samples are collected with a small amount of a much cheaper reagent, sodium fluoride, in the sample-collection vial. Fluoride is a strong competitive inhibitor of enolase, blocking glycolysis and lactate production in the RBC. It is an unusual competitive inhibitor, since fluoride bears little resemblance to 2-phosphoglycerate. In this case, fluoride forms a complex with phosphate and Mg^{2+} in the active site of the enzyme, blocking access of substrate.

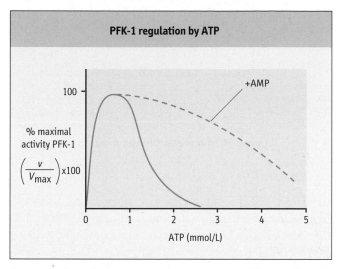

Fig. 11.7 **Allosteric regulation of phosphofructokinase-1 (PFK-1) by ATP.** AMP is a potent activator of PFK-1 in the presence of ATP.

transport of O_2 or CO_2. Glycolysis in red cells appears to be regulated simply by the energy needs of the cell, i.e. the requirement for ATP to maintain ion gradients, which is relatively constant. The balance between ATP consumption and production is controlled allosterically at three sites, the hexokinase, phosphofructokinase-1, and pyruvate kinase reactions (Fig. 11.2). Based on measurements of the V_{max} of the various enzymes in RBC lysates *in vitro*, hexokinase is present at the lowest activity of all glycolytic enzymes. Its maximal activity is only about five times the rate of glucose consumption by the RBC. However, it is also subject to feedback (allosteric) inhibition by its product Glc-6-P, and is rate-limiting for glucose utilization in the RBC – in contrast, the glucose transporter GLUT-1 is present at much higher concentration and activity, representing over 5% of total RBC membrane protein. Hexokinase has 30% homology between its N and C terminal domains, the result of duplication and fusion of a primordial gene; binding of Glc-6-P to the N-terminal domain inhibits the activity of the enzyme and production of Glc-6-P at the active site in the C-terminal domain.

PFK-1 is the primary site of regulation of glycolysis, controlling the flux of Fru-6-P to Fru-1,6-BP and, indirectly through the phosphoglucose isomerase reaction, the level of Glc-6-P and inhibition of hexokinase. Although present at 20 times higher concentration than hexokinase, PFK-1 activity is uniquely sensitive to the energy status of the cell. Amazingly, ATP is both a substrate and an allosteric inhibitor of PFK-1 – a dual function that permits fine control over the activity of the enzyme (Fig. 11.7). AMP and ADP relieve the

inhibition by ATP, so that the overall activity of PFK-1, and thus the rate of glycolysis, depends on the cell's (AMP + ADP)/ATP concentration ratio. These products are interconvertible by the adenylate kinase reaction:

$$2\ ADP \rightleftharpoons ATP + AMP$$

When ATP is consumed and ADP increases, AMP is formed. The increasing ADP and AMP concentrations relieve the inhibition of PFK-1 by ATP, activating glycolysis. The phosphorylation of ADP during glycolysis and then of AMP by the adenylate kinase reaction gradually restores the ATP concentration or *energy charge* of the cell, and, as the AMP concentration declines, the rate of glycolysis decreases to a steady-state level. In general, glycolysis operates at a constant rate in the red cell, where ATP consumption is steady, but the activity of this pathway changes rapidly in response to ATP consumption (and AMP generation) in muscle during exercise.

As shown in Figure 11.7, the concentration of ATP in the RBC (1–2 mmol/L), is poised at the steep point in the concentration-response curve for ATP inhibition of PFK-1. Under normal conditions, the activity of PFK-1 is heavily suppressed by ambient ATP. AMP, which is present at much lower concentration (~0.05 mmol/L), relieves this inhibition. In effect, small fractional conversions of ATP to AMP in the RBC yield large relative increases in AMP concentration. In this way, the activity of PFK-1 in the red cell (and especially muscle) becomes exquisitely sensitive to changes in the energy status of the cell, as measured by the AMP concentration. AMP not only relieves the inhibition of PFK-1 by ATP, but also decreases the K_m for the substrate Fru-6-P, further increasing the catalytic efficiency of the enzyme.

In addition to regulation at hexokinase and PFK-1, pyruvate kinase in liver is allosterically activated by Fru-1,6-BP,

Regulation of glycolysis in the red cell	
Enzyme	**Regulator**
Hexokinase	inhibited by glucose-6-P
Phosphofructokinase-1	inhibited by ATP; activated by AMP
Pyruvate kinase	activated by fructose-1,6-BP

Table 11.1 **Regulation of glycolysis in the red cell.**

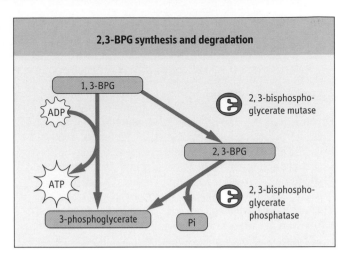

Fig. 11.8 **Pathway for biosynthesis and degradation of 2,3-bisphosphoglycerate (2,3-BPG).** BPG mutase catalyzes the conversion of 1,3-BPG into 2,3-BPG. The same enzyme has bisphosphoglycerate phosphatase activity, which hydrolyzes the 2-phosphate group, yielding 3-phosphoglycerate. Note that this pathway bypasses the phosphoglycerate kinase reaction, so that the overall yield of ATP per mol of glucose is decreased.

the product of the PFK-1 reaction. This process, known as feed-forward regulation, may be important in the RBC to limit the accumulation of reactive triose phosphate intermediates in the cytosol.

Each of the three enzymes involved in regulation of glycolysis – hexokinase, PFK-1, and pyruvate kinase – has characteristic features of regulatory enzymes: they are dimeric or tetrameric enzymes, are present at low V_{max} in comparison with other enzymes in the pathway, and catalyze irreversible reactions. The regulation of glycolysis in liver, muscle, and other tissues is more complicated than in the RBC (Table 11.1), because of greater variability in the rate of fuel consumption and the interplay between carbohydrate and lipid metabolism during aerobic metabolism. In these tissues, the amount and activity of the regulatory enzymes are regulated by other allosteric effectors, by covalent modification, and by induction or repression of enzyme activity.

SYNTHESIS OF 2,3-BISPHOSPHOGLYCERATE

2,3-Bisphosphoglycerate (2,3-BPG) (Fig. 11.8) is an important by-product of glycolysis in the RBC, sometimes reaching 5 mmol/L concentration, comparable with the molar concentration of Hb in the RBC. It is in fact the major phosphorylated intermediate in the erythrocyte, present at even higher concentrations than ATP (1–2 mmol/L) or inorganic phosphate (1 mmol/L). 2,3-BPG is a negative allosteric effector of the O_2 affinity of Hb. It decreases the O_2 affinity of deoxyhemoglobin, promoting the release of O_2 in peripheral tissue. The presence of 2,3-BPG in the RBC explains the observation that the O_2 affinity of purified HbA is greater than that of whole RBCs. 2,3-BPG concentration increases in the RBC during adaptation to high altitude and in anemia, promoting the release of O_2 to tissues when the O_2-tension and saturation of hemoglobin is decreased in the lung. Fetal Hb (HbF) is less sensitive than adult Hb (HbA) to the effects of 2,3-BPG, promoting efficient transfer of O_2 across the placenta from HbA to HbF (see Chapter 4).

THE PENTOSE PHOSPHATE PATHWAY

Overview

The pentose phosphate pathway is a cytosolic pathway present in all cells, so named because it is the primary pathway for formation of pentose phosphates for synthesis of nucleotides for polymerization into DNA and RNA. This pathway branches from glycolysis at the level of Glc-6-P, thus its alternative designation, the hexose monophosphate shunt. The pentose phosphate pathway is also described as a shunt, rather than a pathway, because, when pentoses are not needed for biosynthetic reactions, the pentose phosphate intermediates are recycled to the mainstream of glycolysis by conversion into Fru-6-P and glyceraldehyde-3-phosphate. This rerouting is especially important in the RBC and in non-dividing or quiescent cells, where there is limited need for synthesis of DNA and RNA.

NADPH is a major product of the pentose phosphate pathway in all cells. In tissues with active lipid biosynthesis, e.g. liver, adrenal cortex or lactating mammary glands, the NADPH is used in redox reactions required for biosynthesis of fatty acids, cholesterol, steroid hormones, and bile salts. The liver also uses NADPH for hydroxylation reactions involved in the detoxification and excretion of drugs. The RBC has little biosynthetic activity, but still shunts about 10% of glucose through the pentose phosphate pathway, in this case almost exclusively for the production of NADPH. The NADPH is used primarily for the reduction of a cysteine-containing tripeptide glutathione (GSH), an essential cofactor for antioxidant protection (Chapter 35).

The pentose phosphate pathway is divided into an irreversible redox stage, which yields both NADPH and pentose phosphates, and a reversible interconversion stage, in which excess pentose phosphates are converted into glycolytic intermediates. Both stages are important in the RBC, since it needs NADPH for reduction of glutathione, but has limited need for *de novo* synthesis of pentoses.

The redox stage of the pentose phosphate pathway – synthesis of NADPH

NADPH is synthesized by two dehydrogenases, in the first and third reactions of the pentose phosphate pathway (Fig. 11.9). In the first step of the pathway, the Glc-6-P dehydrogenase (G6PDH) reaction produces NADPH by oxidation of Glc-6-P to 6-phosphogluconic acid lactone, a cyclic sugar ester. The lactone is hydrolyzed to 6-phosphogluconic acid by lactonase. Oxidative decarboxylation of 6-phosphogluconate, catalyzed by 6-phosphogluconate dehydrogenase, then yields the ketose sugar, ribulose 5-phosphate, plus 1 mole of CO_2 and the second and final mole of NADPH.

CONCENTRATIONS OF REDOX COENZYMES IN THE CELL

G6PDH and 6-phosphogluconate dehydrogenase maintain a cytoplasmic ratio of NADPH/NADP⁺ ≈100. Interestingly, because NAD⁺ is required for glycolysis, the ratio of NADH/NAD⁺ in the cytoplasm is nearly the inverse, less than 0.01. Although the total concentrations (oxidized plus reduced forms) of NAD(H) and NADP(H) in the RBC are similar (~25 μmol/L), the cell maintains these two redox systems with similar redox potentials at such different setpoints in the same cell by isolating their metabolism through the specificity of cytoplasmic dehydrogenases. The glycolytic enzymes (G3PDH and LDH) use only NAD(H), while pentose phosphate pathway enzymes use only NADP(H). There are no enzymes in the RBC that catalyze the reduction of NAD⁺ by NADPH, so that high levels of both NAD⁺ and NADPH can exist simultaneously in the same compartment.

The interconversion stage of the pentose phosphate pathway

In cells with active nucleic acid synthesis, ribulose-5-phosphate is isomerized to ribose-5-phosphate for synthesis of ribo- and deoxyribo-nucleotides for RNA and DNA (Fig.

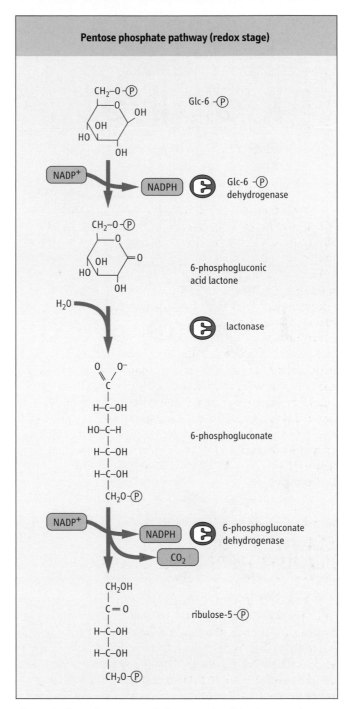

Pentose phosphate pathway (redox stage)

Fig. 11.9 **The redox stage of the pentose phosphate pathway.** A sequence of three enzymes forms 2 moles of NADPH per mole of Glc-6-P, which is converted into ribulose-5-phosphate, with evolution of CO_2.

11.10). In non-dividing cells, the pentose phosphates are routed back to glycolysis. This is accomplished by a series of equilibrium reactions in which 3 moles of ribulose-5-phosphate are converted into 2 moles of Fru-6-P and 1 mole of glyceraldehyde-3-phosphate. Certain restrictions are imposed on the interconversion reactions – they may be

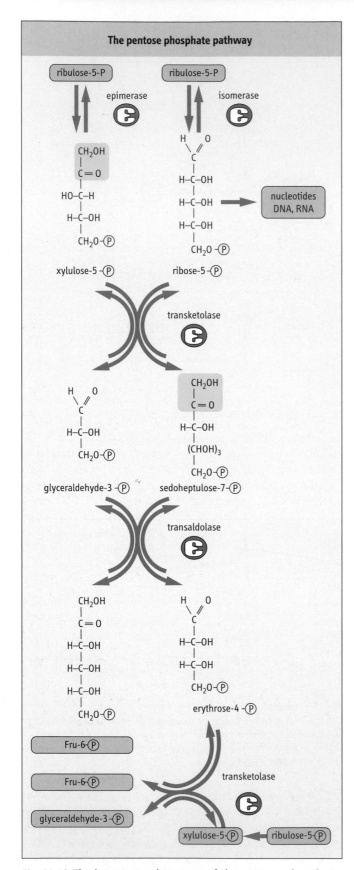

Fig. 11.10 **The interconversion stage of the pentose phosphate pathway.** The carbon skeletons of three molecules of ribulose-5-phosphate are shuffled to form two molecules of Fru-6-P and one molecule of glyceraldehyde 3-phosphate.

The Pentose Phosphate Pathway

Substrate(s)		Product(s)	Enzyme
Ribulose-5-P	⇌	Ribose-5-P	isomerase
2 Ribulose-5-P	⇌	2 Xylulose-5-P	epimerase
Xylulose-5-P + Ribose-5-P	⇌	Glyceraldehyde-3-P + Sedoheptulose-7-P	transketolase
Sedoheptulose-7-P + Glyceraldehyde-3-P	⇌	Erythrose-4-P + Fructose-6-P	transaldolase
Xylulose-5-P + Erythrose-4-P	⇌	Glyceraldehyde-3-P + Fructose-6-P	transketolase
3 Ribulose-5-P	⇌	Glyceraldehyde-3-P + 2 Fructose-6-P	

Table 11.2 **Summary of equilibrium reactions in the Pentose Phosphate Pathway.**

carried out only by transfer of two or three carbon units between sugar phosphates. Each reaction must also involve a ketose donor and an aldose receptor. Isomerases and epimerases provide the five-carbon aldose and ketose phosphate substrates for the interconversion stage. Transketolase, a thiamine-dependent enzyme, catalyzes the two-carbon transfer reactions. Transaldolase acts similarly to the aldolase in glycolysis, except that the three-carbon unit is transferred to another sugar, rather than released as a free triose phosphate into the cytoplasm.

As shown in Figure 11.10 and Table 11.2, two molecules of ribulose 5-phosphate, the first pentose product of the redox stage, are converted into separate products: one molecule is isomerized to the aldose sugar, ribose-5-phosphate, and the other is epimerized to xylulose-5-phosphate. Transketolase then catalyzes transfer of two carbons from xylulose-5-phosphate to ribose-5-phosphate, yielding a seven-carbon ketose sugar, sedoheptulose-7-phosphate, and the three-carbon glyceraldehyde-3-phosphate. Transaldolase then catalyzes a three-carbon transfer between the two transketolase products, from sedoheptulose-7-phosphate to glyceraldehyde-3-phosphate, yielding the first glycolytic intermediate, Fru-6-P, and a residual erythrose-4-phosphate. A second molecule of xylulose-5-phosphate donates two carbons to erythrose-4-phosphate in a second transketolase reaction, yielding a second molecule of Fru-6-P and a molecule of glyceraldehyde-3-phosphate, both of which enter glycolysis.

Thus, the three five-carbon sugar phosphates formed in the redox stage of the pentose phosphate pathway are converted into one three-carbon and two six-carbon glycolytic intermediates. In the RBC, these glycolytic intermediates normally continue through glycolysis to lactate, illustrating that glucose is only temporarily shunted away from the mainstream of glycolysis.

✳ MEASUREMENT OF BLOOD GLUCOSE – REDUCING SUGAR ASSAYS

The original assays for blood glucose measured the reducing activity of blood. These assays work because glucose, at 5 mM concentration, is the major reducing substance in blood. The Fehling and Benedict assays use alkaline cupric salt solutions. With heating, the glucose decomposes oxidatively, yielding a complex mixture of organic acids and aldehydes. Oxidation of the sugar reduces cupric ion (blue-green color) to cuprous ion (orange-red color) in solution. The color yield produced is directly proportional to the glucose content of the sample. Reducing sugar assays do not distinguish between glucose, fructose or galactose. In diseases of fructose and galactose metabolism, such as hereditary fructose intolerance of galactosemia (Chapter 25), these assays could yield positive results for high plasma and urinary sugars, creating the false impression of diabetes.

Function of the pentose phosphate pathway in the red cell

Glutathione (GSH) is a tripeptide γ–glutamyl-cysteinyl-glycine (Fig. 11.11). It is present in cells at 2–5 mmol/L, 99% in the reduced (thiol) form, and is an essential coenzyme for protection the cell against a range of oxidative and chemical insults (Chapter 35). Most of the NADPH formed in the red cell is used by glutathione reductase to maintain GSH in the reduced state. During its function as a coenzyme for antioxidant activities, GSH is oxidized to the disulfide form, GSSG, which is then regenerated by the action of glutathione reductase (Fig. 11.12).

GSH has a range of protective functions in the cell. Glutathione peroxidase (GPx) is found in all cells and uses

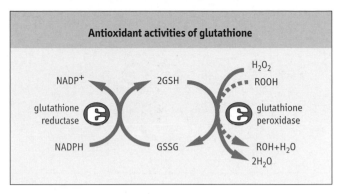

Antioxidant activities of glutathione

Fig. 11.12 **Antioxidant activities of glutathione.** GSH is the coenzyme for glutathione peroxidase which detoxifies hydrogen peroxide and organic (lipid) hydroperoxides. Hydrogen peroxide and lipid peroxides are formed spontaneously in the red cell, catalyzed by side reactions of heme iron during oxygen transport on hemoglobin (Chapter 35).

GSH for detoxification of hydrogen peroxide and organic (lipid) peroxides in the cytosol and cell membranes (Fig. 11.12). Because GPx contains a selenocysteine residue in its active site, selenium, which is required in trace amounts in the diet, is often described as an antioxidant nutrient (see Chapter 10).

GSH also acts as an intracellular sulfhydryl buffer, maintaining exposed –SH groups on proteins and enzymes in the reduced state. Under normal circumstances, when proteins are exposed to O_2, their free sulfhydryl groups gradually oxidize to form disulfides, either intramolecularly or intermolecularly with other proteins. In the red cell, GSH maintains the –SH groups of hemoglobin in the reduced state, inhibiting oxidative crosslinking of the protein.

✳ MEASUREMENT OF BLOOD GLUCOSE – ENZYMATIC ASSAYS

In the clinical laboratory, plasma and urinary glucose are measured by automated enzymatic methods. The most common assay procedure uses a mixture of glucose oxidase and peroxidase (Fig. 11.13). Glucose oxidase is highly specific for glucose, but oxidizes only the β-anomer of the sugar, which represents ~64% of glucose in solution. The assay mixture is therefore supplemented with mutarotase, which rapidly catalyzes the interconversion of the anomers, enhancing assay sensitivity by ~50%. The H_2O_2 produced in the oxidase reaction is then used to oxidize a chromogen to yield a colored chromophore. The color yield is directly proportional to the glucose content of the sample. There are fluorometric versions of this assay for high sensitivity, and one commercial analyzer uses an oxygen electrode to measure the rate of decrease in oxygen concentration in the sample, which is also directly proportional to the glucose concentration.

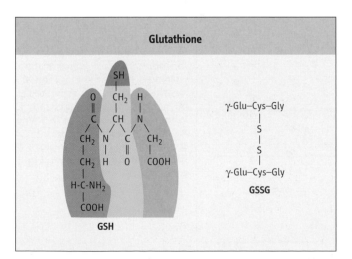

Glutathione

Fig. 11.11 **Glutathione.** Structure of reduced glutathione (GSH) and oxidized glutathione (GSSG).

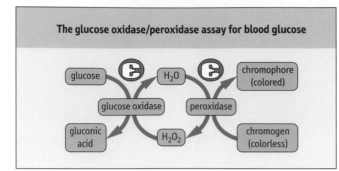

Fig. 11.13 **The glucose oxidase/peroxidase assay for blood glucose.** The color produced in this assay is directly proportional to blood glucose concentration.

 ## MEASUREMENT OF BLOOD GLUCOSE – REAGENT STRIPS AND GLUCOSE METERS

Persons with diabetes normally monitor their blood glucose several times a day using reagent strips and glucose meters. The reagent strips are impregnated with a glucose oxidase-peroxidase reagent. In the manual version of this assay, the extent of color change on a dipstick is related to glucose concentration – typically on a +1 to +4 scale. Glucose meters use a small drop of blood and amperometric electrodes to measure the current produced by the redox reaction catalyzed by glucose oxidase. These assays require only ~5 μL of whole blood. They are not as accurate or precise as laboratory methods, but are commonly used where rapid or frequent measurements of blood glucose are required.

 ## MEASUREMENT OF BLOOD GLUCOSE – KINETIC ASSAYS

In the assay shown in Figure 11.13 and plotted for several glucose concentrations in Figure 11.14A, the reaction is allowed to proceed to its end-point, *i.e.* until all the glucose has been oxidized, then the color change is measured. The color yield is then plotted against a standard to determine blood glucose concentration (Fig. 11.14B). Kinetic analyzers, which are commonly used in clinical chemistry laboratories, estimate the glucose concentration in a sample by measuring the initial rate of the reaction. Analysis of the kinetic plots in Figure 11.14A, for example, indicates that both the end point and the rate of the glucose oxidase assay are dependent on glucose concentration.

Thus, the analyzer can measure the change in absorbance (or some other parameter) during the early stages of the reaction and compare this rate to that of a standard solution to estimate the glucose concentration (Figure 11.14C). These assays are performed on flow-injection or centrifugal analyzers to insure rapid mixing of reagents and sample. Kinetic analyzers are inherently faster than end-point assays because they estimate glucose concentration before the assay reaches its end point. These assays work because glucose oxidase has a high K_m and at concentrations of glucose found in blood, the rate of the oxidase reaction is proportional to glucose concentration, i.e. in the first order region of the Michaelis–Menten equation.

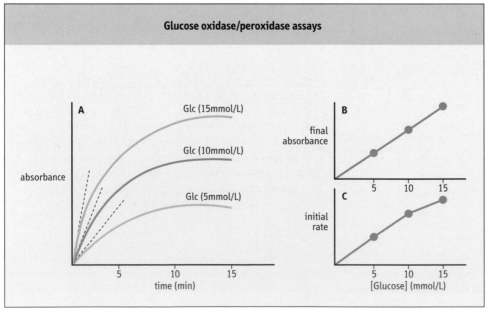

Fig. 11.14 **Glucose oxidase/ peroxidase assays – end-point versus kinetic assays.** (A) Graphical analysis of an end-point assay. (B) The final (end-point) absorbances are plotted as a function of glucose concentration, yielding a straight line. (C) Initial rates of reactions are estimated by multiple measurements early in the assay (dotted lines in frame A), and plotted vs. glucose concentration. Non-linear plots, when obtained, are analyzed by computer.

GLUCOSE-6-PHOSPHATE DEHYDROGENASE DEFICIENCY CAUSES HEMOLYTIC ANEMIA

Just prior to a planned departure to the tropics, a patient visited his physician, complaining of weakness, and noting that his urine had recently become unexplainably dark. Physical examination revealed slightly jaundiced (yellow, icteric) sclera. Laboratory tests indicated a low hematocrit, a high reticulocyte count, and a significantly increased blood level of bilirubin. The patient had been quite healthy during a previous visit a month ago when he received immunizations and prescriptions for antimalarial drugs.

Comment. A number of drugs, particularly primaquine and related antimalarials, undergo redox reactions in the cell, producing large quantities of reactive oxygen species. The ROS cause oxidation of –SH groups in hemoglobin and peroxidation of membrane lipids. Some persons have a genetic defect in Glc-6-P dehydrogenase (Chapter 11), typically yielding an unstable enzyme that has a shorter half-life in the RBC or is unusually sensitive to inhibition by NADPH. In either case, because of the decreased activity of this enzyme and insufficient production of NADPH under stress, the cell's ability to recycle GSSG to GSH is impaired, and drug-induced oxidative stress leads to lysis of RBCs (hemolysis) and hemolytic anemia. Bilirubin, a product of heme metabolism overloads hepatic detoxification pathways, and also accumulates in plasma and tissues, causing jaundice. If the hemolysis is severe enough, Hb spills over into the urine, resulting in hematuria and dark-colored urine. Heinz bodies, disulfide crosslinked aggregates of hemoglobin, are also apparent in blood smears.

Glc-6-P dehydrogenase deficiency is asymptomatic, except in response to an oxidative challenge, which may be induced by drugs (antimalarials, sulfa drugs), diet (fava beans) or severe infection.

There are over 200 known mutations in Glc-6-P dehydrogenase, yielding a wide variation in severity of disease. The RBC appears to be especially sensitive to oxidative stress, because, unlike other cells, it cannot synthesize and replace enzymes. Older cells, which have lower Glc-6-P dehydrogenase activity, are therefore particularly affected. The activity of all enzymes in the RBC declines with the age of the cell, and cell death eventually results from inability of the cells to produce sufficient ATP for maintenance of cellular ion gradients. The gradual increase in cytosolic Ca^{2+} and decline in pentose phosphate activity in older cells is one mechanism leading to crosslinking of membrane proteins and turnover of the RBC in the spleen.

PYRUVATE KINASE DEFICIENCY

A child presented with jaundice and abdominal (splenic) tenderness, which developed following a severe cold. Laboratory tests revealed a low hematocrit and hemoglobin concentration, normochromatic erythrocytes with normal morphology, and mild reticulocytosis. Serum bilirubin was increased.

Comment. Pyruvate kinase deficiency is the most common of the hemolytic anemias that result from a deficiency in a glycolytic enzyme. It is an autosomal recessive disorder that occurs with a frequency of 1/10 000 (~1% gene frequency) in the world population. It is second only to G6PDH deficiency as an enzymatic cause of hemolytic anemia. These diseases are diagnosed by measurement of erythrocyte levels of enzymes or metabolites, by demonstrating abnormalities in enzymatic activities, or by genetic analysis. Enzymatic defects in pyruvate kinase that have been characterized include thermal lability, increased Km for PEP, and decreased activation by Fru-1,6-BP.

Pyruvate kinase deficiency varies significantly in severity, from a mild, compensated condition requiring little intervention to a severe disease requiring transfusions. The anemia results from inability to synthesize ATP, required for maintenance of RBC metabolism, ion gradients and cell shape. Interestingly, patients may tolerate the anemia quite well. The accumulation of 2,3-bisphosphoglycerate in their RBCs decreases the oxygen affinity of hemoglobin, promoting oxygen delivery to muscle during exercise and even to the fetus during pregnancy.

Summary

This chapter describes two ancient metabolic pathways common to all cells in the body, glycolysis and the pentose phosphate pathway. The RBC, which lacks mitochondria and the capability for oxidative metabolism and obtains all of its ATP energy by glycolysis, is used as a model for introducing these pathways. Anaerobic glycolysis in the RBC provides a limited amount of ATP by conversion of the six-carbon sugar, glucose, to two molecules of the three-carbon hydroxyacid, lactate. Through a series of sugar phosphate intermediates, glycolysis provides metabolites for branch points to numerous other metabolic pathways, including the pentose phosphate pathway. This pathway provides pentoses for synthesis of DNA and RNA in nucleated cells, and NADPH for biosynthetic reactions. NADPH is also required for maintenance of reduced glutathione, which is an essential cofactor for antioxidant defense systems that protect the cell against oxidative stress.

ACTIVE LEARNING

1. Why was glucose selected as blood sugar during evolution, rather than other sugars, *e.g.* galactose, fructose or sucrose?
2. Describe coupled enzymatic reactions, using only red cell enzymes, that could be used to measure blood glucose and lactate concentrations.
3. Which test procedure is used for measuring blood glucose in your local hospital? Discuss the principles and normal values for this assay.

Further reading

Arya R, Layton DM, Bellingham AJ. Hereditary red cell enzymopathies. *Blood Reviews* 1995;**9**:165–175.

Brown SP, Keith WB. The effect of acute exercise on levels of erythrocyte 2,3-bisphosphoglycerate: a brief review. *J Sports Med* 1993;11:479–484.

Knull H, Minton AP. Structure within eukaryotic cytoplasm and its relationship to glycolytic metabolism. *Cell Biochemistry and Function* 1996;**14**:237–248.

Mehta A, Mason PJ, Vulliamy TJ. Glucose-6-phosphate deficiency. *Baillière's Clinical Hematology* 2000;**13**:21–38.

McMullin M. The molecular basis of disorders of red cell enzymes. *J Clin Pathol* 1999;**52**:241–244.

Relevant websites

American Society of Hematology: Case Studies on anemia:www.ashteachingcases.org

National Institutes of Health: www.nlm.nih.gov/medlineplus/ency/article/000528.htm

E-Medicine: www.emedicine.com/med/topic1980.htm and topic900.htm

Glucose-6-P dehydrogenase deficiency: www.rialto.com/g6pd/

12. Carbohydrate Storage and Synthesis in Liver and Muscle

J W Baynes

LEARNING OBJECTIVES

After reading this chapter you should be able to:

- Describe the structure of glycogen.
- Identify the primary sites of glycogen storage in the body and the function of glycogen deposits in these tissues.
- Outline the metabolic pathways for synthesis and degradation of glycogen.
- Describe the mechanism by which glycogen is mobilized in liver in response to glucagon and in muscle during exercise and in response to epinephrine.
- Explain the origin and consequences of glycogen storage diseases in liver and muscle.
- Describe the mechanism for counter-regulation of glycogenolysis and glycogenesis in liver.
- Outline the pathway of gluconeogenesis, including substrates, unique enzymes and regulatory mechanisms.

INTRODUCTION

The red cell and the brain have an absolute requirement for blood glucose for energy metabolism. These cells consume about 80% of the 200 g of glucose consumed in the body per day. There is only about 10 g of glucose in the plasma and extracellular fluid volume, so that blood glucose must be replenished constantly. Otherwise, hypoglycemia develops and compromises brain function, leading to confusion and disorientation and possibly life-threatening coma at blood glucose concentrations below 2.5 mmol/L (45 mg/dL). We absorb glucose from our intestines for only 2–3 h following a carbohydrate-containing meal, so there must be a mechanism for maintenance of blood glucose between meals.

Glycogen, a polysaccharide storage form of glucose, is our first line of defense against declining blood glucose concentration. During and immediately following a meal, glucose is converted in liver into glycogen (a process known as glycogenesis). Hepatic glycogen is gradually degraded between meals, by the pathway of glycogenolysis, releasing glucose to maintain blood glucose concentration. However, total hepatic glycogen stores are barely sufficient for maintenance of blood glucose concentration during a 12-h fast.

During sleep, when we are not eating, there is a gradual shift from glycogenolysis to *de novo* synthesis of glucose, also an hepatic pathway, known as gluconeogenesis (Fig. 12.1). Gluconeogenesis is essential for survival during fasting or starvation, when glycogen stores are negligible. The liver uses amino acids from muscle protein as the primary precursor of glucose, but also makes use of lactate from glycolysis and glycerol from fat catabolism. Fatty acids, mobilized from adipose tissue triglyceride stores, provide the energy for gluconeogenesis.

Glycogen is also stored in muscle, but this glycogen is not available for maintenance of blood glucose. Glucose, derived in part from glycogen, especially during bursts of physical activity, is essential for muscle energy metabolism, even though muscle relies primarily on fats as a source of energy. The tissue concentration of glycogen is higher in liver than in muscle, but because of the relative masses of muscle and liver, the majority of glycogen in the body is stored in muscle (Table 12.1).

This chapter describes the pathways of biosynthesis (glycogenesis) and mobilization (glycogenolysis) of glycogen in liver and muscle and the pathway of gluconeogenesis in liver.

STRUCTURE OF GLYCOGEN

Glycogen is a branched polysaccharide of glucose, a homoglucan. It contains only two types of glycosidic linkages, chains of $\alpha 1 \rightarrow 4$-linked glucose residues with $\alpha 1 \rightarrow 6$ branches spaced about every 4-6 residues along the $\alpha 1 \rightarrow 4$ chain (Fig. 12.2). Glycogen is closely related to starch, the storage polysaccharide of plants, but starch consists of a mixture of amylose and amylopectin. The amylose component contains only linear $\alpha 1 \rightarrow 4$ chains; the amylopectin component is more glycogen-like in structure but with fewer $\alpha 1 \rightarrow 6$ branches, about one per 12 $\alpha 1 \rightarrow 4$-linked glucose residues. The gross structure of glycogen is dendritic in nature, expanding from a core sequence bound to a tyrosine residue in the protein glycogenin and developing into a final structure resembling a head of cauliflower. The many glucose molecules on the surface of the glycogen molecule provide ready access for enzymes involved in rapid release of glucose from the glycogen polymer.

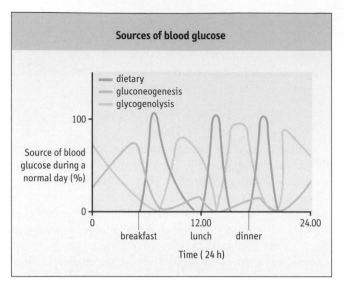

Fig. 12.1 **Sources of blood glucose during a normal day.** Between meals, blood glucose is derived primarily from hepatic glycogen. Depending on the frequency of snacking, glycogenolysis and gluconeogenesis may be more or less active during the day. Late in the night or in early morning, following depletion of a major fraction of hepatic glycogen, gluconeogenesis becomes the primary source of blood glucose.

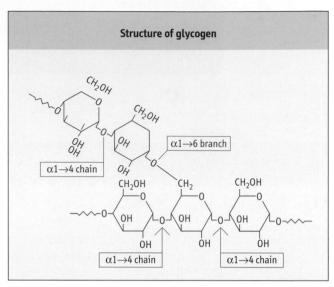

Fig. 12.2 **Close-up of the structure of glycogen.** The figure shows α1→4 chains and an α1→6 branch point. Glycogen is stored as granules in liver and muscle cytoplasm. Most of the glycogenic and glycogenolytic enzymes are bound to these granules, assuring rapid changes in glycogen metabolism in response to allosteric and hormonal stimuli.

Glucose and glycogen stores in the body (70 kg adult)

Tissue	Type	Amount	% of tissue mass	Calories
liver	glycogen	75 g	3–5%	300
muscle	glycogen	250 g	0.5–1.0%	1000
blood and extracellular fluid	glucose	10 g	–	40

Table 12.1 **Tissue distribution of carbohydrate energy reserves (70 kg adult).**

PATHWAY OF GLYCOGENESIS FROM BLOOD GLUCOSE IN LIVER

The liver is rich in the high-capacity, low-affinity (K_m >10 mmol/L) glucose transporter GLUT-2, making it freely permeable to glucose delivered at high concentration in portal blood during and following a meal. The liver is also rich in glucokinase, an enzyme that is specific for glucose and converts it into glucose 6-phosphate (Glc-6-P). Glucokinase (GK) is inducible by continued consumption of a high-carbohydrate diet. It has a high K_m, about 5–7 mmol/L, so that it is poised to increase in activity as portal glucose increases above the normal 5 mmol/L (100 mg/dL) blood glucose concentration. Unlike hexokinase, GK is not inhibited

by Glc-6-P, so that the concentration of Glc-6-P increases rapidly in liver following a carbohydrate-rich meal, forcing glucose into all of the major pathways of glucose metabolism: glycolysis, the pentose phosphate pathway, and glycogenesis. Glucose is channeled into glycogen, providing a carbohydrate reserve for maintenance of blood glucose during the post-absorptive state. Excess Glc-6-P in liver, beyond that needed to replenish glycogen reserves, is then funneled into glycolysis, in part for energy production, but primarily for conversion into triglycerides, which are exported for storage in adipose tissue. Glucose that passes through the liver leads to an increase in peripheral blood glucose concentration following carbohydrate-rich meals. This glucose is used in muscle for synthesis and storage of glycogen and in adipose tissue as a source of glycerol for triglyceride biosynthesis.

The pathway of glycogenesis from glucose (Fig. 12.3A) involves four steps:

- conversion of Glc-6-P into glucose 1-phosphate (Glc-1-P) by phosphoglucomutase;
- activation of Glc-1-P to the sugar nucleotide uridine diphosphate (UDP)-glucose by the enzyme UDP-glucose pyrophosphorylase;
- transfer of glucose to glycogen in α1→4 linkage by glycogen synthase, a member of the class of enzymes known as glycosyl transferases;
- when the α1→4 chain exceeds eight residues in length, glycogen branching enzyme, a transglycosylase, transfers some of the α1→4-linked sugars to an α1→6 branch, setting the stage for continued elongation of

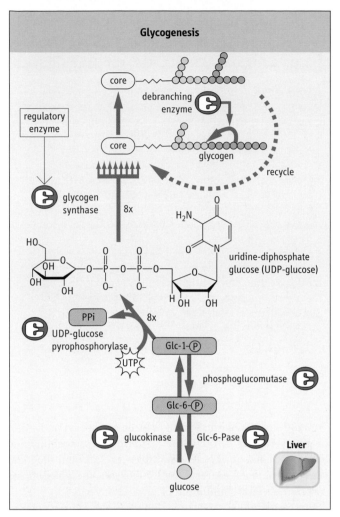

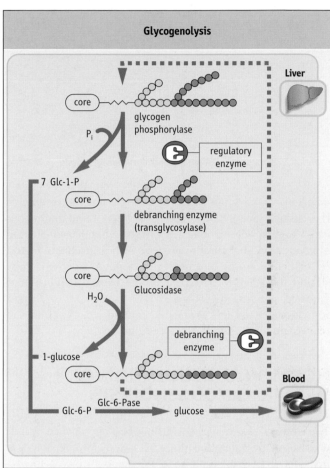

Fig. 12.3 **Pathways of glycogenesis (A) and glycogenolysis (B).** The branching arrays at the top of the figure are meant to illustrate the three-dimensional array of glycogen branching. This branching structure places a substantial fraction of the total glucose molecules on the periphery of the molecule, immediately available for glycogen phosphorylase activity.

both α1→4 chains until they, in turn, become long enough for transfer by branching enzyme.

Glycogen synthase is the regulatory enzyme for glycogenesis, rather than UDP-glucose pyrophosphorylase, because UDP-glucose is also used for synthesis of glycoproteins, glycolipids, and other sugars. Pyrophosphate (PPi), the other product of the pyrophosphorylase reaction, is rapidly hydrolyzed to inorganic phosphate by pyrophosphatase.

PATHWAY OF GLYCOGENOLYSIS IN LIVER

As with most metabolic pathways, separate enzymes, sometimes in separate subcellular compartments, are required for the forward and reverse pathways. The pathway of glycogenolysis (Fig. 12.3B) begins with removal of the abun-

dant, external α1→4 -linked glucose residues in glycogen. This is accomplished not by a hydrolase, but by glycogen phosphorylase, an enzyme that uses cytosolic phosphate and releases glucose from glycogen in the form of Glc-1-P, which is converted into Glc-6-P by phosphoglucomutase. In liver the glucose is released from Glc-6-P by glucose-6-phosphatase (Glc-6-Pase), and the glucose exits via the GLUT-2 transporter into blood. The rate-limiting, regulatory step in glycogenolysis is catalyzed by phosphorylase, the first enzyme in the pathway.

Phosphorylase is specific for α1→4 glycosidic linkages; it cannot cleave α1→6 linkages. Further, this enzyme cannot approach the branching glucose residues efficiently. Thus, as shown in Figure 12.3B, phosphorylase cleaves the external glucose residues until the branches are three or four residues long, then debranching enzyme, which has both transglycosylase and glucosidase activity, moves a short segment of glucose residues bound to the α1→6 branch to the end of an

Hormonal control of glycogenolysis			
Hormone	Source	Initiator	Effect on glycogenolysis
glucagon	pancreatic α-cells	hypoglycemia	rapid activation
epinephrine	adrenal medulla	acute stress, hypoglycemia	rapid activation
cortisol	adrenal cortex	chronic stress	chronic activation
insulin	pancreatic β-cells	hyperglycemia	inhibition

Table 12.2 **Hormones involved in control of glycogenolysis.**

adjacent α1→4 chain, leaving a single glucose residue at the branch point. This glucose is then removed by the exo-1,6-glucosidase activity of branching enzyme, allowing glycogen phosphorylase to proceed with degradation of the α1→4 chain until another branch point is approached, setting the stage for a repeat of the transglycosylase and glucosidase reactions. About 90% of the glucose is released from glycogen as Glc-1-P, and the remainder, derived from the α1→6 branching residues, as free glucose.

HORMONAL REGULATION OF HEPATIC GLYCOGENOLYSIS

The study of glycogen metabolism is best approached by first addressing the regulation of glycogenolysis. Glycogenolysis is activated in liver in response to a demand for blood glucose, either because of its utilization during the post-absorptive state or in preparation for increased glucose utilization in response to stress. There are three major hormonal activators of glycogenolysis: glucagon, epinephrine (adrenaline), and cortisol (Table 12.2).

Glucagon is a peptide hormone (3500 Da), secreted from the α-cells of the endocrine pancreas. Its primary function is to activate hepatic glycogenolysis for maintenance of normoglycemia. It has a short half-life in plasma, about 5 min, as a result of receptor binding, renal filtration, and proteolytic inactivation in liver. Glucagon concentration in plasma therefore changes rapidly in response to the need for blood glucose. Blood glucagon increases between meals, decreases during a meal, and is chronically increased during fasting or on a low-carbohydrate diet.

Glycogenolysis is also activated in response to both acute and chronic stress. The stress may be:

- physiologic, e.g. in response to increased blood glucose utilization during prolonged exercise;
- pathologic, e.g. as a result of blood loss;
- psychological, e.g. in response to acute or chronic threats.

VON GIERKE'S DISEASE: GLYCOGEN STORAGE DISEASE CAUSED BY GLC-6-PASE DEFICIENCY

A baby girl was chronically cranky, irritable, sweaty, and lethargic, and demanded food frequently. Physical evaluation indicated an extended abdomen, resulting from an enlarged liver. Blood glucose, measured 1 h after feeding, was 3.5 mmol/L (70 mg/dL) normal value ~5 mmol/L (100 mg/dL). After 4 h, when the child was exhibiting irritability and sweating, her heart rate was increased (pulse = 110), and blood glucose had declined to 2 mmol/L (40 mg/dL). These symptoms were corrected by feeding. A liver biopsy showed massive deposition of glycogen particles in the liver cytosol.

Comment. This child has a deficiency in glycogen mobilization. Because of the severity of hypoglycemia, the most likely mutation is in hepatic Glc-6-Pase, which is required for glucose production by both glycogenolysis and gluconeogenesis. Treatment involves frequent feeding with slowly digested carbohydrate, e.g. uncooked starch, and nasogastric drip-feeding during the night.

Acute stress, regardless of its source, causes an activation of glycogenolysis through the action of the catecholamine hormone, epinephrine, released from the adrenal medulla. During prolonged exercise, both glucagon and epinephrine contribute to the stimulation of glycogenolysis.

Increased blood concentrations of the adrenocortical steroid hormone cortisol also induce glycogenolysis. Levels of the glucocorticoid cortisol vary diurnally in plasma, but may be chronically elevated under continuously stressful conditions, including psychological and environmental (e.g., cold) stress. Glucagon serves as a general model for the mechanism of action of hormones that act by way of cell-surface receptors. Cortisol, which acts at the level of gene expression, will be discussed later in Chapter 37.

MECHANISM OF ACTION OF GLUCAGON

Glucagon binds to a hepatic plasma-membrane receptor and initiates a cascade of reactions that lead to mobilization of hepatic glycogen (Fig. 12.4). On the inside of the plasma membrane there is a class of signal-transduction proteins, known as G-proteins, that bind guanosine triphosphate (GTP) and guanosine diphosphate (GDP), nucleotide analogs of ATP and ADP. GDP is bound in the resting state. Binding of glucagon to the plasma membrane receptor stimulates exchange of GDP for GTP on the G-protein, and the G-protein

PROTEIN KINASE A IS VERY SENSITIVE TO SMALL CHANGES IN cAMP CONCENTRATION

As illustrated in Figure 12.4, cAMP-dependent PKA is a tetrameric enzyme with two different types of subunits (R_2C_2); a catalytic C-subunit that has protein kinase activity and a regulatory R-subunit that inhibits the protein kinase activity. The R-subunit has a sequence of amino acids that would normally be recognized and phosphorylated by the C-subunit, except that this sequence in R contains an alanine, rather than a serine or threonine, residue. Binding of two molecules of cAMP to each R-subunit results in conformational changes that lead to dissociation of a ($cAMP_2$-R)$_2$ dimer from the C-subunits. The monomeric, active C-subunits then proceed to phosphorylate serine and threonine residues in target enzymes. This is not a typical allosteric regulatory mechanism, but the complete activation of PKA involves cooperative binding of four molecules of cAMP to two R subunits. PKA is fully activated at sub-micromolar concentrations of cAMP, so that it is exquisitely sensitive to small changes in adenylate cyclase activity.

G-PROTEINS

G-proteins are plasma-membrane, guanosine-nucleotide-binding proteins that are involved in signal transduction for a wide variety of hormones (Fig. 12.4; see also Chapter 38). In some cases they stimulate (Gs) and in other cases they inhibit (Gi) protein kinases and protein phosphorylation. G-proteins are closely associated with hormone receptors in plasma membranes and consist of α, β, and γ subunits. The G_α-subunit binds GDP in the resting state. Following hormone binding (ligation), the receptor recruits G-proteins, stimulating exchange of GDP for GTP on the G_α-subunit. GTP binding leads to release of the β- and γ-subunits, and the α-subunit is then free to bind to and activate adenylate cyclase. The hormonal response is amplified following receptor binding, because a single receptor can activate many α-subunits. Hormonal responses are also turned off at the level of receptors and G-proteins by two mechanisms:

- the G_α-subunit has a sluggish guanosine triphosphate phosphatase (GTPase) activity that hydrolyzes GTP, with a half-time measured in minutes, so that it dissociates from, and thereby ceases to activate, adenylate cyclase;
- phosphorylation of the hormone receptor by protein kinases decreases its affinity for the hormone, a process described as desensitization.

These effects dampen the cellular response and require higher levels of extracellular hormone for continued response to the hormone. Chronic high levels of circulating hormone may lead to hormone resistance.

---

then undergoes a conformational change that leads to dissociation of one of its subunits, which then binds to and activates the plasma membrane enzyme, adenylyl cyclase. This enzyme converts cytoplasmic ATP into cyclic-3′,5′-AMP (cAMP), a soluble mediator that is described as the 'second messenger' for action of glucagon (and other hormones). Cyclic AMP binds to the cytoplasmic enzyme protein kinase A (PKA), causing dissociation of inhibitory (regulatory) subunits from the catalytic subunits of the heterodimeric enzyme, relieving inhibition of PKA (see Chapter 38), which then initiates a series of protein-phosphorylation reactions.

The pathway for activation of glycogen phosphorylase (Fig. 12.4) involves phosphorylation of many molecules of phosphorylase kinase by PKA, which then phosphorylates and activates many molecules of glycogen phosphorylase. The net effect of the sequential steps, beginning with activation of many molecules of adenylyl cyclase by G-proteins, is a 'cascade amplification' system, not unlike that of a series of amplifiers in a radio or stereo set, resulting in a massive increase in signal strength within seconds after recognition of glucagon binding to the hepatocyte plasma membrane. Phosphorylation of phosphorylase initiates glycogenolysis, leading to production of Glc-6-P in liver, which is then hydrolyzed to glucose and exported into blood. One other target of PKA is inhibitor-1, a protein phosphatase inhibitor protein, which is activated by phosphorylation. Phosphorylated inhibitor-1 inhibits cytoplasmic phosphoprotein phosphatases, which would otherwise reverse the phosphorylation of enzymes and quench the response to glucagon (see Fig. 12.4).

Glycogenolysis and glycogenesis are opposing pathways. Theoretically, Glc-1-P produced by phosphorylase could be rapidly activated to UDP-glucose and reincorporated into glycogen. To prevent this wasteful or futile cycle, PKA also acts directly on glycogen synthase, in this case inactivating the enzyme. Thus, the activation of glycogenolysis is co-ordinated with inactivation of glycogenesis. Other hepatic pathways, including protein, cholesterol, fatty acid, and triglyceride biosynthesis, and glucose utilization (glycolysis) are also regulated by phosphorylation of key regulatory enzymes, focusing liver metabolism in response to glucagon on the provision of glucose to blood for maintenance of vital body functions (see Chapter 20).

Perhaps in order to balance the cascade of events amplifying the response to glucagon, there are multiple, redundant mechanisms to insure rapid termination of the hormonal response. In addition to the slow GTPase activity of the G_α-subunit, there is also a phosphodiesterase activity in the cell that hydrolyzes cAMP to AMP, permitting reassociation of the inhibitory and catalytic subunits of PKA, decreasing its protein kinase activity. There are also phosphoprotein phosphatases that remove the phosphate groups from the active,

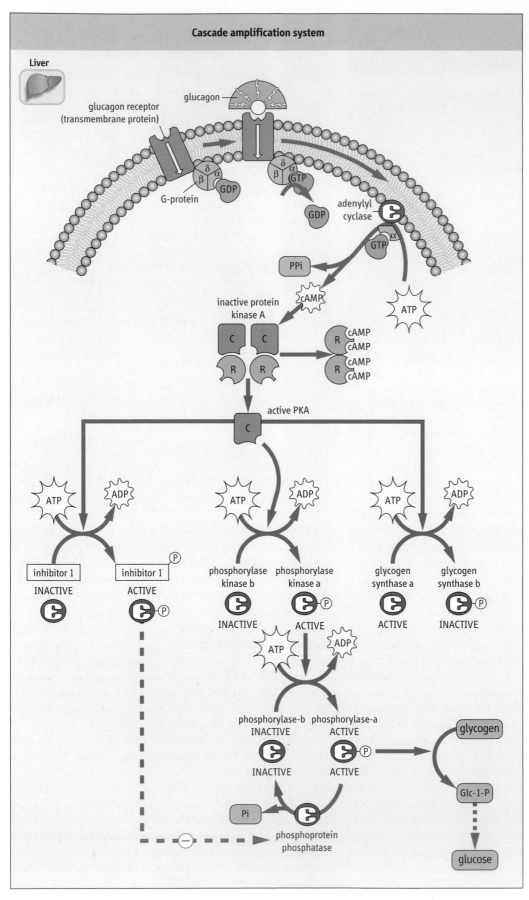

Fig. 12.4 **Cascade amplification system.** Mobilization of hepatic glycogen by glucagon. A cascade of reactions amplifies the hepatic response to glucagon binding to its plasma-membrane receptor. cAMP is known as the second messenger of glucagon action. PKA indirectly activates phosphorylase via phosphorylase kinase and directly inactivates glycogen synthase. C, catalytic subunits; R, regulatory (inhibitory) subunits. PKA, protein kinase A.

phosphorylated forms of phosphorylase kinase and phosphorylase. The decrease in cAMP concentration and PKA activity also leads to decreased phosphorylation of inhibitor-1, permitting increased activity of phosphoprotein phosphatases. Thus, an array of mechanisms act in concert to insure that hepatic glycogenolysis declines rapidly in response to declining blood glucagon concentration (Table 12.3).

There are a number of autosomal recessive genetic diseases affecting glycogen metabolism (Table 12.4). These diseases, known as glycogen storage diseases, are characterized by accumulation of glycogen deposits in tissues, which eventually compromises tissue function. Predictably, glycogen storage diseases affecting hepatic glycogen metabolism are commonly characterized by fasting hypoglycemia and may be life-threatening. Defects in muscle glycogen metabolism are characterized by muscle fatigue during exercise.

Mechanisms of termination of hormonal response to glucagon
Hydrolysis of GTP on G_α-subunit
Hydrolysis of cAMP by phosphodiesterase
Protein phosphatase activity

Table 12.3 **Several mechanisms are involved in terminating the hormonal response to glucagon.**

MAXIMAL INHIBITION OF GLYCOGEN SYNTHASE IS ACHIEVED ONLY THROUGH SEQUENTIAL ACTION OF SEVERAL KINASES

When both glucagon and epinephrine are acting on liver, the activation of glycogenolysis and inhibition of glycogenesis is mediated by at least three kinases: protein kinase A (PKA), protein kinase C (PKC), and Ca^{2+}-calmodulin-activated protein kinase. All three of these protein kinases phosphorylate key serine and threonine residues in regulatory enzymes. These and other protein kinases work in concert with one another in a process known as sequential or hierarchical phosphorylation, leading to phosphorylation of up to nine amino acid residues on glycogen synthase. Maximal inhibition of glycogen synthase is achieved only through the sequential activity of several kinases. In some cases, certain serine or threonine residues must be phosphorylated in a specific sequence by cooperative action of different kinases, i.e. phosphorylation of one site by one enzyme requires prior phosphorylation of another site by a separate enzyme.

MOBILIZATION OF HEPATIC GLYCOGEN BY EPINEPHRINE

Epinephrine works through several distinct receptors on different cells. The best studied of these receptors are the α- and β-adrenergic receptors; they bind epinephrine with different affinities and work by different mechanisms. During severe hypoglycemia, glucagon and epinephrine work together to magnify the glycogenolytic response in liver. However, even when blood glucose is normal, epinephrine is released in response to real or perceived threats, causing an increase in

McARDLE'S DISEASE: A GLYCOGEN STORAGE DISEASE THAT REDUCES CAPACITY FOR EXERCISE

A 30-year-old man consulted his physician because of chronic arm and leg muscle pains and cramps during exercise. He indicated that he had always had some muscle weakness and, for this reason, was not active in scholastic sports, but the problem did not become severe until he recently enrolled in an exercise program to improve his health. He also noted that the pain generally disappeared after about 15–30 min, and then he could continue his exercise without discomfort. His blood glucose concentration was normal during exercise, but serum creatine kinase (MM isoform) was elevated, suggesting muscle damage. Blood glucose declined slightly during 15 min of exercise, but unexpectedly blood lactate also declined, rather than increased, even when he was experiencing muscle cramps. A biopsy indicated an unusually high level of glycogen in muscle, suggesting a glycogen storage disease.

Comment. This patient suffers from McArdle's disease, a rare deficiency of muscle phosphorylase activity. The actual enzyme deficiency must be confirmed by enzyme assay, since a number of other mutations could also affect muscle glycogen metabolism. During the early periods of intense exercise, the muscle obtains most of its energy by metabolism of glucose, derived from glycogen. During cramps, which normally occur during oxygen debt, much of the pyruvate produced by glycolysis is excreted into blood as lactate. In this case, however, the patient did not excrete lactate, suggesting a failure to mobilize muscle glycogen. His recovery after about 0.5 h results from epinephrine-mediated physiologic responses that provide fuels, both glucose and fatty acids, from blood, overcoming the deficit in muscle glycogenolysis. Treatment of McArdle's disease usually involves exercise avoidance or, if necessary, carbohydrate consumption prior to exercise. Otherwise, the course of the disease is uneventful.

Glycogen storage diseases			
Type	Name	Enzyme deficiency	Structural or clinical consequences
I	von Gierke's	Glc-6-Pase	severe postabsorptive hypoglycemia, lactic acidemia, hyperlipidemia
II	Pompe's	lysosomal α-glucosidase	glycogen granules in lysosomes
III	Cori's	debranching enzyme	altered glycogen structure, hypoglycemia
IV	Andersen's	branching enzyme	altered glycogen structure
V	McArdle's	muscle phosphorylase	excess muscle glycogen deposition, exercise-induced cramps and fatigue
VI	Hers'	liver phosphorylase	hypoglycemia, not as severe as Type I

Table 12.4 **Major classes of glycogen-storage diseases.**

blood glucose to support a 'fight or flight' response. Caffeine in coffee and theophylline in tea are inhibitors of phosphodiesterase and also cause an increase in hepatic cAMP and blood glucose. Like epinephrine, caffeine, administered in the form of a few strong cups of coffee, can also make us alert, responsive, and aggressive.

Epinephrine action on hepatic glycogenolysis proceeds by two pathways. One of these, through the epinephrine β-adrenergic receptor, is similar to that for glucagon, involving a plasma-membrane epinephrine-specific receptor, G-proteins, and cAMP. The epinephrine response augments the effects of glucagon during severe hypoglycemia, and also explains, in part, the rapid heartbeat, sweating, tremors, and anxiety associated with hypoglycemia. Epinephrine also works simultaneously through an α-receptor, but by a different mechanism. Binding to α-receptors also involves G-proteins, common elements in hormone signal transduction, but in this case the G-protein is specific for activation of a membrane isozyme of phospholipase C (PLC), which is specific for cleavage of a membrane phospholipid, phosphatidylinositol bisphosphate (PIP$_2$) (Fig. 12.5). Both products of PLC action, diacylglycerol (DAG) and inositol trisphosphate (IP$_3$), act as second messengers of epinephrine action. DAG activates protein kinase C (PKC), which, like PKA, initiates a series of protein-phosphorylation reactions. IP$_3$ promotes the transport of Ca^{2+} into the cytosol. Ca^{2+} then binds to the cytoplasmic protein calmodulin, which binds to and activates phosphorylase kinase, leading to phosphorylation and activation of phosphorylase, providing glucose for blood. A Ca^{2+}-calmodulin-dependent protein kinase and other enzymes are also activated, either by phosphorylation

CHILD BORN OF MALNOURISHED MOTHER MAY HAVE HYPOGLYCEMIA

A baby girl was born at 39 weeks of gestation to a young, malnourished mother. The child was also thin and weak at birth and, within 1 h after birth, was showing signs of distress, including rapid heartbeat and respiration. Her blood glucose was 3.5 mmol/L (63 mg/dL) at birth, and declined rapidly to 1.5 mmol/L (27 mg/dL) by 1 h, when she was becoming unresponsive and comatose. Her condition was markedly improved by infusion of a glucose solution, followed by a carbohydrate-rich diet. She improved gradually over the next 2 weeks before discharge from the hospital.

Comment. During development *in utero*, the fetus obtains glucose exogenously, from the placental circulation. However, following birth, the child relies at first on mobilization of hepatic glycogen, and then on gluconeogenesis for maintenance of blood glucose. Because of the malnourished state of the mother, this child was born with negligible hepatic glycogen reserves. Thus, she was unable to maintain blood glucose homeostasis postpartum and rapidly declined into hypoglycemia, initiating a stress response. After surviving the transient hypoglycemia, she probably still lacked adequate muscle mass to provide a sufficient supply of amino acids for gluconeogenesis. Infusion of glucose, followed by a carbohydrate-rich diet, would address these deficits, but may not correct more serious damage from prolonged malnutrition during fetal development.

or by association with the Ca^{2+}-calmodulin complex. Thus, a range of metabolic pathways is activated in response to stress, especially those involved in the mobilization of energy reserves.

GLYCOGENOLYSIS IN MUSCLE

The tissue localization of hormone receptors provides tissue specificity to hormone action. Only those tissues with glucagon receptors respond to glucagon. Muscle may be rich in glycogen, even during hypoglycemia, but it lacks both the glucagon receptor and Glc-6-Pase. Therefore muscle glycogen cannot be mobilized to replenish blood glucose. Muscle glycogenolysis is activated in response to epinephrine through the β-adrenergic receptor (cAMP-mediated), providing a supply of carbohydrate for the energy needs of muscle. This occurs not only during 'fight or flight' situations, but also during prolonged exercise. There are also two important hormone-independent mechanisms for activation of glycogenolysis in muscle (Fig. 12.6). First, the influx of Ca^{2+} into the muscle cytoplasm in response to nerve stimulation activates the basal, unphosphorylated form of phosphorylase

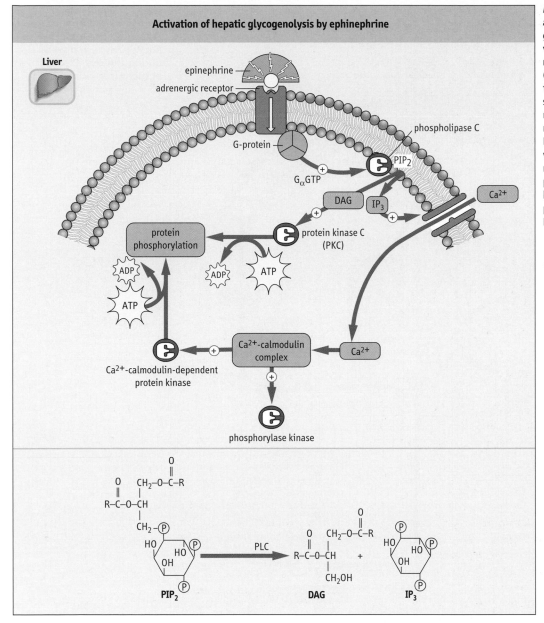

Activation of hepatic glycogenolysis by epinephrine

Fig. 12.5 **Mechanism of activation of glycogenolysis in liver via the α-adrenergic receptor.** Diacylglycerol (DAG) and inositol trisphosphate (IP$_3$) are second messengers mediating the adrenergic response. Both DAG and PKC remain associated with the plasma membrane. PIP$_2$, phosphatidylinositol bisphosphate; PKC, protein kinase C. See also Figures 38.8 and 38.9.

kinase by action of the Ca^{2+}-calmodulin complex. This hormone-independent activation of phosphorylase provides for rapid activation of glycogenolysis during short bursts of exercise, even in the absence of epinephrine action. A second mechanism for activation of muscle glycogenolysis involves direct allosteric activation of phosphorylase by AMP. Increased usage of ATP during a rapid burst of muscle activity leads to rapid accumulation of ADP, which is converted in part into AMP by action of the enzyme myokinase (adenylate kinase), which catalyzes the reaction

$$2\ ADP \rightarrow ATP + AMP$$

AMP activates both the basal and phosphorylated forms of phosphorylase, enhancing glycogenolysis either in the absence or presence of hormonal stimulation. AMP also relieves inhibition of phosphofructokinase-1 (PFK-1) by ATP (see Chapter 11), stimulating the utilization of glucose through glycolysis for energy production. The stimulatory effects of Ca^{2+} and AMP assure that the muscle can respond to its energy needs, even in the absence of hormonal input.

REGULATION OF GLYCOGENESIS

Glycogenesis, and energy storage in general, occurs during and immediately following meals. Glucose and other carbohydrates, rushing into the liver from the intestines via the portal circulation, are efficiently trapped to make glycogen.

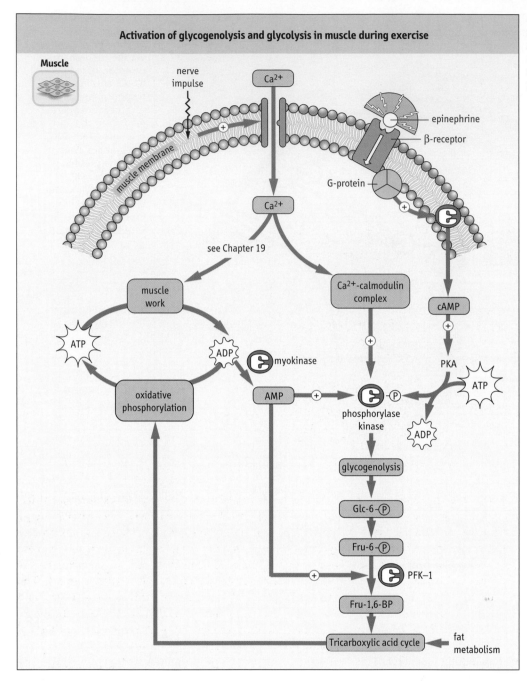

Activation of glycogenolysis and glycolysis in muscle during exercise

Fig. 12.6 **Regulation of protein kinase A in muscle.** Activation of glycogenolysis and glycolysis in muscle during exercise. PFK-1, phosphofructokinase-1.

Excess glucose proceeds to the peripheral circulation, where it is taken up into muscle and adipose tissue for energy reserves or storage. We normally eat sitting down, rather than during exercise, so that the opposing pathways of utilization and storage of energy are temporally compartmentalized functions in our lives. Energy storage is under the control of the polypeptide hormone insulin, which is stored in β-cells in the pancreatic islets of Langerhans. Insulin is secreted into blood following a meal, tracking blood glucose concentration. It has two primary functions in carbohydrate metabolism: first, insulin reverses the actions of glucagon in phosphorylation of proteins, turning off glycogen phosphor-

ylase and activating glycogen synthase, promoting glucose storage; second, it stimulates the uptake of glucose into muscle and adipose tissue, facilitating synthesis and storage of glycogen and triglycerides. Insulin also acts at the level of gene expression stimulating the synthesis of enzymes involved in carbohydrate metabolism and storage and conversion of glucose into triglycerides.

Protein tyrosine phosphorylation, rather than serine and threonine phosphorylation, is a characteristic feature of insulin and growth factor activity. Insulin binding to its transmembrane receptor (Fig. 12.7) stimulates aggregation of receptors and promotes tyrosine kinase activity in the

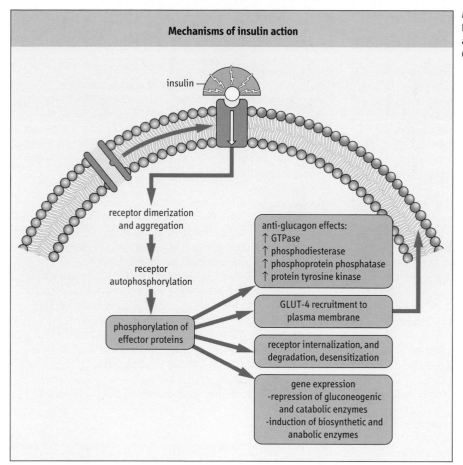

Mechanisms of insulin action

insulin

receptor dimerization
and aggregation

receptor
autophosphorylation

phosphorylation of
effector proteins

anti-glucagon effects:
↑ GTPase
↑ phosphodiesterase
↑ phosphoprotein phosphatase
↑ protein tyrosine kinase

GLUT-4 recruitment to
plasma membrane

receptor internalization, and
degradation, desensitization

gene expression
-repression of gluconeogenic
and catabolic enzymes
-induction of biosynthetic and
anabolic enzymes

Fig. 12.7 **Mechanisms of insulin action.** Regulatory effects of insulin on hepatic and muscle carbohydrate metabolism. (See also Chapter 20.)

intracellular domain of the receptor. The insulin receptor kinase activity autophosphorylates its tyrosine residues, enhancing its protein tyrosine kinase activity and phosphorylating tyrosine residues in other intracellular effector proteins, which then activate secondary pathways. Among these are kinases that phosphorylate serine and threonine residues on proteins, but at sites and on proteins distinct from those phosphorylated by PKA and PKC. Insulin-dependent activation of GTPase, phosphodiesterase and phosphoprotein phosphatases also checks the action of glucagon, which is typically present at high concentration in the blood at mealtimes, i.e. several hours since the last meal.

The liver also appears to be directly responsive to ambient blood glucose concentration, increasing glycogen synthesis following a meal, even in the absence of hormonal input. Thus, the increase in hepatic glycogenesis begins more rapidly than the increase in insulin concentration in blood, and perfusion of liver with glucose solutions *in vitro*, in the absence of insulin, also leads to inhibition of glycogenolysis and activation of glycogenesis. This appears to occur by direct allosteric inhibition of phosphorylase by glucose and secondary stimulation of protein phosphatase activity.

Most, if not all, cells in the body are responsive to insulin in some way, but the major sites of insulin action, on a mass basis, are muscle and adipose tissue. These tissues normally have low levels of cell-surface glucose transporters, restricting the entry of glucose – they rely mostly on lipids for energy metabolism. In muscle and adipose tissue, insulin-receptor tyrosine kinase activity induces movement of glucose transporter-4 (GLUT-4) from intracellular vacuoles to the cell surface, increasing glucose transport into the cell. The glucose is then used in muscle for synthesis of glycogen, and in adipose tissue to produce glyceraldehyde 3-phosphate which is converted to glycerol 3-phosphate for synthesis of triglycerides (Chapter 15).

GLUCONEOGENESIS

During fasting and starvation, when hepatic glycogen is depleted, gluconeogenesis is essential for maintenance of blood glucose homeostasis. Unlike glycogenolysis, which can be turned on rapidly in response to hormonal stimulation, gluconeogenesis is a slower response, reaching maximal activity over a period of hours (Fig. 12.1); it becomes the primary source of our blood glucose concentration about 8 hours into the post-absorbtive state (see also Chapter 20).

Gluconeogenesis requires both a source of energy and a source of carbons for formation of the backbone of the glucose molecule. The energy is provided by metabolism of

EXCESS ALCOHOL CONSUMPTION CAN LEAD TO HYPOGLYCEMIA

A middle-aged, emaciated, chronic alcoholic man collapsed in a bar at about 11 a.m., and was transported to the emergency room by ambulance. Another patron noted that the man had had only a few shots of vodka, and did not appear to be unusually drunk, although he was a little confused, at the time that he fainted. The bartender suggested that the man might have had a heart attack. Physical examination revealed a somewhat clammy skin, unusual for a winter morning, rapid breathing, and a rapid heartbeat. Laboratory tests indicated a blood glucose of 2.5 mmol/L (50 mg/dL), in the hypoglycemic range, and a blood alcohol level of 0.2%, suggesting intoxication. Subsequent tests indicated a normal level of creatine phosphokinase, an enzyme measured for early diagnosis of myocardial infarction, high serum aspartate aminotransferase activity, indicative of ongoing liver damage, a slightly acidic blood pH (7.29 versus normal 7.35), low pCO_2, and high blood lactate. The man responded to an infusion of a glucose solution, regained consciousness, had brunch, and a few hours later, after a miraculous recovery, was referred to a counselor for treatment. What happened?

Comment. This patient probably had not eaten breakfast before starting his morning binge. His glycogen stores were negligible, so he was dependent on gluconeogenesis for maintenance of blood glucose concentration, but gluconeogenesis may be compromised both by liver disease (cirrhosis) and by the limited muscle mass available to mobilize amino acids for gluconeogenesis. The consumption of alcohol places additional stress on gluconeogenesis, since alcohol is metabolized primarily in the liver. The two-step metabolism of alcohol is relatively unregulated, leading to a rapid increase in hepatic NADH:

> Alcohol dehydrogenase:
> $CH_3CH_2OH + NAD^+ + H^+ \rightarrow CH_3CHO + NADH$
> Aldehyde dehydrogenase:
> $CH_3CHO + NAD^+ + H^+ \rightarrow CH_3COOH + NADH$

The increase in hepatic NADH shifts the equilibrium of the LDH reaction toward lactate, limiting gluconeogenesis from pyruvate derived from lactate (or alanine), leading to accumulation of lactic acid in blood (lacticacidemia). It also shifts cytosolic oxaloacetate toward malate, reducing gluconeogenesis from citric acid cycle intermediates, and shifts dihydroxyacetone phosphate toward glycerol-3-phosphate, reducing gluconeogenesis from glycerol. Thus, the redox imbalance induced by alcohol consumption leads to a large increase in NADH in the cytoplasm, inhibiting the flux of all major substrates into gluconeogenesis. The low blood glucose leads to a stress response (rapid heart beat, clammy skin), an effort to enhance stimulation of gluconeogenesis by combined action of glucagon and epinephrine. The rapid breathing is a physiologic response to metabolic acidosis, resulting from the excess of lactic acid.

LARGE CHILD BORN OF A DIABETIC MOTHER

A baby boy, born of a poorly controlled, chronically hyperglycemic, diabetic mother, was large and chubby (macrosomic) at birth (5 kg), but appeared otherwise normal. He declined rapidly, however, and within 1 h showed all of the symptoms of hypoglycemia, similar to the case of the baby girl born of a malnourished mother (p. 164). The difference, in this case, was that the boy was obviously on the heavy side, rather than thin and malnourished.

Comment. This child has experienced a chronically hyperglycemic environment during uterine development. He adapted by increasing endogenous insulin production, which has a growth hormone-like activity, resulting in macrosomia. At birth, when placental delivery of glucose ceases, he has a normal blood glucose concentration and a substantial supply of hepatic glycogen. However, chronic hyperinsulinemia prior to birth probably represses gluconeogenic enzymes, and his high blood-insulin concentration at birth promotes glucose uptake into muscle and adipose tissue. The resultant insulin-induced hypoglycemia leads to a stress response, which was corrected by glucose infusion. After 1–2 days, his ample body mass will provide a good reservoir for synthesis of blood glucose from muscle protein by gluconeogenesis.

fatty acids released from adipose tissue. The carbon skeletons are provided from three primary sources:

- lactate produced in tissues such as the red cell by anaerobic glycolysis;
- amino acids derived from muscle protein;
- glycerol released from triglycerides during lipolysis in adipose tissue.

Among these, muscle protein is the major precursor of blood glucose – the rate of gluconeogenesis is often limited by the availability of substrate, including the rate of proteolysis in muscle or, in some cases, muscle mass. During prolonged fasting, malnutrition or starvation, we lose both adipose and muscle mass. The fat is used both for the general energy needs of the body and to support gluconeogenesis, while most of the amino acids in protein are converted into glucose.

Gluconeogenesis from lactate

Gluconeogenesis is conceptually the opposite of anaerobic glycolysis, but proceeds by a slightly different pathway, involving both mitochondrial and cytosolic enzymes (Fig. 12.8). Lactate is the end product of anaerobic glycolysis – blood lactate is derived primarily from anaerobic glycolysis in red cells and exercising muscle. During hepatic gluconeogenesis lactate is converted back into glucose, using, in part, the

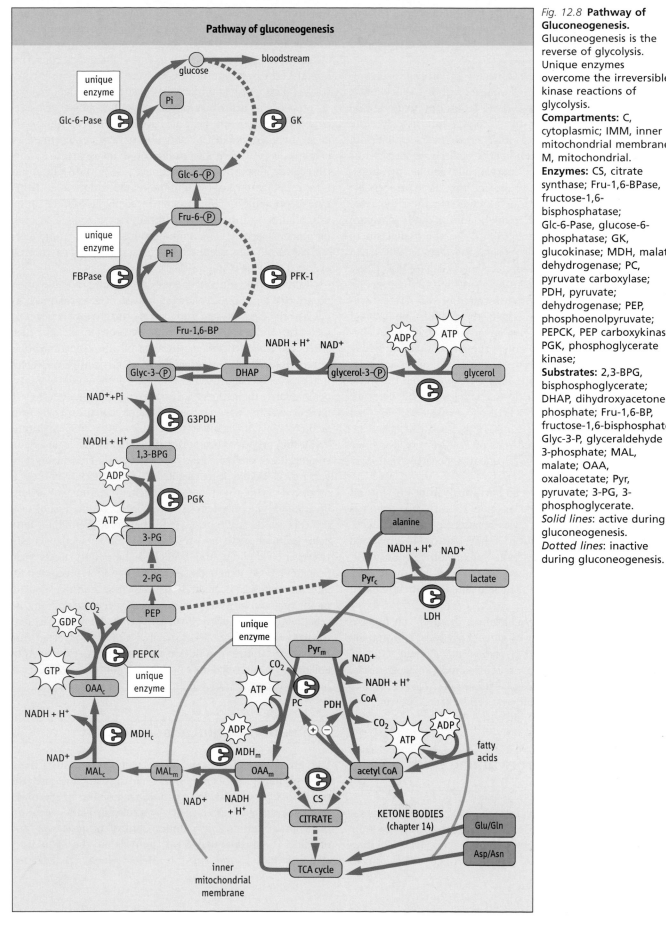

Fig. 12.8 **Pathway of**
Gluconeogenesis.
Gluconeogenesis is the
reverse of glycolysis.
Unique enzymes
overcome the irreversible
kinase reactions of
glycolysis.
Compartments: C,
cytoplasmic; IMM, inner
mitochondrial membrane;
M, mitochondrial.
Enzymes: CS, citrate
synthase; Fru-1,6-BPase,
fructose-1,6-
bisphosphatase;
Glc-6-Pase, glucose-6-
phosphatase; GK,
glucokinase; MDH, malate
dehydrogenase; PC,
pyruvate carboxylase;
PDH, pyruvate;
dehydrogenase; PEP,
phosphoenolpyruvate;
PEPCK, PEP carboxykinase;
PGK, phosphoglycerate
kinase;
Substrates: 2,3-BPG,
bisphosphoglycerate;
DHAP, dihydroxyacetone
phosphate; Fru-1,6-BP,
fructose-1,6-bisphosphate;
Glyc-3-P, glyceraldehyde
3-phosphate; MAL,
malate; OAA,
oxaloacetate; Pyr,
pyruvate; 3-PG, 3-
phosphoglycerate.
Solid lines: active during
gluconeogenesis.
Dotted lines: inactive
during gluconeogenesis.

same glycolytic enzymes involved in conversion of glucose into lactate. The lactate cycle involving the liver, red cells, and muscle, known as the Cori cycle, is discussed in Chapter 20.

A critical problem in the reversal of glycolysis is overcoming the irreversibility of three kinase reactions: glucokinase (GK), phosphofructokinase-1 (PFK-1), and pyruvate kinase (PK). The fourth kinase in glycolysis, phosphoglycerate kinase (PGK), catalyzes a freely reversible, equilibrium reaction, transferring a high-energy acyl phosphate in 1,3-bisphosphoglycerate to an energetically similar pyrophosphate bond in ATP. To circumvent the three irreversible reactions, the liver uses four unique enzymes: pyruvate carboxylase (PC) in the mitochondrion and phosphoenolpyruvate carboxykinase (PEPCK) in the cytoplasm to bypass PK, fructose-1,6-bisphosphatase (Fru-1,6-BPase) to bypass PFK-1, and Glc-6-Pase to bypass GK (see Fig. 12.8). Gluconeogenesis from lactate involves, first, its conversion into PEP, a process requiring investment of two ATP equivalents because of the high energy of the enol-phosphate bond in PEP. Lactate is first converted into pyruvate by lactate dehydrogenase (LDH), and then enters the mitochondrion, where it is converted to oxaloacetate by PC, using biotin and ATP. Oxaloacetate is reduced to malate for export from the mitochondrion, then re-oxidized to oxaloacetate by cytosolic malate dehydrogenase. The cytosolic oxaloacetate is then decarboxylated by PEPCK, using GTP as a co-substrate, yielding PEP. The energy for synthesis of PEP from oxaloacetate is derived from both the GTP and the decarboxylation of oxaloacetate.

Glycolysis may now proceed backwards from PEP until it reaches the next irreversible reaction, PFK-1. This enzyme is bypassed by a simple hydrolysis reaction, catalyzed by Fru-1,6-BPase without production of ATP, as would be required by reversal of the PFK-1 reaction. Similarly, the bypass of GK is accomplished by hydrolysis of Glc-6-P by Glc-6-Pase, without production of ATP. The free glucose is then released into blood.

Gluconeogenesis is fairly efficient – the liver can make a kilogram of glucose per day by gluconeogenesis, and actually does so in poorly controlled, hyperglycemic diabetic patients. Gluconeogenesis from pyruvate is also moderately expensive, requiring a net expenditure of 4 moles of ATP per mole of pyruvate converted into glucose. This ATP is provided by oxidation of fatty acids (Chapter 14).

Gluconeogenesis from amino acids and glycerol

Most amino acids are glucogenic, i.e. following deamination their carbon skeletons can be converted into glucose. Alanine and glutamine are the major amino acids exported from muscle for gluconeogenesis. Their relative concentrations in venous blood from muscle exceed their relative concentration in muscle protein, indicating considerable reshuffling of muscle amino acids to provide gluconeogenic substrates. As discussed in more detail in Chapter 18, alanine is converted directly into pyruvate by the enzyme alanine aminotransferase (alanine transaminase, ALT), and then gluconeogenesis proceeds as described for lactate. Other amino acids are converted into tricarboxylic acid cycle (TCA cycle) intermediates, then to malate for gluconeogenesis. Aspartate, for example, is converted into oxaloacetate by aspartate aminotransferase (aspartate transaminase, AST), and glutamate into α-ketoglutarate by glutamate dehydrogenase. Other glucogenic amino acids are converted by less direct routes into alanine or intermediates in the tricarboxylic acid cycle for gluconeogenesis. The amino groups of these amino acids are converted into urea, via the urea cycle, and the urea is excreted in urine (Chapter 18).

Glycerol enters gluconeogenesis at the level of triose phosphates (see Fig. 12.8). Following release of glycerol and fatty acids from adipose tissue into plasma, the glycerol is taken up into liver and phosphorylated by glycerol kinase, and then enters the gluconeogenic pathway as dihydroxyacetone phosphate. Only the glycerol component of fats can be converted into glucose. As discussed in Chapter 14, metabolism of fatty acids involves their conversion in two carbon oxidation steps to form acetyl CoA, which is then metabolized in the tricarboxylic acid cycle by condensation with oxaloacetate to form citrate. While the carbons of acetate are theoretically available for gluconeogenesis, two molecules of CO_2 are eliminated during conversion of citrate into malate. Thus, although energy is produced during the tricarboxylic acid cycle, the two carbons invested for gluconeogenesis from acetyl CoA are lost as CO_2. For this reason, acetyl CoA, and therefore, even-chain fatty acids, cannot serve as substrates for net gluconeogenesis. However, odd-chain and branched-chain fatty acids yield propionyl CoA, which can serve as a minor precursor for gluconeogenesis. Propionyl CoA is first carboxylated to methylmalonyl CoA, which undergoes racemase and mutase reactions to form succinyl CoA, a tricarboxylic acid cycle intermediate (see Chapter 14). Succinyl CoA is converted into malate, exits the mitochondrion and is oxidized to oxaloacetate. Following decarboxylation by PEPCK, the three carbons of propionate appear intact in PEP for gluconeogenesis.

Regulation of gluconeogenesis

Like glycogen metabolism in liver, gluconeogenesis is regulated primarily by hormonal mechanisms. In this case, the regulatory process involves counter-regulation of glycolysis and gluconeogenesis, largely by phosphorylation/dephosphorylation of enzymes, under control of glucagon and insulin. The primary control point is at the regulatory enzymes PFK-1 and Fru-1,6-BPase, which, in liver, are exquisitely sensitive to the allosteric effector fructose 2,6-bisphosphate (Fru-2,6-BP). Fru-2,6-BP is an activator of PFK-1 and an inhibitor of Fru-1,6-BPase. As shown in Figure 12.9, Fru-2,6-BP is synthesized by an unusual, bifunctional enzyme, phosphofructokinase-2/fructose-2,6-bisphosphatase (PFK-2/Fru-2,6-BPase) which has both kinase and phosphatase activities. In the phosphorylated state, under the influence of glucagon, this enzyme displays Fru-2,6-BPase activity, reducing the level of Fru-2,6-BP, which simultaneously decreases the stimulation of glycolysis at PFK-1 and relieves inhibition of gluconeogenesis at Fru-1,6-BPase. The coordinate, allosterically-mediated decrease in PFK-1 and increase in Fru-1,6-BPase activity ensures that glucose made by gluconeogenesis is not consumed by glycolysis in a futile cycle, but released into blood by Glc-6-Pase. Similarly, any flux of glucose from glycogen, also induced by glucagon, is diverted to blood, rather than to glycolysis, by inhibition of PFK-1. Pyruvate kinase (PK) is also inhibited by phosphorylation by protein kinase A (PKA), providing an additional site for inhibition of glycolysis.

When glucose enters the liver following a meal, insulin mediates the dephosphorylation of PFK-2/Fru-2,6-BPase, turning on its PFK-2 activity. The resultant increase in Fru-2,6-BP activates PFK-1 and inhibits Fru-1,6-BPase activity. Gluconeogenesis is inhibited, and glucose entering the liver is then incorporated into glycogen or routed into glycolysis for lipogenesis. Thus, liver metabolism following a meal is focused on synthesis and storage of both carbohydrate and lipid energy reserves, which it will later use, in the post-absorptive state, for maintenance of blood glucose and fatty acid homeostasis.

Gluconeogenesis is also regulated in the mitochondrion by acetyl CoA. The influx of fatty acids from adipose tissue, stimulated by glucagon to support gluconeogenesis, leads to an increase in hepatic acetyl CoA, which is both an inhibitor of pyruvate dehydrogenase (PDH) and an essential allosteric activator of pyruvate carboxylase (PC) (see Figs 12.8 and Table 12.5). In this way, fat metabolism inhibits the oxidation of pyruvate and favors gluconeogenesis in liver. In muscle, the utilization of glucose is limited both by the low level of

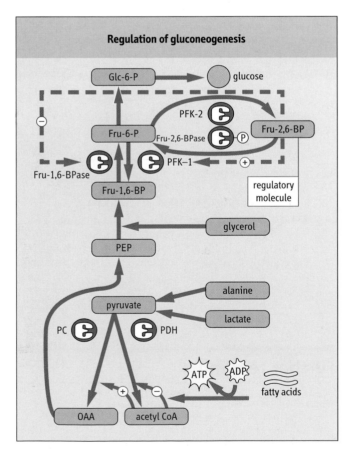

Fig. 12.9 **Regulation of gluconeogenesis.** Gluconeogenesis is regulated by hepatic levels of Fru-2,6-BP and acetyl CoA. The upper part of the diagram focuses on the reciprocal regulation of Fru-1,6-BPase and PFK-1 by Fru-2,6-BP and the lower part on the reciprocal regulation of pyruvate dehydrogenase (PDH) and pyruvate carboxylase (PC) by acetyl CoA.

General features of hormone action

Tissue specificity, determined by receptor distribution
Multistep, cascade amplification
Intracellular second messengers
Coordinate counter-regulation of opposing pathways
Augmentation and/or opposition by other hormones
Multiple mechanisms of termination of response

Table 12.5 **General features of hormone action.** Hormonal regulation of gluconeogenesis illustrates fundamental principles of hormone action.

FRUCTOSE 1,6 BISPHOSPHATASE DEFICIENCY

A three-day-old child was screened for sepsis because of apparent hyperventilation and recurrent apnea spells. Blood glucose was low (2 mmol/L; hypoglycemia), and lactate was grossly elevated at 15 mmol/L. Feeding every 2 hours stopped further attacks, but the liver was noted to be slightly enlarged.

Comment. About half the cases of fructose-1,6-bisphosphatase deficiency present with hypoglycemia and severe lactic acidosis in the first few days of life. Frequent feeding with carbohydrate prevents further problems. The enzyme impairs the formation of glucose from all gluconeogenic precursors, and normoglycemia is dependent on glucose intake, and on degradation of hepatic glycogen. The frequency of attacks decreases with age and the majority of affected children have normal psychomotor development.

GLUT-4 in the plasma membranes (because of the low plasma insulin concentration) and by inhibition of PDH by acetyl CoA. Active fat metabolism and high levels of acetyl CoA in muscle promote the excretion of a significant fraction of pyruvate as lactate, even in the resting state.

Conversion of fructose and galactose to glucose

As discussed in detail in Chapter 24, fructose is metabolized almost exclusively in the liver. It enters glycolysis at the level of triose phosphates, bypassing the regulatory enzyme, PFK-1, so that large amounts of pyruvate may be forced on the mitochondrion for use in energy metabolism or fat biosynthesis. During a gluconeogenic state, this fructose may also proceed toward Glc-6-P, providing a convenient source of blood glucose. Gluconeogenesis from galactose is equally efficient, since Glc-1-P, derived from galactose 1-phosphate (Chapter 25), is readily isomerized to Glc-6-P by phosphoglucomutase. Fructose and galactose are good sources of glucose, independent of glycogenolysis and gluconeogenesis.

Summary

Glycogen is stored in two tissues in the body for different reasons: in liver for short-term maintenance of blood glucose homeostasis, and in muscle as a source of energy. Glycogen metabolism in these tissues responds rapidly to both allosteric and hormonal control. In liver, the balance between glycogenolysis and glycogenesis is regulated by the balance between concentrations of glucagon and insulin in the circulation, which controls the state of phosphorylation of enzymes. Phosphorylation of enzymes under the influence of glucagon directs glycogen mobilization and is the most common condition in the liver, e.g. during sleep. Increases in blood insulin during and after meals promote dephosphorylation of the same enzymes, leading to glycogenesis. Insulin also promotes glucose uptake into muscle and adipose tissue for glycogen and triglyceride synthesis following a meal. Epinephrine controls phosphorylation of liver enzymes, enabling a burst in hepatic glycogenolysis and an increase in blood glucose for stress responses. Muscle is also responsive to epinephrine, but not to glucagon; in this case the glucose produced by glycogenolysis is used for energy metabolism. In addition, muscle glycogenolysis is responsive to intracellular Ca^{2+} and AMP concentrations, providing a mechanism for coupling glycogenolysis to energy consumption during exercise. The actions of insulin, glucagon, and epinephrine illustrate many of the fundamental principles of hormone action (Table 12.5). Gluconeogenesis takes place primarily in liver, and is designed for maintenance of blood glucose during the fasting state. It is essential after 12 h of fasting, when the majority of hepatic glycogen has been consumed. The major substrates for gluconeogenesis are lactate, amino acids, and glycerol; fatty acid metabolism provides the necessary energy. The major control point is at the level of phosphofructokinase-1 (PFK-1), which is activated by the allosteric effector Fru-2,6-BP. The synthesis of Fru-2,6-BP is under control of the bifunctional enzyme, PFK-2/Fru-2,6-BPase, whose kinase and phosphatase activities are regulated by phosphorylation/dephosphorylation, under hormonal control by insulin and glucagon. During fasting and active gluconeogenesis, glucagon mediates phosphorylation and activation of the phosphatase activity of this enzyme, leading to a decrease in the level of Fru-2,6-BP, and a corresponding decrease in glycolysis. Oxidation of pyruvate is also inhibited in the mitochondrion by inhibition of PDH by acetyl-CoA, derived from fat metabolism.

ACTIVE LEARNING

1. The inactivation of glycogenesis in response to epinephrine occurs in a single-step by action of PKA on glycogen synthase, while the activation of glycogenolysis involves an intermediate enzyme, phosphorylate kinase, which phosphorylates phosphorylase. Discuss the metabolic advantages of the two-step activation of glycogenolysis.
2. Investigate the use of inhibitors of glycogenolysis and gluconeogenesis for treatment of type 2 diabetes.
3. Glucose-6-phosphatase is essential for production of glucose in liver, but is not a cytosolic enzyme. Describe the activity and subcellular localization of this enzyme and the final stages of the pathway for production of glucose in liver.

Further reading

Barthel A, Schmoll D. Novel concepts in insulin regulation of hepatic gluconeogenesis. *Am J Physiol Endocrinol Metab* 2003;**285**:E685–692.

Brooks C. Neonatal hypoglycemia. *Neonatal network* 1997;**16**:15–21.

Donovan CM, Sumida KD. Training enhanced hepatic gluconeogenesis: the importance for glucose homeostasis during exercise. *Med Sci Sports Exercise* 1997;**29**:628–634.

Fischer EH. Cellular regulation by protein phosphorylation: a historical review. *Biofactors* 1997;**6**:367–374.

Hargreaves M. Interactions between muscle glycogen and blood glucose during exercise. *Exercise Sports Sci Rev* 1997;**25**:21–39.

Hawley JA, Schabort EJ, Noakes TD, Dennis SC. Carbohydrate loading and exercise performance. An update. *Sports Med* 1997;**24**:73–81.

Kurland IJ, Pilkis SJ. Covalent control of 6-phosphofructo-2-kinase/fructose-2,6-bisphosphatase. *Protein Sci* 1995;**4**:1023–1037.

Melendez R, Melendez-Hevia E, Cascante M. How did glycogen structure evolve to satisfy the requirement for rapid mobilization of glucose? A problem of physical constraints in structure building. *J Mol Evol* 1997;**45**:446–455.

Mizock BA. Alterations in carbohydrate metabolism during stress: a review. *Am J Med* 1995;**98**:75–84.

Tarui S. Glycolytic defects in muscle: aspects of collaboration between basic science and clinical medicine. *Muscle and Nerve* 1995;**3**: S2–9.

Van den Berghe G. Disorders of gluconeogenesis. *J Inh Metab Dis* 1996;**19**:470–477.

Wolfsdorf JI, Weinstein DA.Glycogen storage diseases. *Rev Endocr Metab Disord* 2003;**4**:95–102.

Websites

Glycogen: http://bip.cnrs-mrs.fr/bip10/glycogen.htm; http://www.rpi.edu/dept/bcbp/molbiochem/MBWeb/mb1/part2/9-glycogen.ppt

Gluconeogenesis: http://bioresearch.ac.uk/browse/mesh/detail/C0017715L0017715.html

Glycogen Storage Diseases: http://www.agsd.org.uk/home/; http://www.agsdus.org/

Gestational Diabetes: http://www.umm.edu/diabetes-info/gesta.htm; http://www.fpnotebook.com/OB37.htm

Hypoglycemia: http://diabetes.niddk.nih.gov/dm/pubs/hypoglycemia/index.htm

13. The Tricarboxylic Acid Cycle

L W Stillway

LEARNING OBJECTIVES

After reading this chapter you should be able to:

■ Outline the sequence of reactions in the tricarboxylic acid (TCA) cycle and explain the purpose of the cycle.

■ Identify the four oxidative enzymes in the TCA cycle and their products.

■ Identify the two intermediates required in the first step of the TCA cycle and their metabolic sources.

■ Identify four major metabolic intermediates synthesized from TCA cycle intermediates.

■ Describe how the TCA cycle is regulated by substrate supply, allosteric effectors, covalent modification, and protein synthesis.

■ Explain why there is no net synthesis of glucose from acetyl-CoA.

■ Explain the concept of 'suicide substrate' as applied to the TCA cycle.

INTRODUCTION

The tricarboxylic acid (TCA) cycle is a common pathway for metabolism of all fuels. Located in the mitochondrion, the TCA cycle, also known as the Krebs or citric acid cycle, is a common pathway for metabolism of all fuels. It oxidatively strips electrons from fat, carbohydrate and protein fuels, producing the majority of the reduced coenzymes that are used for the generation of adenosine triphosphate (ATP) in the electron transport chain. Although the TCA cycle does not use oxygen in any of its reactions, it requires oxidative metabolism in the mitochondrion for re-oxidation of reduced coenzymes. The TCA cycle has two major functions, energy production and biosynthesis (Fig. 13.1).

ENERGY PRODUCTION IN THE TCA CYCLE

Four oxidative steps provide free energy for ATP synthesis

A common end-product of carbohydrate, fatty acid and amino acid metabolism, acetyl-CoA is oxidized in the TCA cycle to produce reduced coenzymes by four redox reactions per turn of the cycle. Three produce reduced nicotinamide adenine dinucleotide (NADH) and another produces reduced flavin adenine dinucleotide ($FADH_2$). These reduced nucleotides provide energy for ATP synthesis by the electron transport system (Chapter 8). One high-energy phosphate, guanosine triphosphate (GTP), is also produced in the cycle by substrate-level phosphorylation. Nearly all metabolic carbon dioxide is produced by decarboxylation reactions catalyzed by pyruvate dehydrogenase and TCA cycle enzymes in the mitochondrion.

BIOSYNTHESES LINKED TO TCA CYCLE

The TCA cycle provides a common ground for interconversion of fuels and metabolites

The TCA cycle (Fig. 13.1) participates in the synthesis of glucose from amino acids and lactate during starvation and fasting (gluconeogenesis; see Chapter 12). It is also involved in the conversion of carbohydrates to fat following a carbohydrate-rich meal (Chapter 15). It is a source of nonessential amino acids, such as aspartate and glutamate, which are synthesized directly from TCA cycle intermediates. One TCA cycle intermediate, succinyl-Coenzyme A (succinyl-CoA), serves as a precursor to porphyrins (heme), in all cells, but especially in bone marrow and liver (Chapter 28). Biosynthetic reactions proceeding from the TCA cycle require the input of carbons from intermediates other than acetyl-CoA. Such reactions are known as anaplerotic (building up) reactions.

The TCA cycle is located in mitochondria

Localization of the TCA cycle within mitochondria is important metabolically; this allows identical intermediates to be used for different purposes inside and outside mitochondria. Acetyl-CoA, for example, cannot cross the inner mitochondrial membrane. The main fate of mitochondrial acetyl-CoA is oxidation in the TCA cycle, but in the cytoplasm, it is used for biosynthesis of fatty acids and cholesterol.

Metabolic defects in the TCA cycle are rare

Metabolic defects involving enzymes of the TCA cycle are rare, because normal functioning of the cycle is absolutely essential to sustain life. Products of energy-producing pathways must be metabolized in the TCA cycle for efficient production of ATP. Any defect in the TCA cycle will severely impair ATP

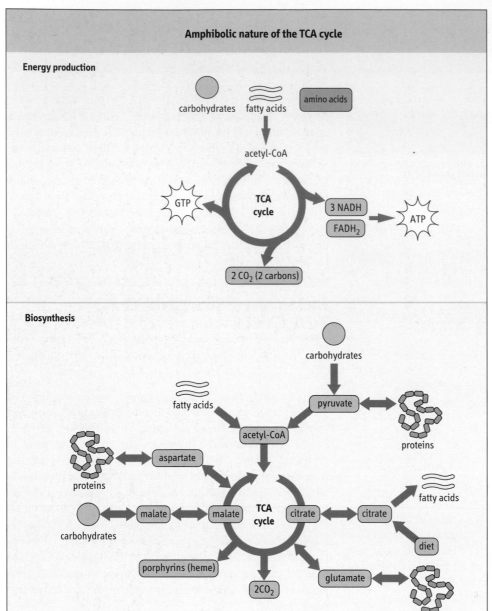

Amphibolic nature of the TCA cycle

Energy production

carbohydrates   fatty acids   amino acids

acetyl-CoA

GTP

TCA cycle

3 NADH
FADH$_2$

ATP

2 CO$_2$ (2 carbons)

Biosynthesis

carbohydrates

fatty acids   pyruvate

acetyl-CoA   proteins

aspartate

proteins

malate   malate   **TCA cycle**   citrate   citrate   fatty acids

carbohydrates

diet

porphyrins (heme)

2CO$_2$ glutamate

Fig. 13.1 **Amphibolic nature of the TCA cycle.** The TCA cycle provides energy and metabolites for cellular metabolism. Because of the catabolic and anabolic nature of the TCA cycle, it is described as amphibolic. FAD, flavin adenine dinucleotide; GDP, guanosine diphosphate; NADH, nicotinamide adenine dinucleotide; Pi, inorganic phosphate.

production, and cells deprived of ATP either die rapidly or are severely impaired functionally. Tissues that use oxygen at rapid rates, such as the central nervous system and muscle, are most susceptible to such defects.

Acetyl-CoA is a common product of many catabolic pathways

The TCA cycle begins with acetyl-CoA, which has three major metabolic precursors (Fig. 13.2). Carbohydrates undergo glycolysis to yield pyruvate (Chapter 11), which can be taken up by mitochondria and oxidatively decarboxylated to acetyl-CoA by the pyruvate dehydrogenase complex. During lipolysis, triacylglycerols are converted to glycerol and free fatty acids, which are taken up by cells and transported into mito-

chondria where they undergo oxidation to acetyl-CoA (Chapter 14). Lastly, proteolysis of tissue proteins releases constituent amino acids, many of which are metabolized to acetyl-CoA and TCA-cycle intermediates (Chapter 18).

The first version of the TCA cycle, proposed by Krebs in 1937, began with pyruvic acid, not acetyl-CoA. Pyruvic acid was decarboxylated and condensed with oxaloacetic acid through an unknown mechanism to form citric acid. The key intermediate, acetyl-CoA, was not identified until years later. It is tempting to begin the TCA cycle with pyruvic acid, unless it is recognized that fatty acids and many amino acids form acetyl-CoA by pathways that bypass pyruvate. It is for this reason that the TCA cycle is said to begin with acetyl-CoA, not pyruvic acid.

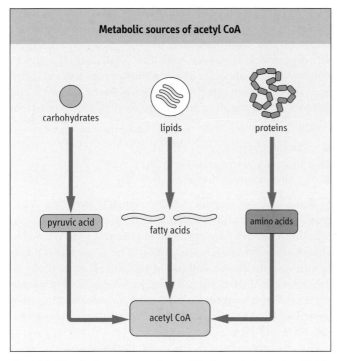

Metabolic sources of acetyl CoA

Fig. 13.2 **Metabolic sources of acetyl-CoA.** Carbohydrates, lipids and amino acids are precursors of mitochondrial acetyl-CoA necessary for operation of the TCA cycle.

PYRUVATE CARBOXYLASE

Pyruvate may be directly converted to four different metabolites

Pyruvate is at a crossroads in metabolism. It may be converted in one step to lactate (lactate dehydrogenase), alanine (alanine aminotransferase, ALT), oxaloacetate (pyruvate carboxylase), and acetyl CoA (pyruvate dehydrogenase complex) (Fig. 13.3). Depending on metabolic circumstances, pyruvate may be routed toward gluconeogenesis (Chapter 12), fatty acid biosynthesis (Chapter 15) or the TCA cycle itself. Pyruvate carboxylase, like most other carboxylases, uses CO_2 and the coenzyme biotin (Fig. 13.4), a water-soluble vitamin and ATP to drive the carboxylation reaction. The enzyme is a tetramer of identical subunits, each of which contains an allosteric site that binds acetyl-CoA, a positive heterotropic modifier. In fact, pyruvate carboxylase has an absolute requirement for acetyl-CoA; the enzyme does not work in its absence. An abundance of mitochondrial acetyl-CoA acts as a signal for the generation of additional oxaloacetate. For example, when lipolysis is stimulated, intra-mitochondrial acetyl-CoA levels rise, which allosterically activates pyruvate carboxylase to produce additional oxaloacetate for gluconeogenesis (Chapter 12).

 MEASURING LACTATE

Lactic acid is measured in a clinical setting, because its accumulation can result in rapid death. Lactic acid is produced metabolically by the reversible reduction of pyruvate with NADH by the enzyme lactate dehydrogenase (LDH). Both lactate and pyruvate coexist in metabolic systems, and the ratio of pyruvate:lactate is roughly proportional to the cytosolic ratio of NAD^+:NADH. Both lactate and pyruvate contribute to the acidity of biological fluid, however, lactate is usually present at higher concentrations and is more easily measured. Blood lactate may increase in chronic obstructive lung disease, and during intense exercise. Its measurement is usually indicated when there is metabolic acidosis, characterized by an elevated anion gap, $\{[Na^+] - ([Cl^-] + [CO_2])\}$, indicating the presence of an unknown anion in plasma. Although rare, lactic acidosis can be caused by metabolic defects in energy-producing pathways, such as some of the glycogen storage diseases or in any enzyme in the pathways from pyruvate to the generation of ATP, including the pyruvate dehydrogenase complex, TCA cycle, electron transport system or ATP synthase.

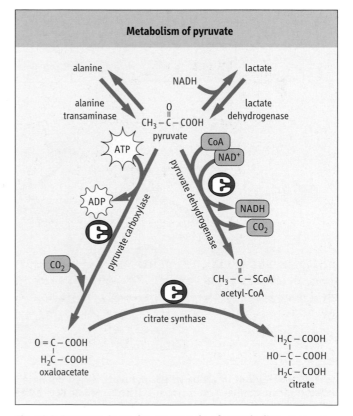

Metabolism of pyruvate

Fig. 13.3 **Pyruvate is at the crossroads of metabolism.** Pyruvate is readily formed from lactate or alanine. Acetyl-CoA and oxaloacetate are derived from pyruvate through the catalytic action of pyruvate dehydrogenase and pyruvate carboxylase, respectively. ADP, adenosine diphosphate.

THE PYRUVATE DEHYDROGENASE COMPLEX (PDC)

The pyruvate dehydrogenase complex (PDC) serves as a bridge between carbohydrates and the TCA cycle (Fig.

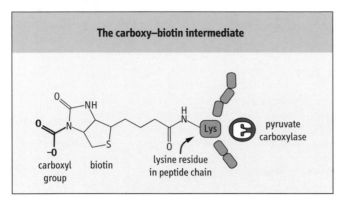

The carboxy–biotin intermediate

Fig. 13.4 **The carboxy-biotin intermediate.** Pyruvate carboxylase catalyzes carboxylation of pyruvate to oxaloacetate. The coenzyme, biotin, is covalently bound to pyruvate carboxylase, and transfers the carbon originating from CO_2 to pyruvate.

13.5). PDC is one of several α-ketoacid dehydrogenases having analogous reaction mechanisms, including α-ketoglutarate dehydrogenase in the TCA cycle and α-ketoacid dehydrogenases associated with the catabolism of leucine, isoleucine and valine. Its irreversibility explains in part why acetyl-CoA cannot yield a net synthesis of glucose. The complex functions as a unit consisting of three principal enzymes:

- pyruvate dehydrogenase (PDH; E_1)
- dihydrolipoyl transacetylase (E_2)
- dihydrolipoamide dehydrogenase (E_3)

Two additional enzymes of the complex, pyruvate dehydrogenase kinase and pyruvate dehydrogenase phosphatase, regulate its activity by covalent modification via reversible phosphorylation/dephosphorylation. There are four known isoforms of the kinase, and two of the phosphatase; the relative amounts of each are cell-specific. Intermediates traverse minimal distances between each catalytic step, because they are tethered to the complex during the reaction sequence (see Figs 13.5 and 13.6).

Five coenzymes are required for PDC activity: thiamine pyrophosphate, lipoamide (lipoic acid bound in amide linkage to protein), CoA, FAD, and NAD^+. For their synthesis, thiamin,

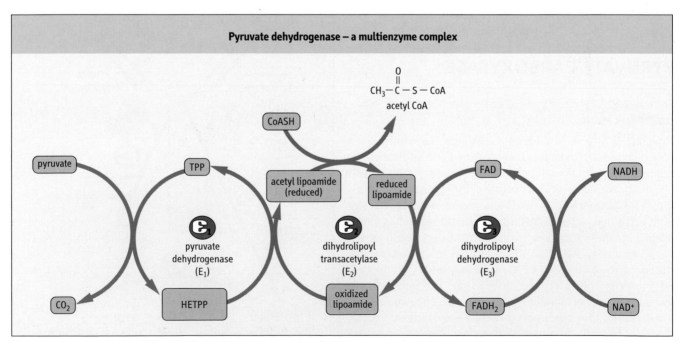

Pyruvate dehydrogenase – a multienzyme complex

Fig. 13.5 **Mechanism of action of the pyruvate dehydrogenase complex.** The three enzyme components of the pyruvate dehydrogenase complex are pyruvate dehydrogenase (E_1), dihydrolipoyl transacetylase (E_2) and dihydrolipoyl dehydrogenase (E_3). Pyruvate is first decarboxylated by the thiamine pyrophosphate-containing enzyme (E_1), forming CO_2 and hydroxyethyl-thiamine pyrophosphate (HETPP). Lipoamide, the prosthetic group on E_2, serves as a carrier in the transfer of the 2-carbon unit from HETPP to coenzyme A (CoA). The oxidized, cyclic disulfide form of lipoamide accepts the hydroxyethyl group from HETPP. The lipoamide is reduced and the hydroxyethyl group converted to an acetyl group during this transfer reaction, forming acetyldihydrolipoamide. Following transfer of the acetyl group to CoA, E_3 reoxidizes the lipoamide, using FAD, and the $FADH_2$ is, in turn, oxidized by NAD^+, yielding NADH.

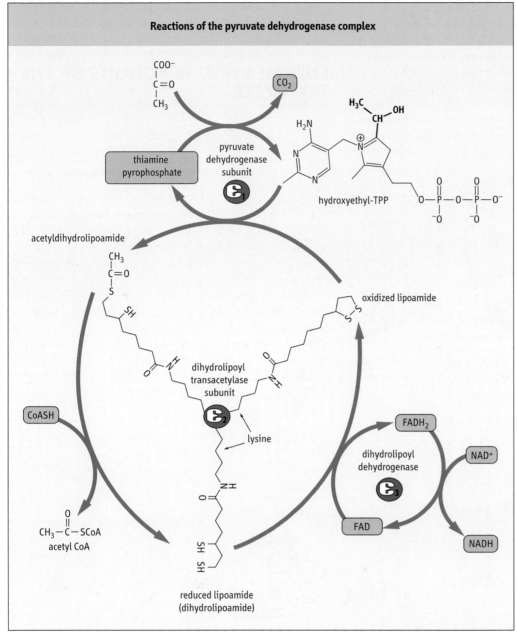

Reactions of the pyruvate dehydrogenase complex

Fig. 13.6 **Lipoic acid in the pyruvate dehydrogenase complex.** The coenzyme lipoamide is attached to a lysine residue in the transacetylase subunit of pyruvate dehydrogenase. Lipoamide moves from one active site to another on the transacetylase subunit in a 'swinging arm' mechanism. The structures of thiamine pyrophosphate (TPP) and lipoamide are shown.

PYRUVATE DEHYDROGENASE COMPLEX DEFICIENCY

Most children with this enzyme deficiency present in infancy with delayed development and reduced muscle tone often associated with ataxia and seizures. Some infants have congenital malformations of the brain.

Comment. Without mitochondrial oxidation, pyruvate is reduced to lactate. The ATP yield from anaerobic glycolysis is less than a tenth of that produced from complete oxidation of glucose via the tricarboxylic acid cycle. The diagnosis is suggested by elevated lactate, but with a normal lactate/pyruvate ratio, i.e. no evidence of hypoxia. A ketogenic diet and severe restriction of protein (<15%) and carbohydrate (<5%) improves mental development. Such treatment ensures that the cells use acetyl-CoA from fat metabolism. A few children show a reduction in plasma lactate on treatment with large doses of thiamine, but the outlook is generally poor.

pantothenic acid, riboflavin and nicotinamide are required. Deficiencies in any of these vitamins have obvious effects on energy metabolism. For example, increases in cellular concentrations of pyruvate and α-ketoglutarate are found in beri-beri because of thiamin deficiency (Chapter 10). In this case, all of the proteins are available, but the relevant coenzyme is not, and the conversions of pyruvate to acetyl-CoA and α-ketoglutarate to succinyl-CoA are significantly reduced. Symptoms include cardiac and skeletal muscle weakness and neurologic disease. Thiamin deficiency is common in alcoholism, because distilled spirits are devoid of vitamins, and symptoms of beri-beri are often observed.

ENZYMES AND REACTIONS OF THE TCA CYCLE

The TCA cycle is a sequence of eight enzymatic reactions (Fig. 13.7), beginning with condensation of acetyl-CoA with

Fig. 13.7 **Intermediates and enzymes of the TCA cycle.**

The TCA cycle

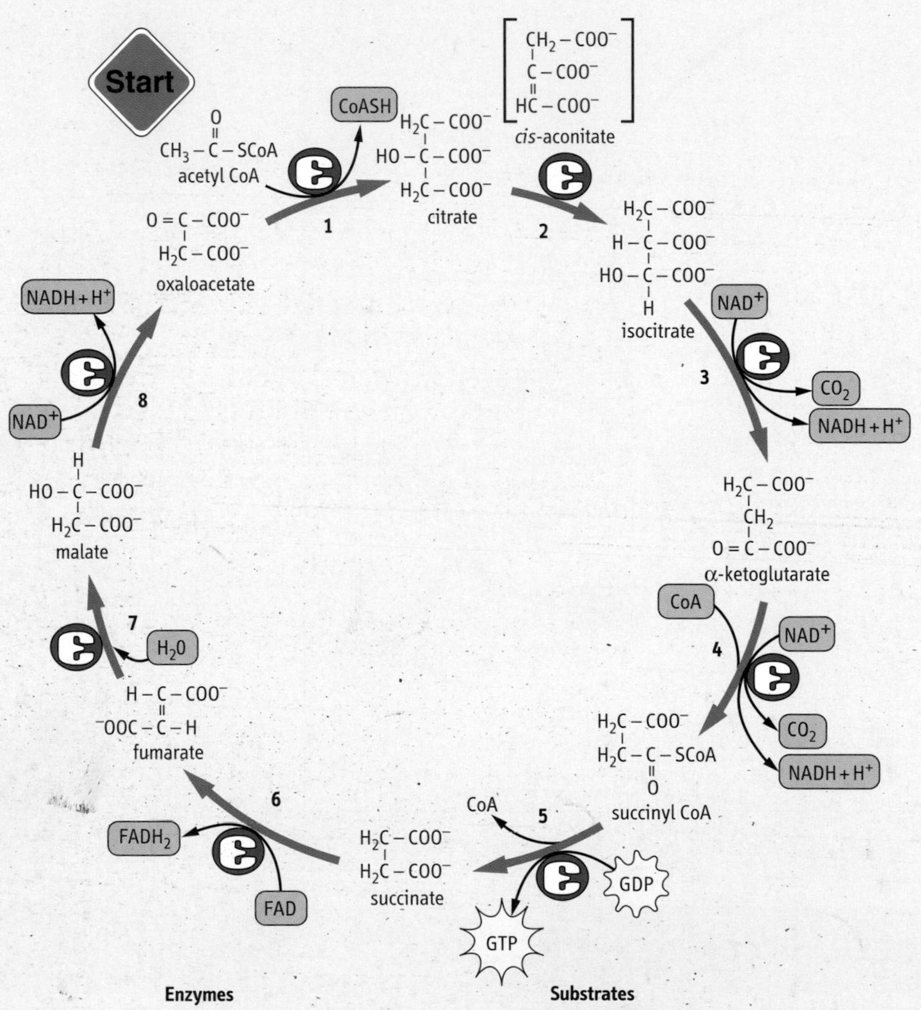

Enzymes

(1) citrate synthase
(2) aconitase
(3) isocitrate dehydrogenase
(4) α-ketoglutarate dehydrogenase
(5) succinyl-CoA synthase (succinate thiokinase)
(6) succinate dehydrogenase
(7) fumarase
(8) malate dehydrogenase

Substrates

1→2 citrate
2→3 isocitrate
3→4 α-ketoglutarate
4→5 succinyl CoA
5→6 succinate
6→7 fumarate
7→8 malate
8→1 oxaloacetate

DEFICIENCES IN PYRUVATE METABOLISM IN THE TCA CYCLE

A 7-month-old-child showed progressive neurologic deterioration characterized by loss of coordination and muscle tone. He was unable to keep his head upright and had great difficulty moving his limbs, which were limp. He also suffered from unrelenting acidosis. Administration of thiamin had no effect. Measurements showed that he had elevated blood levels of lactate, α-ketoglutarate and branched-chain amino acids. Liver, brain, kidney, skeletal muscle, and heart were examined postmortem, and all gluconeogenic enzymes were shown to have normal activities, but both pyruvate dehydrogenase and α-ketoglutarate dehydrogenase were deficient. The defective component was shown to be dihydrolipoyl dehydrogenase (E_3), which is a single gene component required by all of the α-ketoacid dehydrogenases.

Comments. This is an example of one of the many variants of Leigh's disease, which is a group of disorders that are all characterized by lactic acidosis. Lactic acid accumulates under anaerobic conditions or because of any enzyme defect in the pathway from pyruvate to the synthesis of ATP. In this case, there are defects in both the pyruvate dehydrogenase and α-ketoglutarate complexes, as well as other α-keto acid dehydrogenase complexes required for the catabolism of branched-chain amino acids. The failure of aerobic metabolism leads to increases in blood levels of lactate, α-ketoglutarate and branched-chain amino acids. Tissues dependent on aerobic metabolism, such as brain and muscle are most severely affected, so that the clinical picture includes impaired motor function, neurologic disorders and mental retardation. These diseases are rare, but deficiencies in pyruvate carboxylase and all of the components of the pyruvate dehydrogenase complex (PDH) have been described, including the associated kinase and phosphatase enzymes (Fig. 13.12).

oxaloacetate (OAA) to form citrate. The oxaloacetate is regenerated on completion of the cycle. Of the four oxidations in the cycle, two involve decarboxylations. Three produce NADH and one produces $FADH_2$. GTP, a high-energy phosphate, is produced at one step by substrate-level phosphorylation.

Citrate synthase

Citrate synthase begins the TCA cycle by catalyzing the condensation of acetyl-CoA and oxaloacetate to form citric acid. The reaction is driven by cleavage of the high-energy thioester bond of citroyl-CoA, an intermediate in the reaction. A later TCA cycle enzyme, succinyl-CoA synthetase, utilizes the high-energy thioester bond in succinyl-CoA to produce GTP, a high-energy phosphate.

 ## TOXICITY OF FLUOROACETATE – A SUICIDE SUBSTRATE

Fluoroacetate, originally isolated from plants, is a potent toxin. It is activated as fluoroacetyl-CoA and then condenses with oxaloacetate to form fluorocitrate (Fig. 13.8). Death results from inhibition of the TCA cycle by 2-fluorocitrate, a strong inhibitor of aconitase. Fluoroacetate is an example of a 'suicide substrate', a compound that is not toxic *per se*, but is metabolically activated to a toxic product. Thus, the cell is said to commit suicide by converting an apparently harmless substrate to a lethal toxin. Similar processes are involved in the activation of many environmental procarcinogens to carcinogens that induce mutations in DNA.

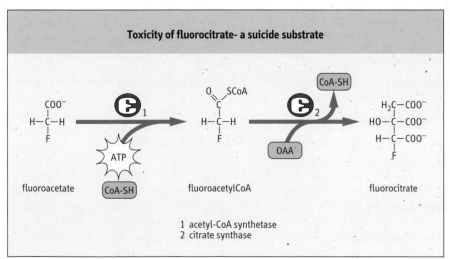

Fig. 13.8 **Toxicity of fluorocitrate – a suicide substrate.** Fluorocitrate is a competitive inhibitor of aconitase. OAA, oxaloacetate.

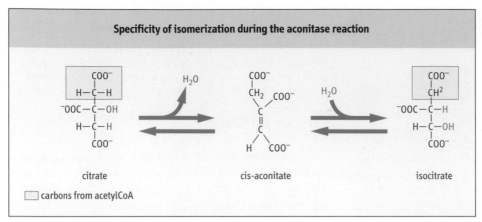

Fig. 13.9 **Specificity of isomerization during the aconitase reaction.**

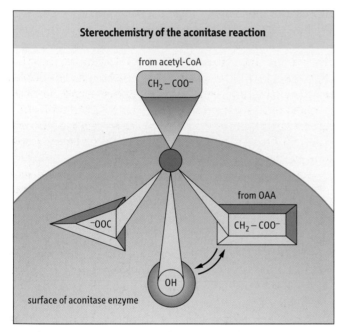

Fig. 13.10 **Stereochemistry of the aconitase reaction.** Aconitase converts achiral citrate to a specific chiral form of isocitrate. Binding of the C-3 hydroxyl (OH) and carboxylate (COO^-) groups of citrate on the enzyme surface places the carboxymethyl (-CH_2-COO^-) group, derived from the oxaloacetate end of the molecule, in touch with the third binding locus in the active site of aconitase. This assures the transfer of the OH group to the CH_2 group derived from oxaloacetate, indicated by arrows, rather than that derived from the acetyl group. OAA, oxaloacetate.

Aconitase

Aconitase is an iron-sulfur protein (Chapter 8) that isomerizes citrate to isocitrate through the enzyme-bound intermediate *cis*-aconitate. The two-step reaction is reversible and involves dehydration followed by hydration. Although citrate is a symmetric molecule, aconitase works specifically on the oxaloacetate end of citrate, not the end derived from acetyl-CoA (Fig. 13.9). Such stereochemical specificity occurs because of the geometry of the active site of aconitase (Fig.

✳ STEREOSPECIFICITY OF ENZYMES

Aconitase catalyzes isomerization at the oxaloacetate end of the citrate molecule. However, citrate has no asymmetric centers; it is achiral. How does aconitase know 'which end is up?' The answer lies in the nature of citrate binding to the active site of aconitase, a process known as three-point attachment. As shown in Figure 13.10, because of the geometry of the active site of aconitase, there is only one way for citrate to bind. This 'three-point binding' places the oxaloacetate carbons in the proper orientation for the isomerization reaction, while the carbons derived from acetyl-CoA are excluded from the active site. Although citrate is a symmetric or achiral molecule, it is termed 'prochiral' because it is converted to a chiral molecule, isocitrate. Similar types of three-point binding processes are involved in transaminase reactions that produce exclusively L-amino acids from ketoacids. The reduction of the nicotinamide ring by NAD(H)-dependent dehydrogenases is also stereospecific. Some dehydrogenases place the added hydrogen exclusively on the front face of the nicotinamide ring (viewed with the amide group to the right), while others add hydrogen only to the back face (see Fig. 13.11).

13.10). A cytosolic aconitase, known as IRE-BP (iron-response element binding protein) functions in the regulation of iron storage.

Isocitrate dehydrogenase and α-ketoglutarate dehydrogenase

Isocitrate dehydrogenase and the α-ketoglutarate dehydrogenase complex catalyze two sequential oxidative decarboxylation reactions in which NAD^+ is reduced to NADH, and CO_2 is released. The first of these enzymes, isocitrate dehydrogenase, catalyzes the conversion of isocitrate to α-ketoglutarate. It is an important regulatory enzyme that is inhibited under

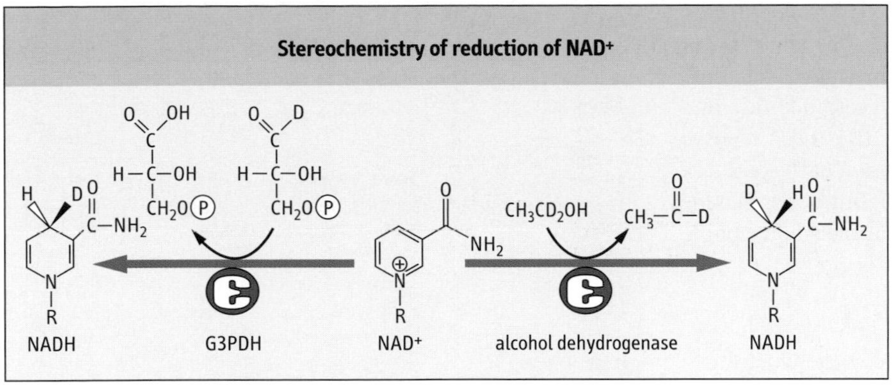

Stereochemistry of reduction of NAD⁺

Fig. 13.11 **Stereochemistry of the reduction of NAD⁺ by dehydrogenases.** Alcohol dehydrogenase places the hydrogen ion on the front face of the nicotinamide ring, while glyceraldehyde-3-phosphate dehydrogenase (G3PDH) places the hydrogen on the back face of the ring. The two positions can be discriminated using deuterated (D) substrates.

THE MALONATE BLOCK

The malate dehydrogenase reaction played an important role in the elucidation of the cyclic nature of the TCA cycle. Addition of tricarboxylic acids (citrate, aconitate) and α-ketoglutarate was known to catalyze pyruvate metabolism – we now know that this is the result of formation of catalytic amounts of oxaloacetate from these intermediates. In 1937, Krebs found that malonate, the 3-carbon dicarboxylic acid homologue of succinate and competitive inhibitor of succinate dehydrogenase, blocked metabolism of pyruvate by minced muscle preparations. He also showed that malonate inhibition of pyruvate metabolism led to accumulation not only of succinate, but also of citrate and α-ketoglutarate, suggesting that succinate was a product of pyruvate metabolism and that the tricarboxylic acids might be intermediates in this process. Interestingly, fumarate and oxaloacetate also stimulated pyruvate oxidation and led to accumulation of citrate and succinate during malonate block, suggesting that the 3- and 4-carbon acids might combine to form the tricarboxylic acids. The experiments with fumarate indicated that there were two paths between fumarate and succinate, one involving reversal of the succinate dehydrogenase reaction, which was inhibited during malonate block, and the other involving conversion of a series of organic acids to succinate. These observations, combined with Krebs' experience a few years earlier in characterization of the urea cycle (Chapter 18), led to the description of the TCA cycle.

energy-rich conditions by high levels of NADH and ATP, and is activated when NAD⁺ and ADP are produced by metabolism. Inhibition of this enzyme following a carbohydrate meal causes intra-mitochondrial accumulation of citrate, which is then exported to the cytosol for lipogenesis (Chapter 15). Citrate is also an important allosteric effector, inhibiting phosphofructokinase-1 (Chapter 11) and activating acetyl-CoA carboxylase.

The second dehydrogenase, α-ketoglutarate dehydrogenase, catalyzes the oxidative decarboxylation of α-keto-

glutarate to NADH, CO_2 and succinyl-CoA, a high-energy thioester compound. Like the pyruvate dehydrogenase complex, this enzyme complex contains three subunits having the same designations as pyruvate dehydrogenase (E_1, E_2 and E_3). E_3 is identical in the two complexes and is encoded by the same gene. The reaction mechanisms and the cofactors thiamine pyrophosphate, lipoate, CoA, FAD and NAD⁺, are the same. Both enzymes begin with an α-keto acid, pyruvate or α-ketoglutarate, and both form the CoA esters, acetyl-CoA or succinyl-CoA, respectively.

At this point, the net carbon yield of the TCA cycle is zero, i.e. two carbons were introduced as acetyl CoA and two carbons were liberated as CO_2. Note, however, that because of the asymmetry of the aconitase reaction, neither of the CO_2 molecules produced in this first round trip through the TCA cycle originates from the carbons of the acetyl-CoA, because they are derived from the oxaloacetate end of the citrate molecule. Both of the carbons that originated from acetyl CoA remain in the TCA cycle intermediates, and may appear in compounds produced in biosynthetic reactions branching from the TCA cycle, including glucose, aspartic acid and heme. However, because of the loss of two CO_2 molecules at this point, there is no net synthesis of these metabolites from acetyl-CoA.

Animals cannot perform net synthesis of glucose from acetyl CoA. This is an especially important concept in the understanding of starvation, diabetes and ketogenesis, because large amounts of acetyl CoA are generated from fatty acids, but it does not yield a net synthesis of glucose. 'Net synthesis' is invoked, because it was clearly shown that labeled carbons of acetyl CoA are incorporated into glucose, making it appear that glucose is synthesized from acetyl CoA.

Succinyl-CoA synthetase

Succinyl-CoA synthetase (succinate thiokinase) catalyzes the conversion of energy-rich succinyl-CoA to succinate and free CoA. The free energy of the thioester bond in succinyl-CoA is conserved by formation of GTP from GDP and inorganic phosphate (Pi). Since the respiratory chain is not involved, this is a substrate-level phosphorylation reaction, like the reactions catalyzed by phosphoglycerate kinase and pyruvate kinase in glycolysis (Chapter 11). GTP is used by enzymes such as phosphoenolpyruvate carboxykinase (PEPCK) in gluconeogenesis (Chapter 12), but is also readily equilibrated with ATP by the enzyme nucleoside diphosphate kinase:

$$GTP + ADP \rightleftharpoons GDP + ATP.$$

The next three reactions in the TCA cycle illustrate a common theme in metabolism for introducing a carbonyl group into a molecule:

- introduction of a double bond
- addition of water across the double bond to form an alcohol
- oxidation of the alcohol to a ketone.

This same sequence occurs in the form of enzyme-bound intermediates during conversion of citrate to α-ketoglutarate and in the oxidation of fatty acids.

Succinate dehydrogenase

Succinate dehydrogenase is a flavoprotein containing the prosthetic group FAD. As described in Chapter 8, this enzyme is embedded in the inner mitochondrial membrane where it is a part of Complex II (succinate-Q reductase). The reaction involves oxidation of succinate to the *trans*-dicarboxylic acid, fumarate, with reduction of FAD to $FADH_2$.

Fumarase

Fumarase stereospecifically adds water across the trans double bond of fumarate to form the α-hydroxy acid, L-malate.

Malate dehydrogenase

Malate dehydrogenase catalyzes the oxidation of L-malate to oxaloacetate, producing NADH, completing one round trip through the TCA cycle. The oxaloacetate may then react with acetyl-CoA, continuing the cycle of reactions.

ENERGY YIELD FROM THE TCA CYCLE

During the course of the TCA cycle, each mole of acetyl-CoA generates sufficient reduced nucleotide coenzymes for

Energetics of glucose oxidation		
Reaction	**Mechanism**	**moles ATP/mol Glc**
hexokinase	phosphorylation	−1
phosphofructokinase	phosphorylation	−1
G3PDH	NADH, oxidative phosphorylation	+6 (+4)*
phosphoglycerate kinase	substrate-level phosphorylation	+2
pyruvate kinase	substrate-level phosphorylation	+2
pyruvate dehydrogenase	NADH, oxidative phosphorylation	+6
isocitrate dehydrogenase	NADH, oxidative phosphorylation	+6
α-ketoglutarate dehydrogenase	NADH, oxidative phosphorylation	+6
succinyl CoA synthetase	substrate-level phosphorylation (GTP)	+2
succinate dehydrogenase	FADH₂, oxidative phosphorylation	+4
malate dehydrogenase	NADH, oxidative phosphorylation	+6
TOTAL		**38 (36)***

Table 13.1 **ATP yield from glucose during oxidative metabolism.** The yields of ATP shown are approximate. Recent work suggests that the actual yields of ATP from NADH and $FADH_2$ are closer to 2.5 and 1.5, respectively, yielding approximately 30 moles of ATP per mole of glucose. The oxidation of glucose in a bomb calorimeter yields 2870 kJ/mol (686 kcal/mol), while the synthesis of ATP requires 31 kJ/mol (7.3 kcal/mol). Aerobic metabolism of glucose is therefore about 40% efficient (2870 kJ/mol glucose / 31 kJ/mole ATP = 93 theoretical moles of ATP/mol glucose; 36/93 = 39%). *Electrons from cytosolic NADH can result in the synthesis of 6 moles of ATP per mole of glucose via the malate-aspartate shuttle, but only 4 via the glycerol 3-phosphate shuttle (see Chapter 8).

synthesis of ~11 moles ATP by oxidative phosphorylation. Note that the ATP yields used here are approximate and are actually slightly less according to recent measurements.

- 3 NADH→9 ATP
- 1 FADH₂→2 ATP

Together with the GTP synthesized by substrate-level phosphorylation in the succinyl-CoA synthetase (succinate thiokinase) reaction, a total of ~12 ATP equivalents are available per mole of acetyl-CoA. Thus, complete metabolism of a mole of glucose through glycolysis and the TCA cycle yields ~36–38 moles ATP (Table 13.1). [The actual ATP yield depends on the route of transport of redox equivalents to the mitochondrion, i.e. six ATP by the malate aspartate shuttle, and four ATP by the glycerol phosphate shuttle (Chapter 8).] In contrast, only 2 moles of ATP (net) are recovered by anaerobic glycolysis in which glucose is converted to lactate.

REGULATION OF THE TCA CYCLE

There are several levels of control of the TCA cycle. In general, the overall activity of the cycle depends on the avail-

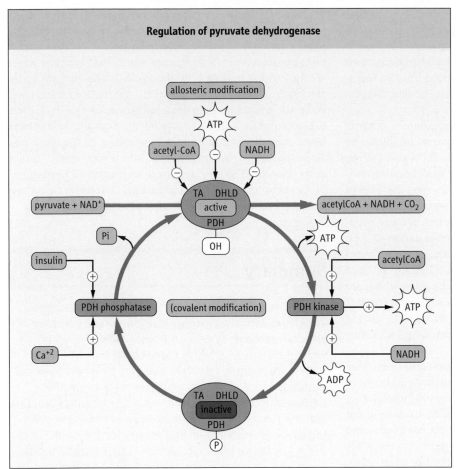

Regulation of pyruvate dehydrogenase

Fig. 13.12 **Regulation of the pyruvate dehydrogenase complex.** The pyruvate dehydrogenase complex regulates the flux of pyruvate into the TCA cycle. NAD(H), ATP and acetyl CoA exert both allosteric and covalent control of enzyme activity. PDH, pyruvate dehydrogenase; TA, dihydrolipoyl transacetylase; DHLD, dihydrolipoamide dehydrogenase subunit.

ability of NAD^+ for the dehydrogenase reactions. This, in turn, is linked to the rate of NADH consumption by the electron transport system, which ultimately depends on the rate of ATP utilization and production of ADP by metabolism (Table 13.1). Thus, as ATP is used for metabolic work, ADP is produced, then NADH is consumed by the electron transport system for ATP production, and NAD^+ is produced. The TCA cycle is activated, fuels are consumed, and more NADH is produced so that more ATP may be made. The mitochondrial level of NAD^+ provides a link between work (ATP utilization) and fuel consumption (Chapter 8).

There are several regulatory enzymes that affect the activity of the TCA cycle. The activity of the pyruvate dehydrogenase complex, and therefore, the supply of acetyl-CoA from glucose, lactate and alanine, is regulated by allosteric and covalent modifications (Fig. 13.12). The products of the pyruvate dehydrogenase reaction, NADH and acetyl-CoA, as well as ATP, act as negative allosteric effectors of the enzyme complex. In addition, the pyruvate dehydrogenase complex has associated kinase and phosphatase enzymes that modulate the degree of phosphorylation of regulatory serine residues in the complex. NADH, acetyl-CoA and ATP activate

the kinase, which phosphorylates and inactivates the enzyme complex. In contrast, when these three compounds are low in concentration, the enzyme complex is activated allosterically and by dephosphorylation by the phosphatase. This is an important regulatory process during fasting and starvation, when gluconeogenesis is essential to maintain blood glucose concentration. Active fat metabolism during fasting leads to increased NADH and acetyl-CoA in the mitochondrion, which leads to inhibition of pyruvate dehydrogenase and blocks the utilization of carbohydrate for energy metabolism. Pyruvate, from such intermediates as lactate and alanine, is directed toward glucose synthesis. Conversely, insulin stimulates pyruvate dehydrogenase by activating the phosphatase when dietary carbohydrates are in excess. This directs carbohydrate-derived carbons into fatty acids via citrate synthase. Ca^{2+} also affects PDC phosphatase activity, in response to changes in intracellular Ca^{2+} during muscle contraction (see Chapter 19).

Oxaloacetate is required for entry of acetyl-CoA into the TCA cycle but, at times, the availability of oxaloacetate appears to regulate the activity of the cycle. This occurs especially during fasting when levels of ATP and NADH, derived from fat metabolism, are increased in the mitochondrion. The increase in NADH shifts the malate:oxaloacetate equilibrium toward malate, directing TCA cycle intermediates toward malate, which is exported to the cytosol for gluconeogenesis (Chapter 12). Meanwhile, acetyl-CoA derived from fat metabolism is directed toward synthesis of ketone bodies (Chapter 14) because of the lack of oxaloacetate.

Isocitrate dehydrogenase is a major regulatory enzyme within the TCA cycle. It is subject to allosteric inhibition by ATP and NADH and stimulation by ADP and NAD+. During consumption of a high carbohydrate diet under resting conditions, the demand for ATP is diminished, and the level of carbohydrate-derived intermediates increases. Under these circumstances, increased insulin levels stimulate the pyruvate dehydrogenase complex and the accumulation of ATP and NADH inhibits isocitrate dehydrogenase, causing a mitochondrial accumulation of citrate. The citrate is then exported to the cytosol for synthesis of fatty acids, which are exported from the liver for storage in adipose tissue as triglycerides. With an increase in energy demand, e.g. during muscle contraction, NAD+ and ADP accumulate, and they stimulate isocitrate dehydrogenase.

Induction and repression, as well as proteolysis of enzyme proteins, such as pyruvate carboxylase and those in the pyruvate dehydrogenase complex and the TCA cycle, clearly play an important regulatory role. In fact, all of the TCA cycle and associated enzymes are synthesized in the cytoplasm and transported through a complex series of steps into the mitochondrion. Regulation can occur at the level of translation, transcription and intracellular transport. Diet, for example, is known to control expression of four pyruvate dehydrogenase kinases; one of them is induced in response to a high fat diet and is repressed in response to a high carbohydrate diet. Unfortunately, the regulation of the TCA cycle at genetic and transport levels is not presently well understood, although it is clearly important for understanding the pathogenesis of a wide-range of contemporary health problems, such as diabetes and obesity.

ANAPLEROTIC ('FILLING UP') REACTIONS

As noted above (Fig. 13.1), TCA cycle intermediates participate in biosynthetic processes, which all require anaplerosis. For example, removal of succinyl-CoA for heme biosynthesis could gradually deplete mitochondrial oxaloacetate. The TCA cycle would cease to function if the intermediates were not replenished, because acetyl-CoA cannot yield a net synthesis of TCA cycle intermediates. Anaplerotic reactions provide the

TCA cycle with intermediates other than acetyl-CoA to maintain activity of the cycle. Pyruvate carboxylase is an example of an enzyme that catalyzes an anaplerotic reaction. It converts pyruvate to malate, a precursor of oxaloacetate, which is required for initiation of the cycle. Malic enzyme in the cytoplasm also converts pyruvate to malate, which can enter the mitochondrion as a substrate for the TCA cycle. α-Ketoglutarate can be produced through an aminotransferase reaction from glutamate, as well as by the glutamate dehydrogenase reaction. Several other 'glucogenic' amino acids (Chapter 18) may also serve as sources of pyruvate or TCA cycle intermediates, guaranteeing that the cycle is never stalled because of a lack of intermediates.

Summary

Located in the mitochondrion, the TCA cycle is closely associated with the pyruvate dehydrogenase complex, the electron transport system and other pathways, all of which function as a highly coordinated unit. The TCA cycle is the central, common pathway by which fuels are oxidized, and it also participates in major biosynthetic pathways. In its oxidative role, its major products are, GTP and the reduced coenzymes NADH and FADH$_2$, which furnish large amounts of free energy for the synthesis of ATP by oxidative phosphorylation. In its biosynthetic role, it provides essential intermediates for the synthesis of glucose, fatty acids, amino acids and heme, as well as the ATP required for their biosynthesis. The activity of the TCA cycle is tightly regulated by substrate supply, by allosteric effectors and control of gene expression so that fuel consumption is coordinated with energy production.

ACTIVE LEARNING

1. In beri-beri, the vitamin thiamine is deficient. Which intermediates would accumulate, and explain why.
2. Based on rates of oxygen consumption, which tissues would be the most critically impaired because of genetically defective enzymes of the TCA cycle?
3. Compare the regulation of the pyruvate dehydrogenase complex to the regulation of cytosolic enzymes by phosphorylation/dephosphorylation reactions.
4. Predict the consequences of deficiencies in TCA cycle enzymes such as succinate dehydrogenase, fumarase or malate dehydrogenase.

Further Reading

De Meirleir L. Defects of pyruvate metabolism and the Krebs cycle. *J Child Neurol* 2002;**17** Suppl 3:3S26–33; discussion 3S33–34.

Haggie PM, Verkman AS. Diffusion of tricarboxylic acid cycle enzymes in the mitochondrial matrix *in vivo*. Evidence for restricted mobility of a multienzyme complex. *J Biol Chem* 2002;**277**(43):40782–8.

McCammon MT, Epstein CB, Przybyla-Zawislak B, McAlister-Henn L, Butow RA. Global transcription analysis of Krebs tricarboxylic acid cycle mutants reveals an alternating pattern of gene expression and effects on hypoxic and oxidative genes. *Mol Biol Cell* 2003;**14**(3):958–72.

Owen OE, Kalhan SC, Hanson RW. The key role of anaplerosis and cataplerosis for citric acid cycle function. *J Biol Chem* 2002;**277**:30409–30412.

Rustin P, Rotig A. Inborn errors of complex II unusual human mitochondrial diseases. *Biochem Biophys Acta* 2002;**1553**(1–2):117–22.

Sheu KFR, Blass JP The α-ketoglutarate dehydrogenase complex. *Ann NY Acad Sci* 1999;**893**:61–78.

Sugden MC, Holness MJ. Recent advances in mechanisms regulating glucose oxidation at the level of the pyruvate dehydrogenase complex by PDKs. *Am J Physiol* 2003;**284**(5):E855–E862.

Relevant websites

A rather complete listing of genetic disorders:
http://www.ncbi.nlm.nih.gov/Omim

TCA Cycle:
http://info.bio.cmu.edu/Courses/BiochemMols/TCACycle/TCAMain.htm

An informational page on causes of Leigh's disease
http://www.ninds.nih.gov/health_and_medical/disorders/leighsdisease_doc.htm

14. Oxidative Metabolism of Lipids in Liver and Muscle

J W Baynes

LEARNING OBJECTIVES

After reading this chapter you should be able to:

■ Describe the pathway for activation and transport of fatty acids to the mitochondrion for catabolism.

■ Outline the sequence of reactions involved in oxidation of fatty acids in the mitochondrion.

■ Describe the general features of pathways for oxidation of unsaturated, odd-chain and branch-chain fatty acids.

■ Explain the rationale for the pathway of ketogenesis and identify the major intermediates and products of this pathway.

■ Describe the mechanism by which hormonal activation of lipolysis in adipose tissue is coordinated with activation of gluconeogenesis in liver during fasting.

INTRODUCTION

Fats are normally the major source of energy in liver and in muscle, and in human tissues in general, except for red cells and brain. Triglycerides are the storage and transport form of fats; fatty acids are the immediate source of energy. They are released from adipose tissue, transported in association with plasma albumin, and delivered to cells for metabolism. The catabolism of fatty acids is entirely oxidative; after they have been transported through the cytoplasm, their oxidation proceeds in both the peroxisome and the mitochondrion, primarily by a cycle of reactions known as β-oxidation. Carbons are released, two at a time, from the carboxyl end of the fatty acid; the major end-products are acetyl-coenzyme A (acetyl-CoA) and the reduced forms of the nucleotides, flavin adenine dinucleotide and nicotinamide adenine dinucleotide ($FADH_2$ and NADH, respectively). In muscle, the acetyl-CoA is metabolized via the tricarboxylic acid (TCA) cycle and oxidative phosphorylation to produce ATP; in liver, it is shunted largely to the synthesis of ketone bodies (ketogenesis), which are water-soluble lipid derivatives that, like glucose, are exported from liver for use in other tissues. Fat metabolism is controlled primarily by the rate of triglyceride hydrolysis (lipolysis) in adipose tissue, regulated by hormonal mechanisms involving insulin and glucagon, epinephrine,

and cortisol. These hormones coordinate the metabolism of carbohydrate, lipid and protein throughout the body (see Chapter 20).

ACTIVATION OF FATTY ACIDS AND THEIR TRANSPORT TO THE MITOCHONDRION

Fatty acids do not exist in free form in the body – they are soaps, and would dissolve membranes. In blood, fatty acids are bound to albumin, which is present at ~0.5 mmol/L concentration (35 mg/mL) in plasma. Each molecule of albumin can bind six to eight fatty acid molecules. In the cytosol, fatty acids are bound to a series of fatty-acid-binding proteins and enzymes. As the priming step for their catabolism, the fatty acids are activated to their CoA derivative, using adenosine triphosphate (ATP) as the energy source (Fig. 14.1). The carboxyl group is first activated to an enzyme-bound, high-energy acyl adenylate intermediate, formed by reaction of the carboxyl group of the fatty acid with ATP. The acyl group is then transferred to CoA by the same enzyme, fatty acyl CoA synthetase. This enzyme is commonly known as fatty acid thiokinase, because ATP is consumed in the formation of the thioester bond in acyl CoA.

The length of the fatty acid dictates where it is activated to CoA

Short- and medium-chain fatty acids (Table 14.1) can cross the mitochondrial membrane by passive diffusion, and are activated to their CoA derivative within the mitochondrion. Very-long-chain fatty acids from the diet are shortened to long-chain fatty acids in peroxisomes. Long-chain fatty acids (16 ± 4 carbons) are the major components of storage triglycerides and dietary fats. They are activated to their CoA derivatives in the cytoplasm and are transported into the mitochondrion via the carnitine shuttle.

The carnitine shuttle

CoA is a large, polar nucleotide derivative, and cannot penetrate the mitochondrial inner membrane. Thus, for the transport of long-chain fatty acids, the fatty acid is first transferred to the small molecule, carnitine, by carnitine palmitoyl transferase-I (CPT-I), located in the outer

PEROXISOMES

Role of peroxisomes in fatty acid oxidation

Peroxisomes are subcellular organelles found in all nucleated cells. They are the principal sites of production of hydrogen peroxide (H_2O_2) in the cell, and account for nearly 20% of oxygen consumption in hepatocytes. They are able to conduct β-oxidation of long and very-long-chain fatty acids by a pathway similar to mitochondrial oxidation, but with some significant differences, e.g. the oxidation of acyl-CoAs is catalyzed by an oxidase, producing H_2O_2, rather than $FADH_2$. Peroxisomes are relatively inefficient at catabolism of short-chain fatty acids, so products such as hexanoyl- and octanoylcarnitine are exported, to be catabolized in the mitochondrion. Peroxisomes are also the primary site of oxidation of branched-chain fatty acids and medium-chain α,ω-dicarboxylic acids produced by microsomal or peroxisomal ω-oxidation of fatty acids. The fibrates are a class of hypolipidemic drugs that act by inducing peroxisomal proliferation in liver.

Peroxisomes are believed to have a role in production of acetyl-CoA for anabolic reactions, e.g. the biosynthesis of cholesterol and polyisoprenoids (Chapter 16). Peroxisomes also have a special role in the metabolism of very-long-chain fatty acids and phytanic acids (see below). Zellweger syndrome, resulting from the absence of peroxisomes, is characterized by accumulation of long-chain fatty acids and branched chain, pristanic acids in plasma and tissues.

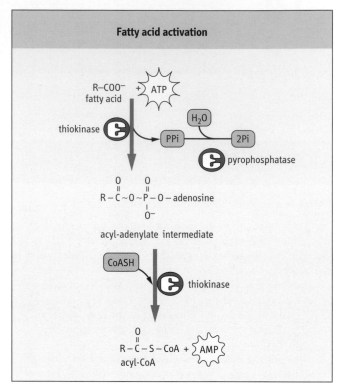

Fig. 14.1 **Activation of fatty acids by fatty acyl-CoA synthetase (thiokinase).** ATP forms an enzyme-bound acyl adenylate intermediate, which is discharged to form acyl CoA. AMP, adenosine monophosphate; CoASH, coenzyme A; PPi, inorganic pyrophosphate.

mitochondrial membrane. An acyl-carnitine transporter or translocase in the inner mitochondrial membrane then mediates transfer of the fatty acid into the mitochondrion, where CPT-II regenerates the acyl-CoA, releasing free carnitine. The carnitine shuttle (Fig. 14.2) operates by an antiport mechanism in which free carnitine and the acyl-carnitine derivative move in opposite directions across the inner mitochondrial membrane. The shuttle is an important site in the regulation of fatty acid oxidation. As discussed in the next chapter, the carnitine shuttle is inhibited by malonyl-CoA after the ingestion of carbohydrate-rich meals. Malonyl-CoA prevents the futile cycle in which newly synthesized fatty acids would be oxidized in the mitochondrion and promotes their export from the liver for storage in adipose tissue.

Metabolism of fatty acids

Size class	Number of carbons	Site of catabolism	Membrane transport
Short-chain	2–4	mitochondrion	diffusion
Medium-chain	4–12	mitochondrion	diffusion
Long-chain	12–20	mitochondrion	carnitine cycle
Very-long-chain	>20	peroxisome	unknown

Table 14.1 **Metabolism of the four classes of fatty acids.**

OXIDATION OF FATTY ACIDS

Mitochondrial β-oxidation

Fatty acyl-CoAs are oxidized in a cycle of reactions involving oxidation of the β-carbon to a ketone; hence the terminology,

β-oxidation (Figs 14.3 and 14.4). The oxidation is followed by cleavage between the α- and β-carbons by a thiolase reaction. One mole each of acetyl-CoA, $FADH_2$, and $NADH + H^+$ is formed during each cycle, along with a fatty acyl-CoA with two fewer carbon atoms. For a 16-carbon fatty acid, such as palmitate, the cycle is repeated seven times, yielding 8 moles of acetyl-CoA (Fig. 14.3, Table 14.1), plus seven moles of $FADH_2$ and 7 moles of $NADH + H^+$. This process occurs in

KETOGENESIS IN LIVER

Deficiencies in carnitine metabolism

The clinical presentation of deficient carnitine metabolism occurs in infancy and is often life threatening. Characteristic features include hypoketotic hypoglycemia, hyperammonemia, and altered plasma free carnitine concentration. Hepatic damage, cardiomyopathy, and muscle weakness are common.

Comment. Carnitine is synthesized from lysine and α-ketoglutarate, primarily in liver and kidney, and is normally present in plasma in a concentration of about 50 mmol/L (0.8 mg/dL). There are high-affinity uptake systems for carnitine in most tissues, including the kidney, which resorbs carnitine from the glomerular filtrate, limiting its excretion in urine. Homozygous deficiencies in carnitine transport, CPTs-I and -II, and the translocase result in defects in long-chain fatty acid oxidation. Plasma and tissue carnitine concentrations decrease to <1 mmol/L in carnitine transport deficiency, because of both defective uptake into tissues and excessive loss in urine. On the other hand, plasma free carnitine may exceed 100 mmol/L (2 mg/dL) in CPT-I deficiency. In both translocase and CPT-II deficiency, total plasma carnitine may be normal, but is mostly in the form of acyl carnitine esters of long-chain fatty acids – in the former case, because they cannot be transported into the mitochondrion, and in the latter because of backflow out from mitochondria. These diseases are treated by carnitine supplementation, by frequent high-carbohydrate feeding, and by avoidance of fasting.

the mitochondrion, and the reduced nucleotides are used directly for synthesis of ATP by oxidative phosphorylation (Table 14.2).

The four steps in the cycle of β-oxidation are shown in detail in Figure 14.3. Note the similarity between the sequence of these reactions and those between succinate and oxaloacetate in the TCA cycle. In common with succinate dehydrogenase, acyl-CoA dehydrogenase uses the prosthetic group FAD as a coenzyme, and is an integral protein in the

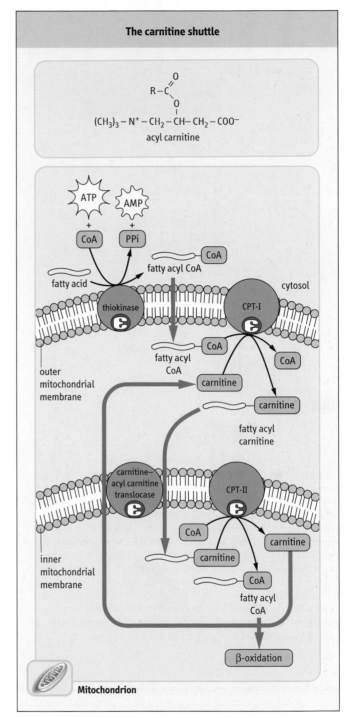

Fig. 14.2 **Transport of long-chain fatty acids into the mitochondrion.** The three components of the carnitine pathway include extra- and intra-mitochondrial CPTs and the carnitine-acyl carnitine translocase.

Caloric value of glucose and palmitate

Substrate	Molecular weight	Net ATP yield (mol/mol)	ATP (mol/g)	Caloric value Cal/g (kJ)
glucose	180	36–38	0.2	4 (17)
palmitate	256	129	0.5	9 (37)

Table 14.2 **Comparative energy yield from glucose and palmitate.**

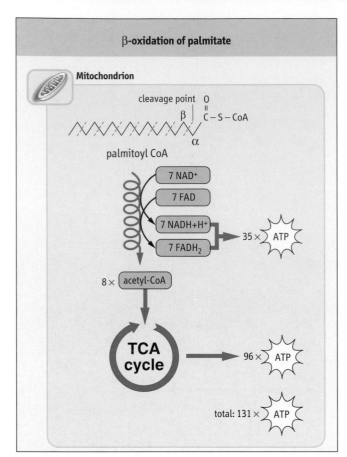

β-oxidation of palmitate

Mitochondrion

Fig. 14.3 **Overview of β-oxidation of palmitate.** In a cycle of reactions, the carbons of the fatty-acyl-CoA are released in two-carbon acetyl-CoA units; the yield of 35 ATP from this β-oxidation is nearly equivalent to that from complete oxidation of glucose. In liver, the acetyl CoA units are then used for synthesis of ketone bodies, and in other tissues they are metabolized in the TCA cycle to form ATP. The complete oxidation of palmitate yields a net 129 moles of ATP, after correction for the 2-mole equivalents of ATP invested at the thiokinase reaction. The overall production of ATP per gram of palmitate is about twice that per gram of glucose, because glucose is already partially oxidized in comparison with palmitate. For this reason, as illustrated in Table 14.2, the caloric value of fats is about twice that of sugars.

inner mitochondrial membrane. Even the *trans* geometry of fumarate and the stereochemical configuration of L-malate in the TCA cycle are mirrored by the trans geometry of the trans-enoyl-CoA and L-hydroxyacyl-CoA intermediates in β-oxidation. The last step of the β-oxidation cycle is catalyzed by thiolase, which traps the energy obtained from the carbon-carbon bond cleavage as acyl-CoA, allowing the cycle to continue without the necessity of reactivating the fatty acid. The cycle continues until all the fatty acid has been converted to acetyl-CoA, the common intermediate in the oxidation of carbohydrates and lipids.

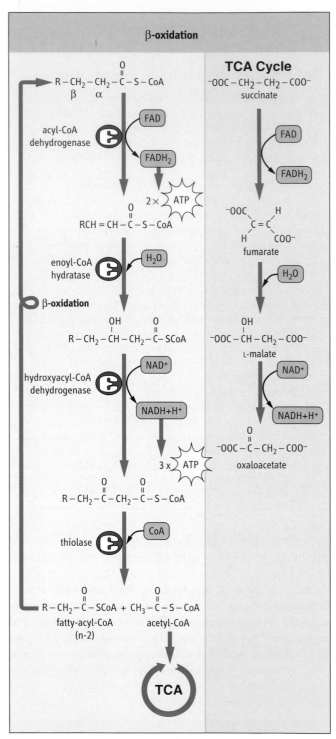

Fig. 14.4 **β-Oxidation of fatty acids.** Oxidation occurs in a series of steps at the carbon that is β to the keto group. Thiolase cleaves the resultant β-ketoacyl-CoA derivative to give acetyl-CoA and a fatty acid with two fewer carbon atoms, which then re-enters the β-oxidation cascade. Note the similarity between these reactions and those of the TCA cycle, shown on the right.

IMPAIRED OXIDATION OF MEDIUM-CHAIN FATTY ACIDS

Fatty acyl CoA dehydrogenase

Fatty acyl CoA dehydrogenase is not a single enzyme, but a family of enzymes with chain-length specificity for oxidation of short-, medium- and long-chain fatty acids; fatty acids are transferred from one enzyme to the other during chain-shortening β-oxidation reactions. Medium-chain fatty acyl CoA dehydrogenase (MCAD) deficiency is an autosomal recessive disease characterized by hypoketotic hypoglycemia. It presents in infancy, and is characterized by high concentrations of medium-chain carboxylic acids, acyl carnitines, and acyl glycines in plasma and urine. Hyperammonemia may also be present, as a result of liver damage. Concentrations of hepatic mitochondrial medium-chain acyl CoA derivatives are also increased, limiting β-oxidation and recycling of CoA during ketogenesis. The inability to metabolize fats during fasting is life threatening because it limits gluconeogenesis and causes hypoglycemia. MCAD deficiency is treated by frequent feeding, avoidance of fasting, and carnitine supplementation. Deficiencies in short- and long-chain fatty acid dehydrogenases have also been described, and have similar clinical features.

Alternative pathways of oxidation of fatty acids

Unsaturated fatty acids yield less FADH$_2$ when they are oxidized

Unsaturated fatty acids are already partially oxidized, so less FADH$_2$, and correspondingly less ATP, is produced by their oxidation. The double bonds in polyunsaturated fatty acids have *cis* geometry and occur at three-carbon intervals, whereas the intermediates in β-oxidation have *trans* geometry and the reactions proceed in two-carbon steps. The metabolism of unsaturated fatty acids therefore requires several additional enzymes, both to shift the position and to change the geometry of the double bonds.

Odd-chain fatty acids gain access to the TCA cycle via propionyl-CoA

The oxidation of fatty acids with an odd number of carbons proceeds from the carboxyl end, like that of normal fatty acids, except that propionyl-CoA is formed by the last thiolase cleavage reaction. The propionyl-CoA is converted to succinyl-CoA by a multi-step process involving three

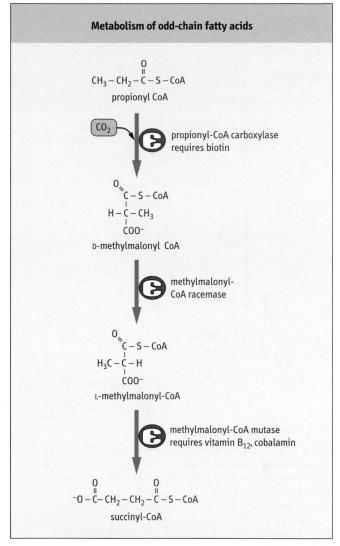

Fig. 14.5 **Metabolism of propionyl-CoA to succinyl-CoA.** Propionyl-CoA from odd-chain fatty acids is a minor source of carbons for gluconeogenesis. The intermediate, methylmalonyl CoA, is also produced during catabolism of branched-chain amino acids. Defects in methylmalonyl-CoA mutase or deficiencies in vitamin B$_{12}$ lead to methylmalonic-aciduria.

enzymes and the vitamins biotin and cobalamin (Fig. 14.5). The succinyl-CoA enters directly into the TCA cycle.

Branched-chain fatty acids must be catabolized, to acetyl CoA and propionyl CoA via α-oxidation

Phytanic acids are branched-chain polyisoprenoid lipids found in plant chlorophylls. Because the β-carbon of phytanic acids is at a branch point, it is not possible to oxidize this carbon to a ketone. The first and essential step in catabolism of phytanic acids is microsomal α-oxidation to pristanic acid,

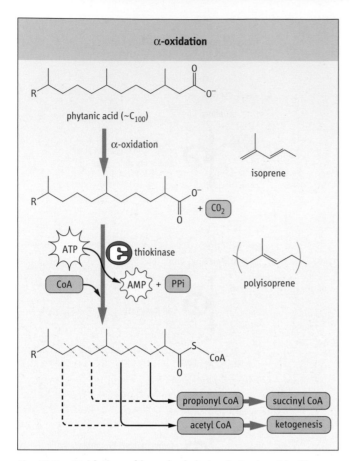

Fig. 14.6 **α-Oxidation of branched-chain phytanic acids.** The first carbon of phytanic acids is removed as carbon dioxide. In subsequent cycles of β-oxidation, acetyl-CoA and propionyl-CoA are released alternately.

releasing the (α-)carbon-1 as carbon dioxide. Thereafter, as shown in Figure 14.6, acetyl-CoA and propionyl-CoA are released alternately and in equal amounts. Refsum's disease is a rare neurologic disorder, characterized by accumulation of phytanic acid deposits in nerve tissues as a result of a genetic defect in α-oxidation.

KETOGENESIS IN LIVER

Gluconeogenesis in fasting and starvation

The liver uses fatty acids as the source of energy for gluconeogenesis during fasting and starvation. Fats are a rich source of energy and, under conditions of fasting or starvation, liver mitochondrial concentrations of fat-derived ATP and NADH are high, inhibiting the isocitrate dehydrogenase reaction and shifting the oxaloacetate-malate equilibrium toward malate. TCA cycle intermediates that are formed from amino acids released from muscle as part of the response to fasting and starvation (see Chapter 19) are converted to malate in the TCA cycle, but the malate then leaves the mitochondrion, to take part in gluconeogenesis. The resulting low level of oxaloacetate in hepatic mitochondria limits the activity of the TCA cycle, resulting in an inability to metabolize acetyl-CoA efficiently in the TCA cycle. The liver, meanwhile, obtains sufficient energy to support gluconeogenesis simply via the enzymes of β-oxidation, which generate both $FADH_2$ and NADH.

BUTTER OR MARGARINE?

There is continuing debate among nutritionists about the health benefits of butter versus those of margarine in foods.

Comments. Butter is rich in saturated fatty acids and cholesterol, which are risk factors for atherosclerosis. Margarine contains no cholesterol, and is richer in unsaturated fatty acids. However, the unsaturated fatty acids in margarine are mostly the unnatural *trans*-fatty acids formed during the partial hydrogenation of vegetable oils. *Trans*-fatty acids affect plasma lipids in the same fashion as long-chain saturated fats, suggesting that there are comparable risks associated with the consumption of butter or margarine. The resolution of this issue is complicated by the fact that various forms of margarine, for example soft-spread and hard-block types, vary significantly in their content of *trans*-fatty acids.

ALTERNATIVE PATHWAYS OF FATTY ACID OXIDATION AND ASSOCIATED DISORDERS

Dicarboxylic aciduria and β-oxidation of fatty acids

Several disorders of lipid catabolism, including alterations in the carnitine shuttle, acyl-CoA dehydrogenase deficiencies, and Zellweger syndrome (a defect in peroxisome biogenesis) are associated with the appearance of medium-chain dicarboxylic acids in urine; both odd- and even-chain dicarboxylic acids may be involved. When fatty acid β-oxidation is impaired, fatty acids are oxidized, one carbon at a time, from the ω-carbon by microsomal cytochrome P_{450}-dependent hydroxylases and dehydrogenases. These dicarboxylic acids are substrates for peroxisomal β–oxidation, which continues to the level of 6–10-carbon dicarboxylic acids, which are then excreted into urine.

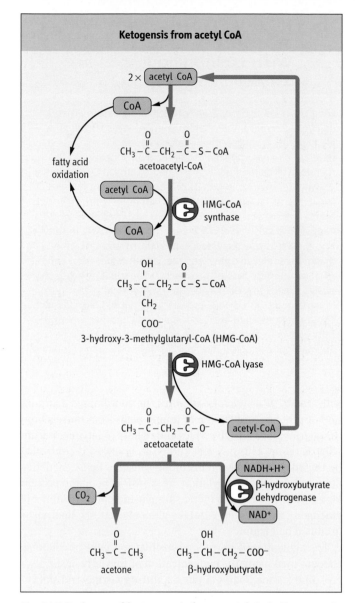

Ketogensis from acetyl CoA

Fig. 14.7 **Pathway of ketogenesis from acetyl-CoA.** Ketogenesis generates ketone bodies from acetyl-CoA, releasing the CoA to participate in β-oxidation. The enzymes involved, HMG-CoA synthase and lyase, are unique to hepatocytes; mitochondrial HMG-CoA is an essential intermediate. The initial product is acetoacetic acid, which may be enzymatically reduced to β-hydroxybutyrate by β-hydroxybutyrate dehydrogenase, or may spontaneously (nonenzymatically) decompose to acetone, which is excreted in urine or expired by the lungs.

What does the liver do with the excess acetyl CoA that accumulates in fasting or starvation?

The problem of dealing with excess acetyl-CoA is a critical one, because CoA is present only in catalytic amounts in tissues, and free CoA is required to initiate and continue the cycle of β-oxidation. To recycle the acetyl-CoA, the liver uses a pathway known as ketogenesis, in which free CoA is regen-

KETONE BODIES IN URINE (KETONURIA) AND WEIGHT-LOSS PROGRAMS

The appearance of ketone bodies in the urine is an indication of active fat metabolism and gluconeogenesis. Ketonuria may also occur normally in association with a high-fat, low-carbohydrate diet. Some weight loss programs encourage gradual reduction in carbohydrate and total caloric intake until ketone bodies appear in urine (measured with Keto-Stix). Dieters are urged to maintain this level of caloric intake, checking urinary ketones regularly to confirm the consumption of body fat.

Comment. Keto-Stix and similar 'dry chemistry' tests are convenient test strips for urinary ketone bodies. They contain a chemical reagent, such as nitroprusside, which reacts with acetoacetate in urine to form a lavender color, graded on a scale with a maximum of '4+' (see Chapter 22 and Fig. 22.11). A reaction of '1+' (representing 5–10 mg ketone bodies/100 mL) or '2+' (10-20 mg/100 mL) on the test strip was established as a goal to assure continued fat metabolism, and therefore weight loss. This type of diet is discouraged today, because the appearance of ketone bodies in the urine indicates greater concentrations in the plasma, and may cause metabolic acidosis.

erated and the acetate group appears in blood in the form of three water-soluble lipid-derived products: acetoacetate, β-hydroxybutyrate, and acetone. The pathway of formation of these 'ketone bodies' (Fig. 14.7) involves the synthesis and decomposition of hydroxymethylglutaryl (HMG)-CoA in the mitochondrion. The liver is unique in its content of HMG-CoA synthase and lyase, but is deficient in enzymes required for metabolism of ketone bodies, which explains their export into blood.

Ketone bodies are taken up in extrahepatic tissues, including skeletal and cardiac muscle, where they are converted to CoA derivatives for metabolism (Fig. 14.8). Ketone bodies are an efficient source of energy (Table 14.3) during fasting and starvation, and appear to be used in muscle in proportion to their plasma concentration. During starvation, the brain also converts to the use of ketone bodies for more than 50% of its energy metabolism, sparing glucose and reducing the demand on degradation of muscle protein for gluconeogenesis (see also Chapter 20).

Mobilization of lipids during gluconeogenesis and work

Insulin, glucagon, epinephrine, and cortisol control the direction and rate of glycogen and glucose metabolism in liver. During fasting and starvation, hepatic gluconeogenesis is

Metabolism of ketone bodies

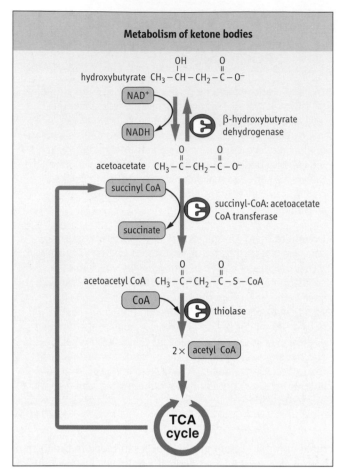

Fig. 14.8 **Catabolism of ketone bodies in peripheral tissues.**
Succinyl-CoA: acetoacetate CoA transferase activates the
transfer of acetoacetate to acetoacetyl CoA. A thiokinase-type
enzyme may also directly activate acetoacetate in some tissues.

Plasma concentrations of fatty acids and ketone bodies

Substrate	Plasma concentration (mmol/L)		
	Normal	Fasting	Starvation
Fatty acids	0.6	1.0	1.5
Acetoacetate	<0.1	0.2	1–2
β-Hydroxybutyrate	<0.1	1	5–10

Table 14.3 **Plasma concentrations of fatty acids and ketone
bodies in different nutritional states.**

HELLP AND AFLP SYNDROMES IN MOTHERS OF CHILDREN BORN WITH LCHAD (incidence 1 in 200,000)

Long chain L-3-hydroxy-acyl-CoA dehydrogenase deficiency
(LCHAD) can present in a wide variety of ways. Those affected
are prone to episodes of non-ketotic hypoglycaemia, but may
develop fulminant hepatic failure, cardiomyopathy,
rhabdomyolysis, and occasionally neuropathy and retinopathy.
As with deficiencies in MCAD or LCAD, treatment involves
avoidance of fasting and diets enriched in medium chain fatty
acids.

Perhaps the most striking feature of this rare defect in fatty
acid metabolism is the association with maternal HELLP
(**h**aemolysis, **e**levated **l**iver enzymes and **l**ow **p**latelets) and
AFLP (**a**cute **f**atty **l**iver of **p**regnancy). These potentially fatal
obstetric emergencies may occur in mothers who are
heterozygotes for LCHAD, especially if the child has LCHAD.
These syndromes are also associated with another recessive
fatty acid defect, carnitine palmitoyl-transferase-I deficiency.
The pathophysiological mechanisms have not been elucidated.

activated by glucagon and requires the coordinated degradation of proteins and release of amino acids from muscle, and
the degradation of triglycerides and release of fatty acids from
adipose tissue. This process, known as lipolysis, is controlled
by the adipocyte enzyme hormone-sensitive lipase, which is
activated by phosphorylation by cAMP-dependent protein
kinase A in response to increasing plasma concentrations of
glucagon (see Chapter 20). Like gluconeogenesis, lipolysis is
inhibited by insulin.

The activation of hormone-sensitive lipase has predictable
effects – increasing the concentration of free fatty acids, glycerol, and ketone bodies in plasma during fasting and starvation (Fig. 14.9); similar effects are observed in response to
epinephrine during the stress response. Epinephrine activates
both glycogenolysis in the liver and lipolysis in adipose tissue,
so that both fuels, glucose and fatty acids, increase in blood
during stress. Cortisol exerts a more chronic effect on lipolysis and also causes insulin resistance. Cushing's syndrome
(see Chapter 37), in which there are high blood concentrations of cortisol, is characterized by hyperglycemia, muscle
wastage, and redistribution of fat from glucagon-sensitive
adipose depots to atypical sites, such as the cheeks, upper
back, and trunk.

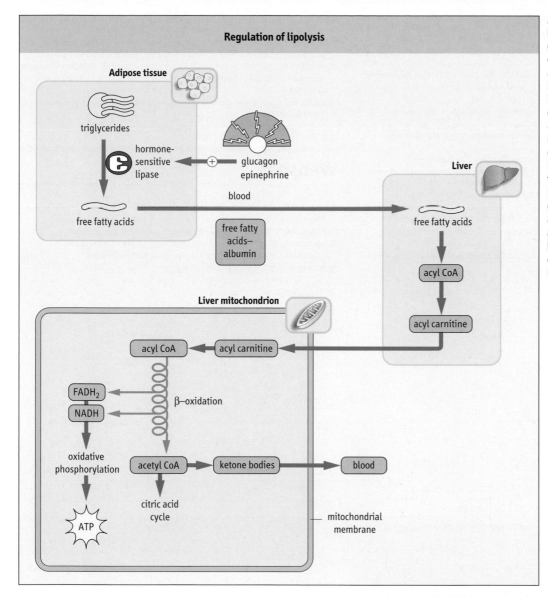

Fig. 14.9 **Regulation of lipid metabolism by glucagon and epinephrine.** Glucagon and epinephrine activate hormone-sensitive lipase in adipose tissue, in coordination with activation of proteolysis in muscle and gluconeogenesis in liver. Metabolism of fatty acids through β-oxidation in liver yields ATP for gluconeogenesis. The acetyl-CoA is converted to and released to blood as ketone bodies. These effects are reversed by insulin following a meal.

Summary

Unlike carbohydrate fuels, which enter the body primarily as glucose or sugars that are readily converted to glucose, lipid fuels are heterogeneous with respect to chain length, branching, and unsaturation. The catabolism of fats is primarily a mitochondrial process, but also occurs in peroxisomes. Using a variety of chain-length-specific transport processes and catabolic enzymes, the primary pathways of catabolism of fatty acids involve their oxidative degradation in two-carbon units – a process known as β-oxidation, which produces acetyl-CoA. In muscle, the acetyl-CoA units are used for ATP production in the mitochondria, whereas in liver the acetyl-CoA is catabolized to ketone bodies, primarily acetoacetate and β-hydroxybutyrate, that are exported for energy metabolism in peripheral tissue.

ACTIVE LEARNING

1. Compare the metabolism of acetyl-CoA in liver and muscle. Explain why the liver produces ketone bodies during gluconeogenesis. What prevents hepatic oxidation of acetyl-CoA?
2. Review the merits of carnitine usage as a performance enhancer during exercise and as a supplement for geriatric patients.
3. Review the current use and mechanism of action of peroxisome proliferator drugs for treatment of dyslipidemia and diabetes.

Further reading

Atar D, Spiess M, Mandinova A, Cierpka H, Noll G, Luscher TF. Carnitine – from cellular mechanisms to potential clinical applications in heart disease. *Eur J Clin Invest* 1997;**27**:973–976.

Depreter M, Espeel M, Roels F. Human peroxisomal disorders. *Microsc Res Tech* 2003;**61**:203–223.

Eaton S, Bartlett K, Pourfarzam M. Mammalian mitochondrial β-oxidation. *Biochem J* 1996;**320**:345–357.

Freeland BS. Diabetic ketoacidosis. *Diabetes Educator* 2003;**29**:384–395.

McGarry JD, Brown NF. The mitochondrial carnitine palmitoyltransferase system. From concept to molecular analysis. *Eur J Biochem* 1997;**244**:1–14.

Mitchell GA, Kassovska-Bratinova S, Boukaftane Y, *et al.* Medical aspects of ketone body metabolism. *Clin Invest Med* 1995;**18**:193–216.

Rinaldo P, Raymond K, al-Odaib A, Bennett MJ. Clinical and biochemical features of fatty acid oxidation disorders. *Curr Opin Pediatr* 1998;**10**: 615–621.

Singh I. Biochemistry of peroxisomes in health and disease. *Mol Cell Biochem* 1997;**167**:1–29.

Swink TD, Vining EP, Freeman JM. The ketogenic diet: 1997. *Adv Pediatr* 1997;**44**:297–329.

Wanders RJ, Jansen GA, Lloyd MD. Phytanic acid alpha-oxidation, new insights into an old problem: a review. *Biochim Biophys Acta* 2003;**163**1:119–135.

Wierzbicki AS, Lloyd MD, Schofield CJ, Feher MD, Gibberd FB. Refsum's disease: a peroxisomal disorder affecting phytanic acid alpha-oxidation. *J Neurochem* 2002;**80**:727–35.

Wood PA. Defects in mitochondrial beta-oxidation of fatty acids. *Curr Opin Lipidol* 1999;**10**:107–112.

Websites

Acyl CoA Dehydrogenase Deficiency: http://www.cdc.gov/genomics/hugenet/reviews/MCAD.htm

Carnitine: http://lpi.oregonstate.edu/infocenter/othernuts/carnitine/

Ketogenesis: http://www.gpnotebook.co.uk/cache/-160759750.htm

Lipids OnLine - Slide Library: http://www.lipidsonline.org/slides/

Peroxisomes: http://www.peroxisome.org/

15. Biosynthesis and Storage of Fatty Acids in Liver and Adipose Tissue

I Broom

LEARNING OBJECTIVES

After reading this chapter you should be able to:

■ Describe the pathway of fatty acid synthesis, and in particular the roles of the malonyl-CoA carboxylase and the multifunctional enzyme fatty acid synthase.

■ Outline short-term and long-term regulation of fatty acid synthesis.

■ Explain the concepts of elongation and desaturation of the fatty acid chain.

■ Describe the synthesis of triglycerides.

■ Discuss endocrine function of adipose tissue.

INTRODUCTION

The majority of fatty acids required by man are supplied in the diet; however, pathways for their *de novo* synthesis (lipogenesis) from 2-carbon compounds are present in many tissues such as liver, brain, kidney, mammary gland, and adipose tissue. In general, the pathway of *de novo* synthesis is used in conditions of excess energy, and in particular, carbohydrate intake. In such conditions carbohydrates are converted to fatty acids in the liver and stored as triacylglycerols (TAG; also known as triglycerides) in the adipose tissue. In man, adipose tissue is not an important site of synthesis of fatty acids; the main organ of lipogenic activity is the liver. Lipogenesis does not appear to be a critical requirement in humans, and no life-threatening illnesses associated with its malfunction have been identified. It does, however, have an important bearing on the development of obesity, and is inhibited in type 1 diabetes mellitus.

The pathway for lipogenesis is not simply the reverse of oxidation of fatty acids (see Chapter 14). Lipogenesis requires a completely different set of enzymes from lipolysis. Also, it is located in a different cellular compartment, the cytosol, and uses nicotinamide dinucleotide phosphate ($NADP^+$) as a source of reductive power, as opposed to the nicotinamide dinucleotide (NAD_+) that is required for β-oxidation of fatty acids.

FATTY ACID SYNTHESIS

The synthesis of fatty acids in mammalian systems can be considered as a two-stage process, both stages requiring acetyl-Coenzyme A (acetyl CoA) and both employing multifunctional proteins (multienzyme complexes):

■ stage 1: involves preparation of the key precursor malonyl-CoA by the acetyl CoA carboxylase,

■ stage 2: involves elongation of the fatty acid chain (in 2-carbon increments) by fatty acid synthase.

Acetyl-CoA carboxylase

Carboxylation of acetyl-CoA to malonyl-CoA is the committed step of fatty acid synthesis

In the first stage of fatty acid biosynthesis, acetyl-CoA, mostly derived from carbohydrate metabolism, is converted to malonyl-CoA under the action of the acetyl-CoA carboxylase (Fig. 15.1). This is a biotin-dependent enzyme with distinct enzymatic functions and a carrier protein function: its subunits serve as a biotin carboxylase, a transcarboxylase, and a biotin–carboxyl-carrier protein. The enzyme is synthesized in an inactive protomer form (each protomer containing the above subunits), a molecule of biotin, and a regulatory allosteric site for the binding of citrate (a Krebs cycle metabolite) or of palmitoyl-CoA (the end-product of the fatty acid biosynthetic pathway). The reaction itself takes place in stages: first there is the carboxylation of biotin, involving adenosine triphosphate (ATP), and this is followed by the transfer of this carboxyl group to acetyl-CoA to produce the end-product of the reaction, the malonyl-CoA. At this stage, the free enzyme–biotin complex is released.

Incidentally, to synthesize fatty acids with an odd-number of carbons, propionyl-CoA is used as a substrate.

This key lipogenic enzyme is subject to both short-term and long-term control

The protomers of the acetyl-CoA carboxylase polymerize in the presence of citrate or isocitrate, producing the active form of the enzyme. The polymerization is also inhibited by palmitoyl-CoA at the same allosteric site. The respective stimulatory and inhibitory effects of citrate and palmitoyl-CoA are

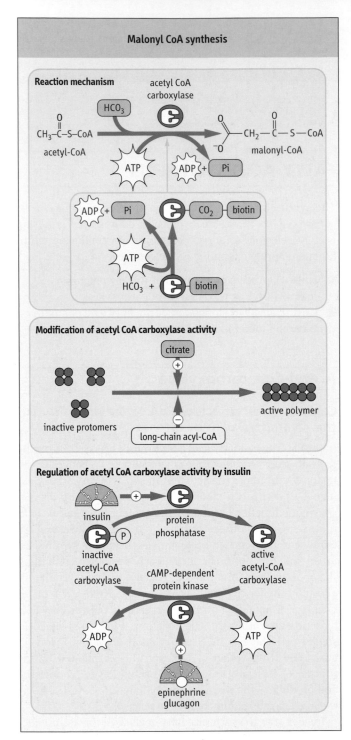

Fig. 15.1 **Conversion of acetyl-CoA to malonyl-CoA.** Acetyl-CoA carboxylase is covalently attached to biotin, which is carboxylated using a molecule of ATP. The enzyme requires the presence of citrate for polymerization to its active form. It is also regulated by insulin, independently of the citrate-stimulated polymerization. cAMP, cyclic adenosine monophosphate.

entirely logical: under conditions of high citrate concentration, energy storage is desirable, but when the product of the pathway (palmitoyl-CoA) accumulates, a decrease in synthesis of fatty acids is appropriate. There is an additional control mechanism: phosphorylation/dephosphorylation of the enzyme molecule. This involves hormone-dependent protein phosphatase/kinase (see Fig. 15.1). Phosphorylation inhibits the enzyme, and dephosphorylation activates it. These effects are independent of the effects of citrate or palmitoyl-CoA. Phosphorylation of the enzyme is stimulated by glucagon and epinephrine, and dephosphorylation by insulin.

The carboxylation of acetyl-CoA to malonyl-CoA is the committed step of fatty acid synthesis. This is why this enzyme is under such strict short-term regulation. Longer-term control also exists and is exerted by the induction or repression of enzyme synthesis effected by diet: synthesis of acetyl-CoA carboxylase is upregulated under conditions of high-carbohydrate/low-fat intake, whereas starvation or high-fat/low-carbohydrate intake leads to downregulation of synthesis of the enzyme.

Fatty acid synthase

The second major step in fatty acid biosynthesis also involves a multienzyme complex, fatty acid synthase.

This enzyme system is more complex than acetyl-CoA carboxylase. The protein contains seven distinct enzyme activities and an acyl-carrier protein (ACP). ACP, a peptide containing 77 amino acids, replaces the CoA as an entity which binds the growing fatty acid chain. It contains a pantetheine residue, the same as CoA. The relatively long pantetheine group acts as a flexible 'arm' which makes the molecule being synthesized available to different enzymes in the fatty acid synthase complex. The structure of the fatty acid synthase is shown in Figure 15.2: it consists of a dimer of large identical polypeptides (260 kDa each) arranged head to tail. Each chain contains all seven enzyme activities grouped into three domains; however, the function in fatty acid synthesis is shared between the two polypeptide chains.

The fatty acid synthase builds up the fatty acid molecule up to the 16-carbon length

The reaction proceeds after an initial priming of the cysteine (–Cys–SH) group with acetyl-CoA under the action of acetyl transacylase (Fig. 15.3). Malonyl-CoA is then transfered to the –SH residue of the pantetheine group attached to the ACP of the other subunit, under the action of malonyl transacylase. Next, 3-ketoacyl synthase (the condensing enzyme) catalyzes the reaction between the previously attached acetyl group and the malonyl residue, liberating carbon dioxide and forming the 3-ketoacyl-enzyme complex. This frees the

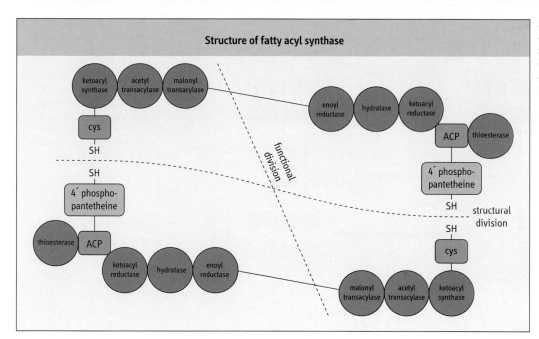

Structure of fatty acyl synthase

Fig. 15.2 **Structure of fatty acyl synthase.** Fatty acid synthase contains seven distinct enzyme activities and an acyl-carrier protein (ACP). Cys, cysteine.

cysteine residue that had been occupied by acetyl-CoA. The 3-ketoacyl group subsequently undergoes sequential reduction, dehydration, and again reduction to form a saturated acyl-enzyme complex. The next molecule of malonyl-CoA then displaces the acyl group from the pantetheine-SH group to the now free cysteine group, and the reaction sequence is repeated through six cycles. Once the 16-carbon chain (palmitate) is formed, the saturated acyl-enzyme complex activates the thioesterase, resulting in the release of palmitate molecule from the enzyme complex. The two —SH sites are now free, allowing another cycle of palmitate synthesis to be initiated.

The synthesis of one molecule of palmitate requires eight molecules of AcCoA, 7 ATP, and 14 NADH according to the formula:

$$8 \text{ Ac CoA} + 7 \text{ ATP} + 14 \text{ NADPH} + 6H^+ = CH_3(CH_2)14COO^-$$
(palmitate) $+ 14 \text{ NADP}^+ + 8 \text{ CoA} = 6 H_2O + 7 \text{ ADP} + 7Pi$

In common with the acetyl CoA carboxylase system, fatty acid synthase activity is also regulated, by substrate flux (the presence of phosphorylated sugars) via an allosteric effect, and by induction and repression of the enzyme.

Alterations in total enzyme protein are effected by the nutritional state of the individual; consequently, this is the main factor controlling the rate of lipogenesis. Rates of fatty acid synthesis are greatest when an individual follows a high-carbohydrate/low-fat diet, and are low during fasting/starvation or when eating high-fat diet. Situations in which there are high circulating concentrations of fatty acids lead to marked inhibition of lipogenesis.

The malate shuttle

Malate shuttle allows the recruitment of 2-carbon units from the mitochondrion to the cytoplasm

The primary molecule required for the synthesis of fatty acids is acetyl-CoA. However, acetyl-CoA is generated in the mitochondria and it cannot freely cross the inner mitochondrial membrane. As said above, fatty acid biosynthesis occurs in the cytosol. The malate shuttle is a mechanism allowing the transfer of 2-carbon units from the mitochondria to the cytosol: it involves the malate-citrate antiporter (Fig. 15.4). Pyruvate derived from glycolysis is decarboxylated to acetyl-CoA in the mitochondria; it subsequently reacts with oxaloacetate in the tricarboxylic acid (TCA) cycle (see Chapter 13) to form citrate. Translocation of a molecule of citrate to the cytosol via the antiporter is accompanied by transfer of a molecule of malate to the mitochondrion. In the cytosol, citrate, in the presence of ATP and CoA, undergoes cleavage to acetyl-CoA and oxaloacetate by citrate lyase. This makes acetyl-CoA available for carboxylation to malonyl-CoA and for the synthesis of fatty acids.The synthesis of fatty acids is also linked to glucose metabolism through the pentose phosphate pathway which is the main provider of NADPH required for lipogenesis. Some NADPH is also generated by the NADP+-linked decarboxylation of of malate to pyruvate by malic enzyme:

$$\text{Malate} + \text{NADP}^+ + \text{pyruvate} + CO_2 + \text{NADPH} + H^+$$

(See also box on p. 100.)

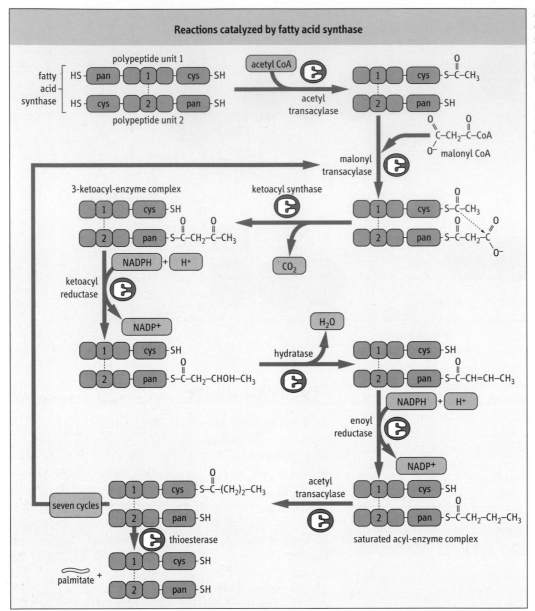

Fig. 15.3 **Reactions catalyzed by fatty acid synthase.** The cyclical part of the fatty acid biosynthesis is completed six times to release one 16-carbon molecule of palmitate. NADPH, reduced nicotinamide dinucleotide phosphate; pan, pantetheine.

FATTY ACID ELONGATION

The elongation of a fatty acid chain beyond 16-carbon length requires another set of enzymes

Palmitate released from fatty acid synthase becomes a substrate for the synthesis of longer-chain fatty acids, with the exception of certain essential fatty acids (see below). Chain elongation occurs by the addition of further 2-carbon fragments derived from malonyl-CoA (Fig. 15.5). This process occurs on the endoplasmic reticulum by the action of yet another multienzyme complex, fatty acid elongase. The reactions occurring during chain elongation are similar to those

involved in fatty acid synthesis, except that the fatty acid is attached to CoA, rather than to the ACP.

The substrates for the cytosolic fatty acid elongase include saturated fatty acids with a chain length from 10-carbon upwards, and also unsaturated fatty acids. Very-long-chain (22–24-carbon) fatty acids are produced in the brain, and elongation of stearoyl-CoA (C_{18}) in the brain increases rapidly during myelination, producing fatty acids required for the synthesis of sphingolipids.

Fatty acids can also be elongated in the mitochondria, where a still different system is used: it is NADH-dependent and uses acetyl-CoA as a source of 2-carbon fragments. It is simply the reverse of β-oxidation (see Chapter 13) and the substrates for chain elongation are short- and medium-chain fatty acids containing fewer than 16 carbon atoms.

LIPID ABNORMALITIES IN ALCOHOLISM

A 36-year-old woman attending a well-woman clinic was found to have serum concentrations of triglyceride 73.0 mmol/L (6388 mg/dL) and cholesterol 13 mmol/L (503 mg/dL). After some initial prevarication she admitted to drinking three bottles of vodka and six bottles of wine per week. When she discontinued alcohol, her triglyceride concentrations decreased to 2 mmol/L (175 mg/dL) and her cholesterol concentration decreased to 5.0 mmol/L (193 mg/dL). Three years later, the woman presented again with an enlarged liver and return of the lipid abnormality. Liver biopsy indicated alcoholic liver disease with steatosis or infiltration of the liver cells with fat.

Comment. In alcoholic individuals, the metabolism of alcohol produces increased amounts of reduced hepatic nicotinamide adenine dinucleotide (NADH⁺). Increased NADH + H₊/NAD₊ ratios inhibit the oxidation of fatty acids. Fatty acids reaching the liver either from dietary sources or by mobilization from adipose tissue are therefore re-esterified with glycerol to form triglycerides. In the initial stages of alcoholism, these are packaged with apolipoproteins and exported as very-low-density lipoproteins (VLDL). Increased concentrations of VLDL, and hence of serum triglycerides, are often present in the early stages of alcoholic liver disease. As the liver disease progresses, there is a failure to produce the apolipoproteins and export the fat as VLDL; accumulation of triglycerides in the liver cells thus ensues.

During fasting and starvation, elongation of fatty acids is greatly reduced.

DESATURATION OF FATTY ACIDS

Desaturation reactions require molecular oxygen

The body has a requirement for mono- and polyunsaturated fatty acids, in addition to saturated fatty acids. Some of these need to be supplied in the diet; these two unsaturated fatty acids, linoleic and linolenic, are known as the essential fatty acids (EFA; see below). The desaturation system requires molecular oxygen, NADH, and cytochrome b₅. The process of desaturation, like that of chain elongation, occurs on the endoplasmic reticulum, and results in the oxidation of both the fatty acid and NADH (Fig. 15.6).

In man, the desaturase system is unable to introduce double bonds between carbon atoms beyond carbon-9 and the ω (terminal methyl) carbon atom. Most desaturations occur between carbon atoms 9 and 10 (annotated as Δ^9 desaturations), e.g. those with palmitic acid producing palmitoleic acid (C-16:1 Δ^9), and those with stearic acid producing oleic acid (C-18:1, Δ^9).

CHANGES IN THE ENZYME EXPRESSION IN RESPONSE TO FOOD INTAKE ARE KEY REGULATORS OF THE STORAGE OF ENERGY SUBSTRATES

The fed state is associated with the induction of enzymes that increase fatty acid synthesis in the liver. A wide range of enzymes are induced, including those involved in glycolysis, e.g. glucokinase (the hepatic form of hexokinase) and pyruvate kinase, as well as enzymes linked to increased production of NADPH (Glc-6-P dehydrogenase, 6-phosphogluconate dehydrogenase, and malic enzyme). Further, there is an increased expression of citrate lyase, acetyl-CoA carboxylase, fatty acid synthase, and Δ_9 desaturase.

Further, in the fed state there is a concomitant repression of the key enzymes involved in gluconeogenesis. Phosphoenolpyruvate carboxykinase, glucose-6-phosphatase (Glc-6-P-ase), and some aminotransferases are reduced in amount, either by reduction in synthesis, or by increased degradation.

ESSENTIAL FATTY ACIDS

As said above the human desaturase is unable to introduce double bonds beyond C-9. On the other hand, two types of fatty acids – those having double bonds 3 carbons from the methyl end (ω-3 fatty acids) and 6 carbons from the methyl end (ω-6 fatty acids) – are required for the synthesis of eicosanoids (C-20 fatty acids), precursors of important molecules such as prostaglandins, thromboxanes and leukotrienes. Therefore, the ω-3 and ω-6 fatty acids (or their precursors) must be supplied with diet. As it happens, they are obtained from dietary vegetable oils which contain the ω-6 fatty acid, linoleic acid (C-18:2, $\Delta^{9,12}$) and the ω-3 fatty acid, linolenic acid (C-18:3, $\Delta^{9,12,15}$). Linoleic acid is converted in a series of elongation and desaturation reactions to arachidonic acid (C-20:4, $\Delta^{5,8,11,14}$), the precursor for the synthesis of other eicosanoids in man. Elongation and desaturation of linolenic acid produces eicosapentaenoic acid (EPA; C-20:5, $\Delta^{5,8,11,14,17}$), which is a precursor of yet another series of eicosanoids.

STORAGE AND TRANSPORT OF FATTY ACIDS: THE SYNTHESIS OF TRIACYLGLYCEROLS

Fatty acids derived from endogenous synthesis or from the diet, are stored and transported as triacylglycerols (triglycerides).

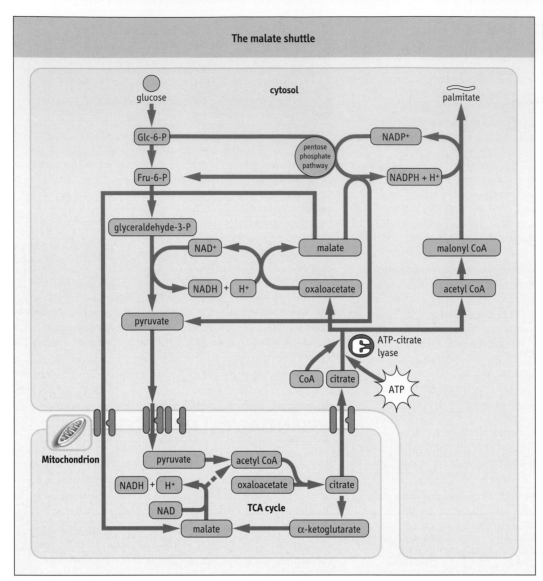

The malate shuttle

Fig. 15.4 **The malate shuttle.** The provision of acetyl-CoA and reducing equivalents for fatty acid biosynthesis and the malate shuttle. Fru-6-P, fructose-6-phosphate; Glc-6-P, glucose-6-phosphate; NADH, reduced nicotinamide dinucleotide. (See also 'Electron shuttles' box on p. 100.)

In both the liver and the adipose tissue, triacylglycerols (TAGs) are produced by a pathway involving glycerol-3-phosphate (glycerol-3-P) and phosphatidic acid as intermediates (Fig. 15.7). However, glycerol-3-P is of different origin in the two tissues: in the liver, glycerol itself provides the source, via the action of glycerol kinase, but in the adipose tissue (which lacks this enzyme), glucose is the source of glycerol-3-P, via glycolysis and its immediate precursor dihydroxy-acetone phosphate (DHAP) (Fig. 15.7). Thus, the storage of fatty acids in the adipose tissue can take place only when glycolysis is activated in the fed state.

The TAG produced in smooth endoplasmic reticulum of the liver is then, together with cholesterol and phospholipids, associated with apolipoprotein B$_{100}$, which is also synthesized on the endoplasmic reticulum, to form very-low-density lipoprotein (VLDL). The VLDL is then processed in the Golgi apparatus and released into the bloodstream, transporting triacylglycerols to other tissues (see Chapter 17). In the bloodstream, VLDL is acted upon by lipoprotein lipase (LPL), an enzyme attached to the basement membrane glycoproteins of the capillary endothelial cells. LPL hydrolyses TAG, releasing fatty acids to tissues. LPL synthesis is induced by insulin (Fig. 15.8 and Chapter 17).

REGULATION OF TOTAL BODY FAT STORES

Adipose tissue is an active endocrine organ

It has been long understood that increased energy intake without appropriate increase in energy expenditure is

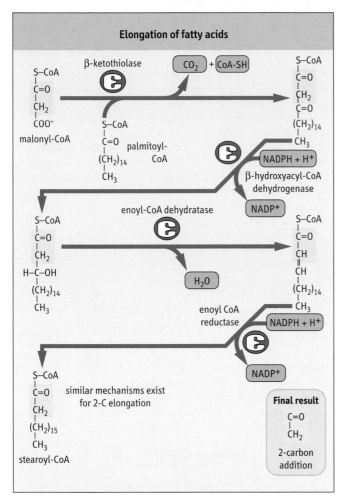

Fig. 15.5 **Elongation of fatty acids.** Fatty acid elongation occurs on the endoplasmic reticulum and is carried out by another enzyme complex, fatty acid elongase.

associated with increased adiposity, in terms both of the numbers of adipocytes and of their fat content – that is, obesity. It is now clear that the adipose tissue is hormonally active. Hormone-like substances such as leptin, adiponectin, and resistin (collectively termed adipokines), growth factors such as vascular endothelial growth factor (VEGF), and pro-inflammatory cytokines (tumor necrosis factor alpha (TNF-α) and interleukin 6 (IL-6)) are all generated by the adipocytes. The main molecules which carry information related to the size of the fat stores (adiposity signals) are leptin, generated in the adipose tissue, and insulin, synthesized in the pancreas. The amount of leptin present in blood is proportional to the body fat content. Leptin regulates food intake and energy expenditure, and also has neuroendocrine function. It decreases appetite and increases thermogenesis. Animals deficient in leptin are hyperphagic and obese. Inefficient leptin action decreases fat oxidation, increases tissue TAG content and increases insulin resistance (Chapter 20). On the other hand, in normal animals, leptin treatment causes hypophagia, leads to increased oxidation of the fatty acid, depletion of tissue TAG, and to an increase in insulin sensitivity. Leptin crosses the blood–brain barrier.

Another adipokine, adiponectin, is specific to the adipose tissue. It has an insulin-sensitizing effect: it decreases glucose and non-esterified fatty acid concentrations in plasma without affecting insulin concentration. (See also Chapter 21.)

Insulin also plays a role in regulating food intake: it decreases appetite; deletion of insulin receptor in experimental animals leads to hyperphagia. Interestingly, both insulin and leptin signalling pathway involves phosphatidyl inositol-3-kinase (PI-3 kinase). This is an example of a pleiotropic (multifunctional) role of key signal transduction molecules. Leptin also signals through the JAK-STAT system (see Chapter 38).

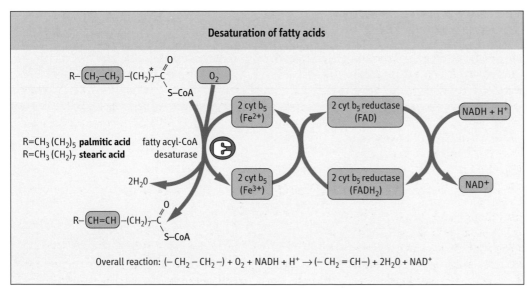

Fig. 15.6 **Desaturation of fatty acids.** Human desaturases cannot introduce a double bond between carbon 9 and the methyl (ω) end of the fatty acid. This $(CH_2)_7$ represents the limit at which a double bond can be introduced. cyt b_5, cytochrome b_5; FAD, flavin adenine dinucleotide; FADH$_2$, reduced flavin adenine dinucleotide; Fe^{3+}, ferric ion.

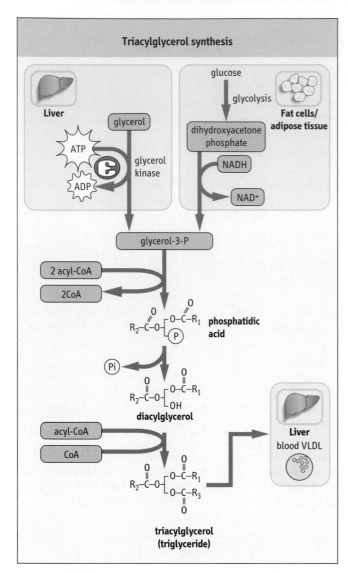

Fig. 15.7 **Triacylglycerol synthesis.** Triacylglycerols (TAGs), also called triglycerides, are synthesized in adipose tissue and the liver. The source of glycerol-3-P is different in the two tissues, because there is no glycerol kinase in adipose tissue.

OBESITY

A 48-year-old ex-Army infantryman (height 1.91 m) presented with the problem of increasing weight over the previous 8 years since leaving the Army. At the time of his retirement from active service, he had weighed 95 kg (209 lb) but at presentation weighed 193 kg (424.6 lb). His current occupation was that of truck driver. He denied any change in food intake since leaving the Army, but admitted to taking little or no exercise. Detailed enquiry indicated that his daily dietary intake provided between 12 600 and 16 800 kJ (3000 and 4000 kcal), with a fat intake approaching 40%. The patient was initially placed on a healthy eating plan, with fat intake reduced to 35% of total calories. He was advised to exercise and proceeded to swim three or four times per week. His weight immediately began to decrease, rapidly at first, and then at 3–4 kg (6.6–8.8 lb) each month until it stabilized at 145–150 kg (319–330 lb). He was then placed on a high-protein/low-carbohydrate/low-fat diet, which induced a return of weight loss that continued for a further year, resulting in a final weight of 93 kg (204.6 lb).

Comment. Obesity is increasingly prevalent in many parts of the world. Clinical obesity is now clearly defined in terms of height and weight through the body mass index (BMI), which is calculated as the weight in kilograms divided by the (height in meters)^2 (see Chapter 12 for details):

$$BMI\ (kg/m^2) = \rightarrow \frac{weight\ (kg)}{(height\ [m])^2}$$

BMI 25–30 kg/m^2 is classified as overweight or grade I obesity, BMI >30 kg/m^2 is clinical or grade II obesity, and BMI >40 kg/m^2 is classified as morbid or grade III obesity. Our patient had a BMI of 53 at presentation falling to 26 after prolonged diet. If energy input exceeds output over time then weight will increase. Obesity predisposes to several diseases. The most important is type 2 diabetes mellitus: 80% of this type of diabetes is associated with the obese state. Other associated illnesses include coronary heart disease, hypertension, stroke, arthritis, and gall bladder disease. (See also Chapter 21.)

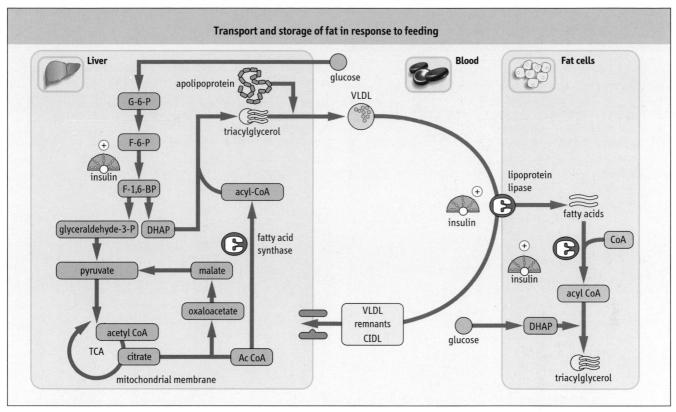

Fig. 15.8 **Transport and storage of fat in response to feeding.** The relationship between the biosynthesis of fatty acids in the liver, their export as VLDL, and increased storage of fat as triacylglycerols (TAGs). Insulin is an important regulator of this pathway. In the liver, it stimulates glycolysis, thereby increasing pyruvate production. It activates the pyruvate dehydrogenase complex (by causing its dephosphorylation), and thus promotes synthesis of acetyl-CoA. This stimulates the TCA cycle and increases the concentration of citrate. Citrate stimulates acetyl-CoA carboxylase, increasing the rate of fatty acid biosynthesis. F-1,6-BP, fructose-1,6 biphosphate; IDL, intermediate-density lipoprotein. (See also Chapter 17 for details of lipoprotein metabolism.)

Summary

- Fatty acid synthesis and storage are essential components of body energy homeostasis.
- Lipogenesis takes place in the cytosol. Its committed step is the reaction catalyzed by acetyl CoA carboxylase.
- The elongation of the fatty acid chain (up to the length of 16 carbon atoms) is carried out by the dimeric fatty acid synthase, which possesses several enzyme activities. Both are subject to a complex regulation.

- The malate shuttle facilitates the transfer of two-carbon units form the mitochondria to cytoplasm for use in lipogenesis.
- The reducing power in the form of NADPH is supplied by the pentose phosphate pathway and also by the malate shuttle.
- The essential unsaturated fatty acids are linoleic and linolenic acid. Linoleic acid is converted to the arachidonic acid, which in turn serves as the precursor of prostaglandins.
- Adiposity signals are provided by adipokines, particularly leptin. Insulin is also important in the regulation of food intake.

ACTIVE LEARNING

1. Describe how a growing fatty acid chain is transferred between the subunits of fatty acid synthase.
2. How are eicosanoids synthesized?
3. Explain why the rate of lipolysis in the fed state is low.
4. What is the role of adipokines?
5. Describe the committed step of lipogenesis and its regulation.
6. What are the sources of acetyl CoA for fatty acid synthesis?
7. Compare and contrast lipogenesis and lipolysis.

Further reading

Kopelman PG. Obesity as a medical problem. Nature 2000;**404**: 635–43.
Semenkovich CF. Regulation of fatty acid synthase (FAS). *Progress in Lipid Research* 1997:**36**:43–53.
Angulo P. Nonalcoholic fatty liver disease. *N Engl J Med* 2002;**346**:1221–31.
Cock T-A, Auverx J. Leptin: cutting the fat off the bone. *Lancet* 2003;**362**:1572–74.

16. Biosynthesis of Cholesterol and Steroids

M H Dominiczak and G Beastall

LEARNING OBJECTIVES

After reading this chapter you should be able to:

■ List the main steps involved in the synthesis of cholesterol molecule.

■ Discuss the regulation of intracellular cholesterol concentration.

■ Describe the sterol signaling involved in regulation of cholesterol synthesis.

■ Explain the mechanisms governing cholesterol metabolism and excretion.

■ Describe bile acids and their enterohepatic circulation.

■ Outline the main pathways of synthesis of steroid hormones.

INTRODUCTION

Cholesterol is one molecule with many functions. It is a lipid that is an essential component of mammalian cell membranes. It is also the most abundant sterol. Cholesterol is the precursor of three important classes of biologically active compounds: the bile acids, the steroid hormones, and vitamin D. Cholesterol metabolism is important in the etiology of cardiovascular disease, and it is a major component of gall stones.

The typical daily Western diet contains approximately 500 mg (1.2 mmol) of cholesterol daily, mainly in meat, eggs, and dairy products (see Chapter 21). Under normal circumstances, 30–60% of this is absorbed from the gut.

After absorption, cholesterol is transported to the liver and to peripheral tissues in the form of chylomicrons. The liver repackages it into another lipoprotein, VLDL (see Chapter 17 and Table 17.3). VLDL subsequently transforms into VLDL remnants (or IDL) and then into LDL. VLDL remnants and LDL can deliver cholesterol to tissues by binding to the apoB/E receptor (LDL receptor).

The sterol ring of cholesterol cannot be degraded in the human body. Therefore it is excreted either in the free form as the biliary cholesterol, or in the form of bile acids. Most of the bile acids are however returned to the liver after reabsorption in the terminal ileum. This is known as the enterohepatic circulation.

Human beings synthesize 1g cholesterol each day, mainly in the liver. The rate of its endogenous synthesis is determined by dietary intake. For this reason both dietary intake and biosynthesis are important in determining its plasma concentration.

CHOLESTEROL STRUCTURE

The structure of cholesterol is shown in Figure 16.1. It has a molecular weight of 386 Da and contains 27 carbon atoms, of which 17 are incorporated into four fused rings (the perhydrocyclopentano-phenanthrene nucleus), two are in angular methyl groups attached at the junctions of rings AB and CD and eight are in the peripheral side chain. Cholesterol is almost entirely composed of carbon and hydrogen atoms; there is a solitary hydroxyl group attached to carbon atom 3. It is also almost completely saturated, having just one double bond between carbon atoms 5 and 6. In three-dimensional terms the ring structure of cholesterol is approximately planar.

THE FREE AND ESTERIFIED CHOLESTEROL

Its structure gives cholesterol a low solubility in water. Only about 30% of circulating cholesterol occurs in the free form, the majority is esterified through the hydroxyl group to a wide range of long-chain fatty acids including oleic and linoleic acids. Cholesterol esters are even less soluble in water than free cholesterol and so it is perhaps surprising to discover cholesterol circulating in plasma in concentrations of about 5 mmol/L (200 mg/dL). The apparent paradox is explained by the presence of a range of lipoproteins which incorporate and thereby solubilize the cholesterol molecule (see Chapter 17). Within these lipoproteins, the hydrophobic cholesterol esters are located in the core of the molecule, with free cholesterol in the outside layer.

The dietary cholesterol brought to the liver is mostly in the form of free cholesterol. On the other hand, the cholesterol present in VLDL and LDL is mostly in the form of cholesteryl esters. Esters are also the tissue storage form of cholesterol

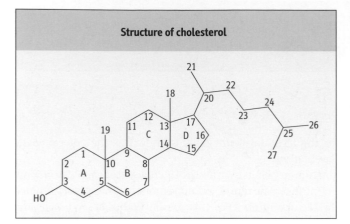

Fig. 16.1 **Structure of cholesterol.** A–D is the conventional notation used to describe the four rings. Numbers 1–27 describe the carbon atoms.

(they are stored in lipid droplets). In the plasma, cholesterol is esterified by the enzyme cholesterol-lecithin acyltransferase (Chapter 17) and in the cells by the acyl-CoA: cholesterol acyltransferase (ACAT, now renamed SOAT) by reacting with fatty acyl-CoA. There are two isoforms of the ACAT present in the endoplasmic reticulum. Sixty to eighty percent of cholesteryl esters present in plasma are taken up by the liver.

CHOLESTEROL BIOSYNTHESIS

Acetyl-coenzyme A is the starting point for the biosynthesis of cholesterol and HMG-CoA reductase is the rate-limiting enzyme in the pathway

Virtually all human cells have the capacity to make cholesterol. In quantitative terms, however, the liver is the major site of cholesterol biosynthesis with the intestine, adrenal cortex and gonads making lesser contributions. An examination of the structure of cholesterol makes it clear that generation of the many carbon–carbon and carbon–hydrogen bonds it contains requires a source of carbon atoms, a source of reducing power and the expenditure of significant amounts of energy. Acetyl-coenzyme A (acetyl-CoA) provides a high-energy starting point. Acetyl-CoA may be derived from several sources, including the β-oxidation of long-chain fatty acids, the dehydrogenation of pyruvate and the oxidation of ketogenic amino acids such as leucine and isoleucine. The reducing power is provided by reduced nicotinamide dinucleotide phosphate (NADPH), which is generated by the enzymes of the pentose phosphate pathway (see Chapter 11).

Additional energy is provided by the breakdown of adenosine triphosphate (ATP). Overall the production of 1 mole of cholesterol requires 18 moles of acetyl-CoA, 36 moles of ATP and 16 moles of NADPH. All the biosynthetic reactions occur

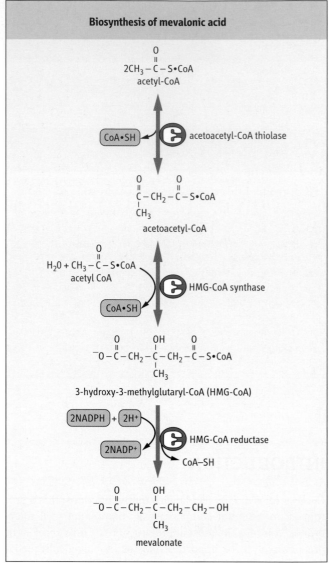

Fig. 16.2 **Biosynthesis of mevalonic acid.** Mevalonic acid contains six carbon atoms, which are derived from three molecules of acetyl CoA.

within the cytoplasm, although some of the enzymes required are bound to membranes of the endoplasmic reticulum.

Mevalonic acid is the first unique compound in the pathway

Three molecules of acetyl-CoA are converted into the six-carbon atom mevalonic acid (Fig. 16.2). The first two steps are condensation reactions leading to the formation of the 3-hydroxy-3-methylglutaryl-CoA (HMG-CoA). These reactions, catalyzed by acetoacetyl-CoA thiolase and HMG-CoA synthase, are common to the formation of ketone bodies, although the latter process occurs within mitochondria rather than the cytosol. These reactions are also favored

HMG-CoA REDUCTASE IS AN EXAMPLE OF A RATE-LIMITING ENZYME IN A PATHWAY

The metabolic regulation of any pathway is usually achieved by modulation of the activity of one key enzyme – known as the rate-limiting enzyme. Such enzyme often catalyzes the committed step – the first one that may be identified as being unique to that pathway. It is of interest that the regulation of cholesterol biosynthesis occurs at a relatively early stage in the process, with the enzyme that uses a six-carbon molecule as its substrate. HMG-CoA reductase is the rate-limiting enzyme that catalyzes the committed step that results in the production of mevalonic acid. Hepatic HMG-CoA reductase synthesis is stimulated by fasting and inhibited by dietary cholesterol intake. HMG-CoA reductase activity is controlled by covalent modification induced by cholesterol feedback and by several hormones.

HMG-CoA REDUCTASE INHIBITORS

Despite strict dietary control a 50-year-old man, from a family with a history of cardiovascular disease, had a serum cholesterol result of 8.0 mmol/L (desirable levels are <5.0 mmol/L, Chapter 17). He started to take one of the statin drugs (statins are inhibitors of HMG-CoA reductase) and 3 months later his cholesterol was 5.5 mmol/L.

Comment. Partial inhibition of the rate-limiting enzyme of cholesterol biosynthesis may be expected to bring about a lowering of plasma cholesterol. This has proved to be the case. A family of competitive inhibitors of HMG-CoA reductase, known as 'statins', have been developed following the original discovery that mevastatin, isolated from *Penicillium citrinum*, had enzyme-inhibiting properties. These drugs bring 20–60% reduction in low density lipoprotein (LDL) cholesterol. The inhibition of HMG-CoA reductase activity leads to the lowering of intracellular cholesterol concentration, to a consequent upregulation of the apo B/E receptor (Chapter 17) and, through that route, to the lowering of the plasma cholesterol concentration.

energetically since they involve cleavage of a thioester bond and liberation of free coenzyme-A. However, the key reaction in the early stages of cholesterol biosynthesis is that catalyzed by the microsomal enzyme HMG-CoA reductase, which leads to the irreversible formation of mevalonic acid. HMG-CoA reductase is a microsomal enzyme with molecular weight of 97.3 kDa; it is active in a non-phosphorylated state and it is inhibited by phosphorylation by a kinase.

THE TRANSMETHYLGLUTACONATE SHUNT – A SECONDARY POINT OF CONTROL

It was once believed that the production of mevalonic acid led to the inevitable formation of farnesyl pyrophosphate. However, it is now known that dimethylallyl pyrophosphate, one of the isoprene units formed from mevalonate (see Fig 16.3), can be dephosphorylated and broken down back into acetoacetate and acetyl-CoA, which may then be diverted into other pathways, such as fatty acid biosynthesis. This mechanism is known as the transmethylglutaconate shunt. Thus, high-energy compounds once destined to be converted into cholesterol may be redeployed to meet a higher priority need.

Farnesyl pyrophosphate is made up of three isoprene units

Figure 16.3 shows how three molecules of mevalonic acid are each decarboxylated into five-carbon atom isoprene units, which are condensed sequentially to produce the 15-carbon atom molecule farnesyl pyrophosphate. The first two reactions require kinase enzymes and ATP to generate the pyrophosphate moiety. Decarboxylation results in the isomeric isoprene units, isopentenyl pyrophosphate and dimethylallyl pyrophosphate, which condense together to form geranyl pyrophosphate. A further condensation with isopentenyl pyrophosphate produces farnesyl pyrophosphate. As well as being an intermediate in cholesterol biosynthesis, farnesyl pyrophosphate is the branching point for the synthesis of dolichol and ubiquinone.

Squalene is a linear molecule capable of folding into a ring formation

Squalene synthase is a complex enzyme present in the endoplasmic reticulum that facilitates the condensation at the pyrophosphate end of two molecules of farnesyl pyrophosphate. Several intermediates are involved and the resulting product is squalene, a 30-carbon atom hydrocarbon containing six double bonds, which enable it to fold into a ring similar to the steroid nucleus (Fig. 16.4).

Squalene cyclizes to lanosterol

Before ring closure, squalene is converted to squalene 2,3-oxide by a mixed-function oxidase in the endoplasmic reticulum. Thereafter, cyclization occurs under the action of the enzyme oxidosqualene: lanosterol cyclase (Fig. 16.5). It is interesting to note that in plants there is a different product of squalene cyclization, known as cycloartenol, which is further metabolized to a range of phytosterols, including β-sitosterol, rather than to cholesterol.

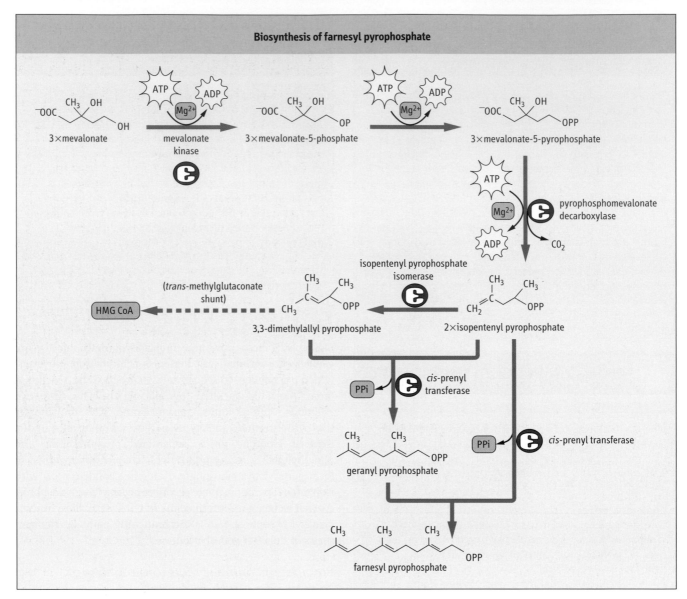

Fig. 16.3 **Biosynthesis of farnesyl pyrophosphate.** Farnesyl pyrophosphate is made up of three isoprene units. ADP, adenosine diphosphate; Mg^{2+}, magnesium; PPi, pyrophosphate. For trans-methylgluconate shunt, see box on p. 211.

The final stages of cholesterol biosynthesis occur on a carrier protein

Squalene, lanosterol and all the further intermediates are hydrophobic molecules. In order for the final steps of the pathway to occur in an aqueous medium, the intermediates react while bound to a squalene and sterol-binding protein. The conversion from the 30-carbon lanosterol into the 27-carbon cholesterol involves three decarboxylation reactions, an isomerization and a reduction (see Fig. 16.5). NADPH is consumed in four of these reactions.

Regulation of cholesterol biosynthesis

Many factors are involved in the regulation of the intracellular concentration of cholesterol (Table 16.1). Under normal circumstances there is an inverse relationship between dietary cholesterol intake and cholesterol biosynthesis. This ensures a relatively constant daily supply of cholesterol but it explains why dietary restriction is only likely to achieve a 15% reduction in circulating cholesterol concentrations.

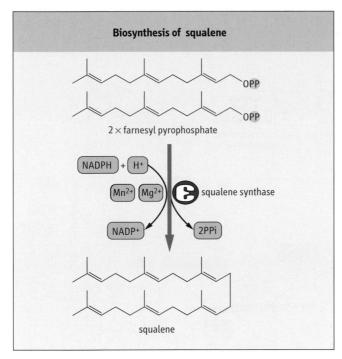

Biosynthesis of squalene

2 × farnesyl pyrophosphate

squalene synthase

squalene

Fig. 16.4 **Biosynthesis of squalene.** The six double bonds enable the structure to fold into a ring similar to the steroid nucleus.

Regulation of intracellular cholesterol

Factors increasing intracellular free cholesterol concentration

de novo biosynthesis
hydrolysis of intracellular cholesterol esters by the enzyme cholesterol ester hydrolase
dietary intake of cholesterol and uptake from chylomicrons
receptor-mediated uptake of cholesterol-containing lipoproteins (LDL)

Factors decreasing intracellular free cholesterol concentration

inhibition of cholesterol biosynthesis
downregulation of the LDL receptor
intracellular esterification of cholesterol by acyl-coenzyme A:cholesterol acyl transferase
release of cholesterol to high-density lipoproteins (HDL)
conversion of cholesterol to bile acids or steroid hormones

Factors influencing the activity of HMG-CoA reductase

intracellular concentration of HMG-CoA
intracellular concentration of cholesterol
hormones: insulin, tri-iodothyronine (+); glucagon, cortisol (–)

Table 16.1 **Regulation of intracellular cholesterol.** (see also Fig. 17.1)

The chylomicron remnants carrying 'fresh' dietary cholesterol might be present in plasma together with the VLDL and LDL containing the 'processed' cholesterol esters. Chylomicron remnants are taken up by the LDL-receptor related protein (LRP) while VLDL remnants and LDL particles bind to

THE MEASUREMENT OF STEROID BY GAS CHROMATOGRAPHY – MASS SPECTROMETRY (GCMS)

In the specialized clinical endocrinology laboratory the measurement of urinary steroid metabolites aids the diagnosis of a number of inherited disorders of the synthesis and metabolism of adrenal steroids, and steroid-producing tumours. It is particularly valuable in identifying the site of the defect in congenital adrenal hyperplasia. These investigations are most often performed in neonates with ambiguous genitalia, children with precocious puberty and in patients with suspected Cushing's syndrome (see Chapter 11). The abnormalities in steroid synthesis are revealed by an alteration in the pattern of urinary steroid metabolites.

The procedure used is gas chromatography–mass spectrometry (GCMS); it is very similar to methods adopted for the identification of anabolic steroids in sport. Current bench-top GCM Spectrometers are compact and reasonably easy to use. Steroid metabolites are excreted in urine mostly as water-soluble sulfate or glucuronic acid conjugates. The first step in the analysis involves enzymatic release of the steroids from these conjugates; this is followed by chemical derivatization to increase their stability and improve separation, which is carried out by gas chromatography on capillary columns at high temperatures. Final detection is by mass fragmentation: for each steroid metabolite a unique ion fragmentation 'fingerprint' is achieved, which allows positive identification and quantitation.

the membrane apoB/E receptor (apoE-containing VLDL remnants bind to the receptor with much higher affinity than apoB-containing LDL; see Chapter 17). The lipoprotein-receptor complex is subsequently internalized in the form of clathrin-coated vesicles.

In the cytoplasm the vesicles which carry internalized lipoprotein-receptor complexes are acted upon by lysosomal enzymes, which separate the LDL from its receptor, and hydrolyze cholesterol esters.

The intracellular free cholesterol can be derived from several different sources:

- it can be newly synthesized within the cell;
- it may be derived from the chylomicron remnants that carry dietary cholesterol;
- it may come from VLDL–LDL pathways.

Intracellular cholesterol concentration is a key factor regulating cellular cholesterol synthesis. The rise in the intracellular free cholesterol concentration results in the following (see Fig. 16.6):

- it causes a reduction both in the activity and expression of HMG-CoA reductase, thus limiting further cholesterol synthesis;

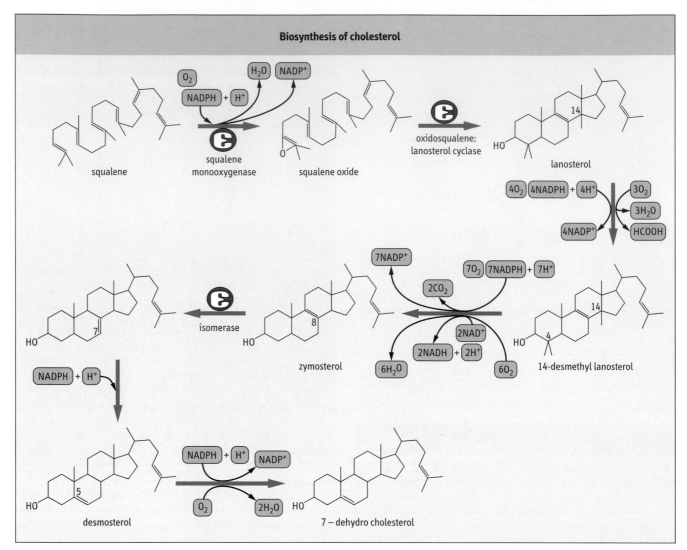

Fig. 16.5 **Biosynthesis of cholesterol**. These reactions occur while bound to a squalene- and sterol-binding protein. FAD, flavin adenine dinucleotide; NADH, reduced nicotinamide adenine dinucleotide.

- it downregulates LDL receptors to limit further entry of cholesterol;
- it increases cholesterol and phospholipid efflux to apoproteins;
- it increases the rate of conversion of cholesterol to bile acids.

Regulation of intracellular cholesterol concentration involves HMG-CoA reductase, LDL receptor and 7α-hydroxylase

LDL receptor (a cell surface glycoprotein containing 839 amino acids) is synthesized in the endoplasmic reticulum from where it moves to the Golgi apparatus and from there transfers to the plasma membrane. It is normally present on the membrane in sites known as coated pits which are lined with a protein, clathrin. The receptor spends some time on the cell surface (its half-time in human beings is 1.5 days and in mice only 1.5 h) and then it recycles back to cytoplasm (irrespectively of whether it bound the LDL). After internalization, the receptor protein dissociates from the LDL particle. The LDL apoprotein is hydrolyzed to its component amino acids. Cholesteryl esters are also hydrolyzed releasing cholesterol to the cytoplasm.

The free cholesterol concentration is sensed by the cytoplasmic regulatory elements

The metabolite of cholesterol which is the signaling species is probably oxysterol. Oxysterol is a ligand of liver X receptors (also called oxysterol receptors) in the cytoplasm, which are sterol-responsive transcription factors that govern the expression of several proteins relevant to the maintenance of normal cholesterol concentration. To act, the X receptors bind to other molecules, retinoid X receptors (RXRs), forming heterodimers. It is probably the X receptors which in turn upregulate the sterol regulatory element-binding proteins (SREBPs). The SREBPs are synthesized as precursors integral to the ER membrane. These precursors are cleaved by a protease to release the transcription factor which translocates to the nucleus and initiates gene transcription. The intermediary there might be another protein, the SREBP cleavage-activating protein (SCAP). SCAP, which possesses sterol-sensing domain, 'brings' SREBP to its active protease, and this step is blocked by sterols. Thus, when the intracellular cholesterol concentration is high, the transcription of genes associated with cholesterol synthesis is repressed. On the other hand, when sterols are absent, SCAP/SREBP complex reaches the protease and the transcription is derepressed.

SREBPs acts on promoter regions of HMG-CoA reductase gene, LDL receptor gene and HMG-CoA synthase gene. Incidentally, one of the SREBPs also affects the enzymes in the fatty acid biosynthesis pathway such as the fatty acid synthetase.

There is a circadian rhythm of cholesterol biosynthesis

Hepatic synthesis of cholesterol is at a peak at about 6 hours after dark and at a minimum some 6 hours after exposure to light. This rhythm is the result of corresponding changes in HMG-CoA reductase activity. Exploiting this, the drugs inhibiting cholesterol synthesis (statins) are usually taken at night to ensure maximal effect. The mechanism of control of HMG-CoA reductase in these circumstances is poorly understood, although dietary pattern plays a part.

Hormones also regulate HMG-CoA reductase activity

Several hormones affect the activity of HMG-CoA reductase and so influence cholesterol biosynthesis. Insulin and tri-iodothyronine increase HMG-CoA reductase activity, while glucagon and cortisol have the opposite effect.

HDL DELIVERS CHOLESTEROL TO THE LIVER AND STEROIDOGENIC TISSUES BY THE SCAVENGER RECEPTOR PATHWAY

The scavenger receptor class B type I (SR-BI) plays an important role in taking the cholesteryl esters back from HDL cholesterol into cells. SR-BI is present in the liver and in steroidogenic tissues such as adrenals. SR-BI acts as a docking site for apo A-I-containing HDL particles. It binds HDL and stimulates the uptake of cholesteryl esters. In contrast to the LDL receptor, the SR-BI-HDL complex is not internalized after the binding. Cholesterol is delivered directly to the membrane. It was suggested that SR-BI acts as a hydrophobic channel transporting cholesterol esters.

Overexpression of SR-BI in mice leads to the increase in the transport of the free cholesterol to bile. The human SR-BI gene expression is regulated by several transcription factors: steroidogenic factor 1 (SF-1), CCAAT/enhancer binding proteins (C/EBP) and SREBP mentioned above.

In the steroidogenic tissues SR-BI is regulated by trophic hormones (for instance, ACTH regulates SR-BI expression in human adrenals), probably through the cAMP/protein kinase A signaling pathway which activates C/EBP and SF-1.

IN THE EXTRACELLULAR SPACE, THE HIGH-DENSITY LIPOPROTEIN (HDL) IS THE MAIN ACCEPTOR OF CHOLESTEROL RELEASED FROM CELLS

The insight into cholesterol efflux from cells came from studies on patients with Tangier disease, which is characterized by the tissue accumulation of cholesterol esters. The cholesterol and phospholipid transport out of cells is controlled by ABC1, a ATP-binding plasma membrane protein which facilitates transport of unesterified cholesterol from cells to the extracellular acceptor, a nascent HDL particle (in effect a lipid-free apolipoprotein A-I). Apparently, first some phospholipids are transferred to lipidate the apolipoprotein, and they determine the subsequent cholesterol efflux. As a result, the nascent HDL transforms into a mature spherical particle (Chapter 8). The cholesterol is subsequently esterified while in the HDL particle by the lecithin-cholesterol acyltransferase enzyme.

BIOSYNTHETIC CHOLESTEROL DEFECT – (INCIDENCE 1 IN 20–40 000)

Smith–Lemli-Opitz syndrome presents at birth with microencephaly, short nasal root, small chin, high arched palate, often with mid-line cleft. There are often accompanying central nervous system (CNS) defects, polydactyly, and in males ambiguous genitalia. Despite the pathway of cholesterol synthesis and metabolism being well understood, a defect in 7-dehydrocholesterol reductase was only identified in 1993.

While some of these children die in infancy, the rest, if assisted in feeding, survive with severe mental retardation (IQ 20–40). Most develop growth retardation. The pathophysiology involves incomplete processing embryonic signaling proteins (HH proteins) resulting in variable defects in different tissues. Treatment involves giving additional cholesterol to the child. This improves growth but it appears to have no CNS benefits, due to the embryonic microencephaly and other CNS defects.

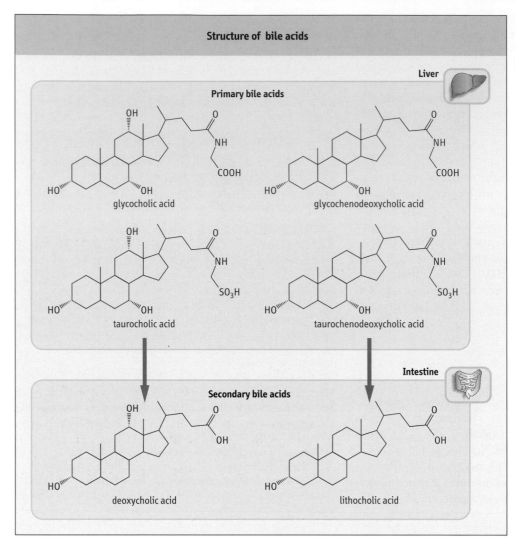

Structure of bile acids

Liver

Primary bile acids

glycocholic acid

glycochenodeoxycholic acid

taurocholic acid

taurochenodeoxycholic acid

Intestine

Secondary bile acids

deoxycholic acid

lithocholic acid

Fig. 16.6 **Structure of bile acids.** Primary bile acids are synthesized in the liver and secondary bile acids in the intestine.

Cholesterol is an essential component of cell membranes

Mammalian cell membranes are composed of lipid and protein with small amounts of complex carbohydrates. The basic structural characteristics of membranes are described in Chapter 7. The protein components of membranes are embedded in and may span a hydrophobic phospholipid bilayer. It is now recognized that membranes are fluid structures in which both the lipid and protein molecules move and undergo conformational change to allow specific transport of molecules, while maintaining a generally impermeable barrier between the intra- and extracellular aqueous phases. The more fluid the phospholipid bilayer becomes, the more permeable is the membrane.

Cholesterol influences membrane fluidity

It is mostly free cholesterol which is the component of biological membranes. At body temperature, the long hydrocarbon chains of the lipid bilayer are capable of considerable motion. Cholesterol is located between these hydrocarbon chains to form a loose crosslink and so reduce fluidity. This relative rigidity is increased still further if cholesterol is adjacent to saturated fatty acids. Cholesterol forms clustered regions within the lipid bilayer. In areas of a cholesterol cluster, there may be 1 mole of cholesterol per mole of phospholipid, while in adjacent areas there may be no cholesterol. Thus, the membrane contains cholesterol-rich impermeable patches and more permeable cholesterol-free areas.

Cholesterol content varies widely in different biological membranes

Cholesterol is found in the highest concentrations in plasma membranes (up to 25% of the lipid content), while it is virtually absent from inner mitochondrial membranes. The cholesterol is held in the lipid bilayer by physical interactions between the planar steroid nucleus and the fatty acid chains.

The absence of covalent bonding means that cholesterol may transfer in and out of the membrane.

BILE ACIDS

The liver secretes cholesterol as free cholesterol or as bile acids

Quantitatively the bile acids are the most important metabolic products of cholesterol. In man there are four main bile acids (Fig. 16.6). They all have 24 carbon atoms with the terminal three carbon atoms of the cholesterol side chain removed during synthesis. They also have a saturated steroid nucleus and differ only in the number and position of the additional hydroxyl groups. It is worthy of note that all these hydroxyl groups have the α-configuration (below the plane of the nucleus) and this means that isomerization of the 3β-hydroxyl group of cholesterol must occur.

Biosynthesis of bile acids occurs within the liver parenchymal cells

Biosynthesis occurs within the liver parenchymal cells to produce cholic and chenodeoxycholic acids. The rate-limiting step in the biosynthesis is the microsomal 7α-hydroxylase

GALL STONES

A 45-year-old woman complained of right upper quadrant abdominal pain and vomiting after eating fatty food. The only biochemical abnormality was a modestly raised alkaline phosphatase at 400 U/L (<280 U/L). An abdominal ultrasound showed that the gallbladder contained gall stones.

Comment. Gall stones occur in up to 20% of the population of Western countries. The condition results from formation of cholesterol-rich stones within the gall bladder. Cholesterol is present in high concentrations in bile, being solubilized in micelles that also contain phospholipids and bile acids. When the liver secretes bile with a cholesterol to phospholipid ratio greater than 1:1 it is difficult to solubilize all the cholesterol in micelles, thus there is a tendency for the excess to crystallize around any insoluble nuclei. This is compounded by further concentration of the bile in the gall bladder by reabsorption of water and electrolytes. The condition may be managed conservatively by reducing the dietary cholesterol and by increasing the availability of bile acids that will assist with cholesterol solubilization in the bile and excretion via the gut. Alternative treatment includes disintegration of stones by shock waves (lithotripsy) and surgery. The elevated alkaline phosphatase is a marker of partial blockage of the bile duct or cholestasis.

enzyme (CYP7A1), which introduces a hydroxyl group at 7α position of cholesterol ring. It is a microsomal monooxygenase which consists of cytochrome P-450 and requires NADPH and molecular oxygen.

Prior to secretion these primary bile acids are conjugated through the carboxyl group forming amide linkages with either glycine or taurine (see Fig. 16.6). In man there is a 3:1 ratio in favor of glycine conjugates. The secreted products are thus principally glycocholic, glycochenodeoxycholic, taurocholic and taurochenodeoxycholic acids. At physiologic pH, the bile acids are mainly ionized and so they occur as sodium or potassium salts. The terms 'bile acids' and 'bile salts' tend to be used interchangeably. As their name suggests, these compounds are secreted from the liver via the bile canaliculi and larger bile ducts, either directly into the duodenum or for storage in the gall bladder. They are an important component of bile, together with water, phospholipids, cholesterol, salts and excretory products such as bilirubin. Cholesterol is pumped into bile by ABCG5 and ABCG8 proteins, the expression of which is regulated by the liver X receptor (their mutations lead to sitosterolaemia).

Secondary bile acids are formed in the intestine

Deoxycholic and lithocholic acids (see Fig. 16.6) are secondary bile acids formed within the intestine through the action of bacterial enzymes on the primary bile acids. Only a proportion of primary bile acids are converted into secondary bile acids, a process which requires hydrolysis of the amide link to glycine or taurine prior to removal of the 7α-hydroxyl group.

Bile acids assist the digestion of dietary fat

The secretion of bile from the liver and the emptying of the bile duct are controlled by the gastrointestinal hormones, hepatocrinin and cholecystokinin, respectively, which are released when partially digested food passes from the stomach to the duodenum. Once secreted into the intestine, possessing polar carboxyl and hydroxyl groups, the bile acids act as detergents assisting the emulsification of ingested lipids into very small globules; this aids the enzymatic digestion and absorption of dietary fat (see Chapter 9).

Bile acids are recirculated via the enterohepatic circulation

Up to 30 g of bile acids pass from the bile duct into the intestine each day and only 2% of this (approximately 0.5 g) is lost through the feces. Most would be deconjugated and reabsorbed. Passive reabsorption of bile acids occurs in the jejunum and colon but the majority takes place in the ileum by active transport. The reabsorbed bile acids are transported in blood via the portal vein, noncovalently bound to albumin, and resecreted into the bile. This is the enterohepatic circulation and it explains why bile contains both primary and secondary bile acids. The total bile acid pool is only 3 g – therefore they have to recirculate 5–10 times a day.

The bile acid flux controls bile acid synthesis; 7α-hydroxylase is under feedback by the amount of bile acids returning to the liver through the portal vein. Biliary secretion is also a major driving force for hepatic secretion of free cholesterol and phospholipids. Dietary bile acids also decrease the expression of 7α-hydroxylase.

Cholestyramine is a bile-acid binding resin which has been used to lower plasma cholesterol

Cholestyramine is a drug which interrupts enterohepatic circulation of the bile acids. It leads to an increased 7α-hydroxylase activity, increased bile acid synthesis and increased bile acid excretion. There also is an increased cholesterol synthesis and increased expression of LDL receptor. Cholestyramine was one of the first effective cholesterol-lowering agents.

The newer preparation is ezetimibe a drug which selectively inhibits absorption of cholesterol in the small intestine by inhibiting the putative cholesterol transporter located within the brush border membrane. Importantly, bile supersaturated with cholesterol facilitates formation of cholesterol gallstones.

Liver X receptors coordinate cholesterol homeostasis

The X receptors coordinate the expression of several genes relevant to cholesterol homeostasis and to lipid metabolism in general. They increase the expression of cholesterol 7α-hydroxylase (CYP7A1) gene. The RXR-LXR heterodimer mentioned above is required for the sterol-mediated upregulation of ABCA1 gene and for the expression of ABCG5 and ABCG8 proteins. The X receptors also also control apoE, lipoprotein lipase, phospholipid transfer protein and cholesteryl ester transfer protein expression. Finally, LXR upregulates SREBP-1c and through this increases triglyceride concentration.

CHOLESTEROL EXCRETION

Cholesterol cannot be metabolized by mammalian cells

Cholesterol cannot be digested in the gut or broken down by mammalian cells into carbon dioxide and water. Removal from the body is thus dependent on transfer into the gut prior to excretion via the feces. As we discussed in the section on bile acids above, there is a considerable flux of cholesterol, either directly or in the form of bile acids, from the liver into bile and then into the duodenum via the common bile duct. About 1g of cholesterol is eliminated from the body each day

STEROID 21-HYDROXYLASE DEFICIENCY

A neonate was born with ambiguous genitalia. Within 48 hours the infant was hypotensive and distressed. Biochemical investigation reveals:

Na$^+$ 115 mmol/L (135–145 mmol/L)

K$^+$ 7.0 mmol/L (3.5–5.0 mmol/L)

17-hydroxyprogesterone 550 nmol/L (<50 nmol/L)

Comment. This baby had a severe form of steroid 21-hydroxylase deficiency, the commonest of a range of conditions that are characterized by defects in the activity of one of the enzymes in the steroidogenic pathway and known as congenital adrenal hyperplasia. The conditions have a genetic basis leading to a failure to produce cortisol (and also possibly aldosterone). As a result there is reduced negative feedback on the pituitary production of ACTH, which then continues to stimulate the adrenal gland to produce steroids upstream of the enzyme block. These include 17-hydroxyprogesterone, which is further metabolized to testosterone (see Fig. 16.7) resulting in androgenization of a female neonate. The renal salt wasting is the result of mineralocorticoid deficiency and requires urgent treatment with fluids and steroids. Long-term maintenance therapy with hydrocortisone and a mineralocorticoid suppresses ACTH and androgen production.

A less severe form of this condition or partial enzyme deficiency occurs in young women who present with menstrual irregularity and hirsutism, as a consequence of excess of adrenal androgens.

through the feces. Approximately 50% is excreted after conversion to bile acids. The remainder is excreted as the isomeric saturated neutral sterols coprostanol (5β-) and cholestanol (5α-) produced by bacterial reduction of the cholesterol molecule.

STEROID HORMONES

Cholesterol is the precursor of all of the steroid hormones

Mammals produce many steroid hormones, some of which differ only by a double bond or by the orientation of a hydroxyl group. Consequently, it has been necessary to employ systematic nomenclature to detail exact structures. There are three broad groups of steroid hormones (Fig. 16.7). The corticosteroids have 21 carbon atoms in the basic pregnane ring structure. Loss of the remaining two carbon atoms from the cholesterol side chain produces the androstane ring structure and the group of hormones known as the androgens. Finally, loss of the angular methyl group at carbon atom

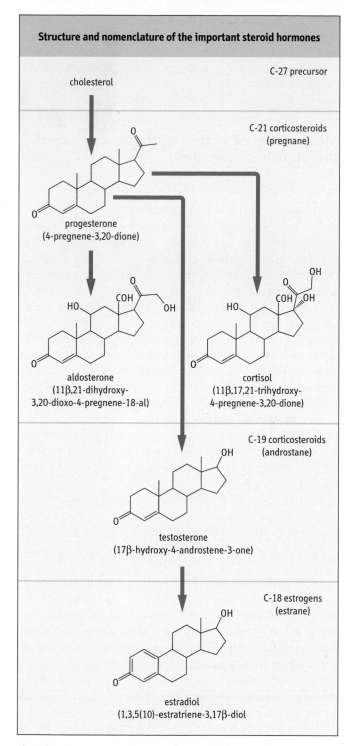

Structure and nomenclature of the important steroid hormones

cholesterol

C-27 precursor

C-21 corticosteroids
(pregnane)

progesterone
(4-pregnene-3,20-dione)

aldosterone
(11β,21-dihydroxy-
3,20-dioxo-4-pregnene-18-al)

cortisol
(11β,17,21-trihydroxy-
4-pregnene-3,20-dione)

C-19 corticosteroids
(androstane)

testosterone
(17β-hydroxy-4-androstene-3-one)

C-18 estrogens
(estrane)

estradiol
(1,3,5(10)-estratriene-3,17β-diol

Fig. 16.7 **Structure and nomenclature of the most important human steroid hormones.** Their trivial and systematic (in parentheses) names are shown. For the biosynthetic pathways, see Fig. 37.7. For numbering of the atoms in a steroid molecule, see Fig. 16.1.

19 as part of the aromatization of the A ring results in the estrane structure found in the estrogens. The presence and position of double bonds and the position and orientation of hydroxyl or other functional groups on the basic nucleus may then be described.

Biosynthesis of the steroid hormones

Conversion of cholesterol into steroid hormones occurs in only three organs: the adrenal cortex, the testis in men and the ovary in women.

It is normal practice to consider the corticosteroids as the products of the adrenal cortex, the androgens as the products of the testis and the estrogens as the products of the ovary. A simplified pathway of the steroid synthesis is shown in Figure 16.7 (see also Chapter 37). The relative activity of the steroidogenic enzymes in each of the three organs determines the major secreted product; however, this is not absolute and all three organs are capable of secreting small amounts of steroids from other groups. In pathologic situations, such as a defect in steroidogenesis or a steroid-secreting tumor, a very abnormal pattern of steroid secretion may be observed.

Cytochrome P450 mono-oxygenase enzymes control steroidogenesis

Most of the enzymes involved in converting cholesterol into steroid hormones are cytochrome P450 proteins that require oxygen and NADPH. In its simplest form, this enzyme complex catalyzes the replacement of a carbon–hydrogen bond with a carbon–hydroxyl bond; hence, the collective term mono-oxygenase. Hydroxylation of adjacent carbon atoms is the forerunner to cleavage of the carbon–carbon bond. Comparison of the structure of cholesterol (see Fig. 16.1) with those of the steroid hormones (see Fig. 16.7) demonstrates that the biosynthetic pathway is largely made up of cleavage of carbon–carbon bonds and hydroxylation reactions. These enzymes have their own nomenclature in which the symbol CYP is followed by a specific suffix. Thus, CYP21A2 refers to the enzyme that hydroxylates carbon atom 21. (See also Chapter 28, p. 408.)

The corticosteroids

The cellular substructure of the adrenal cortex is arranged in three different layers. The inner two layers (zona fasciculata and zona reticularis) are responsible for the synthesis of cortisol, the main glucocorticoid, and the adrenal androgens. The outer layer (zona glomerulosa) is responsible for the synthesis of aldosterone, the main mineralocorticoid (see Chapter 19). Although many of the steps are similar, they are controlled by very different mechanisms and this has led to the suggestion that the adrenal cortex may be considered as two separate endocrine organs.

The biosynthesis of cortisol depends on stimulation by pituitary adrenocorticotropic hormone (ACTH) which binds to its plasma membrane receptor and triggers a range of intracellular events which cause hydrolysis of cholesterol esters stored in lipid droplets and activation of the cholesterol 20,22-desmolase enzyme. This is the rate-limiting step of steroidogenesis which converts C-27 cholesterol into pregnenolone, the first of the C-21 pregnane family of corticosteroids. Thereafter, conversion to cortisol requires a dehydrogenation-isomerization and three sequential hydroxylation reactions at C-17, -21, and -11 under the control of the CYP enzymes. Control of the rate of cortisol biosynthesis is achieved by negative feedback by cortisol on the secretion of ACTH (Chapter 37).

The main stimulus to the synthesis of aldosterone is not ACTH but angiotensin II (see Chapter 22). Potassium is an important secondary stimulus. Angiotensin II, by binding to its receptor, and potassium, work cooperatively to activate the same first step in the pathway: the conversion of cholesterol into pregnenolone. The zona glomerulosa lacks the 17α-hydroxylase but has abundant amounts of 18-hydroxylase which is the first of a two-stage reaction, which yields the 18-aldehyde group found in aldosterone.

The androgens

The conversion of corticosteroids into androgens requires the 17–20 lyase/desmolase enzyme and a substrate that contains a 17α-hydroxyl group. This stimulates the addition of a 17α-hydroxyl group prior to breaking the C-17–C-20 bond to yield the androstane ring structure. This enzyme is abundant in the Leydig cells of the testis and in the granulosa cells of the ovary. In these cases, however, the stimuli to the rate-limiting cholesterol side-chain cleavage step are luteinizing hormone (LH) and follicle-stimulating hormone (FSH), respectively. Thus the same biosynthetic step, is controlled by two different hormones in two different tissues.

The estrogens

The conversion of androgens into estrogens involves removal of the angular methyl group at C-19 under the action of 19-aromatase (see Fig. 37.7). The A ring undergoes two dehydrogenations as part of the reaction, and the characteristic 1,3,5(10)-estratriene nucleus results. This aromatase enzyme is found most abundantly in the granulosa cells of the ovary, although it is worthy of note that an enzyme in adipose tissue can also convert some testosterone into estradiol. The biological actions of the steroid hormones are diverse and are best considered as part of the trophic hormone system to which they belong. This system is described in Chapter 37.

Many genetic defects have been identified in the structure of the CYP enzymes leading to abnormal steroid biosynthesis and characteristic clinical disorders such as congenital adrenal hyperplasia. A genotype:phenotype relationship is becoming established in such conditions and genetic analysis may become routine in these disorders.

Mechanism of action and elimination of the steroid hormones

Steroid hormones act via nuclear receptors

All the steroid hormones act by binding to nuclear receptors and stimulating transcription. which results in specific protein synthesis (see Chapter 33, Fig. 33.4). Steroid hormone receptors belong to a super-family of hormone receptors, which include receptors to the thyroid hormone T3 and the active forms of vitamins A and D. The specificity of each receptor is being achieved through differing hydrophobic pockets in a small hormone-binding domain situated towards the C-terminus of the receptor. Adjacent to the hormone-binding domain is a highly conserved DNA-binding domain, which is characterized by the presence of two zinc fingers (see Fig. 33.3). Binding of the steroid ligand facilitates translocation to the nucleus, dimerization and binding to a specific steroid response element within the nuclear DNA, leading to transcription. Genetic variability in steroid hormone receptors' structure is well described, conveying a variable degree of steroid hormone resistance and diverse clinical presentations.

The biological actions of the steroid hormones are are best considered as part of the trophic hormone system to which they belong. This system is described in Chapter 37.

Steroid hormones are excreted in the urine

Most steroid hormones are excreted via the kidney. In general there are two main steps in this process. First, the biological potency of the steroid must be removed and this is achieved by a series of reduction reactions. Second, the steroid structure must be rendered water-soluble by conjugation to a glucuronide or sulfate moiety, usually through the hydroxyl group at C-3. These steps occur predominantly within the liver. As a result there are many different steroid hormone conjugates in urine, some of them present in high concentrations. Urinary steroid profiling by gas chromatography–mass spectrometry typically identifies more than 30 such steroids and the relative concentrations of these may be used to pinpoint specific defects in the steroidogenic pathway (see box on p. 222).

VITAMIN D$_3$

Vitamin D$_3$ (cholecalciferol) is also derived from cholesterol and plays a very important role in calcium metabolism. Small

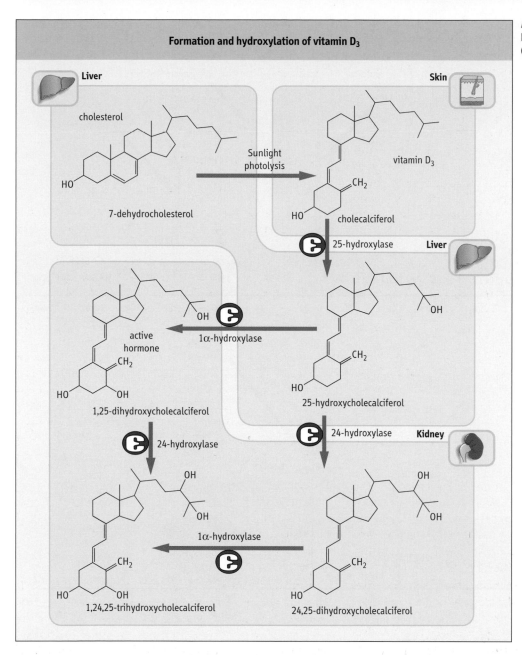

Fig. 16.8 **Formation and hydroxylation of vitamin D₃ (cholecalciferol)**

amounts of the fat-soluble vitamins D occur in food, (e.g. fish liver oil, egg yolk), but the majority of cholecalciferol is manufactured in the Malpighian layer of the epidermis of the skin (Fig 16.8). Cholesterol is converted to 7-dehydrocholesterol, which acts as the substrate for a unique nonenzymatic photolysis reaction in which ultraviolet rays from sunlight mediate the opening of the B-ring of cholesterol so destroying the steroid nucleus (see Chapter 24). The rate of this reaction is inversely related to the amount of pigment in the skin and directly related to the amount of sunlight exposure. Cholecalciferol is transported in plasma bound to a specific vitamin D-binding protein.

In the liver it undergoes hydroxylation at C-25 to produce 25-hydroxycholecalciferol (calcidiol). This step, which is not regulated, is catalyzed by a cytochrome P450 mono-oxygenase in the endo-plasmic reticulum. 25-Hydroxycholecalciferol is then transported in plasma to the kidney, bound to the same specific protein. Production of the potent hormone, 1,25-dihydroxycholecalciferol (cal-citriol), requires the contribution of a 1α-hydroxylase (yet another P450 containing mono-oxygenase) located within the mitochondria of the renal proximal tubule. The actions of 1,25-dihydroxycholecalciferol are discussed in Chapter 24.

SEPARATION OF URINARY STEROIDS

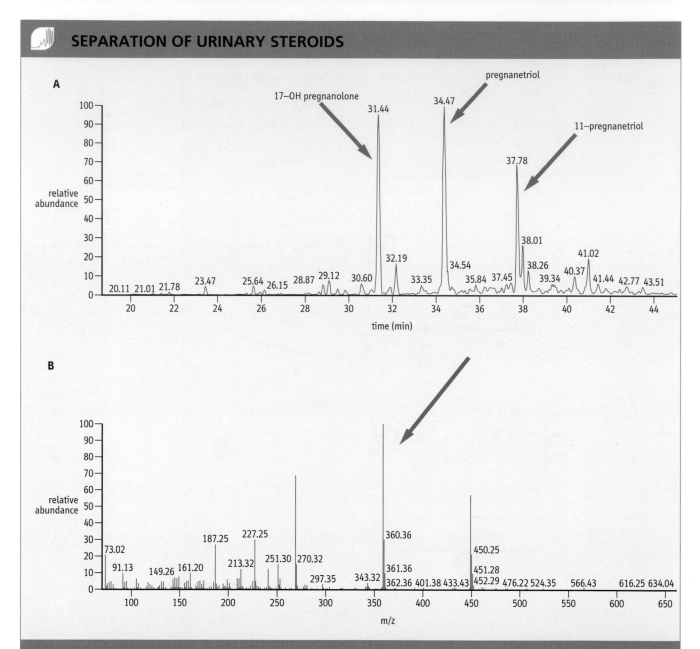

(A) Total ion chromatogram of a urinary steroid metabolite pattern from a patient with 21-hydroxylase deficiency variant of congenital adrenal hyperplasia. In this condition the most prominent steroid metabolites are 17-hydroxypregnanolone, pregnanetriol and 11-oxo-preganetriol.

  x-axis – time in minutes at which the chromatographically separated steroid metabolites are detected by the mass spectrometer. y-axis – relative abundance (quantity of ions)

(B) Complete pattern of ions produced from fragmentation of 11-oxo-pregnanetriol by the mass spectrometry detector.
  x-axis – m/z = mass to charge ratio
  y-axis – relative abundance (quantity of ions)

Summary

- ▪ Cholesterol is a vital constituent of cell membranes and the precursor molecule for bile acids, steroid hormones and vitamin D.
- ▪ Cholesterol is derived both from the diet and also synthesized de novo from acetyl-CoA. Cholesterol biosynthesis is strictly regulated. The rate limiting enzyme is the HMG-CoA reductase.
- ▪ The metabolism of cholesterol into bile acids and steroid hormones involves several hydroxylation reactions catalyzed by cytochrome P450 mono-oxygenase enzymes.
- ▪ Several clinical disorders are associated with abnormalities in the regulation of cholesterol homeostasis or metabolism.

ACTIVE LEARNING

1. Describe the regulation of intracellular cholesterol concentration.
2. How does SR-BI receptor differ from the LDL receptor?
3. Which are the secondary bile acids?
4. Discuss the enterohepatic circulation of bile acids.
5. Discuss the role of monooxygenases in steroid synthesis.

Further reading

1. Sakai J, Rawson RB. The sterol regulatory element-binding protein pathway: control of lipid homeostasis through regulated intracellular transport. *Curr Opin Lipidol* 2001;**12**:261–6.
2. Angelin B, Eriksson M and Rudling M. Bile acids and lipoprotein metabolism: a renaissance for bile acids in the post-statin era? *Curr Opin Lipidol* 1999;**10**:269–74.
3. Repa JJ, Mangelsdorf DJ. The liver X receptor gene team: Potential new players in atherosclerosis. *Nature* 2002;**8**(11):1243–8.
4. Marcil M, Brooks-Wilson A, Clee SM, *et al.* Mutations in the *ABC1* gene in familial HDL deficiency with defective cholesterol efflux. *Lancet* 1999;**354**:1341–6.
5. Janowski BA Willy PJ, Devi TR, Falck JR, Mangelsdorf DJ. An oxysterol signaling pathway mediated by the nuclear receptor LXRa. *Nature* 1996;**383**: 728–31.
6. Thomas MK, Demay MB. Vitamin D deficiency and disorders of vitamin D metabolism. *Endocrinology and Metabolism Clinics of North America* 2000;**29**:611–627.
7. White PC, Speiser PW. Congenital adrenal hyperplasia due to 21hydroxylase deficiency. *Endocrine Reviews* 2000;**21**:245–291.

17. Lipids and Lipoproteins

M H Dominiczak

LEARNING OBJECTIVES

After reading this chapter you should be able to:

- Describe the composition and functions of different lipoproteins present in plasma: chylomicrons, very-low-density lipoproteins, remnant particles, low-density lipoproteins and high-density lipoproteins.
- Describe the fuel transport pathway and the overflow pathway of lipoprotein metabolism.
- Describe the reverse cholesterol transport and its links with other pathways.
- Outline mechanisms and regulation of intracellular cholesterol levels, including the role of relevant genes, transcription factors, and receptor and enzyme proteins.
- Comment on laboratory tests used to assess lipid metabolism and the cardiovascular risk of a person.
- Comment on the relationships between the main component processes of atherogenesis: endothelial dysfunction, arterial deposition of lipids, inflammatory phenomena and their relation to plaque growth and rupture.

STATINS ARE DRUGS WHICH DECREASE PLASMA LDL CONCENTRATION

Statins such as simvastatin, pravastatin, atorvastatin and rosuvastatin are competitive inhibitors of HMG-CoA reductase, the rate-limiting enzyme in the pathway of cholesterol synthesis. The inhibition of this enzyme results in a decrease in intracellular cholesterol levels. This, acting through SREBP (Chapter 16), increases the expression of LDL-receptors on the cell membrane. An increase in the number of cellular receptors leads to increased cellular uptake of LDL and, consequently, to a lower plasma cholesterol concentration. The treatment with statins decreases cholesterol concentration by 30–60% (depending on the preparation), and decreases future cardiovascular events by 20–30%.

INTRODUCTION

Lipoproteins provide means for the transport of triacylglycerols (triglycerides) and cholesterol between organs and tissues. Also, together with defective function of cells lining the arteries (endothelium) and inflammation affecting arterial walls, they play a key role in atherosclerosis, a disease of the cardiovascular system which leads to heart attack (myocardial infarctions), strokes, and peripheral vascular disease. Cardiovascular disease is presently the most frequent cause of death in the industrialized world.

Fatty acids, triacylglycerol, and cholesterol are constantly transported between tissues

Lipoprotein metabolism links closely with the organism's energy metabolism. The lipids which are used for energy production are fatty acids. They are synthesized primarily in the liver and intestine but are stored mainly in adipose tissue as glycerol esters, triacylglycerols (synonymously called triglycerides) (Chapter 15). Fatty acids are released from triglycerides for use in the liver and muscle (see Chapter 20). Also,

fat contained in food needs to be transported from the intestine to the liver and then to the peripheral tissues. Although free (nonesterified) fatty acids travel in plasma bound to albumin, triacylglycerols are too large and too hydrophobic to be transported in this manner. Instead, they are packaged together with cholesterol, phospholipids, and proteins (apoproteins), into particles known as lipoproteins. These are secreted into plasma by liver and intestine. The transported fatty acids are removed from lipoproteins at target tissues by stepwise enzymatic hydrolysis of triacylglycerol. Lipoproteins present in plasma constitute a dynamic system: they exchange their lipid and protein components and as a result change their size, shape, and density. During this process the conformation of constituent apolipoproteins also changes: this is particularly important because their conformation determines how they 'fit' into their cellular receptors, and therefore how 'their' lipoproteins are taken up by cells. Apart from triacylglycerols, cholesterol, and other lipids, lipoproteins also transport fat-soluble vitamins such as vitamin A and vitamin E.

Cholesterol is an essential component of cells

Cholesterol is an essential constituent of cell membranes. It is also a precursor of steroids, including vitamin D, and bile acids. A cell can either synthesize cholesterol or acquire it from the outside. Cholesterol is synthesized from acetyl CoA (see Chapter 16). The rate-limiting step in its synthesis is the reduction of 3-hydroxy-3-methylglutaryl-CoA (HMG-CoA) to

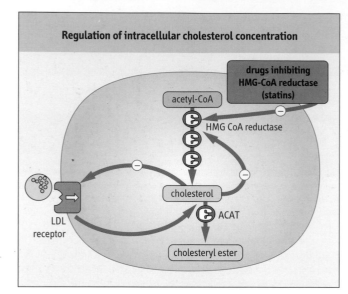

Fig. 17.1 **Regulation of intracellular cholesterol concentration.**
Intracellular cholesterol concentration is stringently regulated.
Intracellular cholesterol regulates the activity of a key enzyme
in its synthesis, HMG-CoA reductase, and also the expression of
LDL receptors on the cell membrane. Statins are the drugs that
inhibit HMG-CoA reductase.

mevalonate by HMG-CoA reductase. The activity of HMG-
CoA reductase is inversely related to the intracellular concentration of cholesterol. Cells acquire cholesterol through
low-density-lipoprotein (LDL) receptors also known as
apoB/E receptors, that mediate lipoprotein uptake into cells.
Thus there is a balance between intracellular synthesis of
cholesterol and its import from plasma (Fig. 17.1).

STRUCTURE AND FUNCTION OF LIPOPROTEINS

Plasma lipoproteins are particles of different size and density

A lipoprotein particle contains a hydrophobic core of cholesterol esters and triacylglycerols (Fig. 17.2). Amphipathic
phospholipids and free cholesterol, together with apoproteins
form an outer layer. Some proteins, such as apoprotein B
(apoB), are embedded in the particles. Others, such as apoC,
are only loosely bound – and can be easily exchanged with
other particles.

Lipoprotein particles present in plasma form a continuum
of size and density (Table 17.1). Their classification is based
on their hydrated density. Thus there are chylomicrons,
very-low-density lipoproteins (VLDL), remnant particles
(which include intermediate-density lipoproteins [IDL]), LDL,
and high-density lipoproteins (HDL). VLDL and remnant particles are triacylglycerol-rich, whereas LDL is cholesterol-rich.

ULTRACENTRIFUGATION IS A POWERFUL SEPARATION METHOD

In the clinical laboratories simple centrifuges are used to
separate serum (or plasma) from red blood cells. These
machines employ a moderate centrifugal force, 2000–3000 g
to sediment the blood cells. However, when much larger
centrifugal forces (40 000–100 000 g) are applied to plasma,
centrifugation, now termed ultracentrifugation, becomes a
powerful separation method for particles and molecules.
Ultracentrifugation is extensively used in lipid research. When
the centrifugal force is applied to a solution, particles that are
heavier than the surrounding solvent sediment, and those
lighter than the solvent float to the surface at a rate
proportional to the applied centrifugal force and to the
particle size. The formula below summarizes factors that
affect the particle movement:

$$v = [d^2(P_p - P_s) - g]/18\mu$$

where v = sedimentation rate, d = diameter,
   Pp = particle density, Ps = solvent density,
   μ = viscosity of the solvent, and g = gravitational force.

In a technique known as flotation ultracentrifugation, plasma
containing lipoproteins are overlayered with a solution of
defined density, e.g. 1.063 kg/L, the density of VLDL. After
several hours of centrifugation (depending on the type of
centrifuge rotor, the rotor speeds would be in the range of
40 000 rev/min), the VLDL float to the surface, where they
can be harvested. Other density solutions can be used to
separate other lipoproteins. Variations of the
ultracentrifugation technique, such as density gradient
centrifugation, can be applied to separate a plasma sample
into several 'bands' containing different lipoprotein fractions.
Ultracentrifugation is also extensively used in protein and
nucleic acid biochemistry.

LABORATORY TESTING FOR LIPID DISORDERS

There are several 'levels' of lipid testing in clinical situations

There are three stages of testing in the diagnosis of
lipoprotein disorders (Fig. 17.5A). The first stage is the
screening for just total cholesterol. This can be done on either
a fasting or nonfasting sample because cholesterol changes
little during the fast-fed cycle. The second stage consists
of measurements of total cholesterol, triacylglycerol
(triglycerides), and HDL-cholesterol in serum. Such
measurements need to be performed after a 12-h fast,
because triacylglycerol concentration increases postprandially.
The LDL concentration is usually calculated from the values of
total cholesterol and HDL-cholesterol (Fig. 17.5B). The final
step performed in specialist laboratories is lipoprotein analysis
by ultracentrifugation.

The lipoprotein classes

Particle	Density (kg/L)	Main component	Apoproteins*	Diameter (µm)
chylomicrons	<0.95	TG	B48 (A, C, E)	75–1200
VLDL	0.95–1.006	TG	B100 (A, C, E)	30–80
IDL	1.006–1.019	TG & cholesterol	B100, E	25–35
LDL	1.019–1.063	Cholesterol	B100	18–25
HDL	1.063–1.210	Protein	AI, AII (C, E)	5–12

Table 17.1 **The characteristics of the main lipoprotein classes.** TG, triacylglycerol (triglyceride); VLDL, very-low-density lipoproteins; IDL, intermediate-density lipoproteins; HDL, high-density lipoproteins. When separated by electrophoresis VLDL are called pre-beta lipoproteins, LDL, beta lipoproteins and HDL alpha lipoproteins. *Main apoproteins present in a given lipoprotein particle are indicated first, with those that are exchanged with other particles in brackets.

Lipoprotein structure

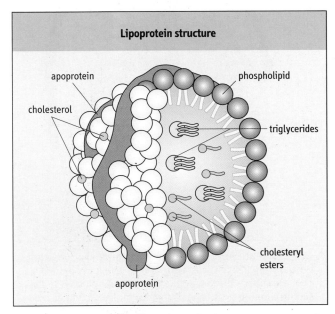

Fig. 17.2 **The lipoprotein particle.** The external monolayer of a lipoprotein particle contains free cholesterol, phospholipids, and apoproteins. Cholesterol esters and triacylglycerols locate in the particle core.

The density of these particles increases and the size decreases with decreasing triacylglycerol content, from chylomicrons (the lightest) through VLDL, remnant particles, IDL, LDL, to HDL (the heaviest). HDL contains several proteins, and some cholesterol and phospholipids, but relatively little triacylglycerol.

One can also characterize lipoproteins by their electrophoretic mobility

On electrophoresis α-lipoproteins (HDL) migrate furthest towards the anode (+electrode), followed by pre-β-lipoproteins (VLDL) and β-lipoproteins (LDL). Chylomicrons remain at the cathodic end, at the origin of the electrophoretic strip. The electrophoretic pattern is the basis for

MUTATION IN APOPROTEIN E GENE CAUSES DYSLIPIDEMIA INVOLVING REMNANT PARTICLES

Apoprotein E plays a key role in the metabolism of lipoprotein remnants. Its synthesis is controled by three major alleles, e2, e3, and e4. It is a relatively small protein, with a molecular mass of 34 kDa. There are three major isoforms: E2, E3, and E4. ApoE is recognized both by the LDL (apo B/E) receptor and by the LRP. The E2 ioform has much lower affinity (1%) to the receptor than other isoforms. This, in homozygotes, slows down the uptake of remnants and results in familial dyslipidemia (also known as type III 3 hyperlipidemia). Also, apoE seems to be important for lipid metabolism in the nervous system where it is synthesized by brain astrocytes. The presence of an e4 allele is associated with Alzheimer's disease, a disorder responsible for at least 50% of all cases of dementia.

the phenotypic classification of dyslipidemias into five types adopted by the WHO (Table 17.2). However, when it became evident that a disorder of lipid metabolism may present with different phenotypic patterns (see Table 17.3) dyslipidemias were re-classified; they are now defined either as separate genetically-determined entities (e.g. familial hypercholesterolemia) or simply classed according to plasma levels of cholesterol, triacylglycerol, and HDL-cholesterol (see below).

Apoproteins (apolipoproteins)

Apoproteins are the protein components of lipoprotein particles

They interact with cellular receptors and thus determine the metabolic fate of lipoproteins. They also serve as activators and inhibitors of enzymes involved in lipoprotein metabolism.

Main apoproteins are listed in Table 17.4. The most important are apoA, apoB, apoC , apoE, and apo(a). Each class of lipoproteins contains a characteristic set of apoproteins. Apoproteins A (AI and AII) are present in HDL. Apoprotein B variant called apoB100 controls the metabolism of LDL, whereas its truncated form, apoB48 (a N-terminal 48% of apoB100), controls the chylomicrons (see Chapter 33, Fig. 33.7). Apoprotein E controls the receptor binding of remnant particles. Apoproteins C act as enzyme activators and inhibitors and they are extensively exchanged between different lipoprotein classes. Lipoprotein (a) [Lp(a)], may have a role in fibrinolysis (see below).

Lipoprotein (a) consists of an LDL particle (containing apoB100) linked through a disulfide bond to another apoprotein, apo(a) (Fig. 17.3). Apo(a) is a glycoprotein with a considerable number of variants of different size (size polymorphism). The molecular mass of these isoforms ranges

between 200 and 800kDa. Apo(a) possesses a protease domain and a number of repeating sequences of approximately 80–90 amino acids in length, stabilized by disulfide bonds into a triple-loop structure. These structures are called kringles (the name of Danish pastry of similar shape). One of the kringles, kringle IV, is repeated 35 times within the apo(a) sequence. The number of kringle IV repeats determines the size of the lipoprotein (a) isoforms.

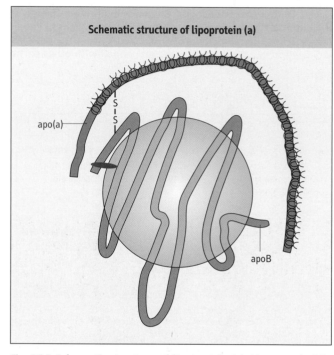

Schematic structure of lipoprotein (a)

Fig. 17.3 **Schematic structure of lipoprotein (a)**. Lipoprotein (a) is essentially an LDL particle, with apo(a) is linked to apoB through a disulfide bridge. Apo(a) is a large molecule containing a number of repeat units (kringles). Kringles have structure similar to plasminogen.

Phenotypic classification of dyslipidemia

Dyslipidemia type (Fredrickson)	Increased electrophoretic fraction (lipoproteins)	Increased cholesterol	Increased triglyceride
I	chylomicrons	yes	yes
IIa	beta (LDL)	yes	no
IIb	pre-beta & beta (VLDL & LDL)	yes	yes
III	'broad beta' band (IDL)	yes	yes
IV	pre-beta (VLDL)	no	yes
V	pre-beta (VLDL) plus chylomicrons	yes	yes

Table 17.2 **Phenotypic classification of dyslipidemia.** This is a phenotypic classification developed by Frederickson and adopted by the WHO; it is based on the electrophoretic separation of serum lipoproteins. For genetic classification refer to Table 17.4.

The most important genetic dyslipidemias

Dyslipidemia	Frequency/inheritance	Defect	Plasma lipid pattern	Increased cardiovascular risk
Familial hypercholesterolemia	1:500 autosomal dominant	LDL receptor deficiency or functional impairment	hypercholesterolemia or mixed hyperlipidemia (IIa or IIb)	yes
Familial combined hyperlipidemia	1:50 autosomal dominant	overproduction of apoB100	hypercholesterolemia or mixed hyperlipidemia (IIa or IIb)	yes
Familial dysbetalipoproteinemia (type III hyperlipidemia)	1:5000 autosomal recessive	presence of E2/E2 isoform defective remnant binding to LDL receptor	mixed hyperlipidemia (III)	yes

Mixed hyperlipidemia = increased plasma cholesterol and triglycerides

Table 17.3 **The most important genetic dyslipidemias.** The three clinically most important dyslipidemias are familial hypercholesterolemia, familial combined hyperlipidemia, and familial dysbetalipoproteinemia.

Apoproteins

Apoprotein	Structural function	Receptor	Effect on enzyme activity
AI	HDL	scavenger receptor B1 (SRB1) putative HDL receptor	LCAT activator
AII	HDL	HDL receptor?	LCAT cofactor
(a)	lp(a)	plasminogen receptor?	probably interferes with fibrinolysis
B48	chylomicrons	LRP	HTGL?
B100	VLDL, IDL, LDL	LDL receptor	–
CI, CII	–	–	LPL activation
CIII	–	–	LPL inhibition
E	remnant particles	LDL receptor	–

Table 17.4 **The function of apoproteins**. Both apoE and apoB bind to LDL (apoB/E) receptor. LCAT, lecithin:cholesterol acyltransferase; LRP, LDL receptor-related protein; HTGL, hepatic triglyceride lipase; LPL, lipoprotein lipase.

 PLASMA HOMOCYSTEINE CONCENTRATION IS ANOTHER NON-LIPID MARKER OF CARDIOVASCULAR RISK

A rare disease, homocystinuria, where homocysteine accumulates, is associated with premature vascular disease. However, it seems that mild increases in plasma homocysteine are also linked to the increased risk of cardiovascular – and also peripheral vascular disease.

Homocysteine metabolism is associated with the metabolism of one-carbon pool. Homocysteine, sulfur-containing amino acid is a product of a metabolism of dietary methionine and is generated as a result of de-methylation of S-adenosyl methionine (Chapter 18, p. 254). Homocysteine can be either metabolized to cystathionine and cysteine, or can be re-methylated to methionine. The re-methylation pathway involves the conversion of $N^{5,10}$-methylene-tetrahydrofolate ($N^{5,10}$-MTHF) to N^5-MTHF by methylene-tetrahydrofolate reductase (MTHFR). Folate is a co-substrate in this reaction. The common cause of hyperhomocysteinemia is folate deficiency, and also a mutation in the MTHFR gene. Proposed mechanisms of homocysteine toxicity include damage to the endothelium and increased oxidation of LDL. Folic acid is effective in lowering homocysteine.

Lipoprotein (a) is assembled in the liver and has a pre-β mobility on electrophoresis. Its density spans the LDL and HDL range (1.04–1.125 g/mL). Its concentration in plasma ranges widely between 0.2 and 120 mg/dL. Apo(a) exhibits a considerable sequence homology with plasminogen. Although it does not possess plasminogen's protease activity, it still may interfere with the action of plasminogen, potentially impairing the process of clot resolution (fibrinolysis) (see Chapter 6).

Functions of lipoproteins

Chylomicrons transport dietary triacylglycerols (triglycerides) from the intestine to the peripheral tissues. Their main apoprotein is apoB48, which is synthesized in the intestine. Chylomicrons also contain apoproteins A, C, and E. After hydrolysis of chylomicrons by the enzyme lipoprotein lipase (LDL), their remnants are taken up by the liver. Their uptake is mediated by apoE binding to the LDL receptor and to the LDL receptor-related protein (LRP).

VLDL transport triacylglycerols from the liver to the periphery. The main apoprotein of VLDL is apoB100. They also contain apoC and apoE. VLDL loses triacylglycerols through the action of the LPL while it transforms into IDL (a remnant particle), which in turn is either taken up by the liver or, by losing more triacylglycerols, transforms further into LDL. These consecutive transformations result in a loss of all the apoproteins except apoB100. The size of particles also successively decreases, and this changes the conformation of apoproteins on their surface. In the relatively large VLDL particles apoB100 and apoE remain 'extended'. Such conformation does not allow binding to the apoB/E receptor. As VLDL shrinks during the transformation into a remnant particle, apoE assumes a conformation that allows its binding to the receptor and liver uptake. Some remnants, instead of being taken up, transform into LDL; in LDL it is apoB100 which assumes receptor-friendly conformation. LDL are the main carrier of cholesterol in plasma.

HDL transport cholesterol centripetally (from the periphery to the liver). This pathway is known as reverse cholesterol transport. The main apoproteins in HDL are apoAI and apoAII. They are synthesized in the intestine and liver. HDL also contains apoC and apoE. HDL participates in the metabolism of other particles (chylomicrons, VLDL, and remnants) through component exchange, exchanging apoproteins, phospholipid, triacylglycerol and cholesteryl ester.

Enzymes and transfer proteins

Two hydrolases, lipoprotein lipase (LPL) and hepatic triglyceride lipase (HTGL), remove triacylglycerols from triacylglycerol – rich lipoprotein particles. LPL binds to heparan sulfate proteoglycans on the surface of the vascular endothelial cells, and HTGL is associated with liver plasma membranes. LPL digests triacylglycerols in chylomicrons and VLDL, and releases fatty acids and glycerol for cell metabolism or storage. LPL may hydrolyze as much as 10 g triacylglycerol per hour. HTGL acts on particles already partially digested by LPL: it facilitates conversion of IDL into LDL.

Lecithin:cholesterol acyltransferase (LCAT) is a glycoprotein enzyme associated with HDL. LCAT esterifies cholesterol acquired by HDL. LCAT is activated by apoAI. Note that inside cells cholesterol is esterified by a different enzyme, acylCoA:acylcholesterol transferase (ACAT).

Cholesterol ester transfer protein (CETP) facilitates the transfer of cholesterol esters from HDL to triacylglycerol-rich lipoproteins in exchange for some of their triacylglycerols and apoproteins. CETP is synthesized in the liver.

LIPOPROTEIN RECEPTORS

Lipoprotein receptors mediate cellular internalization of these particles and allow cells to acquire cholesterol and other lipids from outside. The main lipoprotein receptor is the apo B/E receptor synonymously known as the LDL receptor. This receptor was discovered by Goldstein and Brown, who jointly received the Nobel Prize for this work. As its name implies, it can bind either of the two apoproteins, apoE and apoB100. ApoE binds to LDL receptor with a higher affinity than apoB. The receptor gene is located on chromosome 19; the mature receptor protein is 839 amino acids long and spans the cell membrane (Fig. 17.4). The expression of the receptor gene is regulated by the intracellular cholesterol concentration.

ApoB48 cannot bind to the apoB/E receptor. The metabolism of chylomicron remnants is mediated by apoE binding primarily to the LDL receptor, but also to the LDL receptor-related protein (LRP).

Scavenger receptors

In contrast to the apoB/E receptor which has two well-defined ligands (client molecules) scavenger receptors are membrane receptors with broad specificity. They are present on the phagocytic cells such as macrophages (Fig. 17.4). They also differ from the LDL receptor in that they are not subject to feedback regulation, and therefore they may overload the cell with their ligands. There are classes of scavenger receptor designated A and B, and another known as CD36. Class A receptors contain collagen-like triple-helical structure. Class A scavenger receptor does not bind intact LDL but it readily binds chemically modified (acetylated or oxidized) LDL. Class B receptor participates in HDL metabolism.

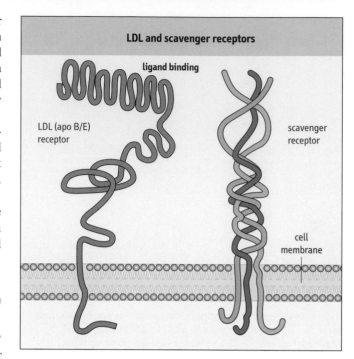

Fig. 17.4 **LDL and scavenger receptors.** While the LDL (apoB/E) receptor mediates the uptake of intact LDL, the scavenger receptor internalizes modified LDL. Both receptors span the cell membranes. The expression of LDL receptor is regulated by the intracellular cholesterol concentration, while the scavenger receptor remains unregulated. The scavenger receptor type A, which is illustrated here, is present on macrophages and has a collagen-like structure. Scavenger receptor type BI participates in HDL-metabolism.

MEASUREMENT OF LIPOPROTEINS

When we measure 'total plasma cholesterol' or 'plasma triglycerides' in clinical laboratories, we measure just one of their components across all classes of lipoproteins. (Note that clinicians use the term 'triglycerides' rather than 'triacylglycerol'; you will have noticed that here we use both to familiarize the reader with both conventions.) It is very difficult to measure the concentration of lipoprotein particles in plasma because of their heterogeneous composition. To get around the problem, we exploit the fact that most of the cholesterol present in plasma is in LDL, and therefore total plasma cholesterol concentration is an approximation of the LDL concentration. Similarly, plasma triacylglycerol (triglyceride) concentration is a marker of the sum total of VLDL and IDL. To obtain a more accurate picture of lipid metabolism we measure, or calculate, the cholesterol present in different lipoprotein fractions that are first separated by precipitation or ultracentrifugation. The results of such measurements are expressed as, e.g., LDL-cholesterol or HDL-cholesterol. Specialist laboratories separate all lipoprotein subfractions employing the technique of ultracentrifugation (see Fig. 17.5).

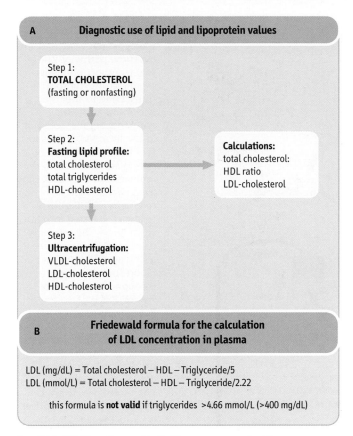

A   **Diagnostic use of lipid and lipoprotein values**

Step 1:
TOTAL CHOLESTEROL
(fasting or nonfasting)

Step 2:
Fasting lipid profile:
total cholesterol
total triglycerides
HDL-cholesterol

Calculations:
total cholesterol:
HDL ratio
LDL-cholesterol

Step 3:
Ultracentrifugation:
VLDL-cholesterol
LDL-cholesterol
HDL-cholesterol

B   **Friedewald formula for the calculation**
of LDL concentration in plasma

LDL (mg/dL) = Total cholesterol − HDL − Triglyceride/5
LDL (mmol/L) = Total cholesterol − HDL − Triglyceride/2.22

this formula is **not valid** if triglycerides >4.66 mmol/L (>400 mg/dL)

Fig. 17.5 **(A) The diagnostic lipid measurements.** The measurement of total cholesterol is a first-line screening test. The next step, fasting lipid profile, provides information about the main lipid markers of cardiovascular risk, i.e the concentrations of of total cholesterol, LDL-cholesterol, and HDL-cholesterol and triacylglycerol (triglycerides). The analysis of lipoprotein subfractions by ultra-centrifugation, and the measurement of apoproteins are specialist tests. The total-cholesterol-to-HDL ratio indicates the balance between cholesterol transport to and from peripheral tissues. A ratio above 5 indicates an increased cardiovascular risk.
(B) The calculation of LDL-cholesterol concentration in plasma. LDL-cholesterol can be calculated from the value of total cholesterol, triglycerides, and HDL-cholesterol using the Friedewald formula.

Please note that the laboratory measurements are made either in plasma or in serum (plasma devoid of fibrinogen, see Chapter 3), depending on the substance measured and the method employed. For the sake of simplicity we will refer here to measurements in plasma.

METABOLISM OF LIPOPROTEINS

The stages of lipoprotein metabolism are as follows:

- Assembly of lipoprotein particles. Chylomicrons are assembled in the intestine, and VLDL in the liver;

- Transfer of fatty acids from lipoproteins to cells. This facilitated by enzymes, LPL and HTGL and transforms chylomicrons and VLDL into the relevant remnant particles (remnants);
- Binding of the remnant particles to membrane receptors and their cellular uptake;
- Transformation of some remnants into LDL, their subsequent receptor binding and cellular uptake.
- Reverse cholesterol transport, i.e. removal of cholesterol from cells by HDL particles, its esterification by LCAT and either transport back to the liver, or CETP-mediated transfer to other lipoproteins by which they re-enter the VLDL-IDL-LDL pathway.

Chylomicrons transport dietary fat

Triacylglycerols contained in food are first acted upon by pancreatic lipases and are absorbed as monoacylglycerols, free fatty acids, and free glycerol (see Chapter 9). In the intestinal cells (enterocytes), triacylglycerols are resynthesized and, together with phospholipids, cholesterol and apoB48, are reassembled into chylomicrons. These are secreted into the lymph and reach plasma through the thoracic duct. They normally appear in plasma only after fat-containing meals, giving plasma a milky appearance. In the peripheral tissues, such as muscle and adipose tissue, chylomicron triacylglycerols are hydrolyzed by LPL. The remaining smaller particles are the chylomicron remnants. The remnants travel to the liver, where they bind to the LDL receptor and the LRP. The half-life of chylomicrons in plasma is less than 1 h (Fig. 17.6).

VLDL transport endogenously synthesized triglycerides

Endogenously synthesized triacylglycerols are transported by VLDL, which are assembled in the liver. There, VLDL are 'built up' around apoB100 molecules. The binding of triacylglycerols to apoB is facilitated by the microsomal triglyceride transfer protein (MTP). Unused ApoB100 is degraded by ubiquitin-dependent protease (see Chapter 32, Fig. 32.10).

In plasma, VLDL acquire cholesteryl esters and apoproteins (including apoE) from HDL. Its triacylglycerols are hydrolyzed by LPL in a way analogous to chylomicrons, and this yields VLDL remnants. At this stage apoE assumes its receptor-binding conformation and it binds to the apoB/E receptor. Most of the remnants are taken up by the liver. The remaining ones are further hydrolyzed by HTGL to yield IDL, which in turn, by losing still more triacylglycerol, transform into LDL. By this stage, all apoproteins except for the apoB100 had been shed from the particle.

LDL is taken up by cells by the same route as remnant particles

By shedding almost all triacylglycerols, LDL becomes relatively rich in cholesterol. The apoB100 now acquires a

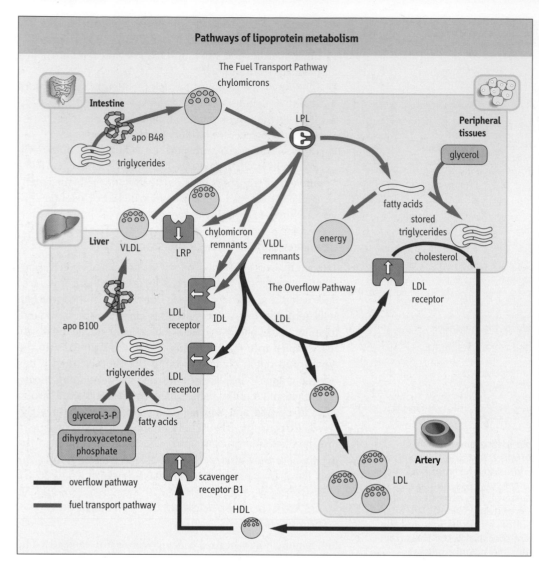

Pathways of lipoprotein metabolism

The Fuel Transport Pathway
chylomicrons

Intestine

apo B48

triglycerides

LPL

Peripheral tissues

glycerol

fatty acids

energy

stored triglycerides

cholesterol

Liver

VLDL

LRP

chylomicron remnants

VLDL remnants

LDL receptor

The Overflow Pathway

apo B100

LDL receptor

IDL

LDL

LDL receptor

triglycerides

glycerol-3-P

fatty acids

dihydroxyacetone phosphate

scavenger receptor B1

HDL

overflow pathway

fuel transport pathway

Artery

LDL

Fig. 17.6 **Lipoprotein metabolism: the fuel transport pathway and the overflow pathway.** The fuel transport pathway: chylomicrons transport triglyceride to the periphery, and their remnants are metabolized in the liver. VLDL transport fuel from the liver to peripheral tissues, and the remnants also return to the liver. Part of VLDL remnants and IDL are further converted into LDL, which enter the overflow pathway. The overflow pathway: LDL travel in blood from the liver through the peripheral tissues and back to the liver. On its way it may enter the arterial wall. The amount of lipids deposited in the arteries is proportional to their plasma concentration. Cholesterol is removed from cells and transported back to the liver by HDL particles. LPL: lipoprotein lipase, LRP: LDL-receptor-related protein.

receptor-binding conformation and begins to control LDL internalization. LDL are taken up by the apoB/E receptor either in the liver (approximately 80% of particles follow this path) or in the peripheral tissues (see Fig. 17.6). Interestingly the apoB-containing LDL particles have lower affinity toward the receptor than apoE-containing remnants.

A sophisticated system controls intracellular cholesterol synthesis and uptake

After internalization, the LDL-receptor complex is digested by lysosomal enzymes and the released cholesterol is esterified within the cell by SOAT. The receptor recycles back to the membrane. The free cholesterol released within the cell regulates the rate of its own endogenous synthesis. The key element in the regulation of intracellular cholesterol concentration are the sterol regulatory element-binding proteins (SREBPs). SREBPs are a family of transcription factors. They regulate

the transcription of genes encoding enzymes responsible for cholesterol synthesis such as 3-hydroxy-3-methylglutaryl coenzyme A synthase and HMG-CoA reductase, and also the gene coding for the apoB/E (LDL) receptor (see also Chapter 16). Thus, depletion of hepatic sterols increases SREBP level, increasing both the cholesterol synthesis, and the expression of LDL receptor. On the other hand, increased intracellular cholesterol concentration inhibits the SREBP pathway and thus represses the receptor gene. It also decreases cholesterol synthesis.

SREBPs are synthesized as integral membrane proteins in a precursor form. SREBP is activated by another protein, the SREBP cleavage-activating protein (SCAP) which has a sterol-sensing domain. Thus, when cell cholesterol concentration is low, SCAP moves together with the membrane-embedded SREBP precursor from the endoplasmic reticulum to the cleaving enzyme (a serine protease) located in the Golgi apparatus. There, the protease cleaves the SREBP precursor and liberates the active transcription factor, which translocates to the nucleus (see also Chapter 16).

Cholesterol is removed from cells by the reverse cholesterol transport

Human beings cannot metabolize the cholesterol ring: it needs to be transported to the liver and excreted either in a free form, or as a bile acid. The system that allows the removal of cholesterol from cells is known as the reverse cholesterol transport. It is mediated by the HDL.

HDL are formed in the liver and intestine as discoidal, lipid-poor particles (pre-β HDL) which contain mainly apoAI: they are partly constructed from the excess phospholipid shed from VLDL during its hydrolysis by LPL. These nascent HDL accept cholesterol from cells.

A membrane protein known as cholesterol efflux regulatory protein (CERP, also called the ATP-binding cassette transporter A1 – see Chapter 7) plays a major role in cholesterol efflux from cells. It uses ATP as a source of energy, CERP is rate-limiting in the efflux of free cholesterol to apoAI. Other ATP-binding cassette transporters, known as ABCG5 and ABCG8, are also involved in cholesterol transport; they reside in the apical membrane of the hepatocyte where they control the movement of cholesterol into bile. The role of CERP in cholesterol efflux was defined as a result of the study of extremely rare dyslipidemia called Tangier disease. Patients suffering from Tangier disease have almost no HDL, and show accumulation of cholesteryl esters in tissues such as tonsils (which acquire a characteristic orange colour), and also in the spleen, intestinal mucosa, and cornea. Patients with Tangier disease suffer from coronary disease more frequently than those without.

After the nascent HDL acquires the free cholesterol, it is esterified by LCAT; the cholesteryl esters move deeper into the HDL particle, and the particle assumes a spherical shape. It is now known as HDL-3. Subsequently, aided by cholesterol ester transfer protein, HDL transfers part of its cholesteryl esters to triglyceride-rich lipoproteins in exchange for triglycerides. At that point it gets even larger, and is now designated HDL-2. This particle now binds to the class B scavenger receptor in the liver. However, binding does not result in HDL internalization, but only in the transfer of cholesterol to the cell membrane. The particle shrinks again, and some of its redundant parts become nascent HDL and participate in the next cycle of transport (Fig. 17.7).

Cholesterol delivered to the liver by the HDL is excreted either as a free sterol or as bile acids. This is controlled by the sterol-responsive transcription factors, termed the liver X receptors (LRX). These receptors form dimers with another class of intracellular receptors, the retinoid X receptors (RXRs) and control the expression of several proteins such as transfer proteins and the enzyme 7α-hydroxylase (CYP7A1), which plays a key role in the biliary cholesterol excretion (see Chapter 16).

PEROXISOME PROLIFERATION ACTIVATING RECEPTORS (PPARS) ARE TRANSCRIPTION FACTORS INVOLVED IN CONTROL OF LIPOPROTEIN METABOLISM AND IN INSULIN ACTION

PPARs are lipid-activated transcription factors (Chapter 33) that regulate the genes controlling lipid and glucose homeostasis. PPARs, similarly to the liver X receptors, form dimers with retinoid X receptor RXR; it is this dimer that subsequently binds to PPAR-response elements.

There are three PPAR proteins: PPARα, PPAR β/δ and PPARγ PPARα is present in liver, kidney, heart, and skeletal muscle and is involved in the control of fatty acid and lipoprotein metabolism. PPARγ is present in the brown and white adipose tissue, and affects cell differentiation, insulin action and fatty acid synthesis. It also stimulates triacylglycerol synthesis and storage. PPARβ/δ participates in brain lipid metabolism and affects proliferation and differentiation of adipocytes. PPARs also regulate reverse cholesterol transport and bile acid synthesis. For instance, PPARα regulates the expression of the AI-CIII-AIV gene cluster; this increases the expression of apoAI and apoAII and reduces the expression of apoCIII gene. It also increases the expression of LPL.

PPARs are important targets of drug action. The commonly used lipid-lowering drugs, derivatives of fibric acid (fibrates) activate PPARα. New antidiabetic drugs, thiazolidinediones, increase insulin sensitivity in insulin-resistant patients (see Chapter 20) activate PPARγ.

The integrated view of lipoprotein metabolism: the two pathways

The metabolism of chylomicrons and VLDL, from their assembly, through hydrolysis of triacylglycerols, to the formation and uptake of remnants, forms a major fuel distribution network in the body. Thus, it could be called the fuel transport pathway (Fig. 17.6). The fuel transport pathway is associated with the reverse cholesterol transport through component exchange.

The fuel transport pathway generates LDL as a byproduct of fuel distribution; further fate of LDL particles is not related to fuel supply. Therefore, the LDL metabolism, from the stage of remnants on, can be called 'the overflow pathway'. The concept of the two pathways is helpful in the understanding of atherogenesis, and the development of disorders of lipoprotein metabolism.

Pathway overload may result either from oversupply or from decreased degradation of a lipoprotein. Normally the apoE-containing remnants are quickly metabolized in the fuel

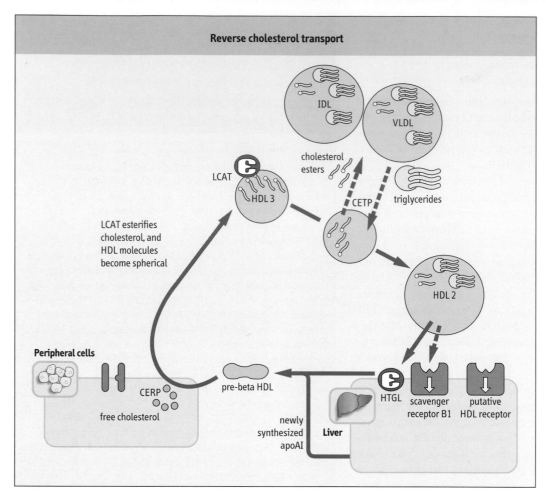

Fig. 17.7 **Reverse cholesterol transport.** HDL are assembled in the liver and intestine as discoidal particles. They acquire cholesterol from cell membranes aided by cholesterol efflux regulatory protein (CERP). LCAT associated with HDL esterifies the acquired cholesterol. The formed cholesteryl esters move to the inside of the particle, and the particle becomes spherical. HDL exchanges apoproteins and cholesteryl esters with triacylglycerol-rich lipoproteins. This is facilitated by cholesterol ester transfer protein (CETP). HDL acquire triacylglycerols in exchange for cholesteryl esters. This increases their size further. However, when cholesterol transfer to the liver mediated by the scavenger receptor BI is completed, the HDL size decreases again: some of the redundant material is used to construct apoAI-rich, lipid-poor particles (pre-beta HDL). These re-enter the cholesterol removal cycle.

transport pathway and no excess LDL appear in the circulation. However, if dietary intake of cholesterol (or VLDL production) is high, or if there is a decrease in the number of apoB/E receptors, more LDL particles enter the overflow pathway.

DYSLIPIDEMIAS

Defects in the lipoprotein metabolism lead to disorders known as hyperlipidemias or, dyslipidemias. Table 17.3 gives the examples of dyslipidemias.

Note that in the western populations, approximately 30% of people have undesirably high plasma cholesterol concentration. The most frequent dyslipidemia (common hypercholesterolemia) is polygenic and is a result of combined genetic and environmental factors such as diet. Then there are rarer disorders with defined genetic background. The most important of these is the familial hypercholesterolemia, a monogenic disorder caused by a mutation in the gene coding for the apoB/E(LDL) receptor. It affects both fuel transport- and overflow pathways, and both remnants and LDL accumulate. The effect on LDL is the most visible. Patients with familial hypercholesterolemia have very high plasma cholesterol and LDL-cholesterol concentrations. There also is a prominent family history of early heart disease, consistent with the autosomal

DYSLIPIDEMIA IS COMMON IN DIABETES MELLITUS

Mr B was 67 years old and had type 2 diabetes and mild hypertension. When he visited the outpatient clinic, his cholesterol was 6.9 mmol/L (265 mg/dL), triacylglycerol (triglycerides) 1.9 mmol/L (173 mg/dL), and HDL 0.9 mmol/L (35 mg/dL). Fasting blood glucose was 8.5 mmol/L (153 mg/dL) and glycated hemoglobin 1c (HbA1c) 6%. He was treated with diet and a sulfonylurea derivative which potentiates glucose-stimulated insulin release and lowers blood glucose concentration.

Comment. Diabetes carries a 2–3 times increased risk of coronary heart disease. This patient's diabetes was well controlled but cholesterol level remained high, so that he required lipid-lowering drug treatment. Low HDL-cholesterol concentration is relatively common in type 2 diabetes. The patient was prescribed a lipid lowering drug in addition to his treatment with a sulfonylurea derivative. Blood pressure responded to treatment with an angiotensin converting enzyme inhibitor (see Chapter 20).

FAMILIAL HYPERCHOLESTEROLEMIA IS A MONOGENIC LIPID DISORDER ASSOCIATED WITH HEART ATTACKS OCCURRING AT YOUNG AGE

A 32-year-old heavy smoker developed a sudden crushing chest pain. He was admitted to the casualty department. Myocardial infarction was confirmed by ECG changes and by high cardiac troponin concentration. On examination the patient had tendon xanthoma on hands and thickened Achilles tendons. There was a strong family history of coronary heart disease (his father had had a coronary bypass graft at the age of 40 and his paternal grandfather died of myorardial infarction in his early fifties). His cholesterol was 10.0 mmol/L (390 mg/dL), triglycerides 2 mmol/L (182 mg/dL) and HDL 1.0 mmol/L (38 mg/dL).

Comment. This patient has familial hypercholesterolemia (FH), an autosomal dominant disorder characterized by a decreased number of LDL receptors. FH carries a very high risk of premature coronary disease, and heterozygotic individuals may suffer heart attacks as early as the 3rd or 4th decade of life. The frequency of FH homozygotes in western populations is approximately 1:500.
This patient was immediately treated with intravenous tissue plasminogen activator. Subsequently he underwent coronary artery bypass graft and was then treated with lipid-lowering drugs. His cholesterol concentration subsequently decreased to 4.8 mmol/L (185 mg/dL) and triglyceride (triacylglycerol) level to 1.7 mmol/L, with HDL-cholesterol increasing to 1.1 mmol/L (42 mg/dL).

dominant inheritance. In addition, some patients develop lipid deposits on hand and knee tendons, and particularly on the Achilles tendon: these are known as tendon xanthomas, and are diagnostic for the disorder. Familial hypercholesterolemia carries a high risk of cardiovascular disease.

Another disorder, similarly inherited dyslipidemia, is the familial combined hyperlipidemia characterized by an overproduction of apoB100 rather than the impairment of receptor-mediated clearance. There is an increased production of VLDL and consequently, increased generation of LDL: again, both the fuel transport- and the overflow pathway become overloaded. This dyslipidemia presents with variable plasma lipid patterns (either hypercholesterolemia or both hypercholesterolemia and hypertriglyceridemia). Familial combined hyperlipidemia is a relatively common cause of premature myocardial infarction (note: premature infarction is defined as one occurring in a man aged below 55 years or a woman below 65 years).

A dyslipidemia affecting primarily fuel transport pathway is the familial dysbetalipoproteinemia caused by a mutation in the apoE gene, yielding apoE isoform with low affinity for the apoB/E receptor (see Box). In this disease the remnants accumulate and there is an increase in both cholesterol and triglycerides in the plasma. Here the characteristic xanthomas occur in palms (palmar xanthoma). Familial dyslipidemia is also associated with early coronary disease.

Dyslipidemia affecting primarily the fuel transport pathway is also characteristic for the type 2 diabetes mellitus. There is the overload of the fuel transport pathway, due to increased VLDL synthesis and a consequent increase in the remnant concentration. Also, there is a decreased concentra-

tion of HDL-cholesterol. The diabetic patients often have normal LDL-cholesterol because the overflow pathway remains quantitatively unaffected; however, it is possible that diabetic LDL are more atherogenic than the non-diabetic particles, because of changes in their size and density.

The instance where glucose intolerance or diabetes, low HDL-cholesterol, abdominal obesity, and hypertension occur together is known as the metabolic syndrome (actually, the presence of any three of these abnormalities is sufficient for diagnosis). The metabolic syndrome is associated with an increased risk of coronary disease.

A very rare dyslipidemia affecting exclusively the fuel transport pathway is caused by the deficiency of LPL. This overloads the 'front end' of the pathway; VLDL metabolism is defective and its accumulation leads to very high triacylglycerol (triglyceride) concentrations. Clinical signs include characteristic, rash-like skin xanthomas. The risk associated with LPL deficiency is primarily that of pancreatic inflammation (pancreatitis, see Chapter 9) caused by the large triacylglycerol load.

ATHEROGENESIS

Normally arterial endothelium repels cells and inhibits blood clotting

The lumen of a healthy artery is lined by a confluent layer of endothelial cells. Normal endothelium forms a surface which repels cells floating in plasma (including platelets), and which is strongly antithrombotic. The arterial wall consists three well-defined layers: the subendothelial layer is called the intima, the middle one, media (this one contains vascular smooth muscle cells, VSMC), and the outer one is adventitia, composed of looser connective tissue and containing relevant nerves.

Substances can penetrate endothelium either through junctions between the endothelial cells, or by transgressing the cells themselves. *An important function, controlled by the endothelium, is the ability of blood vessels to dilate (vasodilatation) and to constrict (vasoconstriction) and thus regulate tissue and organ blood flow.*

The endothelium controls vasodilatation by secreting the endothelium-derived relaxing factor (EDRF), which is a gas, nitric oxide (NO)

Nitric oxide is synthesized from L-arginine by endothelial NO synthase (eNOS).

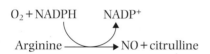

MEASUREMENT OF C-REACTIVE PROTEIN MAY REFLECT INFLAMMATORY PHENOMENA ASSOCIATED WITH ATHEROGENESIS

It has been long known that the inflammatory reaction associated with infection or trauma can be detected by measuring the concentration of plasma C-reactive protein (CRP), a protein produced in the liver in response to stimulation by pro-inflammatory cytokines. Its name comes from its binding to the capsular polysaccharide of bacteria such as *S. pneumoniae* by which way it mediates their clearance. However, measurements of small increases in CRP concentration which require a special, highly sensitive analytical method, demonstrated the association of such and may identify persons at risk who might have normal lipid concentrations. Increased plasma concentrations of other pro-inflammatory molecules such as interleukin-6 (IL-6) and serum amyloid A, have also been associated with coronary heart disease.

The activity of eNOS is controlled by the intracellular calcium concentration. There are two isoenzymes of NOS: eNOS that is constitutively (constantly) expressed in the endothelium, and inducible (iNOS) found in VSMC and in macrophages. Nitric oxide causes vasodilatation via stimulation of guanylate cyclase and cyclic GMP production (see Chapter 38).

Current data suggest that low levels of NO contribute to development of high blood pressure (hypertension). Also, drugs such as glyceryl trinitrate, which relieve chest pain caused by inadequate blood supply to the heart muscle (angina pectoris) by dilating coronary arteries, act by releasing NO.

Atherosclerosis is a disease of the cardiovascular system, affecting the vessel wall and leading to the narrowing of arteries, or to their complete blockage

Clinically this may cause myocardial infarction (resulting from a complete blockage of coronary artery supplying the heart), stroke (a blockage of an artery supplying the brain), or peripheral vascular disease (a condition where narrowing of leg arteries leads to a characteristic pain on walking, known as intermittent claudication). Atherosclerosis is a complex process. Its main components are endothelial dysfunction, lipid deposition, and inflammatory reaction in the vascular wall (Fig. 17.8): all three eventually result, not only in the formation of atherosclerotic plaques, but in the remodeling of the entire arterial wall. The whole process is set in motion, and is maintained, by a intense cross-talk between endothelial cells, VSMC, and plasma-derived inflammatory cells, macrophages, and lymphocytes (Fig. 17.9). The cross-talk involves an array of chemokines, cytokines, and growth factors (see Chapter 37), which cause attraction of cells to the sites of atherosclerotic lesions, induce cell migration, proliferation, apoptosis, and the excess production of extracellular matrix.

The development of atherosclerosis is initiated by endothelial dysfunction

The key early event in atherosclerosis is the damage to the endothelium (Fig. 17.8). This may be caused by excess of lipoproteins, hypertension, diabetes, or the components of cigarette smoke. Initially the damage is functional only. The endothelium becomes more permeable to lipoproteins which move beneath the endothelial layer, in the underlying intima. Also, the endothelium loses its cell-repellent quality, and allows inflammatory cells into the vascular wall. Later, the endothelium may become physically damaged, or even completely destroyed.

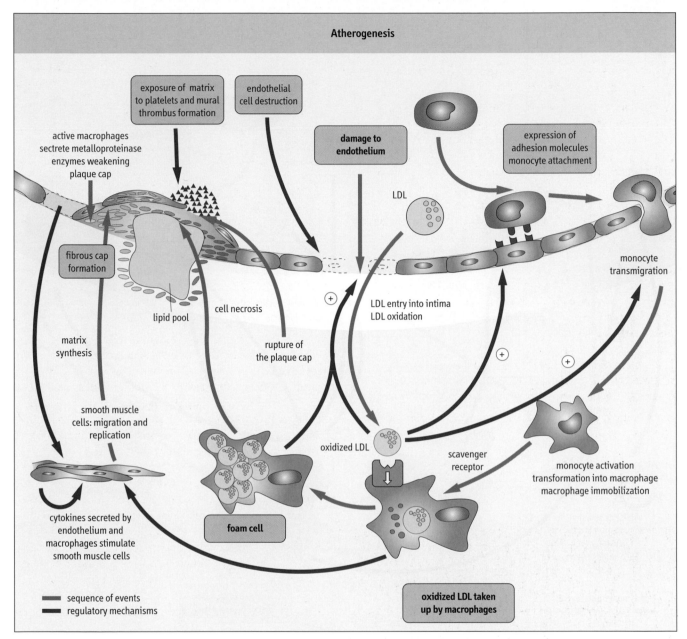

Atherogenesis

exposure of matrix to platelets and mural thrombus formation

endothelial cell destruction

active macrophages sectrete metalloproteinase enzymes weakening plaque cap

damage to endothelium

LDL

expression of adhesion molecules monocyte attachment

fibrous cap formation

monocyte transmigration

lipid pool

cell necrosis

LDL entry into intima LDL oxidation

matrix synthesis

rupture of the plaque cap

smooth muscle cells: migration and replication

oxidized LDL

scavenger receptor

monocyte activation transformation into macrophage macrophage immobilization

cytokines secreted by endothelium and macrophages stimulate smooth muscle cells

foam cell

sequence of events
regulatory mechanisms

oxidized LDL taken up by macrophages

Fig 17.8 **Atherogenesis: the process.** Atherogenesis is driven by signals mediated by cytokines and growth factors generated by all the major types of cells participating in the process: endothelial cells, macrophages, T lymphocytes and vascular smooth muscle cells (VSMC). There are multiple activation paths: for instance, the expression of MCP-1 and VCAM-1 may be stimulated by signals generated macrophages as well as by the oxidized LDL. VSMC may be stimulated by the dysfunctional endothelial cells, by macrophages, and by T lymphocytes (note also the autocrine activation). Note that a hormone, angiotensin II also participates in these processes. MCP-1: monocyte chemoattractant protein 1, VCAM-1: vascular cell adhesion molecule 1, ICAM-1: intracellular cell adhesion molecule 1, TNFβ: tumor necrosis factor beta, TNFα: tumor necrosis factor alpha, IFNγ: interferon gamma, NO: nitric oxide, PDGF: platelet-derived growth factor, bFGF: basic fibroblast growth factor, IGF-1: insulin-like growth factor 1, EGF: epidermal growth factor, TGFβ: transforming growth factor beta, IL-1: interleukin 1.

Dysfunctional endothelium expresses the so-called adhesion molecules on its surface. Molecules called selectins mediate the initial, 'rolling' interaction of cells with the endothelium. The key molecule that promotes adhesion of monocytes (white blood cells that are the precursors of macrophages) and T lymphocytes is the vascular cell-adhesion molecule-1 (VCAM-1) (see also Fig. 25.14). The adhering cells are then stimulated by the monocyte chemoat-tractant protein-1 (MCP-1) to cross the endothelium and lodge in the intima.

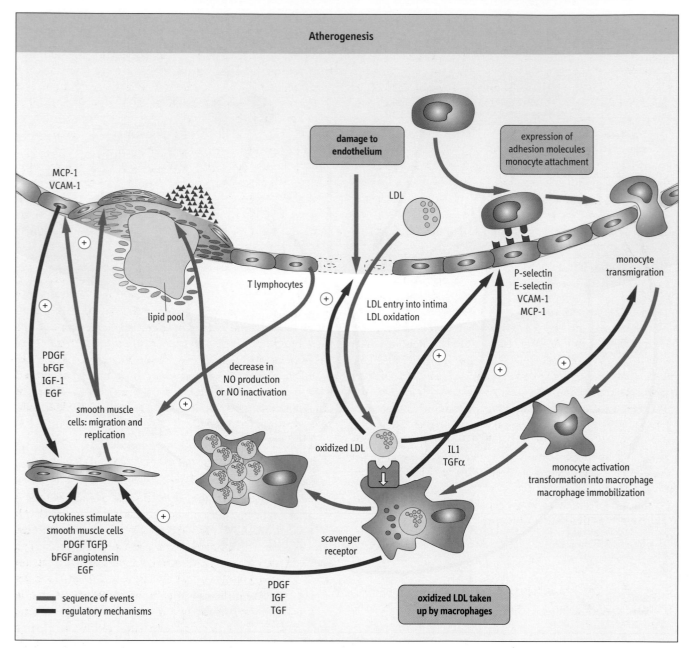

Fig. 17.9 **Atherogenesis: role of growth factors and cytokines.** Atherogenesis involves endothelial dysfunction, arterial deposition of lipids, inflammatory reaction, and the migration and proliferation of the arterial smooth muscle cells. Note the key role of lipid oxidation in the formation of lipid-laden cells and the lipid center of the atherosclerotic plaque. The sequence of events, and their control by cytokines and growth factors are described in the text. (Compare Fig. 17.8.)

In the intima, under the influence of monocyte colony-stimulating factor (M-CSF) secreted by the endothelial cells and VSMC, the monocytes transform into resident macrophages. T lymphocytes also enter the vascular wall at this stage. Macrophages produce reactive oxygen species, which oxidize LDL present in the intima. The expression of macrophage scavenger receptors (such as the scavenger receptor A , and CD36) also increases.

The hormone angiotensin II (see Chapter 22) also contributes to cell entry into intima by contributing to the increased expression of VCAM-1 and MCP-1. In addition, the production of nitric oxide decreases in the damaged endothelium. NO normally reduces monocyte adhesion and VSMC migration and proliferation. Its decrease also shifts the balance between vascular vasodilatation and vasoconstriction towards the latter.

Lipid entry into the arterial wall is a key process in atherogenesis

Another factor which contributes to the induction of VCAM-1 and MCP-1 is hypercholesterolemia. However, it is the physical entry of lipids into the vascular wall, which is another hallmark of atherosclerosis. The lipoproteins of smaller size, the remnants and the LDL, are the most atherogenic partly because they enter the vascular wall more easily. Moreover, after leaving plasma, the LDL are modified in a way which enhances their potential to cause damage: while in plasma they are protected against oxidation by alpha-tocopherol (vitamin E), and ubiquinol, and by plasma antioxidants such as vitamin C and β-carotene. However, that protection does not apply to the extracellular space where the concentration of antioxidants is much lower. Therefore, once LDL exit plasma, their phospholipids and fatty acids oxidize. Enzymes such as lipoxygenases, myeloperoxidase, and NADPH oxidases present in the activated macrophages facilitate LDL oxidation.

Oxidized LDL become yet another factor which stimulates the expression of VCAM-1 and MCP-1. They are also cytotoxic to the endothelial cells and are mitogenic for macrophages. Most importantly though, the LDL 'driver' apolipoprotein, apoB100, once oxidized, binds to the scavenger receptors, and these receptors are not subject to regulation by the intracellular cholesterol level. Therefore, macrophages which take up oxidized LDL overload themselves with lipids. As a result, they change into the so-called foam cells: conglomerates of these cells are visible in the arterial walls as yellow patches, and are called fatty streaks. Dying foam cells release lipid that pools within the intima. These lipid accumulations become centers of the atherosclerotic plaques.

Migration and proliferation of the vascular smooth muscle cells change the structure of the vascular wall

All the above is accompanied by profound changes in the behavior of VSMC. VSMC stimulated by growth factors such as the platelet-derived growth factor (PDGF), the epidermal growth factor (EGF) and the insulin-like growth factor-1 (IGF-1), proliferate and migrate toward the lumen of the arterial wall (see also Chapters 38 and 41). They also secrete adhesion molecules and MCP-1 and, as do the endothelial cells, a range of cytokines and growth factors such as interleukin-1 (IL-1), and tumor necrosis factor (TNF-α). Importantly, activated VSMC also synthesize extracellular matrix, in particular collagen, which is deposited in the forming plaque. As a result, the normally ordered structure of the arterial wall becomes completely disrupted, and the forming plaque may protrude into the lumen of the artery, interfering with the flow of blood.

Inflammation plays a fundamental role in atherogenesis

The exit of monocytes and T leukocytes from plasma and their activation in the intima are parts of the inflammatory response. Normally, such response is initiated by an antigen or trauma. However, no specific antigen capable of intiating atherogenesis has been identified to date.

It is possible that there is a molecular mimicry between the antigens involved in atherosclerosis and the exogenous pathogens (Chapter 36). Such putative antigen(s) might be infectious agents, or molecules modified by reactive oxygen species. For instance, phosphorylcholine group found in the oxidized LDL is also a component of the capsular polysaccharide of bacteria. Indeed, oxidized LDL remains a candidate antigen which could be responsible for the stimulation of inflammatory reaction in atherosclerosis.

Atherogenesis involves both innate and adaptive immunity (see Chapter 36). Innate immunity includes recognition by scavenger receptors A, CD36 (Chapter 36). When molecules which possess patterns encoded in immune memory bind to these receptors, they activate cells through, for instance, the pathway involving the transcription factor NF-κB. We also know that T cells, involved in adaptive immunity, are present in both early and late atherosclerotic lesions. Finally, circulating IgG and IgM-type antibodies against modified LDL have been identified in plasma.

Atherosclerotic plaques grow slowly, but the real danger is their sudden rupture

As we already learned, the foam cells and the lipid pool form the center of developing atherosclerotic plaques. VSMC which had migrated into the intima synthesize new collagenous matrix which now forms a fibrous 'cap' over the lipid pool. This cap, however, is far from an inert structure: it contains VSMC themselves, macrophages, and T lymphocytes. The lipid pool and the cap constitute the mature atherosclerotic plaque, that on the one hand penetrates the arterial wall, and on the other obstructs the arterial lumen (Fig. 17.10). Parts of the more advanced lesions may also become calcified.

A plaque decreases the blood flow to the area supplied by the affected vessel. In the coronary arteries, which supply the blood to the heart muscle, the obstruction by a plaque eventually results in the patient experiencing angina pectoris. If the narrowing occurs in the arteries supplying the legs, it causes intermittent claudication; if it is present in the carotid arteries it may cause the so-called transient ischemic attacks. A plaque may grow slowly and remain stable for long periods of time (in such case the severity of symptoms does not increase: a patient continues to have, for instance, a so-called stable angina). Extensive arteriosclerotic changes can also develop within the arterial wall without much affecting the lumen.

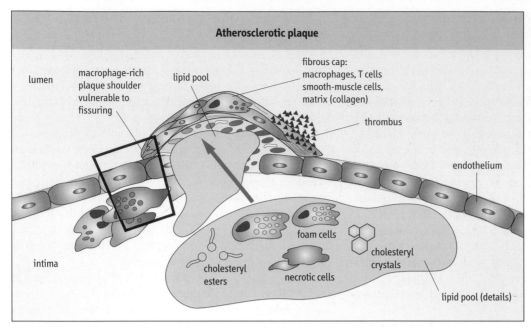

Atherosclerotic plaque

lumen

macrophage-rich plaque shoulder vulnerable to fissuring

lipid pool

fibrous cap: macrophages, T cells smooth-muscle cells, matrix (collagen)

thrombus

endothelium

intima

cholesteryl esters

foam cells

necrotic cells

cholesteryl crystals

lipid pool (details)

Fig. 17.10 **Atherosclerotic plaque.** The lipid center and fibrous cap are the main parts of a mature atherosclerotic plaque which emerges from the structurally changed vascular wall. The so-called vulnerable plaque ruptures easily. This figure illustrates areas vulnerable to breakage and shows the obstructing thrombus formed at the rupture site.

The plaque growth may be periodically accelerated by a cycle of plaque rupture and thrombosis. This is how it happens:

Active macrophages and T lymphocytes preferentially reside at the edges of the plaque (Fig. 17.10). There, macrophages secrete enzymes which degrade extracellular matrix in the plaque cap: these enzymes belong to the metalloproteinase (MMP) family, which includes collagenases, gelatinases, and stromyelysin. In addition, T cells activated by macrophages secrete interferon-γ (IFN-γ) and pro-inflammatory cytokines IL-1, IL-2, and TNF-α. IFN-γ is particularly dangerous because it induces macrophage MMP expression. It also inhibits VSMC proliferation and their collagen synthesis, further weakening the cap. VSMC present in the most vulnerable edge regions of the plaque undergo apoptosis. All this creates a plaque that is prone to rupture.

When such unstable plaque ruptures, it exposes its interior to the blood. The interior is highly thrombogenic due to the presence of the tissue factor, a small-molecular-weight glycoprotein that initiates the extrinsic clotting cascade (see Chapter 6). Tissue factor forms a complex with factor VII/VIIa and this in turn activates factors IX and X. Platelets are also activated, and the thrombus forms quickly on the surface of a ruptured plaque. A thrombus which completely occludes the arterial lumen causes tissue necrosis in the area supplied by the involved artery. In the heart this is a myocardial infarction, and in the brain, a stroke.

Not all instances of plaque rupture result in dramatic, complete lumen blockages. However, even small haemorrhages and thrombi forming either within the plaque, or on its surface, accelerate expansion of the plaque. The plaque grows faster than VSMC proliferation-matrix synthesis mechanism

alone would allow, and may worsen angina. Such stepwise growth is the main mechanism of plaque expansion.

CARDIOVASCULAR RISK AND ITS ASSESSMENT

Plasma concentrations of lipoproteins are one of the important factors in the assessment of the cardiovascular risk of an individual (a probability that that person will suffer from heart attack or stroke in the future). However, there are also other, non-lipid cardiovascular risk factors, and they are listed in Table 17.5.

As far as lipids are concerned, the risk of cardiovascular disease is related to plasma concentrations of total cholesterol (Fig. 17.11), LDL-cholesterol, HDL-cholesterol, and triacylglycerols (triglycerides) The inclusion of triglycerides had been disputed for a long time, and some risk factor lists do not include them to this date. However, recent research made it quite clear that they contribute to risk (Fig. 17.10). The risk increases when the total cholesterol level is above 5.2 mmol/L (200 mg/dL). According to the recommendations of the U.S. National Cholesterol Education Program, the desirable level of total cholesterol is that below 5.2 mmol/L (200 mg/dL) and the optimal level of LDL-cholesterol is below 2.6 mmol/L (100 mg/dL). In contrast to LDL, the relationship between the HDL concentration and cardiovascular risk is inverse: it is the low concentration of HDL which signifies increased risk. The undesirably low concentration of HDL-cholesterol is below 1 mmol/L (40 g/dL) but a concentration above 1.6 mmol/L (60 mg/dL) is regarded as providing some protection against

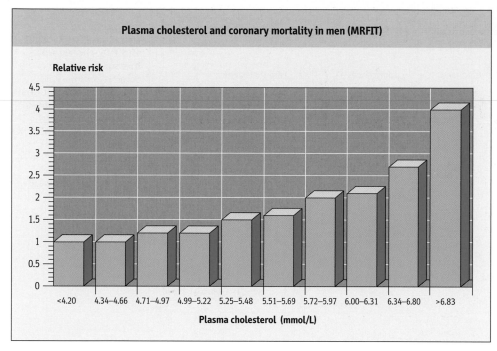

Fig. 17.11 **Plasma cholesterol and coronary mortality in men.** Total cholesterol concentration in plasma in relation to the number of deaths from heart disease in a population. Note: converting plasma lipid values into SI units: cholesterol: to convert mg/dL into mmol/L, mutliply by 0.02586; triglycerides: to convert mg/dL into mmol/L, multiply by 0.01129. The data are from the Multiple Risk Factor Intervention Trial (MRFIT). Stammler *et al. JAMA* 1986;256:2823.

Cardiovascular risk factors and their management

Risk factor	Comment	Remedy
Male sex	the difference in cardiovascular risk between sexes equalizes in postmenopausal women	
Age		
Smoking		smoking cessation
High plasma cholesterol (high LDL-cholesterol)	2–3% decrease in risk for 1% decrease of total plasma cholesterol	diet low in saturated fats and, where appropriate, cholesterol-lowering drugs
Low plasma HDL		smoking cessation, regular exercise
Hypertension	major risk factor for stroke and a risk factor for CHD	control blood pressure: diet and drugs
Obesity		weight reduction
Sedentary lifestyle		regular moderate exercise
Diabetes	cardiovascular disease is the main cause of death in diabetes	diet and drugs (insulin in type 1 diabetes). Lipid-lowering if dyslipidemia present

Table 17.5 **Cardiovascular risk factors and their management.** Plasma lipids are not the only factors that determine the risk of cardiovascular disease. This table lists the most important cardiovascular risk factors and the risk-reducing strategies used in cardiovascular prevention. You will find more on dietary aspects of cardiovascular prevention in Chapter 21.

coronary disease. Clinical interpretation of the fasting lipid profile is summarized in Figure 17.11.

One should remember that the risk associated with lipid concentration can be modified by other factors, such as increased concentration of Lp(a), plasma homocysteine, fibrinogen, or C-reactive protein (CRP; see below). In fact, about 50% of persons who suffer from myocardial infarction have 'average' lipid concentrations. Thus, the search continues for new markers that would more precisely define individual cardiovascular risk. The measurement of substances associated with the inflammatory response, such as small increases in plasma CRP concentration, seem to fulfill this role particularly well.

The risk of an atherosclerotic event such as myocardial infarction or stroke, can be decreased by eliminating risk factors through diet, exercise, smoking cessation, control of

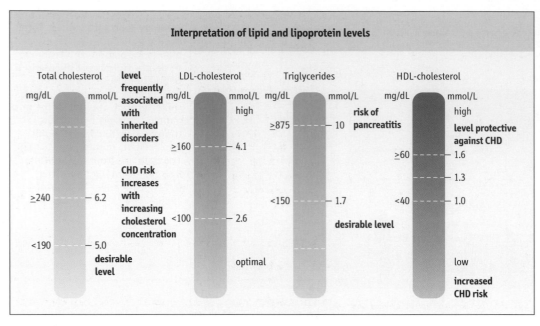

Fig. 17.12 **The interpretation of cholesterol, triglyceride, and HDL-cholesterol measurements.** To convert plasma lipid values into conventional units: total cholesterol, LDL-cholesterol, and HDL-cholesterol: to convert mmol/L into mg/dL: multiply by 38.67; triglycerides: to convert mmol/L into mg/dL, multiply by 87.5. CHD, coronary heart disease.

LIFESTYLE CHANGE IMPROVES PLASMA LIPID PROFILE

A 57-year-old man was referred to the lipid clinic because of hypertriglyceridemia (high triacylglycerol concentration). His triglycerides were 6 mmol/L (545 mg/dL), cholesterol was 5 mmol/L (192 mg/dL), and HDL was 1 mmol/L (39 mg/dL). He was obese, took 30 units of alcohol per week, and led a sedentary lifestyle.
After a hesitant start he eventually managed to lose 7 kg of weight over 6 months, cut drinking to below 20 units per week, and started to exercise regularly. Twelve months later, his triglycerides were 2.5 mmol/L (227 mg/dL), cholesterol 4.8 mmol/L (186 mg/dL), and HDL 1.2 mmol/L (46 mg/dL).

Comment. Lifestyle change may result in appreciable improvements in the lipid profile. To achieve this, the individuals must be committed to changing lifestyle and to maintaining the change over a prolonged period of time. In practice this is often difficult.

Note: 1 unit of alcohol is a one measure (60 mL) of liquor, a one glass (170 mL) of wine, or a half-pint (300 mL) of beer.

lower plasma cholesterol concentration either by inhibiting intracellular cholesterol synthesis (HMG-CoA reductase inhibitors known as statins, which primarily lower plasma cholesterol), by stimulating LPL, decreasing triacylglycerol concentration, and increasing HDL (derivatives of fibric acid, fibrates), or by preventing cholesterol absorption in the intestine (bile acid binding resins, now relatively rarely used, and ezetimibe, an inhibitor of intestinal cholesterol transporter).

In animals, antioxidants such as probucol, vitamin E, or butylated hydroxytoluene inhibit atherosclerotic changes. β-carotene and α-tocopherol protect LDL against oxidation *in vitro* and treatment with antioxidants increases the resistance of LDL to oxidation. Epidemiologic studies have shown that those who take antioxidants such as vitamin E and C or β-carotene have cardiovascular disease less often. However, the puzzling finding is that the prospective clinical trials of antioxidant treatment have failed to confirm their preventive benefit. One tentative explanation for this is that it is the natural antioxidants (such as these contained in fruits) or their combinations, rather than single pure substances which are protective.

The most important, however, is this: since arteriosclerosis is a multifactorial process, the effective cardiovascular prevention needs to involve a comprehensive approach which combines lifestyle modification (smoking cessation, diet and exercise) with appropriate treatment of dyslipidemia, hypertension and diabetes.

high blood pressure, and by lowering undesirably high plasma lipoprotein concentrations (Table 17.5).

The concentration of plasma LDL (and consequently total plasma cholesterol) can decrease when a person follows a low-cholesterol diet. In addition, there are several drugs that

THE PRESENCE OF XANTHELASMA DOES NOT NECESSARILY SIGNIFY A LIPID DISORDER

A 28-year-old lady developed unsightly yellow marks around both eyes, so-called xanthelasma but otherwise she was asymptomatic. Her cholesterol was 5.0 mmol/L (192 mg/dL), triglycerides 0.7 mmol/L (64 mg/dL), and her HDL-cholesterol was 1.4 mmol/L (53 mg/dL). There was no family history of early coronary disease.

Comment. Xanthelasma may occur in individuals with completely normal lipid levels. On the other hand, lipid deposits in tendons (tendon xanthomata) are always diagnostic of familial lipid disorder. The patient was reassured and referred for cosmetic surgery.

ACTIVE LEARNING

1. Compare the composition of VLDL and LDL.
2. What are the differences between the transport of dietary triacylglycerols and triacylglycerols synthesized in the liver?
3. Describe the transport pathway for dietary fatty acids.
4. Give examples of interactions between different cell types in atherogenesis
5. Discuss the mechanism of atherosclerotic plaque rupture.
6. In what way endothelial dysfunction contributes to atherosclerosis?

Further reading

Dominiczak MH. Risk factors for coronary disease: the time for a paradigm shift? *Clin Chem Lab Med* 2001;**39**:907–19.

Expert Panel on Detection, Evaluation and Treatment of High Blood Cholesterol in Adults. Executive Summary of the Third Report of the National Cholesterol Education Program (NCEP) Expert Panel on Detection, Evaluation and Treatment of High Blood Cholesterol in Adults (Adult Treatment Panel III). *JAMA* 2001;**285**:2486–97.

Libby P. Inflammation in atherosclerosis. *Nature* 2002;**420**:868–874.

Libby P, Aikawa M. Stabilization of atherosclerotic plaques: New mechanisms and clinical targets. *Nature Medicine* 2002;**8**:1257–1262.

Prevention of coronary heart disease in clinical practice. Summary of Recommendations of the Second Joint Task Force of European and other Societies on Coronary Prevention, 1998.

Steinberg D. Atherogenesis in perspective: hypercholesterolemia and inflammation as partners in crime. *Nature Medicine* 2002;**8**:1211–17.

Durrington P. Dyslipidaemia. *Lancet* 2003;**362**:717–31.

DeBacker G, Ambrosioni E, Bouch-Johnson K, et al. European guidelines on cardiovascular disease prevention in clinical practice. Third Joint Task Force of European and Other Societies on Cardiovascular Disease Prevention in Clinical Practice. *Eur Heart J* 2003;**24**:1601–10.

Summary

1. Lipoproteins are a transport vehicle for hydrophobic lipids.
2. Chylomicrons mediate the transport of dietary fat.
3. VLDL mediate the transport of endogenously synthesized fat.
4. Chylomicrons, VLDL and remnant lipoproteins are part of the organism's fuel distribution network: the fuel transport pathway.
5. LDL are cholesterol-rich lipoproteins which emerge from the fuel transport pathway. When present in excess their may enter the arterial wall.
6. HDL mediate reverse cholesterol transport, e.g. removal of cholesterol from the peripheral cells to the liver.
7. Atherogenesis is a complex process involving endothelial dysfunction, lipid deposition, inflammatory reaction in the arterial wall, and activation and proliferation of the arterial smooth muscle cells.
8. Interactions between different types of cells participating in atherogenesis are mediated by an array of cytokines, growth factors and adhesion molecules.
9. Atherogenesis results in a gross disruption of the structure of the arterial wall and the formation of atherosclerotic plaque, which narrows the lumen of the affected artery. However, the cause of heart attack is not the slow growth of the plaque, but its sudden rupture.
10. Arteriosclerosis-related diseases are coronary heart disease, stroke and peripheral vascular disease.

Relevant websites

British Heart Foundation: www.bhf.org.uk/
American Heart Association: www.americanheart.org
National Heart, Lung and Blood Institute: www.nhlbi.nih.gov/nhlbi/nhlbi.htm/

18. Biosynthesis and Degradation of Amino Acids

A B Rawitch

LEARNING OBJECTIVES

After reading this chapter you should be able to:

- Describe the three mechanisms used by humans for removal of the nitrogen from amino acids prior to the metabolism of their carbon skeletons.
- Outline the sequence of reactions in the urea cycle and trace the flow of nitrogen from amino acids into and out of the cycle.
- Describe the role of vitamin B_6 in aminotransferase reactions.
- Define the terms, and give examples of a glucogenic and a ketogenic amino acid.
- Summarize the factors that contribute to the input and the depletion of the pool of free amino acids in animals.
- Summarize the sources and use of ammonia in animals and explain the concept of nitrogen balance.
- Identify the essential amino acids and the metabolic sources of the non-essential amino acids.
- Explain the biochemical basis and the therapeutic rationale for treatment of phenylketonuria and maple syrup urine disease.

INTRODUCTION

In addition to their roles as building blocks for peptides and proteins, and as precursors of neurotransmitters and hormones, amino acids are a source of energy from the diet and during fasting. The carbon skeletons of some amino acids can be used to produce glucose through gluconeogenesis, thereby providing a metabolic fuel for tissues that require or prefer glucose; such amino acids are designated as glucogenic or glycogenic amino acids. The carbon skeletons of some amino acids can also produce the equivalent of acetyl-CoA or acetoacetate and are termed ketogenic, indicating that they can be metabolized to give immediate precursors of lipids or ketone bodies (Fig. 18.1). In an individual consuming adequate amounts of protein, a significant quantity of amino acids may also be converted to carbohydrate (glycogen) or fat (triacylglycerols) for storage. Unlike carbohydrates and lipids, amino acids do not have a dedicated storage form equivalent to glycogen or fat.

When amino acids are metabolized, the resulting excess nitrogen must be excreted. As the primary form in which the nitrogen is removed from amino acids is ammonia, and because free ammonia is quite toxic, humans and most higher animals rapidly convert the ammonia derived from amino acid catabolism to urea, which is neutral, less toxic, very soluble, and excreted in the urine. Thus the primary nitrogenous excretion product in humans is urea, produced by the urea cycle in liver. Animals that excrete urea are termed ureotelic. In an average individual, more than 80% of the excreted nitrogen is in the form of urea (25–30 g/24 hours). Small amounts of nitrogen are also excreted in the form of uric acid, creatinine, and ammonium ion.

The carbon skeletons of many amino acids may be derived from metabolites in central pathways, allowing the biosynthesis of some, but not all, the amino acids in humans. Amino acids that can be synthesized in this way are therefore not required in the diet (non-essential amino acids), whereas amino acids having carbon skeletons that cannot be derived from normal human metabolism must be supplied in the diet (essential amino acids). In contrast to the catabolic process, for the biosynthesis of non-essential amino acids, amino groups must be added to the appropriate carbon skeletons. This generally occurs through the transamination of an α-keto acid corresponding to that specific amino acid.

Amino acids from body proteins and the diet

Relationship to central metabolism

Although body proteins represent a significant proportion of potential energy reserves (Table 18.1), under normal circumstances they are not used for energy production. In an extended fast, however, muscle protein is degraded to amino acids for the synthesis of essential proteins and for gluconeogenesis to maintain blood glucose concentration. This accounts for the loss of muscle mass during fasting.

In addition to its role as an important source of carbon skeletons for oxidative metabolism and energy production, dietary protein must provide adequate amounts of those amino acids that we cannot make, to support normal protein synthesis. The relationships of body protein and dietary protein to central amino acid pools and to central metabolism are illustrated in Figure 18.1.

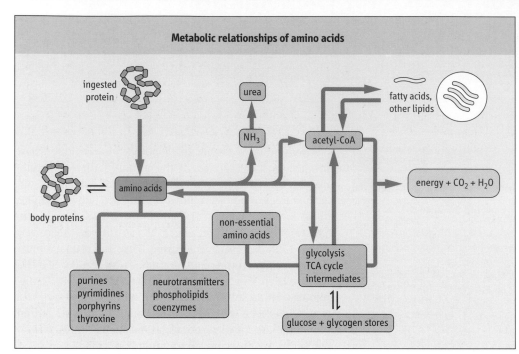

Metabolic relationships of amino acids

Fig. 18.1 **Metabolic relationships of amino acids.** The pool of free amino acids is derived from the degradation and turnover of body proteins and from the diet. The amino acids are precursors of important biomolecules, including hormones, neurotransmitters and proteins, and also serve as a carbon source for central metabolism, including gluconeogenesis, lipogenesis and energy production.

 ## ALANINE AND INTER-ORGAN CARBON AND NITROGEN FLOW

Much of the carbon flow that occurs between skeletal muscle – and several other tissues – and the liver is facilitated by the release of alanine into the blood by peripheral tissues, and its uptake by the liver. The alanine taken into the liver is converted to pyruvate and the nitrogen component is incorporated into urea. The pyruvate can be used for gluconeogenesis to produce glucose, which is released into the blood for transport back to peripheral tissues. This 'glucose-alanine cycle' allows the net conversion of amino acid carbons to glucose, the elimination of amino acid nitrogen as urea, and the return of carbons to the peripheral tissues in the form of glucose. This cycle works in a fashion similar to the Cori cycle (Chapters 12 and 20), in which lactate is released into the blood by skeletal muscle and used for gluconeogenesis in the liver, the key difference being that alanine also carries a nitrogen atom to the liver. It is of significance that alanine and glutamine are released in approximately equal quantities from skeletal muscle and represent almost 50% of the amino acids released by skeletal muscle into the blood – an amount that far exceeds the proportion of these amino acids in muscle proteins. Thus, there is substantial remodeling of protein-derived amino acids by transamination reactions, prior to their release from muscle.

Storage forms of energy in the body

Stored fuel	Tissue	Amount (g)*	Energy (kj)	(kcal)
Glycogen	liver	70	1176	280
Glycogen	muscle	120	2016	480
Free glucose	body fluids	20	336	80
Triacylglycerol	adipose	15 000	567 000	135 000
Protein	muscle	6000	100 800	24 000

*in a 70-kg individual

Table 18.1 **Storage forms of energy in the body.** Proteins represent a substantial energy reserve in the body. (Adapted with permission from Cahill GF Jr, *Clin Endocrinol Metab* 1976;5:398.)

Digestion and absorption of dietary protein

In order for dietary protein to contribute to either energy metabolism or pools of essential amino acids, the protein must be digested to the level of free amino acids or small peptides and absorbed across the gut. Digestion of protein begins in the stomach with the action of pepsin, a protease with an active-site carboxyl group, which is active at the low pH found in the stomach. Digestion continues as the stomach contents are emptied into the small intestine and mixed with pancreatic secretions. These pancreatic secretions are alkaline and contain the inactive precursors of several serine proteases including trypsin, chymotrypsin and elastase along with carboxypeptidases. The digestion process is completed by enzymes in the small intestine (see Chapter 9). After any remaining di- and tripeptides are broken down in enterocytes, the free amino acids are transported to the portal vein and carried to the liver for energy metabolism or biosynthesis, or distributed to other tissues to meet similar needs. Once inside the tissues, those amino acids destined for energy metabolism must be deaminated to yield the carbon skeleton. There are three mechanisms for removal of the amino group from amino acids:

- **Transamination** – the transfer of the amino group to a suitable keto acid acceptor; most often α-ketoglutarate or oxaloacetate; this reaction requires pyridoxal phosphate and involves a pyridoxamine intermediate;
- **oxidative deamination** – the oxidative removal of the amino group, also resulting in keto acids; the amino acid oxidases are flavoproteins, and produce ammonia;
- **removal of a molecule of water by a dehydratase** – e.g. serine or threonine dehydratase; this reaction produces an unstable, imine intermediate that hydrolyzes spontaneously to yield an α-keto acid and ammonia.

Amino acid degradation

Metabolism of the carbon skeleton and the amino group are coordinated

Before the carbon skeletons of most amino acids can be metabolized, the α-amino group must be removed. The principal mechanism for removal of amino groups from the common amino acids is via transamination (above), or the transferring the amino group from the amino acid to a suitable α-keto acid acceptor, most commonly to α-ketoglutarate or oxaloacetate. Several enzymes, called amino transferases (or transaminases), are capable of removing the amino group from most amino acids and producing the corresponding α-keto acid. Aminotransferase enzymes use pyridoxal phosphate, a cofactor derived from the vitamin B_6 (pyridoxine), as a key component in their catalytic mechanism. These structures and the net reaction catalyzed by amino transferases are shown in Figure 18.2.

Nitrogen atoms are incorporated into urea from two sources

The transfer of an amino group from one keto acid carbon skeleton to another may seem to be unproductive and not useful in itself; however, when one considers the nature of the primary keto acid acceptors that participate in these reactions (α-ketoglutarate and oxaloacetate) and their products (glutamate and aspartate), the logic of this metabolism becomes clear. Nitrogen atoms are incorporated into urea exclusively from these two sources (Fig. 18.3), which link amino acid catabolism to energy metabolism. Ammonia produced primarily from glutamate (via the glutamate dehydrogenase (GDH) reaction, see Fig. 18.4) enters the urea cycle as carbamoyl phosphate. The second nitrogen is contributed to urea by aspartic acid. Fumarate is formed in this process and may be recycled via the TCA cycle to oxaloacetate, which can

The catalytic role of pyridoxal phosphate

A

pyridoxal phosphate   Schiff base form   pyridoxamine form

B

amino acid   keto acid   keto acid   amino acid

Fig. 18.2 **The catalytic role of pyridoxal phosphate.** Amino transferases or transaminases use pyridoxal phosphate as a cofactor and involve a pyridoxamine adduct which acts as an intermediate in transfer of an amino group between an α-amino acid and an α-keto acid. (A) Structures of the components involved. The cofactor, pyridoxal phosphate, is used in a variety of enzyme-catalyzed reactions involving both amino and keto compounds, including transamination and decarboxylation reactions. (B) Transamination involves both a donor α-amino acid (R_1), and an acceptor α-keto acid (R_2). The products are an α-keto acid derived from the carbon skeleton of R_1 and an α-amino acid from the carbon skeleton of R_2.

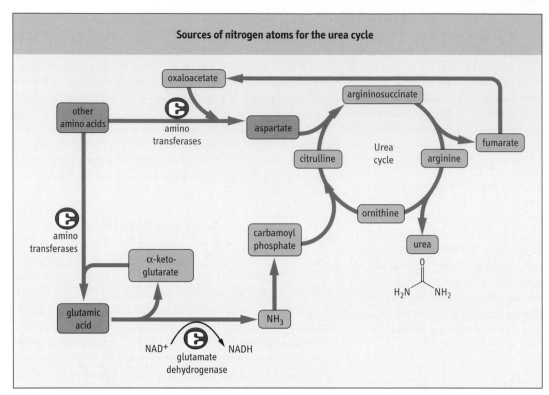

Sources of nitrogen atoms for the urea cycle

Fig. 18.3 **Sources of nitrogen atoms for the urea cycle.** Nitrogen enters the urea cycle from most amino acids via transfer of the α-amino group to either α-ketoglutarate or oxaloacetate, to form aspartate or glutamate, respectively. Glutamate releases ammonia in the liver through the action of GDH. The ammonia is incorporated into carbamoyl phosphate, and the aspartate combines with citrulline to provide the second nitrogen for urea synthesis. Oxaloacetate and α-ketoglutarate can be repeatedly recycled to channel nitrogen into this pathway.

MEASUREMENT OF BLOOD UREA NITROGEN

Blood urea measurements (BUN or blood urea nitrogen) are critical in monitoring patients with a variety of metabolic diseases in which the metabolism of amino acids may be affected, and in tracking the condition of individuals with renal disease. The traditional methodology used for measuring blood urea levels has relied on the action of the enzyme urease which converts urea to CO_2 and ammonia. The resulting ammonia can be detected spectrophotometrically by formation of a colored compound on reaction with phenol or a related compound (the Berthelot reaction). Recently, the direct detection of urea by near infrared spectroscopy and fluorescence coupled assays has been proposed to decrease sample processing and increase sensitivity.

MONOSODIUM GLUTAMATE REACTION

A healthy 30-year-old woman experienced the sudden onset of headache, sweating, and nausea after eating at an oriental restaurant. She felt weak, and experienced some tingling and a sensation of warmth in her face and upper torso. The symptoms passed after about 30 minutes and she experienced no further problems. Upon visiting her doctor the next day, she learned that some individuals react to foods containing high levels of the food additive monosodium glutamate, the sodium salt of glutamic acid.

Comment. The flu-like symptoms that develop, previously described as 'Chinese Restaurant Syndrome', have been attributed to central nervous system (CNS) effects of glutamate or its derivative, the inhibitory neurotransmitter, γ-amino butyric acid (GABA). Interestingly, studies have shown that this phenomenon causes no permanent CNS damage and that, although bronchospasm may be triggered in individuals with severe asthma, the symptoms are generally brief and completely reversible.

accept another amino group to reform aspartate or participate in either the TCA cycle or gluconeogenesis (see Fig. 18.7 and Chapter 12). Thus the funneling of amino groups from other amino acids into glutamate and aspartate provides the nitrogen for urea synthesis in a form appropriate for the urea cycle (see below). The other pathways that lead to the release of amino groups from some amino acids through the action of amino acid oxidases or a dehydratase mechanism (Fig. 18.5) make relatively minor contributions to the flow of amino groups from amino acids to urea.

Glutamine and alanine are key transporters of amino groups between muscle and the liver

In addition to the role of glutamate as a carrier of amino groups to GDH, glutamate serves as a precursor of glutamine, a process that consumes a molecule of ammonia. This is

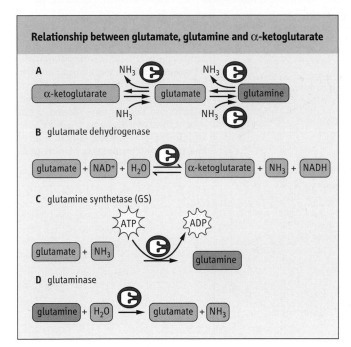

Relationship between glutamate, glutamine and α-ketoglutarate

A

B glutamate dehydrogenase

C glutamine synthetase (GS)

D glutaminase

Fig. 18.4 **Relationship between glutamate, glutamine and α-ketoglutarate.** The several forms of the carbon skeleton of glutamic acid have key roles in the metabolism of amino groups. (A) Three forms of the same carbon skeleton. (B) The GDH reaction is a reversible reaction that can produce glutamate from α-ketoglutarate or convert glutamate to α-ketoglutarate and ammonia. The latter reaction is important in the synthesis of urea because amino groups are fed to α-ketoglutarate via transamination from other amino acids. (C) Glutamine synthetase (GS) catalyzes an energy-requiring reaction with a key role in transport of amino groups from one tissue to another; it also provides a buffer against high concentrations of free ammonia in tissues. (D) The second half of the glutamine transport system for nitrogen is the enzyme, glutaminase, which hydrolyzes glutamine to glutamate and ammonia. This reaction is important in the kidney for management of proton transport and pH control.

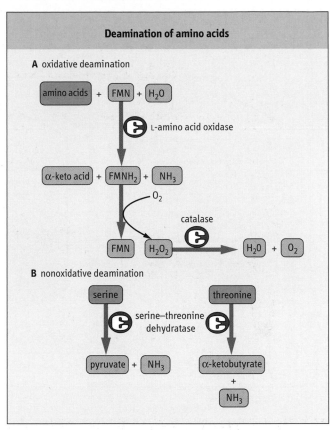

Deamination of amino acids

A oxidative deamination

B nonoxidative deamination

Fig. 18.5 **Deamination of amino acids.** The primary route for amino group removal is via transamination, but there are additional enzymes capable of removing the α-amino group. (A) L-amino acid oxidase produces ammonia and an α-keto acid directly, using flavin mononucleotide (FMN) as a cofactor. The reduced form of the flavin must be regenerated using molecular oxygen; this reaction is one of several that produce H_2O_2. The peroxide is decomposed by catalase. (B) A second means of deamination is possible only for hydroxyamino acids (serine and threonine), through a dehydratase mechanism; the Schiff base imine intermediate hydrolyzes to form the keto acid and ammonia.

important because glutamine, along with alanine (see Chapter 2), is a key transporter of amino groups between various tissues and the liver, and is present in greater concentrations than most other amino acids in blood. The three forms of the same carbon skeleton, α-ketoglutarate, glutamate, and glutamine, are interconverted via amino transferases, glutamate dehydrogenase, glutamine synthetase and glutaminase (Fig. 18.4). Thus glutamine can serve as a buffer for ammonia utilization, as a source of ammonia, and as a carrier of amino groups. Because ammonia is quite toxic, a balance must be maintained between its production and utilization. A summary of the sources and pathways that use or produce ammonia is shown in Figure 18.6. It should be noted that the glutamate dehydrogenase reaction is reversible under physiological conditions if amino groups are required for amino acid and other biosynthetic processes.

The urea cycle and its relationship to central metabolism

The urea cycle (Fig. 18.7 and Table 18.2) was the first metabolic cycle to be well defined; its description preceded that of the TCA cycle. The start of the urea cycle may be considered the synthesis of carbamoyl phosphate from an ammonium ion and bicarbonate in liver mitochondria (Fig. 18.8). This reaction requires two molecules of ATP and is catalyzed by the enzyme, carbamoyl phosphate synthetase I (CPS I), which is found in high concentrations in the mitochondrial matrix.

The mitochondrial enzyme, CPS I, is unusual in that it requires N-acetylglutamate as a cofactor. It is one of two carbamoyl phosphate synthetase enzymes that have key roles in metabolism. The second, CPS II, is found in the cytosol, does

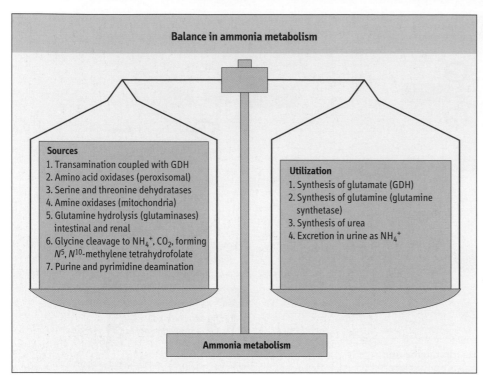

Balance in ammonia metabolism

Sources
1. Transamination coupled with GDH
2. Amino acid oxidases (peroxisomal)
3. Serine and threonine dehydratases
4. Amine oxidases (mitochondria)
5. Glutamine hydrolysis (glutaminases) intestinal and renal
6. Glycine cleavage to NH_4^+, CO_2, forming N^5, N^{10}-methylene tetrahydrofolate
7. Purine and pyrimidine deamination

Utilization
1. Synthesis of glutamate (GDH)
2. Synthesis of glutamine (glutamine synthetase)
3. Synthesis of urea
4. Excretion in urine as NH_4^+

Ammonia metabolism

Fig. 18.6 **Balance in ammonia metabolism.** The balance between production and utilization of free ammonia is critical for maintenance of health. This figure summarizes the sources and pathways that use ammonia. Although most of these reactions occur in many tissues, urea synthesis is restricted to the liver. Glutamine and alanine function as the primary transporters of nitrogen from peripheral tissues to the liver.

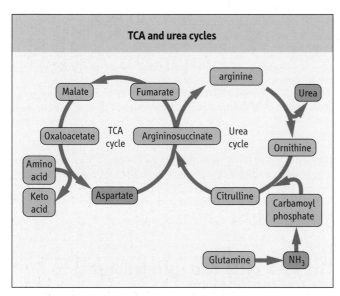

TCA and urea cycles

Fig. 18.7 **TCA and urea cycles.** Analysis of the urea cycle reveals that it is really two cycles: with the carbon flow split between the primary urea synthetic process and the recycling of fumarate to aspartate; the latter cycle occurs in the mitochondrion and involves parts of the citric acid cycle.

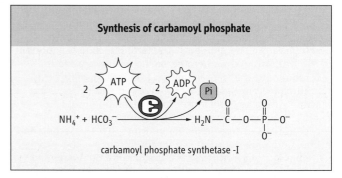

Synthesis of carbamoyl phosphate

carbamoyl phosphate synthetase -I

Fig. 18.8 **Synthesis of carbamoyl phosphate.** Ammonia enters the urea cycle as carbamoyl phosphate, synthesized by carbamoyl phosphate synthetase in liver.

cleaves the ATP to adenosine monophosphate (AMP) and inorganic pyrophosphate (PPi) (2 ATP equivalents). The formation of argininosuccinate brings to the complex the second nitrogen atom destined for urea. Argininosuccinate is in turn cleaved by argininosuccinase, to arginine and fumarate. The arginine produced in this series of reactions is then cleaved by arginase, to a molecule of urea and one of ornithine. The ornithine can then be used to reinitiate this cyclic pathway, while the urea diffuses into the blood, is transported to the kidney, and excreted in urine. The net process of urea synthesis is summarized in Table 18.3.

The urea cycle is split between the mitochondrial matrix and the cytosol

The first two steps in the urea cycle occur in the mitochondrion. The citrulline then diffuses into the cytosol, where the

not require N-acetylglutamate, and is involved in pyrimidine biosynthesis (Chapter 29).

Ornithine transcarbamoylase catalyzes the condensation of carbamoyl phosphate with the amino acid, ornithine, to form citrulline. In turn, the citrulline is condensed with aspartate to form argininosuccinate. This step is catalyzed by argininosuccinate synthetase and requires ATP; the reaction

Enzymes of the urea cycle

Enzyme	Reaction catalyzed	Remarks	Reaction Product
Carbamoyl phosphate synthetase	formation of carbamoyl phosphate from ammonia and CO_2	fixes ammonia released from amino acids, especially glutamine, uses 2 ATP, located in the **mitochondrion**, deficiency leads to high blood concentrations of ammonia and related toxicity	
Ornithine transcarbamoylase	formation of citrulline from ornithine and carbamoyl phosphate	releases P_i, an example of a transferase, located in the **mitochondrion**, deficiency leads to high blood concentrations of ammonia and orotic acid, as carbamoyl phosphate is shunted to pyrimidine biosynthesis	citrulline
Argininosuccinate synthetase	formation of argininosuccinate from citrulline and aspartate	requires ATP, which is cleaved to AMP + PP_i – an example of a ligase, located in the **cytosol**, deficiency leads to high blood concentrations of ammonia and citrulline	arginosuccinate
Argininosuccinase	cleavage of argininosuccinate to arginine and fumarate	an example of a lyase, located in **cytosol**, deficiency leads to high blood concentrations of ammonia and citrulline	fumarate + arginine
Arginase	cleavage of arginine to ornithine and urea	an example of a hydrolase, located in the **cytosol** and primarily in the liver, deficiency leads to moderately increased blood ammonia and high blood concentrations of arginine	urea + ornithine

Table 18.2 **Enzymes of the urea cycle.** Five enzymes catalyze the urea cycle in liver. The first enzyme, CPS-1, which fixes NH_4^+ as carbamoyl phosphate, is the regulatory enzyme and is sensitive to the allosteric effector, N-acetylglutamate.

Urea synthesis

Component reactions in urea synthesis

$CO_2 + NH_3 + 2\ ATP$	$\rightarrow$ carbamoyl phosphate + 2 ADP + Pi
Carbamoyl phosphate + ornithine	$\rightarrow$ citrulline + Pi
Citrulline + aspartate + ATP	$\rightarrow$ arginosuccinate + AMP + PPi
Arginosuccinate	$\rightarrow$ arginine + fumarate
Arginine	$\rightarrow$ urea + ornithine
$CO_2 + NH_3 + 3\ ATP +$ aspartate	$\rightarrow$ urea + 2 ADP + AMP + 2 Pi + PPi + fumarate

Table 18.3 **Urea synthesis.**

cycle is completed with the release of urea and the regeneration of ornithine. Ornithine must be transported back across the mitochondrial membrane to continue the cycle. It is also a precursor of putrescine, spermine and other polyamines found in the cell. These compounds bind to DNA and RNA, and function in cell growth and differentiation. Carbons from fumarate, released in the argininosuccinase step, may also re-enter the mitochondrion after hydration to malate and be

❋ AMMONIA TOXICITY

Ammonia encephalopathy

The mechanisms involved in ammonia toxicity – the encephalopathy in particular – are not well-defined. It is clear, however, that when its concentration builds up in the blood and other biological fluids, ammonia diffuses into cells and across the blood/brain barrier. This increase in ammonia causes an increased synthesis of glutamate from α-ketoglutarate and increased synthesis of glutamine. Although this is a normal detoxifying reaction in cells, when concentrations of ammonia are significantly increased, supplies of α-ketoglutarate in cells of the CNS may be depleted, resulting in inhibition of the TCA cycle and production of ATP. There may be additional mechanisms accounting for the bizarre behavior observed in individuals with high blood concentrations of ammonia. Either glutamate, a major excitatory neurotransmitter, or its derivative, γ-amino butyric acid (GABA), an inhibitory neurotransmitter, may also contribute to the CNS effects.

CARBAMOYL PHOSPHATE SYNTHESIS

The enzyme carbamoyl phosphate synthetase I (CPS I) is found in the mitochondrion and primarily in the liver; a second enzyme, CPS II, is found in the cytosol and in virtually all tissues. Although the product of both these enzymes is the same, namely carbamoyl phosphate, the enzymes are derived from different genes and function in urea synthesis (CPS I) or pyrimidine biosynthesis (CPS II), respectively. Additional differences between the two enzymes include their source of nitrogen (NH_3 in the case of the former and glutamine in the latter) and their requirement for N-acetylglutamate (required by the former, but not by the latter). Under normal circumstances, CPS I and II function independently and in different cellular compartments; however, when the urea cycle is blocked as a result of a deficiency in ornithine transcarbamoylase, the accumulated mitochondrial carbamoyl phosphate spills over into the cytosolic compartment and may stimulate excess pyrimidine synthesis, which is reflected in a build-up of orotic acid in blood and urine.

PARKINSON'S DISEASE

An otherwise healthy, 60-year-old man noticed an occasional tremor in his left arm when relaxing and watching television. He also noticed occasional muscle cramping in his left leg, and his spouse noticed that he would occasionally develop a trance-like stare. A complete physical examination and consultation with a neurologist confirmed a diagnosis of Parkinson's disease. He was prescribed a medication that contained L-dihydroxyphenylalanine (L-DOPA) and a monoamine oxidase inhibitor (MAOI). L-DOPA is a precursor of the neurotransmitter dopamine, while monoamine oxidase is the enzyme responsible for the oxidative deamination and degradation of dopamine. His symptoms improved immediately, but he gradually experienced significant side effects from the medication, especially the occurrence of involuntary movements.

Comment. Parkinson's disease is caused by the death of dopamine-producing cells in the substantia nigra and the locus ceruleus. Although medication can markedly reduce the symptoms, the disease is progressive and may result in severe disability. Dopaminergic agonists often have side effects and also have limited effect on tremor so that other treatments such as deep brain stimulation or ablation are used in selected cases. Monoamine oxidase is also involved in deamination of other amine in the brain, so that MAOIs have many undesirable side effects. Transplantation of dopaminergic fetal tissue is a controversial experimental treatment at present (see Chapter 40).

HEREDITARY HYPERAMMONEMIA

An apparently healthy 5-month-old female infant was brought to a pediatrician's office by her mother, with a complaint of periodic bouts of vomiting and a failure to gain weight. The mother also reported that the child would oscillate between periods of irritability and lethargy. Subsequent examination and laboratory results revealed an abnormal electroencephalogram, a markedly increased concentration of plasma ammonia (323 mmol/L [550 mg/dL]; the normal range is 15–88 mmol/L [25–150 mg/dL]), and greater than normal concentrations of glutamine, but low concentrations of citrulline. Orotate, a pyrimidine nucleotide precursor, was found in her urine.

Comment. The infant was admitted to hospital and treated with intravenous phenylacetate and benzoate along with arginine. The infant improved rapidly, and was discharged from hospital on a low-protein diet with arginine supplementation. Subsequent biopsy of the patient's liver indicated that her hepatic ornithine transcarbamoylase activity was about 10% of normal.

recycled via enzymes in the TCA cycle, to oxaloacetate and ultimately to aspartate (Fig. 18.7), thus completing the second part of the urea cycle. Because the same carbon skeleton of ornithine that begins the cycle is returned after the arginase reaction, this pathway is sometimes also referred to as the ornithine cycle. Urea synthesis occurs virtually exclusively in the liver and the role of the enzyme, arginase, in other tissues is probably related more closely to ornithine requirements in those tissues than to the production of urea.

Regulation of the urea cycle

The primary regulation of the urea cycle appears to be through the control of the concentration of N-acetylglutamate, an essential allosteric activator of CPS-I. High concentrations of arginine stimulate N-acetylation of glutamate. Concentrations of urea cycle enzymes also increase or decrease in response to a high- or low-protein diet. Urea synthesis and excretion is also decreased, and NH_4^+ excretion increased, during acidosis.

Defects in any of the enzymes of the urea cycle (Table 18.2) have serious consequences. Infants born with defects in any of the first four enzymes in this pathway may appear normal at birth, but rapidly become lethargic, lose body temperature, and may have difficulty breathing. Blood concentrations of ammonia increase quickly, followed by cerebral edema. The symptoms are most severe when early steps in the cycle are

SCREENING FOR DEFECTS OF AMINO ACID METABOLISM IN NEWBORNS

In most developed countries today, a spot of the blood of newborn infants is routinely collected on filter paper and tested for a series of compounds which are markers of inherited metabolic disease. The number of markers analyzed may vary from state to state in the US, but generally ranges from 10 to 20. Because of the need for rapid screening, small sample size, and reduced cost, older methodology is rapidly being replaced by technology which uses electrospray tandem mass spectrometry to measure the level of multiple markers simultaneously. The speed and high throughput capacity of this technology allows rapid screening of 20 or more markers from dried blood spots and the identification of infants who are potential victims of these inborn errors of metabolism. This technology can also be applied to urine samples.

affected. However, a defect in any of the enzymes in this pathway is a serious issue and may cause hyperammonemia and lead rapidly to CNS edema, coma and death. Ornithine transcarbamoylase is the most common of these urea cycle defects and shows an X-linked inheritance pattern. The remainder of the known defects associated with the urea cycle are autosomal recessive. A deficiency of arginase, the last enzyme in the cycle, produces less severe symptoms, but is nevertheless characterized by increased concentrations of blood arginine and at least a moderate increase in blood ammonia. In individuals with high blood concentrations of ammonia, hemodialysis must be used, often followed by intravenous administration of sodium benzoate and phenyllactate. These compounds can condense with glycine and glutamine, respectively, trapping ammonia in a nontoxic form that can be excreted in the urine. The enzymes of the urea cycle are listed in Table 18.2.

The concept of nitrogen balance

Because there is no significant storage form of nitrogen or amino compounds in humans, nitrogen metabolism is quite dynamic. A careful balance is maintained between nitrogen ingestion and secretion. In an average, healthy diet, the protein content exceeds the amount required to supply essential and nonessential amino acids for protein synthesis, and the amount of nitrogen excreted is approximately equal to that taken in. Such a healthy adult would be said to be 'in nitrogen balance'. When there is a need to increase protein synthesis, such as in recovering from trauma or in a rapidly growing child, the amount of nitrogen excreted

is less than that consumed in the diet, and the individual would be in 'positive nitrogen balance'. The converse is true in protein malnutrition: because of the need to synthesize essential body proteins, other proteins, such as muscle protein or hemoglobin, are degraded and more nitrogen is lost than is consumed in the diet. Such an individual would be said to be in 'negative nitrogen balance'. Fasting, starvation and poorly controlled diabetes are also characterized by negative nitrogen balance, as body protein is degraded to amino acids and their carbon skeletons are used for gluconeogenesis. The concept of nitrogen balance reminds us of the continuous turnover in the normal human body of amino acids, proteins, and some nucleic acids.

METABOLISM OF THE CARBON SKELETONS OF AMINO ACIDS

Metabolism of amino acids interfaces with carbohydrate and lipid metabolism

When one examines the metabolism of the carbon skeletons of the 20 common amino acids, there is an obvious interface with carbohydrate and lipid metabolism. Virtually all the carbons can be converted into intermediates in the glycolytic pathway, the TCA cycle, or lipid metabolism. The first step in this process is the transfer of the α-amino group by transamination to α-ketoglutarate or oxaloacetate, providing glutamate and aspartate, the sources for the nitrogen atoms of the urea cycle (Fig. 18.3). The exception to this is lysine, which does not undergo transamination. Although the details of pathways for the various amino acids vary, the general rule is that there is loss of the amino group, followed by either direct metabolism in a central pathway (glycolysis, the TCA cycle, or ketone body metabolism), or one or more intermediate conversions to yield a metabolite in one of the central pathways. Examples of amino acids that follow the former scheme include alanine, glutamate, and aspartate, which yield pyruvate, α-ketoglutarate and oxaloacetate, respectively, upon removal of their amino group. The branched-chain amino acids, leucine, valine, and isoleucine, and the aromatic amino acids, tyrosine, tryptophan, and phenylalanine are examples of the latter, more complex scheme.

Amino acids may be either glucogenic or ketogenic

Depending on the point at which the carbons from an amino acid enter central metabolism, that amino acid may be considered to be either glucogenic or ketogenic (i.e. possessing the ability to increase the concentrations of either glucose or ketone bodies, respectively, when fed to an animal). Those

HOMOCYSTINURIA (Incidence 1 in 340 000)

A tall 23-year-old male with wide-span and long 'spidery' fingers and lens dislocation, thought to result from Marfan's syndrome, was admitted with a deep vein thrombosis, following a transatlantic flight. The resident questioned the diagnosis of Marfan's and requested plasma amino acid measurements. These showed elevated methionine and homocysteine dimers, which are diagnostic of homocystinuria.

Comment. The features of Marfan's syndrome and homocystinuria are similar. In Marfan's syndrome, regular echocardiography is appropriate to assess aortic valve and thoracic aortic size to identify risk of rupture. In homocystinuria, there is, in addition, an increased risk of thrombotic events in the arterial or venous system. This can be reduced by a combination of anti-platelet agents (aspirin and dipyridamole) and reduction in plasma homocysteine levels.

The metabolism of methionine is complex involving recycling and desulfuration pathways. Catabolism proceeds by demethylation to homocysteine, which is converted to an intermediate cystathionine by the enzyme cystathionine β-synthase, then to cysteine. Fortunately, approximately half the cases of cystathionine β-synthase deficiency improve on treatment with pharmacological doses of pyridoxine (the enzyme co-factor). In other cases, a combination of protein restriction, amino acid supplementation (excluding methionine) or betaine, which acts as an alternate methyl donor to convert homocysteine into methionine – reduce the homocysteine levels.

amino acids that feed carbons into the TCA cycle at the level of α-ketoglutarate, succinyl-CoA, fumarate, or oxaloacetate, and those that produce pyruvate can all give rise to the net synthesis of glucose via gluconeogenesis and are hence designated glucogenic. Those amino acids that feed carbons into central metabolism at the level of acetyl-CoA or acetoacetyl-CoA are considered ketogenic. Because of the nature of the TCA cycle, no net flow of carbons can occur between acetate or its equivalent to glucose via gluconeogenesis (see Chapter 12).

Several amino acids, primarily those with more complex or aromatic structures, can yield both glucogenic and ketogenic fragments (Fig. 18.9). Only the amino acids, leucine and lysine, are regarded as being exclusively ketogenic and, because of its complex metabolism and lack of ability to undergo transamination, some authors do not consider lysine to be exclusively ketogenic. These classifications may be summarized as follows:

- **glucogenic amino acids** (yield pyruvate, or a TCA cycle intermediate): aspartic acid, glutamic acid, asparagine, glutamine, histidine, proline, arginine, glycine, alanine, serine, cysteine, methionine, valine;
- **ketogenic amino acids** (yield acetoacetate or acetyl-CoA): leucine, lysine;
- **both glucogenic and ketogenic amino acids** (yield pyruvate, or a TCA cycle intermediate, in addition to acetoacetate or acetyl-CoA): phenylalanine, tyrosine, tryptophan, isoleucine, threonine.

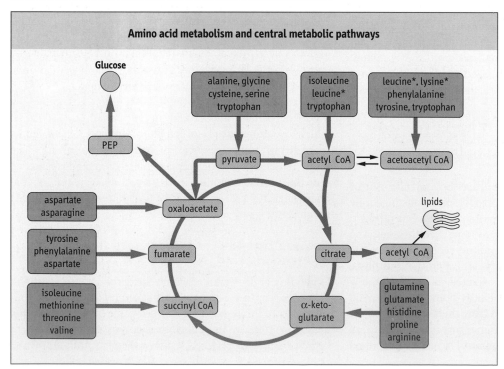

Fig. 18.9 **Amino acid metabolism and central metabolic pathways.** This figure summarizes the interactions between amino acid metabolism and central metabolic pathways. The amino acids marked with an asterisk are ketogenic only. PEP: phosphoenolpyruvate.

Metabolism of the carbon skeletons of selected amino acids

Leucine is an example of a ketogenic amino acid. Its catabolism begins with transamination to produce 2-ketoisocaproate. The metabolism of 2-ketoisocaproate requires oxidative decarboxylation by a dehydrogenase complex to produce isovaleryl-CoA. Further metabolism of isovaleryl-CoA leads to formation of 3-hydroxy-3-methylglutaryl-CoA, a precursor of both acetyl-CoA and the ketone bodies, acetoacetate and 3-hydroxybutyrate. The metabolism of leucine and the other branched-chain amino acids is summarized in

Figure 18.10. Propionyl-CoA derived from either amino acid degradation or odd-chain fatty acid metabolism is converted to succinyl-CoA (see Fig. 14.5).

Alanine, aspartate, and glutamate are examples of glucogenic amino acids. In each case, through either transamination or oxidative deamination, the resulting α-keto acid is a direct precursor of oxaloacetate via central metabolic pathways. Oxaloacetate can then be converted to PEP, and subsequently to glucose via gluconeogenesis. Other glucogenic amino acids reach the TCA cycle or related metabolic intermediates through several steps, after the removal of the amino group (Fig. 18.9).

Tryptophan is a good example of an amino acid that yields both glucogenic and ketogenic precursors. After cleavage of its heterocyclic ring and a complex set of reactions, the core of the amino acid structure is released as alanine (a glucogenic precursor), while the balance of the carbons are ultimately converted to glutaryl-CoA (a ketogenic precursor). Figure 18.11 summarizes key points in the catabolism of the aromatic amino.

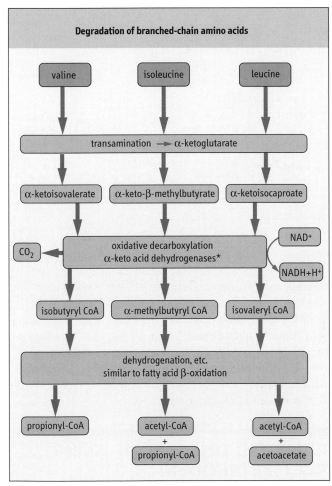

Fig. 18.10 **Degradation of branched-chain amino acids.** Metabolism of the branched-chain amino acids produces acetyl-CoA and acetoacetate. In the case of valine and isoleucine, propionyl-CoA is produced and metabolized, in two steps, to succinyl-CoA (see Fig. 14.5). *The branched chain amino acid dehydrogenases are structurally related to pyruvate dehydrogenase and α-ketoglutarate dehydrogenase, and use the cofactors: thiamine pyrophosphate, lipoic acid, FAD, NAD$^+$ and CoA.

 HOMOCYSTINURIA-2

A 21-year-old male was admitted to the hospital following an episode of loss of speech and severe weakness on his right side. A diagnosis of ischemic stroke was made and the patient was treated with anticoagulant therapy and improved. Laboratory results indicated substantially elevated levels of blood homocysteine. The patient made a significant recovery and was discharged on a modified diet along with supplements of vitamin B$_6$, folic acid, and vitamin B$_{12}$.

Comment. Homocystinuria is a relatively rare autosomal recessive condition (1 in 200 000 births) which results in a variety of symptoms including mental retardation, eye problems and thrombotic strokes and coronary artery disease at a young age. The condition is caused by the lack of an enzyme which catalyzes the transfer of sulfur from homocysteine to serine through the formation of a cystathionine intermediate. Some of these patients improve with vitamin supplementation. Of significant current interest is the role of moderately elevated levels of homocysteine in the development of cardiovascular disease and cerebrovascular ischemic episodes (stroke). Cross-sectional and retrospective studies suggest that even moderately elevated levels of homocysteine may be correlated with increased incidence of heart disease and stroke, but the jury is still out as to whether lowering homocysteine levels will reduce the development of these serious illnesses (see also Chapter 17).

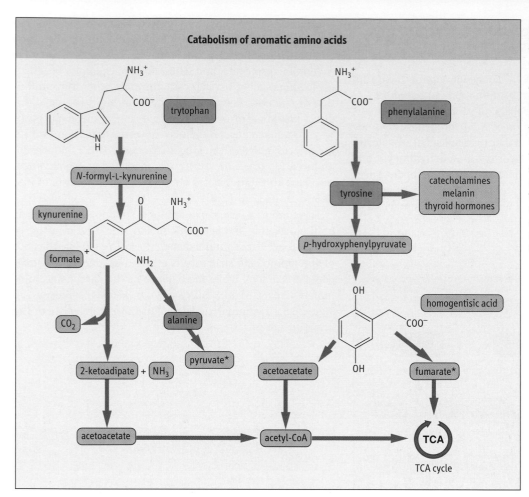

Catabolism of aromatic amino acids

Fig. 18.11 **Catabolism of aromatic amino acids.** This figure summarizes the catabolism of the aromatic amino acids, illustrating the pathways that lead to ketogenic and glucogenic precursors derived from both tyrosine and tryptophan. *Both pyruvate and fumarate link to net glucose synthesis. They constitute the gluconeogenic portions of the metabolism of these amino acids. A small fraction of Trp is converted to nicotinic acid (see Chapter 21).

AMINO ACID BIOSYNTHESIS

Evolution has left our species without the ability to synthesize almost half the amino acids that are essential building blocks and precursors of a variety of critical molecules

Human beings use 20 amino acids to build peptides and proteins that are essential to the many functions of their cells. Biosynthesis of the amino acids involves synthesis of the carbon skeletons for the corresponding α-keto acids, followed by addition of the amino group via transamination. However, humans are capable of carrying out the biosynthesis of the carbon skeletons of only about half of those α-keto acids. Amino acids that we cannot synthesize are termed essential amino acids, and are required in the diet. While almost all of the amino acids can be classified as clearly essential or nonessential, a few require further qualification. For example, although cysteine is not generally considered an essential amino acid because it can be derived from the nonessential amino acid, serine, its sulfur must come from the required or

essential amino acid, methionine. Similarly, the amino acid, tyrosine, is not required in the diet, since it can be derived from the essential amino acid, phenylalanine. This relationship between phenylalanine and tyrosine will be discussed further in considering the inherited disease, phenylketonuria (PKU). Tables 18.4 and 18.5 list the nonessential and essential amino acids, and the source of the carbon skeleton in the case of those not required in the diet.

INHERITED DISEASES OF AMINO ACID METABOLISM

In addition to deficiencies in the urea cycle, specific defects in the metabolism of the carbon skeletons of various amino acids were among the first disease states to be associated with simple inheritance patterns. These observations gave rise to the concept of the genetic basis of inherited metabolic disease states, also known as 'inborn errors of metabolism'. Garrod considered a number of disease states that appeared to be inherited in a Mendelian pattern, and proposed a correlation

Origins of nonessential amino acids

Amino acid	Source in metabolism, etc.
alanine	from pyruvate via transamination
aspartic acid, asparagine, arginine, glutamic acid, glutamine, proline	from intermediates in the citric acid cycle
serine	from 3-phosphoglycerate (glycolysis)
glycine	from serine
cysteine*	from serine; requires sulfur derived from methionine
tyrosine*	derived from phenylalanine via hydroxylation

Table 18.4 **Origins of non-essential amino acids (i.e. those not required in a normal diet).** *These are examples of nonessential amino acids that depend on adequate amounts of an essential amino acid.

Essential amino acids

Mnemonic	Amino acid*	Notes or comments
P	phenylalanine	required in the diet also as a precursor of tyrosine
V	valine	one of three branched-chain amino acids
T	threonine	metabolized like a branched-chain amino acid
T	tryptophan	its complex heterocyclic side chain can not be synthesized in humans
I	isoleucine	one of three branched-chain amino acids
M	methionine	provides the sulfur for cysteine and participates as a methyl donor in metabolism; the homocysteine is recycled
H	histidine	its heterocyclic side chain cannot be synthesized in humans
A	arginine	whereas arginine can be derived from ornithine in the urea cycle in amounts sufficient to support the needs of adults, growing animals require it in the diet
L	leucine	a pure ketogenic amino acid
L	lysine	neither of the nitrogens of lysine can undergo transamination

Table 18.5 **Essential amino acids (i.e. those required in the diet).** *The mnemonic PVT TIM HALL is useful for recalling the names of the essential amino acids.

between these abnormalities and specific genes, in which the disease state could be either dominant or recessive. Dozens of inborn errors of metabolism have now been described, and the molecular defect has been described for many of them. Three classical inborn errors of metabolism will be discussed in some detail here.

METHYLMALONYL-COA MUTASE DEFICIENCY (Incidence 1 in 30 000)

A 4-day-old child became increasingly drowsy and developed tachypnoea. Blood gas analysis demonstrated acidosis. Urine demonstrated gross ketonuria and plasma ammonia was raised at 250 µmol/l (normal range in a term infant of up to 100 µmol/L). The ammonia continued to rise over the following 12 hours to 350 µmol/L.

Comment. This is an emergency situation. The ammonia will cause cerebral edema and brain damage. With the acidosis being present, the most likely defects are in propionyl-CoA carboxylase, methylmalonyl-CoA mutase or holocarboxylase, the enzyme that conjugates biotin to carboxylase enzymes. The appropriate treatment is to stop protein (nitrogen) intake and provide adequate carbohydrates; large doses of bicarbonate and fluids; carnitine to help renal excretion of CoA metabolites, releasing CoA for intermediary metabolism; and biotin which may work on propionic acidaemia and will certainly improve holocarboxylase deficiency. Vitamin B_{12} may also stimulate mutase activity. This child's organic acid profile demonstrated gross elevation of methylmalonate and methylcitrate confirming methylmalonic acidaemia. The hyperammonemia is thought to result from inhibition of carbamoyl phosphate synthetase I by short chain fatty acids and CoA esters, possibly indirectly by inhibiting the synthesis of the allosteric effector, N-acetyl-glutamate.

Phenylketonuria

Phenylketonuria (PKU) results from a deficiency of the enzyme, phenylalanine hydroxylase. The hydroxylation of phenylalanine is a required step in both the normal degradation of the carbon skeleton of this amino acid and the synthesis of tyrosine (Fig. 18.12). When untreated, this metabolic defect leads to excessive urinary excretion of phenylpyruvate and phenyllactate, and severe mental retardation. In addition, individuals with PKU tend to have very light skin pigmentation, unusual gait, stance, and sitting posture, and a high frequency of epilepsy. In the USA, this autosomal recessive defect occurs in about 1 in 30 000 live births. Because of this, and the ability to prevent the most serious consequences of the defect by a low-phenylalanine diet, newborns in most developed countries are routinely tested for blood concentrations of phenylalanine. Fortunately, with early detection and the use of a diet restricted in phenylalanine but supplemented with tyrosine, most of the mental retardation can be avoided. Mothers who are homozygous for this defect have a very high probability of bearing children with congenital defects and mental retardation unless their blood phenylalanine concentrations can be controlled by diet. The developing fetus is very sensitive to the toxic effects of high concentrations of phenylalanine and

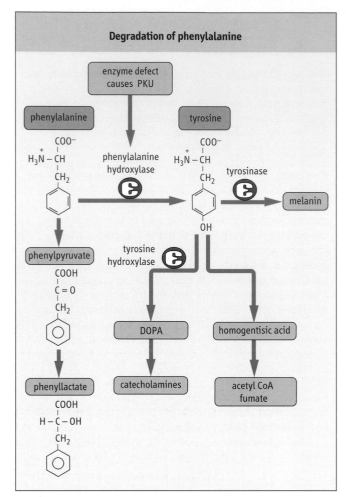

Fig. 18.12 **Degradation of phenylalanine.** In order to enter normal metabolism, phenylalanine must be hydroxylated by the enzyme, phenylalanine hydroxylase. A defect in this enzyme leads to phenylketonuria (PKU). Tyrosine is a precursor of acetyl-CoA and fumarate, catecholamine hormones, the neurotransmitter dopamine, and the pigment melanin. DOPA: dihydroxyphenylalanine.

related phenylketones. Not all hyperphenylalaninemias are caused by a defect in phenylalanine hydroxylase. In some cases, there is a defect in biosynthesis or reduction of a required tetrahydrobiopterin cofactor.

Alkaptonuria (black urine disease)

A second inherited defect in the phenylalanine-tyrosine pathway involves a deficiency in the enzyme that catalyzes the oxidation of homogentisic acid, an intermediate in catabolism of tyrosine and phenylalanine. In this condition, which occurs in 1 in 1 000 000 live births, homogentisic acid accumulates and is excreted in urine. This compound oxidizes on standing or on treatment with alkali, and gives the urine a dark color. Unfortunately, individuals with alkaptonuria

ALBINISM

A full-term infant, born to a normal and healthy mother and father, was observed to have a marked lack of pigmentation. The infant, who appeared to be otherwise normal, had blue eyes and very light blond, almost white, hair. This lack of pigmentation was confirmed as classical albinism on the basis of a family history and the establishment of a lack of the enzyme, tyrosinase, which is responsible for a two-step hydroxylation of tyrosine to dihydroxyphenylalanine (DOPA) and a subsequent further oxidation to a quinone, a precursor of melanin in melanocytes.

Comment. A separate DOPA-producing enzyme, tyrosine hydroxylase, is involved in biosynthesis of the catecholamine neurotransmitters, so albinos do not appear to have neurological deficits. As a result of their lack of pigmentation, however, they are quite sensitive to damage from sunlight and must take added precautions against ultraviolet radiation from the sun. Albinos have normal eyesight, in spite of the lack of pigmentation, but are generally very sensitive to bright light. (See Fig. 18.12.)

PHENYLALANINE HYDROXYLASE

The hydroxylation of phenylalanine is a critical step in the catabolism of that amino acid and its conversion to tyrosine, thyroid hormone and the catecholamine hormones. Phenylalanine hydroxylase is an example of a mixed-function oxidase, an enzyme that uses a reduced cofactor and molecular oxygen to carry out a hydroxylation reaction. The cofactor is tetrahydrobiopterin, which is oxidized to dihydrobiopterin during the hydroxylation reaction. The residual hydrogens and oxygen are released as water. In order for this reaction to continue, the dihydrobiopterin must be reduced to its tetrahydro form, and this requires a second enzyme, dihydrobiopterin reductase, which uses NADH to drive the reduction. The further hydroxylation of tyrosine, in the pathway that leads to catecholamines, requires a similar mixed-function oxidase, tyrosine hydroxylase. (See Fig. 18.12.)

ultimately suffer from deposition of dark (ochre-colored) pigment in cartilage tissue, with subsequent tissue damage, including severe arthritis; the onset of these symptoms is generally in the 3rd or 4th decade of life. This autosomal recessive disease was the first of several that Garrod considered in proposing his initial hypothesis for inborn errors of metabolism. Although alkaptonuria is relatively benign compared with PKU, little is available in the way of treatment, other than symptomatic relief. High doses of ascorbic acid have

SELENOCYSTEINE

In addition to the 20 common amino acids found in proteins, a 21st amino acid has recently been discovered and shown to be an active site amino acid in several enzymes, including the antioxidant enzyme glutathione peroxidase (see Chapter 35) and 5′-deiodinases (Fig. 37.6). Selenocysteine is incorporated into protein by a transfer ribonucleic acid (tRNA) with a UCA anticodon, which is initially aminoacylated with serine. The tRNA is then modified to a selenocysteine-bearing species through the action of selenophosphatase. Selenocysteine has unique properties, and there is at least one report that the substitution of selenocysteine with cysteine resulted in a marked decrease in enzyme activity. It is because of the need for selenocysteine that trace amounts of selenium are required in the diet.

 ## CYSTINURIA

A 21-year-old man came to the emergency room with severe pain in his right side and back. Subsequent investigation indicated a kidney stone, and increased concentrations of cystine, arginine, and lysine in the urine. This patient exhibited the characteristic symptoms of cystinuria.

Comment. Cystinuria is an autosomal recessive disorder of intestinal absorption and proximal tubular reabsorption of dibasic amino acids; it does not result from a defect in cysteine metabolism *per se*. Because of the transport deficiency, cysteine, which is normally reabsorbed in the proximal renal tubule, remains in the urine. The cysteine spontaneously oxidizes to its disulfide form, cystine. Because cystine has very limited solubility, it tends to precipitate in the urinary tract, forming kidney stones. The condition is generally treated by restricting the dietary intake of methionine (a biosynthetic precursor of cysteine), encouraging high fluid intake to keep the urine dilute, and, more recently, with various drugs that may convert urinary cysteine to a more soluble compound that will not precipitate.

been used in some patients, to retard the deposition of pigment on collagen, but the progress of the disease is not significantly affected by this strategy.

Maple syrup urine disease (MSUD)

The normal metabolism of the branched-chain amino acids, leucine, isoleucine, and valine, involves loss of the α-amino group, followed by oxidative decarboxylation of the resulting α-keto acid. This decarboxylation step is catalyzed by branched-chain keto acid decarboxylase, a multienzyme complex, associated with the inner membrane of the mitochondrion. In approximately 1 in 300 000 live births, a defect in this enzyme leads to accumulation of the keto acids corresponding to these branched-chain amino acids in the blood, and then to branched-chain ketoaciduria. When untreated or unmanaged, this condition may lead to both physical and mental retardation of the newborn and a distinct maple syrup odor of the urine. This defect can be partially managed with a low-protein or modified diet, but not in all cases. In some instances, supplementation with high doses of thiamine pyrophosphate, a cofactor for this enzyme complex, has been helpful.

AMINO ACIDS AS PRECURSORS OF SIGNALING MOLECULES

Derivatives of amino acids have important roles as signaling molecules

In addition to their role as building blocks for peptides and proteins, several of the common amino acids serve as precursors of amino acid derivatives that function as neuro-transmitters or hormones. Some of the amino acids may be used as neurotransmitters directly, for example glycine, aspartate, and glutamate, whereas others may be converted to neurotransmitters or hormones through modification. Tyrosine is notable in that it serves as a precursor of several neurotransmitters, the catecholamines, and thyroid hormones (Chapters 37 and 40).

Summary

In this chapter, we have seen that the metabolism of amino acids is integrally related to the mainstream of metabolism. The catabolism of amino acids generally begins with the removal of the α-amino group, which is transferred to α-ketoglutarate and oxaloacetate, and ultimately excreted in the form of urea. The resulting carbon skeletons are converted to an intermediate(s) that enter central metabolism at various points. Because carbon skeletons corresponding to the various amino acids can be derived from or feed into the glycolytic pathway, the TCA cycle, fatty acid biosynthesis and gluconeogenesis, amino acid metabolism should not be considered as an isolated pathway. Although amino acids are not stored like glucose (glycogen) or fatty acids (triacylglycerols), they have an important and dynamic role, not only in providing the building blocks for the synthesis and turnover of protein, but also in normal energy metabolism, providing a carbon source for gluconeogenesis when needed and an energy source of last resort in starvation. In addition, amino acids provide precursors for the biosynthesis of a variety of small signaling molecules, including hormones and neurotransmitters. The severe consequences of abnormal metabolism evident in inherited diseases such as phenylketonuria (PKU) and maple syrup urine disease illustrate the consequences of abnormal amino acid metabolism.

ACTIVE LEARNING

1. Tyrosine is included as a supplement in the diet plan for individuals with phenylketonuria. What is the rationale for this supplement? Compare the therapeutic approaches used for treatment of the various forms of PKU in which phenylalanine hydroxylase is not affected.
2. Review the rationale for use of levodopa, catechol-O-methyl transferase inhibitors and monoamine oxidase inhibitors for treatment of Parkinson's disease.
3. Review the pathways for biosynthesis of the neurotransmitters: serotonin, melatonin, dopamine and the catecholamines. What enzymes are involved in the inactivation of these compounds?
4. Discuss the metabolic fate of lysine in humans.

Further reading

Brusilow SW, Maestri NE. Urea cycle disorders: diagnosis, pathophysiology and therapy. *Adv Pediatr* 1996;**43**:127–170.

Berry GT, Steiner RD. Long-term Management of Patients with Urea Cycle Disorders. *J Pediatr* 2001;**138**(1 Suppl):S56–60.

Cederbaum S. Phenylketonuria: an update. *Curr Opin Pediatr* 2002;**14**:702–706.

Ogier de Baulny H, Saudubray JM. Branched-chain organic acidurias. *Semin Neonatal* 2002;**7**:65–74.

Pitt JJ, Eggington, M. and Kahler, SG. Comprehensive screening of urine samples for inborn errors of metabolism by electrospray tandem mass spectrometry. *Clinical Chemistry* 2002;**48**:1970–1980.

Saudubray JM, Nassogne MC, de Lonlay P, Touati G. Clinical approach to inherited metabolic disorders in neonates: an overview. *Semin Neonatal* 2002;**7**:3–15.

Steiner RD, Cederbaum SD. Laboratory evaluation of urea cycle disorders. *J Pediatr* 2001;**138**(Suppl 1):S21–S29.

Zytkovicz, TH, Fitzgerald EF, Marsden D, *et al.* Tandem mass spectrometric analysis for amino acid, organic and fatty acid disorders in newborn dried blood spots. *Clin Chem* 2001;**47**:1945–1955.

Relevant websites

Amino acid metabolism:
http://bioresearch.ac.uk/whatsnew/detail/3015747.html

Disorders of amino acid metabolism:
www.gpnotebook.co.uk/cache/-1811546080.htm

Urea cycle: www.nucdf.org

PKU: www.pku-allieddisorders.org; www.pkunews.org

MSUD: www.msud-support.org/overv.htm

Parkinson's Disease: www.pdf.org; www.parkinsons.org.uk; www.wpda.org

19. Muscle: Energy Metabolism and Contraction

J A Carson and J W Baynes

LEARNING OBJECTIVES

After reading this chapter you should be able to:

- Compare and contrast the structure, function and metabolism of skeletal, cardiac and smooth muscle.
- Describe the components of the sarcomere in skeletal muscle including the banding pattern and how these change during contraction.
- Outline the mechanisms of mechanochemical coupling and contraction in skeletal muscle, including the roles of Ca^{2+}, ATP, actin and myosin, as described by the sliding filament model.
- Compare substrate utilization for ATP synthesis during short-term high-intensity and long-term low-intensity skeletal muscle contractions.

INTRODUCTION

Muscle is a major determinant of whole-body metabolic activity. The three types of muscle: skeletal, cardiac, and smooth, have both similar and unique biochemical properties related to metabolism and force production. However, the primary function of all muscle is to turn chemical energy into mechanical energy. This is accomplished through the breakdown of ATP. Muscle mass and activity are major determinants of the overall metabolic rate in both the basal and active state. Changes in muscle metabolism occur during prolonged or vigorous physical activity, which affects not only the metabolic rate, but also the relative rate of utilization of glucose and fatty acids as fuels.

Although skeletal muscle is mainly associated with locomotion and heat production, maintenance of skeletal muscle mass is also essential to provide protein reserves for gluconeogenesis during fasting. Muscle is also the major site of glucose and triglyceride disposal in the body following a meal. Through its GLUT-4 transporter and lipoprotein lipase activity, muscle removes excess fuels from the blood. Loss of muscle mass with age or in wasting diseases, such as AIDS and cancer, leads to glucose intolerance and is associated with increased mortality and morbidity.

ATP is used for muscle contraction

Muscle contraction involves the integration of several biochemical processes including: membrane ion flux, calcium release and re-uptake, and ATP hydrolysis and synthesis. ATP is required for the maintenance of ion gradients, restoration of intracellular calcium levels, and for the actual process of muscle shortening. The functional contractile unit of muscle, the sarcomere, relies on the interaction of two filamentous proteins, actin and myosin, for shortening. The head of the myosin protein has ATPase activity that hydrolyzes ATP, and when calcium is present results in sarcomere shortening. Resting ATP stores do not fluctuate a great deal during muscle contraction. Actively contracting muscle relies on the rapid synthesis of ATP from ADP by the creatine phosphate shuttle, with additional ATP production from both anaerobic and aerobic metabolism. This chapter will describe all three types of muscle, focusing primarily on skeletal muscle and pointing out unique features of biochemistry and regulation in cardiac and smooth muscle. Muscle will be examined from three classic points of view: its structure, the mechanism of mechano-chemical coupling, and its energy metabolism.

STRUCTURE OF MUSCLE

Development of Muscle

To understand muscle regulation it is necessary to understand its origin and development. Muscle is derived from proliferating cells that originate from the mesenchyme germ layer in the developing embryo. These cells are 'determined' into the muscle lineage and then become myoblasts. Myoblasts can leave the cell cycle and differentiate into a mature muscle cell phenotype. Differentiation involves the sequential activation of muscle-specific genes including contractile proteins by DNA-binding transcriptional regulator proteins from the family of Myogenic Regulatory Factors (MRFs). Terminally differentiated myoblasts in the heart are called cardiac myocytes; these cells remain single or bi-nucleated throughout life. To date, no myogenic stem cells have been found in cardiac muscle, which may explain the limited regenerative capacity of the heart after injury.

Smooth muscle myoblasts also differentiate into mature smooth muscle cells (SMC), but unlike heart and skeletal muscle they are not terminally differentiated. SMC phenotype also varies, based on its location and function. SMCs are found throughout the body in the vascular wall, and retain the ability to proliferate, e.g. in response to hypertension or during angiogenesis.

Skeletal muscle cells differ from the other muscle types in that they are multi-nucleated. Proliferating myoblasts fuse and terminally differentiate to form a multinucleated myotube. Innervation by a motor nerve end plate induces the myotube to take on mature muscle fiber characteristics. Satellite cells are undifferentiated muscle precursor cells, found only in skeletal muscle. Since muscle fiber nuclei are postmitotic, satellite cell proliferation and differentiation are critical events for postnatal muscle growth and regeneration after damage. Alterations in satellite cell differentiation with advancing age or in wasting syndromes are thought to contribute to skeletal muscle loss under these conditions.

Sarcomere; the functional contractile unit

Unlike other cell types, the unique characteristic of muscle structure is that the cytoplasm is packed full of contractile protein. The arrangement of this contractile protein into sarcomere units gives muscle a striated appearance and has given rise to the classifications of striated (skeletal, cardiac) or non-striated muscle (smooth). Skeletal muscle's hierarchical structure (Fig. 19.1) consists of bundles (fasciculi) of elongated, multinucleated fiber cells (myofibers). The myofiber cells contain bundles of myofibrils, which are, in turn, composed of myofilament proteins that form the sarcomere (Table 19.1). Electron microscopic analysis reveals a repeating pattern of light- and dark-staining regions in the myofibril, which have been defined as specific, named bands (Fig. 19.2).

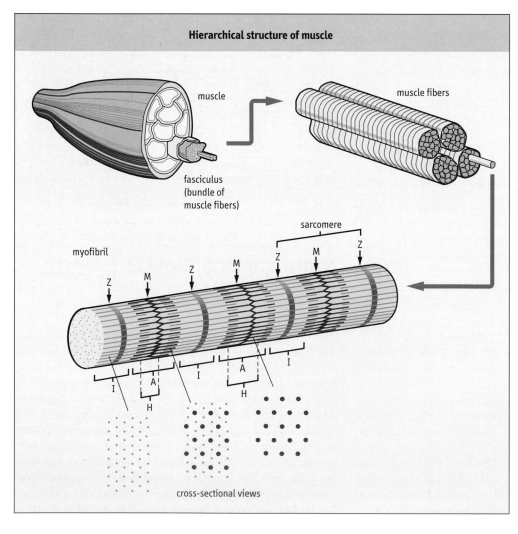

Hierarchical structure of muscle

Fig. 19.1 **Hierarchical structure of muscle.** Hierarchical structure of skeletal muscle, showing an exploding view of fasciculi, myofibers, myofibrils and myofilament proteins. The location of the I-band (thin, actin filaments extending from a Z-line), and the A-band (thick, myosin filaments, extending from the M-line), with darker staining regions of the A-band corresponding to the region of overlap of actin and myosin filaments.

Elements of skeletal muscle structure	
Microscopic unit	**Fasciculus: bundle of muscle cells**
Cellular unit	myofiber cell: long, multinucleated cell
Subcellular unit	myofibril: composed of myofilament proteins
Functional unit	sarcomere: contractile unit, repeating unit of the myofibril
Myofilament components	proteins: primarily actin and myosin

Table 19.1 **The structural elements of skeletal muscle arranged in descending order of size.**

The light- and dark-staining regions are known as the I (isotropic)- and A (anisotropic)-bands, respectively. At the center of the I-band is a discrete, darker staining Z-line, while the center of the A-band has a lighter staining H-zone with a central M-line. The sarcomere, centered on the M-line, extends from one Z-line to the next. Smooth muscle lacks a defined Z-line in its sarcomere structure.

Muscle contraction: The thick and thin filaments

The sarcomere may shorten by as much as 70% in length during muscle contraction (Fig. 19.2; see also Fig. 19.1). The main sarcomere components producing the shortening are the thick and thin filaments. The thick filament is composed of myosin protein, and the thin filament is mainly made up of actin, with associated tropomyosin and the troponin family proteins. Thick and thin filaments extend in opposite directions from both sides of the M- and Z-lines, respectively, and overlap and slide past one another during the contractile process (Fig. 19.2). The M- and Z-lines are, in effect, base plates for anchoring the filaments. In smooth muscle thick and thin filaments are anchored at structures called dense bodies that are further anchored by intermediate filaments. In striated muscle increased thick-thin filament overlap during contraction causes the H-zone (myosin only) and I-bands (actin only) to decrease. Although all three muscle types contain actin and myosin proteins, each muscle type expresses tissue specific protein types or isoforms; the cardiac actin and troponins differ slightly from those in skeletal muscle.

MUSCLE PROTEINS

Myosin

Myosin comprises two heavy and four light chains and contains two hinge regions

Myosin is one of the largest proteins in the body, with a molecular mass of approximately 500 kDa, and accounts for

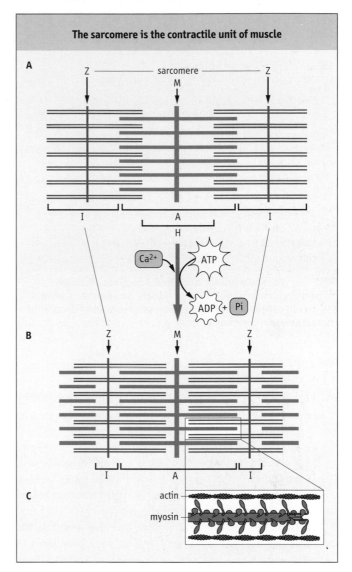

The sarcomere is the contractile unit of muscle

Fig. 19.2 **Schematic structure of the sarcomere, indicating the distribution of actin and myosin in the A- and I-bands.** (A) relaxed sarcomere; (B) contracted sarcomere; (C) magnification of contracted sarcomere, illustrating the polarity of the arrays of myosin molecules. Increased overlap of actin and myosin filaments during contraction, accompanied by a decrease in the length of the I-band, illustrates the sliding-filament model of muscle contraction.

more than half of muscle protein (Table 19.2). Under the electron microscope, myosin appears as an elongated protein with two globular heads. Structurally, it consists of two heavy and four light chains. The myosin head has ATPase activity. The heavy chains form an extended α-helical coiled-coil structure, and the light chains are bound to one end of each heavy chain, forming globular domains. Structural analysis by limited proteolysis indicates that there are two flexible hinge regions in the molecule (Fig. 19.3). One is about

Muscle proteins and their functions

Protein	Function
Myosin	Ca^{2+}-dependent ATPase activity
C-protein	assembly of myosin into thick filaments
M-protein	binding of myosin filaments to M-line
Actin	G-actin polymerizes to filamentous F-actin
tropomyosin	stabilization and propagation of conformational changes of F-actin
troponins-C, I and T	modulation of actin-myosin interactions
α- and β-actinins	stabilization of F-actin and anchoring to Z-line
nebulin	possible role in determining length of F-actin filaments
titin	control of resting tension and length of the sarcomere
desmin	organization of myofibrils in muscle cells
dystrophin	reinforcement of cytoskeleton and muscle cell plasma membrane

Table 19.2 **Muscle proteins and their functions.** Actin and myosin account for over 90% of muscle proteins, but several associated proteins are required for assembly and function of the actomyosin complex.

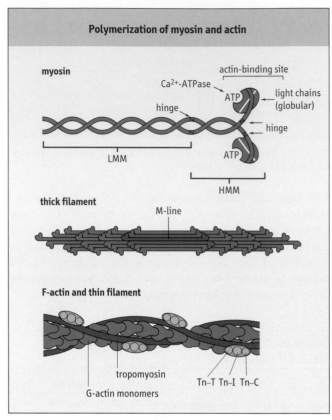

Fig. 19.3 **Polymerization of myosin and actin into thick and thin filaments.** Tn-C, calcium-binding troponin; Tn-I, troponin inhibitory subunit; Tn-T, tropomyosin-binding troponin. LMM: light meromyosin, HMM: heavy meromyosin.

two-thirds of the way along the helical chain and divides the molecule into light meromyosin (LMM: helical region) and heavy meromyosin (HMM: short helical tail plus globular domains). The other hinge is between the short helical and globular domains of HMM. Thick filaments are formed by self-association of LMM helices, up to 400 myosin molecules per thick filament. The filaments extend outward from the M-line toward the Z-line of each myofibril (compare Figs 19.2 and 19.3). Isoforms of actin and myosin are also found in the cytoskeleton of non-muscle cells, where they have roles in diverse processes, e.g. cell migration, vesicle transport during endocytosis and exocytosis, maintenance or changing of cell shape, and anchorage of intracellular proteins to the plasma membrane.

Myosin light chains have Ca^{2+}-dependent ATPase activity and are involved in reversible interactions with actin

The myosin light chains in the globular domain are homologous to calmodulin and have Ca^{2+}-dependent ATPase activity. These chains are also involved in reversible interactions with actin. ATP binding to the myosin head groups reduces their affinity for actin. Hydrolysis of the bound ATP to ADP and inorganic phosphate (Pi), catalyzed by Ca^{2+}, results in structural changes that increase by more than a 1000-fold the binding affinity of the myosin head groups for actin. Rigor mortis sets in after death as a result of the inability of muscle to regenerate ATP, which is required to maintain the low calcium concentration in the sarcoplasm. The increase in sar-

coplasmic Ca^{2+} and hydrolysis of ATP on myosin after death leads to tight interactions between myosin and actin, forming rigid muscle tissue.

Actin

F-actin is a polymer of G-actin subunits; in muscle there are about twice as many actin as myosin chains

Actin is composed of 42 kDa subunits, known as G-actin (globular), but polymerizes spontaneously into a filamentous array (F-actin). The G-actin subunits polymerize in a head-to-tail manner, and two polymer chains coil around one another to form the F-actin myofilament (see Fig. 19.3). The F-actin chains extend in opposite directions from the Z-line, overlapping with the myosin chains extending from the M-line. There are approximately twice as many actin as myosin chains in muscle, yielding an array in which each myosin molecule is associated with six actin molecules and each actin with three myosin molecules (see Fig. 19.1 for a cross-sectional view).

Tropomyosin and troponins

Tropomyosin stabilizes F-actin and coordinates conformational changes among actin subunits during contraction

Tropomyosin is a fibrous protein that extends along the grooves of F-actin, each molecule contacting about seven G-actin subunits. Tropomyosin has a role in stabilizing F-actin and coordinating conformational changes among actin subunits during contraction. In the absence of Ca^{2+}, tropomyosin blocks the myosin binding site on actin. A complex of troponin proteins is bound to tropomyosin: Tn-T (tropomyosin-binding), Tn-C (calcium-binding) and Tn-I (inhibitory subunit). Troponins modulate the interaction between actin and myosin. Calcium binding to Tn-C, a calmodulin-like protein, induces changes in Tn-I, which are then transduced to tropomyosin, moving it out of the myosin-binding site and permitting actin–myosin interactions.

The sliding-filament model of muscle contraction

The general features of the sliding-filament model of muscle contraction are described by a series of chemical and structural changes in the actomyosin complex. The contractile response is powered by reversible 'cross-bridge' interactions between the myosin head and its actin-binding site. A cycle of binding of myosin to actin, conformational changes in the hinge regions of myosin, and release of myosin occurs, with the conformational change providing the 'power stroke' for muscle contraction. This sequence of reactions is summarized in Figure 19.4. The conformational change in the hinge regions of myosin is induced by hydrolysis of ATP and relaxed by dissociation of ADP and Pi. The latter process, the dissociation of ADP and Pi, rather than the hydrolysis of ATP, is the rate-limiting step in myosin ATPase activity and muscle contraction. The stability of the contracted state is maintained by multiple and continuous actin-myosin interactions, so that slippage is minimized until calcium is removed from the sarcoplasm, allowing the muscle to relax.

Excitation-contraction coupling: The calcium trigger

The calcium content of the muscle cytoplasm (sarcoplasm) is normally very low, 10^{-7} mol/L or less, but increases rapidly by ~100-fold in response to neural stimulation, leading to ATP hydrolysis and muscle contraction. Muscle cells have an adapted smooth endoplasmic reticulum organelle, known as the sarcoplasmic reticulum (SR), which serves as the site of calcium sequestration inside the cell. The plasma membrane of the myofiber cell, known as the sarcolemma, invaginates in and around the myofibrils at the Z-lines, forming a series of transverse tubules that indirectly interact with the SR (Fig. 19.5). The muscle cell responds to motor nerve stimulation by initiating a wave of depolarization of the Na^+/K^+-gradient across the muscle plasma membrane, which is transmitted to the SR, causing a voltage-gated opening of SR Ca^{2+}-channels. Calcium is released from the SR, and the influx of Ca^{2+} into the muscle cytoplasm (sarcoplasm) triggers muscle contraction. In striated muscle, calcium interacts with troponin-C on the thin filament to allow actin-myosin interaction. Muscle contraction is mediated by changes in the conformations and

 DUCHENNE MUSCULAR DYSTROPHY

A young boy was brought to the clinic because his mother had noticed that he walked with a waddling gait. Physical evaluation confirmed muscle weakness especially in the legs although his calf muscles were large and firm. There was a 20-fold elevation in serum creatine (phospho) kinase (CK) activity, identified as the MM (muscle) isozyme. Histology revealed muscle loss, some necrosis, and increased connective tissue and fat volume in muscle. A tentative diagnosis of Duchenne muscular dystrophy (DMD) was confirmed by immunoelectrophoretic (Western blot) analysis showing the lack of the cytoskeletal protein dystrophin in muscle.

Comment. Dystrophin is a high-molecular-weight cytoskeletal protein that reinforces the plasma membrane of the muscle cell and mediates interactions with the extracellular matrix. In its absence, the plasma membrane of muscle cells is damaged during the contractile process, leading to muscle cell death. The dystrophin gene is located on the X-chromosome and is unusually long, nearly 2.5×10^6 base pairs. Mutations are relatively common, the frequency of DMD being approximately 1 in 3500 male births. DMD is a progressive myodegenerative disease, commonly leading to confinement to a wheelchair by puberty, with death by age 20 years from respiratory or cardiac failure. Dystrophin is completely absent in DMD patients. A variant of the disease, known as Becker muscular dystrophy, has milder symptoms and is characterized by expression of an altered dystrophin protein and survival into the fourth decade. Although there is currently no treatment, the injection of satellite cells (myogenic stem cell) that express dystrophin protein and incorporate into the dystrophic skeletal muscle has shown promise in animal trials.

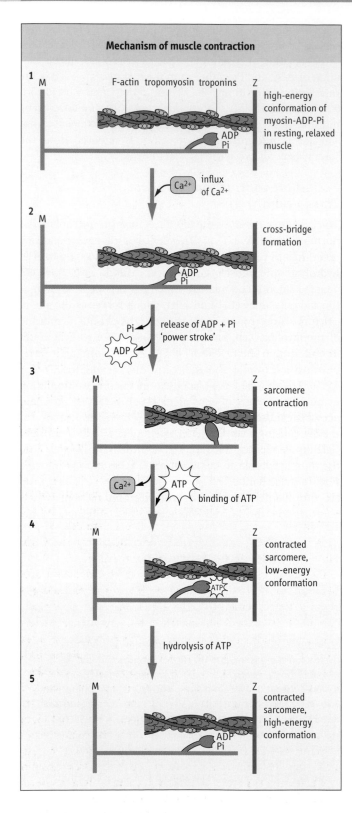

Mechanism of muscle contraction

1 M   F-actin tropomyosin troponins   Z   high-energy conformation of myosin-ADP-Pi in resting, relaxed muscle

ADP Pi

Ca²⁺ influx of Ca²⁺

2 M   cross-bridge formation

ADP Pi

Pi release of ADP + Pi 'power stroke'
ADP

3 M   Z   sarcomere contraction

Ca²⁺   ATP binding of ATP

4 M   Z   contracted sarcomere, low-energy conformation

ATP

hydrolysis of ATP

5 M   Z   contracted sarcomere, high-energy conformation

ADP Pi

Fig. 19.4 Proposed stages in muscle contraction, according to the sliding-filament model.

(1) In resting, relaxed muscle, calcium concentration is ~10^{-7} mol/L. The head group of myosin chains contains bound ADP and Pi, and is extended forward along the axis of the myosin helix in a high-energy conformation. Although the myosin-ADP-Pi complex has a high affinity for actin, binding of myosin to actin is inhibited by tropomyosin, which blocks the myosin-binding site on actin at low calcium concentration.

(2) When muscle is stimulated, calcium enters the sarcoplasm through voltage-gated calcium channels (see Chapter 7). Calcium binding to Tn-C causes a conformational change in Tn-I, which is transmitted through Tn-T to tropomyosin. Movement of tropomyosin exposes the myosin-binding site on actin. Myosin-ADP-Pi binds to actin, forming a cross-bridge.

(3) Release of Pi, then ADP, from myosin during the interaction with actin is accompanied by a major conformational change in myosin, producing the 'power stroke', which moves the actin chain about 10 nm (100 Å) in the direction opposite the myosin chain, increasing their overlap and causing muscle contraction.

(4) The uptake of calcium from the sarcoplasm and binding of ATP to myosin leads to dissociation of the actomyosin cross-bridge.

(5) The ATP is hydrolyzed, and the free energy of hydrolysis of ATP is conserved as the high-energy conformation of myosin, setting the stage for continued muscle contraction in response to the next surge in Ca²⁺ concentration in the sarcoplasm.

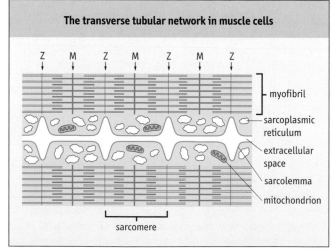

The transverse tubular network in muscle cells

Z M Z M Z M Z

myofibril
sarcoplasmic reticulum
extracellular space
sarcolemma
mitochondrion

sarcomere

Fig. 19.5 Side-view of the transverse tubular network in skeletal muscle cells. Transverse tubules are invaginations of the sarcolemma, which are in intimate contact with the sarcoplasmic reticulum (SR). The SR is a continuous, tubular compartment in close association with the myofibrils. The transverse tubules are extensions of the sarcolemma around the Z-line. They transmit the depolarizing nerve impulse to terminal regions of the SR, coordinating calcium release and contraction of the myofibril.

SARCOPENIA

Sarcopenia is defined as the loss of skeletal muscle mass with age. Sarcopenia is accelerated in humans after the fifth decade of life and can lead to frailty and loss of functional capacity. Besides the basic erosion of quality of life, loss of skeletal muscle mass also increases the risk of mortality and morbidity. The cause of sarcopenia appears to be related to both a biological program of muscle fiber loss and decreased physical activity. Muscle fiber innervation by spinal motor neurons is critical to both development and maintenance of the mature muscle phenotype. Spinal motor neurons decrease in number with advancing age, possibly because of cumulative oxidative damage to these post-mitotic cells. The loss of motor neurons induces muscle fiber loss and an increase in existing motor unit size, which decreases fine motor skill. Sarcopenia has also been linked to age-induced systemic changes to the endocrine, cardiovascular, and immune systems, whose functions are all critical for the maintenance of skeletal muscle mass.

Comment: The scientific evidence is clear that most elder individuals can increase muscle strength and mass with a regular resistance exercise program. Pharmaceutical treatments have also been examined for individuals who cannot regularly exercise. Currently there is no treatment for spinal motor neuron loss. Pharmaceutical treatments targeting muscle have had varying degrees of success, but are usually limited by side-effects. The treatments include endocrine interventions with male or female sex hormone replacement therapy, and growth hormone therapy. Anti-inflammatory medication is also employed to allow individuals to participate in physical activity programs. One of the best defenses from sarcopenia may be regular exercise in order to maintain muscle mass during middle age.

METABOLIC SYNDROME

Metabolic syndrome (Syndrome X), characterized by insulin resistance, hyperinsulinemia, hypertension, and hyperlipidemia, is a major, age-dependent risk factor for diabetes and cardiovascular disease. Loss of muscle mass and insulin sensitivity can dramatically influence the progression from Syndrome X to frank disease through their effect on blood glucose concentration. A half-hour of vigorous physical activity can increase skeletal muscle glucose uptake for up to 24 hours after the exercise period. Regular exercise also reduces the loss of muscle mass, improves muscle perfusion, and enhances the insulin sensitivity of muscle. There is clear evidence that obese people also benefit from regular exercise (see Chapters 20 and 21).

Muscle: An excitable tissue

Muscle has the ability to depolarize upon neural stimulation, and this depolarization is critical for the calcium release that triggers contraction. However, skeletal, cardiac, and smooth muscle receive this neural depolarization in different manners, and have different structural adaptations at the sarcolemma to account for depolarization propagation. Skeletal muscle contraction is volitional and fibers are innervated by motor nerve endplates that originate in the spinal cord. The neuromuscular junction is a special structural feature of skeletal muscle that is not found in cardiac or smooth muscle. Each individual fiber is innervated by only one motor nerve, and all the fibers innervated by one nerve are defined as a motor unit. Motor unit control and synchronization is the basis for coordinated whole muscle contraction.

Cardiac muscle is striated and contracts rhythmically under involuntary control. The general mechanism of contraction of heart muscle is similar to that in skeletal muscle, but the SR is less developed, and the transverse tubule network, an extension of the plasma membrane, is more developed in the heart. Thus, the heart is more dependent on, and actually requires, extracellular calcium for its contractile response. Lacking direct neural contact, cardiac myocytes propagate depolarization from a single node, the SA-node, throughout the myocardium. The depolarization is passed cell to cell along specialized membrane structures called intercalated disks. Cardiac muscle is also more responsive to hormonal regulation. For example, cAMP-dependent protein kinases phosphorylate transport proteins and Tn-I, mediating changes in the force of contraction in response to epinephrine.

Smooth muscle can respond to both neural and circulating factors for the stimulus of depolarization. Unlike skeletal muscle, neural input to smooth muscle innervates bundles of smooth muscle cells that cause both phasic (rhythmic) and tonic contractions of the tissue.

---

interactions of actin and myosin. The actomyosin complex thereby transforms the chemical energy of ATP into the mechanical action of muscle.

Troponin protein is not expressed in smooth muscle. In this case, calcium triggers contraction by calmodulin binding. Calcium-calmodulin binding activates myosin light chain kinase. These events lead to myosin phosphorylation, which allows myosin-actin interaction.

Although muscle contraction is triggered by increased calcium, muscle relaxation is dependent on calcium being pumped back into the SR. The rate of muscle relaxation is directly related to SR-calcium ATPase activity. The SR is rich in a calcium-ATPase, which pumps calcium into the SR, maintaining cytosolic calcium in the muscle cell at sub-micromolar ($\sim 10^{-7}$ mol/L) concentrations. At the same time, the concentration of calcium in the SR is in the mmol/L range, comparable to that in the plasma compartment.

MALIGNANT HYPERTHERMIA

About 1 in 150 000 patients treated with halothane (gaseous halocarbon) anesthesia or muscle relaxants, responds with excessive skeletal muscle rigidity and severe hyperthermia with a rapid onset, up to 2°C (4°F) within 1 hour. Unless treated rapidly, cardiac abnormalities may be life-threatening; mortality from this condition exceeds 10%. This genetic disease results from excessive or prolonged release of Ca^{2+} from the SR, most commonly the result of mutations in the Ca^{2+}-release channels within the SR. Excessive release of Ca^{2+} leads to a prolonged increase in sarcoplasmic Ca^{2+} concentration. Muscle rigidity results from Ca^{2+}-dependent consumption of ATP, and hyperthermia results from increased metabolism to replenish the ATP. As muscle metabolism becomes anaerobic, lacticacidemia, and acidosis may develop. The cardiac abnormalities result from hyperkalemia, caused by release of potassium ions from muscle; as supplies of ATP are exhausted, muscle is unable to maintain ion gradients across its plasma membrane. Treatment of malignant hyperthermia includes use of muscle relaxants, e.g. dantrolene, an inhibitor of the ryanodine-sensitive Ca^{2+}-channel (Chapter 7), to inhibit Ca^{2+}-release from the SR. Supportive therapy involves cooling, administration of oxygen, correction of blood pH and electrolyte imbalances and also treatment of cardiac abnormalities.

MUSCLE ENERGY METABOLISM

Muscle consists of two types of striated muscle cells; fast-glycolytic and slow-oxidative fibers

Striated muscle cells are generally classified by their physiological contractile properties (fast versus slow) that are determined by the level of ATPase activity and the primary metabolic source of ATP synthesis (anaerobic vs. aerobic). The muscle type is closely related to muscle function. In skeletal muscle this comparison is easily seen with muscles whose contraction is necessary to continuously maintaining posture versus muscle contraction for infrequent-burst activities. The two striated muscle types are readily distinguished in skeletal muscle by coloring. Fast-glycolytic muscle is white in appearance because of less blood flow, lower mitochondrial density, and decreased myoglobin content than slow-twitch oxidative muscle, which is red. Fast-glycolytic fibers also have lower fat content and increased glycogen stores. The fast-glycolytic fibers, rely on glycogen and anaerobic glycolysis for short bursts of contraction when additional muscle force is required such as in the 'fight or flight' stress response. These muscle fibers are not capable of sustaining contraction for long periods, when compared to slow-oxidative fibers. In con-

trast, slow-oxidative fibers are well perfused with blood, rich in mitochondria (cytochromes) and myoglobin. This muscle type has the ability to sustain low-intensity contractions for long periods. Slow muscle uses fatty acid oxidation for ATP synthesis, which requires mitochondria. Cardiac muscle, which is continuously contracting, has many contractile and metabolic characteristics that are similar to slow-oxidative skeletal muscle. Cardiac muscle is well perfused with blood, rich in mitochondria, and relies largely on oxidative metabolism of circulating fatty acids.

METABOLISM AND MUSCLE CONTRACTION

Short-duration, high-intensity contractions

For short bursts of energy, skeletal muscle relies on its ATP stores and an additional reserve of the high-energy storage compound, creatine phosphate (creatine-P), to regenerate ATP rapidly during the first minute as glycogenolysis is activated. Creatine is synthesized from arginine and glycine (Fig. 19.6), and is phosphorylated reversibly to creatine-P by

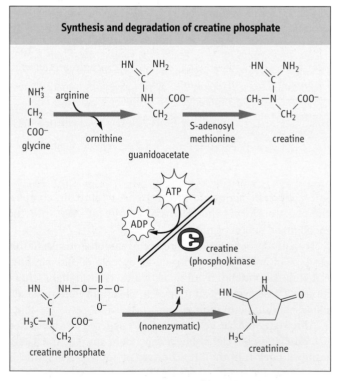

Fig. 19.6 **Synthesis and degradation of creatine phosphate (creatine-P).** Creatine is synthesized from glycine and arginine precursors. Creatine-P is unstable and undergoes slow, spontaneous degradation to Pi and creatinine, the cyclic anhydride form of creatine, which is excreted from the muscle cell into plasma and then into urine.

ASSAY OF CREATININE TO ASSESS RENAL FUNCTION AND URINE DILUTION

Since creatine phosphate concentration is relatively constant per unit muscle mass, the production of creatinine is relatively constant during the day. Creatinine is eliminated in urine at a relatively constant amount per hour, primarily by glomerular filtration, and to a lesser extent by tubular secretion. Since its concentration in urine varies with the dilution of the urine, levels of metabolites in random urine samples are often normalized to the urinary concentration of creatinine. Otherwise, a 24 h collection would be required to assess daily excretion of a metabolite. Normal creatinine concentration in plasma is about 20–80 mmol/L (0.23–0.90 mg/dL). Increases in plasma creatinine concentration are commonly used as an indicator of renal failure. The albumin/creatinine ratio in a random urine sample, an indicator of protein filtration selectivity of the glomerulus, is used as a measure of the microalbuminuria to assess the progression of diabetic nephropathy.

the enzyme creatine (phospho)kinase (CK or CPK). CK is a dimeric protein and exists as three isozymes: the MM (skeletal muscle), BB (brain) and MB isoforms. The MB isoform is enriched in cardiac tissue.

The level of creatine-P in resting muscle is several-fold higher than that of ATP (Table 19.3). Thus, ATP concentration remains relatively constant during the initial stages of exercise. It is replenished not only by the action of CK but also by adenylate kinase (myokinase) as follows:

Creatine phosphokinase: creatine-P + ADP → creatine + ATP

Adenylate kinase: → 2 ADP → ATP + AMP

Changes in energy resources in working muscle

Metabolite	Metabolite concentration (mmol/kg dry weight)		
	resting	3 minutes	8 minutes
ATP	27	26	19
Creatine-P	78	27	7
Creatine	37	88	115
Lactate	5	8	13
Glycogen	408	350	282

Table 19.3 **Changes in energy resources in working muscle.** Concentrations of energy metabolites in human leg muscle during bicycle exercise. These experiments were conducted during ischemic exercise, which exacerbates the decline in ATP concentration. They illustrate the rapid decline in creatine-P and the increase in lactate from anaerobic glycolysis of muscle glycogen. Data are adapted from Timmons JA *et al. J Clin Invest* 1998;101:79–85.

During the initial stages of exercise, muscle glycogenolysis, followed by both anaerobic and aerobic glycolysis, is the major source of energy. Calcium entry into muscle leads to formation of a Ca^{2+}-calmodulin complex, which activates phosphorylase kinase, catalyzing the conversion of phosphorylase b to phosphorylase a. AMP also allosterically activates muscle phosphorylase and phosphofructokinase-1, accelerating glycolysis from muscle glycogen.

Low intensity, long duration contractions

Availability and utilization of oxygen in working muscle are the major limitations for maintaining continuous physical activity. At rest or at low-intensities of physical work, oxygen is readily available and the aerobic oxidation of lipid predominates as the main source of ATP synthesis. However, at higher work intensities oxygen availability and utilization can become limiting, and subsequently the work rate of the muscle decreases. One of the main adaptations to regular vigorous physical activity involves increasing muscle mass and oxygenation (perfusion).

During the first 15–30 minutes of exercise, there is a gradual shift from glycogenolysis and aerobic glycolysis to aerobic metabolism of fatty acids. Perhaps this is an evolutionary response to deal with the fact that lactate, produced by glycolysis, is more acidic and less diffusible than CO_2. In any case, the glycogen reserves in muscle are sufficient to support the energy needs of muscle during exercise for only about 1 hour. As exercise continues, epinephrine contributes to activation of hepatic gluconeogenesis, providing an exogenous source of glucose for muscle. Lipids gradually become the major source of energy in muscle during long-term exercise. The oxidative metabolism of lipids is supported by increased perfusion and delivery of oxygen.

Long-term muscle performance (stamina) depends on levels of muscle glycogen

Marathon runners typically 'hit the wall' when muscle glycogen reaches a critically low level. Glycogen is the storage form of glucose in skeletal muscle, and its muscle concentration can be manipulated by diet. Fatigue occurs when the requirement for ATP exceeds its rate of synthesis. For efficient ATP synthesis, there is a continuing requirement for a basal level of glycogen and carbohydrate metabolism in muscle, even when fats are the primary source of muscle energy. Carbohydrate metabolism is important as a source of pyruvate, which is converted to oxaloacetate by the anaplerotic, pyruvate carboxylase reaction. Oxaloacetate is required to maintain the activity of the TCA cycle – for condensation with acetyl CoA derived from fats. Muscle glycogen can be spared and performance time increased during long-term vigorous physical activity by increasing the availability of circulating glucose, either by gluconeogenesis or by carbohydrate ingestion. Increased utilization of fatty acids is an important

THE MEASUREMENT OF CARDIAC TROPONINS IS THE PRIMARY TEST TO DIAGNOSE MYOCARDIAL INFARCTION

Myocardial infarction (MI) is the result of blockage of blood flow to the heart (see Chapter 17). Tissue damage results in leakage of intracellular enzymes into blood (Fig. 19.7). Among these are glycolytic enzymes, such as LDH (Chapter 11); however, measurements of myoglobin, total plasma CK and CK-MB isozymes are more commonly used for diagnosis and management of MI. Myoglobin is a small protein (17 000 kDa) and rises most rapidly in plasma, within 2 hours following MI. Although it is sensitive, it lacks specificity for heart tissue. It is cleared rapidly by renal filtration and returns to normal within 1 day. Since plasma myoglobin also increases following skeletal muscle trauma, it would not be useful for diagnosis of MI, e.g. following an automobile accident. Total plasma CK and the CK-MB isozyme begin to rise within 3–10 hours following an MI, and reach a peak value of up to 25 times normal after 12–30 hours; they may remain elevated for 3–5 days. Total CK may also increase as a result of skeletal muscle damage but the measurement of CK-MB provides specificity for cardiac damage.

Comment. Enzyme-linked immunosorbent assays (ELISA) for the myocardial troponins are now recommended for the diagnosis and management of MI. These assays depend on the presence of unique isoforms of troponin subunits in the adult heart. Tn-T concentration in plasma increases within a few hours after a heart attack, peaks at up to 300 times normal plasma concentration, and may remain elevated for 1–2 weeks. An assay for a specific isoform in an adult heart, $Tn-T_2$, is essentially 100% sensitive for diagnosis of MI and yields fewer than 5% false-positive results. Significant increases in plasma Tn-T are detectable even in patients with unstable angina and transient episodes of ischemia in the heart. Troponins are commonly used as a component of an algorithm to differentiate high-risk from low-risk patients in terms of need for immediate invasive intervention.

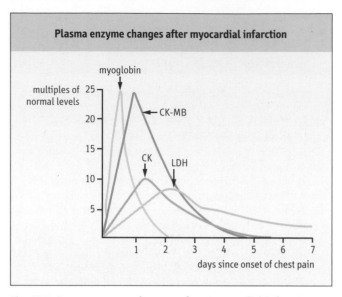

Fig. 19.7 **Serum enzyme changes after myocardial infarction (MI).** Various marker enzymes increase in plasma following MI. LDH, lactate dehydrogenase. These are still used for the diagnosis of MI, but the currently recommended test is the measurement of serum troponin concentration. Adapted from Pettigrew AR, Pacanis A. Diagnosis of myocardial infarction. In: Dominiczak MH, (ed.), Seminars in Clinical Biochemistry. University of Glasgow Computer Publishing Unit, Glasgow, 1997.

training adaptation to regular vigorous physical activity that can also serve to spare glycogen stores (see also Chapter 20).

Summary

Muscle is the major consumer of fuels and ATP in the body. Both glycolysis and lipid metabolism are essential for muscle activity. Reliance on these energy-producing pathways varies with muscle type and its prior contractile activity. The ATP produced in muscle drives the maintenance of ion gradients, restoration of intracellular calcium levels, and the contractile process. Fast, glycolytic muscle relies largely on glycogen and anaerobic glycolysis for short, high intensity bursts of muscle activity. Slow, oxidative muscle is an aerobic tissue; at rest, it uses fats as its primary source of energy. During the initial phases of exercise, it relies on glycogenolysis and glycolysis, but then gradually converts to fat metabolism for long-term energy production.

Skeletal, cardiac, and smooth muscle have a common actomyosin contractile complex, but differ in innervation, contractile protein arrangement, calcium regulation of contraction, and propagation of depolarization from cell to cell. The sarcomere is the fundamental contraction unit of striated muscle and is defined by z-lines and thick and thin filament overlap. Contraction is described by a 'sliding-filament' model in which hydrolysis of ATP is catalyzed by an influx of Ca^{2+} into the sarcoplasm and is coupled to changes in the conformation of myosin. Relaxation of the high-energy conformation of myosin during interaction with actin produces a 'power stroke', resulting in increased overlap of the actin-myosin filaments and shortening of the sarcomere.

ACTIVE LEARNING

1. When chickens are frightened, they squawk a lot, may jump high and fly for short distances, but are unable to take flight and fly for great distances, either normally or to escape danger. In contrast, geese have the ability to fly for great distances, e.g. during semi-annual migrations. Compare the types of muscle fibers and energy resources in the breast of chicken and geese and explain how the differences in fiber type are compatible with the flying capacity of these birds.
2. Discuss the impact of muscle glycogen phosphorylase deficiency (McArdle's disease) and carnitine or carnitine palmitoyl transferase I deficiency on muscle performance during short and long duration exercise.
3. Review the merits of blood doping, carbohydrate loading and creatine supplementation to enhance performance during marathon events.

Further reading

Costelli P, Baccino FM. Mechanisms of skeletal muscle depletion in wasting syndromes: role of ATP-ubiquitin-dependent proteolysis. *Curr Opin Clin Nutr Meta Care* 2003;**6**:407–412.

Greenlund LJ, Nair KS. Sarcopenia – consequences, mechanisms, and potential therapies. *Mech Ageing Dev* 2003;**124**:287–299.
Hawley JA. Adaptations of skeletal muscle to prolonged, intense endurance training. *Clin Exp Pharmacol Physiol* 2002;**29**:218–222.
Henriksen EJ, Saengsirisuwan V. Exercise training and antioxidants: relief from oxidative stress and insulin resistance. *Exerc Sport Sci Rev* 2003;**31**:79–84.
Roberts CK, Vaziri ND, Liang KH, Barnard RJ. Reversibility of chronic experimental syndrome X by diet modification. *Hypertension* 2001;**37**:1323–1328.
Roubenoff R. Catabolism of aging: is it an inflammatory process? *Curr Opin Clin Nutr Metab Care* 2003;**6**:295–299.
Tyska MJ, Warshaw DM. The myosin power stroke. *Cell Motil Cytoskeleton* 2002;**51**:1–15.

Relevant websites

Carnitine deficiency: http://www.emedicine.com/ped/topic321.htm
McArdle's Disease: www.muscular-dystrophy.org/information/KeyFacts/mcardles.html
Muscular Dystrophy: www.ninds.nih.gov/health_and_medical/disorders/md.htm
www.nlm.nih.gov/medlineplus/musculardystrophy.html

20. Glucose Homeostasis, Fuel Metabolism, and Insulin

M H Dominiczak

LEARNING OBJECTIVES

After reading this chapter you should be able to:

- Characterize the main metabolic fuels.
- Outline the actions of insulin and glucagon.
- Describe the metabolism in the fasting and postprandial state.
- Describe the metabolic response to injury and compare it with metabolism in diabetes.
- Characterize the diabetic syndrome.
- Explain the basis of laboratory tests relevant to fuel metabolism and glucose homeostasis.

The existence of an organism depends on the continuous provision of energy to drive metabolic processes. This chapter describes how the body handles energy substrates (metabolic fuels) under different circumstances. It also discusses the most common metabolic disease: diabetes mellitus.

The main metabolic fuels are glucose and fatty acids

Glucose and fatty acids are the most important metabolic fuels. In normal circumstances, glucose is the only fuel which can be used by the brain. Glucose is also preferentially used by muscle during the initial stages of exercise. The amount of glucose present in the extracellular fluid is minute – only about 20 g (<1 oz) (equivalent of 80 kcal) (335 kJ). Therefore, to ensure the continuous provision of glucose to the brain and other tissues, metabolic fuels are stored for use in times of need. Carbohydrates are stored as glycogen. The amount of available glycogen stored is also not large; approximately 75 g (approx 2.5 oz) in the liver and 400 g (<1 lb) in the muscles (about 1900 kcal (7955 kJ) altogether). Liver glycogen can remain the main supplier of glucose for no longer than 16 h. To safeguard the continuous supply of glucose over longer periods, the body needs to transform noncarbohydrate compounds into glucose. This is done through gluconeogenesis.

The esters of glycerol and long-chain fatty acids are the ideal storage fuel

The caloric value of fats 9 kcal/g (37 kJ/g) is higher than that of either carbohydrates 4 kcal/g (17 kJ/g) or proteins (4 kcal/g) (see Table 21.4). The body has a virtually unlimited capacity for the accumulation of fats. A 70 kg (154 lb) man will have approximately 15 kg (33 lb) of fat stored as adipose tissue triacylglycerols (triglycerides), equivalent to over 130 000 kcal (544 300 kJ). Fatty acids can support the body's energy needs over prolonged periods of time. In extreme circumstances, people can fast for as long as 60–90 days and obese persons may survive for over a year without food. Fatty acids are stored in the body as esters of glycerol (triacylglycerols; triglycerides).

Amino acids can be used as a fuel during fasting, illness, or injury

Amino acids normally serve as substrates for the synthesis of the body's own proteins, rather than as a source of energy. However, during a prolonged fast, or after illness or injury, proteins are degraded and the constituent amino acids are converted into glucose. Excess amino acids provided with food are normally converted to carbohydrates either for storage or for energy metabolism. The main metabolic pathways and key metabolites are listed in Table 20.1.

THE ORGAN-FUEL INTERACTIONS

At rest, the brain uses approximately 20% of all oxygen (O_2) consumed by the body. As mentioned above, glucose is normally the brain's only fuel, but during starvation the brain can use ketones as an alternate energy source.

Gluconeogenesis occurs primarily in the liver

When the glucose content of the extracellular fluid decreases, glycogen is mobilized within seconds, providing a short-term supply of endogenous glucose. Subsequently, this supply is complemented by gluconeogenesis, the other source of endogenous glucose. Gluconeogenesis takes place primarily in the liver, with the kidneys contributing during a prolonged fast. The substrates for gluconeogenesis originate from anaerobic glycolysis (lactate) and the breakdown of

Utilization and storage of metabolic fuels

Pathways	Main substrates	End products
Anabolic		
gluconeogenesis	lactate, alanine, glycerol	glucose
glycogen synthesis	G-1-P	glycogen
protein synthesis	amino acids	proteins
lipogenesis	acetyl-CoA,	fatty acids,
	glycerol	triglycerides
Catabolic		
glycolysis	glucose	pyruvate, ATP
tricarboxylic acid cycle	pyruvate	$NADH + H^+$, $FADH_2$,
	acetyl-CoA, pyruvate	CO_2, H_2O, ATP
glycogenolysis	glycogen	G-1-P, glucose
pentose phosphate pathway	G-6-P	$NADPH + H^+$, pentoses, CO_2
lipolysis	triglycerides	glycerol, fatty acids
proteolysis	proteins	amino acids → glucose, amino acids → ketones

Table 20.1 **Principal anabolic and catabolic pathways, and their main substrates and products.** Metabolites, such as pyruvate and acetyl-CoA, link different pathways.

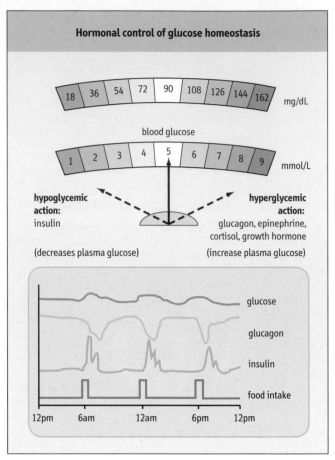

Hormonal control of glucose homeostasis

Fig. 20.1 **Hormonal control of glucose homeostasis.** Plasma glucose concentration reflects the balance between the hypoglycemic action of insulin and the hyperglycemic action of anti-insulin hormones. The lower part of the figure illustrates the daily patterns of insulin, glucagon and plasma glucose concentrations. Glucose concentration throughout the day remains in a relatively narrow range (see also Fig. 12.1). To obtain glucose concentrations in mg/dL, multiply by 18.

either muscle protein (alanine) or adipose tissue triglycerides (glycerol).

Muscle handles carbohydrates quite differently to the liver. In contrast to the liver, it does not have glucose-6-phosphatase (Glc-6-Pase) and therefore cannot release glucose into the circulation. Instead, muscle uses glycogen for its own energy needs. It does, however, contribute to endogenous glucose production by releasing lactate, a product of anaerobic glycolysis. Lactate is transported to the liver, where it enters gluconeogenesis. Muscle can use both glucose and fatty acids as energy sources. During intensive exercise, glucose is the preferred fuel. Fatty acids are the main energy source at rest and during prolonged exercise (see Chapter 19).

GLUCOSE HOMEOSTASIS

In the fasting state, glucose turnover in a 70 kg (154 lb) individual is approximately 2 mg/kg/min (200 g/24 h). The plasma glucose concentration reflects the balance between intake (glucose absorption from the gut), tissue utilization (glycolysis, pentose phosphate pathway, tricarboxylic acid (TCA) cycle, glycogen synthesis) and endogenous production (glycogenolysis and gluconeogenesis). Glucose homeostasis is controlled primarily by the anabolic hormone insulin and also by several insulin-like growth factors. Several catabolic hormones (glucagon, catecholamines, cortisol, and growth hormone) oppose the action of insulin; they are known as anti-insulin or counter-regulatory hormones (Fig. 20.1).

Insulin and glucagon are the main hormones responsible for controlling plasma glucose levels

Insulin is secreted from the pancreas in response to the increase in plasma glucose following a meal. Insulin decreases the plasma glucose concentration by promoting the uptake of glucose into tissues, intracellular glucose metabolism, and glycogen synthesis. Anti-insulin hormones stimulate both the release of glucose from glycogen stores and its *de novo* synthesis, thus causing an increase in glucose concentration in plasma (hyperglycemia). The balance between the effects of insulin and glucagon is a key factor in the control of fuel metabolism. Insulin and glucagon are both secreted from the same anatomic location – the pancreatic islets of Langerhans. Insulin is secreted by β-cells (which constitute approximately 70% of all islet cells) and glucagon is secreted by the α-cells.

INSULIN

Insulin promotes the anabolic state by channeling the metabolism towards storage of carbohydrate and lipids, and synthesis of protein. Insulin acts on three main target tissues – liver, muscle, and adipose tissue (Fig. 20.2).

Insulin secretion

Plasma glucose concentration acts as a signal that initiates the islet hormonal response

Glucose stimulates the secretion of insulin and suppresses the secretion of glucagon. Insulin is synthesized in the rough endoplasmic reticulum of the beta cells and is packaged into the secretory vesicles in the Golgi apparatus. Its secretion is initiated by the increased ATP/ADP ratio within the cell, which closes the membrane ATP-sensitive potassium channel. This depolarizes the cell, and the voltage change opens another ion channel: the calcium channel. The entry of calcium ions stimulates the first short phase of insulin secretion (compare this with the neurosecretory granules, Chapter 39) (Fig. 20.2). The second, more prolonged phase requires other signals such as an increase in the concentration of the cytosolic long-chain acetyl-CoA molecules. It also responds to diacylglycerol (DAG) – protein kinase C signaling (see below).

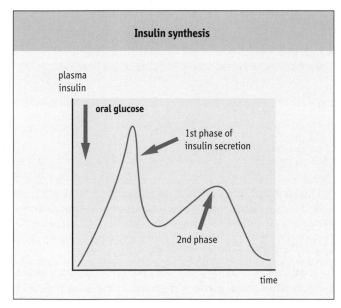

Insulin synthesis

plasma insulin

oral glucose

1st phase of insulin secretion

2nd phase

time

Fig. 20.2 **Secretion of insulin.** Note the biphasic pattern of insulin secretion after glucose load. Glucose is the most important stimulator of insulin secretion. Secretion is also stimulated by some amino acids (branched-chain amino acids – see Chapter 2) and by the stimulation of the vagus nerve.

TREATMENT OF DIABETES WITH INSULIN AND TREATMENT OF DIABETIC KETOACIDOSIS

Insulin is the mainstay of treatment of type 1 diabetes and is also required in some patients with type 2 where glycemic control cannot be achieved by other drugs. Insulin treatment involves daily subcutaneous insulin injections throughout life. Diabetic patients in whom blood glucose is difficult to control are treated with several injections per day, or sometimes, with a constant insulin infusion, delivered by a programmable, portable pump. The rate of infusion is increased at meal times to help with disposal of exogenous glucose. Diet and exercise are also important in the management of diabetes.

Emergency treatment of diabetic ketoacidosis addresses four issues: insulin lack, dehydration, potassium depletion, and acidosis. A ketoacidotic patient requires insulin infusion to reverse the metabolic effect of the excess of anti-insulin hormones, and the infusion of fluids to treat dehydration. Intravenous fluids normally contain potassium supplements to prevent a decrease in plasma potassium hypokalemia. This treatment is usually sufficient to control the metabolic acidosis; however, when the acidosis is severe, infusion of an alkaline solution (sodium bicarbonate) may be required. Type 2 diabetic patients do not usually require insulin treatment because insulin synthesis is at least partly preserved. Instead, the treatment relies on diet and oral hypoglycemic agents. Drugs, such as sulfonylurea derivatives stimulate insulin secretion. Another class of compounds, biguanides (e.g. metformin) reduce hyperglycemia by increasing peripheral glucose uptake. The newest class of drugs are the thiazolidinediones, which also affect the peripheral glucose utilization and improve insulin sensitivity.

Insulin signaling

Insulin signaling involves a membrane receptor, and a multi-step phosphorylation-driven signaling cascades

First, insulin binds to its four-subunit protein membrane receptor on target cells. The β-subunit of the receptor contains a transmembrane protein with an ATP-binding site and has tyrosine kinase activity. The binding of insulin activates the tyrosine kinase, which autophosphorylates the receptor (see Fig. 12.7). Active tyrosine kinase phosphorylates binds other proteins, such as those belonging to the insulin receptor substrate (IRS) family, designated IRS1-4), which are phosphorylated together with other proteins designated Shc, Gab-1 p60^{dok}, APS and Cbl (Cbl is a protooncogene). Subsequently, the IRS protein binds to, and activates, lipid kinase (phosphoinositol kinase) which generates 3′ phosphoinositol (PI) phosphates PI -3,4 -P2 and PI-3,4,5-P3; these act as second messengers (see also Chapter 38) . They in turn activate the phosphoinositide-dependent protein kinase (PDK1) which phosphorylates the serine/threonine kinase designated Akt. Finally, Akt participates in insulin-stimulated GLUT4 translocation, a phenomenon underlying cellular glucose uptake. Insulin also stimulates an alternate, PI3-kinase kinase-independent pathway. The response to insulin is also modulated by protein tyrosine phosphatases, enzymes that dephosphorylate the insulin receptor and other molecules in the signaling cascade. (See also Chapter 38.)

Insulin-dependent glucose transport

Insulin-dependent glucose entry into cells is mediated by glucose transporters, in particular GLUT4 which controls glucose uptake into the skeletal muscle and adipocytes. Insulin stimulates exocytosis of GLUT4 molecules to the surface of the cell membrane. Recruitment of the transporter to the plasma membrane requires insulin binding to its receptor and the operation of signaling cascade described above.

Metabolic effects of insulin

In the liver, insulin stimulates both glycolysis and glycogen synthesis. At the same time, it suppresses lipolysis and promotes the synthesis of the long-chain fatty acids (lipogenesis). Lipids are then packaged into very-low-density lipoproteins (VLDL), which are secreted into the blood. In the peripheral tissues, insulin induces lipoprotein lipase, an enzyme that liberates triacylglycerol from either hepatic VLDL or dietary chylomicrons by hydrolyzing them into glycerol and fatty acids (see Chapter 17). Insulin also stimulates triglyceride synthesis from glycerol-3-phosphate and fatty acids in the adipose tissue. In muscle, insulin stimulates glucose transport, glucose metabolism, and glycogen synthesis. Insulin also increases cellular uptake of amino acids and stimulates protein synthesis (Fig. 20.3).

Metabolic effects of glucagon and anti-insulin hormones

Anti-insulin hormones promote the endogenous production of glucose

Glucagon is a small, single chain, 29-amino-acid peptide, with a molecular weight of 3485 Da. Glucagon focuses energy metabolism on the endogenous production of glucose. Its main effect is the mobilization of the fuel reserves for the maintenance of the blood glucose level between meals. Glucagon inhibits pathways involved in the utilization of glucose and stops the storage of metabolic fuels. It acts rapidly on the liver stimulating glycogenolysis and inhibiting glycogen synthesis, glycolysis, and lipogenesis (Fig. 20.5). In parallel, it stimulates gluconeogenesis and ketogenesis (Table 20.2).

The glucagon, similarly to insulin, binds to a specific membrane receptor (see Chapter 12, Fig. 12.4). The glucagon-receptor complex causes the binding of guanosine 5¢-triphosphate (GTP) to a G-protein complex (for details of this see Chapter 38). G-protein subunits dissociate, and one of them (Ga) activates adenylate cyclase. Adenylate cyclase

PROINSULIN, INSULIN, AND C-PEPTIDE

Insulin consists of two peptide chains linked by two disulfide bonds (Fig. 20.4). The α-chain contains 21 amino acids and the β-chain 30 amino acids. The molecular weight of insulin monomer is 5500 Da. The precursor of insulin within the β-cells of the islet of Langerhans is the single chain preproinsulin. During insulin synthesis a 24-amino-acid signal sequence is first cleaved from preproinsulin by a peptidase, yielding proinsulin.

Proinsulin consists of the insulin sequence interspersed by a connecting peptide (C-peptide). At the final stage of insulin synthesis, proinsulin is split into insulin and C-peptide (Fig. 20.3), both of which are then released from the cell. C-peptide is released in an amount equimolar to insulin. This is exploited in the clinical laboratories to assess β-cell function in patients treated with exogenous (therapeutically injected) insulin. In these patients, endogenous insulin cannot be measured directly, because the exogenous insulin would interfere in the assay. In such circumstances, C-peptide measurement provides an assessment of β-cell function.

Reciprocal effects of insulin and glucagon on key enzymes of carbohydrate metabolism		
Enzyme	**Effect of glucagon**	**Effect of insulin**
Glc-6-Pase	+	−
Fru-1,6-BPase	+	−
PEPCK	+	−

Table 20.2 **Enzyme induction and repression by insulin and glucagon.** The table illustrates reciprocal effects of insulin and glucagon on the key enzymes of gluconeogenesis. Insulin affects the synthesis of key enzymes of glycolysis and gluconeogenesis. On a high-carbohydrate diet, insulin induces gene transcription of the glycolytic enzymes glucokinase, PFK, pyruvate kinase, and glycogen synthase. At the same time, it represses the key enzymes of gluconeogenesis, pyruvate carboxylase (PC), phosphoenolpyruvate carboxykinase (PEPCK), Fru-1,6-BPase, and Glc-6-Pase. Glucagon effects oppose those of insulin. On a high-fat diet, glucagon represses the synthesis of glucokinase, PFK-1, and pyruvate kinase, and induces the transcription of PEPCK, Fru-6-Pase, and Glc-6-Pase.

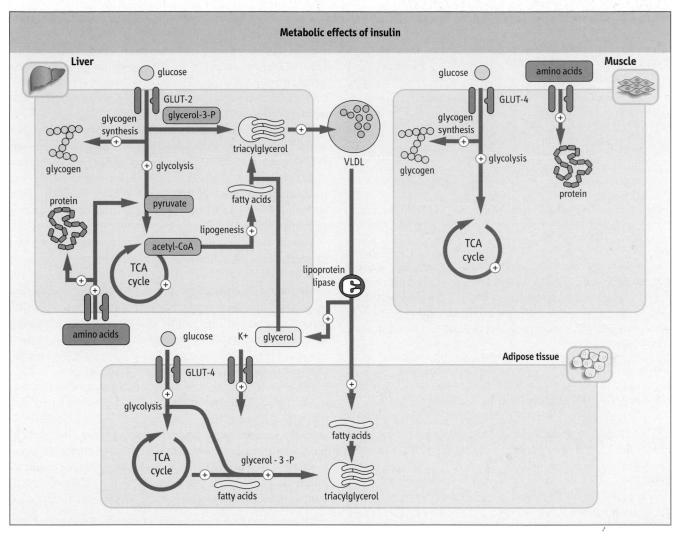

Fig. 20.3 **Metabolic effects of insulin.** Main insulin target tissues are liver, muscle, and adipose tissue. Insulin affects carbohydrate, lipid, and protein metabolism, and also promotes the cellular uptake potassium. Glucose transport mediated by GLUT-4 transporter in muscle and adipose tissue is insulin-dependent. However, the glucose transporter in liver (GLUT-2) is insulin-independent. Triglycerides are transported between tissues incorporated into very low density lipoproteins (VLDL). (See also Chapter 17.)

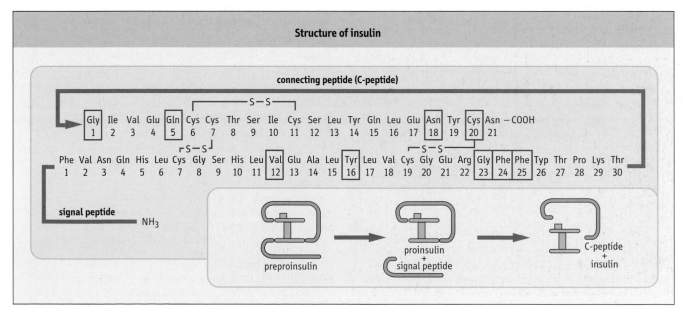

Fig. 20.4 **The insulin molecule.** C-peptide connects the α- and β-chains of insulin. Boxes indicate amino acid residues which participate in the binding to the insulin receptor.

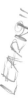

STIMULATION OF INSULIN SECRETION BY GLUCOSE

The glucose concentration in the vicinity of the β-cell is sensed by the β-cell glucose transporter GLUT-2. Glucose is carried into the cell by GLUT-2, where it is phosphorylated to form glucose 6-phosphate (Glc-6-P) by glucokinase which is a part of the glucose-sensing mechanism. Increased availability of Glc-6-P increases the rate of glucose utilization and ATP production in the β-cell. This changes the flux of of ions across the cell membrane, depolarizes the cell and increases the concentration of cytoplasmic free calcium (see text and also Chapter 38). The final result is insulin exocytosis. Insulin secretion from the β-cell after glucose stimulation is biphasic. The first phase of insulin secretion occurs within 10–15 min of stimulation and is the release of preformed insulin. The second phase, which lasts up to 2 hours, is the release of newly synthesized insulin (Fig. 20.4). Insulin secretion is also stimulated by gastrointestinal hormones and some amino acids, such as leucine, arginine, and lysine. Gastrointestinal hormones, such as glucose-dependent insulinotropic peptide (GIP), cholecystokinin, glucagon-like peptide-1 (GLP-1) and vasoactive intestinal peptide (VIP), are secreted following ingestion of foods and potentiate insulin secretion. Thus, the insulin response to orally administered glucose is greater than to an intravenous infusion.

converts ATP into a second messenger – cyclic AMP (cAMP). cAMP in turn activates cAMP-dependent protein kinase which, through phosphorylation of regulatory enzymes, controls the activity of key enzymes in carbohydrate and lipid metabolism (Figs 20.6 and 20.7, Fig. 12.4).

Epinephrine (adrenaline) has effects similar to glucagon in the liver but acts through different receptors (the α- and β-adrenergic receptors – see Chapter 40). Epinephrine promotes an increase in blood glucose in response to stress, even when glucagon concentration is low. This increases the availability of glucose to the red blood cells and the brain during stress (see below).

Muscle does not have glucagon receptors and there glycogenolysis is stimulated primarily by epinephrine in response to stress.

Hormones determine the general direction of metabolism by inducing or suppressing key enzymes (Table 20.2). This mechanism responds to diet as well as to stress and disease; for example, activities of hepatic enzymes differ in persons who eat high-fat diet compared to a high-carbohydrate diet (these changes take days or weeks to take place).

However, the short-term hormonal regulatory mechanism works through phosphorylation/dephospharylation of key molecules. Figure 20.7 illustrates concerted regulation of glycogen breakdown, gluconeogenesis and lipolysis by hormone-driven phosphorylation of key enzymes. Other mechanisms operating in the short term include substrate interactions, allosteric effectors, as well as the cell energy level and redox potential (see also Chapters 11, 12 and 15).

HYPOGLYCEMIA

Hypoglycemia (a low concentration of blood glucose) is defined as a blood glucose concentration below 2.5 mmol/L (45 mg/dL) (see Fig. 20.8). A decrease in plasma glucose concentration stimulates the sympathetic nervous system. Epinephrine and glucagon are released, resulting in a stress response, the manifestations of which may include sweating, trembling, increased heart rate, and a feeling of hunger. If blood glucose continues to fall, brain function is compromised owing to lack of glucose (neuroglycopenia). The patient becomes confused and may lose consciousness. Profound hypoglycemia can be fatal.

Hypoglycemia in healthy individuals is usually mild and may occur during exercise after a period of fasting, or as a result of drinking alcohol. Alcohol increases the intracellular NADH + H+/NAD+ ratio, which favors conversion of pyruvate to lactate and reduces the pool of pyruvate available for gluconeogenesis. Hypoglycemia may also be a feature of endocrine syndromes characterized by a low cortisol concentration caused by an insufficient amount of adrenocorticotrophic hormone (ACTH; see Chapter 37). Another endocrine cause of hypoglycemia is a rare insulin-secreting

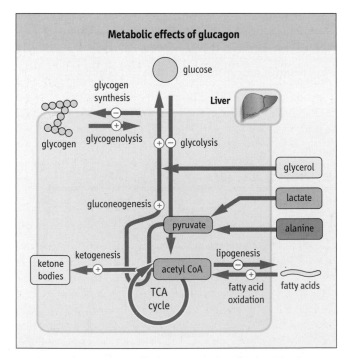

Fig. 20.5 **Metabolic effects of glucagon.** Glucagon mobilizes glucose from every available source; it also increases lipolysis, and ketogenesis from acetyl-CoA.

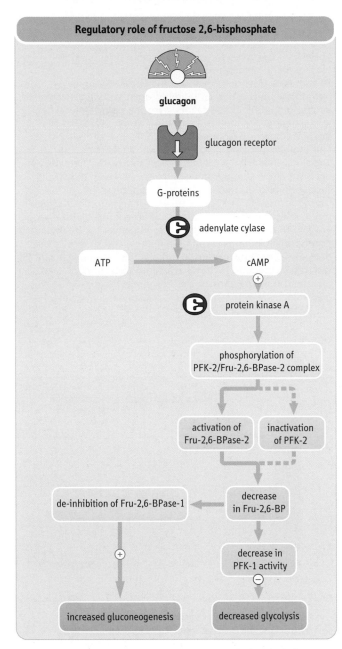

Regulatory role of fructose 2,6-bisphosphate

Fig. 20.6 **Regulation of gluconeogenesis and glycolysis by phosphofructokinase** (see Fig. 20.7). Glucagon regulates gluconeogenesis by controling the bifunctional enzyme complex that contains both phosphofructokinase-2 (PFK-2) and fructose 2,6-biphosphatase-2 (Fru-2,6-BPase-2) activity. This changes the concentration of fructose-2,6-biphosphate (Fru-2,6-BP), which in turn regulates the activity of 'mainline' enzymes: PFK-1 and Fru-2,6-BPase-1. See also Chapters 11 and 12.

 GLYCOGEN STORAGE DISEASES

Glycogen is degraded in response to a falling blood glucose concentration. A defect in the glycogenolytic pathway can lead to insufficient glucose supply and may cause hypoglycemia. This happens in patients with inherited deficiencies of enzymes controling glycogen metabolism. Seven types of glycogen storage disease are known. They are very rare, but provide an excellent insight into human energy metabolism (see Chapter 12). The symptoms of glycogen storage diseases vary and depend on the site of the enzyme defect. For instance, type 1 glycogen storage disease (von Gierke's disease) is a deficiency of Glc-6-Pase, which leads to a fasting hypoglycemia unresponsive to epinephrine and glucagon. On the other hand, patients with type V disease (McArdle's disease), which is caused by muscle phosphorylase deficiency, do not experience hypoglycemia, but have a limited ability to perform strenuous exercise (see clinical box on p. 163).

tumor of β-cells – insulinoma. Other causes are listed in Figure 20.9.

METABOLISM AFTER A MEAL AND IN THE FASTING STATE

Normally an individual oscillates between a high-insulin/low-glucagon state and a low-insulin/high-glucagon state. The high-insulin/low-glucagon state occurs during the ingestion of food and for several hours after a meal (absorptive, postprandial, or fed state). The low-insulin/high-glucagon state occurs on fasting. The early period of fasting, between 6 and 12 h, is called the postabsorptive state. Beyond that, it is either 'prolonged fasting' or 'starvation'.

Postprandial (absorptive) state

Following a meal, insulin release is stimulated and glucagon release is inhibited

Constituents of a meal stimulate insulin release and suppress the secretion of glucagon. This changes the metabolism of the liver, adipose tissue, and muscle (Fig. 20.10). After a meal, glucose utilization by the brain remains unchanged, but there is a large increase in glucose uptake in the insulin-dependent tissues, mainly skeletal muscle. Glucose oxidation and glycogen synthesis are stimulated in the liver, adipose tissue, and muscle; lipolysis is inhibited. Glucose taken up by the liver is immediately phosphorylated by glucokinase into Glc-6-P by an inducible enzyme, glucokinase. Excess glucose is directed

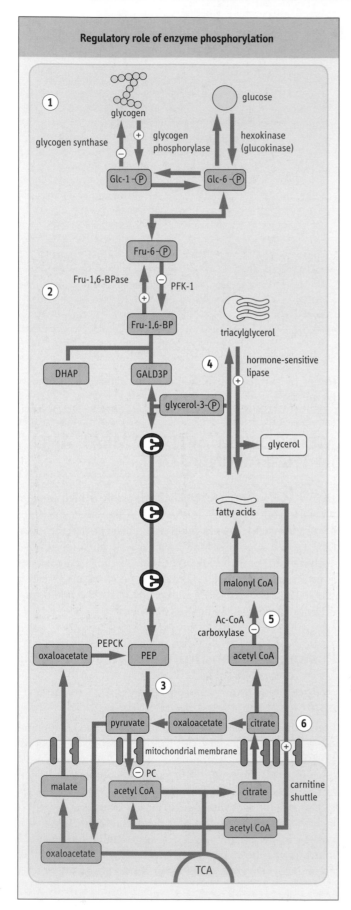

Regulatory role of enzyme phosphorylation

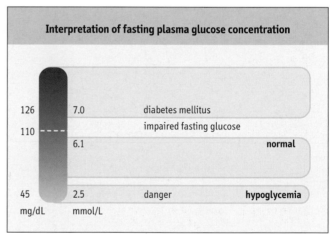

Fig. 20.7 **Regulatory role of enzyme phosphorylation.** Phosphorylation of key enzymes regulates pathways of carbohydrate and lipid metabolism. Phosphorylation of enzymes is triggered by anti-insulin hormones, such as glucagon and epinephrine.
To stimulate glycogen breakdown, hepatic glycogen phosphorylase is activated, and glycogen synthase inactivated by phosphorylation: this favors glycogen degradation (1). In gluconeogenesis, phosphorylation of the PFK-2/Fru-2,6-BPase-2 complex decreases Fru-2,6-BP formation (see Fig. 20.6). This inhibits glycolysis and accelerates gluconeogenesis (2). In addition, since Fru-1,6-BP allosterically activates pyruvate kinase downstream in the glycolytic pathway, decrease in its formation also decreases the rate of glycolysis (3). Glucagon stimulates lipolysis by phosphorylation of hormone-sensitive lipase (4) and by inhibiting acetyl-CoA carboxylase, an enzyme that converts acetyl-CoA to malonyl-CoA (5). Malonyl-CoA normally inhibits carnitine-palmitoyl transferase-1; the decrease in its intracellular de-inhibits the carnitine shuttle (6), facilitating the entry of fatty acids into mitochondria (see also Chapter 14). DHAP, dihydroxyacetone phosphate; GALD3P, glyceraldehyde-3-phosphate; PEP, phosphoenolpyruvate.

Fig. 20.8 **Interpretation of fasting plasma glucose concentration:** the normal level, hyperglycemia, and hypoglycemia. To obtain glucose concentrations in mg/dL, multiply by 18.

into the pentose phosphate pathway to yield NADPH + H+, which is essential for various reductive biosyntheses, such as lipogenesis and cholesterol synthesis.

Intestinal absorption of fat results in the assembly of large chylomicron particles in the enterocytes. Triacylglycerol-rich chylomicrons are released into the lymphatic system and reach the circulation through the thoracic duct. Triacylglycerol is hydrolyzed by lipoprotein lipase, an insulin-inducible enzyme present on the peripheral endothelium, which hydrolyzes it to glycerol and free fatty acids (see Chapter 17). Fatty acids are taken up by adipose tissue and are stored

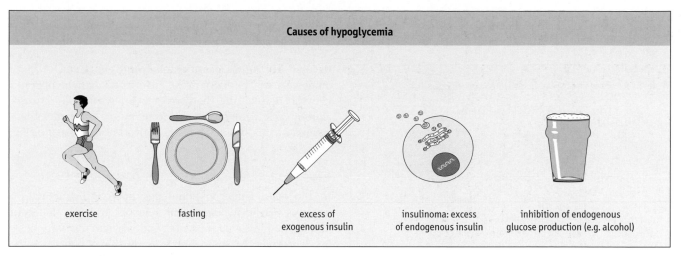

Fig. 20.9 **Causes of hypoglycemia.**

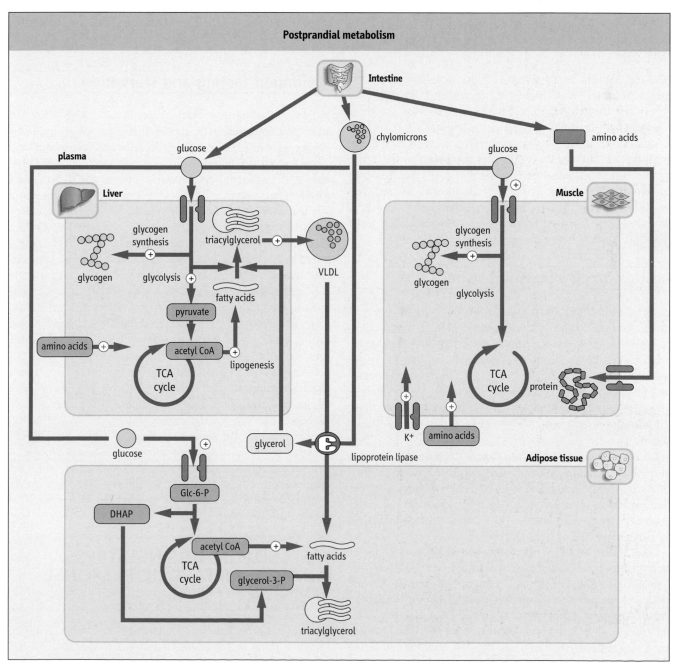

Fig. 20.10 **Postprandial metabolism.** In the postprandial state insulin directs metabolism towards storage and synthesis (anabolism). DHAP, dihydroxyacetone phosphate. Glc-6-P, glucose-6-phosphate.

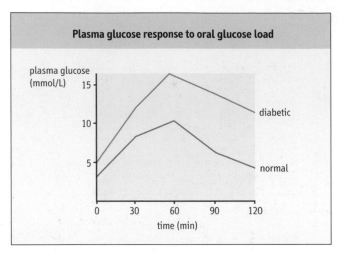

Fig. 20.11 **The oral glucose tolerance test (OGTT).** To obtain glucose concentrations in mg/dL, multiply by 18. (Compare Table 20.5)

reassembled into triacylglycerols. Fatty acids are used as a fuel in muscle. Triose phosphate produced from glycolysis is reduced to glycerol-3-phosphate (glycerol-3-P), which is estrerified to form triacylglycerol. In the liver and adipose tissue, insulin suppresses lipolysis and increases intracellular synthesis of fatty acids. VLDL are assembled to transport lipids synthesized de novo in the liver to the peripheral tissues. Insulin also stimulates amino acid uptake and protein synthesis in the liver, muscle, and adipose tissue. Protein degradation in these tissues decreases. Changes in plasma glucose following glucose ingestion are illustrated in Fig. 20.11.

Postabsorptive (fasting) state

In the clinical jargon the postabsorptive state is often referred to as 'fasting'. During the postabsorptive state, glucose metabolism approaches a steady state (i.e. hepatic glucose production, largely from glycogenolysis, equals its tissue uptake). After an overnight fast, insulin secretion decreases and glucagon secretion increases. This leads to a decrease in glycogen synthesis and to an increase in glycogenolysis (Fig. 20.12); the liver gradually becomes a glucose-producing organ.

In the postabsorptive state, approximately 80% of all glucose is taken up by insulin-independent tissues. Of this, 50% goes to the brain and 20% to the erythrocytes. In the postabsorptive state insulin-dependent tissues use little glucose – muscle and adipose tissue together are responsible for just about 20% of total glucose utilization.

After a 12h fast, 65–75% of endogenous glucose is derived from glycogen, and the rest from gluconeogenesis. The contribution of gluconeogenesis, however, increases. Muscle releases lactate which, after being oxidized to pyruvate, enters gluconeogenesis. Glucose that is formed returns to the skeletal muscle; this is known as the Cori cycle. Low insulin level also stimulates proteolysis. The two main amino acids

released from muscle are alanine and glutamine. A cycle analogous to the Cori cycle, involving alanine, operates between muscle and the liver: it is known as the glucose-alanine cycle. Alanine released from muscle enters gluconeogenesis in the liver after being converted to pyruvate (Fig. 20.13).

Glucagon activates lipolysis in adipose tissue

In the liver, glucagon stimulates lipolysis by acting on hormone-sensitive lipase. This releases glycerol, the third major gluconeogenic substrate, and provides free fatty acids for energy metabolism in muscle. Activation of lipolysis in the liver secondarily stimulates ketogenesis from acetyl-CoA, yielding acetoacetate, hydroxybutyrate, and the product of spontaneous decarboxylation of acetoacetate, acetone. The three metabolites are known as ketone bodies and are oxidized in heart and skeletal muscle.

Prolonged fasting and starvation

Prolonged fasting is a chronic low-insulin, high-glucagon state. The brain adapts to this by using ketone bodies as an energy substrate. There is also a decrease in thyroid hormone levels and, clinically, lethargy. Early in the fasting period, free fatty acid concentrations increase in plasma and they become a major energy source. At the same time oxaloacetate is being directed towards gluconeogenesis and its low concentration in the mitochondria tends to limit TCA cycle activity (see Chapter 13). Consequently, large amounts of acetyl CoA produced by β-oxidation of fatty acids in the liver enter ketogenesis instead of the TCA cycle. There is an increase in the concentration of plasma ketone bodies, which are oxidized in the muscle. Alanine and glutamine released from muscle serve as substrates for gluconeogenesis. During prolonged fasting, gluconeogenesis in the kidney becomes a significant source of endogenous glucose. The body minimizes the use of proteins as a gluconeogenic substrate by becoming almost totally dependent on fat as an energy source (Fig. 20.14). The amount of the GLUT-4 in the adipose tissue and muscle decreases. As the plasma concentrations of ketone bodies continue to rise, the brain uses them as a fuel. Some brain tissue also switches from the complete oxidation of glucose to CO_2, to glycolysis. As the produced lactate enters the Cori cycle operating between the brain and the liver, the requirement for endogenous glucose production decreases; this spares muscle protein.

METABOLISM DURING STRESS, AND THE METABOLIC RESPONSE TO INJURY

Stress is not only 'fight and flight' response but also trauma, injury – particularly burns, surgery, or infection. All are

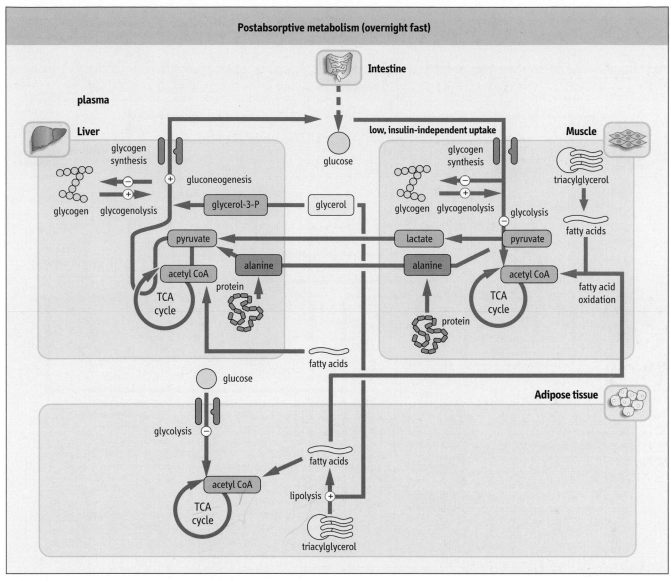

Fig. 20.12 **Postabsorptive metabolism (overnight fast).** In the postabsorptive state, glucose is provided from endogenous sources (glycogenolysis and gluconeogenesis). Alanine and lactate cycles are operative (see Fig. 20.13 for details) There are three main gluconeogenic substrates: alanine, lactate, and glycerol.

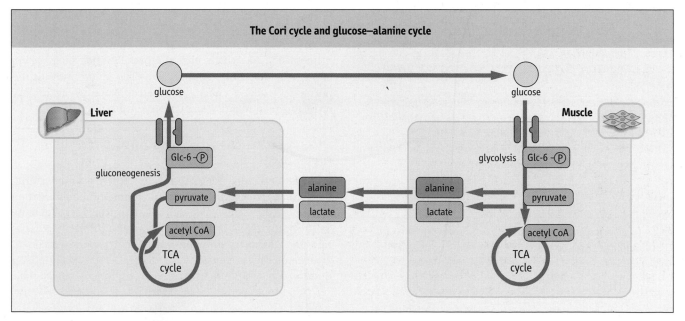

Fig. 20.13 **The Cori cycle and glucose–alanine cycle.** The Cori (glucose-lactate) cycle allows recycling of lactate back to glucose, but does not contribute to the *de novo* synthesis of glucose.

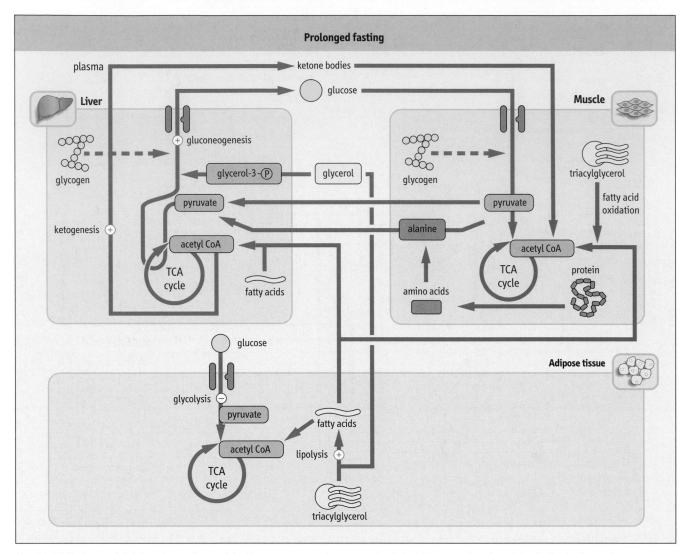

Fig. 20.14 **Prolonged fasting.** In prolonged fasting, glycogen stores are depleted. The supply of metabolic fuels depends on gluconeogenesis and lipolysis. Ketone bodies become an important energy source; their utilization spares muscle protein.

 PLASMA GLUCOSE AFTER MYOCARDIAL INFARCTION 245

A 66-year-old woman was admitted to the cardiology ward after suffering a myocardial infarction. Her random plasma glucose level was 10.5 mmol/L (189 mg/dL). The next day a fasting blood glucose was only slightly raised at 6.5 mmol/L (117 mg/dL). Normal fasting plasma glucose is <6.1mmol/L.

Comment. This patient underwent a major stress, myocardial infarction, which is associated with a counter-regulatory hormone response and this in turn leads to the elevation of the blood glucose concentration. Care is necessary in the interpretation of raised fasting glucose levels or abnormal glucose tolerance tests in the context of acute illness.

associated with a metabolic response characterized by hypermetabolism, in which the sympathetic nervous system plays a major role (Fig. 20.15). The main anti-insulin hormones taking part are catecholamines (primarily epinephrine) and glucagon; cortisol is also important.

During stress the brain has priority for fuel supply

In the first phase of the stress response there is vasoconstriction, which limits blood loss, should it happen. Fuels are then mobilized from all available sources, with provision of glucose for the brain taking priority: high concentrations of epinephrine and glucagon stimulate glycogenolysis and gluconeogenesis to provide endogenous glucose. Decreased peripheral uptake of glucose enhances the hyperglycemic effect. This

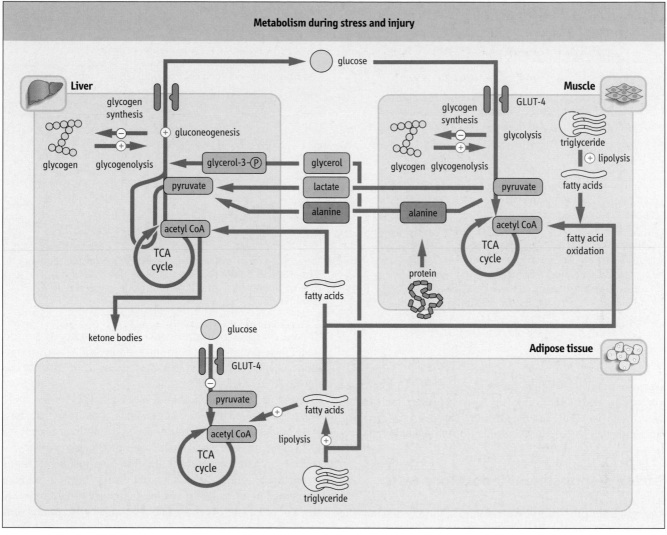

Fig. 20.15 **Metabolism during stress and injury.** First, glucose is mobilized from all available sources. Epinephrine inhibits the secretion of insulin and the effect of anti-insulin hormones prevails. Stress also induces peripheral insulin resistance. Second, metabolic fuels are provided from fatty acids and from protein catabolism. Such metabolic response occurs in injury, trauma, surgery, burns, and infection.

results in moderate, frequently detectable, hyperglycemia. Later, the metabolic rate increases and energy is provided primarily from the oxidation of fatty acids and from protein metabolism. Gluconeogenesis from muscle-derived amino acids increases. A negative nitrogen balance is evident approximately 2-3 days post injury.

Stress induces insulin resistance in muscle, adipose tissue, and liver, probably at a postreceptor level

The insulin-dependent transport of glucose in adipose tissue and skeletal muscle decreases most probably because of the suppression of insulin's effect on GLUT-4-mediated glucose uptake. However, at the same time insulin-independent glucose uptake, particularly in muscle, increases. This is caused by tumor necrosis factor (TNF) and other cytokines, such as interleukin-1 (IL-1) (see Chapter 41). TNF also stimulates muscle glycogen breakdown. Glucocorticoids contribute to the stress response by inhibiting glucose transport in peripheral cells. They also facilitate stimulation of gluconeogenesis by glucagon and catecholamines by inducing Glc-6-Pase and PEPCK genes (see Table 20.2). Cytokines, such as IL-6, also affect PEPCK. They stimulate lipolysis in adipose tissue and contribute to muscle proteolysis.

There is also an increase in lactate concentration. Lactate is converted to pyruvate in the liver via lactate dehydrogenase. Thus, in the metabolic response to stress there is suppression of anabolic pathways (glycogen synthesis, lipogenesis), increased catabolism (glycogenolysis, lipolysis, and proteolysis), increased insulin-independent peripheral

MAJOR STRESS ALSO AFFECTS WATER AND ELECTROLYTE METABOLISM

A 65-year-old woman underwent a partial gastrectomy. After surgery she was given a standard intravenous fluid replacement. The volume of fluids to be replaced was calculated on the basis of fluid lost in urine, through gastric drainage, and included an allowance for an insensible loss (water loss with breath and sweat). In spite of carefully calculated fluid volume and a normal renal function, the patient developed hyponatraemia due to overload with water. Rapid onset of hyponatraemia may cause convulsions or coma due to cerebral edema.

Comment. The response to stress, such as major surgery, includes the stimulation of the secretion of vasopressin (antidiuretic hormone) from the posterior pituitary (see Chapter 35). This causes increased water reabsorption by the kidney and a consequent water retention which needs to be taken into account when prescribing fluid therapy in the postoperative period. (See also Chapters 21 and 22.)

glucose uptake. All this takes place on the background of insulin resistance. Clinically there is fever, tachycardia (increased heart rate), tachypnea (increased respiratory rate), and leukocytosis (increased number of white blood cells).

Stress response and laboratory tests

Understanding of the stress response is important for the physician as it affects the results of laboratory tests. Hyperglycemia observed during stress should not be confused with diabetes mellitus. Stress such as injury, infection, or trauma is also associated with the acute phase response, in which a variety of proteins, such as α_1-antitrypsin, C-reactive protein (CRP), haptoglobin, α_1-acid glycoprotein, complement proteins, and others, are produced. The measurements of CRP are important in the monitoring of the progress of therapy in patients with severe infections and inflammatory disorders. (See Chapter 3.)

DIABETES MELLITUS: THE PRINCIPAL DISORDER OF FUEL METABOLISM

Diabetes mellitus is a heterogeneous metabolic disease characterized by hyperglycemia and by the presence of long-term vascular complications. Diabetes has been defined as 'a lifestyle disorder with the highest prevalence seen in genetically susceptible populations, where the disease is unmasked lifestyle-associated environmental factors'. It is a common

Classification of diabetes	
Syndrome	**Comments**
Type 1	autoimmune destruction of β-cells
Type 2	insulin resistance and β-cell failure
Other types	genetic defects of β-cells (e.g. mutations of glucokinase gene). Rare insulin resistance syndromes. Diseases of exocrine pancreas. Endocrine diseases (acromegaly, Cushing's syndrome). Drugs and chemical-induced diabetes, Infections (e.g. mumps). Rare syndromes with the presence of antireceptor antibodies. Diabetes accompanying other genetic diseases (e.g. Down syndrome)
Gestational diabetes	any degree of glucose intolerance diagnosed in pregnancy

Table 20.3 **Classification of diabetes.** Type 1 (insulin-dependent) diabetes and type 2 (noninsulin-dependent) diabetes. Approximately 90% of all diabetic patients have type 2 diabetes.

disease. Alarmingly, its prevalence has been increasing worldwide. Type 2 diabetes affects approximately 8% of the population of the USA, and in 1995 its worldwide prevalence was approximately 4% (Table 20.3).

There are two main forms of diabetes: type 1 and type 2. Ten percent of all diabetic patients have type 1 and 90% have type 2 diabetes (Table 20.4). While type 1 patients are unable to produce insulin and need exogenous insulin to survive, type 2 patients secrete insulin, but are insulin-resistant. Importantly, some diabetic patients may have no clinical symptoms at all, with the diagnosis made exclusively on the basis of laboratory results. The diagnostic criteria are summarized in Table 20.5.

CATABOLIC STATE AFTER ROAD TRAFFIC ACCIDENT

A 60-year-old man was admitted to an Intensive Care Unit following multiple trauma in a road traffic accident. He developed respiratory failure and was intubated. On the third day he was still unable to eat. His fasting blood glucose was 6.7 mmol/L (121 mg/dL), he had mild ketonuria (+), and his 24-h urine collection revealed the excretion of 600 mg of α-amino nitrogen/24 h (normal 50–300 mg/24 h).

Comment. This patient is hypercatabolic as a result of the stress response to injury. He is not able to take food. His high urinary nitrogen loss indicates excessive catabolism of muscle protein. He requires nutritional support. The patient was prescribed an intravenous nutrition regimen containing 2000 kcal (8374 kJ) as 50% glucose solution, 1000 kcal (4187 kJ) as lipid emulsion, and amino acid solution containing the equivalent of 18 g of nitrogen/day.

Type 1 diabetes

Type 1 diabetes develops in young people, with the peak incidence at approximately 12 years of age. It is caused by autoimmune destruction of pancreatic β-cells. The precipitating cause is still unclear. It could be that a viral infection initiates the autoimmune reaction. Alternatively, a cytokine response to viral infection, or to another insult, could attract monocytes and macrophages that infiltrate and destroy the pancreatic islets. In addition to the inflammatory infiltr of the islets, a proportion of patients have antibodies aga...ist β-cell proteins. These are often present before the diagnosis of diabetes. Circulating autoantibodies to insulin itself are also present in some individuals.

The susceptibility to type 1 diabetes appears to be inherited, however, no 'diabetes gene' has yet been discovered. The best investigated susceptibility gene is located on chromosome 6 in the major histocompatibility complex (MHC) that codes for immune system recognition molecules known as histocompatibility antigens (HLA) (see Chapter 36). Susceptibility to type 1 diabetes is associated with HLA types DR4 and DQw8, whereas DR2 and DQw1.2 appear to suppress the tendency to develop the disease. The sibling of a type 1 diabetic patient has a 10% chance of developing diabetes by the age of 50 years.

Type 2 diabetes

Type 2 diabetes usually develops in patients who are over 40 years old and who frequently are obese. The pathogenesis of type 2 diabetes involves insulin resistance and impairment of insulin secretion. It is unclear which of these mechanisms is primary, because they usually operate together. The response of the diabetic β-cell to the glucose stimulus in type 2 diabetes is suboptimal and, after glucose stimulation, there is no first phase of insulin secretion (see Fig. 20.2).

There is no consistent inheritance pattern in type 2 diabetes. No doubt there is a strong hereditary component; monozygotic twins are 90–95% concordant for type 2 diabetes, and first-degree relatives of diabeteic persons have a 40% chance of developing the disease. By contrast, in people with no diabetic relatives such risk is only 10%.

There is a genetic form of type 2 diabetes, the maturity onset diabetes of the young (MODY); however, it affects only a small minority of patients. MODY results from

Comparison of type 1 and type 2 diabetes mellitus

	Type 1	Type 2
Onset	usually under 20 years of age	usually over 40 years of age
Insulin synthesis	absent: immune destruction of β-cells	preserved: combination of impaired β-cell function and insulin
Plasma insulin concentration	low or absent	low, normal, or high
Genetic susceptibility	inheritance associated with HLA antigens	not associated with HLA, polygenic
Islet cell antibodies at diagnosis	yes	no
Obesity	uncommon	common
Ketoacidosis	yes	possible as a result of major stress

Table 20.4 **Comparison of type 1 and type 2 diabetes.** Type 1 diabetes was formerly known as insulin-dependent diabetes, IDDM, or juvenile diabetes, and type 2 diabetes was described as noninsulin-dependent diabetes, NIDDM, or maturity-onset diabetes.

Diagnosis of diabetes mellitus and glucose intolerance

Condition	Diagnostic criteria (mmol/L)	Diagnostic criteria (mg/dL)	Comments
normal fasting plasma glucose	below 6.1	below 110	
impaired fasting glucose (IFG)	equal or above 6.1 but below 7.0	equal or above 110 but below 126	
impaired glucose tolerance (IGT)	plasma glucose 2 h after 75 g load 7.8 or above, but below 11.1	plasma glucose 2 h after 75 g load 140 or above, but below 200	diagnosed during OGIT
diabetes mellitus*			
criterion 1	random plasma glucose 11.1 or above[†]	random plasma glucose 200 or above[†]	
criterion 2	fasting plasma glucose 7.0 or above	fasting plasma glucose 126 or above	
criterion 3	2 h value during OGTT 11.1 or above	2 h value during OGTT 200 or above	

*If one of the criteria is fulfilled, diagnosis is provisional. The diagnosis needs to be confirmed next day using a different criterion.
[†]If accompanied by symptoms (polyuria, polydypsia, unexplained weight loss). These are the criteria proposed by the American Diabetes Association in 1997 (see Further Reading).

Table 20.5 **Diagnostic criteria for diabetes mellitus and glucose intolerance.**

TYPICAL PRESENTATION OF DIABETIC KETOACIDOSIS

A 15-year-old girl was admitted to the Accident and Emergency department. She was confused and her breath had a smell of acetone. She had signs of dehydration with reduced tissue turgor and dry tongue. She also had rapid pauseless respirations. Her blood glucose was 18.0 mmol/L (324 mg/dL) and ketones were present in the urine. Her serum potassium concentration was 4.9 mmol/L (normal = 3.5–5.0 mmol/L) and her arterial blood pH was 7.20 (normal = 7.37–7.44).

Comment. This is a typical presentation of diabetic ketoacidosis. Hyperventilation is a compensatory response to acidosis (see Chapter 22). A patient like this needs to be treated as a medical emergency. She received an intravenous infusion containing physiologic saline with potassium supplements to replace lost fluid and an infusion of insulin.

mutations of at least six different genes: an enzyme glucokinase (MODY2), and several transcription factors (hepatocyte nuclear factor HNF-4α (MODY1) , HNF-α₁ (MODY3)), insulin promoter factor (IPF-1), HNF-1α and β-cell transcription factor (neuroD1). There is also a mitochondrial DNA mutation that leads to impaired oxidative phosphorylation and to the so-called 'mitochondrial diabetes'.

In most patients the disease has a polygenic background

A large research effort focuses presently on the identification susceptibility genes for type 2 diabetes. The recently discovered such gene is present in NIDDM1 locus on chromosome 2 and codes for calpain-10 (calcium-activated neutral protease). Other susceptibility genes could be coding for any of the components of fuel metabolism described above: the insulin receptor, IRS-1, GLUT4, or enzymes associated with carbohydrate and lipid pathways. Watch this space.

Metabolism in diabetes

Poorly controlled diabetes may lead to life-threatening diabetic ketoacidosis

Ketoacidosis develops predominantly in persons with type 1 diabetes who have no, or very little, insulin in plasma. Because of this they have a low insulin-to-glucagon concentration ratio. Lack of insulin does not allow glucose to enter insulin-dependent tissues, such as adipose tissue and muscle. Glycolysis and lipogenesis are inhibited, and glycogenolysis, lipolysis, ketogenesis, and gluconeogenesis are stimulated (Fig. 20.16). The key phenomenon is that the liver becomes a net producer of glucose. Increased endogenous glucose production, together with impaired glucose transport, lead to

fasting hyperglycemia. Simultaneously, unopposed lipolysis produces an excess of acetyl-CoA. Ketogenesis is stimulated. In a decompensated patient, ketonemia and ketonuria develop (Fig. 20.17). Overproduction of acetoacetic and b-hydroxybutyric acids decrease the pH of blood, and causes metabolic acidosis (see Chapter 23). In a type 1 diabetic patient, ketoacidosis can develop quickly, even after missing a single insulin dose. In type 2 diabetes, ketoacidosis is relatively rare but may be precipitated by a major stress, such as myocardial infarction.

Because glucose is osmotically active, its increased renal excretion causes water loss (osmotic diuresis). Poorly controlled diabetic patients complain of having to drink a lot of fluid (polydypsia) and of passing large volumes of urine (polyuria). The fluid loss eventually leads to dehydration (see Chapter 22).

Hypoglycemia is the most common complication of diabetes

Hypoglycemia, described earlier in this chapter, is the most common acute complication of diabetes. It develops when the balance between insulin dose, carbohydrate supply, and physical activity becomes disrupted. Thus, hypoglycemia may occur as a result of taking too much insulin or missing a meal. Exercise increases tissue glucose uptake independently of insulin; therefore diabetic patients must decrease their insulin dose before strenuous exercise to prevent hypoglycemia. In mild hypoglycemia, having a sweet drink or several lumps of sugar to eat is enough to control it. Many diabetic patients sense the early symptoms of hypoglycemia and should carry sweets to prevent severe events. Severe hypoglycemia, however, is a medical emergency that requires immediate treatment with either intravenous glucose or glucagon.

In diabetes, glucose present in excess is a toxic substrate

Glucose undergoes auto-oxidation yielding reactive oxygen species and intracellular precursors of advanced glycation endproducts (AGE, see below). Also, hyperglycemia alters the cellular redox state by increasing the NADH/NAD⁺ ratio and decreasing NADPH/NADP⁺. This causes increases the flux of substrates through the polyol pathway. The reactive oxygen species create oxidative stress, which damages molecules and activates a number of signaling molecules such as protein kinase C or the transcription factor NFκB (NFκB is a key determinant of inflammatory response). Hyperglycemia itself also activates NFκB pathway.

Inflammatory reaction in diabetes may play a role in the vascular complications

The low grade inflammatory reaction affecting the vascular wall seems to be present not only in atherosclerosis (Chapter

non insulin dependent diabetes mellitus

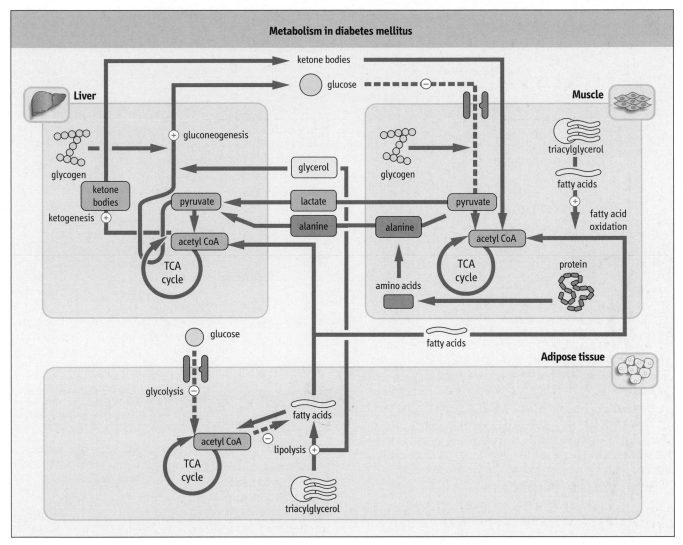

Fig. 20.16 **Metabolism in diabetes mellitus.** Hyperglycemia in diabetes mellitus is caused by the combined effect of the increased endogenous glucose production by the liver and the impaired peripheral glucose uptake.

17) but also in obesity and type 2 diabetes, and leads to increased expression of mediators such as TNF and IL-6. It seems that the deterioration of carbohydrate intolerance leading from obesity to type 2 diabetes is faster if it happens on the background of low-grade inflammation.

Formation of the advanced glycation endproducts is a result of hyperglycemia

Hyperglycemia leads to the formation of glucose adducts with proteins, the AGE (Fig. 20.18). Some AGE function as protein crosslinks and, for instance, increase the ridigity of collagen molecules. They also bind to membrane receptors on the vascular endothelial cells, stimulate the generation of TNF-α, IL1-β and IL-6, and activate NFκB (Chapter 32). They may contribute to the development of atherosclerosis in diabetes.

Toxicity of glucose is associated with long-term complications of diabetes

Slowly developing changes in small (microangiopathy) and large (macroangiopathy) arteries are part of the diabetic syndrome. In the long term these changes lead to kidney failure (diabetic nephropathy), blindness (caused by diabetic retinopathy), and to the impairment of nerve function (diabetic neuropathy). Diabetic patients also develop lens opacities (cataracts). Owing to macroangiopathy, diabetic individuals are at a two to three times greater risk of myocardial infarction than people who are nondiabetic. Finally, the diabetic peripheral vascular disease is a major cause of foot ulcers and lower limb amputations. Currently, cardiovascular disease is the most prevalent complication, and is the main cause of death among people with diabetes. Diabetes is also

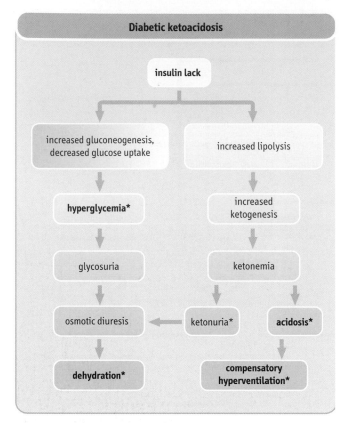

Fig. 20.17 **The development of diabetic ketoacidosis.** The clinical picture of ketoacidosis is a consequence of hyperglycemia (osmotic diuresis, dehydration) and increased lipolysis (ketonemia and acidosis). *Indicates the most important clinical and laboratory findings.

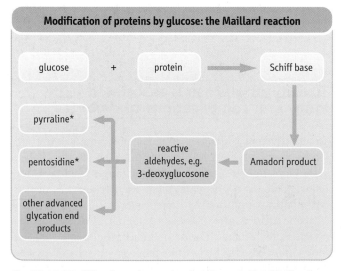

Fig. 20.18 **Modification of proteins by glucose: the Maillard reaction.** The modification of protein structure and function by sugars leads the formation of the advanced glycation end-products (AGE). (See also Chapter 35.)

DIABETIC KETOACIDOSIS AFFECTS BODY POTASSIUM BALANCE

Insulin increases potassium uptake by cells. Lack of insulin leads to release of potassium, particularly from skeletal muscle. Since uncontrolled diabetes is accompanied by an osmotic diuresis, the released potassium is excreted through the kidney. Most diabetic patients admitted to hospital with ketoacidosis are potassium-depleted but often have normal or raised levels of plasma potassium. Exogenous insulin given to such patients stimulates the entry of potassium into cells and can lead to very low plasma potassium levels (hypokalemia). Hypokalemia is dangerous, owing to its effects on cardiac muscle. Thus, except for patients with very high potassium levels, potassium supplementation needs to be considered in the treatment of diabetic ketoacidosis. (See Chapters 21 and 22.)

PROTEIN MODIFICATION BY GLUCOSE

Hyperglycemia promotes the nonenzymatic attachment of glucose to protein molecules (protein glycation). Glucose-protein adducts transform further in a sequence of nonenzymatic reactions (Fig. 20.20), collectively known as the Maillard reaction (so-called after the French chemist, Louis Camille Maillard). Amino acid residues involved include the a-amino terminal amino acid and ε-amino groups of lysine residues. First, a labile Schiff base is formed. This spontaneously transforms to ketoamine through the Amadori rearrangement. Glycated hemoglobin, hemoglobin A1c (HbA1c), is the most widely studied Amadori product. Other proteins, such as albumin and collagen, can also form Amadori products. Glycation changes the electrical charge of proteins and can affect their functions, such as binding to membrane receptors. For instance, glycation of apolipoprotein B slows down the rate of receptor-dependent metabolism of low-density lipoproteins (LDL). (See Chapter 17.)
Amadori products transform further to form protein crosslinks known as advanced glycation end products (AGE). AGE crosslink long-lived body proteins such as tissue collagen or a nerve protein, myelin. AGE formation 'stiffens' the extracellular matrix and decreases the elasticity of, for instance, the arterial wall. Their formation also affects the function of endothelial cells, phagocytes (macrophages), and smooth muscle cells in the wall of blood vessels. Through these mechanisms AGE may contribute to the development of the late complications of diabetes and probably other vascular diseases.

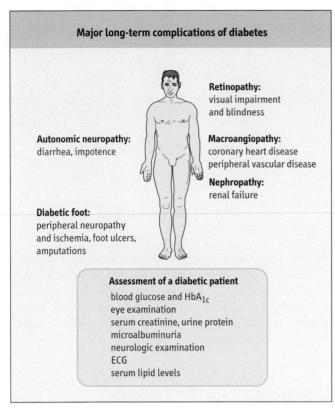

Fig. 20.19 **Major long-term complications of diabetes.** Late complications of diabetes mellitus include abnormalities of small arteries (microangiopathy: diabetic retinopathy and nephropathy), large arteries (diabetic macroangiopathy: coronary heart disease and peripheral vascular disease), and also in diabetic neuropathy, which results from a combination of vascular and structural tissue changes.

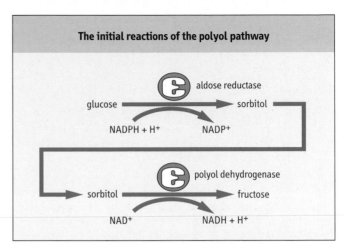
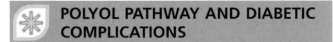

Fig. 20.20 **The polyol pathway.** The polyol pathway contributes to the development of diabetic neuropathy. This pathway may be inhibited by inhibitors of its rate-limiting enzyme, aldose reductase.

POLYOL PATHWAY AND DIABETIC COMPLICATIONS

Glucose can be reduced to sorbitol by aldose reductase (Fig. 20.20). Sorbitol is further oxidized by sorbitol dehydrogenase to fructose. Since aldose reductase has a high Km for glucose, the pathway is not very active at normal glucose levels. When there is hyperglycemia, however, glucose levels in insulin-independent tissues (which glucose enters freely), such as the red blood cells, nerve, and lens, increase and consequently there is an increase in the activity of the polyol pathway. Like glucose, sorbitol exerts an osmotic effect. This is thought to play a role in the development of diabetic cataracts. In addition, the high level of sorbitol decreases cellular uptake of another alcohol, myoinositol, which decreases the activity of plasma membrane Na^+/K^+ ATPase. This in turn affects nerve function and, along with hypoxia and reduced nerve blood flow, contributes to the development of diabetic neuropathy. Drugs inhibiting aldose reductase improve the peripheral nerve function in diabetes.

the main cause of blindness in the Western world and one of the main causes of kidney failure. The late complications are illustrated in Figure 20.19.

Presently considered mechanisms of microvascular complications include the formation of AGE, the oxidative stress, and also the increased substrate flux through polyol pathways (Fig. 20.20). Abnormal activation of the signaling cascades, changing the pattern of synthesis of growth factors and the operation of ion channels emerges as fundamentally important. A recent hypothesis put forward by Michael Brownlee proposes that the production of excess reactive oxygen species by the mitochondrial electron transport chain is the unifying mechanism of diabetic complications (see Further Reading). Hyperglycemia, by affecting the amount of proton donors within the cell, would increase electrochemical potential difference across the inner mitochondrial membrane and would thus lead to an increased production of reactive oxygen species (ROS). ROS would change cellular signaling patterns, leading to the development of insulin resistance and impaired insulin secretion, and in the long-term, the vascular changes.

Insulin resistance

Insulin resistance signifies inadequate tissue response to the hormone

Insulin resistance, mentioned above in the context of development of type 2 diabetes, is a condition where a given amount of insulin produces a less than expected response. In insulin resistant individuals normal plasma glucose

Sites of insulin resistance		
Site of resistance	**Possible defect**	**Role in diabetes**
Prereceptor	insulin receptor antibodies, abnormal molecule	rare
Receptor	decreased number or affinity of insulin receptors	not important in diabetes
Postreceptor	defects in signal transduction: defective tyrosine phosphylation (?), reduced IRS-1 level, decreased phosphatidylinositol-3' kinase decreased activity of key enzymes such as pyruvate dehydrogenase or glycogen synthase	most probable site of insulin resistance in diabetes
Glucose transport	defective translocation of glucose transporters to cell membrane	important

Table 20.6 **Sites of insulin resistance.** Cellular insulin resistance may arise at prereceptor or postreceptor level. Insulin resistance is important in obesity, glucose intolerance and type 2 diabetes mellitus. As a component of the metabolic syndrome it is associated with increased risk of cardiovascular disease.

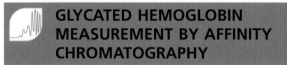

GLYCATED HEMOGLOBIN MEASUREMENT BY AFFINITY CHROMATOGRAPHY

Originally HbA1c has been identified by its electrical charge: it migrated faster than the main HbA1 peak on electrophoresis. An ingenious way of measuring glycated hemoglobin is by boronic acid affinity chromatography. The hydroxyl groups in cis-configuration present in the glycated hemoglobin molecule interact with with m-aminophenylboronic acid immobilized on a chromatographic column. Borate produces a complex with the hydroxyl groups favouring the *cis* configuration. As a result glycated haemoglobin is retained on the column while non-glycated species washes through. Subsequently glycated species is liberated from the columsn and measured spectrophotometrically. Importantly, this method measures all glycated fractions of haemoglobin, not only HbA1c, therefore reference values obtained with this method are different from those obtained by electrophoresis.

insulin receptor signaling: for instance, in persons with type 2 diabetes and those with strong family history of diabetes, abnormal operation of the IRS-phosphoinositol kinase pathway leads to a defective cellular translocation of the GLUT4 transporter, and consequently to the impaired glucose uptake in skeletal muscle and adipose tissue.

Treatment of insulin resistance

Drugs which affect insulin resistance are metformin and recently introduced thiazolidinediones. Thiazolidinediones improve insulin action by binding to the nuclear peroxisome proliferator activator receptor receptor-gamma (PPARγ in the adipose tissue (and, to a lesser extent in muscle), and subsequently increasing transcription of a variety of insulin-sensitive genes responsible for glucose and lipid metabolism. They also activate IRS- phosphoinositol kinase signaling pathway.

There are links between obesity, glucose intolerance, diabetes, and cardiovascular disease

Because diabetes mellitus affects all pathways of fuel metabolism, it should not be just regarded as a discrete, separate disease. First of all, it is closely linked to obesity (obesity is a major risk factor for diabetes). In many obese persons one often observes transition from normal glucose metabolism to impaired glucose tolerance and, subsequently, to diabetes.

Also, it is increasingly clear that there are common denominators in diabetes mellitus and cardiovascular disease such as insulin resistance, the low-grade inflammation affecting vasculature (Chapter 17), and the increased tendency to blood coagulation (hypercoagulable state – Chapter 6). In fact, these observations led to the hypotesis proposing 'common soil' for diabetes and cardiovascular disease. The relationships between obesity diabetes and atherosclerosis are illustrated in Figure 20.21.

concentrations is present together with hyperinsulinemia: this is because more insulin is required to produce the 'normal' effect. Insulin resistance is present not only in overt type 2 diabetes mellitus but also in the two conditions which commonly precede diabetes: obesity and impaired glucose tolerance. It also occurs in children of diabetic parents, certifying to its genetic background.

The genetic component to insulin resistance is also confirmed by studies on several strains of knockout mice lacking genes for insulin receptor, GLUT-4, and IRS-1: they all demonstrate insulin resistance. Within a target cell, the resistance may be caused by defects at several levels (Table 20.6). Insulin-receptor binding could be compromised; very rarely a mutation in the insulin-receptor gene causes an extreme insulin resistance. Resistance is also caused by the presence of antireceptor antibodies. However, probably the most important cause of insulin resistance are the defects in

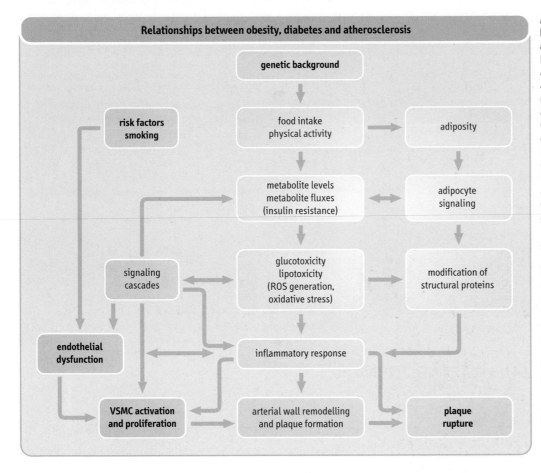

Relationships between obesity, diabetes and atherosclerosis

Fig. 20.21 **Relationships between obesity diabetes and atherosclerosis.** Increased food intake and/or decreased physical activity lead to changed metabolite fluxes and adipocyte signaling. Changed metabolism generates glucose- and lipid-derived molecules (glucotoxicity and lipotoxicity) and reactive oxygen species (ROS). ROS further modify body structure proteins and interfere with cell signaling sytems. A low-grade inflammatory response ensues: it has been observed in obesity and diabetes as well as in atherosclerosis. VSMC: vascular smooth muscle cells. (From Dominiczak MH, Obesity, gludose intolerance and diabetes, and their links to cardiovascular disease. Implications for laboratory medicine. *Clin Chem Lab Med* 2003;**41**:1266–1278, reprinted with permission.)

The metabolic syndrome

Metabolic syndrome links obesity, diabetes, hypertension, and cardiovascular disease

Obesity and insulin resistance resulting in either glucose intolerance or diabetes, may coexist with dyslipidemia and increased arterial blood pressure. Such combination became known as the metabolic syndrome, and is associated with an increased risk of cardiovascular disease.

TREATMENT OF DIABETES

The goals of treatment in diabetes are the prevention of acute and chronic complications

Perhaps the single most important change in the field in the last decade has been the change in therapeutic approach to diabetes from that focused exclusively on the control of glycemia to the parallel management of cardiovascular risk factors.

The maintenance of good glycemic control had been long-recognized as fundamental for diabetes care. Two major clinical trials, the Diabetic control and Complications trial (DCCT) in type 1 diabetes, and the UK Prospective Diabetes Study (UKPDS) in type 2 patients confirmed the long-held view that microvascular complications are associated with the level of glycemia. The results of both trials also suggest that the level of glycaemia is not a major determinant of atherosclerotic disease. On the other hand, there is an increasing evidence that it is the intervention which includes glycemic control and the management of cardiovascular risk that is most effective in the prevention of the long-term complications.

Thus, in addition to striving to maintain the concentration of plasma glucose close to normal, the intensive management of cardiovascular risk factors such as hypertension and dyslipidemia is necessary. This is in line with the recent clinical recommendations such as the JNC 7 Report on treating blood pressure and the recommendations of the Adult Treatment Panel III (ATP III) of the National Cholesterol Education Program on treatment of dyslipidemia (both are included in the Further Reading list at the end of this chapter).

SEVERE HYPOGLYCEMIA IS A MEDICAL EMERGENCY

A 12-year-old diabetic boy was playing with his friends. He received his normal insulin injection in the morning but continued playing through the lunch time without a meal. He became confused and then lost consciousness. He was given an injection of glucagon from the emergency kit his father carried, and recovered within minutes.

Comment. An immediate improvement after glucagon injection confirms that this boy's symptoms were caused by hypoglycemia, caused by the exogenous insulin and insufficient food intake. Recovery from hypoglycemia was due to the action of glucagon. In the hospital, hypoglycemic patients who cannot eat or drink are treated with an intravenous infusion of glucose. An intramuscular glucagon injection is an emergency measure that can be applied at home.

INSULIN RESISTANCE INCREASES THE RISK OF HEART ATTACK

A 45-year-old man was referred to the cardiology outpatient clinic for an investigation of chest discomfort which he felt when climbing steep hills and, in his own words, 'when stressed or excited'. The patient was 170 cm tall and weighed 102 kg (224 lb). His blood pressure was 160/98 mmHg (upper limit of normal = 140/90 mmHg), triglyceride concentration was 4 mmol/L (364 mg/dL) (desirable level <1.7 mmol/L [148 mg/dL]), and fasting plasma glucose was 6.5 mmol/L (117 mg/dL). His resting ECG was normal but an ischemic pattern was observed during exercise. His plasma insulin response to the oral glucose load was higher than normal.

Comment. This obese man presented with arterial hypertension, hypertriglyceridemia, and impaired fasting glucose. The impaired fasting of glucose in this case was due to peripheral insulin resistance. Such a cluster of abnormalities is called metabolic syndrome and carries a high risk of coronary heart disease.

ASSESSMENT OF FUEL METABOLISM

The measurement of plasma glucose is an important clinical test

The most important laboratory test of fuel metabolism is the simple measurement of plasma glucose. We differentiate between the normal glucose concentration (normoglycemia), too high a level (hyperglycemia), and too low a level (hypoglycemia). Because plasma glucose concentration increases after ingestion of food, it is important to relate the time of blood sampling to the last meal.

The definition of diabetes is based on the evidence that people with glucose levels above the diagnostic level are more likely to develop long-term complications.

Refer to Table 20.5 for the summary of the laboratory diagnosis of diabetes

The fasting plasma glucose is relatively stable. Normal fasting (no caloric intake for approx 10 h) plasma glucose remains below 6.1 mmol/L (<110 mg/dL). A concentration above 6.1 mmol/L but below 7.0 mmol/L (126 mg/dL) is defined as impaired fasting glucose (IFG). The level of 7.0 mmol/L (126 mg/dL) or above, if confirmed, indicates diabetes. Plasma glucose measured irrespective of the meal time (random plasma glucose) is useful for diagnosis of hypoglycemia or severe hyperglycemia, but is of little diagnostic use when the abnormality is mild. The criteria for the diagnosis of diabetes described here are those proposed by the American Diabetic Association in 1997 (see Further Reading).

Oral glucose tolerance test assesses the plasma glucose response to the ingestion of glucose

Blood glucose response to a carbohydrate load is the principle behind the oral glucose tolerance test (OGTT). For a meaningful result it is essential that the test is performed under standard conditions. The patient should attend in the morning, after approximately 10 h fast. To avoid stress-, or exercise-related change in plasma glucose, the patient should sit throughout the test. The test should not be performed during or immediately after an acute illness.

Fasting plasma glucose is measured first. Next, the patient is given a standard quantity of glucose to drink (75 g in 300 mL of water) and glucose is measured again after 30, 60, 90, and 120 min (Fig. 20.11).

Normally, plasma glucose rises to a peak concentration after approximately 60 min and returns to a near-fasting state within 120 min. If it remains above 11.1 mmol/L (200 mg/dL/min) in the 120-min sample the patient has diabetes, even if the fasting blood glucose is normal. If fasting blood glucose is normal but postload glucose is between 6.1 and 7.8 mmol/L (100 mg/dL and 140 mg/dL, respectively), the condition is classified as impaired glucose tolerance (IGT). Individuals with IGT are at an increased risk of developing diabetes in the future. The interpretation of the OGTT is summarized in Table 20.5. For many years OGTT used to be regarded as a reference test for the diagnosis of diabetes but current evidence suggests that the simpler measurement of fasting plasma glucose is equally accurate.

Urine glucose is an insensitive indicator of glycemic control

At normal plasma concentration, all the glucose filtered through the renal glomeruli is reabsorbed in the proximal tubule, and none appears in the urine (Chapter 22). The urinary threshold for glucose is approximately 10.0 mmol/L (180 mg/dL). At plasma glucose concentrations higher than that, the capacity of the renal tubular transport system is exceeded, and glucose filters into the urine (glucosuria). Rarely, in a patient with the renal glucose threshold lower than normal, glucosuria can be detected at non-diabetic blood glucose levels. Thus, the measurement of urine glucose is not a sensitive test for diabetes.

Testing for the presence of ketones in urine (ketonuria) is clinically important

A high concentration of ketones in urine signifies a high rate of lipolysis. This may occur in healthy individuals during prolonged fasting or on a high-fat diet (see box in Chapter 17). In a diabetic patient, however, ketonuria is a sign of metabolic decompensation which should not be ignored.

Increased plasma lactate indicates inadequate oxygenation

High plasma lactate level indicates increased anaerobic metabolism, and is usually a marker of inadequate tissue oxygenation (hypoxia; see also Chapter 4). The measurements of

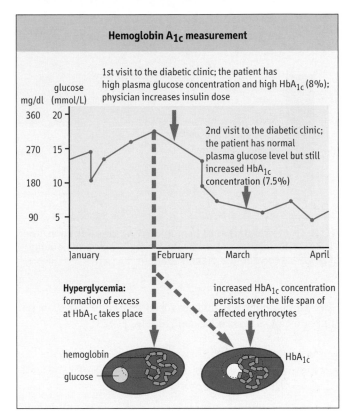

Fig. 20.22 **Hemoglobin A1c measurement assesses time-averaged control of glycemia.** The concentration of HbA1c in blood reflects time-averaged glycemia over the 3–6 weeks preceding its measurement. To obtain glucose concentrations in mg/dL, multiply by 18.

HBA1C IDENTIFIES PATIENTS WHO DO NOT COMPLY WITH TREATMENT OF DIABETES

A 15-year-old insulin-dependent boy visited a Diabetic Clinic for a routine check-up. He told the doctor that he complied with all the dietary advice and never misses insulin. Although his random blood glucose was 6 mmol/L (108 mg/dL), HbA1c concentration was 11% (normal 4–6%). He had no glycosuria or ketones in his urine.

Comment. Blood and urine glucose results indicate good control of this boy's diabetes at the time of measurement, whereas the HbA1c level suggests poor control over the last 3–6 weeks. The probability is that he only complied with treatment days before he was due to come to the clinic. This is not uncommon in adolescents, who find it hard to accept the necessity to adjust their lifestyle to the requirements of diabetes treatment.

plasma lactate are important in rare instances of hyperglycemic nonketotic coma, a life-threatening condition where very high plasma glucose levels, and extreme dehydration, occur in the absence of ketoacidosis.

Glycated hemoglobin (HbA$_{1c}$) reflects average glycemic control

A drawback of the measurement of plasma glucose is that it changes quickly. Therefore, a major advance in the monitoring of diabetic patients has been the measurement of glucose-modified hemoglobin (glycated hemoglobin or HbA$_{1c}$). Native hemoglobin (HbA) can be converted to a glycated form (HbA$_{1c}$); such conversion increases during hyperglycemia (Fig. 20.22) and is proportional to the mean plasma glucose concentration. Because the formation of HbA$_{1c}$ at physiologic pH is virtually irreversible, glycation leaves a 'record' of glycemia throughout the rest of the erythrocyte's life: the HbA1c concentration in blood reflects the time-averaged plasma glucose level over the 3–6 weeks preceding the measurement. The normal concentration of HbA$_{1c}$ is 4–6% of total

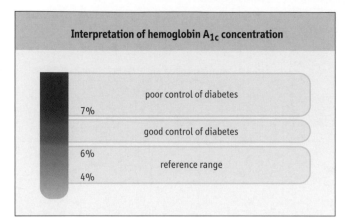

Fig. 20.23 **Interpretation of hemoglobin A₁c concentration.** The HbA₁c concentration allows the physician to assess the quality of glycemic control in a diabetic patient.

HbA. Levels below 7% indicate acceptable control of diabetes. Higher levels suggest poor control (Fig. 20.23).

Testing renal function and urinary albumin excretion is important in the assessment of diabetic kidney disease

Urea and creatinine concentrations in the plasma of diabetic patients (see Chapter 21) are routinely tested in diabetic persons. The presence of minimal amounts of albumin present in urine (microalbuminuria, above 200 mg/day) predicts the development of the diabetic nephropathy, and urinary protein excretion (proteinuria) above 300 mg/day is diagnostic for it. To assess microalbuminuria one needs to use a method of measurement which is more sensitive than the conventional method for the measurement of albumin in serum.

When ordering laboratory tests, remember the fast-feed cycle

Blood sampling during the postabsorptive state provides the best assessment of basal metabolism. This is why patients are often asked not to eat anything 8–12 h before having blood taken for laboratory tests.

Summary

- Glucose homeostasis requires interactions between key tissues and organs – liver, adipose tissue, skeletal muscle and pancreas.
- Stress response involves major changes in fuel metabolism.
- Disruption of this homeostatic system results in potentially life-threatening conditions – hypoglycemia and diabetes mellitus.

- The organism alternates between the fasting and postabsorptive state. Metabolite concentrations in blood change during the fast-feed cycle, and are influenced by stress and disease.
- The measurement of plasma glucose concentration is part of a routine assessment of every patient admitted to hospital. In diabetic patients the measurements of glucose, ketones, HbA₁c, and tests of renal function, including microalbuminuria, are performed.

ACTIVE LEARNING

1. Describe how insulin causes an increase in cellular glucose uptake.
2. What are anti-insulin hormones?
3. Why a non-diabetic patient brought to emergency unit with extensive burns would have an inceased plasma glucose concentration? Describe her metabolic state.
4. You have asked a patient to come to the outpatient clinic to have plasma triglycerides tested. The patient asks whether he needs to be fasting that day. Please provide an answer and explain your reasons.
5. Do people with impaired glucose tolerance develop long-term vascular complications?
6. What do obesity and diabetes mellitus have in common?

Further reading

Diamond J. The double puzzle of diabetes. *Nature* 2003;**423**:599–602.

Zimmet P, Alberti KGMM, Shaw J. Global and societal implications of the diabetes epidemic. *Nature* 2001;**414**:782–787.

Vollenveider P. Insulin resistant states and insulin signaling. *Clin Chem Lab Med CCLM* 2003;**41**:1107–1119.

Service FJ. Hypoglycemic disorders. *New Engl J Med* 1995;**332**:1144–1152.

Schmidt MI, Duncan BB. Diabesity: an inflammatory metabolic condition. *Clin Chem Lab Med* 2003;**41**:1120–1130.

The Expert Committee on the Diagnosis and Classification of Diabetes Mellitus. Report of the Expert Committee on the Diagnosis and Classification of Diabetes Mellitus. *Diabetes Care* 2003;**26**:S4–S20.

Alberti KG, Zimmet. Definition, diagnosis and classification of diabetes mellitus and its complications. Part 1: diagnosis and classification of diabetes mellitus. Provisional report of a WHO consultation. *Diabetic Medicine* 1998;**15**:539–553.

The Diabetes Control and Complications Trial (DCCT) Research Group. The effect of intensive treatment of diabetes on the development and progression of long-term complications in insulin-dependent diabetes mellitus. *N Engl J Med* 1993;**329**:977–986.

U.K. Prospective Diabetes Study (UKPDS) Group. Intensive Blood-glucose control with sulphonylureas or insulin compared with conventional treatment and risk of complications in patients with type 2 diabetes (UKPDS 33). *Lancet* 1998;**352**:837–853.

Chobanian AV, Bakris GL, Black HR, *et al*. The Seventh Report of the Joint National Committee on Prevention, Detection, Evaluation, and Treatment of High Blood Pressure. The JNC 7 Report. *JAMA* 2003;**289**:2560–2572.

Expert Panel on Detection, Evaluation and Treatment of High Blood Cholesterol in Adults. Executive Summary of the Third report of the National Cholesterol education Program (NCEP) Expert Panel on Detection, Evaluation and Treatment of High Blood Cholesterol in Adults (Adult Treatment Panel III). *JAMA* 2001;**285**:2486–2497.

Sacks DB, Bruns DE, Goldstein DE, Maclaren NK, MCDonald JM, Parrott M. Guidelines and recommendations for laboratory analysis in the diagnosis and management of diabetes mellitus. *Diabetes Care* 2003;**25**:750–786.

Brownlee M. Biochemistry and molecular cell biology of diabetic complications. *Nature* 2001;**414**:813–820.

Dominiczak MH. Obesity, glucose intolerance and diabetes and their links to cardiovascular disease. Implications for laboratory medicine. *CCLM* 2003;**41**:1266–1278.

INTRODUCTION

Nutrition is essential for survival; it underpins health and affects susceptibility to disease. Specific nutritional deficiencies arise as a result of particular dietary deficiencies, or are caused by genetically determined metabolic errors.

The major factors which determine the nutritional state are the genetic background, the environment, the phase of the life cycle, the physical activity and the presence of disease (Fig. 21.1).

Importantly, nutrition relates to many other issues discussed in this book. Thus, this chapter covers the elements of nutrition science and focuses on macronutrients; Chapter 10 addresses micronutrients (vitamins and trace elements); Chapter 22 deals with water and main electrolytes, and Chapters 4 and 23 with oxygen delivery and acid base balance, respectively.

KEY DEFINITIONS AND RECOMMENDATIONS USED IN NUTRITION SCIENCE

Diet is the total of all the foods and drinks ingested by an individual. The food or foodstuff is the individual food that is ingested; and nutrients are chemically defined components required by the body.

Recommendations on nutrient intake are based on Dietary Reference Intakes (DRIs)

Dietary intake is not easy to assess in a formal way, particularly when micronutrients are concerned. The available assessments are based on (sometimes incomplete) population data. We currently use sets of values, which describe suggested minimal, average, and adequate intakes. Different values are used in different countries, and there has been a degree of confusion and overlap between definitions (see box on following page). Currently the estimates of nutrient intake are based on the Dietary Reference Intakes (DRI). The DRI are sets of values that describe the intake of a given nutrient in a population (Fig. 21.2). The DRI variables include:

(a) Estimated Average Requirement (EAR)
(b) Recommended Daily Allowance (RDA)
(c) Adequate Intake (AI), and
(d) Tolerable Upper Intake (UL).

A EAR and an RDA values are given for a nutrient or, if these cannot be determined, AI is used. Please see box on p. 300 for the definitions of these variables. There are limitations to the interpretation of DRI. First, they are intended for healthy people. Second, a DRI established for any one nutrient presupposes that requirements for other ones are being met.

NUTRITION AND GENETICS

Individual response to nutrients varies: this variation is to a substantial extent the result of the genetic variation. Genes influence structures and functions associated with the digestion and absorption of nutrients, their metabolism or their excretion. Perceptions such as taste or satiation are also, to an extent, genetically determined. All this has practical implications: because the gene pool varies between populations, it seems that the optimal nutritional guidelines should be population-specific, rather than general.

Nutritional genomics and metabolomics

The ongoing development of nutritional genomics has huge potential implications for future nutritional interventions.

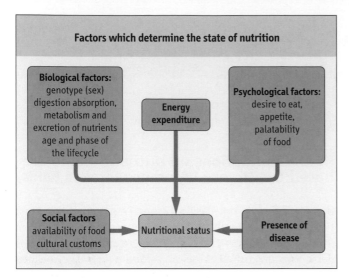

Fig. 21.1 **Factors which determine the state of nutrition.**

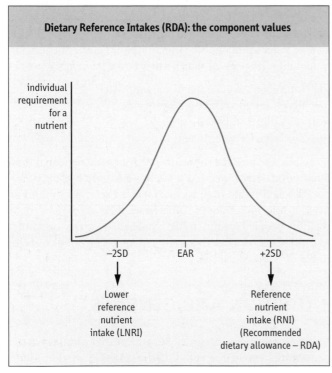

Fig. 21.2 **Dietary Reference Intakes (RDA): the component values.** While the Estimated Average Requirement (EAR) reflects the intake adequate for half of a population, the RNI (or RDA) are values representing intake adequate for the great majority of individuals.

Nutritional genomics is analogous to pharmacogenomics: it aims to exploit the knowledge accumulated by the Human Genome Project, and the ability to monitor the expression of a large number of genes, to devise individual dietary treatments customized to a genetic background. There is more – the monitoring of the patterns of metabolic response (metabolomics) offers further opportunities to determine

DEFINITIONS IN NUTRITION SCIENCE

These are the definitions used by the Food and Nutrition Board, Institute of Medicine (IOM) of the National Academies in the United States:

Estimated Average Requirement (EAR): The average daily nutrient intake level estimated to meet the requirement of half of the healthy individuals in a particular life stage and gender group.

The EAR is bracketed by two other values:

(1) Recommended Daily Allowance (RDA), (in the United Kingdom the Reference Nutrient Intake, RNI). It describes the average daily nutrient intake level sufficient to meet the nutrient requirement of nearly all (97 to 98%) healthy individuals in a particular life stage and gender group.

(2) The lower Reference Nutrient Intake (LNRI) used in the UK: the daily intake observed at the low end of intake distribution in a population (about 2%). Below this intake a deficiency may occur.

Adequate Intake (AI): a recommended average daily nutrient intake level based on observed or experimentally determined approximations or estimates of nutrient intake by a group (or groups) of healthy people that are assumed to be adequate – used when an RDA cannot be determined.

Tolerable Upper Intake Level (UL): The highest average daily intake level likely to pose no risk of adverse health effects to almost all individuals in a particular life stage and gender group. As intake increases above the UL the potential risk of adverse health effects increases.

Note that the currently used Dietary Reference Intakes have replaced the Dietary Reference Values (DRVs) used previously in the UK, and the Recommended Dietary Allowances (RDAs) used in the USA. Refer to Further Reading for details.

individual responses to nutrients and to develop personalized nutrition profiles.

Genotype influences plasma concentrations of nutrients

An example of the effect of genotype on nutrient intake is the response of plasma cholesterol concentration to its dietary content. Approximately 50% of individual variation in plasma cholesterol is genetically determined. Response to cholesterol-containing diet is associated with apoprotein E (apoE) genotype. ApoE is a protein synthesized in the liver, and is the main metabolic driver of the remnant particles (Chapter 17). It occurs in several isoforms coded by alleles designated e2, e3 and e4. It has been demonstrated that plasma cholesterol concentration increases on low fat/high cholesterol diet in persons with E4/4 but not E2/2, phenotype.

There are many examples of nutrients affecting gene expression. For instance, the activities of key hepatic enzymes differ in persons on a long-term high-fat diet compared to a high-carbohydrate diet (see Table 20.2). The amount of dietary cholesterol affects the activity of HMG-CoA reductase. Polyunsaturated fatty acids inhibit the expression of fatty acid synthase and the ω-3 fatty acids (see below) reduce the synthesis of RNA for the platelet-derived growth factor (PDGF) and inflammatory cytokine interleukin 1 (IL-1; Chapter 41). Another example comes from the field of hypertension: thirty to sixty percent of blood pressure variation is genotype-related and only 50% of patients with essential hypertension are salt-sensitive. The sensitivity to dietary salt is controlled, at least to an extent, by the angiotensinogen gene variants. Genetic factors are also fundamental in obesity: more than 50% of variation in weight is associated with the genetic background. Obesity is concordant in 74% between monozygotic- and 32% between dizygotic twins.

Nutrition, life cycle and metabolic adaptation

Physiological states, as well as disease, change the demand for nutrients and the energy expenditure. Pregnancy, lactation, and growth (in particular the intensive growth *in utero*, during infancy and the adolescent growth spurt) are the three most important physiological states associated with increased demand for nutrients.

Pregnancy is an example of the type of metabolic adaptation termed expansive adaptation. Here the body of the mother adapts to carrying the fetus and supplying it with nutrients. Around the time of conception mother's body prepares for the metabolic demands of the fetus. In the early pregnancy the mother sets up the 'supply capacity', and later in pregnancy the actual supply takes place. Ninety percent of fetal weight is gained between the 20th and 40th week of pregnancy and the steepest growth takes place between the 24th and 36th week. The total amount of energy stored during pregnancy is about 70 000 kcal (293 090 kJ), amounting to approx 10 kg of weight.

Nutrient intake changes during the life cycle. After delivery there is a transition from feeding through the placenta to breastfeeding, and then, gradually, to diet. Up to the breastfeeding stage nutrition is controlled by substrates and the infant is entirely dependent on the mother for nutrition. Later, the growth hormone assumes a major role in directing development. At the school age, new eating and activity patterns emerge as a child learns to be independent from parents. This continues during adolescence on the background of the accelerated growth. At this stage, sex hormones begin to play a prominent developmental role.

In adulthood, muscle mass increases between the age of 20 and 30 years, and at that point the level of physical activity stabilizes. Thereafter, muscle mass starts to decline and the fat mass starts to increase. This accelerates after the age of sixty. The bone mass also declines with age.

When nutrients are in short supply, i.e. both in the instances of increased nutritional need and the reduced availability of food, the so-called reductive adaptation occurs. In such instance the metabolic rate falls and the desire to eat increases. This limits the weight loss.

Nutrition and disease

Major illness and trauma are often associated with a degree of starvation and they are also characterised by a specific metabolic response to injury, which is an adaptive response known as the acute-phase reaction. It is characterized by a major shift in the hepatic pattern of protein synthesis: proteins, such as C-reactive protein (CRP), α_1-antitrypsin, haptoglobin, α_1-acid glycoprotein, components of the complement system, and others, are produced at a greater rate (see Chapter 3). The acute phase reaction also results in changes in the plasma concentration of trace elements: for instance, plasma copper concentration increases and zinc concentration decreases (see Chapter 10).

Importantly, surgical procedures performed on the GI tract may affects the nutritional status. There might be an impaired nutrient adsorption after removal of segments of the gut, or nutrient losses induced, for instance, by the drainage of intestinal fistulas. Some radical surgery creates the need for long-term nutritional support.

THE MAIN CLASSES OF NUTRIENTS

The main classes of nutrients are carbohydrates (including fibre), fats, proteins, minerals (including trace metals) and vitamins. Carbohydrates, proteins fat, fibre and some minerals are macronutrients (see Fig. 21.3). Vitamins and trace metals are micronutrients (Chapter 10).

Carbohydrates

Carbohydrates, like fats, are a primary energy source. They also are precursors of glycoproteins, glycolipids, and mucopolysaccharides. Dietary carbohydrates include refined carbohydrates such as sucrose contained in sweets or drinks and fruit juices, and complex carbohydrates such as starch, which are the component of grains and potatoes. Fiber consists of carbohydrates which are indigestible by the human gut and includes cellulose, hemicellulose, lignin, pectin, and beta-glucan. Fibre is present in unprocessed cereals, legumes,

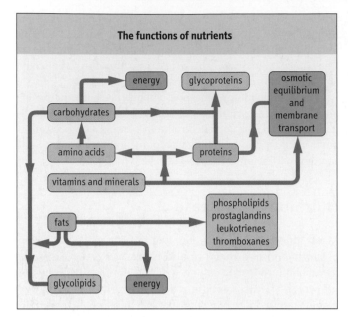

Fig. 21.3 The functions of nutrients. All main classes of nutrients can be used to produce energy, and all contribute to the synthesis of more complex compounds. The main role of vitamins and minerals is participation in enzymatic reactions. Prostaglandins, thromboxanes and leukotrienes: refer to Chapter 38 Glycolypids: Chapter 26. Glycoproteins: Chapter 25.

Daily protein requirements for selected age groups		
Age	g/day males	g/day females
0–3 months	12.5	12.5
10–12 months	14.9	14.9
4–6 years	19.7	19.7
15–18 years	55.2	45
19–50 years	55.5	45
50+ years	53.3	46.5

Table 21.1 **Daily protein requirements for selected age groups.** Protein requirements are age- and sex-dependent. Here we show the reference nutrient intakes (RNI) for selected age groups. Data from Dietary Reference Values for Food Energy and Nutrients for the United Kingdom; Report of the Panel on Dietary Reference Values of the Committee on Medical Aspects of Food Policy, London: TSO 2003.

vegetables, and fruits. The main role of fiber is to regulate gut transit and motility.

Proteins

Dietary proteins are digested to their component amino acids. Aminoacids derived from dietary proteins are used as a material to build, and rebuild, the host's own proteins, and they also serve as a 'last resort' energy substrate. The body proteins are renewed at a different rate. Amino acids are contained in animal and plant proteins. Due to the different composition of animal and plant proteins, eating no animal products at all may lead to nutrient deficiencies such as these of vitamin B_{12}, calcium, iron, and zinc. Similarly to energy requirements, protein requirements change during life cycle (Table 21.1). Increased demand for amino acids (dietary protein) is associated with pregnancy, lactation and the adolescent growth spurt.

Fats

Fats are the main nutrient used for energy storage. Lipids are also essential components of biological membranes and serve as substrates for the synthesis of glycolipids and glycoproteins, and also phospholipids, prostaglandins, leukotrienes, and thromboxane. Lipid-derived molecules have many signaling functions and affect gene transcription. Lipids provide thermal insulation for the body. They are particularly important for the development of brain and retina. Fats are classified into saturated and unsaturated (and within the latter category there is a subdivision into mono-and polyunsaturated fats: see below).

Saturated fats

Long-chain fatty acids are not souble in water but medium-chain fatty acids are. The most common saturated fatty acid is the palmitic acid (C16). Other are stearic (C18), myristic (C14), and lauric (C12) acids. Medium chain saturated fats (C8-C10) are water-soluble and are transported between the tissues in plasma rather than in chylomicrons. All animal fats (beef fat, butterfat, lard) are highly saturated. Saturated fats are also present in palm oil, cocoa butter and coconut oil.

Mono-unsaturated fats

Oleic acid (ω-9) is the only significant dietary monounsaturated fatty acid

Monounsaturated fatty acids are present in all animal and vegetable fats. Olive oil is a particularly rich source of monounsaturated fats. Monounsaturated trans-fatty acids (Fig. 21.4), the isomers of the cis-oleic acid are by-products of the hydrogenation process of liquid vegetable oils.

Polyunsaturated fats

Polyunsaturated fatty acids include ω-6 and ω-3 acids

The ω-6 acids are arachidonic acid (ω-6, C-20:4, $\Delta^{5,8,11,14}$) and its precursor linoleic acid (C-18:2, $\Delta^{9,12}$). They are present in vegetable seed oils. The ω-6 fatty acids are present in soybean

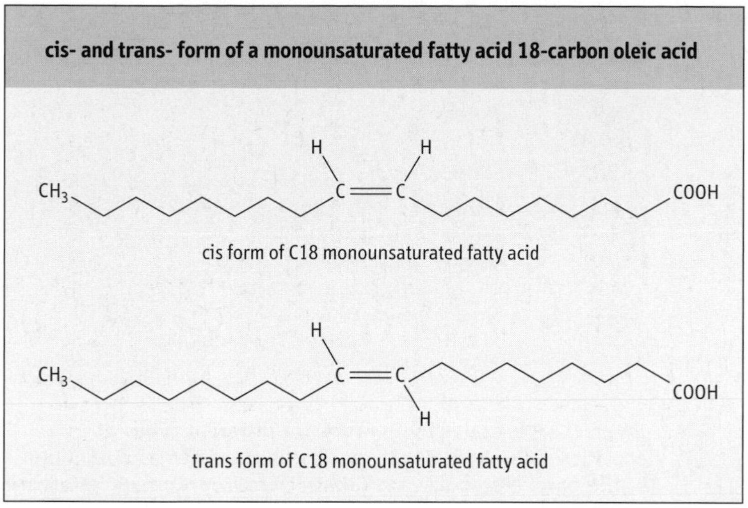

cis- and trans- form of a monounsaturated fatty acid 18-carbon oleic acid

cis form of C18 monounsaturated fatty acid

trans form of C18 monounsaturated fatty acid

Fig. 21.4 **The example of *cis-* and *trans-* form of a monounsaturated fatty acid (18-carbon oleic acid).** Trans fatty acids are produced during the hydrogenation process of liquid vegetable oils.

and canola oils and in fish oils (particularly in fatty fish such as salmon, sardines, and pilchards).

The $\omega 3$ fatty acids are α-linolenic (ω-3, C-18:3, $\Delta^{9,12,15}$), eicosapentaenoic (ω-3, C-20:5, $\Delta^{5,8,11,14,17}$), and docosahexaenoic (ω-3, C-22:6, $\Delta^{4,7,10,13,16,19}$) acids. They are present primarily in fish, shellfish, and phytoplankton and also in some vegetable oils such as olive, safflower, corn, sunflower, and soybean and leafy vegetables.

THE ESSENTIAL (LIMITING) NUTRIENTS

Essential nutrients are nutrients which cannot be synthesized in the human body and therefore need to be supplied from outside. Essential nutrients include essential amino acids, essential fatty acids (EFA), and some vitamins and trace elements. Carbohydrates (glucose and starches) are not essential nutrients.

Essential amino acids

The essential amino acids are phenylalanine (tyrosine can be synthesized from phenylalanine), the branched chain amino acids valine, leucine, isoleucine, threonine; and methionine and lysine. Histidine and arginine are essential for rats. Some plant proteins are relatively deficient in essential amino acids, whereas animal proteins usually contain a balanced mixture. (See Chapter 2.)

Essential lipids

The essential fatty acids (EFA) are linoleic acid and α-linolenic acid. Arachidonic acid, eicosapentaenoic acid, and docosa-

hexaenoic acid can be made in limited amounts from EFA: they become essential nutrients when EFA are deficient.

WATER AND MINERALS

Major minerals are sodium potassium, chloride, calcium, phosphate, and magnesium

With the exception of chloride, deficiencies and excess of these cause clinical symptoms. Sodium is important in the maintenance of extracellular fluid volume (Chapter 22). It participates in electrophysiological phenomena and, together with potassium, is essential in maintaining transmembrane potential. Most of the chloride anion (70%) also resides in the ECF. Sodium (and water) overload is seen in cardiac failure and also in renal disease (Chapter 22) and low sodium intake is recommended in the prevention of hypertension.

Potassium is the main intracellular cation. The maintenance of normal plasma potassium concentration is important because hyperkalemia and hypokalemia lead to arrythmias that may cause cardiac arrest. Also, dietary potassium intake needs to be limited in renal disease because of its impaired excretion and a tendency to hyperkalemia (Chapter 22). Potassium is contained in vegetables and fruit, particularly bananas, and in fruit juices.

Calcium and phosphate balance is important for maintaining bone structure (Chapter 24). Calcium is present in milk and milk products, and in some vegetables. Phosphates are present in plant and animal cells.

Magnesium is important for skeletal development and for the maintenance of electrical potential in nerve and muscle membranes. It is also a co-factor for ATP-requiring enzymes, and it is important for the replication of DNA and for the RNA synthesis. Magnesium deficiency develops in starvation and malabsorption, may be due to the loss from the gastrointestinal tract in diarrhoea and vomiting, and sometimes occurs as a result of diuretic treatment and surgical procedures on the gastrointestinal tract. It is also associated with acute pancreatitis and alcoholism. Hypomagnesemia is often accompanied by hypocalcaemia. Magnesium deficiency leads to muscle weakness and cardiac arrythmias.

Trace metals and vitamins

Vitamins and trace metals are important for the catalysis of chemical reactions. They act as coenzymes and form functionally important prosthetic groups of enzymes. They are discussed in detail in Chapter 10.

ENERGY HOMEOSTASIS

Energy expenditure

Total daily energy expenditure is a sum of basal metabolic rate, the thermic effect of food and the energy used up in physical activity.

Energy expenditure can be measured by direct calorimetry which relies on the measurement of heat production. Indirect calorimetry is based on the measurement of the rate of oxygen consumption (VO_2). The ratio of VCO_2 to VO_2 is known as the Respiratory Exchange Rate (RER) or Respiratory Quotient. For carbohydrates RER = 1 and for fat RER = 0.7.

Energy expenditure required to maintain body function at a complete rest is called the basal metabolic rate (BMR). BMR is sex-, age-, and body weight-dependent. At rest, energy is required for membrane transport (30% of the total), protein synthesis and degradation (30%), and for maintaining temperature, physical activity and growth. Certain organs use particularly high amounts of energy: in a 70-kg person brain metabolism constitutes approximately 20% of basal metabolic demand, liver 25% and muscle 25%. On the other hand, in very-low-birth babies brain is responsible for as much as 60% of the BMR, liver for 20% and muscle for only 5%.

In health, physical activity is the most important changeable component of energy expenditure. It is normally expressed as multiplies of the BMR. Examples of energy expenditure associated with different activities are given in Table 21.2. Energy requirement also depends on sex and age (Table 21.3).

The caloric value of nutrients

The caloric value of the main classes of nutrients is given in Table 21.4. Fat is the most energy-dense substrate yielding

Energy expenditure during physical activity

Physical Activity Ratio	Activity
1.0–1.4	Watching TV, reading, writing
1.5–1.8	Washing dishes, ironing
1.9–2.4	Dusting and cleaning, cooking
2.5–3.3	Dressing and undressing, making beds, walking slowly
3.4–4.4	Cleaning windows, golf, carpentry
4.5–5.9	Volley ball, fast walk, dancing, slow jogging, digging and shovelling
6.0–7.9	Climbing stairs, cycling, football, skiing

Table 21.2 **Physical activity ratios for different types of activities.** The physical activity ratio is expressed as a multiple of the basal metabolic rate (BMR). Data from Dietary Reference Values for Food Energy and Nutrients for the United Kingdom; Report of the Panel on Dietary Reference Values of the Committee on Medical Aspects of Food Policy, London: TSO 2003.

Daily energy requirements for selected age and sex groups

Age	EAR kcal/d (mJ) males	females
0–3 months	545 (2.28)	515 (2.16)
4–6 months	690 (2.89)	645 (2.69)
4–6 years	1,715 (7.16)	1,545 (6.46)
15–18 years	2,755 (11.51)	2,110 (8.83)
19–50 years	2,550 (10.60)	1.940 (8.10)
75+ years	2,100 (8.77)	1.810 (7.61)

Table 21.3 **Estimated average requirements (EAR) for energy for selected age and sex groups.** Data from Dietary Reference Values for Food Energy and Nutrients for the United Kingdom; Report of the Panel on Dietary Reference Values of the Committee on Medical Aspects of Food Policy, London: TSO 2003.

Caloric content of nutrients

Nutrient	Energy kJ	kcal/g
Starch	17	4
Glucose	17	4
Fat	37	9
Protein	17	4
Alcohol	30	7

Table 21.4 **Caloric content of the main classes of nutrients.** (1kJ = 239cal; 1kcal = 4.184kJ).

9 kcal/g (37 kJ) and carbohydrates and proteins yield 4 kcal/g (17 kJ). Note that alcohol also contributes significantly to energy production 7 kcal/g (29 kJ).

REGULATION OF FOOD INTAKE

The nutritional status is determined by a combination of biological, psychological and social factors

It depends on the availability of nutrients and on the rate of their utilization. These in turn are influenced by the availability of food, its palatability and variety, and the absence or presence of illness. The food intake is controlled by hunger (a desire to eat) and appetite (a desire for a particular food).

The brain is the main regulator in energy homeostasis and it is also the primary regulator of the body weight (Fig. 21.5). According to the lipostatic model of energy homeostasis, signals controlling energy intake originate from the adipose tissue and are sent to the central nervous system; in response, the brain sends efferent signals which are mediated by a complex network of neuropeptides. These signals regulate appetite and hunger. The main signals received by the central nervous system (CNS) are mediated by the adipokine leptin and the pancreatic hormone insulin (see Chapters 15 and 20).

Leptin and insulin act directly on the central neurones in the regions of the brain, which control appetite and energy expenditure. These neurones are located in the hypothalamic arcuate nucleus and project throughout hypothalamus. They express two neuropeptides: catabolic proopiomelatocortin (POMC), and anabolic neuropeptide Y/agouti-related protein (NPY/AgRP). POMC is cleaved yielding melanocortins (such

as alpha-MSH), that decrease food intake. NPY/AgRP links to neurons expressing melanin-concentrating hormone (MCH) and orexins A and B. They in turn, by acting on brain stem neurones, are involved in the control of food intake. These neurones connect with the brain cortex (the satiety center) to promote hunger and to stimulate yet another set of hormones such as thyreoliberin (TRH), corticoliberin (CRH) and oxytocin. Thyreoliberin increases thermogenesis and food intake, whereas corticoliberin decreases food intake and increases energy expenditure through the sympathetic activity.

Further signals involved in the control of food intake come from the gastrointestinal tract and are mediated by gastrointestinal peptides such as glucagon, cholecystokinin, glucagon-like peptide, amylin and bombesin-like peptide. Ghrelin, which is secreted by the stomach and stimulates NPY/AgRP-expressing neurons, is the only known appetite-stimulating peptide. Gastric stretch itself also affects the food intake. Finally, hypoglycemia decreases the activity of the satiety centre.

ASSESSMENT OF NUTRITIONAL STATUS

Nutritional assessment includes clinical assessment of the state of nutrition together with the assessment of dietary habits; it includes dietary history, a range of body (anthropometric) measurements, and biochemical and haematological laboratory tests. Nutritional assessment may be carried out either in the community for public health purposes, or in hospitals and outpatient clinics to determine nutritional needs of individual patients. It is important to remember that

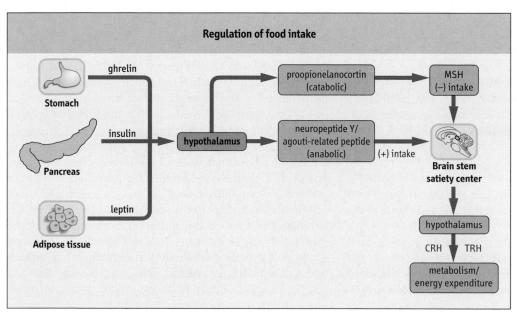

Fig. 21.5 **Regulation of food intake.** The regulation of food intake is accomplished by signals generated in the adipose tissue, pancreas, stomach and brain. The (+) sign means action leading to increase of appetite and food intake, and the sign (–), to a decrease.

NUTRITIONAL NEEDS AND EMERGENCY TREATMENT

Eating and drinking, like breathing, are major routes that connect living organisms with environment. To function we need oxygen, water and nutrients. One can exist without oxygen for minutes only. Without water the survival time is days. With these two supplied, a human being can survive without food for between 60 and 90 days. Importantly, these considerations also determine the urgency of treatment when things go wrong. Thus, re-establishment of the oxygen supply and circulating volume (necessary for adequate oxygen delivery to the tissues) are required right away (Chapter 4). Repletion of lost fluid and electrolytes is also necessary within hours to days, depending on a state of the patient (Chapter 22). Provision of other nutrients is important as soon as the life-saving actions have been taken.

Body mass index (BMI) and nutritional status

BMI	Interpretation
<18.5	malnourished
18.5–20	underweight
21–25	desirable
26–30	overweight
>30	obese

Table 21.5 **Classification of nutritional status based on the body mass index (BMI).**

there is no single definitive marker of the nutritional state. Therefore, nutritional assessment relies on the interpretation of a range of variables.

Body weight and the body mass index

Body weight in relation to height is a most commonly used measurement in nutritional assessment. The relationship between the two is expressed as the body mass index (BMI) calculated according to the formula:

$$BMI = weight\ (kg)/height(cm)^2$$

BMI is used to categorize the nutritional status as shown in Table 21.5. As mentioned above, one should remember that BMI alone should not be used as a definitive indication of the nutritional state.

Other measurements used in the nutritional assessment are the waist-to-hip ratio, the mid-arm circumference and the skinfold thickness measured with carefully calibrated calipers. More detailed analysis includes the assessments of total body water, the analysis of body bioelectrical impedance and the measurements of lean body mass using the dual-energy X-ray absorptiometry (DEXA). Some of these measurements allow to calculate variables such as body fat content and composition. Also, functional measurements such as grip strength or peak expiratory flow are relevant to nutritional state.

Biochemical markers of nutrition

Urinary nitrogen excretion is important in assessing the body nitrogen balance

The nitrogen balance is used to assess the body protein requirements. Nitrogen balance is a difference between the intake of nitrogen and its excretion. The positive nitrogen balance means that the intake exceeds loss. Negative nitrogen balance signifies that the loss exceeds intake.

The quantity of proteins oxidized by the body is estimated by measuring the 24 h urinary nitrogen excretion. Ninety percent of the excreted nitrogen appears in the urine (and 80% of this is present as urea). The rest is excreted in the stool, hair, and sweat. Nitrogen excretion adjusts to protein intake over 2 to 4 days. The measurement of urinary nitrogen (or urea) excretion is the most reliable way of assessing daily protein requirements. Unfortunately the method is tedious, and the test requires the 24 h urine collection. As a guide, most people require 1–1.2 g protein/kg body weight /day. More detailed requirements are listed in Table 21.1.

Several plasma proteins have been used as markers of nutritional state

The concentration of a protein in plasma may reflect the nutritional state, and the time-period such measurement reflects is dependent on the half-life of the particular protein. The proteins which have been most commonly used for this purpose are albumin, transthyretin (prealbumin), and transferrin.

Many studies confirmed the link between liver albumin synthesis (albumin half-life is approximately 20 days) and the nutritional state. Transthyretin, which has a half-life of two days, has been also extensively used in nutritional assessment. Transthyretin is synthesized in the liver and forms a complex with retinal-binding protein in plasma. Transferrin, an iron-binding protein is also synthesized in the liver has a half-life of approximately 10 days. Unfortunately, the interpretation of plasma concentrations of nutritionally-relevant proteins is often difficult, because their concentration is not determined exclusively by the state of nutrition. For instance, although the albumin concentration in plasma reflects the rate of its synthesis in the liver, it is also heavily dependent on the state of hydration; albumin concentration is low in over-hydrated patients. In addition, albumin, transthyretin and transferrin are all affected by the acute phase response (transferrin and transthyretin concentrations increase during the acute-phase reaction and albumin concentration decreases:

albumin is called a negative acute-phase reactant). All this means that, as many other biochemical variables, they cannot be interpreted in isolation; still, they are helpful when seen as a part of the entire clinical/laboratory picture.

Full nutritional assessment also involves measurements of vitamins and trace metals. This is particularly important in patients who remain on long-term parenteral nutrition. With regard to these measurements, the interpretation of laboratory results is complicated by the fact that their concentration in blood may not reflect the status of body stores (see Chapter 10).

General laboratory tests provide useful supplementary information related to the nutritional status

Other laboratory tests provide important supplementary information during a nutritional assessment of hospitalized patients, and particularly those who are candidates for parenteral nutrition (see below). For instance, the measurement of haemoglobin may uncover iron deficiency. Testing the liver (Chapter 28) and kidney function (Chapter 22), the measurements of serum electrolytes such as sodium, potassium chloride, bicarbonate, calcium, phosphate and magnesium, and the assessment of iron metabolism, provide useful information. Finally, assessing daily fluid intake and loss is essential in patients who are being considered for nutritional support.

A WOMAN WITH RENAL FAILURE AND WEIGHT LOSS

A 59-year-old lady was admitted to the Renal Unit with recurrent infections and recurrent endocarditis. She had been treated with hemodialysis for 5 years and over a period of 2 years had lost 33% of her body weight. She had a very poor appetite and had been taking two cartons (1.5 kcal/ml) of milkshake sip feeds daily. She was anuric and her fluid intake was restricted to 1000 ml daily. Her height was 1.68 m and she weighted 52.7 kg: the BMI was 18. Her most recent biochemistry results revealed persistent hyperkalaemia ranging between 5.7 and 6.2 mmol.

Comment. Because of her poor nutritional status and continuous weight loss she needs to continue taking nutritional supplements to minimize further weight loss. However, due to hyperkalaemia, a low-electrolyte sip feed should be considered. She was initially taking 22 mmol of potassium from the 1.5kcal/ml milkshake. Subsequently this was changed to a low electrolyte sip feed, which provided only 12 mmol in total. The UK Renal Nutrition Group Standards recommend that daily potassium intake in this type of patient should be less than 1 mmol/kg/body weight. Low electrolyte/volume sip feeds should always be considered for renal patients and the serum concentration needs to be closely monitored. (See Chapter 22.)

MALNUTRITION

Malnutrition is a gradual decline in the nutritional status, which in its more advanced stages leads to a decrease in functional capacity and to medical complications. Protein energy malnutrition (PEM) is defined as poor nutritional status due to inadequate nutrient intake.

Reduced food intake leads to reductive adaptation which includes a decrease in nutrient stores, changes in body composition and the more efficient use of fuels such as the use of ketone bodies by the brain (the metabolic changes in starvation are described in more detail in Chapter 20).

Malnutrition is one of the key problems faced by public health in the developing world and needs to be viewed from not only medical, but also social and economic perspective. Mortality in malnourished patients (BMI between 10 and 13) is four times higher compared to well-nourished ones. The effects of malnutrition are summarized in Table 21.6. Worldwide, malnutrition contributes to 54% of 11.6 million deaths annually among children below 5 years of age.

In the developed world, malnutrition is a problem in hospitalized patients who are unable to eat because of their disease such as, for instance, stroke or cancer. Gastrointestinal problems, particularly the colon pathology and coeliac disease (see case, Chapter 9), or post-operative conditions, are associated with specific nutritional problems. Malnutrition also affects a large group of elder individuals who might have problems with, for instance, access to food. In the UK, up to 40% of patients admitted to hospitals are undernourished. In addition to malnutrition, specific deficiencies such as those of vitamin D, iron, and vitamin C occur.

Effects of protein-calorie malnutrition
Effects of protein-calorie malnutrition
Decreased protein synthesis
Decreased activity of Na$^+$/K$^+$ ATPase
Decreased glucose transport
Fatty liver, liver necrosis, liver fibrosis
Depression, apathy, mood changes
Hypothermia
Compromised ventilation
Compromised immune system: impaired wound healing.
Risk of wound breakdown
Decreased cardiac output
Decreased renal function
Loss of muscle strength
Anorexia
Decreased mobility

Table 21.6 **The effects of protein-calorie malnutrition.** Malnutrition affects multiple organs and systems.

Classification of malnutrition			
	Moderate	Severe	Complicated
Weight for height (% of median)	70–80	<70	<80
– or pitting oedema	no	yes	yes
– or mild upper arm circumference	110–125	<110 mm	<110 mm
Appetite, clinically well, alert	yes	yes	no*

Table 21.7 **Classification of malnutrition.** Note that, in the classical classification of malnutrition, the presence of edema is also the main differentiating feature between marasmus and kwashiorkor. *Patients with complicated malnutrition may develop anorexia, high fever, anemia and dehydration. After Collins S, Yates R. The need to update the classification of acute malnutrition *Lancet* 2003;**362**:249.

There are two types of protein-calorie malnutrition: marasmus and kwashiorkor

Marasmus results from a prolonged inadequate intake of calories and protein. It is a chronic condition, which develops over months or years. It is characterized by loss of muscle tissue and subcutaneous fat with the preservation of the synthesis of visceral proteins such as albumin. There is a clear loss of weight.

Kwashiorkor is a more acute form of undernutrition, which may also occur on the background of marasmus. It also develops because of inadequate nutrient intake after trauma or infection. In kwashiorkor, in contrast to marasmus, visceral tissues are not spared: the hallmark of kwashiorkor is oedema due to the low concentration of plasma albumin and the loss of oncotic pressure (Chapter 22). Such edema may mask the weight loss. Complications of kwashiorkor are dehydration, hypoglycemia, hypothermia, electrolyte disturbances and septicemia. These patients have impaired immunity and wound healing, and are prone to infection. The WHO classification of malnutrition is based on anthropometry and the presence of bilateral pitting edema. A classification has been proposed recently which distinguishes complicated from uncomplicated malnutrition (Table 21.7). Marasmus and kwashiorkor are the terms rarely used in the hospital practice in the developed countries: malnutrition and complicated malnutrition are probably more appropriate terms.

Inappropriate treatment of a malnourished person may lead to refeeding syndrome

The inpatient treatment of malnutrition in the famine areas includes standard preparations such as the Formula 100 therapeutic milk (F100). F100 is a liquid diet with an energy content 100kcal/100 ml. It includes dried skimmed milk, oil, sugar and a mix of vitamins and minerals (without iron). In the areas of famine, community feeding programs use the

AN OBESE MAN WITH TYPE 2 DIABETES, CORONARY DISEASE, AND ARTHRITIS

Mr K is a 55-year-old gentleman with type 2 diabetes and coronary disease. He gets angina on effort and also suffers from severe arthritic knee pain. When he initially presented to the outpatient clinic his weight was 140 kg and his height 1.80 m (BMI 43). Within a year he managed to lose 12 kg by dieting. Subsequently, he was prescribed a lipase inhibitor, which he tolerated well. However, his arthritis worsened and he was increasingly less able to exercise. As a result his weight increased again to 137 kg. He was referred to the surgeons and is now being considered for gastric banding surgery.

Comment. This patient illustrates multiple problems associated with obesity and in particular the way disease may interfere with weight reduction programs. Weight loss is, to a substantial extent, dependent on the level of exercise. This patient lost weight initially but the maintenance of lower body weight was compromised by decreased mobility caused by arthritis.

so-called life-sustaining general rations (at least 2100 kcal; 8786 kJ/day) containing grains, legumes, and vegetable oil. During the treatment of malnutrition, this needs to be combined with providing adequate water, sanitation, and basic health care.

It is important to take time to replete nutritionally a starved person. Too quick a replacement may be dangerous due to a major fluid shifts between intracellular and extracellular fluid. This is known as the refeeding syndrome, characterized by low concentrations of serum magnesium, phosphate and potassium (the latter because of the stimulation of insulin secretion). Also, if thiamin deficiency is present, carbohydrate feeding can precipitate the Wernicke-Korsakoff syndrome (see Chapter 10). Frequent simple meals at short intervals are recommended during famine relief and, in a hospital setting a gradual introduction of nutritional support and close monitoring are required.

OBESITY

Obesity has emerged as a major health problem worldwide

Worldwide obesity increased by more than 70% since 1980. In the USA, 61% of adults are overweight and 26% are obese (USA National Center for Health Statistics Report 2002). The main causes of this seem to be the availability of highly caloric food, and the decrease in physical activity both at work

Diseases associated with obesity
Diseases associated with obesity
Type 2 diabetes
Hypertension and stroke
Dyslipidemia
Gallstones, particularly in women
Some cancers: breast, endometrial, ovarian, gallbladder, colon
Respiratory disorders
Musculoskeletal disorders (however, reduction of risk of osteoporosis)
Psychological problems

Table 21.8 **Diseases associated with obesity.** Obesity is associated with an increased risk for several diseases. This is, at least partially, preventable by weight loss. (See also Fig. 20.21.)

and during leisure time. There is a genetic predisposition to obesity, although in a great majority of cases it appears to be polygenic: as many as 59 chromosomal regions were quoted to contain obesity-related genes. Also rare mutations in at least six human genes, including leptin, were found to underlie morbid obesity.

Obesity is associated with an increased risk of several diseases

The reason why obesity is regarded as a health problem is that it is associated with an increased risk of several diseases (Table 21.8). In particular, it is a risk factor for type 2 diabetes mellitus; the increased incidence of diabetes worldwide parallels that of obesity. Insulin resistance, which develops in obesity, is an important common denominator between obesity and diabetes (see Chapter 20). The closely associated with obesity metabolic syndrome (Chapter 17) is associated with an increased risk of cardiovascular disease. (See also clinical box on p. 206.)

DIET IN HEALTH AND DISEASE

Dietary history should include more than the details of food intake

'Dietary habits' include the pattern of meals, and the amount and composition of eaten food. Individual diet is determined by biological, psychological, sociological and cultural factors. The biological factors involved are essentially the state of the systems responsible for the intake, digestion, absorption and and metabolism of nutrients. Enzyme deficiencies such as, for instance, that of lactase (Chapter 9) cause impaired absorption of foodstuffs (in this case, milk).

Psychological factors play an important role in determining food ingestion patterns; eating disorders such as anorexia nervosa and bulimia nervosa may lead to severe malnutri-

tion. The sociological factors include availability and price of food, and measures taken by the society to improve diets such as, for instance, school meals or subsidized meals for the elder or disabled persons. Cultural factors also determine eating pattern and the type of preferred foodstuffs. All the above are important when taking the nutritional/dietary history as part of the nutritional assessment. Individual food intake is assessed by food frequency questionnaires, 24-hour dietary recalls, food records, and also by direct analysis of foods and by metabolic balance studies. The newer method of diet research is the so-called structured assessment of dietary patterns.

Diets in health

Current dietary recommendations for the general population focus on balanced eating

The example of dietary recommendations for a healthy population is the Food Pyramid developed by the US Department of Agriculture (Fig. 21.6). These recommendations promote eating a variety of foods. They stress the balance between food intake and physical activity. They recommend diet containing plenty of complex carbohydrates in the form of grain products, vegetables and fruits. The recommended diet is low in saturated fat and cholesterol and moderate in sugars, salt and sodium. Alcohol needs be taken in moderation. The Food Pyramid consists of several groups of foodstuffs which need to be taken daily in a decreasing number of daily servings:

- Bread, pasta, and cereal group forms the basis of nutrition with the 6–11 recommended servings
- Fruit (2–4 servings) and vegetable (3–5 servings) groups
- Milk, yoghurt, and cheese – and meat, poultry, fish, dry beans, eggs, and nuts group (both 2–3 servings)
- Fats, oils, and sweets group (to be used sparingly)

Weight reduction

Losing weight increases life expectancy, decreases blood pressure, decreases visceral fat deposition, improves plasma lipid concentrations, increases insulin sensitivity and normalizes glycemia, improves clotting and platelet function, and enhances the quality of life.

To lose weight one needs to change the balance between energy intake and expenditure; i.e between food intake and physical activity. However, the process involves many other factors, such as motivation, available time, cost, and access to the appropriate programs. Low calorie diets contain approximately 1200–1300 kcal/day and the very low calorie diets around 800 kcal/day. Generally, a combination of diet and exercise is more effective in inducing weight loss than diet

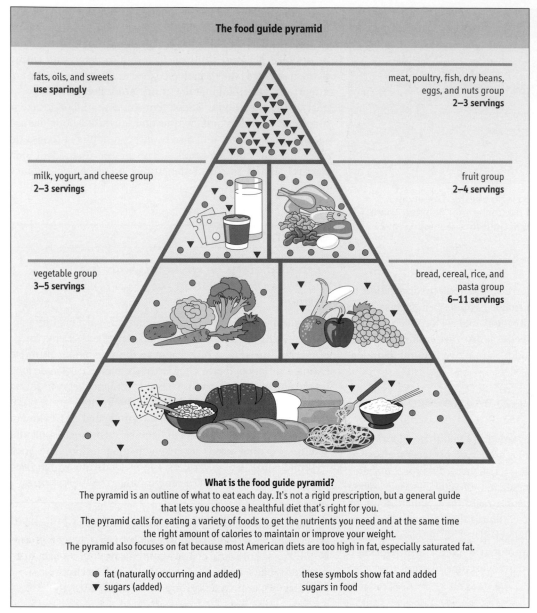

The food guide pyramid

fats, oils, and sweets
use sparingly

meat, poultry, fish, dry beans, eggs, and nuts group
2–3 servings

milk, yogurt, and cheese group
2–3 servings

fruit group
2–4 servings

vegetable group
3–5 servings

bread, cereal, rice, and pasta group
6–11 servings

What is the food guide pyramid?
The pyramid is an outline of what to eat each day. It's not a rigid prescription, but a general guide
that lets you choose a healthful diet that's right for you.
The pyramid calls for eating a variety of foods to get the nutrients you need and at the same time
the right amount of calories to maintain or improve your weight.
The pyramid also focuses on fat because most American diets are too high in fat, especially saturated fat.

● fat (naturally occurring and added)
▼ sugars (added)

these symbols show fat and added
sugars in food

Fig. 21.6 **The Food Guide Pyramid.** The Food Pyramid forms a basis for current recommendations on healthy eating. (US Department of Agriculture.)

alone (see Chapter 15, clinical box on p. 206). In extreme obesity, the treatment with appetite suppressants and, more recently, fat absorption inhibitors has been used. Also, surgical treatments such as gastric plication (banding) and jejuno-ileal bypass surgery can be considered in severe obesity (see Fig. 21.7).

Low-carbohydrate, high-fat diet and associated controversies

American physician, Robert Atkins devised a weight reducing diet, which developed a large following worldwide. It is based on a 2-week period of lipolysis- and ketosis-inducing, very- low-carbohydrate, high-fat, and high-protein diet. After this short, intensive period there is a more prolonged transition to the so-called maintenance phase, which includes titration of carbohydrate intake to maintain weight. The program recommends avoidance of refined carbohydrates and strongly promotes regular exercise. This diet was devised primarily for healthy, severely obese persons. Its authors stress that persons with renal disease or diabetes can only consider it under medical supervision.

This diet appears to be effective in weight reduction. As many other aspects of dietary management, it is not completely evidence-based. The persisting concerns about the low carbohydrate, high-fat diets include the potential risk of abnormalities of liver and kidney function, and the long-term

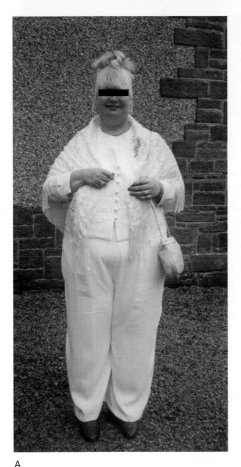

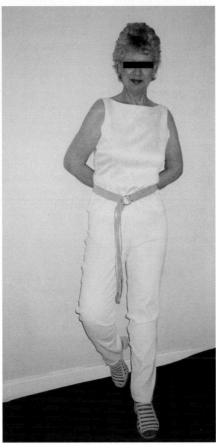

A   B

Fig. 21.7 **Surgical treatment such as gastric banding is used in severe cases of obesity.** These photographs show the same patient before and after gastric banding surgery. Her weight before surgery was 136.1 kg; within three years it decreased to 63 kg.

effects of the high-fat diet on cardiovascular risk. In any case, the impact the Atkins diet made on a general population is likely to stimulate research in the field.

NUTRITION AND CHRONIC DISEASE

The major groups of diseases, which are affected by diet, are coronary heart disease and cancer. They are also the two main causes of death in the developed world.

Diet plays an important role in the prevention of coronary disease

Nutrients which affect atherosclerosis are dietary cholesterol, saturated fat and trans-fatty acids. Excessive caloric intake and consequent obesity also facilitate atherosclerosis. High dietary cholesterol and high saturated fat decrease the LDL receptor expression mediated through an increase in the intracellular cholesterol content in the hepatocytes: this leads to an increase in plasma cholesterol concentration (Chapter 17). Foods containing saturated fatty acids (full-fat milk, cheese,

butter, and red meats) are atherogenic in excess. The rationale behind the low-cholesterol diets is that LDL receptor expression can be increased if dietary cholesterol content is sufficiently low. The typical Western diet contains approximately 400–500 mg of cholesterol daily. The intake required to achieve reduction in plasma cholesterol is much lower: below 200 mg or even below 100 mg daily (incidentally, when the intake is above 500 mg, further increase in intake does not necessarily lead to further increase in cholesterol concentration).

Nutrients that seem to be protective against atherosclerosis include polyunsaturated ω-6-rich fatty acids (contained in vegetable oils) and ω-3-rich fish and fish oils, monounsaturated fat, and soluble fibre such as beta-pectin. Polyunsaturates reduce plasma cholesterol concentration. The ω-3 fatty acids reduce triglycerides by decreasing VLDL synthesis and increasing its catabolism. They are also antithrombotic: fish oil inhibits thromboxane and PDGF synthesis, reduces blood viscosity and enhances fibrinolysis. Monounsaturated fats increase the concentration of HDL, increase insulin sensitivity and decrease plasma triacylglycerol (triglyceride) concentration.

Diets low in fat and cholesterol have been a hallmark of cardiovascular prevention for decades

These diets normally result in approximately 10% decrease in serum cholesterol if applied during clinical trials and, unfortunately, to a much lesser decrease (usually below 5%) when applied in general population. Alcohol seems to be protective against coronary disease but if taken in excess it carries multiple other risks, obesity included. Unfortunately, the low fat diets, if the protein content is kept constant, need to be high in carbohydrates. High-carbohydrate low-fat diet is, however, not without problems. The main practical problem is that, in spite of recommendations to use predominantly complex carbohydrates, in many populations refined sugars constitute too high a proportion of carbohydrate intake, and this promotes obesity. High carbohydrate diets may also lead to hypertriglyceridemia. Finally, low-fat diets seem to decrease HDL-cholesterol by 10–20%.

Diabetes mellitus

The management of diabetes is closely linked to nutrition

To ensure optimal glycemic control, not only the quality and quantity of food, but also timing and regularity of meals are important. Importantly, in persons with glucose intolerance, the comprehensive approach including weight reduction, reduction of fat intake, increase in fiber intake, and increase in physical activity decreases the risk of developing diabetes.

Cancer

Lifestyle and diet may influence the incidence of cancer

High intake of fruit and vegetables seems to be protective against cancer, possibly due to the presence of antioxidants and fiber. Dairy products seem also to be protective. There were suggestions that high-fat diets may increase cancer risk, but epidemiological evidence for this is weak. In clinical studies beta-carotene, retinoids (see Chapter 10), fiber, and calcium were not found to be effective in cancer prevention. However, coincidental findings suggest that vitamin E prevents the development of prostate cancer; and selenium is beneficial in prostate and colorectal cancers.

Renal disease

The factors contributing to the development of malnutrition in renal failure (uremia, see Chapter 22) include, in addition to nutrient intake, increased catabolism, chronic inflammation, and endocrine changes.

Levels of nutritional support
Levels of nutritional support
Special diets
Assistance with eating
Enteral nutrition (feeding through different feeding tubes: nasogastric, nasoduodenal; gastrostomy and jejunostomy)
Parenteral nutrition

Table 21.9 **The levels of nutritional support.** Nutritional support ranges from simple measures such as assistance with meals, to an intravenous provision of all nutrients. The higher level of support should only be instituted if the lower level is not effective.

Maintaining adequate protein and energy intake is important and low-potassium, low-phosphate diet is recommended due to the tendency to retain potassium and phosphate when renal function deteriorates.

Nutritional support

Nutritional support is required for a substantial number of hospitalized patients and ranges from a simple assistance with meals, through enriched- or special-consistency diets, to enteral nutrition and total parenteral nutrition (Table 21.9).

Enteral nutrition entails feeding through special tubes placed in the stomach or jejunum, and parenteral nutrition is essentially intravenous feeding. Enteral nutrition is appropriate when there are difficulties with taking food orally but when the gastrointestinal tract functions properly.

When the gastrointestinal tract does not function because of, for instance, intestinal obstruction, or when large parts of it have been surgically removed, total parenteral nutrition is appropriate (see clinical box on p. 286).

Total parenteral nutrition, while in many instances lifesaving, is a procedure potentially associated with complications caused by delivery (which requires strict sterility) as well as metabolic problems. For this reason, parenteral nutrition in hospitals is managed by multidisciplinary teams that include specialist nurses, surgeons, gastroenterologists, dieticians, pharmacists, and laboratory medicine physicians.

Summary

- Appropriate nutrition underpins health and well being, and poor nutrition increases susceptibility to disease.
- Nutrition is considered at a population level and at individual level.

- Genotype, food availability, state of health, and physical activity are factors which determine nutritional status.
- Nutritional needs change during life cycle.
- Main categories of nutrients are carbohydrates, fats, proteins, and vitamins and minerals. Water balance is closely associated with nutrition.
- Food intake is controlled by a complex neuroendocrine system responding to primary signals generated in adipose tissue.
- Malnutrition affects large areas of the developing world, and in the developed world is an issue among disadvantaged social groups and also in hospitalized persons.
- Obesity has become a major health problem worldwide.
- Nutritional support includes graded assistance with nutrient intake, ranging from assistance with meals to total parenteral nutrition.
- The assessment of nutritional status is an important part of general assessment of persons visiting outpatient clinics or admitted to a hospital. It includes the assessment of current diet, dietary history, clinical examination and a range of biochemical and hematological tests.

ACTIVE LEARNING

1. Outline the neuroanatomical basis for energy homeostasis.
2. Describe the role of different classes of fatty acids in nutrition.
3. List the principles of a weight reduction programme.
4. Discuss instances when increased nutritional demand can precipitate malnutrition.
5. How can the developments in genomics and proteomics be applied to nutrition science?
6. What diet would you recommend for a diabetic patient?

Further Reading

Dietary Reference Values for food energy and nutrients for the United Kingdom. Report of the Panel on Dietary reference Values of the Committee on Medical Aspects of Food Policy Department of Health, London: TSO 2003.

Moore, MC. Nutritional Care. St Louis: Mosby's Pocket Guide Series. 2001; 532pp.

Kopelman PG. Obesity as a medical problem. *Nature* 2000; **404**:635–43.

Dr Atkins new diet revolution. London: Vermillion 2003.

Collins S Yates R. The need to update the classification of acute malnutrition *Lancet* 2003;**362**:249.

Collins S. Changing the way we address severe malnutrition during famine. *Lancet* 2003;**358**:498–501.

WHO. Management of severe malnutrition: a manual for physicians and other senior health workers. Geneva: World Health Organization 1999. ISBN 92 4 154511 9. (Available online at *www.who.int/nut/documents/manage_severe_malnutrition_eng.pdf*)

Gidden F, Shenkin A. Laboratory support of the clinical nutrition service. *Clin Chem Lab Med* 2000;**38**:693–714.

Websites

Report: Dietary Reference Intakes: Applications in Dietary Planning (2003)

Food and Nutrition Board, Institute of Medicine (IOM) of the National Academies http://www.iom.edu (accessed October 2003)

The UK Food Standards Agency website: www. Foodstandards.gov.uk (accessed October 2003)

American Dietetic Association www.eatright.org

The Food Pyramid www.nal.usda.gov

22. Water and Electrolyte Balance: Kidney Function

M H Dominiczak and M Szczepanska-Konkel

LEARNING OBJECTIVES

After reading this chapter you should be able to:

- Describe the body water compartments in the adult and the composition of the main body fluids.
- Explain the role of albumin in movement of water between plasma and interstitial space, including the consequences of proteinuria.
- Describe how sodium influences the movement of water between the extracellular and intracellular space.
- Explain why sodium-potassium pump is essential for normal cell hydration, and comment on the consequences of its inhibition.
- Describe factors affecting plasma potassium concentration.
- Outline the process of urine formation and the mechanism of renal reabsorption of sodium and water.
- Discuss relations between sodium and water homeostasis.
- Describe the basics of the clinical assessment of water and electrolyte status.

INTRODUCTION

Water is an essential constituent of the human body, accounting for approximately 60% of the body weight in the adult. This changes with age: it is about 75% in the newborn and decreases to less than 50% in older individuals. Water content is greatest in brain tissue (about 90%) and least in adipose tissue (10%).

Both a relative deficiency and an excess of water impair the function of tissues and organs because the stability of sub-cellular structures and activities of numerous enzymes are dependent on adequate cell hydration. Water balance, and the distribution of water between the extracellular (vascular and interstitial) and cellular compartments are closely controlled.

Distribution of water within the body depends on hydrostatic and osmotic forces acting across biological membranes. Osmotic activity depends on the concentration gradients of electrolytes and other substances that cannot freely diffuse through cell membranes. Sodium is the most abundant extracellular cation and, with its associated anions such as chlor-ide and bicarbonate, is fundamental for determining water distribution across cell membranes.

An imbalance between the amounts of water and sodium in the extracellular fluid leads to changes in osmolality. The consequent movement of water is associated with contraction or expansion of the cell volume and underlies many clinical disorders.

The total amount of water and electrolytes in the body depends on the balance between their intake and loss. The kidneys are a major regulator of this balance because they control the loss of body water and electrolytes. Consequently, impaired renal function leads to the water and electrolyte imbalance. This chapter describes the aspects of the water and electrolyte balance which are most relevant to clinical practice.

Note that water and electrolyte balance is closely linked to nutrition (Chapter 21), and particularly to the issues associated with enteral and parenteral feeding.

WATER, SODIUM, AND POTASSIUM METABOLISM

Body water compartments

Approximately two-thirds of total body water is in the intracellular fluid (ICF), and one-third remains in the extracellular fluid (ECF). ECF consists of interstitial fluid and lymph (15% body weight), plasma (3% body weight), and transcellular fluids, which include gastrointestinal fluid, urine, CSF, and others (Fig. 22.1).

The capillary wall, which separates plasma from the interstitial fluid, is freely permeable to water and electrolytes, but restricts the flow of proteins

These properties of the capillary wall mean that, whereas ions and low-molecular-weight molecules are similarly distributed in the ECF and plasma, the concentration of protein is four to five times greater in plasma than in the interstitial fluid.

The total plasma concentration of cations is about 150 mmol/L, of which sodium is approximately 140 mmol/L and potassium 4 mmol/L. The most abundant plasma anions are chloride and bicarbonate, with average concentrations

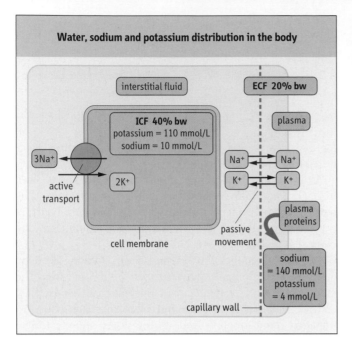

Water, sodium and potassium distribution in the body

Fig. 22.1 **Water, sodium and potassium distribution in the body.** The main water compartments in the body are the intracellular fluid (ICF) and the extracellular fluid (ECF). ECF includes interstitial fluid and plasma. A gradient of sodium and potassium concentration is maintained across cell membranes by Na^+/K^+-ATPase, which pumps sodium ions from ICF to the ECF, and potassium ions in the opposite direction. Sodium is a major contributor to the osmolality of the ECF, and a main determinant of the distribution of water between ECF and ICF. On the other hand, the distribution of water between plasma and interstitial fluid is determined by the oncotic pressure exerted by plasma proteins. bw, body weight.

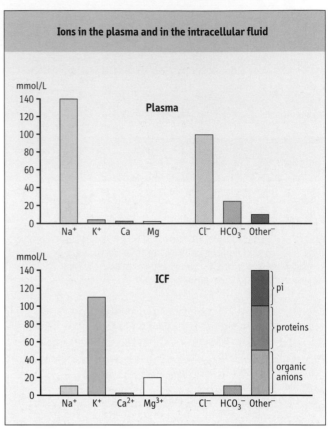

Ions in the plasma and in the intracellular fluid

Fig. 22.2 **Ions in the plasma and in the intracellular fluid.** The most important ions in plasma are sodium, potassium, calcium, chloride, phosphate, and bicarbonate. Sodium chloride, in a concentration close to 0.9%, is the main ionic component of the ECF. Potassium is the main intracellular cation.

In addition to the electrolytes shown here, glucose and urea contribute to plasma osmolality. Normally their contribution is small, because they are present in plasma at relatively low molar concentrations (about 5 mmol/L each). The contribution of glucose to osmolality becomes important in diabetes, when its concentration increases: because glucose is confined to the ECF, glucose excess induces movement of water from the cells to the ECF. The plasma concentration of urea increases in renal failure; however, because it can cross cell membranes freely, it does not contribute to water movement between ECF and ICF.

The main intracellular cation is potassium. There is also a substantial amount of magnesium in cells. The main anions in the ICF are phosphates and proteins.

100 mmol/L and 25 mmol/L, respectively (Fig. 22.2). The rest of the anions are, for the purposes of electrolyte balance, considered together as constituting the so-called anion gap which is calculated as follows:

$$\text{anion gap} = \{[Na^+] + [K^+]\} - \{[Cl^-] + [HCO^{3-}]\}$$

'Anion gap' is a somewhat artificial term which came into existence because anions, which include phosphate, sulfate, protein, and organic anions such as lactate, citrate, pyruvate, acetoacetate, and 3-hydroxybutyrate, are not measured by the clinical laboratories as frequently as the 'main' electrolytes. The anion gap is normally about 10 mmol/L. It may increase several-fold in conditions where inorganic and organic anions accumulate, e.g., in renal failure or diabetic ketoacidosis, and for this reason it is diagnostically important.

In the intracellular fluid (ICF), the main cation is potassium. Its concentration in this fluid is about 110 mmol/L, which is almost 30-fold greater than that in the ECF. The concentrations of sodium and chloride in the ICF are only

10 mmol/L and 4 mmol/L, respectively. Anions present in the ICF include proteins, phosphate, and other substances that cannot diffuse freely through the cell membranes.

Water diffuses freely across most cell membranes, but the movement of ions and neutral molecules is restricted

The transport of small molecules across otherwise impermeable membranes is made possible because of the existence

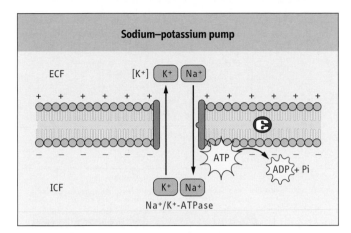

Sodium–potassium pump

Fig. 22.3 **Sodium-potassium pump.** The enzyme, Na$^+$/K$^+$-ATPase, is responsible for maintaining sodium and potassium concentration gradients across cell membranes. It also has a key role in the reabsorption of sodium in the kidney tubules.

of specific transport proteins, including ion pumps. Of the several ion pumps, the sodium/potassium ATPase (Na$^+$/K$^+$ATPase), also referred to as the sodium-potassium pump, shows the greatest transport activity. Its hydrolyzes one ATP molecule, and the released energy drives the transfer of three sodium ions from the cell to the outside, and, in turn, two potassium ions from the outside into the cell. Thus this pump maintains chemical and electrical potential gradients between the inside and the outside of the cell (Fig. 22.3). For most cells, the membrane potential ranges from 50 to 90 mV, being negative inside the cell. The electrochemical gradient is a source of energy for the transport of many substances, in particular for the cotransport of sodium ions with glucose, amino acids, and phosphate (see Chapter 7; the role of ion gradients in nerve transmission is described in Chapter 39).

OSMOLALITY AND VOLUME OF ECF AND ICF

The relative volumes of ECF and ICF depend on the amount of osmotically active substances in each of these compartments

All molecules dissolved in the body water contribute to the osmotic pressure, which is proportional to the molal concentration of the solution. One millimole of a substance dissolved in 1 kg H$_2$O at 37°C exerts an osmotic pressure of approximately 19 mmHg. Under physiologic conditions, the average concentration of all osmotically active substances in the ECF is 290 mmol/kg H$_2$O, and this remains in equilibrium with the ICF.

A change in the concentration of osmotically active ions in either of the compartments creates a gradient of osmotic

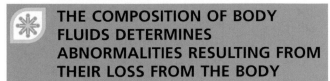

THE COMPOSITION OF BODY FLUIDS DETERMINES ABNORMALITIES RESULTING FROM THEIR LOSS FROM THE BODY

Clinical problems caused by the loss of body fluids

It is possible to predict problems that may arise from the loss of body fluids. For instance, sweat contains less sodium than extracellular fluid, therefore excessive sweating leads to a predominant loss of water, and 'concentrates' extracellular fluid sodium, leading to increased plasma sodium. In contrast, the sodium content of the intestinal fluid is similar to that of plasma; it contains considerable amounts of potassium. Thus the loss of intestinal fluid (for instance, in severe diarrhea) results in dehydration and hypokalemia, but may not affect plasma sodium concentration (Table 22.1).

Electrolyte content of body fluids				
	Sodium (mmol/L)	Potassium (mmol/L)	Bicarbonate (mmol/L)	Chloride (mmol/L)
Plasma	140	4	25	100
Gastric juice	50	15	0–15	140
Small intestinal fluid	140	10	variable	70
Feces in diarrhea	50–140	30–70	20–80	variable
Bile, pleural, and peritoneal fluids	140	5	40	100
Sweat	12	10	–	12

Table 22.1 **The electrolyte composition of body fluids.** Loss of fluid that has an electrolyte content similar to that of plasma leads to dehydration with normal plasma electrolyte concentrations. In contrast, dehydration may be accompanied by hypernatremia when the sodium content of the lost fluid is less than that of plasma (e.g. sweat). Overhydration is usually accompanied by hyponatremia. (Adapted with permission from Dominiczak MH, ed. Seminars in clinical biochemistry, 2nd ed. Glasgow: Glasgow University, 1997.)

pressure and, consequently, induces a movement of water between compartments. Water diffuses from a compartment of low osmolality to one of high osmolality until the osmotic pressures are identical in both of them (i.e. until iso-osmolality is achieved). Thus the relative volumes of ECF and ICF are reflected in the amount of osmotically active substances in these compartments; the sodium ion is the most important in the ECF. Glucose, which is normally present in plasma in a concentration about 5 mmol/L (90 mg/dL), does not contribute much to osmolality, but it may reach very high concentrations in diabetes (in extreme circumstances above

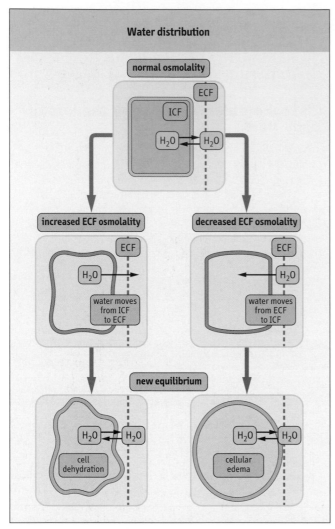

Fig. 22.4 **Water redistribution.** Osmotic pressure controls the movement of water between different compartments. An increase in ECF osmolality leads to movement of water from the cells into the ECF, and to cellular dehydration. In contrast, when ECF osmolality decreases, water moves from the ECF into the cells. This leads to expansion of the cell volume (edema). Arrows indicate the direction of water movement.

50 mmol/L [900 mg/dL]) and that profoundly affects the osmolality (see Chapter 20) (Fig. 22.4).

Within the ECF, the distribution of water between intravascular and extravascular compartments depends on the concentration of plasma proteins

In the plasma, proteins, particularly albumin, exert osmotic pressure (about 3.32 kPa [25 mmHg]), which retains water in the vascular bed; it is known as the oncotic pressure. This is balanced by the hydrostatic pressure, which forces fluid out of the capillaries. In the arterial part of capillaries, the hydro-

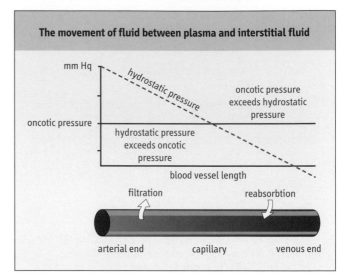

Fig. 22.5 **The movement of fluid between plasma and interstitial fluid is determined by the balance between oncotic and hydrostatic pressures.**

static pressure prevails over the oncotic pressure. As a result, water and low-molecular-weight substances filter out into the extravascular space. In contrast, in the venous part of capillaries, oncotic pressure prevails over hydrostatic pressure, and fluid is drawn into the vascular lumen (Fig. 22.5). A reduction in plasma oncotic pressure, which occurs, for instance, when the plasma concentration of albumin decreases, results in the movement of fluid into the extravascular space; clinically this causes edema.

Regulation of cell osmolality and volume

The cellular mechanism responsible for maintaining its volume is the sodium–potassium pump. The inhibition of the pump, for example by a poisonous glycoside such as ouabain, results in a decrease of intracellular potassium concentration and an increase in sodium. This decreases the membrane potential (depolarizes the cell membrane). To maintain electrical neutrality, chloride ions also enter the cells as counterions to sodium.

Intracellular sodium concentration regulates the activity of the sodium-potassium pump

When the intracellular concentration of sodium increases, the activity of the sodium–potassium pump also increases, and sodium ions are extruded from the cell. In this way, cells protect themselves from changes in the fluid volume. Another mechanism which protects cell volume is the intracellular generation of osmotically active substances. For instance, the brain cells adapt to the increased ECF osmolality by increas-

EDEMA RESULTS FROM A LOSS OF PROTEIN

An 8-year-old girl was referred to a nephrologist after she had been noticed to have puffiness of her face and swollen ankles over a period of about 2 weeks. Dipstick test for urine protein yielded a strongly positive (++++) result and measurement in a 24-hour collection showed protein excretion of 7g/day. Reference value for urinary protein excretion is less than 0.15g/day.

Comment. Renal biopsy showed so-called minimal change disease. The damage to the renal filtration barrier was the cause of the proteinuria, with the urinary protein loss causing in turn a decrease in the plasma oncotic pressure and retention of water in the ECF, leading to edema. The condition went into remission after therapy with a glucocorticoid.

ing their amino acid concentration, and cells in the renal medulla exposed to a hyperosmotic environment (see below) produce an osmotically active alcohol, sorbitol, and increase the concentration of an amino acid taurine.

THE WATER BALANCE

The body constantly exchanges water with the environment. In a steady state, the intake of water equals its loss. The main source of water intake is oral and the main source of loss is the urine. We also lose water through the lungs, sweat and feces: this is called the 'insensible' water loss and amounts to approximately 500 mL daily (Fig. 22.6). Importantly, the insensible loss can increase substantially with high temperatures, during intensive exercise, and also as a result of diarrhea or fever.

THE KIDNEY

The main functions of the kidneys are to maintain the composition, osmolality, and volume of the ECF and also to control the acid–base balance (see Chapter 23). Kidneys remove products of metabolism such as urea, uric acid, and creatinine, and retain valuable substances such as glucose, amino acids, and proteins. They also metabolize and remove drugs and toxins. Kidney function is regulated hormonally by vasopressin (antidiuretic hormone; ADH) and renin–angiotensin system. The kidneys themselves produce renin involved in the regulation of blood pressure, calcitriol (also known as 1α-25-dihydroxycholecalciferol; $1,25(OH)_2D_3$) involved in calcium homeostasis, (see Chapter 24), and ery-

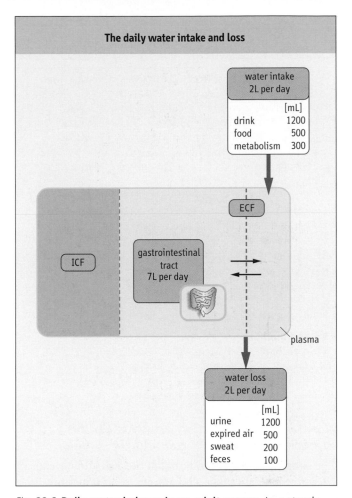

Fig. 22.6 **Daily water balance in an adult person.** In a steady state, intake of water equals output: water is obtained from the diet and from oxidative metabolism, and is lost through the kidneys, skin, lungs, and intestine. Note how much water enters and leaves the gastrointestinal tract daily; this explains why severe diarrhea leads to dehydration (see above).

thropoetin which controls the production of erythrocytes (see Chapter 3).

The nephron is the functional unit of the kidney

Each kidney consists of approximately 1 million tiny structures called nephrons (Fig. 22.7). Glomeruli located in the kidney cortex connect the cardiovascular system to the excretory tubules. An incoming small artery (afferent arteriole) branches out inside the glomerular capsule (Bowman's capsule) into bundles of capillary vessels that combine again into the outgoing (efferent) arteriole. The glomerular capsule itself transforms into a long tube, the renal tubule; the first part of this is the proximal tubule, which becomes the thin loop of Henle; further along its length it thickens again to form the distal tubule and the collecting duct.

DIARRHEA MAY LEAD TO SEVERE FLUID LOSS

A 4-year-old child was admitted to the Pediatric Unit after 2 days of severe diarrhea. The child had tachycardia and low blood pressure. Her serum sodium concentration was 145 mmol/L, creatinine concentration 50 mmol/L (0.57 mg/dL), and urea concentration 5.2 mmol/L (31 mg/dL). Treatment with an intravenous infusion of sodium chloride and antibiotics was started, and the girl recovered within 2 days.

Comment. This child was quite severely hypovolemic, but there was little evidence of abnormality in her biochemistry tests. This was because she lost fluid having an electrolyte concentration similar to that of plasma. Therefore, in spite of volume loss, there was no change in electrolyte concentrations.

Children may have slightly different reference values than the adult values given here:

- **sodium:** 133–145 mmol/L
- **creatinine:** 20–80 mmol/L (0.23–0.90mg/dL)
- **urea:** 2.5–6.5 mmol/L (16.2–39 mg/dL)

Normal kidney function depends on the integrity of the glomeruli and the tubular cells

The nephron twists around, so that the distal tubule ends up close to the glomerulus. This results in an important functional junction formed by a group of cells in the distal tubule, known as the macula densa, and the so-called juxtaglomerular cells of the afferent arteriole. Together they form the juxtaglomerular apparatus, which secretes a proteolytic enzyme, renin (see below) in response to a decrease in blood pressure in the afferent arteriole. The macula densa also senses sodium chloride concentration in the distal tubule, participating in the so-called tubulo-glomerular feedback mechanism (TGF). Macula densa sends vasoconstriction signals to the afferent arteriole in response to an increase in the solute concentration in the distal tubule; this way TGF modulates glomerular perfusion and filtration rate in each nephron.

Energy metabolism and transport function of the kidney

The kidney consumes large amounts of oxygen, mainly to support active sodium transport

Most of the metabolic processes in the kidneys are aerobic, and consequently oxygen consumption in the kidneys is high: it approximately equals that of the cardiac muscle, and is three times greater than that of the brain. Such high metabolic activity is required to maintain tubular reabsorption:

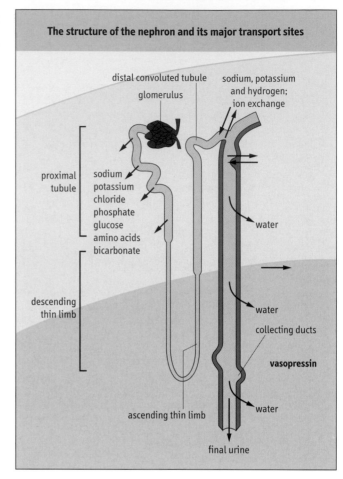

Fig. 22.7 **The structure of the nephron and of its major transport sites.**

about 70% of the consumed oxygen is used to support active sodium transport, which in turn determines the reabsorption of glucose and amino acids. The partial pressure of oxygen (pO_2) is greater in the kidney cortex than in the medulla; because of the relatively low pO_2, and the concurrent high activity of Na^+/K^+-ATPase; therefore, the distal segments of the nephron are particularly vulnerable to a decreased oxygen supply.

Main energy substrates in the renal cortex are fatty acids, lactate, glutamate, citrate, and ketone bodies. Renal tubular cells with a high Na^+/K^+-ATPase activity possess multiple mitochondria close to the plasma membrane, so that the ATP released to the cytosol is easily accessible.

The glomerulus

The excretory function of the kidneys includes filtration of the plasma in the glomeruli, transport of water and solutes from the tubular lumen back to the blood (tubular reabsorp-

amount of filtered water and solute, but not the composition of the filtrate.

The glomerular filtrate

The volume, composition, and osmolality of the glomerular filtrate all change during its flow through the renal tubules. Approximately 80% of the filtrate is reabsorbed at the early stage, in the proximal tubule. Sodium is reabsorbed in the tubule by several mechanisms: through specific ion channels, in exchange for the hydrogen ion, and in cotransport with glucose, amino acids, phosphate, and other anions. The entry of sodium into the proximal tubular cells is passive which is possible because of its low concentration in the cytoplasm of tubular cells which is maintained by the Na^+/K^+-ATPase localized on the 'blood side' (basolateral membrane) of the tubular cells. Na^+/K^+-ATPase catalyzes active extrusion of sodium to the interstitial fluid. The sodium transport causes reabsorption of water from the tubule lumen to the surrounding extracellular space.

Because of the equal reabsorption of sodium and water, the fluid leaving the proximal tubule is isotonic. Further along, in the descending limb of the loop of Henle, water diffuses from the tubules to the hyperosmotic renal medulla, and some sodium and chloride diffuse back into the tubular lumen. In contrast, the ascending limb is impermeable to water, but actively reabsorbs sodium and chloride. This generates hyperosmolality in the surrounding medulla. The different permeability characteristics of the descending and ascending limbs of the loop of Henle maintain the high osmolality of the medulla essential for the efficient reabsorption of water later; this is known as the countercurrent system (Fig. 22.9). Countercurrent multiplication builds up an osmotic gradient in the medulla through the different permeability characteristics of descending and ascending loop of Henle.

Because of the relatively greater absorption of sodium than water, the tubular fluid that leaves the loop of Henle is hypotonic. In the distal tubule and in the collecting duct, still more sodium is reabsorbed in exchange for potassium or hydrogen ion. This is controlled by the hormone aldosterone (Fig. 22.10). Further in the distal tubule and in the collecting duct water is reabsorbed along the osmotic gradient created by countercurrent multiplication; this is known as the countercurrent exchange. The water reabsorption in the collecting duct is controlled by vasopressin (see below).

The urine

Kidneys excrete from 0.5 L to more than 10 L of urine daily; the average daily volume is 1–2 L. The minimum volume necessary to remove the products of metabolism (mainly

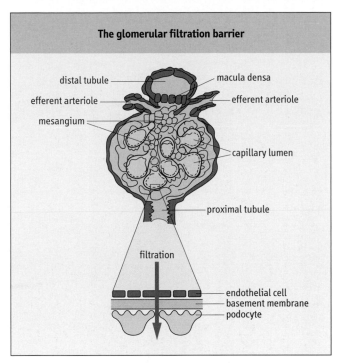

The glomerular filtration barrier

distal tubule

macula densa

efferent arteriole

efferent arteriole

mesangium

capillary lumen

proximal tubule

filtration

endothelial cell
basement membrane
podocyte

Fig. 22.8 **The glomerular filtration barrier.** This consists of the endothelial cells, the basement membrane, and the podocytes. Macula densa cells are a part of the juxtaglomerular apparatus and sense the chloride concentration in the distal tubule and adjust the diameters of different arterioles accordingly, thus regulating the glomerular blood flow.

tion), and secretion of different substances from the tubular cells into the lumen.

Plasma from the glomerular capillaries is filtered into the Bowman's space. Glomerular filtration depends on the filtration surface and on the permeability of the filtration barrier, which includes the layer of endothelial cells with characteristic pores (fenestrations) that line the glomerular blood vessels, the basement membrane, and epithelial cells (podocytes) with characteristic foot processes (Fig. 22.8). The fenestrations in the endothelial layer and the spaces between foot processes of the podocytes form a sieve that filters water and small molecules. Filtration of larger molecules through this barrier is limited by their size, shape, and electric charge. For instance, at pH 7.4, most plasma proteins are negatively charged, and so is the filtration barrier; this hinders filtration of even the smallest proteins such as myoglobin (molecular mass 17 kDa), and prevents almost completely filtration of the larger (69 kDa) albumin.

Glomerular filtration is driven by the hydrostatic pressure in the glomerular capillaries, which is approximately 50 mmHg. The hydrostatic pressure is counteracted by the oncotic pressure of the plasma and the back-pressure (approximately 10 mmHg) of the filtrate in the glomerular capsule. Changes in glomerular filtration rate alter the total

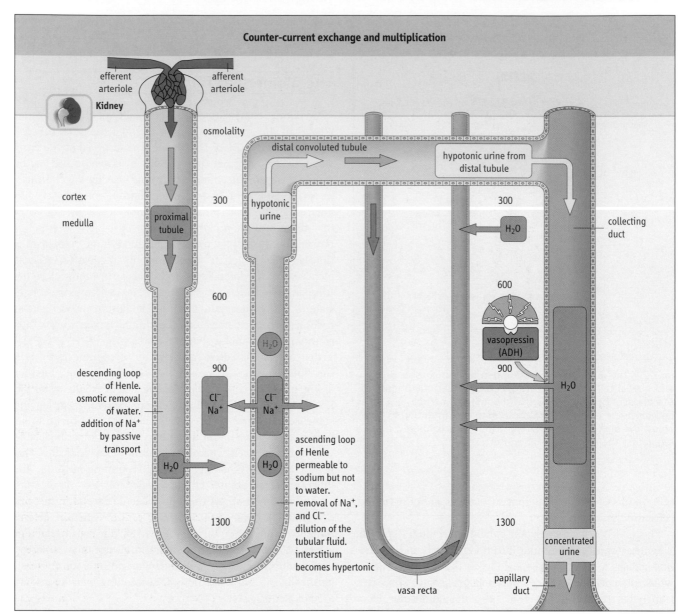

Fig. 22.9 **Counter-current exchange and multiplication.** The counter-current mechanism is essential for the formation of urine, and for the efficient reabsorption of water in the distal tubule: it enables the kidney to maintain high osmolality in the medulla. The descending and ascending arms of the loop of Henle have different permeability characteristics. In the ascending arm, sodium and chloride ions are pumped out into the interstitial fluid. They then diffuse freely into the lumen of the descending limb, creating a functional 'loop', which perpetuates the increase in osmolality of the filtrate reaching the ascending limb. This is known as counter-current multiplication.

As a result of this, the osmolality of the renal cortex is similar to that of plasma (300 mmol/L), whereas in the medulla it might be as high as 1300 mmol/L. High osmolality of the medulla facilitates reabsorption of water in the collecting ducts. This is known as counter-current exchange. Reabsorbed water diffuses into the medullary blood vessels (vasa recta). The amount of water absorbed is controlled by vasopressin.

Counter-current multiplication and counter-current exchange act in concert to enable efficient reabsorption of water in the collecting duct.

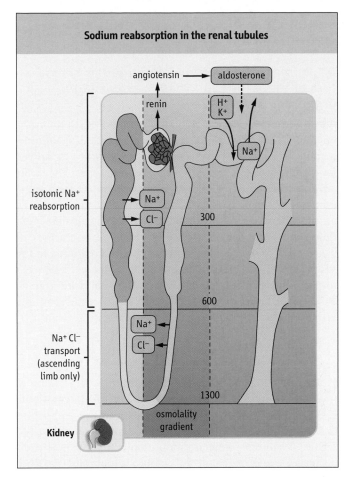

Sodium reabsorption in the renal tubules

Fig. 22.10 Sodium reabsorption in the renal tubules. More than 80% of filtered sodium is actively reabsorbed in the proximal tubule. In addition, sodium and chloride ions are reabsorbed in the ascending limb of the loop of Henle (see also Fig. 22.9). A different mechanism operates in the distal tubule, where sodium reabsorption is stimulated by aldosterone and is coupled with the secretion of hydrogen and potassium ions. Aldosterone causes sodium retention and an increased secretion of potassium.

DIABETES OFTEN LEADS TO THE IMPAIRMENT OF RENAL FUNCTION

A 37-year-old woman with a 12-year history of type 1 diabetes came for a routine visit to the Diabetic Clinic. She had poor diabetic control and a glycated hemoglobin (HbA$_{1c}$) value of 8%. Blood pressure was mildly raised at 138/88 mm Hg. A quantitative measurement of albumin in urine revealed protein concentration of 40 mg/L, indicating microalbuminuria. Reference values are:

- **HbA$_{1c}$:** desirable value below 6%.
- **Microalbuminuria:** less than 30 mg/L.

Comment. This patient had mildly impaired renal function and raised blood pressure as a result of glomerular damage from diabetes. The presence of microalbuminuria predicts future overt diabetic nephropathy. Blood pressure should be maintained at <130/80 mmHg preferably with an angiotensin converting enzyme inhibitor drug.

mulation of amino acids such as phenylalanine, leucine, isoleucine, and valine in the plasma.

Analysis of urine (urinalysis) is important in the diagnosis of renal disease, diabetes, and jaundice and helps to diagnose hereditary defects of amino acid transport

The analysis of urine carried out in clinical laboratories includes testing for the presence of protein, glucose, ketone bodies, bilirubin, and urobilinogen, and looking for traces of blood. Urinary osmolality is checked to assess the concentrating capacity of the kidney. Specialist investigations include the analysis of urinary amino acids. The urine is also tested for the presence of leukocytes and various crystals and deposits (Fig. 22.11).

Protein is normally detectable in the urine in trace amounts only, but this increases significantly when the glomeruli are damaged; the presence of significant amounts of protein in urine is an important sign of renal disease. Even minimal amount of albumin in the urine (microalbuminuria) predicts the development of diabetic nephropathy (see Chapter 20). Larger proteins such as immunoglobulins appear in the urine when the glomerular damage is more extensive: the immunoglobulin light chains (Bence–Jones protein) are present in urine in multiple myeloma (see Chapter 3). In hemolytic anemia, the urine may contain free hemoglobin and urobilinogen. Myoglobin is present in urine in cases of widespread muscle damage (rhabdomyolysis). The measurement of glucose and ketones in the urine, together with their measurements in blood, is important in monitoring the glycemic control (Chapter 20). The measurements

nitrogen excreted as urea) is approximately 0.5 L/24 h. Urine osmolality varies from about 80 to 1200 mmol/L. The osmolality of the glomerular filtrate is about 300 mmol/L, therefore the maximal urine concentration is approximately fourfold. The ability to form concentrated urine in response to fluid deprivation depends on normal tubular function and on the presence of vasopressin.

Only small amounts of amino acids (0.7 g/24 h), and almost no glucose, are normally present in the urine. Each substance reabsorbed in the renal tubules has its own renal transport maximum (T_{max}). T_{max} can be exceeded either when the load of a substance becomes too large to handle, swamping the transport system, or when the tubular cells themselves do not function properly. Thus, aminoaciduria may result from an impaired tubular function or from the accu-

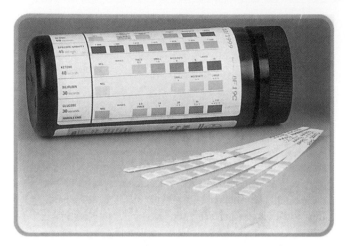

Fig. 22.11 **The urine testing (urinalysis) is performed using ready-made dry tests;** these are strips coated with reagents immobilized on a plastic support. Dipping the strip in the urine initiates a reaction yielding a colored product. The readout is against a standardized color scale.

of urobilinogen and bilirubin in urine help to assess liver function (see Chapter 28).

Assessment of renal function

Renal clearance and the glomerular filtration rate are important characteristics of kidney function

The renal clearance is the volume of plasma (in milliliters) that the kidney clears of a given substance per unit of time (minutes). The concept of glomerular filtration rate (GFR) is derived from this and is the most important characteristic describing kidney function. GFR could be estimated by measuring the clearance of a substance, such as polysaccharide inulin, that is removed from the body only through the kidneys, and that is neither secreted nor reabsorbed in the renal tubules. The amount of inulin filtered from plasma (plasma concentration, P_{in}, multiplied by GFR) equals the amount recovered in urine (i.e. the urinary concentration, U_{in}, times the rate of urine formation rate, V). One can present this in the form of an equation:

$$P_{in} \times GFR = U_{in} \times V$$

From this the GFR can be calculated as:

$$GFR = \frac{U_{in} \times V}{P_{in}}$$

The expression $\frac{U \times V}{P}$ is called the renal clearance and the renal clearance of inulin equals the GFR. The average GFR is 120 mL/min for men and 100 mL/min for women.

Serum creatinine concentration and creatinine clearance

Measurement of serum creatinine is a simple test of renal function that does not require urine collection

Administering inulin intravenously to assess the GFR is quite impractical. Instead, we calculate the clearance of creatinine, a compound normally detected in plasma which is derived from phosphocreatine present in skeletal muscles. The clearance of creatinine is similar to that of inulin. There is some tubular reabsorption of creatinine, but this is compensated by an equivalent degree of tubular secretion. To calculate creatinine clearance, one needs a sample of blood, and urine collected over 24 hours. The concentration of creatinine in the serum and the urine is measured. The urine excretion per unit of time is calculated by dividing the total urine volume by the collection time (V, above). The clearance of creatinine is then calculated according to the formula:

$$creatinine\ clearance = \frac{U_{creatinine} \times V}{P_{creatinine}}$$

The concentration of creatinine in serum is 20–80 mmol/L (0.28–0.90 mg/dL). The measurement of serum creatinine is the simplest test of renal function. An increase in serum creatinine concentration is a marker of a decrease in GFR: serum creatinine concentration doubles when the GFR decreases to approximately 50% of its original value. Another test that is used to assess kidney function is the measurement of serum urea. However, because urea is an end product of protein catabolism, its amount in plasma, apart from renal function, is also dependent on factors such as the amount of protein in the diet (Chapter 18) and the rate of tissue breakdown (Fig. 22.12).

The newest test to measure renal function is the assessment of cystatin C concentration which seems to provide accurate assessment of moderate decreases in the glomerular filtration rate

Cystatin C is a 122-amino acid, 13 kDa protein belonging to the family of cysteine proteinase inhibitors. It is a product of the 'housekeeping' gene expressed in all nucleated cells, and is produced at a constant rate. Because of its small size and its basic pI, cystatin C is freely filtered through the glomerulus. It is not secreted by the tubules but it is reabsorbed and subsequently catabolized, therefore it does not return to blood. The use of serum cystatin C to estimate GFR follows the same logic as the use of serum creatinine.

The measurements of serum creatinine and urea concentration are performed as first-line tests and are essential for the diagnosis of renal failure. In renal failure one observes a decrease in urine volume, an increase in serum concentra-

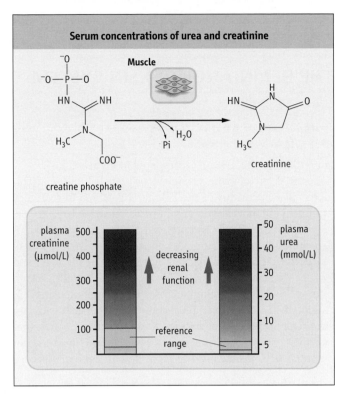

Fig. 22.12 **Serum levels of urea and creatinine.** The most important biochemical markers of renal function are serum urea and serum creatinine. The upper panel shows the conversion of muscle phosphocreatine into creatinine. Loss of 50% of nephrons results in approximate doubling of serum creatinine concentration.

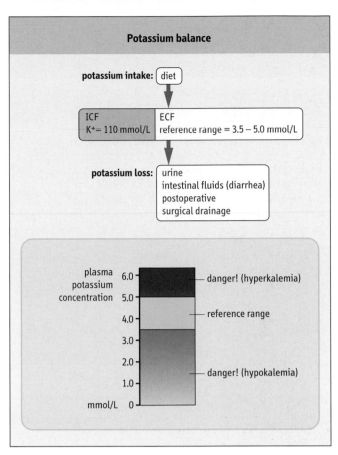

Fig. 22.13 **Potassium balance.** Plasma potassium concentration is maintained within narrow limits. Both low (hypokalemia) and high (hyperkalemia) concentrations may be dangerous, because of the effect of potassium on the contractility of heart muscle. The upper panel shows the main sources of potassium loss from the body.

tions of urea and creatinine, and a decrease in creatinine clearance.

THE IMPORTANCE OF PLASMA POTASSIUM CONCENTRATION

Potassium affects the contractility of the heart, and both high (hyperkalemia) and low concentration (hypokalemia) can be life threatening

The measurement of serum potassium concentration is a very important laboratory test (Fig. 22.13). The serum concentration of potassium is 3.5–5 mmol/L. Because the intracellular concentration of potassium is much higher than in the ECF and plasma, a relatively minor movement of potassium between ECF and ICF may result in large changes in the serum potassium concentration. A potassium value of less than 2.5 mmol/L or greater than 6.0 mmol/L is dangerous, and therefore maintenance of the potassium concentration close to normal is fundamentally important.

DISORDERS OF VASOPRESSIN SECRETION

Diabetes insipidus and the syndrome of inappropriate secretion of vasopressin

Deficiency of vasopressin causes the condition known as diabetes insipidus, in which large amounts of dilute urine are lost. In contrast, an uncontrolled, excessive secretion of vasopressin may take place following major trauma or surgery. This is known as the syndrome of inappropriate antidiuretic hormone secretion (SIADH), and leads to water retention.

The most common cause of severe hyperkalemia is renal failure: in this condition potassium cannot be excreted in the urine. On the other hand, low serum potassium usually results from its excessive losses, either in urine or through the gastrointestinal tract. Importantly, changes in serum

DIURETICS ARE DRUGS USED FOR TREATMENT OF EDEMA, CARDIAC FAILURE AND HYPERTENSION

Diuretics are drugs that stimulate water and sodium excretion. Diuretics act by inhibiting the reabsorption of sodium and chloride in the renal tubules. Thiazide diuretics, e.g., bendrofluazide, decrease sodium reabsorption in the distal tubules by blocking sodium and chloride cotransport. Loop diuretics, such as frusemide, inhibit sodium reabsorption in the ascending loop of Henle. Spironolactone, a potassium-sparing diuretic, is a competitive inhibitor of aldosterone, inhibits sodium–potassium exchange in the distal tubules, and also decreases potassium excretion. Finally, an osmotic diuresis may be induced by the administration of the sugar alcohol, mannitol. The net effect of diuretics is to increase urine volume and induce the loss of water and sodium. They are important in the treatment of edema associated with circulatory problems such as heart failure, in which impaired cardiac function may lead to a severe breathlessness caused by pulmonary edema. They are also essential in the treatment of hypertension.

potassium concentration are also associated with the acid–base disorders (see Chapter 23).

THE RENIN-ANGIOTENSIN SYSTEM

The renin-angiotensin system is important in the control of blood pressure and the vascular tone

An outline of this system is presented in Figure 22.14.

Renin is an enzyme produced principally in the juxtaglomerular apparatus of the kidney; it is stored in secretory granules and released in response to decreased renal perfusion pressure. Renin is a protease that uses angiotensinogen as its substrate. Angiotensinogen is a glycoprotein of more than 400 amino acids, is synthesized in the liver, and has a variable structure and molecular weight. Renin cleaves the decapeptide angiotensin I from angiotensinogen. Angiotensin I is a short, 10-amino-acid peptide. It is a substrate for peptidyl-dipeptidase A (angiotensin converting enzyme; ACE). ACE removes two amino acids from angiotensin I, producing the most potent known vasocon-

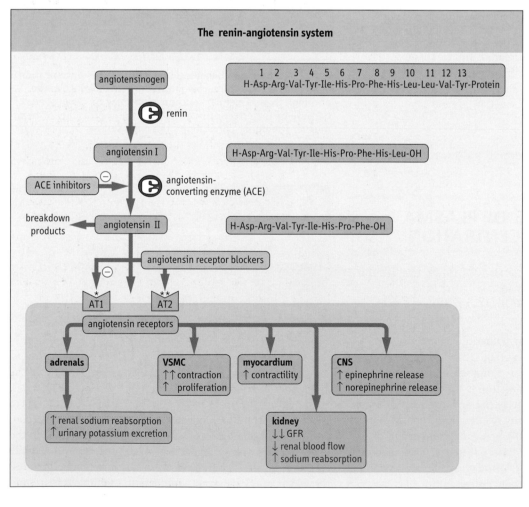

Fig. 22.14 **The renin–angiotensin system.** VSMC, vascular smooth muscle cells; CNS, central nervous system. *AT-1 receptor blocked by e.g. losartan. **AT-2 receptor blocked by saralasin.

RENIN–ANGIOTENSIN SYSTEM AND CARDIAC FAILURE

A 65-year-old man with a previous anterior myocardial infarction presented with increasing fatigue, shortness of breath and ankle edema. Physical examination showed mild tachycardia, a raised jugular venous pressure and some ankle oedema. An echocardiogram showed that the function of the left ventricle during systole was very poor. The patient's serum measurements revealed: sodium 140 mmol/L, potassium 3.5 mmol/L, protein 34 (normal 35-45), g/dL, creatinine 80 µmol/L (0.90 mg/dL), and urea 7.5 mmol/L (45 mg/dL).

Comment. This man presents with symptoms and signs of cardiac failure. The impaired function of the heart leads to a decreased blood flow through the kidney, activation of the renin–angiotensin system and stimulation of aldosterone secretion. Aldosterone causes an increased renal reabsorption of sodium and water retention, thereby increasing extracellular fluid volume and causing edema.

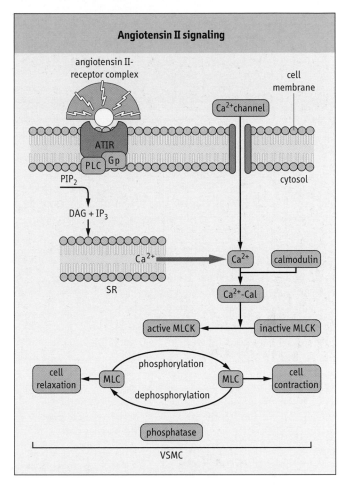

Fig. 22.15 Cellular mechanism of Angiotensin II-induced vasoconstriction. The angiotensin receptor (AT1) is linked to G-proteins. The binding of angiotensin II to the receptor leads to phospholipase C-mediated formation of inositol 1,4,5-trisphosphate (IP₃) and 1,2-diacylglycerol (DAG). This results in the mobilization of Ca^{2+} from the sarcoplasmic reticulum (SR), and to the cell entry of the extracellular Ca^{2+} which takes place as a result of the activation of calcium channels. The increase in the cytosolic Ca^{2+} initiates the contractile response of the vascular smooth muscle cells (VSMC) and Ca^{2+} subsequently binds to calmodulin (Cal). The Ca^{2+}-calmodulin complex activates myosin light-chain kinase (MLCK) which phosphorylates myosin light chains and elicits muscular tension. This effect is terminated by the dephosphorylation of myosin (see also Chapter 19). AT1 receptor antagonists, such as losartan, inhibit the vasoconstrictor effects of angiotensin II and are used in the treatment of hypertension.

strictor molecule, angiotensin II. ACE is particularly abundant in the pulmonary blood vessels where it is bound to the luminal surface of the endothelial cells. Drugs that inhibit ACE are now extensively used in the treatment of hypertension and in cardiology (Fig. 22.15).

Angiotensin II constricts vascular smooth muscle, thereby increasing blood pressure and reducing renal blood flow and glomerular filtration rate. It also stimulates aldosterone secretion. These actions of angiotensin II are mediated through membrane receptor (AT1) which signals through G-proteins and phospholipase C. This action is antagonized through the AT2 receptor class which promotes vasodilatation and renal sodium loss.

Apart from the classical pathway of production of angiotensin II from angiotensin I by the action of ACE, there is an alternative pathway leading directly from angiotensinogen to angiotensin II. Substantial amounts of angiotensin II are formed in the kidney. Juxtaglomerular cells contain ACE, angiotensin I and angiotensin II. Angiotensin II is also synthesized in the glomerular and tubular cells and is secreted into the tubular fluid and interstitial space. Angiotensin II receptors are present on the tubular and renal vascular cells: therefore locally produced angiotensin II probably influences tubular reabsorption and renal vascular tone through autocrine and paracrine action.

Aldosterone regulates sodium reabsorption

Aldosterone is produced in the adrenal cortex, and is a major mineralocorticosteroid hormone in man. Aldosterone regulates the extracellular volume and controls potassium

homeostasis. These effects are mediated by binding to the cytosolic mineralocorticoid receptor in the epithelial cells, principally in the renal collecting duct. The receptor moves to the nucleus and binds to specific domains on targeted genes, altering gene expression. This leads to modification of the activities of the sodium channel and the Na⁺/K⁺-ATPase, resulting in increased sodium transport across the cell membrane. Aldosterone increases sodium reassertion,

ACUTE RENAL FAILURE LEADS TO A STEEP FALL IN OUTPUT OF URINE, AND CAUSES HIGH SERUM UREA AND CREATININE CONCENTRATIONS

A 25-year-old man was admitted to hospital unconscious after a motorcycle accident. He had evidence of shock with hypotension and tachycardia, a fractured skull and multiple injuries to his limbs. Despite treatment with intravenous colloid and blood he showed persistent oliguria (5–10ml/hour: oliguria is <20ml/hour). Oliguria due to acute tubular necrosis may be distinguished from prerenal azotemia by measuring urine osmolality (>500mOsm/kg in prerenal azotemia and <350 mOsm/kg in acute renal failure) also urine sodium concentration (<20mmol/L in prerenal azotemia and >40 mmol/L in acute renal failure). On the third day, his serum creatinine concentration had risen to 300 μmol/L (3.9 mg/dL) and his urea concentration is to mmol/L (132 mg/dL). Reference values are:

- **creatinine:** 20–80 μmol/L (0.23–0.90 mg/dL)
- **urea:** 2.5–6.5 mmol/L (16.2–39 mg/dL)

Comment. This young man has developed acute renal failure due to acute tubular necrosis as a consequence of hypovolaemic shock. He subsequently underwent emergency haemofiltration. Renal function started to recover after 2 weeks with an initial increased urine volume, the so-called 'diuretic phase'.

- **urea** mg/dL = mmol/L × 6.02
- **creatinine** mg/dL = μmol/L × 0.0113

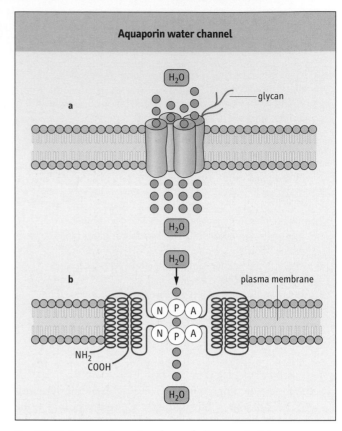

Fig. 22.16 **Aquaporin water channel.** Aquaporin-1 is a multisubunit water channel with a glycan unit attached to one of the subunits (A). Each of the two monomers has two tandem repeat structures each consisting of three membrane-spanning regions (B) and connecting loops containing asn-pro-ala (NPA) sequences embedded in the membrane bilayer.

and potassium and hydrogen ion excretion in the distal tubule.

WATER REABSORPTION IN THE DISTAL TUBULE AND THE COLLECTING DUCT

Aquaporins are a family of membrane channel proteins which enable rapid transport of water through biological membranes.

Aquaporin 0 (AQPOP) gene is expressed in lens cells and the mutations of its gene are associated with congenital cataracts. AQP1 is expressed in erythrocytes, renal proximal tubular cells, and in the capillary endothelium. AQP2 is principally expressed in the renal collecting ducts. Mutations in AQP2 gene and in the vasopressin receptor gene lead to dif-

ferent types of the so-called nephrogenic diabetes insipidus, a condition associated with passing large amounts of urine and dehydration (Fig. 22.16).

Vasopressin (antidiuretic hormone, ADH) controls water reabsorption in the collecting ducts of the kidney

Vasopressin is synthesized in the supraoptic and paraventricular nuclei of the hypothalamus and transported along axons to the posterior pituitary where it is stored before being further processed and released. The binding of vasopressin to its receptor located on the membranes of tubular cells in the collecting ducts leads to the synthesis of a variety of proteins, including aquaporin-2, which facilitates passage of water through the membrane (Fig. 22.17). The action of vasopressin determines the final volume and concentration of the urine (see Fig. 22.18).

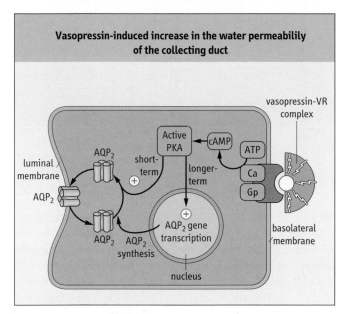

Vasopressin-induced increase in the water permeabilily of the collecting duct

Fig. 22.17 **Vasopressin-induced increase in the water permeability of the collecting duct.** Aquaporins regulate transport of water across cell membrane. Aquaporin-2 (AQP2) water channel is regulated by vasopressin. Vaspopressin binds to its receptor (VR) and through the activation of G-protein stimulates the production of cAMP which activates protein kinase A (PKA) activity. PKA phosphorylates cytoplasmic AQP2 and induces its translocation to the cell membrane, increasing capacity for water transport. Vasopressin also regulates the expression of the AQP2 gene.

POOR FLUID INTAKE LEADS TO DEHYDRATION

An 80-year-old man had been admitted to hospital after a prolonged period on the floor at home as a result of an acute stroke. He had poor tissue turgor, dry mouth, tachycardia and hypotension. Serum measurements revealed: sodium 150 mmol/L, potassium 5.2 mmol/L, bicarbonate 35 mmol/L, creatinine 110 µmol/L (1.13 mg/dL), and urea 19 mmol/L (90.3 mg/dL).
Reference values are:

- **sodium:** 135–145 mmol/L
- **potassium:** 3.5–.0 mmol/L
- **bicarbonate:** 20–25 mmol/L
- **creatinine:** 20–80 µmol/L (0.28–0.90 mg/dL)
- **urea:** 2.5–6.5 mmol/L (16.2–39mg/dL)

Comment. This patient presents with dehydration, indicated by the high sodium and urea values. He was treated with intravenous fluid predominantly in the form of 5% dextrose to replace the water deficit. The water deficit can be calculated from tables which give estimates of total body water based on age and leanness. In the adult, total body water is usually about 60% of body weight.

The renal reabsorption and excretion of water

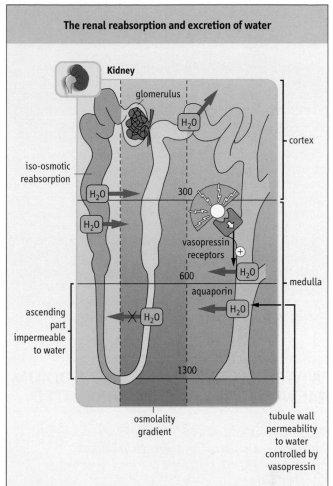

Fig. 22.18 **The renal reabsorption and excretion of water.** The permeability of the tubular walls to water differs along the nephron. About 80% of filtered water is reabsorbed in the proximal tubule, by iso-osmotic reabsorption. The ascending loop of Henle is impermeable to water; sodium is reabsorbed there, creating high osmolality in the medulla. In the collecting duct, vasopressin controls the reabsorption of water through aquaporin water channels.

ENDOCRINE CAUSES OF HYPERTENSION

Disorders of aldosterone secretion

Hyperaldosteronism is a common finding in hypertension. Primary hyperaldosteronism occurs as a result of abnormal adrenal activity and is rare. It may be a result of a single adrenal tumor, adenoma (Conn's syndrome). The more common secondary hyperaldosteronism is due to an increased secretion of renin. Pheochromocytomas are catecholamine-secreting tumors that cause hypertension in about 0.1% of hypertensive patients. It is important to correctly diagnose pheochromocytoma, because it can be surgically removed (see Chapter 40, clinical box on p. 576).

ARTERIAL HYPERTENSION IS A COMMON DISEASE

Hypertension is inappropriately increased arterial blood pressure above the desirable level of systolic blood pressure 140 mmHg and diastolic pressure 90 mmHg (normal below 140/90 mmHg, optimal below 120/80 mmHg). According to the World Health Organization, up to 20% of the population of the developed world may suffer from the condition. Hypertension causes one in every eight deaths worldwide. Traditionally, arterial hypertension has been classified as 'essential' (primary) or 'secondary'. A cause of essential hypertension has not yet been identified, although it is known to involve multiple genetic and environmental factors including neural, endocrine, and metabolic components. Hypertension is associated with an increased risk of stroke and myocardial infarction. A range of drugs is used in the modern treatment of hypertension. These include diuretics such as bendrofluazide, the drugs blocking adrenoreceptors, the inhibitors of the angiotensin converting enzyme and the antagonists of angiotensin receptors.

WATER METABOLISM AND SODIUM METABOLISM ARE INTERRELATED

The actions of aldosterone and vasopressin comprise a control system that directs the handling of both water and sodium by the kidney

Normally, despite large variations in fluid intake, plasma osmolality is maintained within narrow limits (280–295 mmol/kg H_2O). Vasopressin contributes to the control of plasma osmolality by regulating water metabolism. It responds to both osmotic and volume signals. On the one hand its secretion, and thirst, are stimulated by signals from osmoreceptors which respond to even minute (about 1%) increase in plasma osmolality. On the other, vasopressin release is stimulated by a decrease (more than 10%) in circulating volume which triggers receptors sensitive to pressure.

Vasopressin and the renin–angiotensin system in water and electrolyte disorders

Water excess increases plasma volume, renal blood flow, and GFR

In the condition of water excess the production of rennin, and thus the whole renin-angiotensin–aldosterone axis, is suppressed. The low concentration of aldosterone causes urinary sodium loss. Also, the excess of water 'dilutes' plasma, and plasma osmolality decreases. The decrease in osmolality also suppresses thirst and the secretion of vaso-

DIAGNOSTIC UTILITY OF BNP PROPEPTIDES

Instead of measuring the active forms of natriuretic peptides in plasma, it is more convenient to measure the pro-peptides which are present in plasma in equimolar amounts to the active species. Thus proBNP (1-76) reaches higher levels in cardiac failure than BNP 32. Similarly, proANP (1-98) has a longer half-life in plasma than biologically active 1-28 ANP and therefore is present in the circulation in higher concentrations.

pressin through the action of hypothalamic osmoreceptors. The suppression of vasopressin leads to increased urinary loss of water. The overall response to water excess is therefore a compensatory increase of water and sodium excretion.

On the other hand, water deficit (dehydration) leads to a decrease in plasma volume and thus in renal blood flow and GFR. This stimulates the renin–angiotensin system and the production of aldosterone which inhibits urinary sodium excretion. In addition, because of the loss of water, the plasma osmolality increases and this stimulates vasopressin secretion, with a consequent decrease in the urine volume. Thus the response to water deficit is the retention of sodium and water by the body (Fig. 22.19).

Natriuretic peptides are important markers of heart failure

Another family of peptides, the natriuretic peptides, is involved in the regulation of fluid volume. The two main peptides are the atrial natriuretic peptide (ANP) and the brain natriuretic peptide (BNP). The ANP is synthesized predominantly in the cardiac atria as a 126 amino acid pro-peptide (pro-ANP). It is then cleaved into a smaller 98 amino acid propeptide and the biologically active 28-amino acid ANP. The BNP is synthesized in the cardiac ventricles as 108-amino acid propeptide, and is cleaved into a 76-amino acid propeptide and a biologically active 32-amino acid BNP. BNP 32, and another peptide CNP (22 amino acids long) were also isolated from the porcine brain, thus the name. All natriuretic peptides possess a ring-type structure due to the presence of a disulfide bond.

Natriuretic peptides promote sodium excretion and induce a decrease blood pressure. ANP and BNP are secreted in response to atrial stretch and ventricular volume overload. They act on the specific receptors which signal through guanyl cyclase and cGTP: the A type receptors are located predominantly in the endothelial cells and the B-type receptors in the brain. There is cross-reactivity between different natriuretic receptors with regard to these peptides. Importantly for clinical diagnosis, the levels of ANP and BNP are increased in heart failure and therefore their measurements are used as biochemical markers of this

Close links between water and sodium metabolism

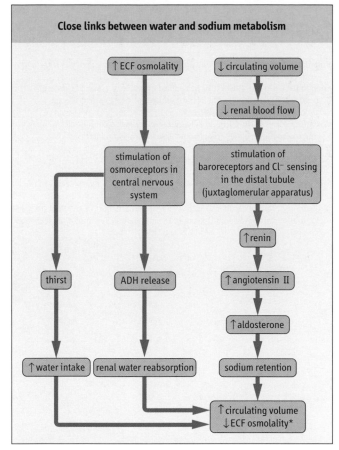

Fig. 22.19 **Close links between water and sodium metabolism.** The metabolism of water and that of sodium are closely interrelated. An increase in ECF osmolality by only as much as 2% stimulates secretion of vasopressin. Vasopressin increases the renal reabsorption of water through aquaporin-2 water channel. This leads to 'dilution' of the ECF and a decrease in osmolality. This response is reinforced by the stimulation of thirst. Water retention can be induced, not only by an increase in osmolality, but also by a decrease in the volume of circulating plasma, through stimulation of the pressure-sensitive receptors (baroreceptors) in the juxtaglomerular apparatus in the kidney. *Osmolality will decrease if the degree of water retention is relatively greater than sodium retention.

condition. These measurements are particularly useful for excluding the presence of mild heart failure in patients who present with nonspecific symptoms such as shortness of breath.

The assessment of water and electrolyte status is an important part of clinical practice

The assessment of water and electrolyte balance is an important part of the general examination of a patient. In addition to the physical examination and medical history, the following measurements are required:

SERUM SODIUM CONCENTRATION IN DISORDERS OF FLUID AND ELECTROLYTE BALANCE

Disorders of water and electrolyte metabolism

Water and electrolyte disturbances may result from an imbalance between the intake of fluids and electrolytes and their loss through either renal or extrarenal routes, a movement of water and electrolytes between body compartments, or both. A decreased sodium concentration (hyponatremia) usually indicates that the extracellular fluid is being 'diluted', whereas an increasing sodium concentration means that the extracellular fluid is being 'concentrated'. Hyponatremia may result from either excess of water in the system (common), or from the loss of sodium (rare). Conversely, hypernatremia results from either loss of water (common) or excess of sodium (rare).

- serum electrolyte concentrations: the profile commonly requested a physician includes sodium, potassium, chloride and bicarbonate and also:
  - serum creatinine and urea concentration
  - urine volume, osmolality and sodium concentration
  - serum osmolality

Importantly, patients who stay on a hospital ward and who have or are expected to have abnormal water or electrolyte balance need a fluid chart – that is, a daily record of fluid intake and loss.

Summary

- Both the deficit of body water (dehydration) and its excess (overhydration) lead to potentially serious clinical problems. The assessment of water and electrolyte balance is an important part of clinical examination.
- Body water balance is closely linked to the balance of dissolved ions (electrolytes), the most important of which are sodium and potassium.
- The movement of water between ECF and ICF is controlled by osmotic gradients.
- The movement of water between the lumen of a blood vessel and the interstitial fluid is controlled by the balance between the osmotic and hydrostatic pressures.
- The main regulators of water and electrolyte balance are vasopressin (water excretion and intake) and aldosterone (sodium and potassium excretion).

■ The renin–angiotensin system is the principal regulator of blood pressure and vascular tone.

■ The measurements of natriuretic peptides help to diagnose cardiac failure.

■ Kidney is the key organ controlling the water and electrolyte balance. Serum concentrations of urea and creatinine, and creatinine clearance, are the key tests performed to assess the renal function.

ACTIVE LEARNING

1. Comment on the role of Na^+K^+-ATPase in maintaining the ion gradients across cell membrane.
2. Describe the role of counter-current multiplication in the renal water reabsorption.
3. Explain the role of renin–angiotensin system in the maintenance of blood pressure.
4. Describe water movements between ECF and ICF which take place in water deprivation.
5. Why does the low concentration of albumin in plasma lead to edema?

Further reading

Rubattu S, Volpe M. The atrial natriuretic peptide: a changing view. *J Hypertens* 2001;**19**:1923–1931.

Shapiro BP, Chen HH, Burnett JC Jr, Redfield MM. Use of plasma brain natriuretic peptide concentration to aid in the diagnosis of heart failure. *Mayo Clinic Proceedings* 2003;**78**:481–486.

Kozono, D, Yasui M King L S, Agre P. Aquaporin water channels: atomic structure and molecular dynamics meet clinical medicine. *J Clin Invest* 2002;**109**:1395–1399.

Adrogue, H J.; Madias NE. Hyponatremia. *The N Engl J Med* 2000;**342**:1581–1589.

Manohar P, Pina IL. Therapeutic role of angiotensin II receptor blockers in the treatment of heart failure. *Mayo Clinic Proceedings* 2003;**78**:334–338.

Chobanian A, Bakris GL, Black HR *et al.* The Seventh Report of the Joint National Committee on Prevention, Detection, Evaluation and Treatment of High Blood Pressure. *The JNC7 Report. JAMA* 2003;**289**:2560–2572.

Lung and Kidney: The Control of Acid–Base Balance

M H Dominiczak and M Szczepanska-Konkel

LEARNING OBJECTIVES

After reading this chapter you should be able to:

- Explain the nature of the bicarbonate buffer.
- Describe the gas exchange occurring in the lungs.
- Describe the respiratory and metabolic components of the acid-base balance.
- Define and classify acidosis and alkalosis.
- Comment on clinical conditions associated with disturbances of the acid-base balance.

The two gases, oxygen and carbon dioxide are key elements of metabolism. While oxygen is used by the body to sustain energy production, metabolism generates carbon dioxide (and hydrogen ion). There is large daily flux of oxygen, carbon dioxide, and hydrogen ion through the human body. Carbon dioxide generated in tissues dissolves in H_2O to form carbonic acid, which in turn dissociates releasing hydrogen ion. Metabolism also generates strong acids such as sulfuric acid, and organic acids such as uric acid, lactic acid and others; all are a source of hydrogen ion in the extracellular fluid. Despite large variations in generation of CO_2 and acids, for example during exercise, the blood concentration of hydrogen ion (or its negative logarithm, the pH), is surprisingly constant: it remains between 36 and 46 nmol/L (pH 7.36–7.46). Changes in pH profoundly affect the ionization of proteins and, consequently, the activity of many enzymes. Also, a decrease in pH decreases cardiac output and blood pressure, whereas an increase in pH causes constriction of small arteries and may lead to arrhythmia. Also, changes in pH together with the partial pressure of carbon dioxide (pCO_2) affect tissue oxygenation by changing the shape of the hemoglobin saturation curve, and thus the ease with which hemoglobin gives up its oxygen to the tissues (see Chapter 4).

This chapter describes how the regulation of extracellular and intracellular pH (the acid–base balance) is closely linked with gas exchange, and now problems with gas exchange and acid–base balance underlie many of diseases of the respiratory system and kidney.

Maintaining the acid–base balance involves lungs, blood, and kidneys

Organs and tissues involved in the maintenance of the acid–base balance are the lungs, the erythrocytes, and the kidneys (Figure 23.1). The lungs control the exchange of carbon dioxide and oxygen between the blood and the external atmosphere; the erythrocytes transport gases between lungs and tissues; and the kidneys control plasma bicarbonate concentration and excrete the hydrogen ion in urine.

THE BODY BUFFER SYSTEMS

Substantial quantities of inorganic and organic acids are generated from the dissolving of metabolically produced CO_2 in water, and the metabolism of sulfur-containing amino acids and phosphorus-containing compounds. Lactic acid and ketoacids (acetoacetate and hydroxybutyrate) are also produced. The excess of lactic acid is the hallmark of hypoxic conditions and the accumulation of ketoacids becomes clinically important in diabetes (see Chapter 20). Acids derived from sources other than CO_2 are known as nonvolatile; by definition, they cannot be removed through the lungs, and must be excreted via the kidney. The net production of nonvolatile acids is in the order of 50 mmol/24 h.

Blood and tissues contain buffer systems to minimize changes in hydrogen ion concentration

These systems are summarized in Table 23.1 (see also Chapter 2). The main buffer that neutralizes hydrogen ions released from cells is bicarbonate. Hemoglobin also plays an important role in buffering hydrogen generated from the carbonic anhydrase reaction (see below). Hydrogen ion is also buffered by intracellular buffers, mainly proteins and phosphates.

The bicarbonate buffer

The bicarbonate buffer is unique, because it remains in equilibrium with atmospheric air, creating an open system with

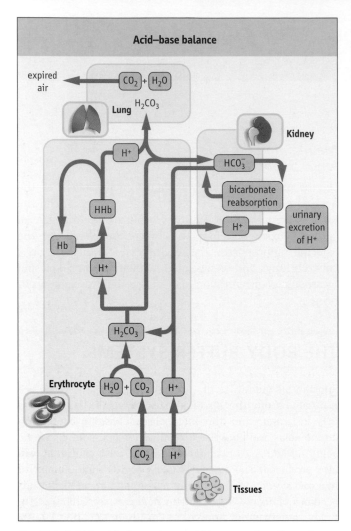

Fig. 23.1 **Acid-base balance.** Lungs, kidneys, and erythrocytes contribute to the maintenance of acid–base balance. The lungs control gas exchange with the atmospheric air. Carbon dioxide generated in tissues is transported in plasma as bicarbonate; the erythrocyte hemoglobin (Hb) also contributes to CO_2 transport. Hemoglobin buffers hydrogen ion derived from carbonic acid. The kidneys reabsorb filtered bicarbonate in the proximal tubules and generate new bicarbonate in the distal tubules, where there is a net secretion of hydrogen ion.

 ## RESPIRATORY AND METABOLIC COMPENSATION IN ACID-BASE DISORDERS

Respiratory and metabolic components of the acid–base balance adjust to maintain optimal blood pH. When the primary disorder is respiratory, the accumulation of CO_2 leads to a compensatory increase in bicarbonate reabsorption by the kidney. Conversely, a decrease in pCO_2 decreases bicarbonate reabsorption. In the event that the primary disorder is metabolic, a decrease in bicarbonate concentration and resulting decrease in pH stimulate the respiratory center to increase the ventilation rate: CO_2 is blown off and pCO_2 in plasma decreases. This is why patients with metabolic acidosis hyperventilate. Conversely, an increase in plasma bicarbonate concentration, leads to an increase in pH and to a decrease in the ventilation rate: CO2 is retained, and the pH returns towards normal.

Buffers in the human body			
Buffer	**Acid**	**Conjugate base**	**Main buffering action**
Hemoglobin	HHb	Hb^-	erythrocyles
Proteins	HProt	$Prot^-$	intracellular
Phosphate buffer	$H_2PO_4^-$	HPO_4^{2-}	intracellular
Bicarbonate	$CO_2 \rightarrow H_2CO_3$	HCO_3^-	extracellular

Table 23.1 **Main buffers in the human body.** (For the principles of buffering action see Chapter 2)

many times greater capacity than that of any of the 'closed' buffer systems. This is how it works:

Carbon dioxide produced in tissues diffuses through cell membranes and dissolves in plasma. The solubility coefficient of CO_2 in plasma is 0.23 if pCO_2 is measured in kPa (or 0.03 if pCO_2 is measured in mmHg; 1 kPa = 7.5 mmHg or 1 mmHg = 0.133 kPa). Thus, at normal pCO_2 of 5.3 kPa (40 mmHg), the concentration of dissolved CO_2 (dCO_2) is:

$$dCO_2 \text{ (mmol/L)} = 5.3 \text{ kPa} \times 0.23 = 1.2 \text{ mmol/L}$$

This CO_2 equilibrates with H_2CO_3 in plasma in the course of a very slow, nonenzymatic reaction. As a result there is only very little, about 0.0017 mmol/L, of H_2CO_3 normally present in plasma. However, because of equilibrium between the formed H_2CO_3 and dissolved CO_2 (theoretically all dissolved CO_2 could eventually convert into H_2CO_3), we take the 'acid' component of the bicarbonate buffer as being equal to the plasma concentration of dissolved CO_2.

The Henderson–Hasselbalch equation (see Chapter 2) expresses the relationship between pH and the components of the bicarbonate buffer. It reads:

$$pH = pK + \log [\text{bicarbonate}]/pCO_2 \times 0.23$$

Thus the plasma pH is determined by the ratio between the concentrations of plasma bicarbonate (the 'base' component of the buffer) and the dissolved CO_2 (the 'acid' component).

Normally, at a plasma pCO_2 of 5.3 kPa (dCO_2 concentration 1.2 mmol/L), the erythrocytes and renal tubular cells maintain the plasma bicarbonate concentration at about 24 mmol/L. The pK (see Chapter 2) of the bicarbonate buffer is 6.1, and if we insert the concentrations of buffer components into the Henderson–Hasselbalch equation above the pH is very near 7.40 (hydrogen ion concentration 40 nmol/L)

$$pH = 6.1 + \log (24/1.2); pH = 7.40$$

Thus, pH 7.40 is the average pH of the extracellular fluid at a normal concentration of bicarbonate and normal partial pressure of CO_2.

The bicarbonate buffer minimizes changes in hydrogen ion concentration when either acid or alkali are added to blood. This is how it works: When an acid (H^+) is added, it reacts with bicarbonate; this leads to a release of CO_2. Thus pCO_2 in blood increases slightly and excess of CO_2 is subsequently eliminated through the lungs:

$$H^+ + HCO_3^- \rightleftharpoons H_2CO_3 \rightleftharpoons CO_2 + H_2O$$

When alkali (OH^-) is added, carbonic acid/CO_2 neutralizes it to water, and the bicarbonate concentration in plasma increases slightly.

$$OH^- + H_2CO_3 \rightleftharpoons H_2O + HCO_3^-$$

as a consequence of a decrease in the H_2CO_3 concentration; the reaction

$$CO_2 + H_2O \rightleftharpoons H_2CO_3$$

proceeds to the right, decreasing pCO_2

The depletion of CO_2 is subsequently compensated by a decreased ventilation rate and its resulting retention in blood. The above shows that the denominator in the Henderson–Hasselbalch equation is controlled by the lungs. This is why we call pCO_2 'the respiratory component of the acid–base balance'.

On the other hand, plasma bicarbonate concentration is controlled by the kidneys and erythrocytes (therefore we call the bicarbonate concentration 'the metabolic component of the acid-base balance'). Erythrocytes and renal tubular cells contain a high activity of a zinc-containing enzyme, carbonic anhydrase (CA; also known as carbonic dehydratase), which catalyses the conversion of dissolved CO_2 into carbonic acid:

$$CO_2 + H_2O \rightleftharpoons H_2CO_3 \rightleftharpoons H^+ + HCO_3^-$$

However, the carbonic acid dissociates, forming the hydrogen and bicarbonate ions. Renal tubular cells and erythrocytes are therefore sources of bicarbonate. Through this reaction the kidneys control plasma bicarbonate concentration by regulating its reabsorption and synthesis, and the erythrocytes make fine adjustments to the plasma bicarbonate concentration in response to changes in pCO_2.

Intracellular buffering

Hydrogen ion is also buffered by the intracellular buffers, mainly proteins and phosphates

The hydrogen ion enters cells in exchange for potassium, therefore buffering of hydrogen ion may result in an increase in plasma potassium concentration. Conversely, low concentration of hydrogen ion in plasma, and an excess of bicarbonate, can be buffered by cell-derived hydrogen ion. In this case, hydrogen ion enters plasma in exchange for potassium, and the plasma potassium concentration decreases.

Thus, and this is important to recall again, the excess of hydrogen ions in plasma (acidemia, low plasma pH) may be associated with efflux of potassium from cells and therefore hyperkalemia. On the other hand, a low hydrogen ion concentration in plasma (alkalemia, high blood pH), is often associated with an entry of potassium into cells and thus hypokalemia (Fig. 23.2).

Classification of the acid–base disorders

The concept of respiratory (CO_2) and metabolic (bicarbonate) components of acid–base balance described above, provides a key to the classification of the clinical disorders of acid–base balance (Fig. 23.3). The primary classification of these disorders is into acidosis or alkalosis. Acidosis denotes a process that leads to the accumulation of hydrogen ion in the body. Alkalosis, on the other hand, is a process leading to a decrease in hydrogen ion concentration in the body. (Note again: acidemia and alkalemia are terms which simply describe the blood pH status. Acidosis and alkalosis are pathological processes which result in either alkalemia or acidemia).

Depending on the primary cause, acidosis and alkalosis can each be divided into either respiratory or metabolic. Thus there are four main disorders of acid–base balance: respiratory acidosis, metabolic acidosis, respiratory alkalosis, and metabolic alkalosis (Fig. 23.4). However, and this complicates things a little, as mixed disorders can also develop; we consider them later in the chapter.

The measurement of blood gases

The so-called 'blood gas measurement' is an important first-line investigation performed whenever there is a suspicion of respiratory failure or acid–base disorders such as diabetic ketoacidosis (see Chapter 20). In respiratory failure, the results of such measurements are also an essential guide to oxygen therapy and assisted ventilation.

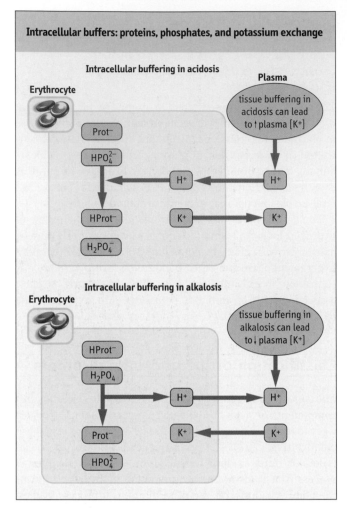

Fig. 23.2 **Intracellular buffers: proteins, phosphates, and potassium exchange.** In contrast to blood, intracellular buffers are primarily proteins and phosphates. Hydrogen ion from the plasma enters cells in exchange for potassium. Therefore, an accumulation of the hydrogen ion in the plasma (acidemia) and the entry of large amounts of hydrogen ion into cells lead to increased plasma potassium concentration. Conversely, a deficit of hydrogen ion in plasma (alkalemia) may lead to a low plasma potassium concentration.

Prot, protein.

These measurements are performed by taking a sample of arterial blood, usually from the radial artery in the forearm or, less commonly, from the femoral artery in the leg. The jargon term 'blood gases' means the measurements of pO_2, pCO_2, and pH (or hydrogen ion concentration) from which the concentration of bicarbonate is calculated using the Henderson–Hasselbalch equation. Several other indices are also computed: they include the total amount of buffers in the blood (so-called buffer base) and the difference between the desired (normal) amount of buffers in the blood and the actual amount (base excess). The acid–base analysers used in the hospitals are programmed to perform these calculations.

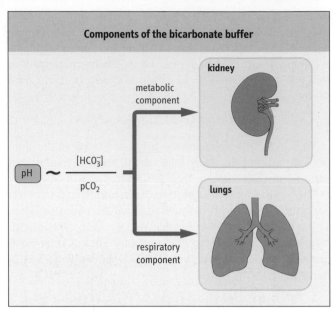

Fig. 23.3 **Components of the bicarbonate buffer.** Blood pH is proportional to the ratio of plasma bicarbonate to the partial pressure of carbon dioxide in blood (pCO_2). Carbon dioxide and bicarbonate are the components of the bicarbonate buffer. The pCO_2 is called 'the respiratory component of the acid–base balance' because it depends on the rate of respiration. Bicarbonate is called 'the metabolic component of the acid base balance' because its concentration is affected by the nonvolatile acids produced in tissues.

The reference values for pH, pCO_2, and O_2 are given in Table 23.2.

THE LUNGS AND THE GAS EXCHANGE

The lungs supply oxygen necessary for tissue metabolism and remove the produced CO_2; CO_2 removal is essential for maintenance of blood pH

Approximately 10 000 L of air pass through the lungs of an average person each day. Anatomically, the lungs belong to the lower respiratory tract (as opposed to the upper respiratory tract which comprises nose, pharynx, and larynx) and lie in the thoracic cavity. They are surrounded with the pleural sac, a thin 'bag' of tissue that lines the thoracic cage at one end, and attaches to the external surface of the lungs at the other. When the thoracic cage (chest cavity) expands during inspiration, the negative pressure created in the expanding pleural sac inflates the lung.

The airways are a set of tubes of progressively decreasing diameter. They consist of the trachea, large and small bronchi, and even smaller bronchioles (Fig. 23.5). At the end

Acid–base disorders

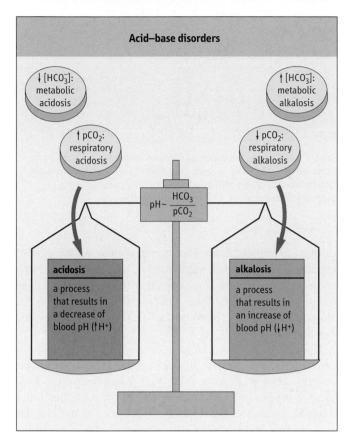

Fig. 23.4 **The acid–base disorders.** A primary increase in pCO_2, or a decrease in plasma bicarbonate concentration, leads to acidosis. A decrease in pCO_2, or an increase in plasma bicarbonate, leads to alkalosis. If the primary change is in pCO_2, the disorder is called respiratory, and if the primary change is in plasma bicarbonate it is called metabolic.

Oxygen, CO$_2$, and control of respiration

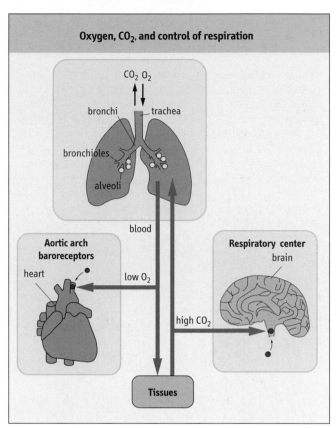

Fig. 23.5 **The structure of the lungs and the regulation of the respiratory rate by pCO_2 and pO_2.** Lung ventilation and perfusion are the main factors controlling gas exchange. The pCO_2 affects the ventilation rate through the central chemoreceptors in the brainstem. However, when pO_2 decreases, the control switches to pO_2-sensitive peripheral receptors in the carotid bodies and in the aortic arch.

Reference range for blood gas results

	Arterial	Venous
[H⁺]	36–43 mmol/L	35–45 mmol/L
pH	7.37–7.44	7.35–7.45
pCO_2	4.6–6.0 kPa	4.8–6.7 kPa
pO_2	10.5–13.5 kPa	4.0–6.7 kPa
bicarbonate	23–30 mmol/L	

Table 23.2 **The reference (normal) values for blood gases.** The key clinically used parameters are pH, pCO_2 and pO_2; the bicarbonate concentration is calculated from pH and pCO_2 values; pH below 7.0 or above 7.7 is life threatening. (Adapted with permission from Hutchinson AS. In: Dominiczak MH, ed. Seminars in clinical biochemistry. Glasgow: Glasgow University Press, 1997.)

RESPIRATORY ALKALOSIS IS CAUSED BY HYPERVENTILATION

A 25-year-old man was admitted to hospital with an asthmatic attack. Peak expiratory flow rate was, measured at 75% of his best. His blood gas values were pO_2 9.3 kPa (70 mmHg) and pCO_2 4.0 kPa (30 mmHg), with pH 7.50 (hydrogen ion concentration 42 nmol/L). He was treated with nebulized salbutamol, a β_2-adrenergic stimulant (see Chapter 39) which is a bronchodilator, and made a good recovery.

Comment. This man's blood gases show a mild degree of respiratory alkalosis caused by hyperventilation and 'blowing off' the CO_2. Respiratory alkalosis causes reduction in serum levels of ionized calcium leading to neuromuscular irritability. Only in severe asthma does the ventilatory impairment lead to CO_2 retention and respiratory acidosis. Reference ranges are given in Table 23.2.

RESPIRATORY ACIDOSIS OCCURS IN CHRONIC LUNG DISEASES

A 56-year-old woman was admitted to a general ward with increasing breathlessness. She had smoked 20 cigarettes a day for the previous 25 years and reported frequent attacks of 'winter bronchitis'. Blood gas measurements revealed a pO_2 of 6 kPa (45 mmHg), pCO_2 of 8.4 kPa (53 mmHg), and pH 7.35 (hydrogen ion concentration 51 nmol/L); bicarbonate concentration was 35 mmol/L (for reference ranges, refer to Table 23.2).

Comment. This patient had an exacerbation of chronic obstructive pulmonary disease and a respiratory acidosis. Her pCO_2 was high, and her ventilation was probably dependent on hypoxia, the so-called 'hypoxic drive'. Her bicarbonate was also increased, as a result of metabolic compensation of the respiratory acidosis. It is necessary to be careful when treating such patients with high concentrations of oxygen, because the increased pO_2 may remove hypoxic drive and cause respiratory depression. Monitoring of arterial pO_2 and pCO_2 after oxygen treatment is mandatory. This patient was successfully treated with a 28% concentration of oxygen.

Partial pressure gradients determine diffusion of gases through the alveolar-blood barrier

	Dry air	Alveoli	Systemic arteries	Tissue
pO_2	21.2 kPa	13.7 kPa	12 kPa	5.3 kPa
pCO_2	<0.13 kPa	5.3 kPa	5.3 kPa	6 kPa
water vapor		6.3 kPa		

Table 23.3 **Partial pressures of oxygen and carbon dioxide in atmospheric air, lung alveoli, and the blood.** Partial pressure gradients determine diffusion of gases through the alveolar/blood barrier. (1 kPa = 7.5 mmHg)

the lungs, the blood flows through pulmonary veins to the left atrium. In the alveolar capillaries of the lungs, the blood accepts oxygen which diffuses through the alveolar wall from the inspired air; at the same time the CO_2 diffuses from the blood into the alveoli (see Fig. 23.5) to be removed with the expired air.

The rate of diffusion of gases in and out of the blood is determined by the partial pressure gradient between alveolar air and the arterial blood. Table 23.3 shows the partial pressures of oxygen (pO_2) and carbon dioxide (pCO_2) in the lungs. Compared with the atmospheric air, the pCO_2 in the alveolar air is slightly higher and pO_2 slightly lower (this is due to the water vapor pressure). Carbon dioxide is much more soluble than oxygen in water, and equilibrates with blood much more rapidly. Therefore, when problems develop, one first notices a decrease in blood pO_2 (hypoxia). An increase in pCO_2 (hypercapnia) occurs later and usually indicates a more severe disease.

The other major factor determining gas exchange is the rate at which the blood flows through the lungs (the perfusion rate). Normally, the ratio of ventilation to perfusion (Va/Q) is 0.8: the alveolar ventilation rate is approximately 4 L/min and the perfusion 5 L/min. Table 23.4 shows problems which may develop with gas exchange. Some parts of the lung may be well-perfused, but poorly ventilated. This occurs when some alveoli collapse and are unable to exchange gases. As a result, the pO_2 in the outflowing blood is low, because there is no diffusion of oxygen from the alveolar air. The appearance of oxygen-poor blood in the arterial circulation is known as a 'shunt' condition. When ventilation is adequate but perfusion is poor, gas exchange cannot take place: in such cases, part of the lung behaves as if it had no alveoli at all; forming the 'physiologic dead space'.

In general then, the respiratory problems may be related to poor ventilation, poor perfusion, or the combination of both, and some examples are given below:

■ rib-cage deformities impair ventilation by limiting the movement of lungs;

of the bronchioles, there are pulmonary alveoli – structures lined with endothelium and covered with a film of surfactant – the main component of which is dipalmitoylphosphatidylcholine (see Chapter 26). Surfactant decreases the surface tension of the alveoli. The epithelium in the bronchi and bronchioles purifies the air by removal of organic and particulate matter. The gas exchange takes place in the alveoli.

The rate of respiration is controlled by the respiratory center in the brainstem. Both pO_2 and pCO_2 affect respiratory control and thus the ventilation rate: the respiratory center located in the medulla oblongata has chemoreceptors sensitive to pCO_2 and to pH. Under normal circumstances, an increase in pCO_2 or a decrease in pH (and not the pO_2), stimulate ventilation. However, when as the pO_2 falls and hypoxia develops, the pO_2 begins the control of ventilation through a set of receptors located in the carotid bodies in the aortic arch. When the arterial pO_2 decreases to less than 8 kPa (60 mmHg), this 'hypoxic drive' becomes the main mechanism controlling ventilation. Importantly, persons who suffer from long-term hypoxia due to chronic lung disease depend on hypoxic drive to maintain their ventilation rate.

Main factors that determine gas exchange are ventilation and perfusion of the lungs

The blood supply to the alveoli is provided by the pulmonary arteries, blood vessels that carry deoxygenated blood from the periphery through the right ventricle. After oxygenation in

Blood pCO_2 and pO_2 are affected by the perfusion and ventilation of the lungs					
	Alveolar pO_2	Alveolar pCO_2	Arterial pO_2	Arterial pCO_2	Comment
poor ventilation, adequate perfusion	decreased	increased	decreased	normal	physiologic shunt
adequate ventilation, poor perfusion	increased	decreased	decreased*	increased*	physiologic dead space

Table 23.4 **Blood partial pressures of oxygen and carbon dioxide depend on lung perfusion and ventilation.** *Depending on a degree of shunt.

- chest trauma may decrease ventilation as a result of lung collapse; alveoli may be actually destroyed in pulmonary emphysema; inadequate synthesis of surfactant leads to the collapse of alveoli and to the respiratory distress syndrome;
- the bronchial tree may be mechanically obstructed by inhaled objects, or narrowed by a growing tumor: this impairs ventilation or makes it entirely impossible;
- constriction of the bronchi occurs in asthma;
- the ventilatory efficiency may be reduced by impaired elasticity of the lung or the poor function of ventilatory muscles (the diaphragm and intercostal muscles of the chest wall);
- diffusion of gases is more difficult in the presence of fluid in the alveoli (pulmonary edema);
- lung movement is affected by defects in the neural control;
- circulatory problems such as shock and heart failure impair lung perfusion.

ANEMIA IS A CAUSE OF SHORTNESS OF BREATH AND TIREDNESS

A 35-year-old man presented with shortness of breath after climbing two flights of stairs. His chest radiograph was normal, as were examination of the heart and the electrocardiogram; blood gases were normal. He was taking a non-steroidal anti-inflammatory agent (NSAID) for joint pain. His blood cell count revealed a hemoglobin value of 10 g/dL (reference range for men 13-18 g/dL) and a reduced mean corpuscular volume of 72 dL (reference range 80–100). Serum ferritin concentration was low at 10 ug/L (reference range 30–280).

Comment. This person had chronic iron deficiency anaemia. Anemia can present with general symptoms such as tiredness or breathlessness. The patient had a gastric ulcer caused by the NSAID with increased loss of blood from the gastrointestinal tract.

The handling of carbon dioxide

The body produces CO_2 at a rate of 200–800 mL/min. As described above, the CO_2 dissolves in water and generates carbonic acid, which in turn dissociates into hydrogen and bicarbonate ions:

$$CO_2 + H_2O \rightleftharpoons H_2CO_3 \rightleftharpoons H^+ + HCO_3^-$$

Thus, CO_2 generates acid (large amounts of hydrogen ion).

Erythrocytes play an important role in the transport of CO_2 between the tissues, and the lungs

We already know that in plasma, the above reaction is nonenzymatic and proceeds slowly, generating very small amounts of carbonic acid, which remain in equilibrium with a substantial amount of dissolved CO_2. The same, but much faster, reaction occurs in the erythrocytes. Here the reaction is catalyzed by the carbonic anhydrase, which 'fixes' CO_2 as bicarbonate. The hydrogen ion resulting from the dissociation of carbonic acid is buffered by hemoglobin.

The bicarbonate produced by carbonic anhydrase in the erythrocytes moves to plasma in exchange for the chloride ion (this is known as 'chloride shift') (Fig. 23.6). Approximately 70% of all CO_2 produced in tissues becomes bicarbonate; approximately 20% is carried as carbamino groups on hemoglobin molecules; and only 10% travels simply dissolved in plasma.

In the lungs, the dissolved CO_2 diffuses into the alveolar space

In the lungs, the increased pO_2 facilitates the dissociation of CO_2 from hemoglobin. This is known as the Haldane effect. In parallel, hemoglobin releases its hydrogen ion, which reacts with bicarbonate and forms carbonic acid which then releases CO_2.

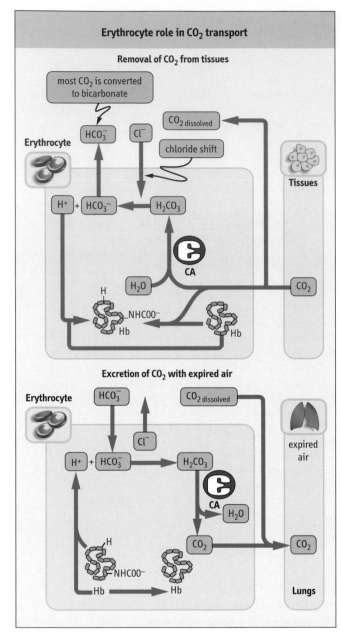

Fig. 23.6 **Erythrocyte role in CO$_2$ transport.** Most of the CO$_2$ produced in tissues is converted to bicarbonate for transport to the lungs: approximately 20% of the total amount is transported bound to hemoglobin as carbamino groups, and small amounts are transported as a dissolved gas in plasma.

KIDNEYS AND THE HANDLING OF BICARBONATE

The kidneys control plasma bicarbonate concentration and the excretion of hydrogen ion from the body

The kidneys play an essential role in the control of plasma bicarbonate concentration and in the removal of hydrogen

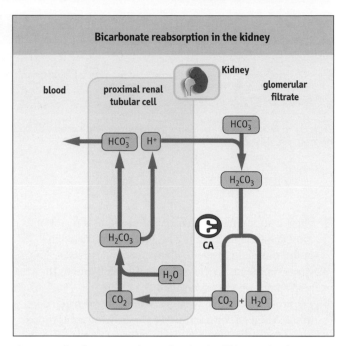

Fig. 23.7 **Bicarbonate reabsorption in the kidney.** Bicarbonate reabsorption takes place in the proximal tubule. At this stage, there is no net excretion of hydrogen ion. Carbonic anhydrase (CA) is present on the luminal side of the tubular cells (see text for details).

ion from the body. In common with erythrocytes, the renal (proximal and distal) tubular cells contain carbonic anhydrase which plays a major role in the handling of hydrogen ion.

Bicarbonate reabsorption takes place in the proximal tubule

Normally, urine is almost bicarbonate free; an amount equivalent to that filtered by glomeruli is returned to the plasma by the proximal tubular cells. The surfaces of the renal tubular cells facing the tubule lumen (the luminal surfaces) are impermeable to bicarbonate. However, the filtered bicarbonate ion combines with the hydrogen ion secreted by the proximal tubular cells to form carbonic acid, and this is then converted to freely diffusible CO$_2$ and H$_2$O by carbonic anhydrase located on the luminal membrane. Thus the CO$_2$ diffuses into cells where it is re-converted by carbonic anhydrase into carbonic acid dissociating back into hydrogen and bicarbonate ions. The two ions are now moved in opposite directions: bicarbonate is returned to the plasma, completing the reabsorption process and hydrogen ion is secreted into the lumen of the tubule, to combine with another filtered bicarbonate ion. Therefore in this process hydrogen ion is used exclusively to aid bicarbonate reabsorption, and no net excretion of hydrogen ion takes place (Fig. 23.7).

Bicarbonate generation and hydrogen ion excretion take place in the distal tubule

The situation is different in the distal tubules where bicarbonate generation takes place. The mechanism is identical to that of bicarbonate reabsorption but this time there is both a net loss of hydrogen ions from the body and a net gain of bicarbonate. This is how it happens: CO_2 diffuses freely into cells. In the distal tubule, carbonic anhydrase converts it into carbonic acid which dissociates into hydrogen ion and bicarbonate. As in the proximal tubule, bicarbonate is transported to the plasma and hydrogen ion is secreted into the tubule lumen (in exchange for sodium). However, since normally no bicarbonate is present in the lumen of the distal tubule (all has been reabsorbed earlier), the hydrogen ion is buffered instead by the filtered phosphate ions and by ammonia synthesized by the proximal tubule cell. It is subsequently excreted in the urine (Fig. 23.8).

The ammonia derives from the transformation of glutamine into glutamic acid by the enzyme glutaminase. Ammonia diffuses freely through the luminal membrane and the hydrogen ion is trapped inside the tubule as the ammonium ion (NH^{4+}) to which the membrane is impermeable.

Problems with renal handling of bicarbonate and hydrogen ion lead to a group of relatively rare disorders known as renal tubular acidoses (RTA). The distal RTA is due to the impairment of hydrogen ion excretion in the collecting duct, and the proximal RTA to the impaired reabsorption of bicarbonate. Proximal RTA usually occurs together with other defects in proximal transport mechanisms in the so-called Fanconi syndrome.

RESPIRATORY AND METABOLIC DISORDERS OF ACID–BASE BALANCE CAN OCCUR TOGETHER

During resuscitation of a 60-year-old man from a cardiorespiratory arrest, the blood gas analysis revealed pH 7.00 (hydrogen ion concentration 100 nmol/L) and pCO_2 7.5 kPa (52 mmHg). His bicarbonate concentration was 11 mmol/L. pO_2 was 12.1 kPa (91 mmHg) during treatment with 48% oxygen.

Comment. This patient had a mixed disorder: a respiratory acidosis caused by lack of ventilation, and metabolic acidosis caused by the hypoxia that had occurred before oxygen treatment was instituted. The acidosis was probably caused by an accumulation of lactic acid: the measured lactate concentration was 7 mmol/L (reference range is 0.7–1.8 mmol/L [6-16 mg/dL]). The terms acidosis and alkalosis do not just describe blood pH changes: they relate to the processes that result in these changes. Therefore, in some instances, two independent processes may occur: for example a patient may be admitted to hospital with diabetic ketoacidosis and coexisting emphysema causing respiratory acidosis. The final result could be a more severe change in pH than would have resulted from a simple disorder (Table 23.5). Any combination of disorders can occur; the skills of an experienced physician are usually required to diagnose this.

THE CLINICAL DISORDERS OF THE ACID–BASE BALANCE

The lung and the kidney work in a concerted way to minimize changes in plasma pH, and can compensate for each other when problems occur

Disturbances of acid–base balance may be caused by primary problems affecting the regulation of pCO_2 (the respiratory component) or bicarbonate concentration (the metabolic component). Returning to the Henderson–Hasselbalch

Mixed metabolic and respiratory acidosis			
Disorder	**pH**	**pCO₂**	**Bicarbonate**
metabolic acidosis	decrease	decrease (respiratory compensation)	decrease (primary change)
respiratory acidosis	decrease	increase (primary change)	increase (metabolic compensation)
mixed respiratory and metabolic acidosis	large decrease	increase (respiratory acidosis)	decrease (metabolic acidosis)

Mixed metabolic and respiratory alkalosis (rare)			
Disorder	**pH**	**pCO₂**	**Bicarbonate**
metabolic alkalosis	increase	increase (respiratory compensation)	increase (primary change)
respiratory alkalosis	increase	decrease (primary change)	decrease (metabolic compensation)
mixed respiratory and metabolic alkalosis	large increase	decrease (respiratory alkalosis)	increase (metabolic acidosis)

Table 23.5 **Mixed metabolic and respiratory acidosis and alkalosis.** Mixed acid-base disorders result in a greater change in blood pH than simple disorders; they may pose diagnostic difficulties.

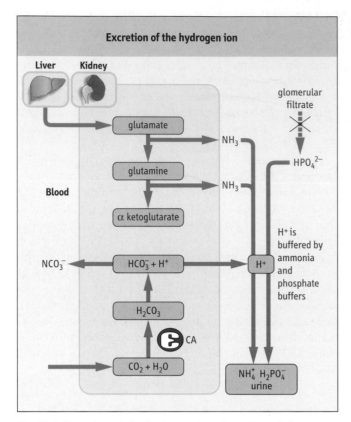

Excretion of the hydrogen ion

Fig. 23.8 **Excretion of the hydrogen ion.** Excretion of the hydrogen ion takes place in the distal tubules of the kidney. Hydrogen ion reacts with ammonia forming the ammonium ion which is excreted. Hydrogen ion is also buffered by phosphate. The daily excretion of hydrogen ion is approximately 50 mmol. CA, carbonic anhydrase.

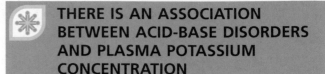

THERE IS AN ASSOCIATION BETWEEN ACID-BASE DISORDERS AND PLASMA POTASSIUM CONCENTRATION

Plasma potassium concentration is one of the more important clinical laboratory tests. This is because potassium affects the contractility of the heart and either a too high or too low plasma concentration (hyperkalemia and hypokalemia, respectively) can be life threatening. The effects of potassium on heart function can be observed on the electrocardiogram. Hypokalemia leads to an increased excretion of hydrogen ion and, consequently, to metabolic alkalosis. The converse is also true: metabolic alkalosis leads to an increased renal excretion of potassium, and hypokalemia. Plasma potassium concentration needs to be checked whenever a disorder of acid–base balance is suspected (see Fig. 22.13, and Chapter 21).

Respiratory and metabolic compensation of acid–base disorders

Acid/base disorder	Primary change	Compensatory change	Timescale of compensatory change
metabolic acidosis	decrease in plasma bicarbonate concentration	decrease in pCO_2 (hyperventilation)	minutes/hours
metabolic alkalosis	increase in plasma bicarbonate concentration	increase in pCO_2 (hypoventilation)	minutes/hours
respiratory acidosis	increase in pCO_2	increase in renal bicarbonate reabsorption: increase in plasma bicarbonate concentration	days
respiratory alkalosis	decrease in pCO_2	decrease in renal bicarbonate reabsorption: decrease in plasma bicarbonate concentration	days

Table 23.6 **Respiratory and metabolic compensation in the acid base disorders minimizes changes in the blood pH.** A change in the respiratory component leads to metabolic compensation, and a change in the metabolic component stimulates respiratory compensation. Metabolic compensation involves a change in renal bicarbonate handling, and respiratory compensation means changes in the ventilation rate. A compensatory increase or decrease in the rate of ventilation (hyper- or hypoventilation) is seen within minutes, however, an adjustment of the rate of bicarbonate reabsorption may take days.

Clinical causes of acid–base disorders

Metabolic acidosis	Respiratory acidosis	Metabolic alkalosis	Respiratory alkalosis
diabetes mellitus (ketoacidosis)	chronic obstructive airways disease	vomiting (loss of hydrogen ion)	hyperventilation (anxiety, fever)
lactic acidosis (lactic acid)	severe asthma	nasogastric suction (loss of hydrogen ion)	lung diseases associated with hyperventilation
renal failure (inorganic acids)	cardiac arrest	hypokalemia	anemia
severe diarrhea (loss of bicarbonate)	depression of respiratory center (drugs, e.g. opiates)	intravenous administration of bicarbonate (e.g. after cardiac arrest)	salicylate poisoning
surgical drainage of intestine (loss of bicarbonate)	weakness of respiratory muscles (e.g. poliomyelitis, multiple sclerosis)		
renal loss of bicarbonate (renal tubular acidosis type 2 – rare)	chest deformities		
impairment of renal H$^+$ excretion (renal tubular acidosis type 1 – rare)	airway obstruction		

Table 23.7 **The clinical causes of acid–base disorders.** Disorders of the acid-base balance are acidosis and alkalosis: each of them can be either respiratory or metabolic. Respiratory acidosis is common and is caused primarily by diseases of the lung that affect gas exchange. Respiratory alkalosis is rarer and is caused by hyperventilation, which decreases pCO_2. Metabolic acidosis is common and results from either overproduction or retention of nonvolatile acids in the circulation. Metabolic alkalosis is rarer: its most common causes are vomiting and gastric suction, both causing loss of hydrogen ion from the stomach.

equation, please note that the increased ratio of plasma bicarbonate to pCO_2 indicates acidosis, and the decreased ratio, alkalosis.

Acidosis

Clinically, acidosis is a much more common disorder than alkalosis (Table 23.6) and it can be sub-classified into either respiratory or metabolic.

Respiratory acidosis

Respiratory acidosis occurs most often in lung disease and results from decreased ventilation

The most common cause is the chronic obstructive airways disease (COAD). Severe asthmatic attack can also result in respiratory acidosis because of bronchial constriction. Respiratory acidosis often accompanies hypoxia (respiratory failure); in such a case, an increase in pCO_2 occurs together with the decrease in pO_2.

Metabolic acidosis

Metabolic acidosis results from the excessive production, or inefficient metabolism or excretion, of nonvolatile acids

A classic example of metabolic acidosis is the diabetic ketoacidosis, when ketoacids, acetoacetic acid, and α-

 VOMITING CAN LEAD TO METABOLIC ALKALOSIS

A 47-year-old man came to the outpatient clinic with a history of intermittent profuse vomiting and loss of weight. He had tachycardia, reduced tissue turgor, hypotension and an abdominal succussion splash. His blood pH was 7.55 (hydrogen ion concentration 28 nmol/L) and pCO_2 was 6.4 kPa (48 mmHg). His bicarbonate concentration was 35 mmol/L and then was also hyponatraemia and hypokalaemia. Despite the systemic alkalosis urine pH was only 3.5.

Comment. This patient presents with metabolic alkalosis caused by the loss of hydrogen ion through vomiting. Investigations showed gastric outlet obstruction of the stomach entrance due to scarring from chronic peptic ulceration. He subsequently underwent surgery for pyloric stenosis, with a good outcome. Note the increased pCO_2 as a result of respiratory compensation of metabolic alkalosis. The paradoxical acid urine is probably due to depletion of chloride which then limits reabsorption of sodium in the thick ascending limb of the loop of Henle so that sodium is then exchanged for hydrogen ions and potassium in the distal nephron.

hydroxybutyric acid accumulate in the plasma (see Chapter 20). Acidosis may also occur during extreme physical exertion, when there is accumulation of lactate generated from muscle metabolism; in normal circumstances, this lactate would be quickly metabolized after cessation of exercise.

However, when large amounts of lactate are generated as a consequence of hypoxia, lactic acidosis may become life-threatening, as happens, for instance, in shock.

Excretion of nonvolatile acids is also impaired in kidney disease (renal failure) and this also causes metabolic acidosis. Renal failure develops when the perfusion of the kidneys is inadequate (e.g. in trauma, shock, or dehydration) or if there is an intrinsic kidney disease such as glomerulonephritis (inflammatory reaction in the renal tubular tissue; see Chapter 22).

Excessive loss of bicarbonate can also be a cause of metabolic acidosis. This may occur when renal reabsorption mechanism is defective, but is more common when bicarbonate present in the intestinal fluid is lost as a result of severe diarrhea or surgical drainage after bowel surgery.

Alkalosis

Alkalosis is rarer than acidosis
(see Tables 23.6 and 23.7)

A mild respiratory alkalosis is a consequence of hyperventilation during exercise, anxiety attack, or fever. It also occurs in pregnancy.

Metabolic alkalosis is often associated with abnormally low potassium concentration in plasma, as a result of cellular buffering. As mentioned above, the cellular entry or exit of potassium ion is associated with the movement of hydrogen ion in an opposite direction. Thus, alkalosis can cause hypokalemia, and primary hypokalemia (see Chapter 22) may lead to alkalosis. Finally severe metabolic alkalosis may also occur as a result of the massive loss of hydrogen ion from the stomach in severe vomiting, or as a result of nasogastric suction after surgery. Rarely, it occurs when too much bicarbonate is given intravenously, for instance, during resuscitation after cardiac arrest.

Summary

- Maintenance of the hydrogen ion concentration within a narrow range is vital for cell survival.

- The acid–base balance is regulated by the concerted action of lungs and kidneys. The erythrocytes play a key role not only in the transport of oxygen, but also in the transport of carbon dioxide in blood.
- The main buffers in blood are hemoglobin and bicarbonate, whereas in the cells they include proteins and phosphate. The bicarbonate buffer system is unique in that it communicates with atmospheric air.
- Acid-base disorders are acidosis and alkalosis and each of them may be either metabolic or respiratory. The determination of pH, pCO_2 and bicarbonate, and pO_2, is a first line investigation frequently required in emergencies.

ACTIVE LEARNING

1. Describe how does the bicarbonate buffer cope with an addition of acid to the system.
2. Discuss bicarbonate handling by the kidney and characterize differences between processes occurring in the proximal and distal renal tubule.
3. Outline the role of ventilation in acid-base disorders.
4. Which disorders of the acid base balance may be associated with gastrointestinal surgery?
5. Discuss the association between acid-base disorders and plasma potassium concentration.

Further reading

Androgue HJ, Madias NE. Management of life-threatening acid–base disorders (first of two parts). *N Engl J Med* 1998;**338**:26–34.

Androgue HJ, Madias NE. Management of life-threatening acid–base disorders (second of two parts). *N Engl J Med* 1998;**338**:107–111.

Thomson WST, Adams JF, Cowan RA. *Clinical acid–base balance*. Oxford: Oxford University Press; 1997.

Dominiczak MH, ed. *Seminars in clinical biochemistry*. Glasgow: University of Glasgow 1997.

Gluck SE. Electrolyte quintet: Acid–base. *Lancet* 1998;**352**:474–79.

24. Calcium and Bone Metabolism

W D Fraser

LEARNING OBJECTIVES

After reading this chapter you should be able to:

- Describe the chemical composition of bone, and the process of mineralization.
- Recognize the major cells in bone and their interactions in the bone remodeling cycle.
- Understand the role of major factors contributing to the regulation of serum calcium concentration.
- Know the causes of hypercalcaemia and hypocalcaemia.
- Explain the pivotal role of parathyroid hormone related protein in hypercalcaemia of malignancy.
- Understand the role of vitamin D and its metabolism in health and disease.
- Define osteoporosis, its causes and treatment.
- Recognize the causes and presentation in adults of osteomalacia.

Bone is a specialized connective tissue that, along with cartilage, forms the skeletal system. In addition to serving a supportive and protective role, bone is the site of substantial metabolic activity. Two types of bone are recognized: the thick, densely calcified external bone (cortical or compact bone), and a thinner, honeycomb network of calcified tissue on the inner aspect of bone (trabecular or cancellous bone).

Collagen and hydroxyapatite are the main components of the bone matrix

Within the bone matrix, type 1 collagen is the major protein (90%) and calcium-rich crystals of hydroxyapatite ($Ca_{10}[PO_4]_6[OH]_2$) are found on, within, and between the collagen fibers. The attachment of hydroxyapatite to collagen and the calcification of bone are, in part, controlled by the presence of glycoproteins and proteoglycans with a high ion-binding capacity. Collagen fibers orientate so that they have the greatest density per unit volume and are packed in layers, giving the lamellar structure observed on microscopy. Post-translational modifications of collagen occur that result in the formation of intra- and intermolecular pyridinoline and pyrrole crosslinks, which have an important role in fibril strength and matrix mineralization. This microarchitecture allows bone to function as the major reservoir of calcium for the body. The noncalcified organic matrix within bone, known as osteoid, becomes mineralized through two mechanisms.

Within the bone extracellular space, plasma-membrane-derived matrix vesicles act as a focus for deposition of calcium phosphate, the lipid-rich inner membrane of these vesicles being the nidus for the formation of hydroxyapatite crystals. Crystallization proceeds rapidly, eventually obliterating the vesicle membrane and leaving a collection of clustered hydroxyapatite crystals. Within this environment, osteoblasts (bone-forming cells) can also secrete pre-organized packets of matrix proteins that rapidly mineralize, and these combine with matrix-vesicle-derived crystals to form a continuous mineralized tissue within the matrix space. Molecules that inhibit this process – for example pyrophosphate – exist within the matrix environment, but the secretion of alkaline phosphatase by osteoblasts destroys pyrophosphate, allowing mineralization to occur.

Within lamellar bone, collagen fibrils are tightly packed and matrix vesicles are rarely seen. Mineralization occurs in association with matrix fibrils, especially at the spaces between collagen molecules, and is controlled by noncollagenous proteins (e.g. proteoglycans and osteonectin).

These processes of mineralization are highly dependent on an adequate supply of calcium and phosphate. When mineral deprivation exists, there is an increase in the percentage of osteoid (the non-mineralized organic matrix) within bone, resulting in the clinical condition of osteomalacia.

Bone remodeling is a coupled process of resorption by osteoclasts and formation by osteoblasts

Small amounts of calcium are exchanged daily between bone and the extracellular fluid (ECF) as a result of constant bone remodeling, i.e. coupled processes of resorption by osteoclasts and formation by osteoblasts (Fig. 24.1). This exchange maintains a relative calcium balance between newly formed bone and older resorbed bone. Calcium flux takes place across the bone-lining cell layer and within bone into the ECF of the periosteocytic space.

Osteocytes are found in osteocytic lacunae and are believed to be derived from osteoblasts trapped during production of bone matrix

Cellular processes extend between osteocytes and from osteocytes to bone-lining cells, forming a network of canaliculi throughout the bone matrix. These cells may contribute to

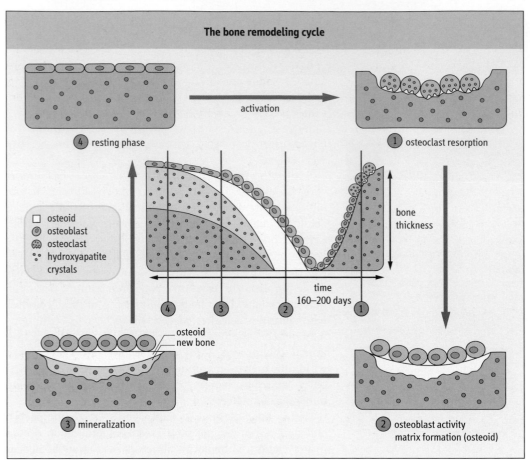

The bone remodeling cycle

activation

(4) resting phase

(1) osteoclast resorption

osteoid
osteoblast
osteoclast
hydroxyapatite crystals

bone thickness

time
160–200 days

4   3   2   1

osteoid
new bone

(3) mineralization

(2) osteoblast activity
matrix formation (osteoid)

Fig. 24.1 **Maintaining bone mass – the bone remodeling cycle.** Resorption and formation of bone by osteoclasts and osteoblasts is coupled.

the maintenance of calcium homeostasis by resorbing bone, and they may have a role in activating bone turnover.

Osteoclasts

Osteoclasts are multinucleated giant cells found on the endosteal surface of bone, in Haversian systems and periosteal surfaces

They are in contact with a calcified surface generated by their resorptive activity and contain between four to 20 nuclei, pleomorphic mitochondria, and a ruffled cell border. Osteoclasts are derived from pluripotent hematopoietic mononuclear cells in the bone marrow.

Generation, maturation, and regulation of osteoclasts are controlled by the macrophage colony-stimulating factor (MCSF) and the receptor activator for nuclear factor kappa beta ligand (RANKL). RANKL markedly stimulates osteoclast activity and this effect is regulated in part by a decoy receptor, osteoprotegrin (OPG), produced by osteoblasts. Genetic manipulation of animals producing targeted disruption of the OPG gene, results in profound osteoporosis, and RANKL knockout mice lack osteoclasts and suffer osteopetrosis with excessively thickened bone. Parathyroid hormone (PTH) activates osteoclasts indirectly via osteoblasts and calcitonin is a

potent direct inhibitor of osteoclast activity, decreases proliferation of the progenitor cells, and inhibits differentiation of precursors. Local factors such as the cytokines interleukin-1 (IL-1), tumor necrosis factor (TNF), transforming growth factor-β (TGF-β) and interferon-γ (INF-γ) are important regulators of osteoclasts and act through changes in RANKL and OPG. Osteoclast resorption of bone releases collagen peptides, pyridinoline crosslink fragments, and calcium from the bone matrix through the production, secretion, and action of lysosomal enzymes, collagenases, and cathepsins at an acidic pH. Collagen breakdown products in serum and urine (e.g. hydroxyproline) and collagen fragments (amino or carboxy telopeptides NTX and CTX, respectively) can be measured as surrogate biochemical markers of bone metabolism.

Osteoblasts

Osteoblasts are metabolically active bone-forming cells

The precursor cell is the committed progenitor cell, or preosteoblast, which is derived from a pluripotent stromal mesenchymal cell. Mature osteoblasts synthesize type 1 collagen, osteocalcin (also known as bone Gla protein), cell attachment proteins (thrombospondin, fibronectin, bone sialoprotein, osteopontin), proteoglycans, and growth-related proteins, and they control bone mineralization. Osteoblast function and activity are altered by several hormones and growth factors. PTH binds to a specific receptor, stimulating production of cyclic adenosine monophosphate (cAMP), ion and amino acid transport, and collagen synthesis. 1,25-dihydroxycholecalciferol ($1,25(OH)_2D_3$; calcitriol) stimulates synthesis of alkaline phosphatase, matrix, and bone-specific proteins, and can decrease osteocalcin secretion. Growth factors TGF-β, insulin-like growth factors (IGFs)-I and -II, and platelet-derived growth factor (PDGF) serve as autocrine regulators of osteoblast function. Serum biochemical markers reflecting osteoblast function are bone-specific alkaline phosphatase, osteocalcin, and markers of collagen formation: carboxy-terminal procollagen extension peptide (ICTP) and amino or carboxy-terminal procollagen extension peptide (PINP, P1CP).

CALCIUM METABOLISM

Bone serves as a store of calcium

A complex calcium homeostatic mechanism utilizes bone as the reservoir of calcium when deficiency exists, and as a store of calcium when the body is replete.

The skeleton contains 99% of calcium present in the body in the form of hydroxyapatite; the remainder is distributed in the soft tissues, teeth, and ECF. Many cell and organ functions are dependent on the tight control of extracellular calcium concentration; these include neural transmission, cellular secretion, contraction of muscle cells, cell proliferation, the stability and permeability of cell membranes, blood clotting, and the mineralization of bone. Total serum calcium is maintained between 2.2 and 2.60 mmol/L (8.8–10.4 mg/dL).

Hormonal control of circulating calcium involves bone, kidneys, and the gastrointestinal tract

Hormonal control of circulating calcium involves bone, kidneys, and the gastrointestinal tract: if plasma calcium decreases, PTH is released from the parathyroid glands, stimulating osteoclast-mediated bone resorption, reabsorption of calcium at the kidney, and absorption of calcium at the small intestine (mediated by $1,25(OH)_2D_3$); increasing calcium decreases PTH secretion and stimulation of calcitonin release from the thyroid, which inhibits osteoclast resorption of bone (Fig. 24.2).

Calcium exists in the circulation in three forms (Fig. 24.3):

- **ionized Ca^{2+}:** the most important, physiologically active form (50% of total calcium).
- **protein-bound:** the majority of the remaining calcium, mainly bound to negatively charged albumin (40%);
- **complexed to substances such as citrate and phosphate:** a smaller fraction (10%).

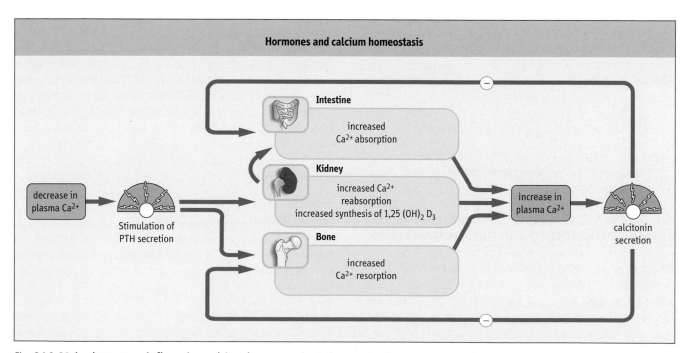

Fig. 24.2 **Major hormones influencing calcium homeostasis.** A decrease in plasma ionized calcium stimulates release of PTH; this promotes Ca^{2+} reabsorption from the kidney, resorption from bone, and absorption by the gut via increased production of $1,25(OH)_2D_3$. As a result, plasma calcium increases. Conversely, an increase in plasma ionized calcium stimulates release of calcitonin, which inhibits reabsorption of calcium by the kidney and osteoclast-mediated bone resorption.

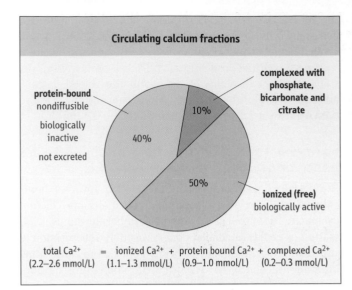

Circulating calcium fractions

protein-bound
nondiffusible

biologically
inactive

not excreted

complexed with phosphate, bicarbonate and citrate

10%

40%

50%

ionized (free)
biologically active

total Ca^{2+}	=	ionized Ca^{2+}	+	protein bound Ca^{2+}	+	complexed Ca^{2+}
(2.2–2.6 mmol/L)		(1.1–1.3 mmol/L)		(0.9–1.0 mmol/L)		(0.2–0.3 mmol/L)

Fig. 24.3 **Circulating calcium fractions.** The three forms of circulating calcium.

If serum protein concentration increases (as in dehydration and after prolonged venous stasis), protein-bound calcium and total serum calcium increase. In conditions of reduced serum proteins (e.g. liver disease, nephrotic syndrome, malnutrition), the protein-bound calcium concentration is reduced, decreasing the total calcium, although ionized calcium is maintained within the reference range 1.1–1.3 mmol/L (4.4–5.2 mg/dL). Many acute and chronic illnesses decrease serum albumin concentration, which consequently decreases serum total calcium. Because of this, in clinical situations it is important to calculate the 'adjusted calcium' – total serum calcium, adjusted for the patient's prevailing albumin concentration. This is achieved by means of a formula utilizing the population mean albumin concentration 40 g/L (4 g/dL):

$$\text{adjusted } Ca^{2+} = \text{measured Ca (mmol/L)} + 0.02$$
$$(40 - \text{albumin [g/L]})$$

Factors influencing calcium homeostasis

Calcium-sensing receptor is a cell-surface G-protein receptor

Ionized calcium is maintained within a narrow range through an extracellular calcium-sensing receptor (CaSR) that is a cell surface G-protein coupled receptor present in the chief cells of the parathyroid gland, the thyroidal C-cells and along the kidney tubules. Minute changes in ionized calcium modulate cellular function to maintain normocalcaemia.

PARATHYROID HORMONE MEASUREMENT

Intact $PTH_{(1-84)}$ is the most important biologically active form of PTH, and can be measured by specific immunoradiometric assays (IRMAs) without interference from its amino- or carboxy-terminal fragments. These assays utilize a double-antibody technique, with a capture antibody directed against one end of the intact molecule, and the labeled detection antibody directed against the opposite end of the molecule. Only the full-length, 1–84-amino acid molecule can bind to the two antibodies, which means that fragments of PTH produced during its metabolism (see Fig. 24.3) are not measured by these assays.

Parathyroid hormone (PTH)

Parathyroid hormone responds to changes in ionized calcium and phosphate

PTH is an 84-amino-acid, single-chain peptide hormone secreted by the chief cells of the parathyroid glands. A decrease in extracellular ionized calcium or an increase in serum phosphate concentration stimulates its secretion, chronic severe magnesium deficiency can inhibit its release from secretory vesicles, and low concentrations of $1,25(OH)_2D_3$ interfere with its synthesis. $PTH_{(1-84)}$ is mainly metabolized into a biologically active $PTH_{(1-34)}$ amino-terminal fragment and an inactive carboxy-terminal fragment, $PTH_{(35-84)}$ (Fig. 24.4).

PTH regulates serum calcium concentrations by direct actions on bone and kidney, and indirect actions on the intestine by increasing the synthesis of $1,25(OH)_2D_3$ (see Fig. 24.2). Most of the classical cellular actions of PTH are mediated by cAMP, which is generated through G-protein-stimulated adenylyl cyclase.

Vitamin D

Vitamin D is synthesized in the skin by UV radiation

The synthesis and metabolism of vitamin D are illustrated in Figure 24.6. Vitamin D_2 (ergocalciferol) is synthesized in the skin by UV radiation of ergosterol. Vitamin D_3 (cholecalciferol) is derived also by UV irradiation from 7-dehydrocholesterol in the skin of animals. Vitamin D_3 and its hydroxylated metabolites are transported in the plasma bound to a specific globulin, vitamin D-binding protein (DBP). The affinity of cholecalciferol for DBP is low but that for D_3 is high, thus ensuring the movement of D_3 from the skin to the circulation. Vitamin D_3 is also found in the diet where its absorption is associated with other fats (see Chapter 9), and it is

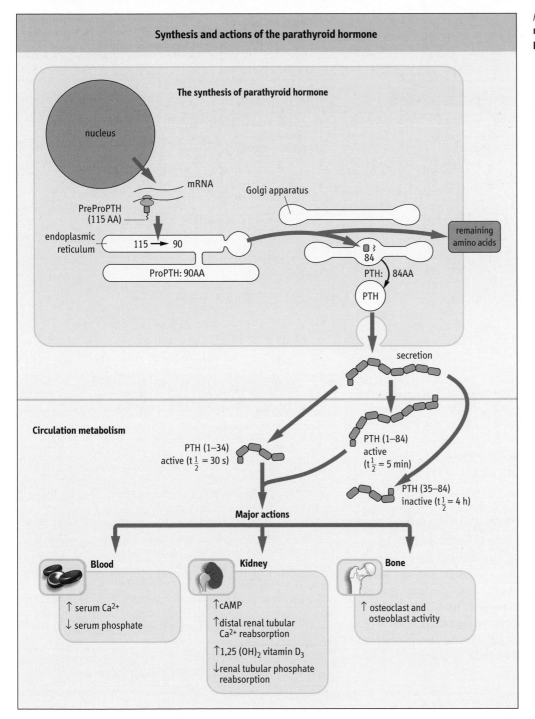

Fig. 24.4 **Synthesis and major actions of parathyroid hormone (PTH).**

Synthesis and actions of the parathyroid hormone

The synthesis of parathyroid hormone

nucleus

mRNA

Golgi apparatus

PreProPTH
(115 AA)

remaining
amino acids

endoplasmic
reticulum

115 → 90

84

ProPTH: 90AA

PTH: 84AA

PTH

PTH

secretion

Circulation metabolism

PTH (1–34)
active ($t\frac{1}{2}$ = 30 s)

PTH (1–84)
active
($t\frac{1}{2}$ = 5 min)

PTH (35–84)
inactive ($t\frac{1}{2}$ = 4 h)

Major actions

Blood

↑ serum Ca^{2+}

↓ serum phosphate

Kidney

↑cAMP

↑distal renal tubular
Ca^{2+} reabsorption

↑1,25 $(OH)_2$ vitamin D_3

↓renal tubular phosphate
reabsorption

Bone

↑ osteoclast and
osteoblast activity

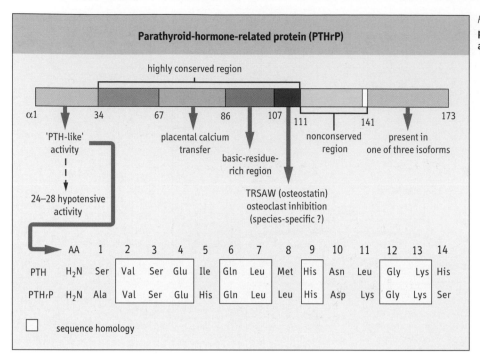

Fig. 24.5 **Parathyroid-hormone-related protein (PTHrP) synthesis, structure, and functional relationships.**

transported to the liver in chylomicrons. It is released from chylomicrons in the liver by DBP and hydroxylated at the 25-position forming 25-hydroxycholecalciferol ((25(OH)D$_3$; calcidiol).

25-hydroxycholecalciferol (25(OH)D$_3$) is the main liver storage form of vitamin D

The 25-hydroxylation step is carried out by a hepatic microsomal enzyme and is the rate-limiting step in conversion of vitamin D$_3$ to its active metabolite. The hepatic content of 25(OH)D$_3$ regulates the rate of 25-hydroxylation. 25(OH)D$_3$ is the major form of the vitamin found in both the liver and in the circulation, in each case bound to DBP, and its levels in the circulation reflect the hepatic stores of the vitamin. A significant proportion of 25(OH)D$_3$ is subject to an enterohepatic circulation, being excreted in the bile and reabsorbed in the small bowel. Disturbance in the enterohepatic circulation can lead to deficiency of this vitamin.

The active metabolite of vitamin D is 1α,25-dihydroxycholecalciferol (1,25-(OH)$_2$D$_3$)

The main site for further hydroxylation at the 1-position are the renal tubules, although bone and the placenta can also carry out this reaction. The 25(OH)D$_3$ 1α-hydroxylase is a mitochondrial enzyme. 1,25(OH)$_2$D$_3$; calcitriol is the most potent of the vitamin D metabolites and the only naturally occurring form of vitamin D that is active at physiologic concentrations. The 1α-hydroxylase activity is stimulated by PTH, low serum concentrations of phosphate or calcium, vitamin D deficiency, calcitonin, growth hormone, prolactin,

 PARATHYROID-HORMONE-RELATED PROTEIN (PTHrP)

PTHrP is synthesized as three isoforms containing 139, 141, and 173 amino acids, as a result of alternative differential splicing of RNA. There is amino-terminal sequence homology with PTH: eight of the first 13 amino acids are identical in PTHrP and PTH, three are identical within residues 14–34, and a further three are identical within residues 35–84. Activation of the classical PTH receptor is by the amino-terminal portion of both PTH and PTHrP, and there is a common α-helical secondary structure in the binding domain of both peptides. As a result of this structural similarity, PTHrP possesses many of the biological actions of PTH.

There is, to date, little evidence to suggest that PTHrP has a role in normal adult calcium homeostasis, but evidence from animal models indicates that it is important in regulating fetal skeletal development and calcium homeostasis. Deletion of the PTHrP gene results in either severe skeletal abnormalities (heterozygote) or a lethal mutation (homozygote). PTHrP has an important role in the etiology of hypercalcemia associated with malignancy (HCM) (see below). PTHrP is subject to post-translational processing, producing fragments with biological activities that have yet to be characterized. The structural and functional relationships of PTHrP as they are currently understood are summarized in Figure 24.5.

and estrogen. Conversely, the activity of 1α-hydroxylase is feedback-inhibited by 1,25(OH)$_2$D$_3$, hypercalcemia, high phosphate and hypoparathyroidism.

The renal tubules, cartilage, intestine, and placenta also contain a 24-hydroxylase, producing the inactive

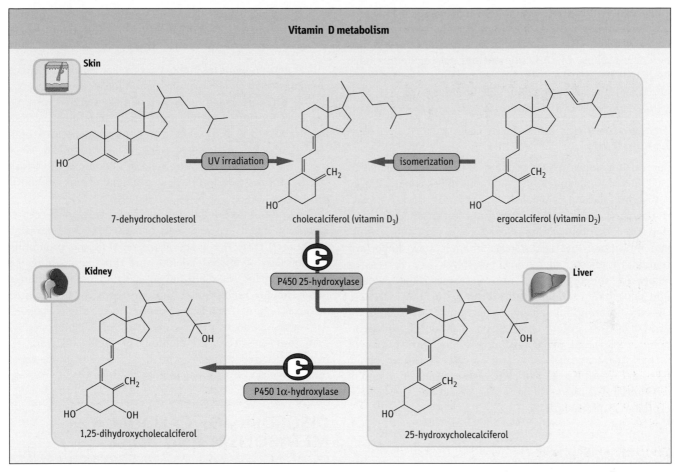

Fig. 24.6 Vitamin D metabolism and its action. Vitamin D is mainly synthesized in response to the action of sunlight on the skin; a smaller component comes from the diet. Normal liver and kidney function are essential to the formation of the active form 1,25(OH)$_2$D$_3$. Plasma calcium concentration controls the level of 125 (OH$_2$)D$_3$ through the parathyroid hormone. PTH: parathyroid hormone. DBP: vitamin D-binding protein.

24,25-dihydroxycholecalciferol (24,25[OH]$_2$D$_3$; 24(R)-hydroxycalcidiol). The level of the 24,25[OH]$_2$D$_3$ in the circulation is reciprocally related to the level of the 1,25(OH)$_2$D$_3$.

1,25(OH)$_2$D$_3$ is transported in plasma, also bound to DBP. Since it affects Ca^{2+} transport and metabolism at a distance, vitamin D may be described as a hormone. In the intestinal epithelial cells it binds to a cytoplasmic receptor like other steroid hormones (see Chapter 16) and this ligand–protein complex is transported to the nucleus where 1,25(OH)$_2$D$_3$ induces gene expression affecting calcium metabolism.

1,25(OH)$_2$D$_3$ increases serum concentrations of calcium and phosphate

1,25(OH)$_2$D$_3$ increases the absorption of calcium and phosphate from the gut via active transport by calcium-binding proteins. Together with PTH, it stimulates bone resorption by osteoclasts. These effects increase serum calcium and phosphate concentrations. Low 1,25(OH)$_2$D$_3$ causes abnormal mineralization of newly formed osteoid. This is a result of low calcium and phosphate availability and reduced osteoblast function, which result in rickets (in infants and children) or osteomalacia (in adults).

Calcitonin inhibits osteoclastic bone resorption

Calcitonin is a 32-amino-acid peptide synthesized and secreted primarily by the parafollicular cells of the thyroid gland (C-cells). Its secretion is regulated acutely by serum calcium through the CaSR: an increase in serum calcium results in a proportional increase in calcitonin, and a decrease elicits a corresponding reduction in calcitonin. Chronic stimulation results in exhaustion of the secretory reserve of the C-cells. The precise biological role of calcitonin is not known, but the main effect is inhibition of osteoclastic bone resorption. There is significant species homology for calcitonin, with a 1–7 amino-terminal disulfide bridge, a glycine residue at position 28, and a carboxy-terminal proline amide residue. Basic amino acid substitutions enhance potency; because of this, salmon and eel calcitonins have increased biological activity in mammalian systems, compared with that of endogenous calcitonin.

Other hormones also affect calcium homeostasis

Several hormones whose primary action is not related to calcium regulation directly or indirectly affect calcium homeostasis and skeletal metabolism.

Thyroid hormone stimulates osteoclast-mediated resorption of bone. Adrenal and gonadal steroids, particularly estrogen in women and testosterone in men, have important regulatory effects, increasing osteoblast and decreasing osteoclast function. They also decrease renal calcium and phosphate excretion and intestinal calcium excretion. Growth hormone has anabolic effects on bone, promoting growth of the skeleton. These effects of growth hormone on bone are believed to be mediated by insulin-like growth factors (IGF-I and IGF-II) acting on cells of the osteoblast lineage. Growth hormone increases the urinary excretion of calcium and hydroxyproline, whilst decreasing the urinary excretion of phosphate.

Calcium is absorbed in the small intestine and is excreted in urine and feces

Calcium is absorbed predominantly in the proximal small intestine; this is regulated through the quantity of calcium ingested in the diet, and two cellular calcium transport processes:

- active saturable transcellular absorption which is stimulated by $1,25(OH)_2D_3$;

- nonsaturable paracellular absorption which is controlled by the concentration of calcium in the intestinal lumen relative to the serum concentration.

In a normal adult taking a Western diet, calcium balance is maintained: the amount of calcium intake and its deposition in bone are exactly matched by the excretion in urine and feces. During growth, a child will be in positive calcium balance, whereas in the elderly and in several diseases, individuals may be in negative calcium balance. Reduced or increased calcium absorption reflects alterations in dietary calcium intake, intestinal calcium solubility, and vitamin D metabolism.

Generally, as serum calcium increases, calcium excretion increases. When hypercalcemia is caused by hyperparathyroidism (HPT), PTH will act on the renal tubule, promoting reabsorption of filtered calcium and thus diminishing the effects of the increased filtration of calcium and inhibition of renal tubular reabsorption that are caused by increased serum calcium. Decreasing serum calcium is associated with a reduction in urinary excretion of calcium, mainly as a result of decreased amounts of filtered calcium. In hypoparathyroid patients, who lack PTH secretion, renal tubular reabsorption of calcium is reduced.

DISORDERS OF CALCIUM METABOLISM AND BONE

Hypercalcemia

Hypercalcemia is most commonly caused by primary hyperparathyroidism and malignancy

There is a wide individual variation in the development symptoms and signs of hypercalcemia (Fig. 24.7). In general, the higher the adjusted calcium, and the more rapid the increase

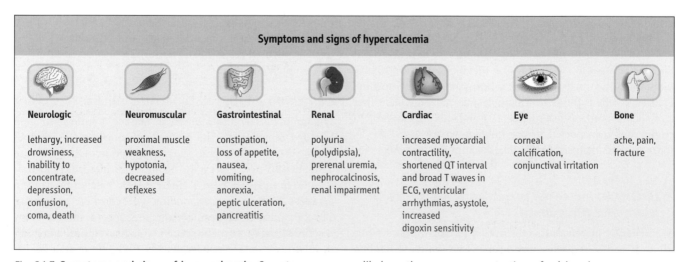

Symptoms and signs of hypercalcemia

Neurologic	Neuromuscular	Gastrointestinal	Renal	Cardiac	Eye	Bone
lethargy, increased drowsiness, inability to concentrate, depression, confusion, coma, death	proximal muscle weakness, hypotonia, decreased reflexes	constipation, loss of appetite, nausea, vomiting, anorexia, peptic ulceration, pancreatitis	polyuria (polydipsia), prerenal uremia, nephrocalcinosis, renal impairment	increased myocardial contractility, shortened QT interval and broad T waves in ECG, ventricular arrhythmias, asystole, increased digoxin sensitivity	corneal calcification, conjunctival irritation	ache, pain, fracture

Fig. 24.7 **Symptoms and signs of hypercalcemia.** Symptoms are more likely as the serum concentration of calcium increases.

Causes of hypercalcemia	
Common causes	primary hyperparathyroidism
	malignant disease
	iatrogenic – vitamin D or vitamin D analogs
Uncommon causes	thyrotoxicosis
	multiple myeloma
	sarcoidosis
	drug-induced:
	thiazide diuretics
	lithium
	renal failure (acute and chronic)
	familial hypocalciuric hypercalcemia

Table 24.1 **Common and uncommon causes of hypercalcemia.**

PRIMARY HYPERPARATHYROIDISM (HPT)

A 52-year-old woman presented to the Accident and Emergency Department of her local hospital with severe right-sided flank pain. Blood was detected on stick testing of urine and radiography revealed the presence of kidney stones. The pain settled with opiate analgesia. Further questioning revealed a history of recent depression, generalized weakness, recurrent indigestion, and aches in both hands. Serum adjusted calcium was 3.20 mmol/L (12.8 mg/dL; normal range 2.2–2.6 mmol/L [8.8–10.4 mg/dL]), serum phosphate 0.65 mmol/L (2.0 mg/dL; normal range 0.7–1.4 mmol/L [2.2–5.6 mg/dL]), and PTH 16.9 pmol/L (169 pg/mL); normal range 1.1–6.9 pmol/L (11-69 pg/mL).

Comment. Most patients with primary HPT are now identified when asymptomatic hypercalcemia is discovered on 'routine' biochemical testing or during investigation of nonspecific symptoms. When symptomatic, primary HPT classically affects the skeleton, kidneys, and gastrointestinal tract, resulting in the well-recognized triad of complaints described as: 'bones, stones, and abdominal groans'. Renal stone disease is now the most common presenting complaint.

in calcium, the more likely are symptoms to be present. In practice, 90% of cases are due to either primary HPT or malignancy; a greater diagnostic challenge is presented when it becomes necessary to differentiate occult malignancy from the less common causes of hypercalcemia (Table 24.1).

Investigation of hypercalcemia

In the majority of cases, the cause of hypercalcemia will be identified by obtaining an accurate history, by clinical exami-

nation, and by appropriate biochemical tests. In some cases, however, additional valuable information on causation may be obtained from radiologic investigations and tissue biopsies. The development and ready availability of specific, sensitive, and reliable assays for intact PTH has enabled the clinician to discriminate primary HPT from non-parathyroid causes of hypercalcemia (particularly malignancy): an increased or inappropriately detectable intact PTH in the presence of hypercalcemia is observed in primary HPT, whereas an intact PTH below the limit of detection of the assay (undetectable) is usually observed in non-parathyroid causes of hypercalcemia.

Several laboratory tests may be required to differentiate the various non-parathyroid causes of hypercalcemia

In a high percentage of cases, HCM is caused by tumors secreting parathyroid-hormone-related protein (PTHrP). Vitamin D excess or overdose may be obvious from the history, but sometimes only becomes apparent after measurement of the concentrations of vitamins D_3 (cholecalciferol), D_2 (ergocalciferol), and $1,25(OH)_2D_3$. Measurement of serum electrolytes, urea, and creatinine will confirm renal failure, and estimation of protein, albumin, and immunoglobulins may indicate the presence of myeloma (Chapter 3), which should be investigated by both serum and urine electrophoresis. Thyroid function tests (measurement of thyroid-stimulating hormone, total thyroxine, and total tri-iodothyronine, or estimation of free thyroid hormone (see Chapter 37) enable diagnosis of thyrotoxic hypercalcemia. Rare causes of hypercalcemia may be diagnosed by estimation of lithium (toxicity or overdose), growth hormone (acromegaly), vitamin A (toxicity), and urine catecholamines (pheochromocytoma, see Chapter 40).

Primary hyperparathyroidism is relatively common

Primary HPT is a relatively common endocrine disease, characterized by hypercalcemia associated with an increased or inappropriate intact PTH. It has an incidence ranging from 1 in 500 to 1 in 1000 of the population. In 80–85% of patients, a solitary parathyroid gland adenoma is present, and the condition is curable by successful removal of the adenoma.

Hypercalcemia associated with malignancy (HCM) is a poor prognostic sign

Hypercalcemia tends to occur late in the course of malignant disease, and is usually a poor prognostic sign. Effective and relatively innocuous treatment for HCM is now available, and can markedly improve the quality of life of these patients, by relieving the symptoms of hypercalcemia.

HYPERCALCEMIA ASSOCIATED WITH MALIGNANCY (HCM)

Treatment of HCM

Treatment of hypercalcemia can greatly improve the quality of life of patients. Symptomatic hypercalcemia or serum calcium concentrations exceeding 3.00 mmol/L (12 mg/dL) would merit treatment. Dehydration results from hypercalcemia-induced polyuria, reduced fluid and food intake, associated vomiting, decreased arginine-vasopressin, AVP (also known as ADH) activity at the distal tubule, and reduced renal perfusion. Fluid replacement corrects hypovolemia and provides a moderate sodium load, which will cause a concomitant increase in calcium excretion. Bisphosphonates (Fig. 24.8) have improved the management of HCM, and are the most effective drugs available for treating hypercalcemia. This group of drugs have their major effects by inhibiting osteoclast activity immediately when infused, and then exert a more prolonged effect by being incorporated into bone matrix in a position normally occupied by pyrophosphate. Calcitonin also inhibits osteoclast activity directly, and decreases renal tubular reabsorption of calcium; downregulation of calcitonin receptors subsequently occurs, and so the calcium-decreasing effect lasts only 4–5 days.

HYPOCALCAEMIA IN THE NEONATE

A healthy full-term boy aged 7 days and weighing 3.5 kg was noted by the community midwife to be jittery and feeding poorly at home. On review by the paediatrician, the blood calcium was measured and found to be 1.55 mmol/L. The child responded to calcium supplementation and vitamin D.

Comment. Postnatal hypocalcaemia is common, with most levels being above 1.75 mmol/L. In the first thirty-six hours of life, calcium levels fall as the relatively higher maternal levels switch the foetal parathyroid gland off. After 2 days, the concentration increases again.

Where a more profound drop in calcium is present, and particularly when it is at the end of the first week of life, other causes may be found. Here the possibilities include primary hypoparathyroidism, maternal hyperparathyroidism with hypercalcaemia, and maternal vitamin D deficiency. Thus, investigations on the neonate and mum are required.

Pyrophosphate and bisphosphonates

$$O = P - O - P = O$$

pyrophosphate

etidronate

alendronate

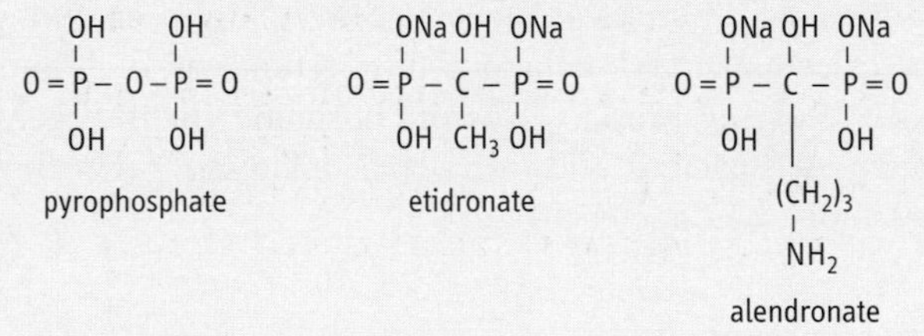

Fig. 24.8 Structural formulae of pyrophosphate and bisphosphonates. The P-C-P bonds of the biphosphonates can resist enzymatic cleavage, and the potency of these drugs is determined by the chemical sequence attached to the carbon molecule.

Two major mechanisms of HCM are recognized

Calcium reabsorption by the kidney is often enhanced in HCM, interfering with the ability of the kidneys to limit the increased release of serum calcium that results from increased osteoclast activity. There are two main sources of stimulation of the osteoclasts:

- a circulating humoral factor secreted by the tumor;
- a locally active secretory factor(s) produced by the tumor or metastases in bone.

Current evidence indicates that the most common cause of HCM is the production, by tumors or their metastases, of a humoral factor, PTHrP (see above), that can circulate in blood and exert its effects on the skeleton and kidneys. Production of PTHrP is common in breast, lung, kidney, or other solid tumors, but is more rare in hematologic, gastrointestinal, and head and neck malignancies. The amino-terminal portion of PTHrP possesses PTH-like activity that results in hypercalcemia, hypophosphatemia, phosphaturia, increased renal calcium reabsorption, and osteoclast activation.

The second type of hypercalcemia is the result of increased bone resorption by osteoclasts stimulated by factors produced by the primary tumor or, more usually, by metastases, that stimulate osteoclasts by alteration of the RANKL/OPG balance. Mediators such as PTHrP, cytokines, and growth factors (e.g. IL-1, TNF-α, lymphotoxin, and TGF-α) have all been shown to possess osteoclast-stimulating activity that results in significant bone resorption. Production of prostaglandins, especially those of the E series (PGE$_2$), has been demonstrated in several classes of tumor, particularly breast cancer. Prostaglandins stimulate osteoclastic bone resorption, and infusion of high concentrations of prostaglandins results in hypercalcemia.

Excess of vitamin D is toxic

Increasing therapeutic use of potent vitamin D analogs, hydroxylated at position 1 or at positions 1 and 25, made vitamin D toxicity the third most common cause of hypercalcemia.

Hypocalcemia

It is important to adjust serum calcium concentration for the concentration of albumin

Many acute and chronic illnesses lead to a decrease in serum albumin, which in turn decreases serum total calcium concentration. It is important that adjusted calcium is calculated in clinical situations. A serum-adjusted calcium that is below the reference range (<2.20 mmol/L; 8.8 mg/dL) may occur commonly in clinical practice. Changes in ionized calcium can result from pH changes in plasma – particularly alkalemia (Chapter 23), which increases the protein binding of calcium, causing decreased concentrations of ionized calcium.

Clinical signs of hypocalcemia are, in the main, due to neuromuscular irritability and are more obvious and severe when the onset of hypocalcemia is acute. In some cases, this irritability may be demonstrated by eliciting specific clinical signs. Chvostek's sign is the presence of twitching of the muscles around the mouth (circumoral muscles) in response to tapping the facial nerve anterior to the ear, and Trousseau's sign is the typical contraction of hand in response to reduced blood flow in the arm induced by inflation of a blood-pressure cuff. Numbness, tingling, cramps, tetany and even seizures may be stimulated by hypocalcemia.

Hypocalcemia may be due to a low PTH concentration, secondary hyperparathyroidism or to tissue resistance to PTH

Causes of hypocalcemia can be divided into those associated with low $PTH_{(1-84)}$, those in which the decreased serum calcium results in secondary HPT, and rare cases in which there is PTH resistance (Table 24.2). Development of hypocalcemia indicates that the normal physiologic compensatory mechanisms controlled by PTH have failed and there are disturbed fluxes of calcium between bone, kidney, and intestine.

Hypoparathyroidism

The most common cause of hypoparathyroidism is as a complication of neck surgery, particularly that for pharyngeal or laryngeal tumors, thyroid disease, or parathyroid disease.

Pseudohypoparathyroidism

The group of pseudohypoparathyroidism syndromes is characterized by hypocalcemia, hyperphosphatemia, and increased concentrations of $PTH_{(1-84)}$ (markedly increased in some patients).

The classical type of pseudohypoparathyroidism (PHP) is due to end-organ resistance to PTH, caused by a genetic defect resulting in an abnormal regulatory subunit of the G-protein of the adenylate cyclase complex. Confirmation of the diagnosis is made by demonstrating a lack of increase in plasma or urinary cAMP in response to the infusion of PTH.

Abnormal metabolism of vitamin D

Hypocalcemia resulting from abnormalities in vitamin D metabolism can be due to vitamin D deficiency, acquired or inherited disorders of vitamin D metabolism, and vitamin D resistance.

In addition, tissue insensitivity to $1,25(OH)_2D_3$ results in the characteristic findings of hypocalcemia, secondary HPT, and increased $11,25(OH)_2D_3$. Individually or in combination, the most common causes of vitamin D deficiency are:

- **reduced exposure to sunlight:** this is common in institutionalized elderly persons and immigrants to western Europe from the Middle East or Indian subcontinent who wear traditional dress;

Causes of hypocalcemia

Hypoparathyroid	Nonparathyroid	PTH resistance
postoperative	vitamin D deficiency	pseudohypoparathyroidism
idiopathic	malabsorption	hypomagnesemia
acquired hypomagnesemia	liver disease	
neck irradiation	renal disease	
anticonvulsant therapy	vitamin D resistance	
	hypophosphatemia	

Table 24.2 **Causes of hypocalcemia.**

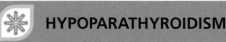

HYPOPARATHYROIDISM

Magnesium in hypoparathyroidism

Patients with a low plasma magnesium concentration develop a state of functional hypoparathyroidism and end-organ resistance to PTH; these patients tend not to respond to treatment with calcium supplementation alone. Secretion of PTH from the parathyroid gland requires a finite amount of magnesium to allow fusion of the secretory granules with the membrane and release of PTH (see Fig. 24.3); thus, in order to restore normal parathyroid gland function and normocalcemia, magnesium supplementation is essential.

METABOLIC BONE DISEASE

Prevention and treatment of osteoporosis

Estrogen has a pivotal role in the maintenance of bone mass in women. An increased rate of osteoclast-mediated bone loss is observed immediately after the menopause, as a result of ovarian failure and the decrease in estrogen secretion. This can be prevented by HRT, which can be given as cyclical or continuous combined estrogen and progesterone in women with an intact uterus, or as estrogen alone in women who have had their uterus surgically removed (by hysterectomy). The Women's Health Initiative (WHI) trial established an excess of adverse events including increased breast cancer, thromboembolic disease, stroke and cardiovascular events in women receiving greater than 5 years of continuous combined HRT. Although short-term therapy is valuable for menopausal symptoms long-term use of this type of HRT is no longer recommended as prophylaxis or treatment for osteoporosis.

Other treatments that are recommended are bisphosphonates, selective estrogen receptor modulators (SERMs), nightly injections of PTH, calcitonin, and, in elderly patients, calcium with vitamin D supplementation.

- **poor dietary intake:** most Western diets contain sufficient vitamin D, but diets such as strict vegetarian or lactovegetarian have inadequate vitamin D content and, in the long term, may result in deficiency;
- **malabsorption** of vitamin D may be caused by celiac disease, Crohn's disease, pancreatic insufficiency, inadequate bile-salt secretion, and nontropical sprue (see Chapter 9).

Abnormalities of vitamin D metabolism are observed, among others, in patients with liver disease (deficient 25-hydroxylation, malabsorption), and renal failure (1α-hydroxylase deficiency).

Genetics of calcium disorders

The calcium-sensing receptor (CaSR) is pivotal in regulating responses to alterations in calcium and genetic abnormalities altering CaSR function result in both hyper and hypocalcaemia. In subjects heterozygous for an inactivating mutation of the CaSR a state of relative 'resistance' to the effects of ionized calcium exists producing a condition known as familial hypocalciuric hypercalcaemia (FHH). Homozygous inactivating mutations cause neonatal severe hyperparathyroidism (NSHPT) which can be fatal if parathyroidectomy is not performed in early life. When an activating mutation of the CaSR is present, varying degrees of hypocalcaemia are observed depending on the severity of the mutation and this accounts for some of the cases of familial hypocalcaemia described.

METABOLIC BONE DISEASE

Osteoporosis is a common age-related disease of bone

Osteoporosis can be defined as 'a significant reduction of bone mineral density compared with age- and sex-matched norms, with an increased susceptibility to fractures'. Osteoporosis is associated with aging and, with increasing longevity, a greater percentage of the population will become susceptible to osteoporosis and its sequelae. Bone density decreases from a peak achieved by the age of 30 years in men and women, and the rate of bone loss is accelerated in women after loss of estrogen secretion at the menopause. The progressive loss of bone that takes place with aging is a result of uncoupling of bone turnover over a prolonged period of time, with a relative increase of bone resorption or decrease in bone formation. A number of factors have been recognized as contributing to an increased risk of osteoporosis (Fig. 24.9).

There is much debate on the best therapeutic approach to osteoporosis, and many questions are raised about the possibility of detecting 'fast bone-losers' by measuring biochemical markers of bone metabolism. Most of the available treatments decrease osteoclast activity, and are therefore anti-resorptive, but new therapies are available such as nightly sub-cutaneous injections of PTH$_{(1-34)}$ that have an anabolic action stimulating osteoblast activity and new bone formation.

Paget's disease of bone is a disorder characterized by areas of accelerated bone turnover initiated by increased osteoclast-mediated bone resorption

Osteoclasts in Paget's disease are large, numerous, and multinucleate (up to 100 nuclei); their activity is coupled to increased osteoblast number and activity. A common biochemical abnormality of the disease is increased alkaline phosphatase, which is indicative of increased osteoblast activity. Increased collagen breakdown by osteoclasts results in a high serum and urine concentration of hydroxyproline, pyridinolines, and telopeptides. The bisphosphonates (see Fig. 24.8) have significant antiosteoclastic activity, and are the drugs of first choice for treating Paget's disease.

Osteomalacia

The characteristic pathology in osteomalacia is the defective mineralization of osteoid in mature bone. When this occurs in the growing skeleton, there is also loss of maturation and mineralization of the cartilage cells at the growth plate; the

Factors increasing the risk of osteoporosis

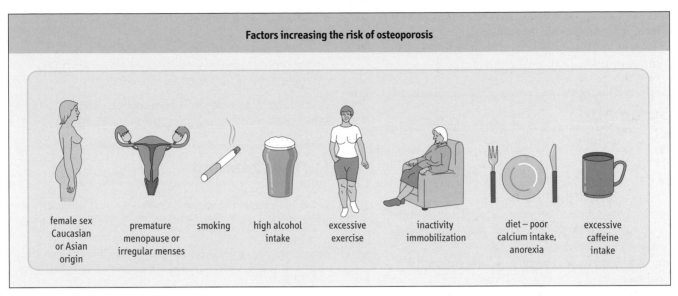

female sex Caucasian or Asian origin | premature menopause or irregular menses | smoking | high alcohol intake | excessive exercise | inactivity immobilization | diet – poor calcium intake, anorexia | excessive caffeine intake

Fig. 24.9 **Risk factors and secondary causes of osteoporosis.**

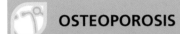 OSTEOPOROSIS

A 62-year-old woman was admitted to hospital because of sudden onset of severe back pain between the shoulder blades after a fall in her bathroom. Radiography detected a wedge fracture of two thoracic vertebrae reduced bone density. A bone density scan or dual energy X-ray absorptiometry (DEXA) scan showed severely reduced density in femur and spine. She had experienced the menopause after a hysterectomy at age 41 years but had been unable to tolerate hormone replacement therapy (HRT). Biochemical investigations were all within normal limits.

Comment. Symptoms of osteoporosis develop at a late stage of the disease, and are often caused by the presence of fracture(s). Hip, vertebral, and wrist fractures are common in patients with osteoporosis, and result in significant mortality and morbidity. HRT can be used to prevent the development of bone loss in postmenopausal women but slightly increases the risk of stroke, heart attack and breast cancer.

OSTEOMALACIA

A 60-year-old woman who had become increasingly infirm and housebound was referred to the Metabolic Outpatient Clinic. She had experienced a gradual onset of diffuse aches and pains throughout her skeleton but especially around the hips. She was having difficulty walking, had generalized weakness, and had recently experienced sudden severe pain in her ribs and pelvis. Radiography detected fractured ribs. Adjusted serum calcium was 2.1 mmol/L (8.4 mg/dL; normal range 2.2–2.6 mmol/L [8.8–10.4 mg/dL]), serum phosphate 0.56 mmol/L (1.7 mg/dL; normal range 0.7–1.4 mmol/L [2.2–4.3 mg/dL]), alkaline phosphatase 300 IU/L (normal range 50–260 IU/L) and PTH 12.6 pmol/L (normal range 1.1–6.9 pmol/L [11–69 pg/mL]).

Comment. In severe forms of osteomalacia, biochemical abnormalities are commonly seen, including low serum adjusted calcium, low serum phosphate, increased alkaline phosphatase and increased $PTH_{(1-84)}$. Clinically, patients may have diffuse bone pain or more specific pain related to a fracture, lateral bowing of the lower limbs, and a distinctive waddling gait. Ethnic groups with dark skin are particularly at risk in countries with low-average sunlight, as the majority of vitamin D in the body comes from synthesis by the action of UV light on 7-dehydrocholesterol. This may be exacerbated by traditional dress and a diet that is high in phytates (unleavened bread) and low in calcium and vitamin D.

term 'rickets' is used to describe the clinical, radiologic, and pathologic findings seen in children. There are several diverse causes of osteomalacia, many related to abnormalities of vitamin D metabolism.

Summary

- Bone is a metabolically active tissue that undergoes constant remodeling.
- The major cells involved in the remodeling process are the osteoclast and osteoblast.
- Bone metabolism is closely interrelated with the metabolism of calcium which also involves the intestine and kidney.
- A calcium sensing receptor is present on the parathyroid, thyroid and kidney cells that is pivotal in calcium regulation.
- The calcium balance is hormonally regulated by parathormone, vitamin D metabolites and calcitonin.
- The measurement of calcium in serum is an important test in the clinical laboratories, because both hypercalcemia and hypocalcemia lead to clinical symptoms.
- Main causes of hypercalcaemia are primary hyperparathyroidism, malignancy and vitamin D excess.

Osteoporosis, a decrease in bone density leading to bone fractures, is a major health problem.

Further reading

Buckley KA, Fraser WD. Receptor activator for nuclear factor kappaB ligand and osteoprotegrin: regulators of bone physiology and immune responses/potential therapeutic agents and biochemical markers. *Ann Clin Biochem* 2002;**39**:551–556.

Favus MJ, ed. *Primer on the metabolic bone disease and disorders of mineral metabolism*, 5th ed. Washington DC: American Society for Bone and Mineral Research; 2003.

Fraser WD. Paget's disease of bone. *CPD Rheumatology* 2001;**2**:8–13.

Fleisch H. *Bisphosphonates in bone disease. From the laboratory to the patient*, 5th ed. New York, London: The Parthenon Publishing Group; 2001.

Mundy GR. *Bone remodelling and its disorders*. 2nd ed. London: Martin Dunitz; 1999.

Nissenson RA. Parathyroid hormone-related protein. *Rev Endocr Metab Disord* 2000;**1**:343–352.

Complex Carbohydrates: Glycoproteins

A D Elbein

LEARNING OBJECTIVES

After reading this chapter you should be able to:

■ Describe the general structures of the various types of N-linked oligosaccharides, i.e., high mannose, biantennary, triantennary and tetraantennary complex chains.

■ Outline the sequence of reactions involved in biosynthesis and processing of N-linked oligosaccharides to produce the various types of oligosaccharide chains.

■ Distinguish between co-translational and post-translational glycosylation and pruning reactions.

■ Explain how N-linked oligosaccharides are involved in protein folding and in cell recognition, and why O-linked oligosaccharides are so important in mucin function.

■ Describe how each of the monosaccharides involved in biosynthesis of N-linked and O-linked oligosaccharides are synthesized from glucose and activated for synthesis of glycoconjugates.

■ Distinguish lectins from other types of proteins and describe their role in cell function and the reasons for their toxicity.

■ Describe several diseases that are associated with deficiencies in enzymes involved in synthesis, modification or degradation of complex carbohydrates.

Most mammalian proteins contain covalently attached sugars – i.e., they are glycoproteins. There are two distinct types of sugar-containing proteins that occur in animal cells: glycoproteins and proteoglycans. Along with glycolipids, which are discussed in the next chapter, they are part of the group of sugar-containing molecules that are called glycoconjugates. Figure 25.1 presents models of the structure of glycoproteins and proteoglycans in order to demonstrate the differences between them: glycoproteins have short oligosaccharide (glycan) chains (1–20 sugars in length); they are highly branched and generally do not have a repeating sequence. In contrast, proteoglycans are long, linear, unbranched glycans that have a disaccharide-repeating unit. This chapter will focus on the glycoproteins; Chapter 26 will address glycolipids, and Chapter 27 will consider the proteoglycans.

The class of glycoproteins includes most of the proteins that are integral components of the plasma membrane, that function as receptors for hormones or other molecules in the circulation, or that mediate interactions between cells. In addition, many of the proteins of the endoplasmic reticulum, Golgi apparatus and lysosome, and those that are secreted by cells, including serum and mucous proteins, are glycoproteins. Indeed, glycosylation is the major post-synthetic modification of proteins; it occurs either during the course of protein synthesis in the endoplasmic reticulum or once the protein has been synthesized and transported to the Golgi apparatus. The functions of the carbohydrate chains of glycoproteins are diverse: they may stabilize the protein against denaturation, protect it from proteolytic degradation, enhance its solubility, or serve as recognition signals for transport or cell-cell interactions.

GLYCOPROTEINS: STRUCTURES AND LINKAGES

Sugars are attached to specific amino acids in proteins

Sugars may be attached to protein in either N-glycosidic or O-glycosidic linkage. N-linked oligosaccharides, characteristic of plasma and membrane proteins, are always attached by a glycosylamine linkage of N-acetylglucosamine (GlcNAc) to the amide nitrogen of an asparagine residue (Fig. 25.2A). The asparagine at the site of glycosylation must be in an Asn-X-Ser (Thr)-consensus sequence in order to undergo glycosylation. However, not all asparagine residues present in that consensus sequence are glycosylated, indicating that other factors, such as the conformation of the protein around the glycosylation site, are also important.

Mucins, collagens, and cytoplasmic proteins may be glycosylated

Many membrane proteins and proteins in mucous secretions (mucins) contain oligosaccharides linked by a glycosidic linkage between N-acetylgalactosamine (GalNAc) and the hydroxyl group of serine or threonine residues (Fig. 25.2B). There is no known consensus sequence that indicates which serine residues are to be glycosylated.

A glucosyl-galactose disaccharide may be linked to the hydroxyl group of hydroxylysine residues in collagen (Fig.

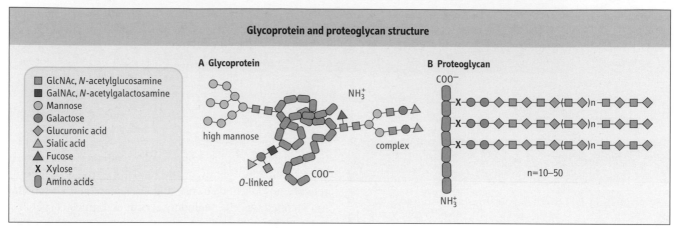

Fig. 25.1 **Generalized model of the structure of glycoproteins and proteoglycans.**

25.2C). Hydroxylysine is an unusual amino acid that occurs in mammalian collagens; it is formed by hydroxylation of lysine after this amino acid has been incorporated into the collagen chain. Collagen is first synthesized in the cell in a precursor form called procollagen. Procollagens are usually N-glycosylated glycoproteins, but peptide segments containing N-linked oligosaccharides are removed during maturation of the protein, and only the O-linked glycans remain in mature collagen. The less glycosylated collagens tend to form ordered, fibrous structures, such as occur in tendons; the more heavily glycosylated collagens are found in meshwork structures, such as basement membranes (Chapter 27).

Finally, a recently discovered structure found in many cytoplasmic proteins involves a single GlcNAc that is O-glycosidically linked to serine residues in protein (Fig. 25.2D). This GlcNAc appears to be attached to the same serine residues that become phosphorylated as part of regulatory and signal transduction processes. The GlcNAc may represent a means by which the cell blocks or controls the phosphorylation of certain proteins, while allowing others to be phosphorylated.

Structures of the oligosaccharides attached to proteins

Sugars are linked to each other in glycosidic linkages. Two identical hexose residues can be linked together in many different ways ($\alpha1,2$; $\alpha1,3$; $\alpha1,4$; $\alpha1,6$; $\beta1,2$; $\beta1,3$; $\beta1,4$; $\beta1,6$), yielding distinct disaccharides; in contrast, two identical amino acids can only be combined in one way – two alanine residues can form only one dipeptide, alanyl-alanine. Thus carbohydrate structures have greater structural diversity, and therefore have the potential to contain more information than proteins of similar size. Nevertheless, although there are

a large number of structures produced by living cells, most of the oligosaccharides on glycoconjugates have many sugars and linkages in common.

N-*linked oligosaccharides have either 'high-mannose' or 'complex' structures built on to a common core of mannose and GlcNAc*

All the N-linked oligosaccharide chains that are found on proteins are, typically, branched structures having a common core structure of two GlcNAc and three mannose residues (shown by the boxed areas in Fig. 25.3). Beyond this core region, the oligosaccharides can be very different from each other, giving rise to a vast array of structures. Thus, oligosaccharides may be either 'high-mannose' structures containing only two GlcNAc residues and up to nine mannose units (Fig. 25.3A), or they may consist of 'complex' chains (Fig. 25.3B), so named because of their more complex composition. All the N-linked chains are initially assembled as the high-mannose structure, which is then modified to give rise to different types of complex oligosaccharides. High-mannose oligosaccharides are found to a limited extent in animal glycoproteins; they are more common in glycoproteins of lower eukaryotes and in viral envelope glycoproteins. Complex oligosaccharides are common in animals, but are generally not present in lower eukaryotes.

Complex oligosaccharides have the same core structure as the high-mannose oligosaccharides, but have terminal trisaccharide sequences composed of sialic acid-galactose-GlcNAc attached to the core mannose structure. Fucose may be found in the core (see Fig. 25.1A) or in place of sialic acid in complex oligosaccharides. In common with sialic acid, fucose is usually a terminal sugar on oligosaccharides – that is, no other sugars are attached to it. Some complex oligosaccharides have two of the terminal trisaccharide sequences (one

same or different types of antennary structures. Generally, oligosaccharides located near the amino terminus are more highly processed (complex types) whereas those near the carboxy terminus are more likely to be high-mannose types. More than 100 different complex oligosaccharide structures have now been identified, giving carbohydrates great diversity as mediators of chemical signaling and recognition events.

The viscous properties of mucins derive from their content of negatively charged sialic acid

In mucins, the O-linked oligosaccharides are usually short, branched structures containing sialic acid (N-acetylneuraminic acid), galactose, and GalNAc, and sometimes other sugars such as GlcNAc and L-fucose (Fig. 25.4). Salivary mucin contains an unusually large number of serine or threonine residues, and many of these serines or threonines are glycosylated with a sialic acid-galactose-GalNAc trisaccharide. The O-linked oligosaccharides are negatively charged because of the presence of the sialic acid residues, and when they occur in clusters and in close proximity to each other, they repel each other and prevent the protein from folding. As a result, the protein assumes an extended state, yielding a highly viscous (mucous) solution. Mucins form a protective barrier on the surface of epithelial cells, provide lubrication between surfaces, and facilitate transport processes – for example, the movement of food through the gastrointestinal tract.

General structures of glycoproteins

A glycoprotein may contain a single N-linked oligosaccharide chain, or it may have several of these types of oligosaccharides. Furthermore, the N-linked oligosaccharides may all have identical structures, or they may be quite different in structure; such a glycoprotein may also contain O-linked oligosaccharide chains. Alternatively, a glycoprotein may contain only N-linked oligosaccharides, or only O-linked oligosaccharides. The total number of oligosaccharide chains may also vary considerably, depending on the protein and its function. For example, the low-density lipoprotein receptor that is found in plasma membranes of smooth muscle cells and fibroblasts contains two N-linked biantennary complex chains, in addition to a cluster of O-linked chains. This receptor has a membrane-spanning region of hydrophobic amino acids, an extended region on the external side of the plasma membrane that contains the O-linked, negatively charged oligosaccharides, and a functional domain that is involved in binding serum low-density lipoprotein (Fig. 25.5). The two N-linked oligosaccharides are near the functional domain. It remains unclear what role these N-linked chains play in the function of this receptor, but the O-linked oligosaccharides are believed to keep the molecule in an extended state.

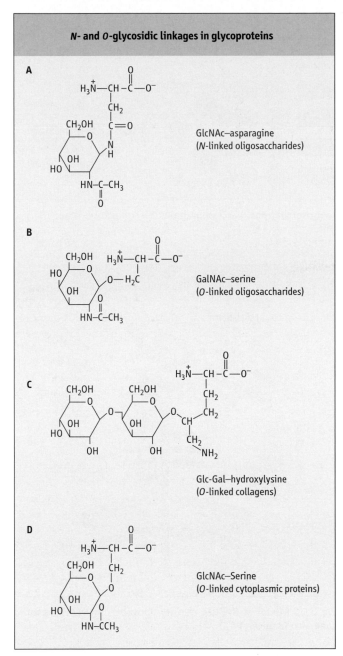

N- and O-glycosidic linkages in glycoproteins

A GlcNAc–asparagine (N-linked oligosaccharides)

B GalNAc–serine (O-linked oligosaccharides)

C Glc-Gal–hydroxylysine (O-linked collagens)

D GlcNAc–Serine (O-linked cytoplasmic proteins)

Fig. 25.2 **Various linkages of sugars to amino acids in glycoproteins.** GlcNAc, N-acetylglucosamine.

attached to each mannose) and are called 'biantennary' complex chains, whereas others have tri- or tetra-antennary structures (Fig. 25.3B). 'Microheterogeneity' of oligosaccharide structure results from the fact that the basic structure is often found in an incomplete form on glycoproteins, e.g. a missing terminal sialic acid or sialyl-galactose residues on one or more of the antennae. A given glycoprotein may also have several N-linked oligosaccharides and these may have the

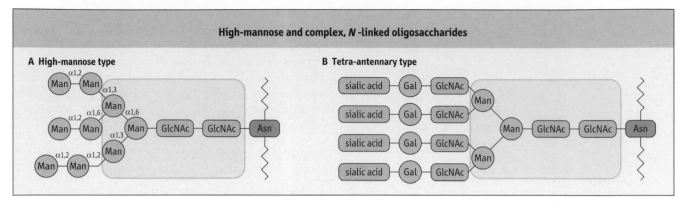

Fig. 25.3 **Typical structures of high-mannose and complex, *N*-linked oligosaccharides.** Asn, asparagine; Gal, galactose; Man, mannose. The core structure (shaded area) is common to both structures.

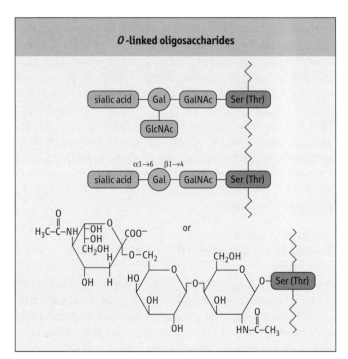

Fig. 25.4 **Typical structures of *O*-linked oligosaccharides.**

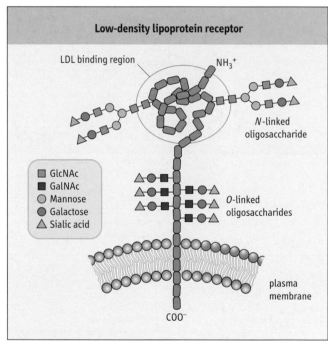

Fig. 25.5 **Model of the low density lipoprotein (LDL) receptor.** (See also Chapter 17.)

INTERCONVERSIONS AND ACTIVATION OF DIETARY SUGARS

Glucose is a precursor of all sugars in the body

Humans have a requirement for some essential amino acids and fatty acids, but all the sugars in glycoconjugates can be synthesized from D-glucose. Figure 25.6 shows the reactions that occur in animal cells to convert glucose to mannose or galactose. The latter is achieved by epimerization of the nucle-

oside diphosphate sugar, uridine diphosphate-glucose (UDP-Glc) (see Fig. 25.8), to UDP-galactose (UDP-Gal) by UDP-Gal 4-epimerase, providing a source of UDP-Gal for glycoconjugate biosynthesis. Glucose-6-phosphate (Glc-6-P), which is an early intermediate in that pathway, may also be converted to fructose-6-phosphate (Fru-6-P) by the glycolytic enzyme, phosphoglucose isomerase, and Fru-6-P can then be isomerized to mannose-6-phosphate (Man-6-P) by phosphomannose isomerase. Man-6-P is then converted by a mutase to mannose-1-phosphate (Man-1-P), which reacts with guanosine triphosphate (GTP) in a pyrophosphorylase reaction to form guanosine diphosphate-mannose (GDP-Man), the activated form of mannose. Mannose also occurs in the diet,

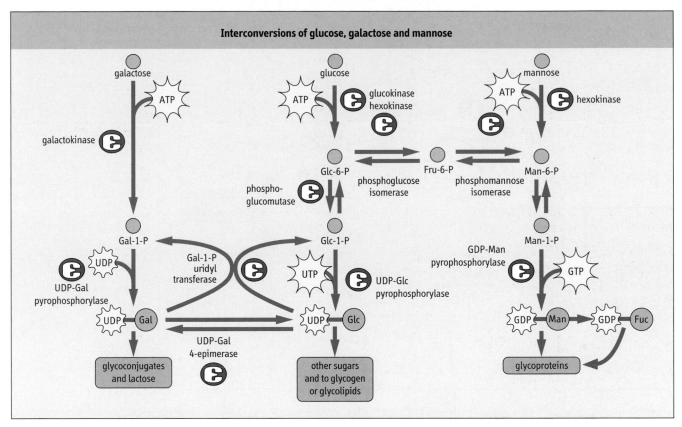

Interconversions of glucose, galactose and mannose

Fig. 25.6 **Interconversions of glucose, mannose, galactose, and their nucleotide sugars.** Fuc, fucose.

although in small amounts; it is phosphorylated by hexokinase and enters metabolism through phosphomannose isomerase.

Galactose

Galactose is an important component of our diet, because it is one of the sugars in the milk disaccharide, lactose. The pathway of galactose metabolism and its conversion to glucose is fairly complex (see Fig. 25.6). Galactose is first phosphorylated by a specific hepatic kinase, galactokinase, to form galactose-1-phosphate (Gal-1-P). The conversion of Gal-1-P to Glc-1-P involves the nucleoside diphosphate sugar intermediate, UDP-Glc. The enzyme Gal-1-P uridyl transferase catalyzes an exchange between UDP-Glc and Gal-1-P to form UDP-Gal and Glc-1-P – that is, the Glc-1-P part of UDP-Glc is replaced with Gal-1-P, to give UDP-Gal and Glc-1-P. This enzyme is absent in individuals with galactosemia (see box).

The Glc-1-P arising from galactose metabolism can be converted to Glc-6-P by phosphoglucomutase, and thus enter glycolysis. UDP-Glc is present at only micromolar concentrations in cells, so that its availability for galactose metabolism would

be quickly exhausted were it not for the presence of UDP-Gal 4-epimerase. This enzyme catalyzes the equilibrium between UDP-Glc and UDP-Gal, providing a constant source of UDP-Glc during galactose metabolism. UDP-Gal 4-epimerase is actually a dehydrogenase, a redox enzyme, requiring NAD^+ as a coenzyme. In this reaction, UDP-Gal is first oxidized to the achiral intermediate, UDP-4-ketogalactose, with the reduction of NAD^+ to NADH. The 4-keto intermediate is then reduced by the enzyme-bound NADH, but with a change in the stereochemistry of the 4-hydroxyl group, producing UDP-Glc and regenerating NAD^+.

Fructose

Fructose is a component of the disaccharide sucrose, table sugar; it is also found in the diet in the form of common sweetener, high-fructose corn syrup. Fructose is metabolized by two pathways in cells (Fig. 25.7). It may be phosphorylated by hexokinase, an enzyme that is present in all cells; however, hexokinase has a strong preference for glucose, and glucose, which is present at about 5 mmol/L (100 mg/dL) concentration in blood, is a strong competitive inhibitor of the phosphorylation of fructose. The major pathway of

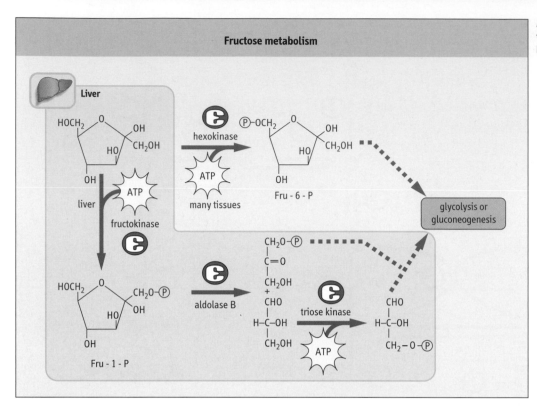

Fig. 25.7 **Metabolism of fructose by fructokinase or hexokinase.**

GALACTOSEMIA

An apparently normal baby began to vomit and develop diarrhea after breast feeding. These problems, together with dehydration, continued for several days, when the baby began to refuse food and developed jaundice, indicative of liver damage, followed by hepatomegaly, and then lens opacification (cataracts). Measurement of glucose in the blood and urine by a specific enzymatic technique indicated that concentrations of glucose were low, consistent with the failure to absorb foods. However, glucose measured by a colorimetric test that determined total reducing sugar indicated that the concentration of sugar was quite high in both blood and urine. The reducing sugar was eventually identified as galactose, indicating an abnormality in galactose metabolism known as galactosemia. This finding was consistent with the observation that, when milk was removed from the diet and replaced with an infant formula containing sucrose rather than lactose, the

vomiting and diarrhea stopped, and hepatic function was gradually restored.

Comment. The accumulation of galactose in the blood is most often a result of a deficiency of Gal-1-P uridyl transferase, which prevents the interconversion of galactose and glucose and leads to the accumulation of galactose and Gal-1-P in tissues. Accumulation of the latter interferes with phosphate and glucose metabolism, leading to widespread tissue damage, organ failure, and mental retardation. In addition, accumulation of galactose in tissues results in galactose conversion via the polyol pathway to galactitol, and the accumulation of galactitol in the lens results in osmotic stress and formation of cataracts. A milder form of galactosemia is caused by galactokinase deficiency.

fructose metabolism in liver involves fructokinase, and this pathway is especially important after a meal. Thus, in liver, fructose is phosphorylated to fructose-1-phosphate (Fru-1-P) by fructokinase, and the liver aldolase, called aldolase B, can cleave Fru-1-P, as well as fructose-1,6-bisphosphate (Fru-1,6-BP). In contrast, muscle aldolase, called aldolase A, is specific for Fru-1,6-BP. The products of aldolase B are dihydroxyacetone phosphate and glyceraldehyde (not glyceraldehyde phosphate). The glyceraldehyde must then be phosphorylated by

triose kinase in order to be metabolized in the glycolytic pathway.

It should be noted that in the liver, fructose enters glycolysis at the level of triose phosphate intermediates, i.e. after the control points for the regulatory enzymes, hexokinase and phosphofructokinase-1 (PFK-1). By circumventing these two rate-limiting and regulatory enzymes, fructose provides a rapid source of energy for both aerobic and anaerobic cells. This is part of the rationale behind the development

BIOSYNTHESIS OF LACTOSE

Lactose synthase α-lactalbumin

Lactose (galactosyl-β1,4-glucose) is synthesized from UDP-Gal and glucose in mammary glands during lactation. Lactose synthase is formed by the binding of α-lactalbumin to the galactosyl transferase that normally participates in biosynthesis of N-linked glycoproteins. α-Lactalbumin, which is expressed only in the mammary glands during lactation, converts galactosyl transferase to lactose synthase by lowering the enzyme's Km for glucose by about three orders of magnitude, from 1 mol/L to 1 mmol/L, leading to preferential synthesis of lactose. α-Lactalbumin is the only known example of a 'specifier' protein that alters the substrate specificity of an enzyme.

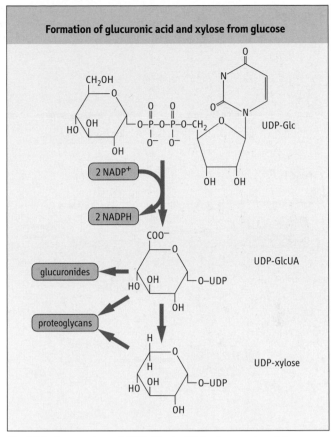

Fig. 25.8 **Conversion of UDP-Glc to UDP-glucuronic acid (UDP-GlcUA) and UDP-xylose.** Note that oxidation of UDP-Glc is a two-step reaction, from alcohol to aldehyde, then to an acid. Both reactions are catalyzed by UDP-Glc dehydrogenase.

of high-fructose drinks, such as 'Gatorade'. The significance of the fructokinase, as opposed to the hexokinase, pathway of fructose metabolism is indicated by the pathology associated with genetic defects in fructokinase or aldolase B. Fructokinase deficiency leads to a relatively asymptomatic condition, fructosuria. However, a defect in aldolase B causes accumulation of Fru-1-P in the liver, leading to problems similar to those seen in galactosemia. Fortunately, both galactosemia and hereditary fructose intolerance can be managed by removing galactose or fructose, respectively, from the diet.

OTHER PATHWAYS OF SUGAR NUCLEOTIDE METABOLISM

UDP-glucose

UDP-Glc is the precursor of other essential sugars, such as glucuronic acid and xylose, which are required for proteoglycan biosynthesis. The reactions that lead to the formation of these sugars are outlined in Figure 25.8. Oxidation of UDP-Glc by UDP-Glc dehydrogenase leads to the activated form of glucuronic acid, i.e. UDP-glucuronic acid (UDP-GlcUA). This nucleotide is the donor of glucuronic acid both for the formation of proteoglycans (see Chapter 27) and for conjugation and detoxification reactions that occur in the liver. In that organ, glucuronic acid is conjugated to steroid hormones, bilirubin (a degradation product of heme), and many drugs. The conjugation reaction increases the water solubility of hydrophobic compounds, facilitating their excretion in urine. UDP-GlcUA undergoes a decarboxylation reaction to form UDP-xylose, the activated form of xylose, the pentose sugar that serves as the link between

protein and glycan in proteoglycans. UDP-GlcUA is also a precursor of ascorbate (vitamin C) in most mammals, except primates and guinea pigs.

Guanosine diphosphate-mannose

GDP-Man is not only the mannose donor for glycoprotein synthesis, but it is also the precursor of L-fucose, a deoxyhexose that is an important recognition signal in many glycoproteins and glycolipids. The conversion of GDP-D-Man to GDP-L-fucose involves a complex series of oxidative and reductive steps, as well as epimerizations. Failure of this pathway causes leukocyte adhesion deficiency disease (LAD).

Fructose-6-phosphate (Fru-6-P)

Fru-6-P is the common precursor of amino sugars, which are found in almost all glycoconjugates. Figure 25.9 shows the pathway of formation of GlcNAc, GalNAc, and sialic acid. The initial reaction involves transfer of an amino group

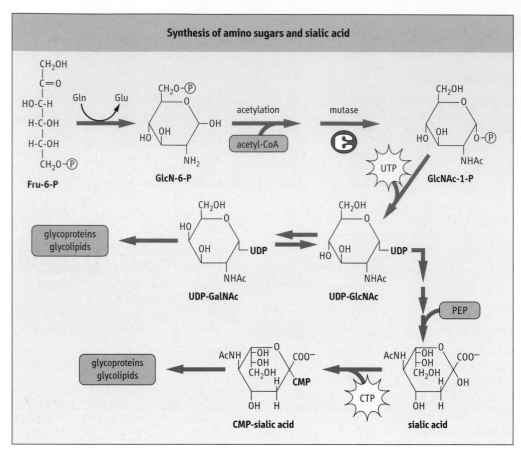

Synthesis of amino sugars and sialic acid

Fig. 25.9 **Synthesis of amino sugars and sialic acid.** Acetyl CoA, acetyl Coenzyme A; GlcN-6-P, glucosamine-6-phosphate; GlcNac-6P, N-acetylglucosamine-6-phosphate; GalNAc, acetylgalactosamine; HNAc, AcHN, acetamide group; PEP, phosphoenolpyruvate.

from glutamine to Fru-6-P, to form glucosamine-6-phosphate (GlcN-6-P). This is followed by transfer of acetate from acetyl-CoA to the amino group to form N-acetylglucosamine-6-phosphate (GlcNAc-6-P). GlcNAc-6-P is converted to its activated form, UDP-GlcNAc, by mutase and pyrophosphorylase reactions. In addition to its role as a GlcNAc donor, UDP-GlcNAc can also be epimerized to UDP-GalNAc.

N-Acetyl-neuraminic acid (sialic acid)

UDP-GlcNAc is the precursor of N-acetyl-neuraminic acid (NANA) or sialic acid. These are 9-carbon sugar acids that are common components of N- and O-linked oligosaccharides. Sialic acid is produced by the condensation of an amino sugar with phosphoenolpyruvate. Cytidine monophosphate (CMP)-sialic acid is the sugar nucleotide donor for glycoconjugate biosynthesis. It is formed by reaction of free sialic acid with cytidine triphosphate (CTP) (see Fig. 25.9). CMP-sialic acid (CMP-NANA) is the only nucleotide-monophosphate sugar donor in glycoconjugate metabolism. In microorganisms, keto-deoxy-octulosonic acid, a component of the cell wall, is activated as CMP-KDO. With few exceptions, all amino sugars

in eukaryotic glycoconjugates are acetylated; thus, they are neutral and do not contribute charge to glycoconjugates.

BIOSYNTHESIS OF OLIGOSACCHARIDES

N-linked oligosaccharides

The assembly of the N-linked oligosaccharide chains begins in the endoplasmic reticulum

The pathway of assembly of N-linked oligosaccharides involves the participation of a lipid carrier to form an activated oligosaccharide, which is then transferred *en bloc* to specific asparagine residues on the protein (Fig. 25.10). The lipid carrier is a long-chain polyisoprenol of about 120 carbon atoms, with a phosphate group esterified to the terminal isoprene unit. This molecule, called dolichol phosphate (Dol-P), is an integral lipid of the endoplasmic reticulum. The individual sugars – GlcNAc, mannose and glucose – are added to Dol-P, one at a time, to form $Glc_3Man_9GlcNAc_2$-PP-Dol, which then donates the oligosaccharide to protein. For

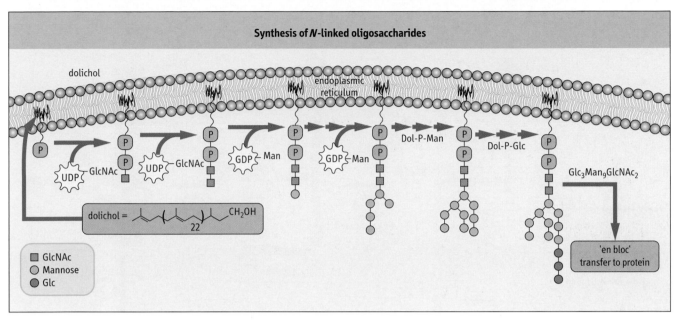

Fig. 25.10 **Synthesis of N-linked oligosaccharides in the endoplasmic reticulum.** GlcNAc, acetylglucosamine; Dol, dolichol; Man, mannose.

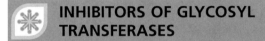

INHIBITORS OF GLYCOSYL TRANSFERASES

Several inhibitors of the biosynthesis of N-linked oligosaccharides have become valuable reagents for understanding the role of specific carbohydrate structures in glycoprotein function. Tunicamycin is a glycoside antibiotic that inhibits the first step in synthesis of N-linked oligosaccharides – formation of Dol-PP-GlcNAc (see Fig. 25.10). It has varied effects on the synthesis and function of glycoproteins. Some proteins are insoluble without their carbohydrate, and aggregate in the cell. Others do not fold correctly, or may fail to function in recognition reactions. Tunicamycin is quite toxic to animals, as animal cells need N-linked oligosaccharides for essential functions.

N-linked oligosaccharides, glycosylation is co-translational, which means that it occurs while the peptide chain is still being synthesized on the membrane-bound ribosome (see Chapter 32).

The first GlcNAc residue is added with its phosphate residue, so that the core structure is dolichyl pyrophosphate-GlcNAc (Dol-PP-GlcNAc), a hydrophobic, membrane-bound analogue of a sugar nucleotide. The remaining GlcNAc and five mannose units are transferred from their sugar nucleotides (UDP-GlcNAc and GDP-Man), whereas the next four mannose and three glucose residues are donated from lipid precursors (Dol-P-mannose and Dol-P-glucose). Each of the sugars that are added to the Dol-PP carrier is transferred by a specific enzyme; these enzymes are members of the class of enzymes known as glycosyl transferases. The completed oligosaccharide is finally transferred from its Dol-PP derivative to an asparagine residue in an Asn-X-Ser(Thr) sequence in a protein.

The function of the glucoses on the initial oligosaccharide is to expedite oligosaccharide transfer from lipid to protein. Oligosaccharyl transferase, the transferring enzyme, has a preference for oligosaccharides that contain three glucose units. In addition, as indicated below, the glucose residues are important for expediting the folding of the protein.

Intermediate processing continues in the endoplasmic reticulum

Once the oligosaccharide chain has been transferred to the protein, various glycosidases (enzymes that remove specific sugars, including the glucosidases that are specific for glucose) act on the protein-bound oligosaccharide. In a series of processing or 'pruning' reactions, the three glucose residues are removed in the endoplasmic reticulum, and up to six mannose residues in the Golgi apparatus. These trimming reactions give rise to a core structure of two GlcNAc and three mannose residues, and this core oligosaccharide is elongated to form complex oligosaccharides. The elongation reactions involve the addition of one or more of the sugars, GlcNAc, galactose, sialic acid, and L-fucose. The reactions involved in the modification of the oligosaccharide chains are outlined in Figure 25.11.

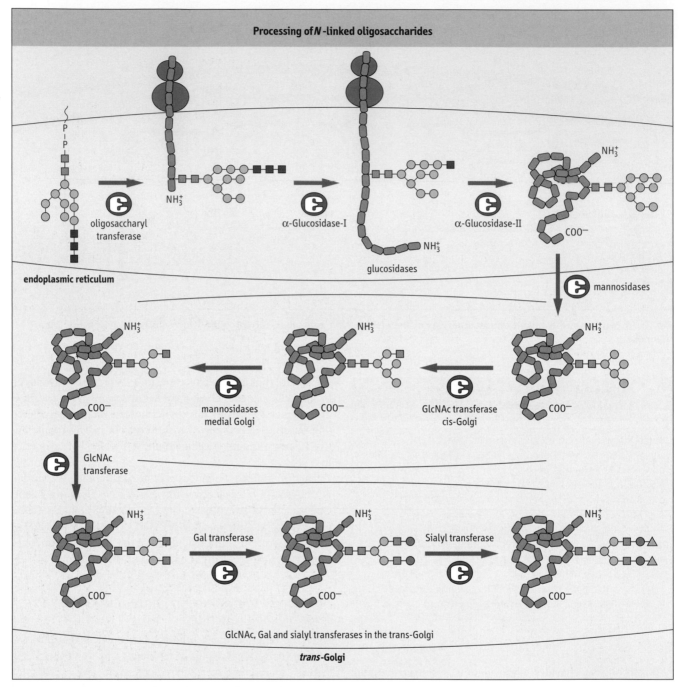

Fig. 25.11 **Processing of *N*-linked oligosaccharides from high-mannose to complex forms.** Glycoproteins are transported between the endoplasmic reticulum and Golgi compartments in vesicles. GlcNAc, acetylglucosamine.

Final modifications to the glycoprotein take place in the Golgi apparatus

When the glucose residues have been removed and the protein has folded into its correct conformation, the glycoprotein with one or more $Man_9GlcNAc_2$ oligosaccharides is transported from the endoplasmic reticulum to the Golgi apparatus, where other modification reactions can occur. Usually, in the *cis* and *medial* regions of the Golgi, six of the mannose residues are removed by several different α-mannosidases. The exact role of each of the mannosidases is not known, but they produce glycoproteins with oligosaccharide chains having variable numbers of mannose residues. If the oligosaccharide is trimmed to its core structure, it may then be converted to a complex structure by glycosyl transferases in the *trans*-Golgi apparatus (Fig. 25.11), which add GlcNAc, Gal, sialic acid and fucose residues.

O-linked oligosaccharides

The biosynthesis of *O*-linked oligosaccharides occurs in the Golgi apparatus by the stepwise addition of sugars from their sugar nucleotide donors. No lipid intermediates are involved. Figure 25.12 describes the straightforward sequence of reactions for assembly of the oligosaccharide chains of salivary mucins. GalNAc is first transferred from UDP-GalNAc to serine or threonine residues on the protein by a GalNAc transferase in the Golgi apparatus. The GalNAc-serine-(protein) serves as the acceptor for galactose and then sialic acid, transferred from their sugar nucleotides by Golgi galactosyl and sialyl transferases, to form the final trisaccharide sequence on the mucin. Other Golgi glycosyl transferases are involved in the stepwise biosynthesis of oligosaccharides on proteoglycans and collagen. There are more than 100 glycosyl transferases involved in glycoconjugate biosynthesis in a typical cell.

FUNCTIONS OF THE OLIGOSACCHARIDE CHAINS OF GLYCOPROTEINS

N-linked oligosaccharides

N-*linked oligosaccharides have an important role in protein folding*

Resident proteins in the endoplasmic reticulum, known as chaperones, assist newly synthesized membrane proteins to fold into their correct conformations. Two of these chaperones, calreticulin and calnexin, bind to unfolded glycoproteins by recognition of high-mannose oligosaccharides that have a single glucose remaining on their structure. These two chaperones are examples of a class of carbohydrate-binding

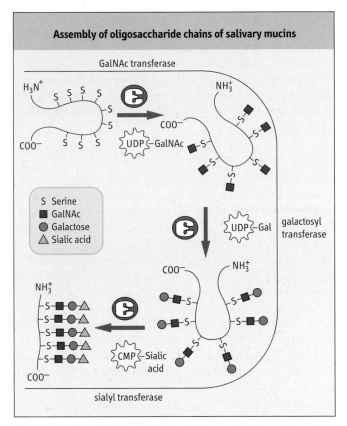

Fig. 25.12 **Biosynthesis of O-linked oligosaccharides of mucins in the Golgi apparatus.** GalNAc, acetylgalactosamine.

INHIBITORS OF GLYCOSIDASES

Several plant alkaloids are potent glycosidase inhibitors, and some of these compounds inhibit the 'pruning' enzymes shown in Figure 25.11. Castanospermine inhibits glucosidases I and II, blocking the removal of the glucose residues from the $Glc_3Man_9GlcNAc_2$-protein. Many proteins, including the AIDS virus envelope glycoprotein, are assisted in folding by interacting with chaperone proteins such as calnexin. Calnexin binds to glycoproteins in which the oligosaccharide has been trimmed to contain a single glucose (that is, $Glc_1Man_9GlcNAc_2$). If removal of glucose is inhibited by castanospermine, the protein does not fold correctly. Other plant alkaloids inhibit the mannosidases required for synthesis of complex oligosaccharides (see Fig. 25.11). Swainsonine inhibits mannosidase II, yielding oligosaccharides with only a partial complex chain; this alkaloid is of considerable interest, as plants that contain it (commonly known as locoweed in the USA) are quite toxic to animals and cause the disease known as locoism.

proteins known as lectins – proteins that have a recognition and binding site for specific carbohydrate structures. Not all the proteins synthesized in the cell require assistance in folding; for those that do, the rate of folding is greatly increased by the chaperones. Incorrectly folded or unfolded proteins do not undergo normal transport to the Golgi apparatus, and are frequently degraded in the endoplasmic reticulum.

High-mannose oligosaccharides target some proteins to specific sites in the cell

Lysosomes are involved in the hydrolysis and turnover of many cellular components, and contain a variety of degradative hydrolytic enzymes, including proteases, lipases, and glycosidases. Most of these lysosomal enzymes are *N*-linked glycoproteins. The 'sorting' of lysosomal enzymes occurs in the *cis*-Golgi region. Those enzymes destined for the lysosomes have a cluster of lysine residues formed by folding of the protein. As outlined in Figure 25.13, these lysine residues serve as a docking site for an *N*-acetylglucosamine-1-phosphate (GlcNAc-1-P) transferase that binds to the lysosomal enzyme and transfers GlcNAc-1-P from UDP-GlcNAc to the terminal mannose residue on the high-mannose chains of these proteins. A hexosaminidase then removes the GlcNAc residues to expose Man-6-P structures, which are recognized by a Man-6-P receptor in the Golgi; the receptor

binds to the modified glycoproteins and directs them to the lysosomes. The Man-6-P receptor is also present on the cell surface, so that even extracellular enzymes containing this signal are endocytosed and transferred to lysosomes.

The oligosaccharide chains of glycoproteins increase the solubility and stability of proteins

Because of the increased solubility conferred by oligosaccharide chains, most proteins secreted from cells into the environment, such as plasma proteins, or degradative enzymes released by yeast and fungi, are glycoproteins. These enzymes have high stability to heat, detergents, acids, and bases. Enzymatic removal of the carbohydrate greatly reduces their stability. Indeed, when glycoproteins are synthesized in cells in the presence of glycosylation inhibitors such as tunicamycin, which inhibits the synthesis of Dol-PP-GlcNAc, many of these proteins precipitate in the endoplasmic reticulum because of a combination of incorrect folding or processing, or decreased solubility.

Both N- and O-linked glycan structures are involved in recognition processes

N-linked glycoproteins are frequently present at the animal cell surface and have important roles in cell-cell interactions. One cell may contain on its cell surface a recognition protein – that is, a specific lectin – that binds to specific carbohydrate

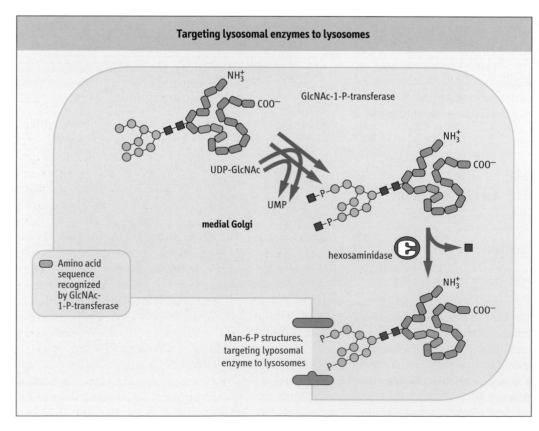

Fig. 25.13 **Targeting of lysosomal enzymes to lysosomes.** GlcNAc, acetylglucosamine; Man, mannose.

DEFICIENCIES IN GLYCOPROTEIN SYNTHESIS

The carbohydrate-deficient glycoprotein syndromes (CDGSs) are a newly described group of rare genetic diseases. All patients show multisystem pathology, with severe involvement of the nervous system. Three distinct variants have been identified and are characterized by a deficiency of the carbohydrate moiety of secretory glycoproteins, lysosomal enzymes, and, probably, membrane glycoproteins. The diagnosis is made by electrophoresis of serum transferrin. In CDGS, the transferrin contains less sialic acid and migrates more slowly.

Comment. The basic defects in this group of diseases appear to be in the synthesis or processing of N-linked oligosaccharides. Defects in GlcNAc transferase I and mannosidase II have been identified, and it seems likely that defects in each of the enzymes depicted in Figure 24.11 will eventually be demonstrated, giving rise to a family of related diseases.

TOXICITY OF RICIN AND OTHER LECTINS

Many plant lectins are toxic to animal cells. In edible plants, these may be less of a problem if the foods are cooked, since the lectins are denatured and therefore susceptible to intestinal proteases. On the other hand, lectins in uncooked plants are very stable to proteases and can therefore cause serious problems. For example, raw soybean lectin and wheat germ lectin can apparently affect gastrointestinal function since they cause the release of cholecystokinin. Raw navy beans alter the intestinal microflora and cause intestinal dysfunction.

Ricin, produced by the castor bean plant, is among the most poisonous proteins known to man. These types of toxic lectins are usually composed of several subunits, one of which is the carbohydrate recognizing or binding site, while the other subunit is an enzyme that can catalytically inactivate ribosomes. Thus a single molecule of this catalytic subunit entering a cell can completely block protein synthesis in that cell. Other toxic lectins include modeccin, abrin and mistletoe lectin I.

I-CELL DISEASE

I-cell disease (mucolipidosis II) and pseudo-Hurler polydystrophy (mucolipidosis III) are rare inherited diseases that are due to deficiencies in the machinery that targets lysosomal enzymes to lysosomes.

Comment. I-cell disease results from a deficiency of the enzyme, GlcNAc-1-P transferase, such that lysosomal enzymes do not acquire the targeting signal (Man-6-P residues on their N-linked oligosaccharides). As a consequence, these enzymes are secreted from cells, rather than transported to lysosomes. Fibroblasts from individuals with this disease have dense inclusion bodies (hence the term 'I-cell') and are deficient in many lysosomal enzymes. The lysosomes become engorged with undigested substrates, leading to death in infancy.

oligosaccharides obtained from ZP3 also have sperm-binding activity and inhibit fertilization *in vitro*. Differences between the *O*-glycan structures of cytotoxic lymphocytes and helper cells involved in the immune response are also believed to be important in mediating cellular interactions during the immune response.

Lectins – plant and animal carbohydrate-binding proteins

Lectins are defined as proteins that do not have enzymatic activity but that reversibly bind monosaccharides and oligosaccharides with high specificity. They can be present either in the soluble fraction of cells or in the membranes. Lectins were first discovered in the seeds of various plants because extracts of these seeds caused the agglutination of specific types of red blood cells (hemagglutination reaction). This activity was later shown to result from the interaction of the lectin with a glycan on the surfaces of the red blood cells. Some of the well-known plant lectins are Concanavalin A which recognizes mannose and specifically binds high-mannose types of oligosaccharides, phytohemagglutinin which recognizes galactose and GalNAc and binds to complex types of glycans such as those on brush border membranes, and peanut lectin which also recognizes galactose and binds to complex oligosaccharides.

The function of plant lectins are unknown, but some of them such as ricin are highly toxic to animal cells as well as to insects (see box). In fact, one function that has been

structures on the surface of the complementary cell. This interaction provides for specific cell recognition, and is a key factor in fertilization, inflammation, development and differentiation (see box).

Variations in mucin structure appear to have a role in the specificity of fertilization, cell differentiation, development of the immune response, and virus infectivity. Glycoprotein ZP3, present on the zona pellucida of the mouse egg, functions as a receptor for sperm during fertilization. Enzymatic removal of *O*-linked oligosaccharides from ZP3 results in loss of sperm receptor activity, whereas removal of the N-linked oligosaccharides has no effect on sperm binding. The isolated *O*-linked

proposed for plant lectins is that they provide a defense for the plant against predators or against bacterial or fungal pathogens. Plant lectins have been very useful to researchers in many areas of biology since they provide valuable tools for the isolation and/or detection of specific carbohydrate structures as well as glycoproteins (via their specific carbohydrate structure) or glycolipids. They have been used for blood typing because of their ability to distinguish carbohydrate determinants in human blood cells, and for histochemical studies in lectin-blotting assays, as well as for chromatographic separations of various structures.

Carbohydrate-binding proteins are also present in animal cells, as well as in the microbial world. In animal cells, they were first noticed for their role in reaggregation of dissociated sponge (algae) cells, and this phenomenon was proposed to involve cell–cell recognition. Sometime later, lectins were proposed to be involved in homing of cells such as leukocytes to different internal organs (see box). The first direct evidence for lectins in mammalian cells was the isolation of a receptor protein from hepatocytes that bound circulating blood glycoproteins that had either lost or had the terminal sialic acids removed from their N-linked oligosaccharides. This 'lectin' was referred to as the asialoglycoprotein receptor and was shown to be a galactose-binding lectin.

Animal lectins were originally classified according to the carbohydrate structures that they recognized. However, now, with the potential for molecular cloning of proteins, they can be classified on the basis of amino acid sequence homologies and their relation by evolutionary classification. Thus the family of C-type lectins include some 20 members that share a common lectin sequence motif and require Ca^{++} for binding but have a variable carbohydrate recognition domain. On the other hand the S-type lectin family all recognize β-galactoside structures and do not require Ca^{++} for binding. Other families of lectins include P-types, I-types, and so on.

Several of the animal lectins have been crystallized, permitting study of the molecular interactions of protein and carbohydrate at the level of atomic resolution. Several principles have evolved concerning the N and O-glycans and their lectins. First, the binding sites are generally of low affinity and occur in shallow indentations at the protein surface. A second point is that selectivity or specificity is achieved by a combination of hydrogen bonding, van der Waals forces and hydrophobic interactions between the sugars and the side chains on the amino acids. Finally, the region of contact between the carbohydrate and the protein usually involves only one to three monosaccharide residues. Although the binding sites are generally of low affinity, they are quite specific in terms of carbohydrate structures recognized.

The S-type lectins, recently termed galectins, represent a family of proteins that bind β-galactoside terminal glycoconjugates, and within the family they share structural homo-

INFLAMMATION

An important example of carbohydrate-dependent cell-cell interactions occurs during inflammation. Injury to vascular endothelial cells elicits an inflammatory response that causes the release of cytokines (proteins affecting cell migration) from the injured tissue. The cytokines attract leukocytes to the site of the injury or infection to remove the invading organisms or damaged tissue. These leukocytes must be able to exit from the blood flow and attach to the injured tissue. They are able to do this because they have a tetrasaccharide, known as sialyl Lewis-X antigen, as a component of a membrane glycoprotein or glycolipid. The sialyl Lewis-X antigen is recognized by a lectin, E-selectin, that is present on the surface of the endothelial cells. The interaction between E-selectin and the sialyl Lewis-X antigen enables the leukocytes to adhere to the vascular wall even under the shear forces of the circulation. Figure 25.14 presents a model demonstrating the chemistry of this important interaction. Selectins mediate the initial adhesive step, which is described as tethering, then a 'rolling' of leukocytes along the endothelial cell surface. In fact, leukocytes also contain a selectin, L-selectin, that probably interacts with a saccharide structure on the endothelial cells. These weak binding interactions enable leukocytes to penetrate the interstitial layer and clean up the site of injury. (See also Chapter 36.) While adherence of leukocytes to endothelial cells is important in fighting infection, it can be dangerous. In coronary disease, the leukocytes contribute to the development of atherosclerotic plaque, leading to ischemia (see also Chapter 17). Because of the significance of this interaction, many laboratories are seeking to develop novel chemicals, known as glycomimetics, that mimic the sialyl Lewis-X structure. Administration of these drugs to patients who have suffered a heart attack should theoretically block the selectin sites, inhibiting the binding of leukocytes to the vascular wall and diminishing the probability of further ischemia.

logy in their carbohydrate recognition domains (CRD). Galectins are widely distributed throughout the animal kingdom and play a key role in many cell–cell interactions. Some galectins can induce apoptosis or programmed cell death; others induce metabolic changes such as cellular activation and mitosis.

Summary

Sugars are common components of proteins, added during the synthesis and transport of proteins in the rough endoplasmic reticulum and Golgi apparatus. Individual glycoproteins may have multiple types of

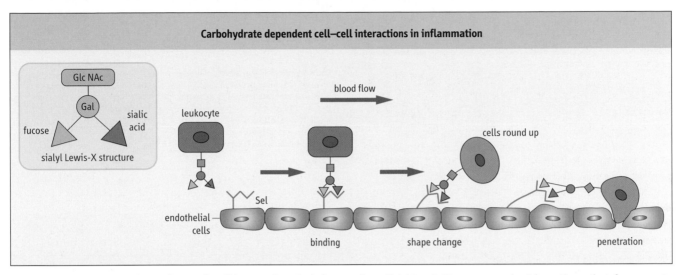

Fig. 25.14 **Carbohydrate dependent cell–cell interactions in inflammation.** Sialyl Lewis-X, a tetrasaccharide antigen that forms part of the membrane structure of leukocytes, is recognized by a carbohydrate-binding protein, E-selectin (Sel), on the surface of endothelial cells. Leukocytes are first retarded by, then roll along, and eventually penetrate the endothelial monolayer. In addition, leukocytes contain L-selectins, proteins that recognize saccharide structures on endothelial cells. Multiple copies of both carbohydrates and receptors participate in and strengthen these cell:cell interactions.

LECTIN-CARBOHYDRATE INTERACTIONS AND INFECTION

Some lectin-carbohydrate interactions may be harmful to animal cells. Many bacterial pathogens use this type of interaction to allow them to bind to specific host cells and gain entry into the body. One example is the influenza virus, which uses a hemagglutinin protein on its surface to bind sialic acid residues on target cells.

Comment. Pathogenic enteric bacteria, such as Enterobacter cloacae, have surface structures called pili (or fimbriae) that contain a protein subunit with lectin activity. This protein binds to high-mannose oligosaccharides that are components of N-linked glycoproteins on the surface of intestinal epithelial cells. This binding frequently leads to infection and, in some cases, severe disease.

oligosaccharides, linked to asparagine (in *N*-linked, plasma-type glycoproteins), or serine, threonine (in *O*-linked, mucin-type glycoproteins) or hydroxylysine (in collagen) residues in the proteins. The oligosaccharides are synthesized by glycosyl transferases, using sugar nucleotide or dolichol-phosphate-sugar donors; all of these activated forms of sugars can be derived from glucose. Oligosaccharides on glycoproteins display characteristic structural motifs, but the structures may vary

in completeness, i.e. they are microheterogeneous in nature. The carbohydrates serve a number of different functions in glycoproteins, including modification of the physical properties of the protein (solubility, stability, viscosity), and assisting in its folding, processing, transport, and targeting. Because sugars are located on the surfaces of cells, they are in an excellent position to act as informational molecules, mediating recognition reactions between cells or with other molecules in the environment.

Further reading

Asano N. Glycosidase inhibitors: update and perspectives on practical use. *Glycobiology* 2003;**13**:93R–104R.

Boehncke WH, Schon MP. Interfering with leukocyte rolling – a promising therapeutic approach in inflammatory skin disorders? *Trends Pharmacol Sci* 2003;**24**:49–52.

Elbein AD. Glycosylation inhibitors. *Annu Rev Biochem* 1987;**56**:497–534.

Gorelik E, Galili U, Raz A. On the role of cell surface carbohydrates and their binding proteins (lectins) in tumor metastasis. *Cancer Metastasis Rev* 2001;**20**:245–277.

Marquardt T, Denecke J. Congenital disorders of glycosylation: review of their molecular bases, clinical presentations and specific therapies. *Eur J Pediatr* 2003;**162**:359–379.

Mouricout M. Interactions between the enteric pathogens and the host. An assortment of bacterial lectins and a set of glycoconjugate receptors. *Adv Exp Med Biol* 1997;**412**:109–123.

Novelli G, Reichardt JK. Molecular basis of disorders of human galactose metabolism: past, present, and future. *Mol Genet Metab* 2000;**71**:62–65.

Rubin BK. Physiology of airway mucus clearance. *Respir Care* 2002;**47**:761–768.

ACTIVE LEARNING

1. Why do eukaryotic cells use lipid-linked oligosaccharides as intermediates in synthesis of *N*-linked oligosaccharides but not *O*-linked oligosaccharides?
2. Do animal cells need amino sugars in the diet in order to synthesize complex carbohydrates? If not, why not? Review the use of glucosamine-chondroitin supplements for the treatment of arthritis.
3. Why are sugars converted to nucleoside diphosphate sugars before they are polymerized?

Websites

Carbohydrate-deficient glycoprotein syndrome:
  http://www.familyvillage.wisc.edu/lib_cdgs.htm
Galactosemia: http://www.galactosemia.org; http://www.galactosemia.com/
Hereditary Fructose Intolerance: http://www.bu.edu/aldolase/HFI/
I-Cell Disease: http://www.emedicine.com/ped/topic1150.htm;
www.mpssociety.org/images/pdfs/ booklets/I-Cell%20final.pdf
Lectins: http://www.dadamo.com/lectin-kb.htm

26. Complex Lipids

A D Elbein

LEARNING OBJECTIVES

After reading this chapter you should be able to:

- Classify the major phospholipids and explain their function in the cell.
- Describe how the various glycerol-based phospholipids are synthesized and how they are inter-converted.
- Describe the multiple roles of cytidine nucleotides in activation of intermediates in phospholipid synthesis.
- Describe the various types of sphingolipids and glycolipids that occur in mammalian cells and their functions.
- Explain the etiology of lysosomal storage diseases, their pathology, and the rationale for enzyme replacement therapy for treatment of these diseases.

INTRODUCTION

The term 'complex lipids' refers to a diverse group of water-insoluble compounds found in biological membranes. They are characterized by the following general properties:

- **They are water insoluble**, but soluble in nonpolar organic solvents, such as chloroform, ether, or benzene;
- **they may be polar or nonpolar** triacylglycerols and cholesterol esters are nonpolar, while phospholipids and sphingolipids are polar;
- **they may be saponifiable:** the ester bonds of glycerophospholipids are saponifiable, while the amide bonds of sphingolipids are not saponifiable.

Polar lipids are amphipathic, meaning that they contain both a hydrophobic domain that forms the membrane environment and a hydrophilic domain that interacts with the aqueous environment. Polar lipids are the major components of all biological membranes, and have other, diverse functions in the cell. This chapter discusses the structure, biosynthesis, and function of the two major classes of polar lipids: glycerophospholipids and sphingolipids.

GLYCEROPHOSPHOLIPIDS (PHOSPHOLIPIDS)

Structure of phospholipids

The term 'phospholipid', introduced in Chapter 7, commonly refers to the major class of membrane lipids, glycerophospholipids, or phosphoglycerides. They contain a diacylglycerol (DAG) phosphate (phosphatidic acid) backbone. In addition to phosphatidylcholine, phosphatidylethanolamine, and phosphatidylserine, there are a number of more complicated structures, such as phosphatidylglycerol and diphosphatidylglycerol (cardiolipin), which are found in mitochondrial membranes, and phosphatidylinositol, which has a role in signal transduction and in anchoring proteins in the plasma membrane (Fig. 26.1).

Phospholipids from any natural source contain a spectrum of fatty acids. For example, phosphatidylcholine usually contains palmitic acid (C-16:0) or stearic acid (C-18:0) at its carbon-1 position and an 18-carbon, unsaturated fatty acid (e.g. oleic, linoleic, or linolenic) at its carbon-2 position (C-16:0 represents a 16-carbon fatty acid with no double bonds, while C-18:1 represents an 18-carbon fatty acid with one unsaturated (C=C) bond). Phosphatidylethanolamine usually has a longer-chain fatty acid at carbon-2, such as arachidonic acid (C-20:4). In addition to forming the backbone of the membrane, these complex lipids contribute charge to the membrane: phosphatidylcholine and phosphatidylethanolamine are zwitterionic at physiologic pH and have no net charge, but the other glycerophospholipids and the major species of sphingolipids are anionic in nature.

Biosynthesis of precursors: phosphatidic acid and diacylglycerol (DAG)

All animal cells, except for erythrocytes, are able to synthesize phospholipids *de novo*, whereas triglyceride synthesis occurs mainly in liver, adipose tissue, and intestinal cells. As shown in Figure 26.2, phosphatidic acid and 1,2-DAG are common intermediates in the synthesis of both triacylglycerols and phospholipids. Glycerol-3-phosphate is the primary starting material for synthesis of phosphatidic acid;

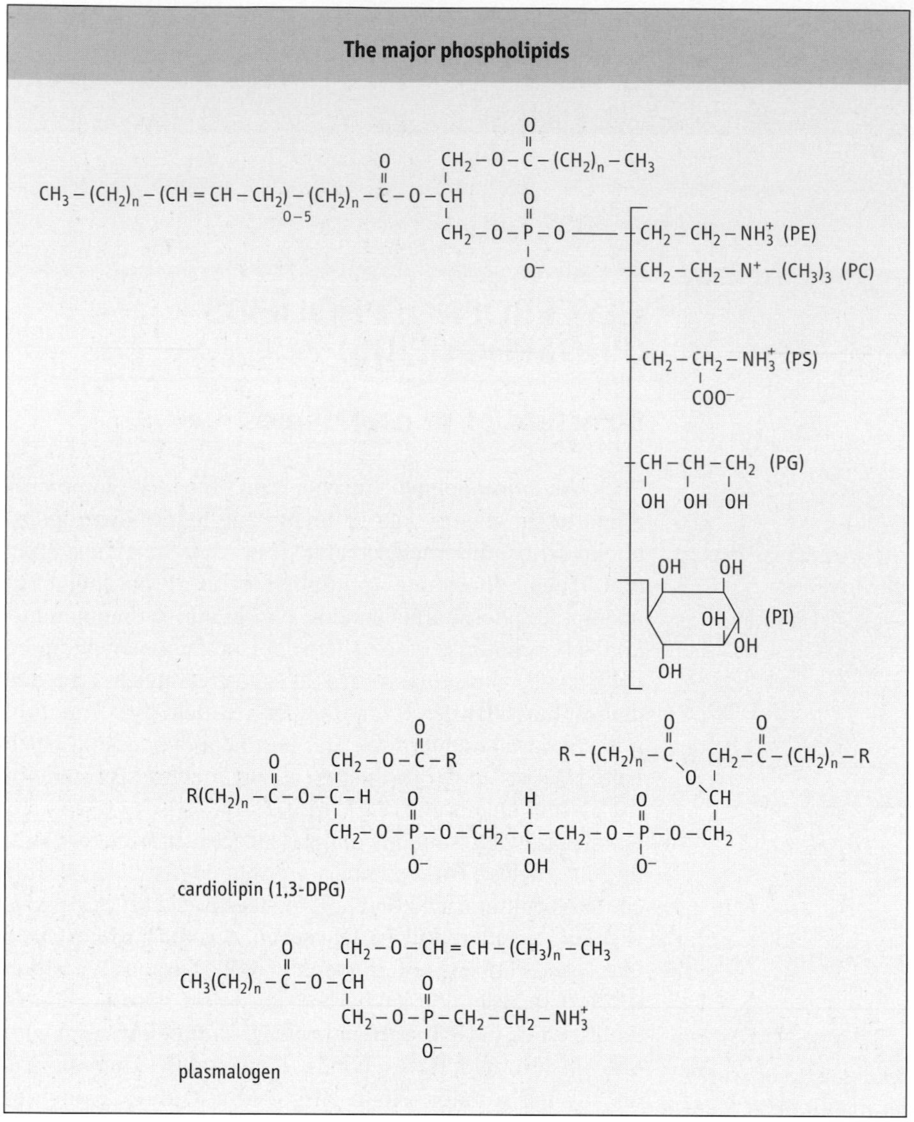

The major phospholipids

Fig. 26.1 **Structure of the major phospholipids of animal cell membranes.** DPG, diphosphatidylglycerol; PC, phosphatidylcholine; PE, phosphatidylethanolamine; PG, phosphatidylglycerol; PI, phosphatidylinositol; PS, phosphatidylserine.

it is formed in most tissues by reduction of the glycolytic intermediate, dihydroxyacetone phosphate (DHAP). In liver, kidney, and intestine, glycerol-3-P can also be formed directly via phosphorylation of glycerol by a specific kinase.

Glycerol-3-P is acylated by transfer of two long-chain fatty acids from fatty acyl-CoA to the hydroxyl groups at carbons 1 and 2, producing phosphatidic acid. The first fatty acid – usually a saturated fatty acid – is added to carbon-1, forming lysophosphatidic acid; the prefix 'lyso' indicates that one of the hydroxyl groups is not acylated. Then, a second fatty acid – usually an unsaturated fatty acid – is added to carbon-2 to form phosphatidic acid. DHAP may also be acylated by addition of a fatty acid to the 1-hydroxyl group, and this intermediate is then reduced and acylated to phosphatidic acid. Phosphatidic acid is converted to DAG by a specific cytosolic phosphatase.

Biosynthesis of phospholipids

The biosynthesis of lecithin (phosphatidylcholine) from DAG requires activation of choline to a cytidine diphosphate (CDP) nucleotide derivative. In this series of reactions, shown in Figure 26.4, the choline 'head-group' is converted to phosphocholine, and then activated to CDP-choline by a pyrophosphorylase reaction. The pyrophosphate bond is cleaved, and phosphocholine is then transferred to DAG to form lecithin. This reaction is analogous to the transfer of glucose from UDP-glucose to glycogen, except that both the choline and phosphate groups are transferred to DAG. Phosphatidylethanolamine is formed by a similar pathway using cytidine triphosphate (CTP) and phosphoethanolamine, to form CDP-ethanolamine.

Formation and conversion of phosphatidic acid

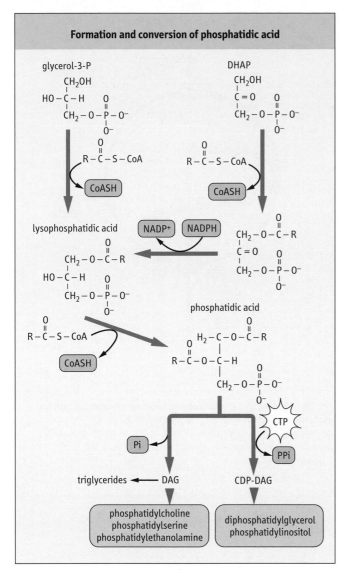

Fig. 26.2 **Pathway of formation of phosphatidic acid and its conversion to diacylglycerol (DAG) and major phospholipids.** CDP, cytidine diphosphate; CTP, cytidine triphosphate; CoASH, coenzyme A; DHAP, dihydroxyacetone phosphate; Pi, inorganic phosphate; PPi, inorganic pyrophosphate.

 ## PLATELET ACTIVATING FACTOR AND HYPERSENSITIVITY

Platelet activating factor (PAF; Fig. 26.3) contains an acetyl group at carbon-2 of glycerol and a saturated 18-carbon alkyl ether group linked to the hydroxyl group at carbon-1, rather than the usual long-chain fatty acids of phosphatidylcholine. It is a major mediator of hypersensitivity reactions, acute inflammatory reactions, and anaphylactic shock, and affects the permeability properties of membranes, increasing platelet aggregation and causing cardiovascular and pulmonary changes, including edema and hypotension. In allergic persons, cells involved in the immune response become coated with immunoglobulin E (IgE) molecules that are specific for a particular antigen or allergen, such as pollen or insect venom. When these individuals are re-exposed to that antigen, antigen-IgE complexes form on the surface of the inflammatory cells and initiate the synthesis and release of PAF.

Platelet activating factor and hypersensitivity

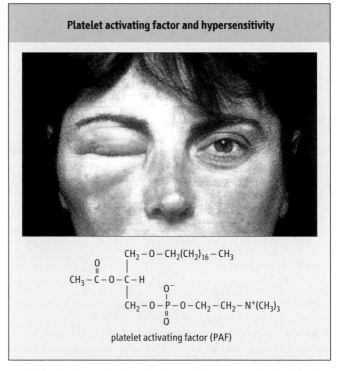

platelet activating factor (PAF)

Fig. 26.3 **Platelet activating factor and hypersensitivity.** PAF is a major mediator of acute inflammatory reactions, such as the anaphylactic response to bee venom seen in this patient. (Courtesy of Professor Jonathan Brostoff.)

Both phosphatidylcholine and phosphatidylethanolamine can react with free serine by an exchange reaction to form phosphatidylserine and the free base, choline or ethanolamine (Fig. 26.5). In a secondary pathway, phosphatidylcholine can also be formed by methylation of phosphatidylethanolamine with the methyl donor, S-adenosylmethionine (SAM) (Fig. 26.6). The methylation pathway involves the sequential transfer of three activated methyl groups from three different molecules of SAM. Liver also has another route to phosphatidylethanolamine, involving decarboxylation of phosphatidylserine by a specific mitochondrial decarboxylase.

Phospholipids that have an alcohol as the head group, e.g. phosphatidylglycerol and phosphatidylinositol, are synthesized by an alternative pathway, which also involves activation by cytidine nucleotides. In this case, the phosphatidic acid is activated, rather than the head group, yielding

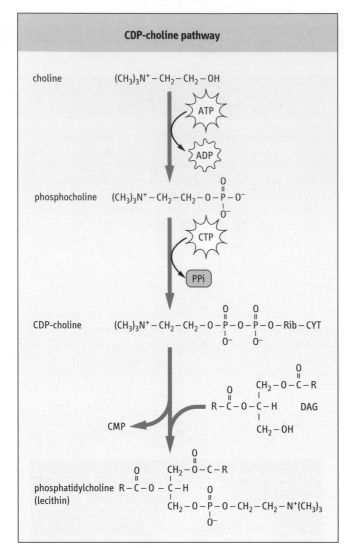

Fig. 26.4 **Formation of phosphatidylcholine by the CDP-choline pathway.** CYT, cytosine; CDP, cytidine diphosphate, CMP, cytidine monophosphate; DAG, diacyl glycerol; Rib, ribose. CTP, cytidine triphosphate.

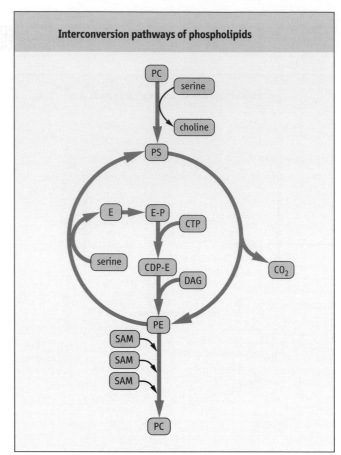

Fig. 26.5 **Pathways of interconversion of phospholipids by exchange of head groups, by methylation or by decarboxylation.** E, ethanolamine, DAG, diacylglycerol; PC, phosphatidylcholine; PS, phosphatidylserine; SAM, S-adenosylmethionine.

SURFACTANT FUNCTION OF PHOSPHOLIPIDS

Acute respiratory distress syndrome (ARDS) accounts for 15–20% of neonatal mortality in Western countries. The disease affects only premature infants and its incidence is directly related to the degree of prematurity.

Comment. Immature lungs do not have enough type II epithelial cells to synthesize sufficient amounts of the phospholipid, dipalmitoylphosphatidylcholine (DPPC). This phospholipid makes up more than 80% of the total phospholipids of the extracellular lipid layer that lines the alveoli of normal lungs. DPPC decreases the surface tension of the aqueous surface layer of the lungs, facilitating opening of the alveoli during inspiration. Lack of surfactant causes the lungs to collapse during the expiration phase of breathing, leading to ARDS. The maturity of the fetal lung can be determined by measuring the lecithin:sphingomyelin ratio in amniotic fluid. If there is a potential problem, a mother can be treated with a glucocorticoid to accelerate maturation of the fetal lung. ARDS is also seen in adults in whom the type II epithelial cells have been destroyed as a result of the use of immunosuppressive drugs or certain chemotherapeutic agents.

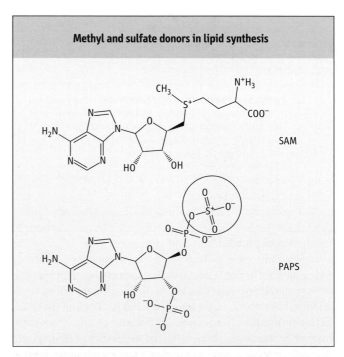

Fig. 26.6 **Structures of the methyl and sulfate donors involved in the synthesis of membrane lipids.**
SAM, S-adenosylmethionine; PAPS, 3'-phosphoadenosine-5'-phosphosulfate (active sulfate).

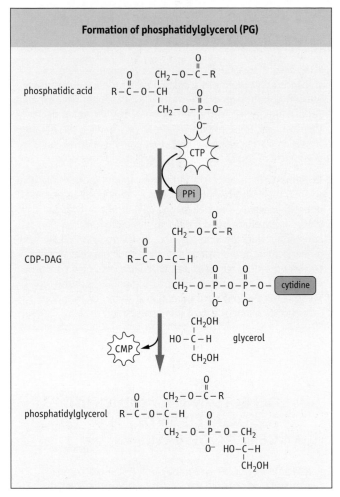

Fig. 26.7 **Formation of phosphatidylglycerol by activation of phophatidic acid to form CDP-DAG, and transfer of DAG to glycerol.** CMP, cytidine monophosphate; CTP, cytidine triphosphate.

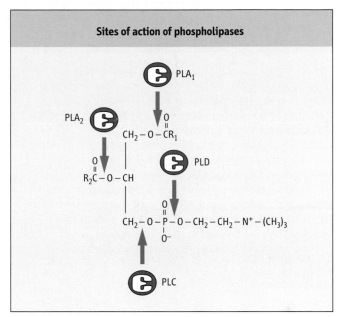

Fig. 26.8 **Sites of action of phospholipases on phosphatidylcholine.** PLA_1, PLA_2, PLC, PLD are phospholipases A_1, A_2, C, and D, respectively.

tection against oxidative stress in tissues with active aerobic metabolism.

Turnover of phospholipids

Phospholipids are in a continuous state of turnover in most membranes. This occurs as a result of oxidative damage, during inflammation, and through activation of lipases, particularly in response to hormonal stimuli. As shown in Figure 26.8, there are number of phospholipases that act on specific bonds in the phospholipid structure. Phospholipases A_2 (PLA_2) and C (PLC) are particularly active during the inflammatory response and in signal transduction. Phospholipase B (not shown) is a lysophospholipase that removes the second acyl group after action of PLA_1 or PLA_2. The lysophospholipids and other products are recycled by scavenger pathways.

CDP-DAG (Fig. 26.7). The phosphatidic acid group is then transferred to free glycerol or inositol, to form phosphatidylglycerol or phosphatidylinositol, respectively. A second phosphatidic acid may also be added to phosphatidylglycerol to form diphosphatidylglycerol (DPG) (see Fig. 26.1).

Plasmalogens

Plasmalogens are a subclass of glycerophospholipids that have a 1-alkenyl ether linked to the carbon-1 of glycerol (see Fig. 26.1). They are a major class of mitochondrial lipids, and are enriched in nerve and muscle tissue – in the heart they may account for nearly 50% of total phospholipids. Their function in relation to that of diacylphospholipids is not clear, but there is some evidence that they are more resistant to oxidative degradation, which may provide pro-

SPHINGOLIPIDS

Structure and biosynthesis of sphingosine

Sphingolipids are a complex group of amphipathic, polar lipids. They are built on a core structure of the long-chain amino alcohol, sphingosine, which is formed by oxidative decarboxylation and condensation of palmitate with serine. In all sphingolipids, the long-chain fatty acid is attached to

GLYCOSYLPHOSPHATIDYLINOSITOL MEMBRANE ANCHORS

Phosphatidylinositol is an integral component of the glycosylphosphatidylinositol (GPI) structure that anchors various proteins to the plasma membrane (Fig. 26.9). In contrast to other membrane phospholipids, including most of the membrane phosphatidylinositol, GPI has a glycan chain containing glucosamine and mannose attached to the inositol. Ethanolamine connects the GPI-glycan to the carboxyl terminus of the protein. Many membrane proteins in eukaryotic cells are anchored by a GPI structure, including alkaline phosphatase and acetylcholinesterase. In contrast to integral or peripheral membrane proteins, GPI-anchored proteins may be released from the cell surface by phospholipase C in response to regulatory processes.

VARIABLE SURFACE ANTIGENS OF TRYPANOSOMES

The parasitic trypanosome that causes sleeping sickness, *Trypanosoma brucei*, has a protein called the variable surface antigen bound to its cell surface by a GPI anchor. This variable surface antigen elicits the formation of specific antibodies in the host, and these antibodies can attack and kill the parasite. However, some of the parasites evade immune surveillance by shedding this antigen, as if they were shedding a coat.

Comment. Trypanosomes and some other pathogens are able to shed their surface antigens because they have an enzyme, phospholipase C, that cleaves the GPI anchor at the inositol-phosphate bond, releasing the protein-glycan component into the external fluid. Surviving cells rapidly make a new coat with a different antigenic structure that will not be recognized by the antibody. Of course, this new coat will elicit the formation of new specific antibodies, but the parasite can again shed this coat, and so on, in a random sequence to evade the host immune system.

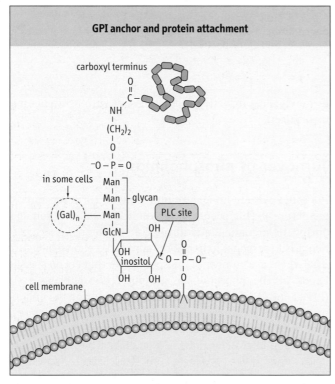

Fig. 26.9 **Structure of the glycosylphosphatidylinositol (GPI) anchor and its attachment to proteins.** Gal, galactose; GlcN, glucosamine; Man, mannose; PLC, phospholipase C.

DEFECTS IN GPI ANCHORING ASSOCIATED WITH GENETIC DISEASE

Paroxysmal nocturnal hemoglobinuria (PNH) is a complex hematologic disorder characterized by hemolytic anemia, venous thrombosis in unusual sites, and deficient hematopoiesis. The diagnosis of this disease is based on the unusual sensitivity of the red blood cells to the hemolytic action of Complement (Chapter 36), because red cells from patients with PNH lack several proteins that are involved in regulating the activation of Complement at the cell surface.

Comment. One of these cell-surface proteins is decay accelerating factor, a GPI-anchored protein that inactivates a hemolytic complex formed during Complement activation; in its absence, there is increased hemolysis. There are several genetic variants of PNH. One of these involves a defect in the GlcNAc transferase that adds *N*-acetylglucosamine to the inositol moiety of phosphatidylinositol, the first step in GPI anchor formation (Fig. 26.2).

the amino group of the sphingosine in an amide linkage (Fig. 26.10). Because of the alkaline stability of amides, compared to esters, sphingolipids are non-saponifiable, which facilitates their separation from alkali-labile glycerophospholipids.

The synthesis of the sphingosine base of sphingolipids involves condensation of palmitoyl-CoA with serine, in

which the carbon-1 of serine is lost as carbon dioxide. The product of this reaction is converted in several steps to sphingosine, which is then *N*-acylated to form ceramide (*N*-acylsphingosine). Ceramide (see Fig. 26.10) is the precursor and backbone structure of both sphingomyelin and glycosphingolipids.

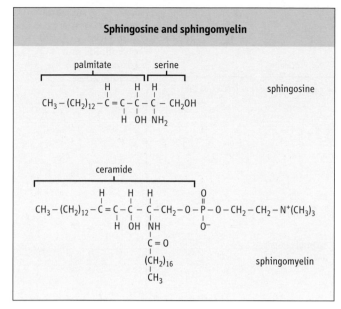

Sphingosine and sphingomyelin

palmitate   serine

sphingosine

$$CH_3-(CH_2)_{12}-\overset{\underset{|}{H}}{C}=\overset{\underset{|}{C}}{C}-\overset{\underset{|}{C}}{\underset{OH}{C}}-\overset{\underset{|}{C}}{\underset{NH_2}{C}}-CH_2OH$$

ceramide

$$CH_3-(CH_2)_{12}-\overset{\underset{|}{H}}{C}=\overset{\underset{|}{C}}{C}-\overset{\underset{|}{C}}{\underset{OH}{C}}-\overset{\underset{|}{C}}{\underset{NH}{C}}-CH_2-O-\overset{\overset{O}{||}}{\underset{O^-}{P}}-O-CH_2-CH_2-N^+(CH_3)_3$$

C = O
|
(CH_2)_{16}   sphingomyelin
|
CH_3

Fig. 26.10 Structures of sphingosine and sphingomyelin.

Sphingomyelin

Sphingomyelin (Fig. 26.10) is found in plasma membranes, subcellular organelles, endoplasmic reticulum, and mitochondria. It comprises 5–20% of the total phospholipids in most cell types, and is mostly localized in the plasma membrane. It is the only sphingolipid that contains phosphorus, and is the major phospholipid of the myelin sheath of nerves. The phosphocholine group in sphingomyelin is transferred to the terminal hydroxyl group of sphingosine from phosphatidylcholine. The fatty acid composition varies, but long-chain fatty acids are common, including lignoceric (C-24:0), cerebronic (2-hydroxylignoceric) and nervonic (24:1) acids.

Glycolipids

Sphingolipids containing covalently bound sugars are known as glycosphingolipids, or glycolipids. The cell's complement of carbohydrate structures on glycolipids (and glycoproteins) does not depend on a template mechanism for synthesis, as do nucleic acids and proteins. Instead, it is determined by the enzymatic makeup of the cell (that is, its content of glycosyltransferases), and on how these various enzymes are expressed with respect to each other. The glycosyltransferase distribution and glycosphingolipid content of cells

varies during development and in response to regulatory processes.

Glycolipids can be classified into four different groups: cerebrosides, sulfatides, globosides, and gangliosides. In all of these compounds, the polar head-group – comprising the sugars – is attached to ceramide by a glycosidic bond at the terminal hydroxyl group of sphingosine; Figure 26.11 illustrates this, together with the pathways involved in the biosynthesis of some of the more complex members of the group. The simplest of the glycosphingolipids are the gluco- and galacto-cerebrosides (glucosyl and galactosyl ceramides), which have a single sugar attached to sphingosine. Sulfatides are formed by addition of sulfate from the sulfate donor, 3'-phosphoadenosine-5'-phosphosulfate (PAPS) (see Fig. 26.6), yielding, for example, galactocerebroside 3-sulfate. When the carbohydrate portion of the cerebroside contains two or more neutral sugars plus an N-acetyl-galactosamine (GalNAc), it is referred to as a globoside. Finally, glycolipids containing sialic acids (N-acetylneuraminic acid, NANA) are termed gangliosides.

Structure and nomenclature of gangliosides

The term 'ganglioside' refers to glycolipids that were originally identified in high concentrations in ganglionic cells of the central nervous system. In cells of the nervous system in general, more than 50% of the sialic acid in the cell is present in gangliosides, and the other 50% is in glycoproteins. Gangliosides are also found in the surface membranes of cells of most extraneural tissues, but in these tissues they account for less than 10% of the total sialic acid.

The nomenclature used to identify the various gangliosides is based on the number of sialic acid residues contained in the molecule, and on the sequence of the carbohydrates (Fig. 26.12). 'GM' means a ganglioside with a single (mono) sialic acid, whereas GD, GT and GQ would indicate two, three and four sialic acid residues in the molecule, respectively. The number after the GM, e.g. GM_1 refers to the structure of the oligosaccharide. These numbers were derived from the relative mobility of the glycolipids on thin layer chromatograms; the larger, GM_1, gangliosides migrate the most slowly. These complex structures are built up, one sugar residue at a time, in the Golgi apparatus, and are degraded by a series of exoglycosidases in lysosomes (Fig. 26.13). Defects in sequential degradation of glycolipids lead to a number of lysosomal storage diseases, known as cerebrosidoses and gangliosidoses (see box on p. 384).

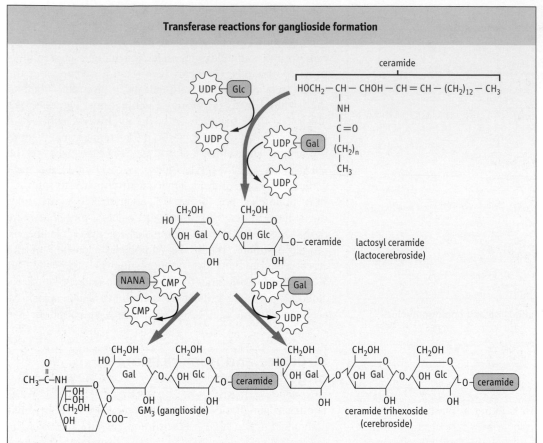

Transferase reactions for ganglioside formation

Fig. 26.11 **An outline of transferase reactions for elongation of glycolipids and formation of gangliosides.**

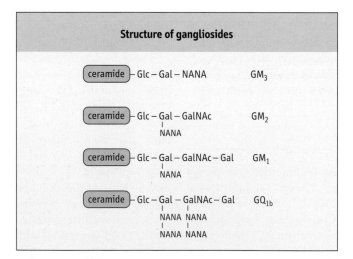

Structure of gangliosides

ceramide — Glc – Gal – NANA		GM₃

ceramide — Glc – Gal – NANA   GM$_3$

ceramide — Glc – Gal – GalNAc   GM$_2$
                              |
                            NANA

ceramide — Glc – Gal – GalNAc – Gal   GM$_1$
                              |
                            NANA

ceramide — Glc – Gal – GalNAc – Gal   GQ$_{1b}$
                              | |
                            NANA   NANA
                              | |
                            NANA   NANA

Fig. 26.12 **Generalized structures of gangliosides.** Glc, glucose; Gal, galactose; NANA, N-acetyl neuraminic acid; GalNAc, N-acetylgalactosamine.

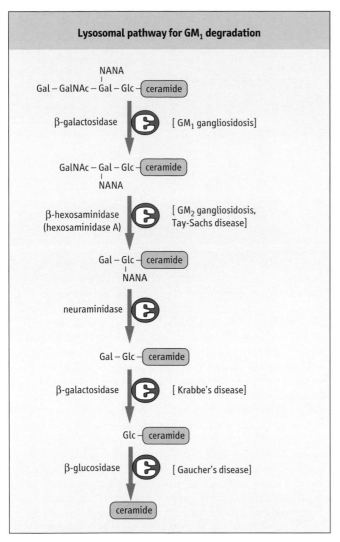

Lysosomal pathway for GM₁ degradation

Fig. 26.13 **Lysosomal pathway for turnover (degradation) of ganglioside GM1 in human cells.** Various enzymes may be missing in specific lipid storage diseases, as indicated in Table 26.1. Gal, galactose; GalNAc, N-acetylgalactosamine; Glc, glucose; NANA, N-acetyl neuraminic acid.

LYSOSOMAL STORAGE DISEASES RESULTING FROM DEFECTS IN SPHINGOMYELIN DEGRADATION

Niemann–Pick syndrome is a lysosomal storage disease characterized by the formation of lipid-laden phagocytes, known as 'foam cells', that are engorged with sphingomyelin. There is no treatment for this disease, but its inheritance is autosomal recessive and, if carriers are identified, prenatal diagnosis is possible by amniocentesis and assay of sphingomyelinase activity in fetal fibroblasts.

Comment. Niemann–Pick syndrome results from a deficiency in the activity of the enzyme, acid sphingomyelinase. In one of the final steps in sphingolipid turnover, this enzyme cleaves the sphingolipid to release choline phosphate and ceramide. Absence of this enzyme leads to accumulation of sphingomyelin in lysosomes.

GAUCHER'S DISEASE-A MODEL FOR ENZYME REPLACEMENT THERAPY

Gaucher's disease is a lysosomal storage disease in which afflicted individuals are missing the enzyme glucocerebrosidase. This enzyme removes the final sugar from the ceramide, allowing the lipid portion to be further degraded in the lysosomes. This disease is characterized by hepatomegaly and neurodegenerative disease, but there are milder variants that are amenable to treatment by enzyme replacement therapy.

For treatment of Gaucher's disease, exogenous β-glucosidase was successfully targeted to the lysosomes of macrophages using a cell surface mannose receptor. In order to do this successfully, it was necessary to produce the recombinant replacement enzyme with N-glycan chains containing terminal mannose residues. This was done by cleaving the glycans of the enzyme produced in mammalian cells with a combination of sialidase (neuraminidase), β-galactosidase and β-hexosaminidase to trim the complex chains down to the mannose core. An alternative recombinant glucosidase has been produced in a baculovirus-infected insect cell system. In this case, the enzyme has a high mannose oligosaccharide that is not processed to complex chains. The recombinant enzymes are administered intravenously. The success in using glucocerebrosidase for treatment of Gaucher's disease has stimulated the development of other lysosomal hydrolases for treatment of lysosomal storage diseases. In a recent study, the lysosomal enzyme, acid lipase, inhibited the progression of atherosclerosis in a hyperlipidemic mouse model.

FABRY'S DISEASE – (INCIDENCE 1 IN 100,000)

A 30-year-old man is found to have proteinuria at an insurance medical examination. He had been seen over a number of years from around age 10 with headaches, vertigo and shooting pains in his arms and legs. No diagnosis was made and he had grown accustomed to these problems. The physician carefully examined his perineum and scrotum identifying small, raised, red angiokeratoma.

Comment. This gentleman has Fabry's disease, which often takes years before a diagnosis is confirmed by measuring α-galactosidase A activity. His insurance was declined as proteinuria is expected to progress to renal failure within 15 years.

The principal endothelial depositions of globotriaosylceramide occur in the kidney (leading to proteinuria and renal failure), the heart and brain (leading to myocardial infarction and stroke), and around blood vessels supplying nerves (leading to painful paresthesiae). Recombinant enzyme replacement therapy appears to clear the deposited globotriaosylceramide and initial studies suggest that renal function is maintained.

Lipid storage diseases			
Disease	Symptoms	Major storage product	Deficient enzymes
Tay-Sachs	blindness, mental retardation, death between 2nd and 3rd year	GM$_2$ ganglioside	hexosaminidase A
Gaucher's	liver and spleen enlargement, mental retardation in infantile form	glucocerebroside	β-glucosidase
Fabry's	skin rash, kidney failure, pain in lower extremities	ceramide trihexoside	α-galactosidase
Krabbe's	liver and spleen enlargement, mental retardation	galactocerebroside	β-galactosidase

Table 26.1 **Some lipid storage diseases.**

CEREBROSIDOSES AND GANGLIOSIDOSES

Tay–Sachs disease is a gangliosidosis in which GM$_2$ accumulates as a result of an absence of hexosaminidase A. Individuals with this disease usually have mental retardation and blindness and die between 2 and 3 years of age. Fabry's disease is a cerebrosidosis resulting from deficiency of α-galactosidase and accumulation of ceramide trihexoside. The symptoms of Fabry's disease are skin rash, kidney failure, and pain in the lower extremities. Patients with this condition benefit from kidney transplants and usually live into early to mid-adulthood. Most of these lysosomal storage diseases appear in several forms (variants), resulting from different mutations in the genome; some variants are more severe and debilitating than others. Although lysosomal storage diseases are relatively rare, they have had a major impact on our understanding of the function and importance of lysosomes.

Comment. When cells die, their components, including glycosphingolipids and glycoproteins, are degraded to their individual components. Figure 26.13 presents the pathway for the degradation of a ganglioside such as GM1 in the lysosomes. These organelles contain a number of exoglycosidases and other necessary enzymes that function in a prescribed sequence to degrade complex glycolipids. A number of lysosomal diseases result from the absence of one of these essential glycosidases (Table 26.1). The sphingolipidoses are characterized by lysosomal accumulation of the substrate of the missing enzyme. This either causes lysosomes to lyse and release their hydrolytic enzymes into the cell, or prevents the lysosome from functioning normally.

ABO BLOOD-GROUP ANTIGENS ARE GLYCOSPHINGOLIPIDS

Blood transfusion replenishes the oxygen-carrying capacity of blood in persons who suffer from blood loss or anemia. The term 'blood transfusion' is something of a misnomer, because it involves only the infusion of washed and preserved red cells. The membranes of the human red blood cells contain a number of blood group antigenic determinants (as many as 100), of which the ABO blood-group system is the best understood and most widely studied. The antigens in this group are derived from a common precursor, called the H substance, and an individual may have type A, type B, type AB, or type O blood. Individuals with type A cells develop natural antibodies in their plasma that are directed against, and will agglutinate type B and type AB red blood cells; whereas those with type B red cells develop antibodies against A substance and will agglutinate type A and type AB blood. Persons with type AB blood have neither A nor B antibodies, and are called 'universal recipients', as they can be transfused with cells of either blood type. Individuals with type O blood have only H substance, not A or B substance, on their red blood cells, and are 'universal donors', as their red blood cells are not agglutinated with either A or B antibodies; they may accept blood only from a type O donor. The ABO blood-group antigens are complex carbohydrates present as components of glycoproteins or glycosphingolipids of red cell membranes. The precursor of the ABO types is the H substance (Fig. 26.14); the H locus codes for a fucosyltransferase. Individuals with type A blood have, in addition to the H substance, an A gene that codes for a specific GalNAc transferase that adds GalNAc α1,3 to the galactose residue of H substance, to form the A-type glycolipid. Individuals with type B blood have a B gene that codes for a galactosyl transferase that adds galactose α1,3 to the galactose residue of H substance, to form the B-type glycolipid. Individuals with type AB blood have both the GalNAc and the galactosyl transferases, and their red blood cells contain both the A and the B substances. Those with type O blood, and only H substance on their red cell glycosphingolipids, do not make either enzyme. Enzymes such as coffee bean α-galactosidase can remove the galactose from type B red cells, an approach that may be tested for increasing the supply of type O red cells.

OTHER BLOOD GROUP SUBSTANCES ARE ALSO CARBOHYDRATES

The Lewis blood group antigens correspond to a set of $\alpha1,3(4)$-fucosylated glycan structures. The Lewis A antigen (Le^a) is synthesized by fucosyltransferase encoded by the *Lewis (Le)* blood group locus. The Lewis B antigen (Le^b) is synthesized by the concerted action of a second fucosyltransferase encoded by the *Se* (secretor) blood group locus. The nature of the alleles at an individual's *Le* and *Se* loci determines the complement of Lewis-active oligosaccharides that that individual will produce.

The P blood group antigens are membrane glycosphingolipids on red cells and on other tissues. Again, the glycans in this blood group are synthesized by the sequential action of distinct glycosyltransferases, but so far relatively little is known about the enzymes or genes involved. The physiological function for blood groups is unknown, but the P antigens are associated with the pathophysiology of urinary tract infections and parvovirus infections. The basis for implicating P antigens in urinary tract infections is that uropathogenic strains of *E. coli* express lectins that bind to the Gal$\alpha1,4$Gal moiety of the P^k and P$_1$ antigens. Clearly more work is necessary to understand the genetics and biochemistry of these and other blood group antigens as well as their roles in physiology and disease.

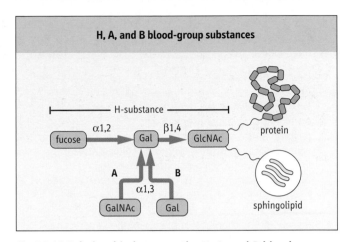

Fig. 26.14 **Relationship between the H, A, and B blood-group substances.** The terminal oligosaccharide is linked through other sugars to proteins and lipids of the red cell membrane. GlcNAc, N-acetylglucosamine; GalNAc, N-acetylgalactosamine; Gal, galactose.

GANGLIOSIDES

Ganglioside receptor for cholera toxin

The galactose-containing cerebrosides and globosides in the plasma membranes of intestinal epithelial cells are binding sites for bacteria. The glycolipids appear to assist in retention of normal intestinal flora (symbionts) in the intestine but, conversely, binding of pathogenic bacteria to these and other glycolipids is believed to facilitate infection of the epithelial cells. The difference between symbiotic and parasitic bacteria depends, in part, on their ability to secrete toxins or to penetrate the host cell after the binding reaction.

Intestinal mucosal cells contain ganglioside GM1 (see Fig. 26.12). This ganglioside serves as the receptor to which cholera toxin binds as the first step in its penetration of intestinal cells. Cholera toxin is a hexameric protein secreted by the bacterium *Vibrio cholerae*. The protein is composed of one A subunit and five B subunits. The protein binds to gangliosides through the B subunits, which enables the A subunit to enter the cell and activate adenylate cyclase on the inner surface of the membrane. The cyclic AMP that is formed then stimulates intestinal cells to export chloride ions, leading to osmotic diarrhea, electrolyte imbalances, and malnutrition. Cholera remains the number one killer of children in the world today.

Summary

Complex polar lipids are essential components of all living cell membranes. Phospholipids are the major structural lipids of all membranes, but they also have important functional properties as surfactants, as cofactors for membrane enzymes, as mediators of hypersensitivity, and as components of signal transduction systems. The primary route for *de novo* biosynthesis of phospholipids involves the activation of one of the components (either DAG or the head group) with CTP to form a high-energy intermediate, such as CDP-diglyceride or CDP-choline. In addition, there are exchange and modification reactions by which the animal cell interconverts various phospholipids. The other major types of membrane lipids are the sphingolipids, including sphingomyelin and various glycolipids. These lipids function as receptors for cell-cell recognition and interactions, and as binding sites for symbiotic and pathogenic bacteria and for viruses. Furthermore, various carbohydrate structures on the glycosphingolipids of red cell membranes are also the antigenic determinants responsible for the ABO and other blood types. Glycosphingolipids are degraded in the lysosomes by a complex sequence of reactions that involve a stepwise removal of sugars from the non-reducing end of the molecule, with each step involving a specific lysosomal exoglycosidase. A number of inherited lipid-storage diseases result from defects in degradation of glycosphingolipids.

ACTIVE LEARNING

1. Describe the role of plasmalogens vs. diacylglycerol-phospholipids in cell membrane structure and function.
2. Discuss the challenges in development of a vaccine to protect against trypanosomiasis.
3. Review current therapeutic approaches for treatment of acute respiratory distress syndrome (ARDS).
4. In addition to the glycosphingolipidoses and mucopolysaccharidoses, what other lysosomal storage diseases might be treated by enzyme replacement therapy?
5. Review the mechanisms of host-pathogen interaction, focusion on the role of lectins in microbial pathogenicity.

Further reading

Barranger JA, O'Rourke E. Lessons learned from the development of enzyme therapy for Gaucher disease. *J Inherit Metab Dis* 2001;**24** Suppl 2:89–96; discussion 87–8.

Brady RO. Enzyme replacement therapy: conception, chaos and culmination. *Philos Trans R Soc Lond B Biol Sci* 2003;**358**:915–919.

Dowhan W. Molecular basis for membrane phospholipid diversity: why are there so many lipids? *Annu Rev Biochem* 1997;**66**:199–232.

Garratty G, Telen MJ, Petz LD. *Red cell antigens as functional molecules and obstacles to transfusion.* Hematology (Am Soc Hematol Educ Program) 2002:445–462.

Hall C, Richards SJ, Hillmen P. The glycosylphosphatidylinositol anchor and paroxysmal nocturnal haemoglobinuria/aplasia model. *Acta Haematol* 2002;**108**:219–230.

Sandhoff K, Kolter T. Biosynthesis and degradation of mammalian glycosphingolipids. *Philos Trans R Soc Lond B Biol Sci* 2003;**358**:847–861.

Whitsett JA, Weaver TE. Hydrophobic surfactant proteins in lung function and disease. *N Engl J Med* 2002;**347**:2141–2148.

Websites

Acute Respiratory Distress Syndrome: http://www.ards.org/; http://hedwig.mgh.harvard.edu/ardsnet/

Blood Groups: http://www.people.virginia.edu/~rjh9u/abo.html; http://www.bloodbook.com/type-sys.html

Enzyme Replacement Therapy: http://www.gaucher.org.uk/tenyearsapr03.htm

Gaucher's disease: http://www.ninds.nih.gov/health_and_medical/disorders/gauchers_doc.htm http://www.gaucher.org.uk/wraith99.htm; http://www.encyclopedia.com/html/G/Gaucher.asp

Paroxysmal nocturnal hemoglobinuria: http://www.hosppract.com/genetics/9709gen.htm; http://www.emedicine.com/med/topic2696.htm

Tay-Sachs Disease: http://www.ninds.nih.gov/health_and_medical/disorders/taysachs_doc.htm; http://www.ntsad.org/pages/t-sachs.htm

27. The Extracellular Matrix

G P Kaushal and A D Elbein

LEARNING OBJECTIVES

After reading this chapter you should be able to:

■ Describe the composition, structure and function of the extracellular matrix (ECM) and its components, including collagens, elastin, noncollagenous proteins and proteoglycans.

■ Outline the role of the ECM in regulating basic cellular processes, including attachment, proliferation, differentiation, migration and cell-cell interactions.

■ Outline the sequence of steps in the biosynthesis and post-translational modification of collagens and elastin, including the structure and synthesis of crosslinks.

■ Describe the pathways of biosynthesis and turnover of proteoglycans.

■ Describe the pathology of genetic diseases resulting from errors in the synthesis or turnover of ECM components.

INTRODUCTION

The extracellular matrix (ECM) is a complex network of secreted macromolecules located in the extracellular space. The ECM of skin and bone provides the structural framework of the body; however, in all tissues it has a central role in regulating basic cellular processes, including proliferation, differentiation, migration and cell–cell interactions. The macromolecular network of the ECM is made up of collagens, elastin, glycoproteins, and proteoglycans, secreted by connective tissue cells such as fibroblasts, chondrocytes, and epithelial cells. The components of the ECM are in intimate contact with their cells of origin and form a three-dimensional gelatinous bed in which the cells thrive. Proteins in the ECM are also bound to the cell surface, so that they transmit signals resulting from stretching and compression of tissues. The relative abundance, distribution of proteins, and molecular organization of ECM components vary enormously among tissues, depending on their structure and function. Changes in the composition and turnover of the ECM are associated with chronic diseases, such as arthritis, atherosclerosis, cancer, and fibrosis.

COLLAGENS

Collagens are the major proteins in the ECM

The collagens are a family of proteins that comprise about 30% of total protein mass in the body. As the primary structural components of the ECM in connective tissues, collagens have an important role in tissue architecture and integrity, and a wide variety of cell–cell and cell–matrix interactions. To date, more than 20 different types of collagens have been identified. They are composed of related, but distinct, peptide chains and vary greatly in their distribution, organization, and function in tissues.

Triple-helical structure of collagens

The structural hallmark of collagens is their triple-helical structure, formed by folding of three peptide chains. These chains vary in size from 600–3000 amino acids. X-ray diffraction analysis indicates that three left-handed helical chains are wrapped around one another in a rope-like fashion, to form a right-handed superhelix structure (Fig. 27.1). The left-handed helix is more extended than the α-helix of globular proteins (Fig. 2.10), having nearly twice the rise per turn and only three, rather than 3.6, amino acids per turn. Every third amino acid is glycine, because only this amino acid, with the smallest side chain, fits into the crowded central core. The characteristic, repeating sequence of collagen is Gly-X-Y, where X and Y can be any amino acid, but most often X is proline and Y is hydroxyproline. Because of their restricted rotation and bulk, proline and hydroxyproline confer rigidity to the helix. The intra- and inter-chain helices are stabilized by hydrogen bonds, largely between peptide NH and C=O groups. The side chains of the X and Y amino acids point outward from the helix, and thus are on the surface of the protein, where they form lateral interactions with other triple helices or proteins.

Types of collagen

Some representative collagens are listed in Table 27.1. The collagen family of proteins can be divided into two main

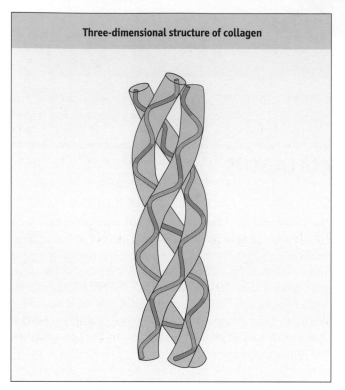

Fig. 27.1 **Three-dimensional structure of collagen.** Collagen monomer strands assume a left-handed, α-helical tertiary structure. They then associate to form a triple-stranded, right-handed superhelical quarternary structure.

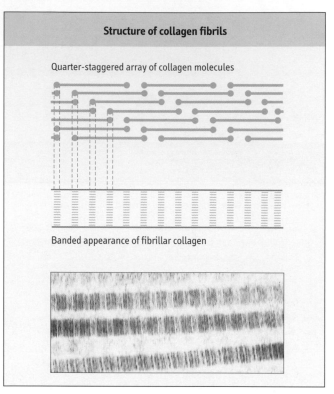

Fig. 27.2 **Formation of the quarter-staggered array of collagen molecules in a fibril.** The regular overlap of the short, nonhelical termini of the collagen chains yields a regular, banded pattern in the collagen fiber. (Electron micrograph courtesy of Dr Trevor Gray.)

types: the fibril-forming (fibrillar) and the nonfibrillar collagens.

Fibril-forming collagens

Fibril-forming collagens include type I, -II, -III, -V, and -XI collagens (Table 27.1). Collagen fibrils can be formed from a mixture of different fibrillar collagens. Dermal collagen fibrils are hybrids of type I and type III collagen, and fibrils in corneal stroma are hybrids of type I and type IV collagen. Type I is the most abundant fibrillar collagen and occurs in a wide variety of tissues; others have a more limited tissue distribution (see Table 27.1). Type I and related fibrillar collagens form well-organized, banded fibrils and provide high tensile strength to skin, tendons, and ligaments. These collagens are composed of two different α-helical peptide chains, known as α1(I) and α2(I), each containing about 1000 amino acids per chain and having a triple-helical domain structure, $[\alpha 1(I)]2\alpha 2(I)$, along almost the entire length of the molecule. The collagen fibrils are formed by lateral association of triple helices in a 'quarter-staggered' alignment in which each molecule is displaced by about one-quarter of its length relative to its nearest neighbor (Fig. 27.2); the quarter-

Type	Class	Distribution
I	fibrillar	skin and tendon
II	fibrillar cartilage	developing cornea and vitreous humor
III	fibrillar	extensible connective tissue, e.g. skin, lung and vascular system
IV	network	basement membranes, kidney, vascular wall
V	fibrillar	liver, cornea and mucosa
VI	beaded filament	most connective tissue
IX	FACIT	cartilage, vitreous humor
XI	fibril forming	cartilage, bone, placenta
XII	FACIT	embryonic tendon and skin
XIII	transmembrane domain	widely distributed
XIV	FACIT	fetal skin and tendons

Members of the collagen family

Table 27.1 **Classification and distribution of representative collagens.** FACIT, fibril-associated collagen with interrupted triple helices.

staggered array is responsible for the banded appearance of collagen fibrils in connective tissues. The fibrils are stabilized by both noncovalent forces and interchain crosslinks derived from lysine residues (see below).

OSTEOGENESIS IMPERFECTA – (INCIDENCE 1 IN 30 000–50 000)

A six-year-old boy was seen in the casualty department with broken tibia and fibula occurring during a soccer game. His 6-foot-tall father explained that he had broken his legs four times while at school. The father's teeth were slightly transparent and discoloured.

Comment. Osteogenesis imperfecta (OI), also called brittle-bone disease, is a congenital disease caused by multiple genetic defects in the synthesis of type I collagen. It is characterized by fragile bones, thin skin, abnormal teeth and weak tendons. The majority of the individuals with this disease have mutations in genes encoding α1(I) and α2(I) chains. Many of these mutations are single-base substitutions that convert glycine in the Gly-X-Y repeat to bulky amino acids, preventing the correct folding of the collagen chains into a triple helix and their assembly to form collagen fibrils. The dominance of type 1 collagen in bone explains why bones are predominantly affected. However, there is remarkable clinical variability characterized by bone fragility, osteopenia, variable degrees of short stature, and progressive skeletal deformities. The most common form of OI, with a presentation that is sometimes mistaken for child abuse, has a good prognosis, with fractures decreasing after puberty, though the general reduction in bone mass ensures lifetime risk remains high. Patients frequently develop deafness due to osteosclerosis, partly from recurrent fractures of the stapes. Bisphosphonate drugs, which inhibit osteoclast activity and thereby inhibit normal bone turnover, have reduced the incidence of fractures. Long-term follow-up studies are underway.

Nonfibrillar collagens

Nonfibrillar collagens are a heterogeneous group containing triple-helical segments of variable length, interrupted by one or more intervening nonhelical (noncollagenous) segments. This group includes basement membrane collagens (the type IV family), fibril-associated collagens with interrupted triple helices (FACITs), and collagens with multiple triple-helical domains with interruptions, known as multiplexins. Nonfibrillar collagens associate with the fibrillar collagens, forming microfibrils and network or mesh-like structures.

Type IV collagen, with the composition $[\alpha1(IV)]2\alpha2(IV)$, is the major structural component of all basement membranes, where it assembles into a flexible network structure. It contains a long triple-helical domain interrupted by short non-collagenous sequences; these interruptions in the helical domain block continued association of two triple helices, oblige them to find another partner, and thus form the meshwork of interactions. Anomalies in type IV collagen in the glomerular basement membrane (GBM) result in several glomerular diseases including Goodpasture's syndrome (GP). GP is caused by anti-GBM antibodies that specifically binds to type IV collagen of the GBM. Type VI collagen is widely distributed in connective tissues, where it assembles to form beaded filaments or microfibrillar meshwork structures. Each of its three chains contains a short triple-helical domain and large amino (N)-terminal and carboxyl (C)-terminal globular domains. Collagens of the FACIT group have short triple-helical domains interspersed by nonhelical domains. They do not assemble to form fibrils, but associate with the fibrillar collagens.

Synthesis and post-translational modification of collagens

Collagen synthesis begins in the rough endoplasmic reticulum (RER)

After synthesis in the RER, the nascent collagen polypeptide undergoes extensive modification, first in the RER, then in the Golgi apparatus, and finally in the extracellular space, where it is modified to a mature extracellular collagen fibril (Fig. 27.3). A nascent polypeptide chain, preprocollagen, is synthesized initially with a hydrophobic signal sequence that facilitates binding of ribosomes to the endoplasmic reticulum (ER) and directs the growing polypeptide chain into the lumen of the ER. Post-translational modification of the protein begins with removal of the signal peptide in the ER, yielding procollagen. Three different hydroxylases then add hydroxyl groups to proline and lysine residues, forming 3- and 4-hydroxyprolines and δ–hydroxylysine. These hydroxylases require ascorbate (Vitamin C) as a cofactor. Vitamin C deficiency leads to scurvy (Chapter 10) as a result of alterations in collagen synthesis and crosslinking.

O-linked glycosylation occurs by the addition of galactosyl residues to hydroxylysine by galactosyl transferase; a disaccharide may also be formed by addition of glucose to galactosyl hydroxylysine by a glucosyl transferase (Chapter 25). These enzymes have strict substrate specificity for hydroxylysine or galactosyl hydroxylysine, and they glycosylate only those peptide sequences that are in noncollagenous domains. N-linked glycosylation also occurs on specific asparagine residues in nonfibrillar domains. The nonfibrillar collagens, with a greater extent of nonhelical domains, are more highly glycosylated than fibrillar collagens. Thus, the extent of glycosylation may influence fibril structure, interrupting fibril formation and promoting interchain interactions required for a meshwork structure. Intra- and inter-chain disulfide bonds are formed in the C-terminal domains by a protein disulfide isomerase, facilitating the association and folding of peptide chains into a triple helix. At this stage, the procollagen is still soluble, and contains additional, nonhelical extensions at its N- and C- terminals.

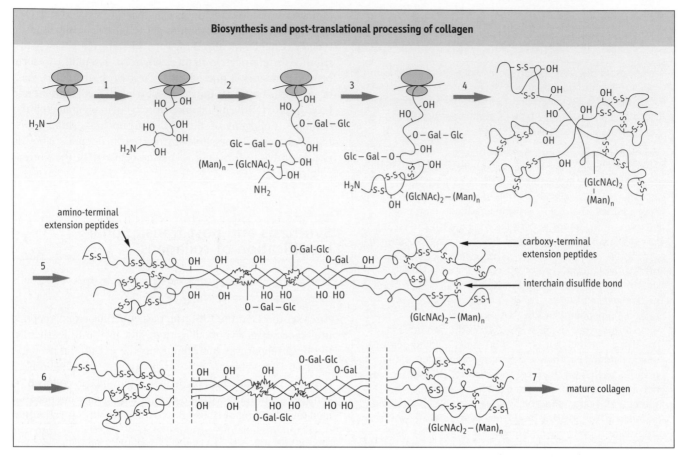

Fig. 27.3 Biosynthesis and post-translational processing of collagen. Collagen is synthesized in the RER, post-translationally modified in the Golgi apparatus, then secreted, trimmed of extension peptides, and finally assembled into fibrils in the extracellular space. (1) Hydroxylation of proline and lysine residues. (2) Addition of *O*-linked and *N*-linked oligosaccharides. (3) Formation of intrachain disulfide bonds at the N-terminal of the nascent polypeptide chain. (4) Formation of interchain disulfides in the C-terminal domains, which assist in alignment of chains. (5) Formation of triple-stranded, soluble tropocollagen, and transport to Golgi vesicles. (6) Exocytosis and removal of N- and C-terminal propeptides. (7) Final stages of processing, including lateral association of triple helices, covalent crosslinking and collagen fiber formation. Gal, galactose; Glc, glucose; GlcNAc, *N*-acetylglucosamine; Man, mannose.

Procollagen is finally modified to collagen in the Golgi apparatus

After assembly into the triple helix, the procollagen is transported from the rough endoplasmic reticulum (RER) to the Golgi apparatus, where it is packaged into cylindrical aggregates in secretory vesicles, then exported to the extracellular space by exocytosis. The nonhelical extensions of the procollagen are now removed in the extracellular space, by specific N- and C-terminal procollagen proteinases. The 'tropocollagen' molecules then self-assemble into insoluble collagen fibrils, which are further stabilized by the formation of aldehyde-derived intermolecular crosslinks. Lysyl oxidase – not to be confused with lysyl hydroxylase involved in formation of hydroxylysine – oxidatively deaminates the amino group from the side chains of some lysine and hydroxylysine residues, producing reactive aldehyde derivatives, known as allysine and hydroxyallysine. The aldehyde groups now form

aldol condensation products with neighboring aldehyde groups, generating crosslinks both within and between triple-helical molecules. They may also react with the amino groups of unoxidized lysine and hydroxylysine residues to form Schiff base (imine) crosslinks (Fig. 27.4). The initial products may rearrange, or be dehydrated, or reduced to form stable crosslinks, such as lysinonorleucine.

NONCOLLAGENOUS PROTEINS IN THE EXTRACELLULAR MATRIX

Elastin

The flexibility required for function of our blood vessels, lungs, ligaments and skin is contributed by a network of

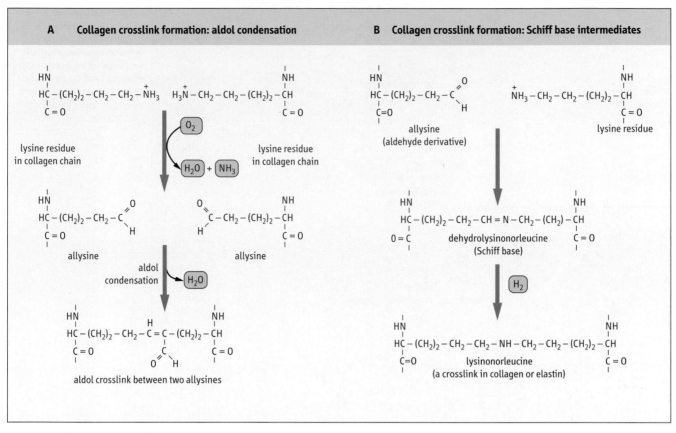

Fig. 27.4 **Collagen crosslink formation.** Allysine (and hydroxyallysine) are precursors of collagen crosslink formation by (A) aldol condensation and (B) Schiff base (imine) intermediates.

elastic fibers in the ECM of these tissues. The predominant protein of elastic fibers is elastin. Unlike the multigene collagen family, there is only one gene for elastin – a polypeptide about 750 amino acids long. In common with collagens, it is rich in glycine and proline residues, but elastin is more hydrophobic: one in seven of its amino acids is a valine. Unlike collagens, elastin contains little hydroxyproline and no hydroxylysine or carbohydrate chains, and does not have a regular secondary structure. Its primary structure consists of alternating hydrophilic and hydrophobic, lysine, and valine-rich domains. The lysines are involved in intermolecular crosslinking, while the weak interactions between valine residues in the hydrophobic domains impart elasticity to the molecule.

Elastin can stretch in two dimensions

The soluble monomeric form of elastin initially synthesized on the RER is called tropoelastin. Except for some hydroxylation of proline, tropoelastin does not undergo post-translational modification. During the assembly process in the extracellular space, lysyl oxidase generates allysine in specific sequences: -Lys-Ala-Ala-Lys- and -Lys-Ala-Ala-

Ala-Lys-. As with collagen, the reactive aldehyde of allysine condenses with other allysines or with unmodified lysines. Allysine and dehydrolysinonorleucine on different tropoelastin chains also condense to form pyridinium crosslinks – heterocyclic structures known as desmosine or isodesmosine (Fig. 27.5). Because of the way in which elastin monomers are crosslinked in polymers, elastin can stretch in two dimensions.

Fibronectin

Fibronectin is a glycoprotein present in the ECM and also in plasma as a soluble protein. It is involved in a large number of biological activities, including cell adhesion, cell migration, cell morphology, embryonic differentiation, and cytoskeletal organization. It has a central role in binding together the many structures of the ECM, including collagens, proteoglycans, and the cell surface. Fibronectin is a dimer of two identical subunits, each of 230 kDa, joined by a pair of disulfide bonds at their C-terminals. Each subunit is organized into domains, known as type I, II, and III domains,

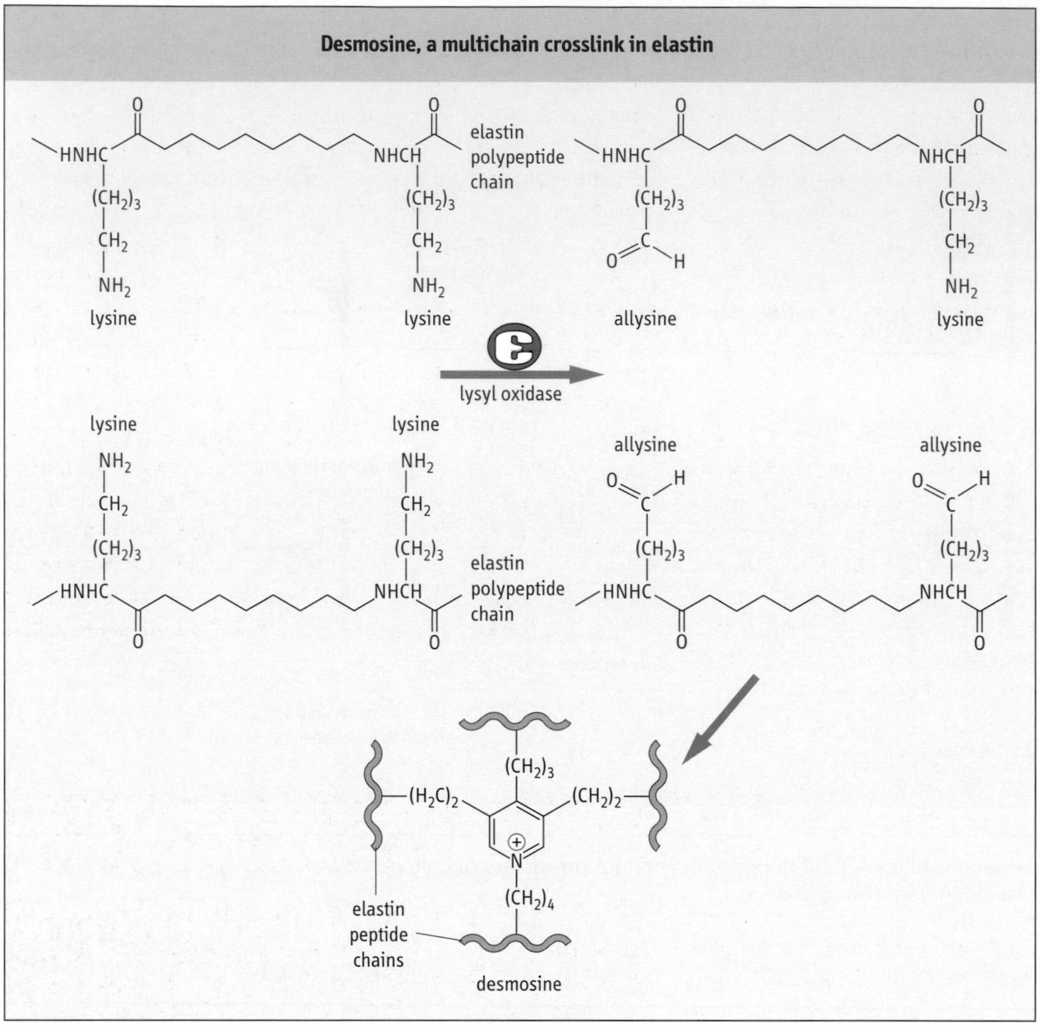

Desmosine, a multichain crosslink in elastin

Fig. 27.5 **Desmosine – a multichain crosslink in elastin.** Allysine and dehydrolysinonorleucine residues in adjacent elastin chains react to form the three-dimensional elastic polymer, crosslinked by desmosine.

EPIDERMOLYSIS BULLOSA

Epidermolysis bullosa is a rare heritable disorder characterized by severe blistering of the skin and epithelial tissue. Three kinds are known:

- **simplex:** blistering in the epidermis, caused by defects in keratin filaments;
- **junctional:** blistering in the dermal-epidermal junction, caused by defects in laminin;
- **dystrophic:** blistering in the dermis, caused by mutations in the gene encoding type VII collagen.

Epidermolysis bullosa illustrates the multifactorial nature of connective tissue diseases that have similar clinical features.

LATHYRISM

Lathyrism is a diet-induced disease characterized by deformation of the spine, dislocation of joints, demineralization of bones, aortic aneurysms, and joint hemorrhages. These problems develop as a result of inhibition of lysyl oxidase, an enzyme required for the crosslinking of collagen chains. Lathyrism can be caused by chronic ingestion of the sweet pea, *Lathyrus odoratus*, the seeds of which contain β-aminopropionitrile, an irreversible inhibitor of lysyl oxidase. Penicillamine, a sulfhydryl agent used for chelation therapy in heavy-metal toxicity, also causes lathyrism, because of either chelation of copper required for lysyl oxidase activity or reaction with aldehyde groups of (hydroxy)allysine, inhibiting collagen crosslinking reactions.

and each of these has several homologous repeating units or modules in its primary structure (Fig. 27.6): there are 12 type I repeats, 2 type II repeats, and 15–17 type III repeats. Each module is independently folded, forming a 'string of beads' type of structure. At least 20 different tissue-specific isoforms of fibronectin have been identified, all produced by alternative splicing of a single precursor messenger ribonucleic acid (mRNA). The alternative splicing is regulated, not only in a tissue-specific manner, but also during embryogenesis, wound healing, and oncogenesis. Plasma fibronectin, secreted mainly by liver cells, lacks two of the type III repeats that are found in cell- and matrix-associated forms of fibronectin.

Functional domains in fibronectin have been identified by their binding affinity for other ECM components, including collagen, heparin, fibrin, and the cell surface. The type I modules interact with fibrin, heparin, and collagen, type II modules have collagen-binding domains, and type III modules are involved in binding to heparin and the cell surface. The specific interactions have been further mapped to short stretches of amino acids. A short peptide containing Arg-Gly-Asp (RGD), present in the tenth type III repeat of fibronectin, binds to the integrin family of proteins present on cell surfaces; this sequence is not unique to fibronectin, but is also found in other proteins in the ECM. Another sequence, Pro-X-Ser-Arg-Asn (PXSRN), present in the ninth type III repeat, is implicated in integrin-mediated cell attachment. The integrins are a family of transmembrane proteins that bind extracellular proteins on the outside and cytoskeletal proteins, such as actin, on the inside of the cell, providing a mechanism for communication between the intracellular and extracellular environments of the cell. The loss of fibronectin from the surface of many tumor cells may contribute to their release into the circulation and penetration through the ECM, one of the first steps in tumor metastasis.

Laminins

Laminins are a family of noncollagenous glycoproteins in basement membranes, expressed in variant forms in different tissues. They are large (850 kDa), heterotrimeric molecules, composed of α-, β-, and γ-chains. The three chains are arranged in an asymmetric cruciform molecule, held together by disulfide linkages. Laminins undergo reversible self-assembly in the presence of calcium, to form polymers. Biochemical and electron microscopic studies indicate that all full-length short arms of laminin are required for self-assembly and that the polymer is formed by joining the ends of the short arms in a polymeric network. Like fibronectin, laminins interact with cells through multiple binding sites in several domains of the molecule. The α-chains have binding sites for integrins, dystroglycan (Chapter 25), heparin, and heparan sulfate (below). Laminin polymers are also connected to type IV collagen by a single-chain protein, nidogen/entactin, which has a binding site for collagen and, in common with fibronectin, also has an RGD sequence for integrin binding. Nidogen also binds to the core proteins of proteoglycans (below). It has a central role in formation of crosslinks between laminin and type IV collagen, generating a scaffold for anchoring of cells and ECM molecules in the basement membranes.

 ## MARFAN SYNDROME

The ultrastructure of elastic fiber reveals elastin as an insoluble, polymeric, amorphous core covered with a sheath of microfibrils that contribute to the stability of the elastin fiber. The predominant constituent of microfibrils is the glycoprotein, fibrillin. Marfan syndrome is a relatively rare genetic disease of connective tissues caused by mutations in the fibrillin gene (frequency: 1 in 10000 births). People with this disease have typically tall stature, long arms and legs, and arachnodactyly (long, 'spidery' fingers). The disease in a mild form causes loose joints, deformed spine, floppy mitral valves (leading to cardiac regurgitation), and eye problems such as lens dislocation. In severely affected individuals, the aorta wall is prone to rupture because of defects in elastic fiber formation.

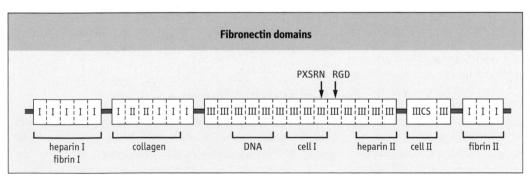

Fig. 27.6 **Structural map of fibronectin.** This shows various globular domains and domains involved in binding to various molecules in the cell and ECM. RGD, Arg-Gly-Asp; PXSRN, Pro-X-Ser-Arg-Asn.

The proteoglycans			
Proteoglycan	**Characteristic disaccharide**	**Sulfation**	**Tissue location**
Hyaluronic acid	[4GlcUAβ1–3GlcNAcβ1]	none	joint and ocular fluids
Chondroitin sulfates	[4GlcUAα1–3GalNAcβ1]	GalNAc	cartilage, tendons, bone
Dermatan sulfate	[4IdUAα1–3GalNAcβ1]	IdUA, GalNAc	skin, valves, blood vessels
Heparan sulfate	[4IdUAα1–4GlcNAcβ1]	GlcNAc	cell surfaces
Heparin	[4IdUAα1–4GlcNAcβ1]	GlcNH₂, IdUA	mast cells, liver
Keratan sulfates	[3Galβ1–4GlcNAcβ1]	GlcNAc	cartilage, cornea

Table 27.2 **Structure and distribution of the proteoglycans.** GalNAc, *N*-acetylgalactosamine; $GlcNH_2$, glucosamine; GlcUA, D-glucuronic acid; IdUA, L-iduronic acid.

PROTEOGLYCANS

Proteoglycans are gel-forming components of the ECM. Some proteoglycans are located on the cell surface, where they bind growth factors and other ECM components. They are composed of peptide chains containing covalently bound sugars (see Fig. 25.1). However, the peptide chains of proteoglycans are usually more rigid and extended than the protein portion of the glycoproteins, and the proteoglycans contain much larger amounts of carbohydrate – typically >95% carbohydrate. The sugar chains are linear, unbranched oligosaccharides that are much longer than those of the glycoproteins, and may contain more than 100 sugar residues in a chain. Furthermore, the oligosaccharide chains of proteoglycans have a repeating disaccharide unit, usually composed of an amino sugar and a uronic acid. Proteoglycan oligosaccharide chains are polyanionic because of the many negative charges of the carboxyl groups of the uronic acids, and from sulfate groups attached to some of the hydroxyl or amino groups of the sugars.

Structure of proteoglycans

The general structures of the glycosaminoglycans (GAGs), the carbohydrate part of the proteoglycans, are shown in Table 27.2. The disaccharide repeat is different for each type of GAG, but is usually composed of a hexosamine and a uronic acid residue, except in the case of keratan sulfate, in which the uronic acid is replaced by galactose. The amino sugar in GAGs is either glucosamine ($GlcNH_2$) or galactosamine ($GalNH_2$), both of which are present mostly in their *N*-acetylated forms (GlcNAc and GalNAc), although in some of the GAGs (heparin, heparan sulfate) the amino group is sulfated, rather than acetylated. The uronic acid is usually D-glucuronic acid (GlcUA), but in some cases (dermatan sulfate, heparin) it may be L-iduronic acid (IdUA). With the exception of hyaluronic acid and keratan sulfate, all of the GAGs are attached to protein by a core trisaccharide, Gal-Gal-Xyl, attached to a serine or threonine residue of a core protein. Keratan sulfate is also attached to protein, but in that case the linkage is either through an *N*-linked oligosaccharide

(keratan sulfate I), or an *O*-linked oligosaccharide (keratan sulfate II). Hyaluronic acid, which has the longest polysaccharide chains, is the only GAG that does not appear to be attached to a core protein.

Hyaluronic acid

Hyaluronic acid is composed of repeating units of GlcNAc and GlcUA. This polysaccharide chain is the longest of the GAGs, with molecular weight of 10^5-10^7 Da (250–25 000 repeating disaccharide units), and is the only nonsulfated GAG.

The chondroitin sulfates

The chondroitin sulfates are major components of cartilage. They contain GalNAc rather than GlcNAc as the amino sugar, and their polysaccharide chains are shorter: $2-5 \times 10^5$ Da. The chondroitin chains are attached to protein via the trisaccharide linkage region (Gal-Gal-Xyl), and they contain sulfate residues linked to either the 4- or 6-hydroxyl groups of GalNAc.

Dermatan sulfate

Dermatan sulfate was originally isolated from skin, but is also found in blood vessels, tendon and heart valves. This GAG is similar in structure to chondroitin sulfate, but has a variable amount of L-IdUA, the C-5-epimer of D-GlcUA, formed in an unusual reaction by epimerization of GlcUA after it has been incorporated into the polymer. Dermatan sulfate has a higher charge density than the chondroitin sulfates, as it contains sulfate residues on the C-2 position of some IdUA residues, and on the 4-hydroxyl groups of GalNAc.

Heparin and heparan sulfate

Heparin and heparan sulfate consist primarily of repeating disaccharide units of $GlcNH_2$ with IdUA or GlcUA, respectively. The linkage between the amino sugar and the uronic acid is uniformly 1–4, rather than the alternating 1–4/1–3 linkages seen in other GAGs. Most of the $GlcNH_2$ units of heparin are *N*-sulfated, whereas many of the IdUA residues are sulfated at the C-2 hydroxyl group, and the $GlcNH_2$ residues at the C-6 hydroxyl group. Heparin and heparan sulfate are the most highly charged of the GAGs. Although the structures of these two polymers are closely related, their distribution in the body and their functions are quite different: heparin is a small microheterogeneous molecule (~3,000–30 000 Da), found intracellularly as a proteoglycan. It is released into the extracellular space as a glycosaminoglycan, and has strong anticoagulant activity. In contrast, heparan sulfate is bound in the ECM or on the surface of cells, and has only weak anticoagulant activity.

Keratan sulfate

The final GAG structure shown in Table 27.2 is keratan sulfate (KS). This is a rather unusual GAG because it is linked to protein either by an *N*-linked (KS I), or by an *O*-linked (KS II) oligosaccharide. Thus it has features common to both proteoglycans and glycoproteins. It is considered to be a proteoglycan, however, because the glycan portion has a repeating disaccharide unit and a long, linear chain. The repeating unit is composed of GlcNAc and galactose in place of the uronic acid. Both the GlcNAc and the galactose are generally sulfated on the C-6 hydroxyl groups.

Synthesis and degradation of proteoglycans

Proteoglycans are synthesized by a series of glycosyl transferases, epimerases and sulfotransferases, beginning with the synthesis of the core oligosaccharide while the core protein is still in the RER. Synthesis of the repeating oligosaccharide and other modifications takes place in the Golgi apparatus. As with the synthesis of glycoproteins and glycolipids, separate enzymes are involved in individual steps. For example, there are separate galactosyl transferases for each of the galactose units in the core, a separate GlcUA transferase for the core and repeating disaccharides, and separate sulfotransferases for the C-4 and C-6 positions of the GalNAc residues of chondroitin sulfates. Phosphoadenosine phosphosulfate (PAPS) (see Fig. 26.6) is the sulfate donor for the sulfotransferases. These pathways are illustrated in Figure 27.7, for chondroitin-6-sulfate.

Defects of proteoglycan degradation lead to mucopolysaccharidoses

The degradation of proteoglycans occurs in lysosomes. The protein portion is degraded by lysosomal proteases, and the GAG chains are degraded by the sequential action of a

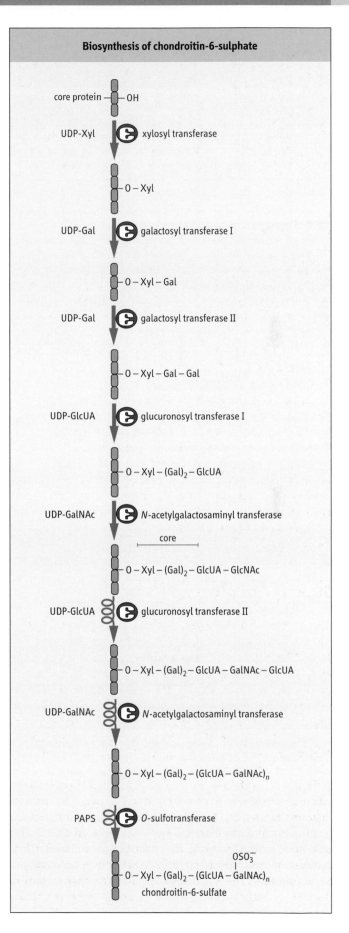

Biosynthesis of chondroitin-6-sulphate

core protein — OH

UDP-Xyl — xylosyl transferase

— O – Xyl

UDP-Gal — galactosyl transferase I

— O – Xyl – Gal

UDP-Gal — galactosyl transferase II

— O – Xyl – Gal – Gal

UDP-GlcUA — glucuronosyl transferase I

— O – Xyl – (Gal)$_2$ – GlcUA

UDP-GalNAc — *N*-acetylgalactosaminyl transferase

core

— O – Xyl – (Gal)$_2$ – GlcUA – GlcNAc

UDP-GlcUA — glucuronosyl transferase II

— O – Xyl – (Gal)$_2$ – GlcUA – GalNAc – GlcUA

UDP-GalNAc — *N*-acetylgalactosaminyl transferase

— O – Xyl – (Gal)$_2$ – (GlcUA – GalNAc)$_n$

PAPS — *O*-sulfotransferase

$$OSO_3^-$$
— O – Xyl – (Gal)$_2$ – (GlcUA – GalNAc)$_n$

chondroitin-6-sulfate

Fig. 27.7 **Synthesis of the proteoglycan, chondroitin-6-sulfate.**
Several enzymes participate in this pathway. Xyl, xylose.

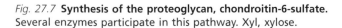

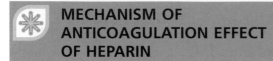

MECHANISM OF ANTICOAGULATION EFFECT OF HEPARIN

Heparin is heterogeneous (3,000–30,000 kDa), polyanionic oligosaccharide activator of antithrombin III (AT). AT is a slow, but quantitatively important inhibitor of thrombin (Factor X) and other factors (IX, XI, XII) in the blood-clotting cascade. When heparin binds to AT, it converts AT from a slow inhibitor to a rapid inhibitor of coagulating enzymes. Heparin interacts with a lysine residue in AT and induces a conformational change that promotes covalent binding of AT to the active serine centers of coagulating enzymes, inhibiting their pro-coagulant activity. Heparin then dissociates from the ternary complex and can be recycled for anticoagulation. The smallest, most active component of heparin is a pentasaccharide that has a Kd of ~10 μmol/L: GlcN-(N-sulfate-6-O-sulfate)-α1,4-GlcUA-β1,4-GlcN-(N-sulfate-3,6-di-O-sulfate)-α1,4-IdUA-(2-O-sulfate)-α-1,4-GlcN-(N-sulfate-6-O-sulfate-). Heparin has an average half-life of 30 min in the circulation, so that it is commonly administered by infusion. Heparin does not have fibrinolytic activity; therefore, it will not lyse existing clots. In addition to its anticoagulant activity, heparin also releases several enzymes from proteoglycan binding sites on the vascular wall, including lipoprotein lipase, which is often assayed as heparin-releasable plasma lipoprotein lipase activity. Lipoprotein lipase is inducible by insulin, and decreased activity of this enzyme delays plasma clearance of chylomicrons and VLDL, contributing to hypertriglyceridemia in diabetes.

The mucopolysaccharidoses

Syndrome		Deficient enzyme	Product accumulated in lysosomes and secreted in urine
Hunter's		iduronate sulfatase	heparan and dermatan sulfate
Hurler's		α-iduronidase	heparan and dermatan sulfate
Morquio's	A	galactose-6-sulfatase	keratan sulfate
	B	β-galactosidase	keratan sulfate
Sanfilippo's	A	heparan sulfamidase	heparan sulfate
	B	N-acetylglucosaminidase	
	C	N-acetylglucosamine-6-sulfatase	

Table 27.3 **Enzymatic defects characteristic of various mucopolysaccharidoses.**

dermatan sulfate. As with degradation of glycosphingolipids, if one of the enzymes involved in the stepwise pathway is missing, the entire degradation process is halted at that point, and the undegraded molecules accumulate in the lysosome. The lysosomal storage diseases resulting from accumulation of GAGs are known as mucopolysaccharidoses (Table 27.3), because of the original designation of GAGs as mucopolysaccharides. There are more than a dozen such mucopolysaccharidoses, resulting from defects in degradation of GAGs. In general, these diseases can be diagnosed by the identification of specific GAG chains in the urine, followed by assay of the specific hydrolases in leukocytes or fibroblasts. Although they are rare genetic diseases, the mucopolysaccharidoses have been important in the elucidation of the role of lysosomes in health and disease, and the mechanisms involved in biosynthesis of lysosomes and targeting of lysosomal enzymes.

Functions of the proteoglycans

Bottlebrushes, silly putty and reinforced concrete

Proteoglycans are found in association with most tissues and cells. One of their major roles is to provide structural support to tissues, especially cartilage and connective tissue. In cartilage, large aggregates, composed of chondroitin sulfate and keratan sulfate chains linked to their core proteins, are non-covalently associated with hyaluronic acid via link proteins, forming a jelly-like matrix in which the collagen fibers are embedded. This macromolecule of macromolecules, a 'bottlebrush' structure known as aggrecan (Fig. 27.9), provides both rigidity and stability to connective tissue.

Because of their negative charge, the GAGs bind large amounts of monovalent and divalent cations: a cartilage proteoglycan molecule of 2×10^6 Da would have an aggregate negative charge of about 10 000. The maintenance of

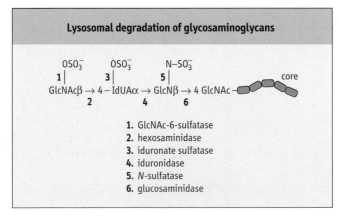

Fig. 27.8 **Degradation of heparan sulfate.** This proceeds by a defined sequence of lysosomal hydrolase activities.

number of different lysosomal acid hydrolases. The stepwise degradation of GAGs involves exoglycosidases and sulfatases, beginning from the external end of the glycan chain. This may involve the removal of sulfate by a sulfatase, then removal of the terminal sugar by a specific glycosidase, and so on. Figure 27.8 shows the steps in the degradation of

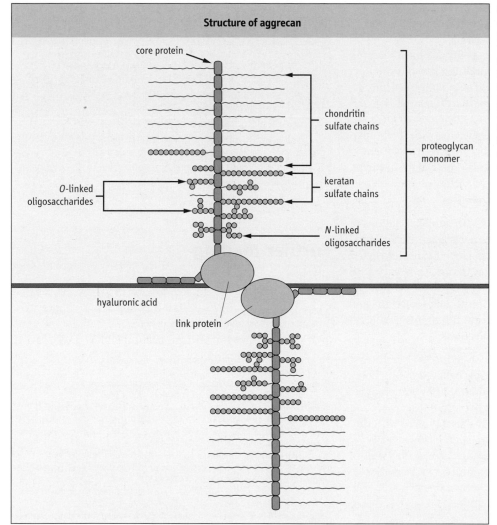

Structure of aggrecan

core protein

chondritin
sulfate chains

proteoglycan
monomer

O-linked
oligosaccharides

keratan
sulfate chains

N-linked
oligosaccharides

hyaluronic acid

link protein

Fig. 27.9 **Structure of aggrecan.** Associations between proteoglycans and hyaluronic acid form an aggrecan structure in the extracellular matrix (ECM). The extension of this structure yields a three-dimensional array of proteoglycans bound to hyaluronic acid, which creates a stiff matrix or 'bottlebrush' structure in which collagen and other ECM components are embedded.

electrical neutrality consequently requires a high concentration of counterions. These ions draw water into the ECM, causing swelling and stiffening of the matrix, the result of tension between osmotic forces and binding interactions between proteoglycans and collagen. The structure and hydration of the ECM allows for a degree of rigidity, combined with flexibility and compressibility, enabling the tissue to withstand torsion and shock. The hyaluronic acid-proteoglycan-collagen aggregates in vertebral and articular disks have some of the viscoelastic properties of 'silly putty', bounce plus resilience, cushioning the impact between bones. These discs compress during the course of the day, expand elastically during the course of night, and deform gradually with age.

The overall structure of cartilage can be likened to that of the vertical reinforced-concrete slabs poured during the construction of large buildings, in which steel rods (collagen fibers) are embedded in an amorphous layer of cement (the

proteoglycan aggregates). Collagen stabilizes the network of proteoglycans in cartilage in much the same way that the reinforcing rods in the concrete provide structural strength for the cement walls. The structure of earthquake-resistant buildings, like the ECM, provides a balance between integrity and flexibility.

Although the amounts involved are low compared with those in skin and cartilage, organs such as the liver, brain, or kidney also contain a variety of proteoglycans:

■ **hepatocytes:** heparan sulfate is the principal GAG; it is present both intracellularly and on the cell surface of the hepatocyte, and the attachment of hepatocytes to their substratum in cell culture is mediated, at least in part, by this proteoglycan;

■ **kidney:** changes in both the collagen and proteoglycan content of the renal basement membrane are associated with diabetic renal disease. In this case, the change in structure and charge of the proteoglycans aggregate, known as perlecan, is associated with a change in the filtration selectivity of the glomerulus;

- **cornea:** two populations of proteoglycans have been identified in the cornea, one containing keratan sulfate and the other dermatan sulfate. These molecules have a much smaller hydrodynamic size than the large cartilage proteoglycans, which may be required for interaction of the corneal proteoglycans with the tightly packed and oriented collagen fibers in this transparent tissue. Corneal clouding in macular corneal dystrophy is associated with undersulfation of keratan sulfate I proteoglycan.

Other complex glycan aggregates with subtle variations in core protein structure and glycan composition are distributed in intracellular compartments, plasma membranes and in the extracellular space in a tissue-specific manner and vary with age and disease.

Some proteoglycans or GAGs, especially heparin and heparan sulfate, probably have important physiologic roles in binding proteins or other macromolecules:

- **mast cells** (granulated cells involved in the inflammatory response): heparin is believed to function as an intracellular binding site maintaining proteinases in secretory granules in an inactive state.
- **the vascular wall:** proteoglycans are involved with the binding of proteins and enzymes, such as low-density lipoprotein and lipoprotein lipase, to the vascular wall (see Chapter 17). They may also inhibit clot formation on the vascular wall by surface activation of antithrombin III (Chapter 6).

Summary

The ECM contains a complex array of fibrillar and network-forming collagens, elastin fibers, a stiff gelatinous matrix of proteoglycans, and a number of glycoproteins that mediate the interaction of these molecules with one another and with the cell surface. These molecules and their interactions afford structure, stability, and elasticity to the ECM, and provide a route for communication between the intra- and extra-cellular environments in tissues. The heterogeneity of both the protein and the carbohydrate components of these molecules provides for the great diversity in the structure and function of the ECM in various tissues.

ACTIVE LEARNING

1. Compare the structure of heparin, its mechanism of action, its route and frequency of administration to that of other common anticoagulants, such as aspirin and coumarin derivatives.
2. Discuss factors that promote the turnover of ECM components, as part of normal growth and development and in diseases, such as rheumatoid arthritis.
3. Review the consequences of genetic defects in sulfation of proteoglycans.

Further reading

Hulmes DJ. Building collagen molecules, fibrils, and suprafibrillar structures. *J Struct Biol* 2002;**137**(1–2):2–10.

Aumailley M, Gayraud B. Structure and biological activity of the extracellular matrix. *J Mol Med* 1998;**76**:253–265.

Myllyharju J, Kivirikko KI. Collagens and collagen-related diseases. *Ann Med* 2001;**33**(1):7–21.

Brown JC, Timpl R. The collagen superfamily. *Int Arch Allergy Immunol* 1995;**107**:484–490.

Bosman FT, Stamenkovic I. Functional structure and composition of the extracellular matrix. *J Pathol* 2003;**200**(4):423–428.

Clark EA, Bruggse JS. Integrins and signal transduction pathways: the road taken. *Science* 1995;**268**:233–239.

Fraser JR, Laurent TC, Laurent UB. Hyaluronan: its nature, distribution, functions and turnover. *J Int Med* 1997;**242**:27–33.

Mewer UM, Engvall E. Domains of laminin. *J Cell Biochem* 1996;**61**:493–501.

Prockop DJ, Kivirikko KI. Collagens: molecular biology, diseases and potentials for therapy. *Annu Rev Biochem* 1995;**64**:403–434.

Rosenbloom J, Abrams WR, Mecham R. Extracellular matrix 4: the elastic fiber. *FASEB J* 1993;**7**:1208–1218.

Timpl R, Brown JC. Supramolecular assembly of basement membranes. *Bioessays* 1996;**18**:123–132.

Tilstra DJ, Byers PH. Molecular basis of hereditary disorders of connective tissue. *Annu Rev Med* 1994;**45**:149–163.

Relevant websites

Ehrlers-Danlos syndrome:
http://www.nlm.nih.gov/medlineplus/ehlersdanlossyndrome.html
www.ehlers-danlos.org; www.ednf.org

Extracellular matrix: http://www.teaching-biomed.man.ac.uk/lawson/ECM.HTM

Heparin: www.amhrt.org
http://www2.kumc.edu/wichita/meded/cvresource/antithrombotic/heparin/

Marfan's syndrome: www.marfan.org; www.marfan.org.uk
http://www.nlm.nih.gov/medlineplus/marfansyndrome.html

Mucopolysaccharidoses:
http://www.ninds.nih.gov/health_and_medical/pubs/mps.htm
http://www.ninds.nih.gov/health_and_medical/disorders/mucopolysaccharidoses.htm

28. Special Liver Function

A F Jones

LEARNING OBJECTIVES

After reading this chapter you should be able to:

- Discuss the participation of the liver in carbohydrate metabolism and in particular its role in the endogenous glucose production.
- Discuss the role of the liver in lipid metabolism.
- Outline the changes in the hepatic protein synthesis which take place during the acute phase reaction and comment on the mechanisms of proteolysis.
- Describe the pathway of heme synthesis.
- Describe the metabolism of bilirubin and the main types of jaundice.
- Comment on the mechanism of hepatotoxicity of drugs and alcohol.

INTRODUCTION

The liver has a central role in metabolism, because of both its anatomical placement and its many biochemical functions. It receives venous blood from the intestine, and thus all the products of digestion, in addition to ingested drugs and other xenobiotics, perfuse the liver before entering the systemic circulation. The hepatic parenchymal cells, the hepatocytes, have an immensely broad range of synthetic and catabolic functions, which are summarized in Table 28.1. The liver has important roles in the regulation of carbohydrate and lipid metabolism, in amino acid metabolism, in the synthesis and breakdown of plasma proteins, and in the storage of vitamins and metals; it also has the ability to metabolize, and so detoxify, an infinitely wide range of xenobiotics. The liver also has an excretory function, in which metabolic waste products are secreted into a branching system of ducts known as the biliary tree, which in turn drains into the small intestine; the biliary constituents are then excreted in feces.

The liver has a substantial reserve metabolic capacity; mild liver disease may cause no symptoms, and be detected only as biochemical changes in the blood. However, the patient with severe liver disease has a yellow pigmentation of the skin (jaundice), bruises readily, may bleed profusely, has an abdomen distended with fluid (ascites), and may be confused or unconscious (hepatic encephalopathy) (Fig. 28.1). This chapter will describe the specialized metabolic functions of the liver and the abnormalities that occur in liver disease.

STRUCTURE OF THE LIVER

The liver is the largest solid organ in the body and, in adults, weighs about 1500g. It occupies the right upper quadrant of the abdominal cavity, lying below the diaphragm and protected by the rib cage. Approximately 75% of the blood flow to the liver is supplied by the portal vein, which arises from the intestine. Blood leaving the liver enters the venous system through the hepatic vein. The biliary component of the liver comprises the gall bladder and bile ducts.

The microscopic structure of the liver facilitates the exchange of metabolites between hepatocytes and plasma

Under the microscope, the substance of the liver is composed of a very large number of lobules, each of which is polyhedral in shape (Fig. 28.2). Blood sinusoids arise from the terminal branches of the portal vein and interconnect and interweave through these sheets of hepatocytes before joining the central lobular vein.

Sinusoids are lined by two cell types. The first are vascular endothelial cells, which are loosely connected one with another, leaving numerous gaps, and thus form a net-like lining to the sinusoids. Moreover, there is no basement membrane between the endothelial cells and the hepatocytes. This structural arrangement facilitates the exchange of metabolites between hepatocyte and plasma. The second type of sinusoidal cell, known as Kupffer cells, are mononuclear phagocytes; they are generally found in the gaps between adjacent endothelial cells.

PARTICIPATION OF THE LIVER IN CARBOHYDRATE METABOLISM

The liver has a central role in glucose metabolism, specifically in maintaining the circulating concentration of glucose on which a number of tissues, most importantly the brain, are dependent as a source of fuel. This function depends upon the ability of the liver both to store a supply of glucose in a polymerized form as glycogen, and to synthesize

Hepatic function

Function	Markers of impairment in plasma
Heme catabolism	↑ bilirubin
Carbohydrate metabolism	↓ glucose
Protein synthesis	↓ albumin
	↑ prothrombin time
Protein catabolism	↑ ammonia
	↓ urea
Lipid metabolism	↑ cholesterol
	↑ triglycerides
Drug metabolism	↑ drug $t_{\frac{1}{2}}$
Bile acid metabolism	↑ bile acids

Table 28.1 **Hepatic function.** Functions of hepatic parenchymal cells and their disturbances in liver disease. $t_{\frac{1}{2}}$ = biological half-time.

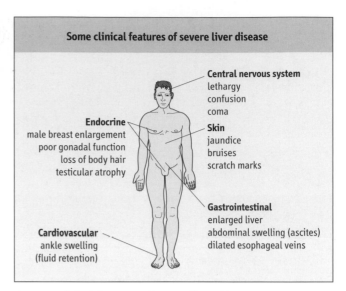

Some clinical features of severe liver disease

Central nervous system
lethargy
confusion
coma

Endocrine
male breast enlargement
poor gonadal function
loss of body hair
testicular atrophy

Skin
jaundice
bruises
scratch marks

Cardiovascular
ankle swelling
(fluid retention)

Gastrointestinal
enlarged liver
abdominal swelling (ascites)
dilated esophageal veins

Fig. 28.1 **Clinical features of severe liver disease.**

Fig. 28.2 **Structure of the liver.** (A) Schema of the structure. (B) A histological slide of a normal liver. (Courtesy Dr J Newman, Birmingham Heartlands and Solihull NHS Trust, UK)

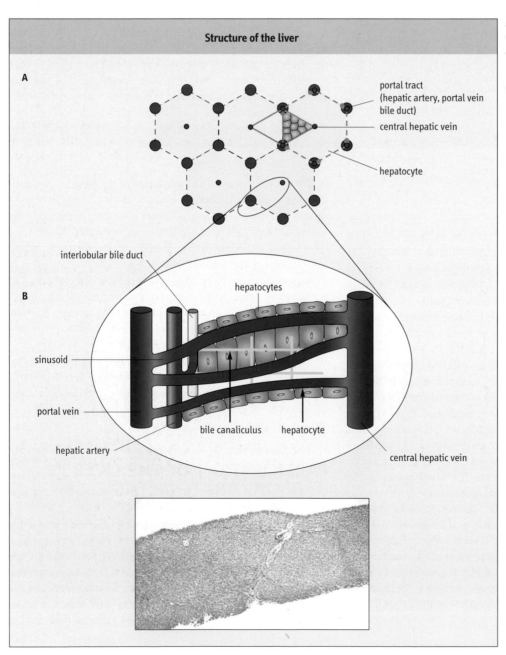

Structure of the liver

A

portal tract (hepatic artery, portal vein bile duct)

central hepatic vein

hepatocyte

B

interlobular bile duct

hepatocytes

sinusoid

portal vein

hepatic artery

bile canaliculus

hepatocyte

central hepatic vein

glucose from non-carbohydrate sources in the process of gluconeogenesis. Importantly the liver also possesses glucose-6-phosphatase which permits the dephosphorylation of glucose-6-phosphate, produced as a result of glycogen breakdown (glycogenolysis) or gluconeogenesis, which is a necessary prerequisite to the release of glucose to the blood (the process of glucose release to blood is also called 'endogenous glucose production'). Although muscle stores more glycogen than the liver, it has no glucose-6-phosphatase activity and hence cannot directly contribute glucose to the blood; the kidney also has both gluconeogenetic enzymes and glucose-6-phosphatase activities but they are quantitatively much smaller than the liver's activities: moreover the kidney does not store glycogen.

On average, the adult liver stores about 80 g of glycogen, and in the fasting (post-absorptive) state releases 9 g of glucose each hour to the blood to maintain the peripheral glucose concentration. The brain extracts approximately half of this glucose, and skeletal muscle most of the rest. Clearly the amount of glucose which can generated by glycogenolysis is limited, and after an overnight (12 h) fast, approximately half of the hepatic glucose production (HGP) derives from gluconeogenesis rather than glycogenolyis. The contribution from gluconeogenesis increases progressively with fasting as glycogen stores become further depleted at the rate of 11% per hour. The carbon substrates for gluconeogenesis are derived from both lactate released by glycolysis in the peripheral tissues (the 'glucose-lactate' or 'Cori' cycle) and from hepatic deamination of amino acids (mainly alanine, the 'glucose-alanine' cycle) from the proteolysis of skeletal muscle (Chapter 20). Energy for gluconeogenesis comes from the β-oxidation of fatty acids. The end product of this process, acetyl-CoA, also stimulates the activity of the first committed enzyme of gluconeogenesis, pyruvate carboxylase.

On feeding, hepatic glucose production from gluconeogenesis is suppressed by insulin, which is carried directly from the pancreas to the liver by the portal vein. Glucose entering the circulation after feeding enters cells by specific transporters of differing kinetic properties. The glucose transporter 1 (GLUT1) present in brain is not sensitive to insulin and has a low Michaelis constant (Km), of the order of 1 mmol/L, and a low maximal velocity, around 3 mmol/L. Hence the GLUT1 transporters are saturated at most prevailing plasma glucose concentrations, and allow the brain to extract glucose at a steady rate which is unlikely to be influenced by feeding or fasting and also prevents excessive glucose uptake which could lead to cerebral oedema. The activity of the GLUT2 transporter, present in both liver and pancreas, is again independent of insulin, but has a very high Km, of the order of 15 to 20 mmol/L. These tissues take up glucose at a rate which is proportional to the plasma glucose concentration, and in the liver glucose is converted to glycogen. Glucose uptake by the pancreas determines β-cell insulin secretion and the GLUT2 transporter and/or the associated hexokinase which then phosphorylates glucose, act as glucose sensors.

Indeed, mutations in this pancreatic hexokinase, termed glucokinase, are the cause of some cases of the so-called 'maturity onset' diabetes in young people (MODY) (see Chapter 20). The majority of ingested glucose, however, is disposed of by muscle and fat tissue that possess another glucose transporter, GLUT4, which, because it has a Km similar to average plasma glucose concentrations of around 5 mmol/L and is sensitive to insulin, becomes the most important glucose sink in the fed state.

The liver, due to its specialized enzymatic properties, has a key role in glucose metabolism, which for glucose production is insulin-dependent, but for glucose consumption is insulin-independent.

LIVER AND PROTEIN METABOLISM

Hepatic protein synthesis is important, as the majority of plasma proteins are synthesized in the liver, and hepatocellular disease may alter protein synthesis both quantitatively and qualitatively.

Albumin is the most abundant protein in blood, and is synthesized exclusively by the liver (see Chapter 3). Low plasma albumin concentrations occur commonly in liver disease, but a better index of hepatocyte synthetic function is the production of the coagulation factors, II, VII, IX, and X (Chapter 6), which all undergo post-translational γ-carboxylation of specific glutamyl residues, allowing them to bind calcium. As a group, their functional concentration can be readily assessed in the laboratory by measurement of the prothrombin time (PT) (see Chapter 6).

The liver also synthesizes most of the plasma α and β-globulins. Plasma concentrations of these globulins change in hepatic disease and in systemic illness; in the latter case, the changes form part of the important acute phase response to the illness (Chapter 3).

Acute phase proteins

The acute phase response is a term which encompasses all of the systemic changes which occur in response to infection or inflammation.

As part of this reaction, the liver synthesizes a number of 'acute phase proteins', which have been defined as those hepatically-derived proteins whose plasma concentrations change by more than 25% within 1 week of the inception of the inflammatory or infective insult. The production of these proteins is stimulated by pro-inflammatory cytokines released by macrophages, and of these interleukin-1 (IL-1), interleukin-6 (IL-6), and tumor necrosis factor (TNF) have a central role in the induction of the acute phase response. The acute phase proteins have a number of different functions in the response to inflammation. Binding proteins, opsonins, such as C-reactive protein (CRP), bind to macromolecules released by damaged tissue or infective agents and promote their phagocytosis. Complement factors promote the phagocytosis of foreign molecules. Protease inhibitors, such as α1-antitrypsin and α1-antichymotrypsin inhibit proteolytic enzymes. These latter two acute phase proteins also promote fibroblast growth and the production of connective tissue required for the repair and resolution of the injury.

A substantial supply of amino acids is required as substrates for this increase in hepatic protein synthesis and these are derived from the proteolysis of skeletal muscle.

TNF and IL-1 again are involved by stimulating the breakdown of specific intracellular proteins by the ubiquitin-proteosome mechanism (see below).

The magnitude of the acute phase protein response often shows a quantitative relationship to the severity of the inflammatory/infective process, such that serial measurements of the serum acute phase proteins by clinical laboratories give useful information about the progress of the disease and its response to treatment. Changes in the serum concentration of CRP are quantitatively the most marked of all the acute phase proteins. Concentrations may increase by one or two orders of magnitude, the response is rapid and CRP has a short half-life. These properties and the relative ease with which it can be measured, have lead to CRP being widely used in clinical practice as a laboratory marker of infection/inflammation (see also Chapter 36).

Clinical conditions associated with abnormal plasma concentrations of specific liver proteins

Genetic deficiency of α1-antitrypsin presents in infancy as liver disease, or in adulthood as lung disease

Hepatic α1 antitrypsin, belongs to serpins, one of the family of serine protease inhibitors, and has, contrary to its name, macrophage-derived elastase as its predominant target protease. Genetic deficiency of α1-antitrypsin presents in infancy as liver disease, or in adulthood as lung disease caused by elastase-mediated tissue destruction; the severity of the liver disease associated with α1-antitrypsin deficiency is variable. Several isoforms of α1-antitrypsin exist as a result of allelic variation: the normal isoform is known as M, and the two common defective isoforms as S and Z; the null allele produces no α1-antitrypsin.

Genetic deficiency of ceruloplasmin itself leads to Wilson's disease, a condition associated with damage to both the liver and the CNS

Ceruloplasmin is the major copper-containing protein of the liver and plasma, and functions as an iron oxidizing (ferroxidase) enzyme: oxidation of Fe^{2+} to Fe^{3+} is necessary for the mobilization of stored iron, and nutritional copper deficiency

produces anemia. Genetic deficiency of ceruloplasmin itself leads to Wilson's disease, a condition associated with damage to both the liver and the CNS. The liver also synthesizes proteins responsible for storage (ferritin) and transport (transferrin) of iron (see Chapter 3).

Particularly high plasma concentrations of α-fetoprotein are associated with liver cancer

α-fetoprotein (AFP) and albumin have considerable sequence homology, and appear to have evolved by reduplication of a single ancestral gene. In the fetus, AFP appears to serve physiologic functions similar to those performed by albumin in the adult; furthermore, by the end of the first year of life, AFP in the plasma is entirely replaced by albumin. During hepatic regeneration and proliferation, AFP is again synthesized: particularly high plasma concentrations of AFP are associated with liver cancer.

Proteolysis

Hepatic protein turnover is highly regulated, which allows the activity of metabolic pathways to adapt to alterations in physiologic circumstances. Mammalian cells possess several proteolytic systems. Plasma proteins and membrane receptors are endocytosed, to be hydrolyzed by acid proteases within intracellular organelles known as lysosomes; intracellular proteins are degraded within structures known as proteasomes. These are large protein complexes that are present in the cytosol. Each proteasome which consists of four rings of protein subunits, the rings being stacked on top of one another to form a hollow cylindrical structure within which the intracellular proteins are hydrolyzed to small peptides of six to 12 amino acids. These peptides are released into the cytoplasm, where they are further degraded to their constituent amino acids by peptidases.

The intracellular proteins intended for proteasomal degradation are marked by conjugation with a small protein, ubiquitin

Ubiquitin is coupled to the amino groups of protein lysyl residues, and this conjugation reaction is repeated to form chains of five or more ubiquitin molecules linked to the protein. Ubiquitin-bound proteins are targeted for degradation. The specificity of the proteasomal degradation relies on the specificity of the enzymes responsible for the ligation of ubiquitin to the protein substrate, without which the protein will not enter the proteasome.

The urea cycle and ammonia

Catabolism of amino acids generates ammonia (NH_3) and ammonium ions (NH_4^+). Ammonia is toxic, particularly to the central nervous system (CNS). Most ammonia is detoxified at its site of formation, by amidation of glutamate to glutamine, which is mainly derived from muscle and used as an energy source by enterocytes. The remaining nitrogen enters the portal vein either as ammonia or as alanine, both of which are used by the liver for the synthesis of urea.

The impaired clearance of ammonia and other nitrogenous waste products is an important cause of brain damage

The urea cycle is the major route by which waste nitrogen is excreted, and is described in Chapter 18. In neonates, inherited defects of any of the enzymes of the urea cycle lead to hyperammonemia, which impairs the function of the brain and causes a clinical condition known as encephalopathy. Such problems arise within the first 48 hours of life, and inevitably are made worse by protein-rich foods such as milk.

HEME SYNTHESIS

Heme, a constituent of hemoglobin, myoglobin, and cytochromes is synthesized in most cells of the body. The liver is the main nonerythrocyte source of its synthesis. Heme is a porphyrin, a cyclic compound which contains four pyrrole rings linked together by methenyl bridges. It is synthesized

 ## PORPHYRIAS

Defects in the heme synthetic pathway lead to rare disorders known as porphyrias. Different forms of porphyrias are caused by defects in enzymes starting from 5-ALA synthase and ending with ferrochelatase. Porphyrias are classified as hepatic or erythropoietic depending on the primary organ affected.

Three porphyrias are known as acute porphyrias and can be a cause of emergency admissions with abdominal pain (which needs to be differentiated from various surgical causes). They also cause neuro-psychiatric symptoms. Acute intermittent porphyria (AIC) is caused by the deficiency of hydroxymethylbilane synthase: an enzyme converting PBG to a linear tetrapyrrole: in this disorder the concentrations of 5-ALA and PBG increase in plasma and urine.

Hereditary coproporphyria is due to the defect in the conversion of coproporphyrinogen III to protoporphyrinogen III (copro-oxidase). The third form of acute porphyria is the variegate porphyria, the clinical manifestations of which are very similar to AIC. Other porphyrias, such as porphyria cutanea tarda, present clinically as the sensitivity of skin to light (photosensitivity) which may cause disfiguration and scarring. Also, the pathway is inhibited by lead at the stage of porphobilinogen synthase.

from glycine and succinyl-Coenzyme A, which condense to form 5-aminolevulinate (5-ALA). This reaction is catalyzed by 5-ALA synthase, located in mitochondria and is the rate-limiting step in heme synthesis. Subsequently, in the cytosol, two molecules of 5-ALA condense to form a molecule containing a pyrrole ring, porphobilinogen (PBG). Then, four PBG molecules combine to form a linear tetrapyrrole compound which cyclizes to yield uroporphyrinogen III and then coproporphyrinogen III. Final stages of the pathway occur again in the mitochondria where a series of decarboxylation and oxidation of side chains in uroporphyrinogen III yield protoporphyrin IX. At the final stage, iron (Fe^{2+}) is added by ferrochelatase to protoporphyrin IX to form heme. Heme controls the rate of its synthesis by inhibiting 5-ALA synthase (Fig. 28.3).

BILIRUBIN METABOLISM

In excess bilirubin imparts a yellow color to the skin. This is called jaundice.

Bilirubin is a catabolic product of heme. About 75% is derived from the hemoglobin of senescent red blood cells, which are phagocytosed by mononuclear cells of the spleen, bone marrow, and liver; in normal adults, this contributes a daily load of 250–350 mg of bilirubin. The ring structure of heme is oxidatively cleaved to biliverdin by heme oxygenase, a P450 cytochrome. Biliverdin is, in turn, enzymatically reduced to bilirubin (Fig. 28.4). The normal plasma concentration of bilirubin is less than 17 μmol/L (1.0 mg/dL); however, increased concentrations (more than 50 μmol/L or 3 mg/dL) are readily recognized clinically, because bilirubin imparts a yellow color to the skin (jaundice). Abnormalities in bilirubin metabolism are important pointers in the diagnosis of liver disease.

Bilirubin is metabolized by the hepatocytes and excreted by the biliary system

Whereas biliverdin is water soluble, bilirubin, paradoxically, is not, and so must be further metabolized before excretion (Fig. 28.5). This occurs in the liver, to which bilirubin is transported as a complex with plasma albumin; the hepatic uptake of bilirubin is mediated by a carrier, and this process may be competitively inhibited by other organic anions. The hydrophilicity of bilirubin is increased by esterification of one or both of its carboxylic acid side chains with glucuronic acid, xylose, or ribose. The glucuronide diester is the major conjugate, and its formation is catalyzed by a uridine diphosphate (UDP)-glucuronyl transferase. Conjugated bilirubin is then secreted by the hepatocyte into the biliary canaliculi.

Conjugated bilirubin in the gut is catabolized by bacteria to form stercobilinogen, also known as fecal urobilinogen,

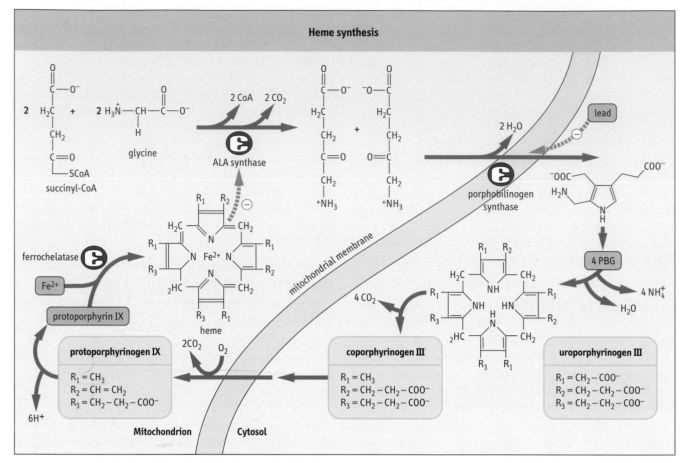

Heme synthesis

Fig. 28.3 **The pathway of heme synthesis.** Part of the pathway is located in the mitochondria and part in the cytosol. ALA, aminolevulinate, PBG, porphobilinogen. Hemoglobin is discussed in Chapter 4.

which is a colorless compound. On oxidation, however, stercobilinogen forms stercobilin (otherwise known as fecal urobilin), which is colored; most stercobilin is excreted in the feces, and is responsible for the color of feces. Some stercobilin may be reabsorbed from the gut and, being water soluble, can then be re-excreted by either the liver or the kidneys.

Bile acid metabolism

Bile acids are key elements in fat metabolism

Bile acids have a detergent-like effect, solubilizing biliary lipids and emulsifying dietary fat in the gut to facilitate its digestion (Chapters 9 and 16). They are synthesized by hepatocytes, which hydroxylate cholesterol at the carbon-7 position to produce the primary bile acids, cholic acid and chenodeoxycholic acid. These are conjugated with glucuronic acid, or with the amino acids taurine or glycine, and secreted in bile. In the intestine, the primary bile acids are

dehydroxylated by bacteria to form the secondary bile acids: cholic acid is converted to deoxycholic acid, and chenodeoxycholic acid to lithocholic acid. Both primary and secondary bile acids are also deconjugated by bacteria.

Intestinal bile acids are reabsorbed and returned to the liver for re-secretion – a process known as the enterohepatic circulation. Elevated plasma, bilirubin levels (levels which occur in liver disease) cause itching.

The liver is the major site of both synthesis and catabolism of cholesterol

Indeed, the chenodeoxycholic acid/lithocholic acid pathway is the major route by which cholesterol is excreted. Consequently, the rate of production of bile acids from cholesterol can affect the plasma concentration of low-density lipoprotein (LDL) cholesterol. Increasing the rate of bile acid production lowers the intracellular concentration of cholesterol, upregulates hepatic cell membrane LDL receptors, and enhances the clearance of LDL from plasma. Interrupting the enterohepatic circulation of bile acids by the use of a

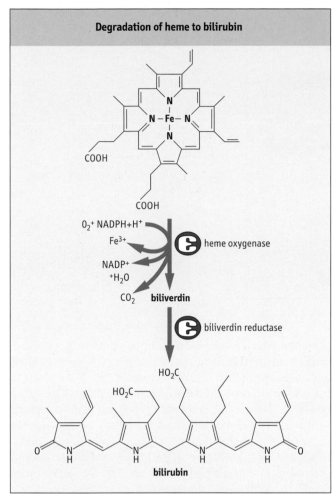

Fig. 28.4 **Degradation of heme to bilirubin.**

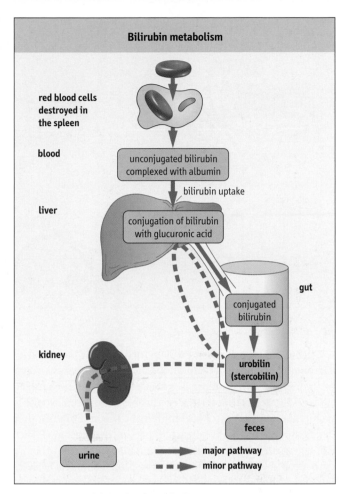

Fig. 28.5 **Normal bilirubin metabolism.**

nonabsorbable drug that binds them in the gut has the effect of decreasing plasma LDL, and was of therapeutic benefit in hypercholesterolemia (see Chapters 16 and 17).

DRUG METABOLISM

Low substrate specificity of hepatic enzymes produces a wide-ranging capability for drug metabolism

Most drugs are metabolized by the liver. Among other effects, this hepatic metabolism usually increases the hydrophilicity of drugs, and therefore their ability to be excreted. Generally, the metabolites that are produced are less pharmacologically active than the substrate drug; however, some inactive prodrugs are converted to their active forms as a result of processing in the liver. It is necessary for the hepatic drug-metabolizing systems to act on an infinite range of molecules; this is achieved by the enzymes involved having low substrate specificity. Metabolism proceeds in two phases:

■ **phase I**: the polarity of the drug is increased by oxidation or hydroxylation catalyzed by a family of microsomal cytochrome P450 oxidases;
■ **phase II**: cytoplasmic enzymes conjugate the functional groups introduced in the first phase reactions, most often by glucuronidation or sulfation.

Three of the 12 cytochrome P450 gene families share the responsibility for drug metabolism

The cytochrome P450 enzymes are heme-containing proteins that co-localize with reduced nicotinamide adenine dinucleotide phosphate (NADPH) cytochrome P450 reductase. The reaction sequence catalyzed by these enzymes is shown in Figure 28.6. There are 12 cytochrome P450 gene families, of which three, designated *CYP1*, *CYP2*, and *CYP3*, are mainly responsible for drug metabolism. Each gene locus has multiple alleles, and the P450 enzyme encoded by the *CYP3A4* gene appears to be involved in the metabolism of most drugs. Liver disease is likely to impair drug metabolism, and so drugs must be prescribed carefully for such patients.

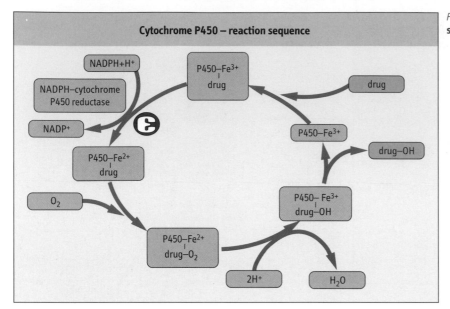

Fig. 28.6 **The role of cytochrome P450 system in the metabolism of drugs.**

The hepatic synthesis of P450 cytochromes is increased by certain drugs and other xenobiotic agents – a process known as 'induction', which increases the rate of phase I reactions. Conversely, drugs that form a relatively stable complex with a particular cytochrome P450 inhibit the metabolism of other drugs that are normally substrates for that cytochrome P450. Allelic variation that affects the catalytic activity of a cytochrome P450 will also affect the pharmacologic activity of drugs. The best described example of such polymorphism is that of the P450 cytochrome *CYP2D6*, which was recognized initially in the 5–10% of normal individuals who were noted to be slow to hydroxylate debrisoquine, a now little-used blood-pressure-lowering drug. *CYP2D6* also metabolizes a significant number of other commonly used drugs, so that 'debrisoquine polymorphism' remains clinically significant.

Drug hepatotoxicity

Drugs that exert their toxic effects on the liver may do so through the hepatic production of a toxic metabolite. Drug toxicity may occur in all individuals exposed to a sufficient concentration of a particular drug. A drug may even be toxic in some individuals at concentrations normally tolerated by most patients prescribed the drug. This phenomenon is known as idiosyncratic drug toxicity, and may be due to a genetic or immunologic cause.

Commonly prescribed drug, acetaminophen (paracetamol) is hepatotoxic toxic in excess

Acetaminophen is widely used as a painkiller. Taken in the usual therapeutic doses, it is conjugated with glucuronic acid or sulfate, which is then excreted by the kidneys. In overdose, the capacity of these conjugation pathways is overwhelmed, and acetaminophen is then oxidized by a liver P450 cytochrome to *N*-acetyl benzoquinoneimine (NABQI), which can cause a free-radical-mediated peroxidation of membrane lipids, and thereby hepatocellular damage. NABQI may be detoxified by conjugation with glutathione, but in acetaminophen overdose these glutathione stores also become exhausted, and hepatotoxicity ensues (Fig. 28.7). Therapeutically, the sulfhydryl compound, *N*-acetyl cysteine (NAC), which promotes detoxification of NABQI by the glutathione pathway and also scavenges free radicals, is routinely used as an antidote to acetaminophen poisoning. The risk of hepatotoxicity can be reliably predicted from measurement of the plasma concentration of acetaminophen, and then NAC can be given to those patients at risk of liver damage.

Alcohol

Excess intake of alcohol remains the most common cause of liver disease in the Western world

Excess intake of alcohol remains the most common cause of liver disease in the Western world and may cause alcoholic hepatitis, steatosis due to deposition of fat or finally fibrosis (known as cirrhosis) which in turn leads to liver failure. The microscopic features of alcoholic cirrhosis are shown in Figure 28.8.

Alcohol is oxidized in the liver, mainly by alcohol dehydrogenase, to form acetaldehyde, which is in turn oxidized by aldehyde dehydrogenase (ALDH) to acetate. Nicotinamide adenine dinucleotide (NAD$^+$) is the cofactor for both these

Products of acetaminophen metabolism

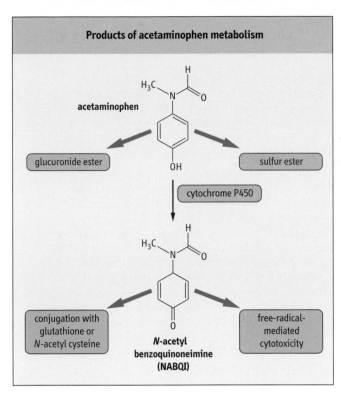

Fig. 28.7 **Metabolism of acetaminophen (paracetamol).**

 ## ACETAMINOPHEN AND HEPATIC FAILURE

A 22-year-old woman was admitted to hospital in a semiconscious state. She had been found with a suicide note and empty acetaminophen containers. Tests revealed: aspartate aminotransferase (AST) 5500 U/L, alkaline phosphatase (ALP) 125 U/L, bilirubin 70 μmol/L (4.1 mg/dL), prothrombin time 120 s (normal value 10–15 s), creatinine 350 μmol/L (4.0 mg/dL) (normal range 20–80 μmol/L [0.28–0.90 mg/dL]), glucose 2.6 mmol/L (47 mg/dL) (normal range 4.0–6.0 mmol/L [72–109 mg/dL]), and blood pH 7.1. No acetaminophen was found in her plasma.

Comment. The patient had acute hepatic failure, most probably caused by acetaminophen poisoning. Blood acetaminophen may be undetectable if the patient first comes to medical attention more than 24 hours after an overdose. The hepatocellular damage worsens over the first 72 hours, but may improve spontaneously after that, as a result of regeneration of hepatocytes. However, in patients with a metabolic acidosis, markedly increased prothrombin times or serum creatinine >300 μmol/L (3.4 mg/dL), mortality is very high, and liver transplantation may be necessary. For reference ranges see Table 28.2.

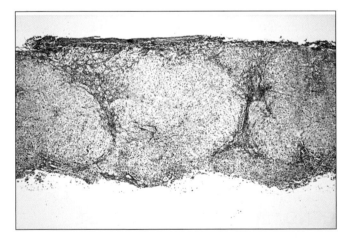

Fig. 28.8 **A histological slide of a cirrhotic liver.** (Courtesy Dr J Newman, Birmingham Heartlands and Solihull NHS Trust, UK).

oxidations, being reduced to NADH. A P450 cytochrome, *CYP2E1*, also contributes to ethanol oxidation, but is quantitatively less important than the alcohol dehydrogenase/ALDH pathway. Liver damage in patients who are abusers of alcohol may arise from the toxicity of acetaldehyde, which forms Schiff base adducts with other macromolecules.

The redox potential of the hepatocyte is altered by ethanol oxidation, as a result of the increased ratio of NADH to NAD$^+$.

This inhibits the oxidation of lactate to pyruvate – a step that requires NAD$^+$ as a cofactor. There is the potential for lactic acidosis and, because hepatic gluconeogenesis requires pyruvate as a substrate, there is also a risk of hypoglycemia. The likelihood of hypoglycemia is also increased in alcoholics when they fast, as they often have low hepatic stores of glycogen because of poor nutrition. The shift in the NADH/NAD$^+$ ratio also inhibits β-oxidation of fatty acids and promotes triglyceride synthesis; this increases hepatic synthesis of very-low-density lipoprotein, and the excess is deposited in the liver (hepatic steatosis) and secreted into plasma (see clinical boxes on p. 203 and p. 408). Hepatic steatosis is often associated with changes in the serum levels of the transaminase enzymes (see below) which are used by the clinical laboratory to monitor liver disease, but can be readily diagnosed by ultrasonography of the liver when one sees a uniform increased echogenicity (see Fig. 28.9).

The unpleasant symptoms of alcohol intolerance are exploited to reinforce abstinence

Both alcohol dehydrogenase and ALDH are subject to genetic polymorphisms, which have been investigated as a potential inherited basis of susceptibility to alcoholism and alcoholic liver disease. Possession of the ALDH2^2 allele, which encodes an enzyme with reduced catalytic activity, leads to increased plasma concentrations of acetaldehyde after the ingestion of

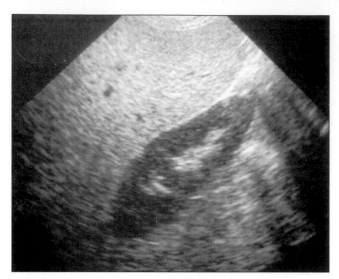

Fig. 28.9 **An ultrasound scan of a liver showing steatosis.** (courtesy Dr A Bannerjee, Birmingham Heartlands and Solihull NHS Trust, UK).

ALCOHOL-RELATED LIVER DISEASE

A 45-year-old businessman had a routine medical examination, at which he was found to have a slightly enlarged liver. Tests reveal: bilirubin 15 μmol/L (0.9 mg/dL), AST 434 U/L, ALT 198 U/L, ALP 300 U/L, γ-glutamyl transpeptidase (γGT) 950 U/L, and albumin 40 g/L (4 g/dL). He seemed perfectly well.

Comment. The patient has liver disease. On the basis of the biochemical tests there is evidence of hepatocellular damage. The increased γGT concentration is one of the most sensitive indices of excessive intake but there may also be enlarged red blood cells (macrocytosis) and an increased serum uric acid concentration. Patients may deny alcohol abuse. Needle biopsy of the liver may be necessary for diagnosis. In this patient microscopic examination of the tissue revealed characteristic changes of alcoholic steatosis, hepatitis and central fibrosis. This may be the forerunner of cirrhosis and the patient should abstain from alcohol. Other causes, such as chronic viral infection of the liver or an autoimmune active chronic hepatitis can be detected by blood tests. For reference ranges see Table 28.2.

alcohol. This causes the individual to experience unpleasant flushing and sweating, which discourages alcohol abuse. Disulfiram, a drug that inhibits ALDH, also leads to these symptoms when alcohol is taken, and may be given to reinforce abstinence from alcohol. (See also box on p. 242.)

PHARMACOGENOMICS

The response to any particular drug will be influenced by the kinetic properties of the drug (pharmacokinetics) and its effects (pharmacodynamics). Genes which code for drug-metabolizing enzymes, receptors and transporters can influence the individual's response to the drug and any variability in these genes may lead to inter-individual differences in response to that drug.

Pharmacogenomics studies the effects of genetic heterogeneity on drug responsiveness

Since the liver has a central role in drug metabolism, the pharmacogenomics of some hepatic drug-metabolizing enzymes, specifically the cytochrome P450 oxidases, is clinically relevant.

CYP2D6 is responsible for the metabolism of more than 100 pharmaceuticals, and a polymorphism of this enzyme is responsible for the long-established variation in the metabolism of debrisoquine, mentioned above. Patients are classified as ultra-rapid, extensive, intermediate and poor metabolizers of debrisoquine. There is one *CYP2D6* genetic locus, and individuals may have two, one or no functional alleles, corresponding to extensive, intermediate and poor metabolizers respectively: gene multiplication can lead to three functional alleles and the ultra-rapid metabolizer

phenotype. Seventy five *CYP2D6* alleleic variants have been identified and pharmacogenetic techniques can identify the metabolize phenotype, thereby predicting clinical response to treatment. Although debrisoquine is now obsolete, the *CYP2D6* polymorphism is relevant for some drugs used in cardiac and psychiatric practice, since poor metabolizers are more likely than other individuals to experience drug toxicity, and less likely to gain benefit from the analgesic codeine, a pro-drug which is metabolized by *CYP2D6* to morphine, the active drug. A polymorphism of *CYP2C19*, again leading to extensive and poor metabolize phenotypes, affects the metabolism of the proton pump inhibitor drugs used to gastro-esophageal reflux disease and the cure rate of treatment.

GENOMICS OF LIVER DISEASE

A few hepatic diseases arise due to single gene disorders and as such genetic techniques can identify those with a propensity to develop that disease or confirm the diagnosis in affected individuals.

Hereditary haemochromatosis is a genetically based disorder of iron metabolism, and is extremely common in northern Europeans, with a population prevalence of 1 in 200 to 1 in 300. Patients chronically absorb excessive amounts of iron from the gut, and tissue iron overload leads to multiorgan dysfunction, including cirrhosis of the liver. A transmembrane glycoprotein, known as HFE, modulates iron uptake and mutations in the genetic locus which encodes this protein, the HFE gene, underlie hereditary haemochromatosis. Two point mutations, *C282Y* and *H63D* are found in the majority of those with hereditary haemochromatosis and can be identified easily by PCR-based assays. Alpha-1 antitrypsin (AA1T) deficiency leads to early onset lung disease and to liver cirrhosis. More than 90 allelic variants of the AA1T gene, at the so-called Pi or proteinase inhibitor locus, have been described, the majority of which do not affect plasma levels or activity of AA1T. Phenotypic variants in AA1T were initially described by their relative mobility on electrophoresis, with the most common variant, M, having medium mobility. The Z and S variants are most frequently associated with AA1T deficiency, and are both due to point mutations which can also be detected by PCR assays. Wilson's disease, another hereditary cause of cirrhosis due to excess copper deposition in the liver, is also caused by a single gene defect, but multiple mutations have been found in affected patients no routine assay is available for diagnosis.

Gilbert's disease (see below) is caused by a dinucleotide polymorphism in the TATA box promoter of the bilirubin UDP-glucuronyl transferase gene which impairs the hepatic uptake of unconjugated bilirubin.

BIOCHEMICAL TESTS OF LIVER FUNCTION

A panel of biochemical measurements are routinely performed in the clinical laboratories on plasma or serum specimens (Table 28.2). This group of tests are usually, and incorrectly, described as liver 'function' tests, which commonly include the measurements of:

- bilirubin,
- albumin,
- transaminases: aspartate aminotransferase (AST) and alanine aminotransferase (ALT).
- alkaline phosphatase (ALP), sometimes in conjunction with:
- γ-glutamyl transferase (γGT).

(Reference ranges for these tests are given in the legend to Table 28.2).

Transaminases

Aspartate amino transferase (AST) and alanine transaminase (ALT) are involved in the interconversion of amino and ketoacids, and are therefore required for hepatic metabolism of nitrogen and carbohydrates. Both these transaminases are located in the mitochondria; ALT is also found in the cytoplasm. The serum activity of ALT is a better marker of liver disease than that of AST, which is also present in muscle and red blood cells. In more severe liver disease, the synthetic functions of the hepatocytes are likely to be affected, and so

Differential diagnosis of jaundice

Test	Prehepatic	Intrahepatic	Posthepatic
Conjugated bilirubin	absent	increased	increased
AST or ALT	normal	increased	normal
ALP	normal	normal	increased
Urine bilirubin	absent	present	present
Urine urobilinogen	present	present	absent

Table 28.2 **Differential diagnosis of jaundice based on laboratory tests.** The reference ranges for liver function tests are as follows:
AST (aspartate aminotransferase) 5–45 U/L,
ALT (alanine aminotransferase) 5–40 U/L,
ALP (alkaline phosphatase) 50–260 (ALP is physiologically elevated in children and adolescents).
Bilirubin <17 μmol/L (<1.0 mg/dL),
Albumin 35–45 g/L (3.5–4.5 g/dL),
γ-glutamyl transpeptidase: men <90 U/L, women <50 U/L.
See also box on p. 422.

The causes of jaundice

Type	Cause	Clinical example	Frequency
Prehepatic	hemolysis	autoimmune	uncommon
		abnormal hemoglobin	depends on region
Intrahepatic	infection	hepatitis A, B, C	common/very common
	chemical/drug	acetaminophen	common
		alcohol	common
	genetic errors: bilirubin metabolism	Gilbert's syndrome	1 in 20
		Crigler–Najjar syndrome	very rare
		Dubin–Johnson syndrome	very rare
		Rotor's syndrome	very rare
	genetic errors: specific proteins	Wilson's disease	1 in 200 000
		α₁ antitrypsin	1 in 1000 with genotype
	autoimmune	chronic active hepatitis	uncommon/rare
	neonatal	physiologic	very common
Posthepatic	intrahepatic bile ducts	drugs	common
		primary bilary cirrhosis	uncommon
		cholangitis	common
	extrahepatic bile ducts	gall stones	very common
		pancreatic tumor	uncommon
		cholangiocarcinoma	rare

Table 28.3 **Causes of jaundice.**

the patient would be expected to have a prolonged prothrombin time and low serum albumin concentration.

Alkaline phosphatase (ALP)

ALP is synthesized both by the biliary tract and by bone, but the two tissues contain different ALP isoenzymes. Thus, the origin of the ALP may be determined from the isoenzyme pattern. Alternatively, the plasma activity of another enzyme, such as γ-glutamyl transpeptidase (GGP), which also originates in the biliary tract, may be measured.

CLASSIFICATION OF LIVER DISORDERS

Hepatocellular disease

Inflammatory disease of the liver is termed hepatitis, and may be of short (acute) or long (chronic) duration. Viral infections, particularly hepatitis A, B, and C, are common infectious causes of acute hepatitis, whereas alcohol and acetaminophen are the most common toxicologic causes. Chronic hepatitis, defined as inflammation persisting for more than 6 months, may also be due to the hepatitis B and C viruses, alcohol, and immunologic diseases in which the body produces antibodies against its own tissues (autoimmune diseases, Chapter 36). Cirrhosis is the result of chronic hepatitis, and is characterized microscopically by fibrosis of the hepatic lobules. The term 'hepatic failure' denotes a clinical condition in which the biochemical function of the liver is severely, and potentially fatally, compromised.

Cholestatic disease

Cholestasis is the clinical term for biliary obstruction, which may occur in the small bile ducts in the liver itself, or in the larger extrahepatic ducts. Biochemical tests cannot distinguish between these two possibilities, which generally have radically different causes; imaging techniques such as ultrasound are required.

Jaundice

Jaundice is clinically obvious when plasma bilirubin concentrations exceed 50 μmol/L (3 mg/dL) (see Table 28.2). Hyperbilirubinemia occurs when there is an imbalance between production and excretion. The causes of jaundice (Table 28.3) are conventionally classified as:

- **prehepatic:** increased production of bilirubin (Fig. 28.10),
- **intrahepatic:** impaired hepatic uptake, conjugation, or secretion of bilirubin (Fig. 28.11),
- **posthepatic:** obstruction to biliary drainage (Fig. 28.12).

Prehepatic jaundice results from excess production of bilirubin after hemolysis, or a genetic abnormality in the

THE SIGNIFICANCE OF NEONATAL JAUNDICE

A normal, term baby developed jaundice on the third day of life, with a bilirubin concentration of 150 μmol/L (8.8 mg/ dL), predominantly of the indirect form. The baby was otherwise well.

Comment. About 50% of normal babies become jaundiced 48 hours after birth. This physiologic jaundice is caused by temporary inefficiency in bilirubin conjugation, and resolves in the first 10 days. The hyperbilirubinemia is unconjugated in nature; if severe, it may require phototherapy (ultraviolet light to photoisomerize bilirubin into a nontoxic form) or exchange blood transfusion to prevent damage to the brain (kernicterus). Bruising from delivery, infection, or poor fluid intake may exaggerate the hyperbilirubinemia. Jaundice in the first 24 hours of life is abnormal and requires investigation to exclude hemolysis, as does physiologic jaundice severe enough to require phototherapy. Jaundice that presents later – after 10 days – is always abnormal, and is likely to indicate an inborn error of metabolism or structural defects of the bile ducts.

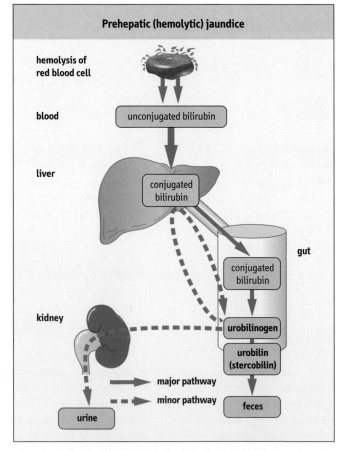

Fig. 28.10 **Prehepatic (hemolytic) jaundice.** There is an increased concentration of plasma total bilirubin due to the excess of the unconjugated fraction (see Table 28.2 for details).

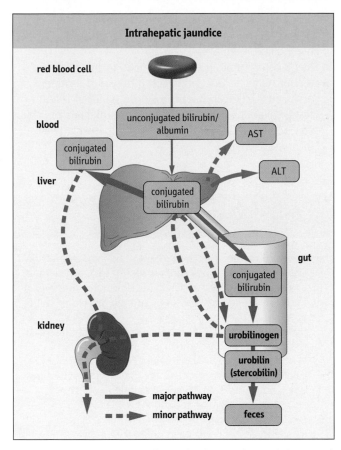

Fig. 28.11 **Intrahepatic jaundice.** Bilirubin in plasma is increased due to an increase in the conjugated fraction. Increased serum enzyme activities signify hepatocyte damage. See Table 28.2 for details.

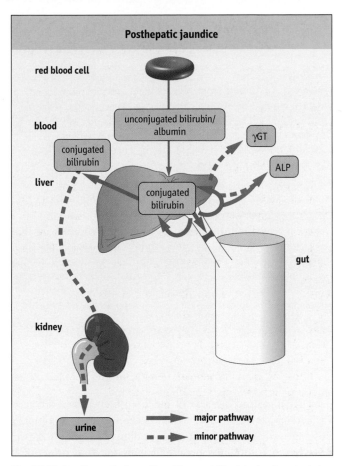

Fig. 28.12 **Posthepatic jaundice.** Plasma bilirubin is elevated due to an increase in the conjugated fraction. Obstruction of the bile duct does not allow passage of bile to the gut. Stools are characteristically pale in color. See Table 28.2 for details. γGT-γ-glutamyl transpeptidase; ALP, alkaline phosphatase.

hepatic uptake of unconjugated bilirubin. Hemolysis is commonly the result of immune disease, structurally abnormal red cells, or breakdown of extravasated blood. Intravascular hemolysis releases hemoglobin into the plasma, where it is either oxidized to methemoglobin or complexed with haptoglobin. More commonly, red cells are hemolyzed extravascularly, within phagocytes, and hemoglobin is converted to bilirubin; such bilirubin is unconjugated. Unconjugated and conjugated bilirubin can be chemically distinguished.

Intrahepatic jaundice reflects a generalized hepatocyte dysfunction. Hyperbilirubinemia is usually accompanied by other abnormalities in biochemical markers of hepatocellular function.

In neonates, transient jaundice is common, particularly in premature infants, and is due to immaturity of the enzymes involved in bilirubin conjugation. Unconjugated bilirubin is toxic to the immature brain, and causes a condition known as kernicterus. If plasma bilirubin concentrations are judged to be too high, phototherapy with blue-white light – which isomerizes bilirubin to more soluble pigments that might be excreted with bile – or exchange blood transfusion to remove the excess bilirubin are necessary to avoid kernicterus.

Posthepatic jaundice is caused by obstruction of the biliary tree. The plasma bilrubin is conjugated, and other biliary metabolites, such as bile acids, accumulate in the plasma. The clinical features are pale-colored stools, caused by the absence of fecal bilirubin and urobilin, and dark urine as a result of the presence of water-soluble conjugated bilirubin. In complete obstruction, urobilinogen/urobilin is absent from urine, as there can be no intestinal conversion of bilirubin to urobilinogen/urobilin, and hence no renal excretion of reabsorbed urobilinogen/urobilin.

Genetic causes of jaundice

There are a number of genetic disorders (Fig. 28.9) that impair bilirubin conjugation or secretion. Gilbert's syndrome, affecting up to 5% of the population, causes a mild unconjugated hyperbilirubinemia that is harmless and asymptomatic. It is due to a modest impairment in uridine diphosphate (UDP) glucuronyl transferase activity.

OBSTRUCTIVE LIVER DISEASE CAUSED BY PANCREATIC CANCER

A 65-year-old man was admitted to hospital because of jaundice. There was no abdominal pain, but he had noticed dark urine and pale stools. The gallbladder appeared palpable but not tender. Liver function tests showed: bilirubin 230 μmol/L (13.5 mg/dL), AST 32 U/L, and ALP 550 U/L. Dipstick urine testing revealed the presence of bilirubin, but no urobilin.

Comment. The patient had a history typical of obstructive jaundice. The increased ALP and normal AST concentrations were consistent with this, and the absence of urobilin in the urine indicated that the biliary tract was obstructed. It was important to carry out liver imaging investigations, to find the site of the obstruction; the absence of pain suggested that gallstones were not the cause. Ultrasound showed dilatation of the bile duct, and a computed tomography scan showed a mass in the head of the pancreas. At operation, cancer of the pancreas was confirmed.

Other inherited diseases of bilirubin metabolism are rare. Crigler–Najjar syndrome, which is the result of a complete absence or marked reduction in bilirubin conjugation, causes a severe unconjugated hyperbilirubinemia that presents at birth; when the enzyme is completely absent, the condition is fatal. The Dubin–Johnson and Rotor's syndromes impair the biliary secretion of conjugated bilirubin, and therefore cause a conjugated hyperbilirubinemia, which is usually mild.

Summary

The liver:

- has a central role in human metabolism;
- is extensively involved in the synthesis and catabolism of carbohydrate, lipids and proteins;
- synthesizes an array of acute phase proteins in response to inflammation and infection, and laboratory measurements of such proteins are clinically useful in monitoring disease progress;
- is specifically involved in the metabolism of bilirubin derived from the catabolism of heme;

- when affected by a variety of disease processes often causes the patient to present with jaundice due to hyperbilirubinemia;
- has a central role in the detoxification of drugs;
- its biochemical function is commonly and routinely assessed in clinical practice using a panel of blood tests, called liver function tests, abnormalities of which can point to disease affecting the hepatocelluar or biliary systems.

ACTIVE LEARNING

1. Discuss how the anatomical position and structure of the liver allows it to absorb and metabolize lipid, protein and carbohydrate, as well as xenobiotics from the intestine, before releasing such molecules or their derivatives to the systemic circulation.
2. Describe the function of the liver in protein synthesis and the systemic response to inflammation.
3. Outline how the liver processes bilirubin, derived from the catabolism of haem, and describe the biochemical causes of hyperbilirubinemia (jaundice) and its classification.
4. How does the liver metabolize drugs?
5. Discuss the biochemical tests used by the clinical laboratory in the investigation of liver disease.

Further reading

Van der Weide J, Steijns LSW. Cytochrome P450 enzyme system: genetic polymorphisms and impact on clinical pharmacology. *Ann Clin Chem* 1999;**36**:722–29.

Dennery PA, Seidman DS, Stevenson DK Neonatal hyperbilirubinaemia. *N Engl J Med* 2001;**344**:581–90.

Riordan SM, Williams R. Fulminant hepatic failure. *Clinics in Liver Disease* 2000;**4**:25–45.

Zakim D, Boyer TD (eds). *Hepatology. A Textbook of Liver Disease*. 4th edition. Philadelphia: Saunders; 2002.

Websites

http://www.nlm.nih.gov/medlineplus/liverdiseasesgeneral.html
http://www.labtestsonline.org/understanding/conditions/liver_disease.html

29. Biosynthesis and Degradation of Nucleotides

R Thornburg

LEARNING OBJECTIVES

After reading this chapter you should be able to:

- Compare and contrast the structure and biosynthesis of purines and pyrimidines, highlighting the differences between *de novo* and salvage pathways.
- Describe how cells meet their requirements for nucleotides at various stages in their cell cycle, at rest and during cell division.
- Describe the metabolic basis and therapy for classic disorders in nucleotide metabolism: Lesch-Nyhan syndrome, gout and SCIDS.
- Explain the biochemical rationale for using methotrexate in chemotherapy.
- Describe several metabolic conditions that result in accumulation of orotic acid in urine.

INTRODUCTION

Nucleotides are intimately involved in the normal physiology of cells. As nucleoside triphosphates, they constitute the currency of energy within cells. In other forms they participate at multiple levels in intermediary metabolism, from nucleotide and macromolecule biosynthesis to the biosynthesis of complex carbohydrates and the regulation of metabolism. Because nucleotides are involved in so many levels of metabolism they are important targets for chemotherapeutic agents used in treatment of microbial and parasitic infections and cancer.

This chapter will discuss the structure and metabolism of the two classes of nucleotides, purines and pyrimidines. The metabolic pathways are divided into four sections:

- *de novo* synthesis of nucleotides from basic metabolites, which provides a source of nucleotides from basic building blocks in growing cells;
- salvage pathways that recycle preformed bases and nucleosides and provide an adequate supply of nucleotides in cells at rest;
- catabolic pathways for excretion of nucleotide degradation products, a process that is essential to limit the accumulation of toxic levels of nucleotides within cells;
- biosynthetic pathways for conversion of the ribonucleotides into the deoxyribonucleotides, providing precursors for deoxyribonucleic acid (DNA) synthesis.

Purines and pyrimidines

Nucleotides are formed from three components: a nitrogenous base, a five-carbon sugar, and a phosphate moiety. The nitrogenous bases found in nucleic acids belong to one of two heterocyclic groups, either purines or pyrimidines (Fig. 29.1). The major purines of both DNA and ribonucleic acid (RNA) are guanine and adenine.

In DNA the major pyrimidines are thymine and cytosine, while in RNA the major pyrimidines are uracil and cytosine; thymine is unique to DNA, and uracil is unique to RNA. When the nitrogenous bases are combined with a five-carbon sugar, they are known as nucleosides. When the nucleosides are phosphorylated, the compounds are known as nucleotides. The phosphate can be attached either at the 5'-position or the 3'-position of ribose, or both. Table 29.1 gives the names and structures of the most important purines and pyrimidines.

PURINE METABOLISM

De novo synthesis of purine ring: inosine monophosphate (IMP)

The *de novo* synthesis of IMP provides the cell with the capacity to construct the purine ring *ab initio*, thereby insuring a source of nucleotides for cellular processes. Figure 29.2 shows portions of the pathway of purine biosynthesis along with the metabolic origin of each of the atoms in the purine ring. Synthesis is an energy-demanding process. Adenosine 5'-triphosphate (ATP) is required at each of the kinase, synthetase, and ring-closure steps. The starting material for purine biosynthesis is ribose 5-phosphate, a product of the pentose phosphate pathway.

The first step, catalyzed by ribose phosphate pyrophosphokinase (PRPP synthetase), generates the activated form of pentose phosphate by transferring a pyrophosphate group from ATP to form 5-phosphoribosyl-pyrophosphate (PRPP).

Classification of nucleotides

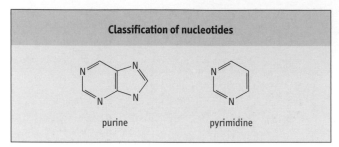

purine   pyrimidine

Fig. 29.1 **Classification of nucleotides.** Basic structure of purines and pyrimidines.

Names and structures of purines and pyrimidines

Structure	Free base	Nucleoside	Nucleotide
adenine structure	adenine	adenosine	AMP ADP ATP cAMP
guanine structure	guanine	guanosine	GMP GDP GTP cGMP
hypoxanthine structure	hypoxanthine	inosine	IMP
uracil structure	uracil	uridine	UMP UDP UTP
cytosine structure	cytosine	cytidine	CMP CDP CTP
thymine structure	thymine	thymidine	TMP TDP TTP

Table 29.1 **Names and structures of important purines and pyrimidines.** The designation NTP refers to the ribonucleotide. The prefix d, as in dATP, is used to identify deoxyribonucleotides. dTTP is usually written as TTP, with the d-prefix implied.

PRPP is also used in other biosynthetic reactions including nucleotide salvage and the biosynthesis of tryptophan and histidine.

In the second step, catalyzed by amidophosphoribosyl transferase, an amino group from glutamine displaces the pyrophosphate group. In a reaction that is similar to the for-

mation of a peptide bond, glycine is added to the β-5-phosphoribosylamine to yield glycinamide ribonucleotide (GAR), catalyzed by GAR synthetase. The free amino group of GAR is then modified by addition of a formyl group by GAR transformylase to make formylglycinamide ribonucleotide (FGAR). The formyl group comes from N^{10}-formyl tetrahydrofolate.

In step 5, a second amino group is added onto FGAR to form formylglycinamidine ribonucleotide (FGAM). As for other amino group additions, the donor is glutamine. The enzyme catalyzing this addition is termed FGAM synthetase. The imidazole ring is now closed to form 5-aminoimidazole ribonucleotide (AIR) by action of AIR synthetase.

The second 6-member ring is built by adding the three atoms, followed by cyclization. The first atom to be added is the C-6 carbon forming carboxyaminoimidazole ribonucleotide (CAIR). In an unusual reaction, catalyzed by AIR carboxylase, this carbon atom arises directly from CO_2, without involvement of biotin. The nitrogen atom at position 1 of the mature purine ring is now added in a two-step reaction, using aspartate as the nitrogen donor. The first step is the formation of an aspartate-CAIR covalent intermediate termed 5-aminoimidazole-4-(N-succinylocarboxamide) ribonucleotide (SACAIR), catalyzed by SACAIR synthetase. The four-carbon dicarboxylic acid, fumarate, is then released from SACAIR by the action of adenylosuccinate lyase to form 5-aminoimidazole-4-carboxamide ribonucleotide (AICAR).

The last purine-ring carbon is added as a formyl group from N^{10}-formyl tetrahydrofolate, by AICAR transformylase; the product is 5-formylaminoimidazole-4-carboxamide ribonucleotide (FAICAR). Finally, IMP synthase catalyzes closure of the second purine ring to form IMP.

Synthesis of purine nucleotides, ATP, and guanosine triphosphate (GTP) from IMP

IMP is the precursor of other purine nucleotides; it does not accumulate significantly within the cell. As shown in Figure 29.3, IMP serves as the starting material for both adenosine and guanosine monophosphate (AMP and GMP). Two enzymatic reactions are required to convert the ring system of IMP into that of AMP. In reactions similar to those in steps 8 and 9 for addition of the N^6 purine nitrogen to CAIR, aspartate is added at C-6 of IMP to form the adenylosuccinate intermediate by adenylosuccinate synthetase. Adenylosuccinate lyase then catalyzes hydrolysis of adenylosuccinate, yielding fumarate and AMP.

The formation of GMP from IMP is also a two-step process. The C-2 carbon is oxidized by IMP dehydrogenase by sequential hydration and oxidation reactions to yield xanthine monophosphate (XMP). XMP is then converted into GMP by GMP synthetase, using glutamine as the nitrogen donor (Fig. 29.3).

Portions of the purine biosynthetic pathway

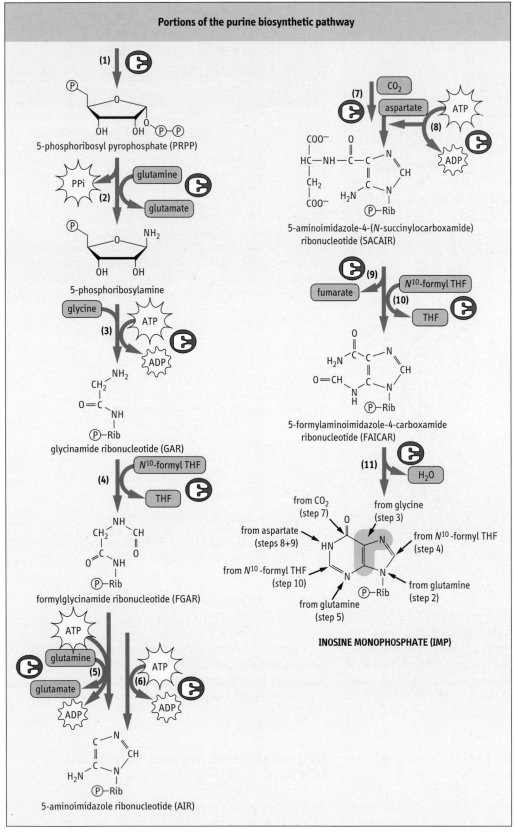

Fig. 29.2 **Portions of the purine biosynthetic pathway.** Enzymes for indicated steps:
(1) PRPP synthetase;
(2) amidophosphoribosyl-transferase;
(3) GAR synthetase;
(4) GAR transformylase;
(5) FGAM synthetase;
(6) AIR synthetase;
(7) AIR carboxylase;
(8) SACAIR synthetase;
(9) adenylosuccinate lyase;
(10) AICAR transformylase;
(11) IMP synthase.

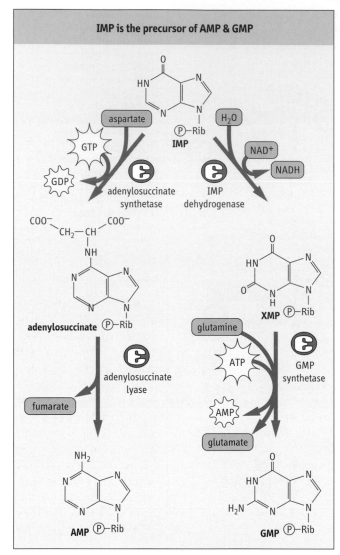

IMP is the precursor of AMP & GMP

Fig. 29.3 **The conversion of IMP into AMP and GMP.** Two enzymatic reactions are needed for each branch of the pathway.

Adenylate kinase and guanylate kinase use ATP to synthesize the nucleotide diphosphates from the nucleotide monophosphates. Finally, a single enzyme, termed nucleotide diphosphokinase, converts diphosphonucleotides into triphosphonucleotides. This enzyme has activity towards all nucleotide diphosphates, regardless of the base or sugar.

Preformed nucleotides can be recycled by salvage pathways

In addition to *de novo* synthesis, cells can use preformed nucleotides obtained from the diet or from the breakdown of endogenous nucleic acids through salvage pathways. In

FOR MANY ORGANISMS SALVAGE PATHWAYS ARE THE PRINCIPAL SOURCE OF NUCLEOTIDES

The observation that organisms blocked in the *de novo* biosynthetic pathways can survive and grow if a source of nucleotides is available from the diet indicates the strategic importance of the nucleotide-salvage pathways. The salvage pathways are especially important for many parasites. These organisms prey metabolically on their host, using preformed metabolites, including nucleotides. Some parasites, such as *Mycoplasma*, *Borrelia*, and *Chlamydia*, have lost the genes required for the *de novo* synthesis of nucleotides; they obtain these important components from their host.

Even in humans, resting T lymphocytes, immune-system cells produced in the thymus, meet their metabolic requirements for nucleotides through the salvage pathway, but *de novo* synthesis is required for lymphocyte proliferation. The salvage of nucleotides is especially important in HIV-infected T lymphocytes. In asymptomatic patients, resting lymphocytes show a block in *de novo* pyrimidine biosynthesis, and correspondingly reduced pyrimidine pool sizes. Following activation of the T-lymphocyte population, these cells cannot synthesize sufficient new DNA. The activation process leads to cell death, contributing to the decline in the T-lymphocyte population during the late stages of HIV infection.

mammals, there are two enzymes in the purine salvage pathway. Adenine phosphoribosyltransferase (APRT) converts free adenine into AMP:

$$\text{Adenine} + \text{PRPP} \rightarrow \text{AMP} + \text{PP}_i$$

Hypoxanthine-guanine phosphoribosyltransferase (HG-PRT) catalyzes a similar reaction for both hypoxanthine and guanine:

$$\text{Hypoxanthine} + \text{PRPP} \rightarrow \text{IMP} + \text{PPi}$$

$$\text{Guanine} + \text{PRPP} \rightarrow \text{GMP} + \text{PPi}.$$

Purine nucleotides are synthesized preferentially by salvage pathways, so long as hypoxanthine is available. This preference is mediated by hypoxanthine inhibition of amidophosphoribosyl transferase, step 2 in the *de novo* pathway (Fig. 29.2).

Degradation of purines in humans to uric acid

Each of the purine monophosphates (IMP, AMP, XMP, and GMP) can be converted into their corresponding nucleosides by 5′-nucleotidase. The enzyme, purine nucleoside phosphorylase, then converts the purine nucleoside (inosine, xanthosine or guanosine) into free purine base. This enzyme, however, does not function on adenosine. Two other enzymes, AMP deaminase and adenosine deaminase, convert the amino group of AMP and adenosine into the carbonyl group of IMP and inosine respectively.

Once the various free bases have been formed, they are catabolized to the common base xanthine. The enzyme guanine deaminase converts the amino group of guanine into a carbonyl group, yielding xanthine. Xanthine oxidase (XO) oxidizes hypoxanthine, the free base derived from adenine via inosine, to xanthine, and this same enzyme oxidizes xanthine to uric acid (Fig. 29.4). Uric acid is the final

metabolic product of purine catabolism in primates, birds, reptiles, and many insects. Other organisms, including most mammals, fish, amphibians, and invertebrates metabolize uric acid to simpler forms.

PYRIMIDINE METABOLISM

Uridine monophosphate (UMP) is the precursor of all pyrimidine nucleotides within a cell. The *de novo* pathway ends with the synthesis of UMP, and which is then converted to cytidine triphosphate (CTP) and thymidine triphosphate (TTP). Several salvage pathways also exist for cells to use preformed pyrimidines.

De novo pathway

The pathways of pyrimidine biosynthesis (Fig. 29.5) are invariant in all organisms that have been examined to date. The first step, catalyzed by the enzyme carbamoyl phosphate synthetase, uses bicarbonate, glutamine, and 2 moles of ATP to form carbamoyl phosphate. Carbamoyl phosphate is also used in the synthesis of arginine and in the urea cycle (Chapter 18). Most of the atoms required for formation of the pyrimidine ring are derived from aspartate, added in a single step by aspartate transcarbamoylase (ATCase). Carbamoyl aspartate is then cyclized to dihydroorotic acid by the action of the enzyme dihydroorotase. Dihydroorotic acid is oxidized to orotic acid by a mitochondrial enzyme, dihydroorotate dehydrogenase, which is linked to the electron-transport system through ubiquinone. Leflunomide, a specific inhibitor of this enzyme, is used for treatment of rheumatoid arthritis

LESCH-NYHAN SYNDROME RESULTS FROM HYPOXANTHINE-GUANINE PHOSPHORIBOSYL TRANSFERASE (HGPRT) DEFICIENCY

The gene encoding HGPRT is located on the X chromosome. Its deficiency results in a rare, X-linked recessive disorder termed Lesch–Nyhan syndrome. The lack of HGPRT causes an over-accumulation of PRPP, which is also the substrate for the enzyme amidophosphoribosyl transferase (see Fig. 29.2). This stimulates purine biosynthesis by up to 200-fold. Because of increased purine synthesis, the degradation product, uric acid, also accumulates to high levels. Elevated uric acid leads to a crippling gouty arthritis and severe neuropathology resulting in mental retardation, spasticity, aggressive behavior, and a compulsion towards self-mutilation by biting and scratching.

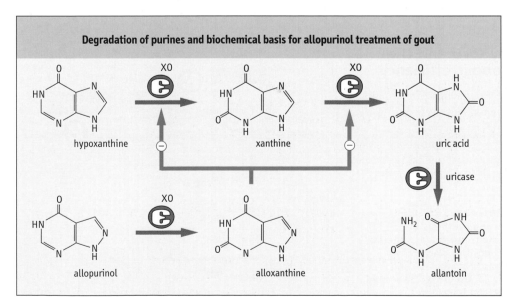

Degradation of purines and biochemical basis for allopurinol treatment of gout

hypoxanthine   xanthine   uric acid

allopurinol   alloxanthine   allantoin

Fig. 29.4 **Degradation of purines and biochemical basis of allopurine treatment of gout.** Inhibition of xanthine oxidase (XO) by alloxanthine is the mechanism involved in allopurinol treatment of gout. The enzyme uricase is missing in primates (including humans), but is commonly used for measurement of serum uric acid levels in humans.

GOUT RESULTS FROM TISSUE ACCUMULATION OF URIC ACID

Gout is a disease caused by accumulation of excess uric acid in body fluids (normal range = 0.1–0.5 mmol/L = 2.5–8.0 mg/dL). Uric acid and its urate salts have a low solubility in water, and excessive accumulation of urates results in the precipitation of needle-shaped sodium urate crystals. These crystals are frequently deposited in the soft tissues, particularly in joints. The toxicity of uric acid can be exacerbated by a variety of biochemical defects, including decreased renal clearance, HGPRT deficiency, and glucose-6-phosphatase deficiency. Glucose-6-phosphatase deficiency causes a stimulation of the pentose phosphate pathway, which increases the synthesis of ribose 5-phosphate and consequently PRPP, resulting in overproduction of purines. The over-production of the purines, and their subsequent turnover, leads to an increase in serum uric acid concentration. Gout is often treated with allopurinol, an inhibitor of xanthine oxidase (Fig. 29.4). Xanthine oxidase catalyzes the two-step oxidation of hypoxanthine to uric acid. Allopurinol undergoes the first oxidation to yield alloxanthine, but cannot undergo the second oxidation. Alloxanthine remains bound to the enzyme, thereby inactivating it. This leads to reduced accumulation of uric acid and accumulation of xanthine and hypoxanthine, which are more soluble and are excreted in urine. Increased dietary fiber also appears to suppress serum and urine levels of uric acid by inhibiting the digestion and promoting the excretion of dietary nucleic acids in feces.

because blockage of this step inhibits lymphocyte activation and thereby limits inflammation. The ribosyl-5'-phosphate group from PRPP is transferred onto orotic acid to form orotate monophosphate (OMP). Finally, OMP is decarboxylated to form UMP.

Metabolic channeling by CAD and UMP synthase improves metabolic efficiency

In bacteria and in some fungi, the six enzymes of pyrimidine biosynthesis exist as distinct proteins. However, during the evolution of mammals the first three enzymatic activities have been fused together into a single multifunctional polypeptide. This multifunctional protein, termed CAD for the first letter of each enzyme activity (see legend to Fig. 29.5), is

Fig. 29.5 **The metabolic pathway for the synthesis of pyrimidines.** This pathway has two multi-functional proteins. The first, CAD, has three enzymatic activities: **C**arbamoyl phosphate synthetase, **A**spartate transcarbamoylase, and **D**ihydroorotase (therefore the abbreviation CAD). The second, UMP synthase, has two enzymatic activities: orotate phosphoribosyl transferase and OMP decarboxylase.

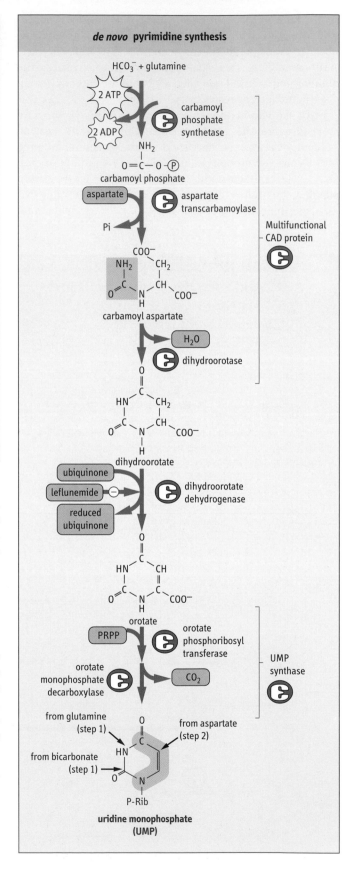

encoded by a single gene. Similarly, the polypeptides having the final two enzymatic activities of pyrimidine biosynthesis, orotate phosphoribosyl transferase and orotidylate decarboxylase, have also been fused into a single polypeptide, UMP synthase, which is also encoded by a single gene.

The advantage of such multifunctional proteins is that one protein can have multiple sequential enzymatic activities. In such enzymes, the products from the first reaction remain bound to the enzyme and are directed to the second enzymatic center. As with the fatty acid synthase complex, this avoids the diffusion of the metabolic intermediates into the intracellular milieu, thereby improving the metabolic efficiency of the individual steps.

CTP is synthesized from UTP

UTP is synthesized in two enzymatic phosphorylation steps by the actions of UMP kinase and nucleotide diphosphokinase.

SEVERE COMBINED IMMUNODEFICIENCY SYNDROMES (SCIDS)

SCIDS are a group of fatal disorders resulting from defects in both cellular and humoral immune function (see Chapter 36). SCIDS patients cannot efficiently produce antibodies in response to an antigenic challenge. Approximately 50% of patients with the autosomal recessive form of SCIDS have a genetic deficiency in the purine salvage enzyme, adenosine deaminase. The pathophysiology involves lymphocytes of both thymic and bone-marrow origin (T and B lymphocytes), as well as 'self-destruction' of differentiated cells following antigen stimulation. The precise cause of cell death is not yet known, but may involve accumulation in lymphoid tissues of adenosine, deoxyadenosine and dATP, accompanied by ATP depletion. The finding that deficiency of the next enzyme in the purine salvage pathway, nucleoside phosphorylase, is also associated with an immune-deficiency disorder suggests that integrity of the purine salvage pathway is critical for normal differentiation and function of immunocompetent cells in man.

Treatment of SCIDS patients has focused on two regimens. First, allogeneic bone marrow transplantation is generally successful. However the severe complications of graft-versus-host disease (GVHD) caused by non-identical donors coupled with only partial restoration of function in treated patients has led to the development of gene replacement therapies. Trials during the 1990s on correction of adenosine deaminase deficiencies in T lymphocytes or in stem cells with retroviral mediated gene transfer met with limited success. However, more recent results using improved techniques coupled with a better understanding of stem cell biology have resulted in successful gene transfer to patients with results comparable or better than can be achieved by bone marrow transplant.

UMP kinase can convert both UMP and CMP into UDP and CDP respectively. Again, as with the purines, nucleotide diphosphokinase converts the diphosphates into triphosphates. CTP synthetase converts UTP into CTP by amination of UTP. The nitrogen group is donated from glutamine in mammals. In bacteria, the nitrogen comes directly from ammonia (Fig. 29.6).

Pyrimidine-salvage pathways

As with the purines, free pyrimidine bases, available from the diet or from the breakdown of nucleic acids, can be salvaged by a series of enzyme reactions. The first of these operates on uracil and is similar to the purine-salvage systems:

$$\text{uracil} + \text{PRPP} \rightarrow \text{UMP} + \text{PP}_i.$$

The enzyme uracil phosphoribosyl transferase (UPRTase) is also required to activate some chemotherapeutic agents such as 5-fluorouracil (FU) or 5-fluorocytosine (FC). A second salvage reaction that is catalyzed by thymidine kinase is relatively specific for thymidine. It converts nucleosides into nucleotides by direct phosphorylation using ATP as the phosphate donor:

$$\text{thymidine} + \text{ATP} \rightarrow \text{TMP} + \text{ADP}.$$

OROTIC ACIDURIA

Orotic aciduria is a very rare genetic condition characterized by anemia resulting from defects in red cell maturation, accompanied by orotic aciduria. Orotic acid crystals form in urine on standing, but may also precipitate *in vivo*, causing obstruction of the urinary tract. The most severe form of orotic aciduria (Type 1) results from a deficiency of the enzyme UMP synthase. These patients are unable to convert orotic acid into UMP. The accumulated orotic acid is excreted in the urine. UMP synthase is a multifunctional protein containing both orotate phosphoribosyltransferase and OMP decarboxylase activity. The Type 1 form results from a complete loss of both activities. A second, rarer form of hereditary orotic aciduria (Type 2) is deficient in only OMP decarboxylase. This deficiency has been successfully treated with chronic uridine therapy.

Other metabolic disorders such as ornithine transcarbamoylase deficiency or argininosuccinic acid synthetase deficiency that result in abnormally high ratios of uridine to adenosine nucleotides in liver can also produce elevated levels of orotic acid in urine.

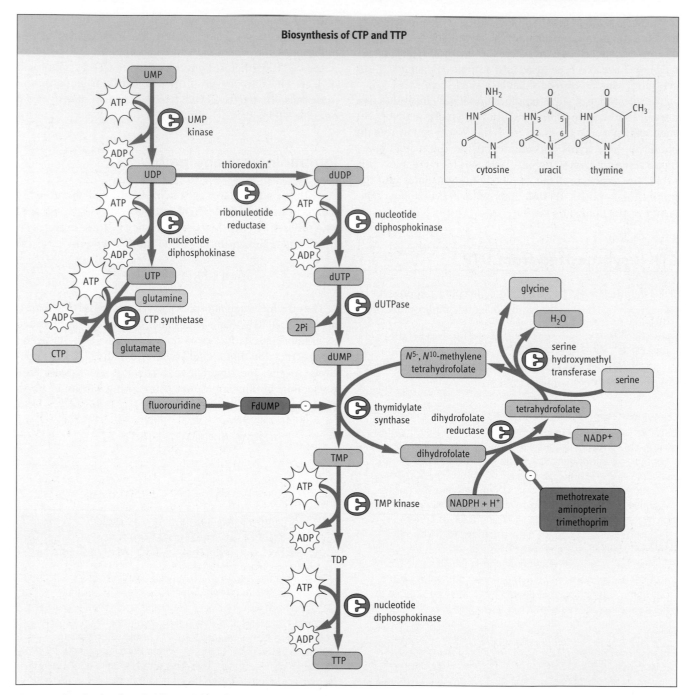

Fig. 29.6 **Synthesis of pyrimidine triphosphates.** Synthesis of thymidine is inhibited by fluorodeoxyuridylate (FdUMP), methotrexate, aminopterin, and trimethoprim at the indicated sites. *Thioredoxin restores sulfhydryl residues on ribonucleotide reductase, regenerating the active enzyme (see p. 422).

Cytosine deaminase

In bacteria and some fungi, there is an additional salvage enzyme, cytosine deaminase, that converts cytosine into uracil, which is salvaged by UPRTase. Cytosine deaminase is not found in most higher eukaryotes, including humans. Therefore, cytosine is not salvaged in humans. Because of this, fluorocytosine is a potent antimicrobial compound. The microbial enzyme converts fluorocytosine into fluorouracil, which is toxic (see below).

Degradation of pyrimidines is essentially the reverse of synthesis

The pyrimidine monophosphates, CMP, UMP, and TMP, are dephosphorylated to form their respective nucleosides. Cytidine is converted into uridine by action of cytidine deaminase. The ribose moiety of both uridine and thymidine (5-methyl uracil) is removed by action of an enzyme, uridine phosphorylase. The next three steps in the degradation of

MEASUREMENT OF OROTIC ACID IN URINE

Orotic aciduria is a symptom of several different metabolic disorders. Urinary orotic acid is usually measured by high performance liquid chromatography (HPLC) with detection at 275 nm; however, this method suffers from a lack of sensitivity and selectivity, i.e., other endogenous components can also absorb at this wavelength. A new analytical method uses liquid chromatography coupled with electrospray ionization tandem mass spectrometry (LC/MS/MS). Instead of measuring the absorbance of orotic acid, the mass spectrometer measures products of fragmentation of the orotate molecule, and provides excellent sensitivity and specificity. Although the instrumentation is expensive, sample preparation is simple and inexpensive, and multiple analytes can be measured simultaneously for diagnosis of a wide range of diseases.

pyrimidines are essentially the reverse of the synthetic pathway. The double bond between carbons 5 and 6 is reduced by dihydrouracil dehydrogenase to form dihydrouracil or dihydrothymine. Next the ring is opened by the action of hydropyrimidine hydratase to form β-ureidopropionate or β-ureidoisobutyrate. The enzyme β-ureidopropionase removes ammonia and carbon dioxide to form β-alanine or β-aminoisobutyrate. Finally, following an amino transfer of the β-amino group to α-ketoglutarate, the resulting malonic semialdehyde or methylmalonic semialdehyde can be condensed with CoA for further metabolism.

FORMATION OF DEOXYNUCLEOTIDES

Because DNA uses deoxyribonucleotides instead of the ribonucleotides found in RNA, cells require pathways to convert ribonucleotides into the deoxy forms. The adenine, guanine and uracil deoxyribonucleotides are synthesized from their corresponding ribonucleotides by direct reduction of the 2′-hydroxyl by the enzyme ribonucleotide reductase.

The nucleotide deoxy-TMP, abbreviated as TMP because it is unique to DNA, is synthesized by a special pathway involving methylation of the deoxyribose form of uridylate, dUMP. However, reduction of ribonucleotides to deoxyribonucleotides occurs only as diphosphates, not as monophosphates. Thus, the TMP biosynthetic pathway leads from UMP to UDP to dUDP (see Fig. 29.6). dUDP is then phosphorylated to dUTP, which creates an unexpected biochemical problem. DNA polymerase does not effectively discriminate between dUTP and TTP and can incorporate dUTP into DNA, which would lead to high rates of mutagenesis. Therefore, cells limit the concentration of dUTP by rapidly hydrolyzing dUTP to dUMP with the enzyme dUTP diphosphohydrolase. This enzyme releases pyrophosphate, which is rapidly hydrolyzed

SOME CHEMOTHERAPEUTIC AGENTS BLOCK PYRIMIDINE BIOSYNTHESIS

When DNA synthesis is blocked, cells cannot divide. Because of this, several important anticancer drugs that block the synthesis of TMP are widely used as chemotherapeutic agents (see Fig. 29.6). These include pyrimidine analogs such as fluorouridine and fluorocytosine, as well as the antifolates: aminopterin, methotrexate, and trimethoprim.

One of the unique steps in DNA biosynthesis is the formation of TMP from dUMP by the enzyme thymidylate synthase. During the process of catalysis, thymidylate synthase forms a covalent bond with its substrate, dUMP. The enzyme-substrate complex then forms a complex with N^5,N^{10}-methylene-THF. Once this ternary complex is formed, the methyl transfer occurs.

Fluorodeoxyuridylate (FdUMP) is a specific, suicide inhibitor of thymidylate synthase. In FdUMP, a highly electronegative fluorine replaces the carbon-5 proton of uridine. This compound can begin the enzymatic conversion into dTMP by forming the enzyme-FdUMP covalent complex; however, the covalent intermediate cannot accept the donated methyl group from methylene THF, nor can it be broken down to release the active enzyme. The result is a suicide complex in which the substrate is covalently locked at the active site of thymidylate synthase. The drug is frequently administered as fluorouridine (Adrucil, Efudex, Fluracil), and the body's normal metabolism converts the fluorouridine into FdUMP. Fluorouridine is used against breast, colorectal, gastric, and uterine cancers.

Fluorocytosine (Flucytosine, Alcobon, Ancotil) is a potent antimicrobial agent. Its mechanism of action is similar to that of FdUMP; however, it must first be converted into fluorouracil by the action of cytosine deaminase. The fluorouracil is subsequently converted into FdUMP, which blocks thymidylate synthase as above. While cytosine deaminase is present in most fungi and bacteria, it is absent in animals and plants. Therefore, in humans, fluorocytosine is not converted into fluorouracil and is nontoxic, while in the microbes, metabolism of fluorocytosine results in cell death. Aminopterin and methotrexate are folic acid analogs that bind about 1000-fold more tightly to dihydrofolate reductase (DHFR) than does dihydrofolate. See Figure 29.6 for the sites of action of these drugs. Antifolates effectively block the synthesis of tetrahydrofolate, which in turn limits the formation of N^5,N^{10}-methylene-THF. In this manner, they block the synthesis of dTMP. Further, these compounds are competitive inhibitors of other THF-dependent enzyme reactions used in the biosynthesis of purines, histidine, and methionine. Trimethoprim binds to DHFR, and binds more tightly to bacterial DHFRs than it does to mammalian enzymes, making it an effective antibacterial agent. Folate analogs are relatively nonspecific chemotherapeutic agents. They poison rapidly dividing cells, including those in hair follicles and gut endothelia, causing the loss of hair and gastrointestinal side-effects of chemotherapy.

to phosphate, pulling the reaction towards the formation of dUMP. The dUMP then serves as the substrate for thymidylate synthase, which transfers a methyl group from N^5,N^{10}-methylene tetrahydrofolate to make TMP. The folate is released as dihydrofolate. Two rounds of phosphorylation using ATP as phosphate donor yield TDP and subsequently TTP. The synthesis of TTP is a roundabout pathway, but does provide opportunities for chemotherapy through inhibition of TMP biosynthesis.

Regeneration of the methyl donor is accomplished in two steps. First, dihydrofolate is reduced to tetrahydrofolate, a step that is inhibited by several important chemotherapeutic agents. Then the amino acid, serine, is degraded to produce formaldehyde and glycine. The formaldehyde reacts with the N^5,N^{10}-imine groups of tetrahydrofolate to yield N^5,N^{10}-methylene tetrahydrofolate.

Feedback control of ribonucleotide reductase maintains similar amounts of all four deoxynucleotides

The reduction of the 2'-hydroxyl of ribose uses a pair of protein-bound sulfhydryls (cysteine residues). The hydroxyl group is released as water, and the cysteines are oxidized to cystine during the reaction. To regenerate an active enzyme, the disulfide must be reduced back to the original sulfhydryl pair by disulfide exchange; this is accomplished by reaction with a small protein, thioredoxin (see Fig. 29.6). Thioredoxin, a highly conserved Fe-S protein, is in turn reduced by the flavoprotein, thioredoxin reductase. The dNTPs are produced by phosphorylation of the dNDPs, using ATP as the phosphate donor.

Because a single enzyme is responsible for the conversion of all ribonucleotides into deoxyribonucleotides, this enzyme is subject to a complex network of feedback regulation. The enzyme contains several allosteric sites for metabolic regulation. Levels of the different dNTPs modify the enzyme activity toward the different NDPs. By regulating the enzymatic activity of deoxyribonucleotide synthesis as a function of the concentration of the different dNTPs, the cell insures that the proper ratios of the different deoxyribonucleotides are produced for normal growth, protein synthesis, and cell division.

De novo nucleotide metabolism is highly regulated

Because nucleotides are required for mammalian cells to proliferate, the de novo pathways of nucleotide metabolism are inducible both transcriptionally and post-transcriptionally. Genes encoding a number of nucleotide biosynthetic enzymes for both purines and pyrimidines are transcriptionally upregulated following growth factor treatment. Post-transcriptional regulation also plays an important role in nucleotide synthesis. The multimeric protein, CAD is activated by phosphorylation by both mitogen-activated protein kinase (MAPK) and protein kinase A (PKA). MAPK phosphorylation increases the binding of PRPP by CAD and decreases the inhibition of UTP. Both of these allosteric regulatory changes favor biosynthesis of pyrimidines for growth. PKA phosphorylation reduces the response to both allosteric effectors on the CAD enzyme activity. The phosphorylation of CAD is also regulated during in the cell cycle, with phosphorylated forms accumulating just before the onset of S-phase, and these changes are reversed when cells emerge from S-phase (see Chapter 41). Recently, this enzyme has also been shown to be degraded by capsase-3 proteolysis during the initial stages of apoptosis. Thus, the pyrimidine biosynthetic pathway is selectively and efficiently inactivated during the process of apoptosis.

MEASUREMENT OF SERUM URIC ACID CONCENTRATION

Hyperuricemia is seen under a variety of conditions characterized by increased cell turnover, e.g. severe infection and inflammation. Diabetic ketoacidosis and renal failure also produce elevated serum uric acid levels. The common analytical method for uric acid utilizes a spectrophotometric test that relies of the enzyme uricase. Because most mammals, with the exception of primates (including humans), express uricase, allantoin is the end degradation product of purines in most mammals. Uricase oxidizes uric acid to allantoin, producing hydrogen peroxide, which is measured in a chromogenic reaction. These assays are generally performed on discrete, random-access, automated autoanalyzers.

PLASMA NUCLEOTIDASE ACTIVITY INCREASES IN HEPATOBILIARY DISEASE

The enzyme, 5'-nucleotidase, catalyzes the conversion of nucleotide monophosphates to nucleosides and inorganic phosphate. This enzyme is distributed in the membranes of liver cells, as well as in other tissues. Serum levels of nucleotidase are low in children, rise gradually during adolescence and reach a plateau at ~50 years of age. Serum levels of nucleotidase increase during hepatobiliary disease, along with other liver enzymes such as alkaline phosphatase. The elevation of both of these enzymes is specific for hepatobiliary disease. Nucleotidase is also elevated in women during the third trimester of pregnancy.

Summary

Nucleotides are synthesized primarily from amino acid precursors and phosphoribosylpyrophosphate by complex, multistep pathways. Not surprisingly therefore, salvage pathways therefore play a prominent role in nucleotide metabolism. *De novo* nucleotide metabolism is required for cell proliferation. Both classes of nucleotides (purines and pyrimidines) are synthesized as precursors (IMP, UMP), which are then converted into the DNA precursors (dATP, dGTP, dCTP, TTP). With the exception of TTP, ribonucleotides are converted to deoxyribonucleotides by ribonucleotide reductase. TTP is synthesized from dUMP by a special pathway involving folates. The salvage pathways have proven useful for the activation of pharmaceutical agents, while the uniqueness of the pathway for synthesis of TTP has provided a special target for chemotherapeutic inhibition of DNA synthesis and cell division in cancer cells.

ACTIVE LEARNING

1. Compare the roles of *de novo* synthesis and salvage pathways of nucleotide synthesis in various cell types, e.g. erythrocytes, lymphocytes, muscle and liver.
2. In addition to its activity as a xanthine oxidase inhibitor, what other activities of allopurinol might contribute to its efficacy for treatment of gout?
3. Discuss the use of thymidylate synthetase inhibitors for treatment of diseases other than cancer, e.g. arthritis and Crohn's disease.

Further reading

Rott KT, Agudelo CA. Gout. *JAMA* 2003;289:2857–2860.

Huennekens FM. The methotrexate story: a paradigm for development of cancer chemotherapeutic agents. *Adv Enz Reg* 1994;34:379–419.

Kinsella AR, Smith D, Pickard M. Resistance to chemotherapeutic antimetabolites: a function of the salvage pathway involvement and cellular response to DNA damage. *Br J Cancer* 1997;75:935–945.

Nyhan WL. The recognition of Lesch-Nyhan syndrome as an inborn error of purine metabolism. *J Inherited Metab Dis* 1997;**20**:171–178.

Rustum YM, Harstrick A, Cao S, Vanhoefer U, Yin M, Wilke H, Seeber S. Thymidylate synthase inhibitors in cancer therapy: direct and indirect inhibitors. *J Clin Oncol* 1997;**15**:389–400.

Sigoillot FD, Berkowski JA, Sigoillot SM, Kotsis DH, Guy HI. Cell cycle-dependent regulation of pyrimidine biosynthesis. *J Biol Chem* 2003;**278**:3403–3409.

Aiuti A. Advances in gene therapy for ADA-deficient SCID. *Curr Opin Mol Ther* 2002;**4**:515–522.

Websites

Purine and pyrimidine disorders: www.amg.gda.pl/~essppmm/index.html;

Gout: www.nlm.nih.gov/medlineplus/goutandpseudogout.html; www.niams.nih.gov/hi/topics/gout/gout.htm; ww.nhsdirect.nhs.uk/en.asp?TopicID=221

Lesch Nyhan Syndrome: www.icondata.com/health/pedbase/files/LESCH-NY.HTM; www.emedicine.com/neuro/topic630.htm

SCIDS: www.scid.net

30. Deoxyribonucleic acid (DNA)

R Thornburg

LEARNING OBJECTIVES

After reading this chapter you should be able to:

■ Describe the composition and structure of DNA, based on the Watson–Crick model, including the concepts of directionality and complementarity in DNA structure.

■ Outline the process for packaging of DNA in the nucleus.

■ Explain how replication of DNA is achieved with high fidelity in a bidirectional manner and in a semi-conservative fashion.

■ Discuss the enzymes involved, the activities at replication forks, and the structures and intermediates participating in the replication process.

■ Describe the mechanism by which replication is controlled in the eukaryotic cell.

■ Describe the nature of the damage and mechanisms involved in the repair of damage to DNA.

■ Explain the mechanism of action of AZT for treatment of AIDS.

XERODERMA PIGMENTOSUM

Xeroderma Pigmentosum (XP) is a group of rare, life-threatening, autosomal recessive disorders (incidence = 1/250 000) that are marked by extreme sensitivity to sunlight. Upon exposure to sunlight or ultraviolet radiation, the skin of XP patients erupts into pigmented spots, resembling freckles. Multiple carcinomas and melanomas appear early in life, exacerbated by sun exposure, and the majority of patients succumb to cancer before reaching adulthood.

XP is the result of a defect in repair of UV-induced thymine dimers in DNA. There are at least eight genes that are involved in repair of UV-induced thymine dimers. Patients with XP must avoid direct sunlight, fluorescent light, halogen light, or any other source of ultraviolet light. An experimental form of protein therapy, currently undergoing clinical evaluation, involves application of a skin lotion containing the missing protein or enzyme. Ideally, this protein will enter the skin cells and stimulate the repair of UV damaged DNA. However, protection occurs only where the lotion can be applied. For example, this treatment does not address the neurological problems that affect about 20% of XP patients.

INTRODUCTION

Cellular nucleic acids exist in two forms, deoxyribonucleic acid (DNA) and ribonucleic acid (RNA). Approximately 90% of the nucleic acid within cells is RNA, and the remainder is DNA. DNA is the repository of genetic information within the cell. This chapter deals with the structure of DNA, the manner in which it is stored in chromosomes in the nucleus, and the mechanisms involved in its biosynthesis and repair.

STRUCTURE OF DNA

DNA is an anti-parallel dimer of nucleic acid strands. It is composed of nucleotides containing the sugar deoxyribose. Deoxyribose is missing the hydroxyl group at the 2′-position. The chains of DNA are polymerized through a phosphodiester linkage from the 3′-hydroxyl of one subunit to the 5′-hydroxyl of the next subunit (Fig. 30.1A). Thus, DNA is a linear deoxyribose phosphate chain with purine and pyrimidine bases attached to carbon-1 of the deoxyribose subunit.

Using X-ray diffraction photographs of DNA taken by Rosalind Franklin, a structure for DNA was proposed by James Watson and Francis Crick in 1953. This model proposed that DNA was composed of two intertwined complementary strands with hydrogen bonds holding the strands together (Fig. 30.1B). The basic simplicity of this structure led to its rapid acceptance. While some of the details of the model have been modified, its essential elements have remained unchanged since originally proposed.

Watson and Crick model of DNA

As originally presented by Watson and Crick, DNA is composed of two strands, wound around each other in a right-handed, helical structure with the base pairs in the middle and the deoxyribosylphosphate chains on the outside. The orientation of the DNA strands is anti-parallel (i.e. the strands run in opposite directions). The nucleotide bases on each

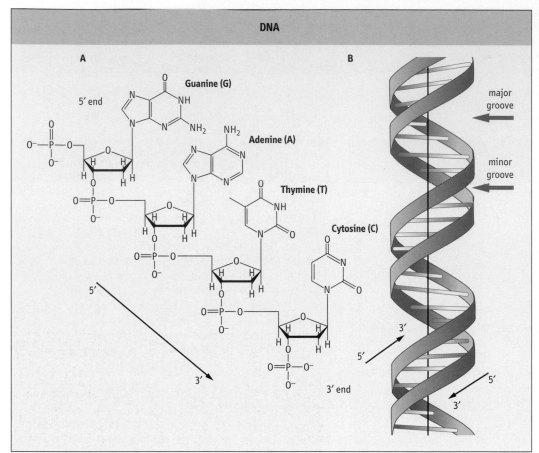

Fig. 30.1 **Structure of DNA.** (A) A tetranucleotide sequence of DNA showing each of the nucleotides normally found in DNA. The deoxyribose sugars are missing the 2'-hydroxyl that is present in the ribose sugars found in RNA. By convention, DNA is read from the 5' to 3' end, so the sequence of this tetranucleotide is 5'-GATC-3'. (B) A graphic representation of the structure of B-DNA, the major form of DNA in the cell. The base pairs in the middle are aligned nearly perpendicular to the helical axis. The major groove and the minor groove are shown. Note that the strands are antiparallel.

strand interact with the nucleotide bases on the other strand to form base pairs (Fig. 30.2). The base pairs are planar and are oriented nearly perpendicular to the axis of the helix. Each base pair is formed by hydrogen bonding between a purine and a pyrimidine. Guanine forms three hydrogen bonds with cytosine, and adenine forms two with thymine. Because of the specificity of this interaction between purines and pyrimidines on the opposite strands, the opposing strands of DNA are said to have complementary structures. The composite strength of the numerous hydrogen bonds formed between the bases of the opposite strands is responsible for the extreme stability of the DNA double helix. While the hydrogen bonds between strands are affected by temperature and ionic strength, stable complementary structures can be formed at room temperature with as few as six to eight nucleotides.

Three-dimensional DNA

The three-dimensional structure of the DNA double helix is such that the deoxyribosyl phosphate backbones of the two strands are slightly offset from the center of the helix. Because of this, the grooves between the two strands are of different sizes. These grooves are termed the major groove and the

minor groove (see Figs 30.1B and 30.2). The major groove is more open and exposes the nucleotide base pairs. The minor groove is more constricted, being partially blocked by the deoxyribosyl moieties linking the base pairs. Binding of proteins to DNA frequently occurs in the major groove and is specific for the nucleotide sequence of DNA.

Alternate forms of DNA may help to regulate gene expression

Although the majority of DNA within a cell exists in the form described above (the B-form), alternative forms of DNA also exist. When the relative humidity of B-form DNA falls to less than 75%, the B-form undergoes a reversible transition into the A-form of DNA. In the A-form of DNA, the nucleotide base pairs are tilted 20°relative to the helical axis and the helix diameter is increased, compared to the B form (Fig. 30.3). When the DNA strands consist of polypurine and polypyrimidine tracks, the DNA helix shows different properties. Polypurine regions are A-like, while polypyrimidine regions are B-like. These regions do not efficiently bind histones and are therefore unable to form nucleosomes (see

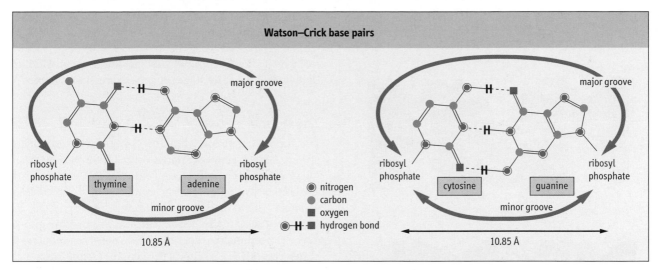

Fig. 30.2 **Watson–Crick base pairing of nucleotides in DNA.** The AT base pairs form two hydrogen bonds and the GC base pairs form three hydrogen bonds. Thus, GC-rich regions are more stable than AT-rich regions.

below), resulting in nucleosome-free (exposed) regions of DNA.

Another unique form of DNA exists when the sequence of nucleotides consists of alternating purine/pyrimidine stretches. This form, termed Z-DNA, is also favored at high ionic concentrations. In Z-DNA, the base pairs flip 180° relative to the sugar nucleotide bond. This results in a novel conformation of the base pairs relative to sugar–phosphate backbones, yielding a form of DNA with a zigzag configuration (hence the name Z-DNA) along the sugar phosphate backbone. Surprisingly, this change in conformation leads to the formation of a left-handed DNA helix. While the Z-DNA form is favored at high ionic concentrations, it can also be induced at normal ionic concentrations by DNA methylation. The positioning of these alternate forms of DNA throughout the genome participates in the regulation of gene expression.

Separated DNA strands can reassociate to form duplex DNA

Because the DNA strands are complementary and are held together only by noncovalent forces, they can be separated into individual strands. This strand separation or denaturation of DNA is commonly induced by heating the solution. The dissociation is reversible, and on cooling, the interactions between the complementary nucleotide sequences reassociate or reanneal to re-form their original base pairs. This is the basis for one of the primary methods for DNA analysis, Southern hybridization (Chapter 34). Because adenine and thymine interact through two hydrogen bonds and guanine and cytosine through three (Fig. 30.2), AT-rich regions melt at lower temperatures than G:C-rich regions in DNA. The

 DNA PATERNITY TESTING

Establishing the paternity of children can often be a divisive issue for families. In the past, this was legally settled by establishing the husband of the mother as the biological father. However, with modern DNA technology, paternity can be firmly established.

DNA samples should ideally be provided from both parents and offspring. If the DNA of the parent and offspring match, then paternity can be established with greater than 99.999% assurance. If there is no match, then the probability of paternity is 0.

The DNA collection method is straightforward. A cotton swab is rubbed on the inside of the cheek to collect epithelial cells, providing a source of the DNA. The DNA is then evaluated for the presence or absence of marker alleles using PCR methods (see Figure 34.11). The FBI uses 13 probes for routine identification of individuals. Even in the case where the father is unavailable or deceased, paternity testing can often be successfully performed. If the father is deceased, a medical examiner's office or hospital may have retained a blood sample that can be used for testing. A personal sample such as a cigarette butt, chewed gum, hair clippings, or electric razor shavings, a licked envelope, or other source of DNA may also be used. The absent parent's DNA type can also be partially reconstructed using that parent's biological parents. Prenatal parentage can also be established after amniocentesis (>12 weeks gestation) or by chorionic villi sampling (CVS) between 9 and 12 weeks gestation. DNA paternity tests have also been legally utilized by persons seeking entry into the US on the grounds that s/he is a biological relative of a citizen, by persons seeking to establish Native American tribal rights, by persons seeking to establish decendency from famous individuals, or by persons seeking to establish biological relationships with long-lost siblings.

B-, A-, and Z-forms of DNA

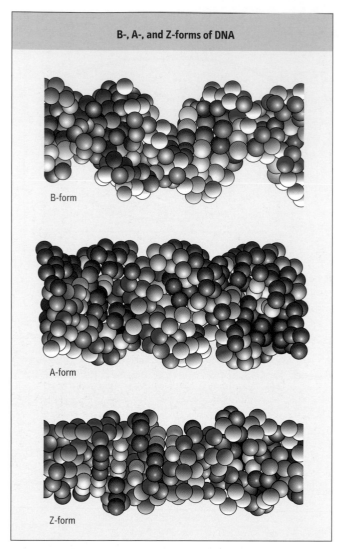

B-form

A-form

Z-form

Fig. 30.3 **The structures of different forms of DNA include the B-, A-, and Z-forms.** The sugar phosphate backbone of the DNA strands is colored blue. The nucleotide bases forming the internal base pairs are yellow for pyrimidines (thymine and cytosine) and red for purines (adenine and guanine).

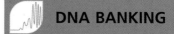 **DNA BANKING**

Knowledge of a person's genetic background provides valuable information for predicting risk for, and susceptibility to, disease for both the individual and his/her descendants. Like a family medical history, this information may be transmitted verbally from previous generations; however this history is often woefully incomplete or even absent in the case of adoptees or children of sperm donors. The process of DNA banking allows an individual to store a sample of DNA for future access. Possible uses include paternity testing, identification of abducted children, and validation of estate claims.

denaturation of DNA can also be induced locally by enzymes or DNA binding proteins. The promoter region of DNA contains a TATA sequence (the TATA box – see Fig. 33.1), an easily melted region of DNA that facilitates the unwinding of DNA during the early stages of gene expression (Chapter 33).

The human genome

The human genome contains 35 000–40 000 different protein coding genes scattered over 23 chromosome pairs. These different genes represent unique DNA sequences that are present in single copies or at most only a few copies per genome. There are also several types of repeated DNA sequences within the genome. These are divided into two major classes: middle repetitive (<10 copies per genome) and highly repetitive (>10 copies per genome) sequences.

Some middle repetitive DNA consists of genes that specify transfer RNAs, ribosomal RNAs, or histone proteins that are required in large amounts in the cell. Other middle repetitive DNA sequences have no known useful function, but may participate in DNA strand association and chromosomal rearrangements during meiosis. The best-characterized repetitive sequence in humans is known as the Alu sequence. Between 300 000 and 500 000 Alu I repeats of about 300 base pairs are scattered throughout the human genome, comprising 3–6% of total DNA. Individual repeats of the Alu sequence may vary by 10–20% in identity. Alu sequences also occur in monkeys and rodents, and similar sequences occur in slime molds and other animal phyla. In addition to the Alu family, there are several other families of middle repetitive DNA, mostly of unknown function, in the human genome.

Satellite DNA

Satellite DNA is highly repetitive DNA that was originally identified because it has a slightly different buoyant density from the main band of DNA when centrifuged through a CsCl gradient. Satellite DNA consists of clusters of short, species-specific, nearly identical sequences that are tandemly repeated hundreds of thousands of times. These clusters are deficient in protein-coding genes and are found principally near the centromeres of chromosomes, suggesting that they may function to align the chromosomes during cell division to facilitate recombination. Because these repetitive sequences cover long stretches of chromosomes (100s to 1000s of kilobase pairs; kbp), determining the sequence of satellite DNA and sequencing the centromere region of DNA are major challenges to completing the sequence of eukaryotic genomes.

Mitochondrial DNA

The nucleus of eukaryotic cells contains the majority of the DNA in the cell – genomic DNA. However, DNA is also found in mitochondria and in plant chloroplasts, which is consistent with current 'endosymbiont' theories for the origins of these cellular organelles. The mitochondrial genome is small in size, circular, and encodes relatively few proteins. In human beings, the mitochondrial genome encodes 22 tRNAs, 2 rRNAs, and 13 proteins. All of the mitochondrial encoded proteins are involved in the respiratory apparatus. The mitochondrial-encoded proteins are cytochrome b, three subunits of cytochrome oxidase, one of the subunits of ATPase, and seven subunits of NADH dehydrogenase.

The remainder of the proteins that are found in mitochondria (about 1000) are produced from nuclear genes, synthesized in the cytoplasm on 'free' ribosomes, then imported into the mitochondrion. This import process requires a special *N*-terminal 'mitochondrial-import' sequence of about 25 amino acids in length that forms an amphipathic helix capable of interacting with receptors on the mitochondrial surface.

Those few proteins that are encoded by the mitochondrial genome are also translated on mitochondrial ribosomes that are assembled on the two mitochondrial rRNAs after import of the nuclear-encoded ribosomal proteins into the mitochondria. Because there are only 22 tRNA genes encoded by the mitochondrial genome, yet 61 potential amino acid codons, there has been a dramatic simplification of the genetic code in the mitochondrion. Thus the genetic code of mitochondria has a restricted set of codons, compared to the universal (nuclear) genetic code (Chapter 32).

DNA is compacted into chromosomes

In eukaryotes, DNA is arranged in linear segments termed chromosomes. Each chromosome contains between 48 million and 240 million base pairs. The B-form of DNA has a contour length of 3.4 Å per base pair. Therefore, chromosomes have contour lengths of 1.6–8.2 cm, which is much larger than a cell. To fit within the nucleus, DNA is precisely condensed (>8000–fold).

In the native chromosome, DNA is complexed with RNA and an approximately equal mass of protein. These DNA–RNA-protein complexes are termed chromatin. The majority of the proteins in chromatin are histones. Histones are a highly conserved family of proteins that are involved in the packing and folding of DNA within the nucleus. There are five classes of histones, termed H1, H2A, H2B, H3, and H4. They are all rich (>20%) in positively charged, basic amino acids (lysine and arginine). These positive charges interact with the negatively charged, acidic phosphate groups of the DNA strands to reduce electrostatic repulsion and permit tighter DNA packing.

Nucleosomes

The histone proteins associate into a complex termed a nucleosome (Fig. 30.4). Each of these complexes contain two

BIOCHEMISTRY OF DNA POLYMERASES

There are several different DNA polymerases in the cell. DNA polymerase III, the principal DNA-replication enzyme, has the highest rate of DNA polymerization. DNA polymerase I is involved in excision repair and in the removal of RNA primers from Okazaki fragments.

DNA polymerase III is a complex protein, with at least 10 distinct subunits, ranging in size from 12 kDa to 130 kDa. The action of DNA polymerase III requires a single-stranded template and a primer, either DNA or RNA. After binding to the template-primer complex, the enzyme first determines which nucleotide is complementary to the next available template nucleotide and allows that nucleotide to bind to the active site. The elongation reaction occurs when the 3'-hydroxyl of the previous base attacks the 5'-phosphate of the incoming deoxynucleotide triphosphate (dNTP). Pyrophosphate is released. This process results in an elongation of the DNA strand by one nucleotide. Then, in a process termed proof-reading, the enzyme checks whether the newly incorporated base can form an allowed Watson–Crick base pair (i.e. AT, TA, CG, or GC) with the opposing base on the template strand. If the base pair is not allowed, the enzyme removes the last added nucleotide and repeats the process. If the base pair is allowed, the enzyme advances one nucleotide along the template strand and repeats the process. The ability of DNA polymerase III to proofread DNA sequences and replace mismatched nucleotides serves to maintain the high fidelity of DNA replication.

molecules each of H2A, H2B, H3, and H4 and one molecule of H1. The nucleosome protein complex is encircled with about 200 base pairs of DNA that form two coils around the nucleosome core. The H1 protein associates with the outside of the nucleosome core to stabilize the complex. By forming nucleosomes, the packing density of DNA is increased by a factor of about seven-fold.

The nucleosome particles themselves are also organized into other, more tightly packed structures, termed 300 Å chromatin filaments. These filaments are constructed by winding the nucleosome particles into a spring-shaped solenoid structure with about six nucleosomes per turn (Fig. 30.4). The solenoid is stabilized by head-to-tail associations of the H1 histones.

Finally, the chromatin filaments are compacted into the mature chromosome that is associated with a nuclear scaffold. The nuclear scaffold is about 0.4 mm in diameter and forms the core of the chromosome. The filaments are dispersed around the scaffold to form radial loops about 0.3 mm in length. The final diameter of a chromosome is about 1 mm.

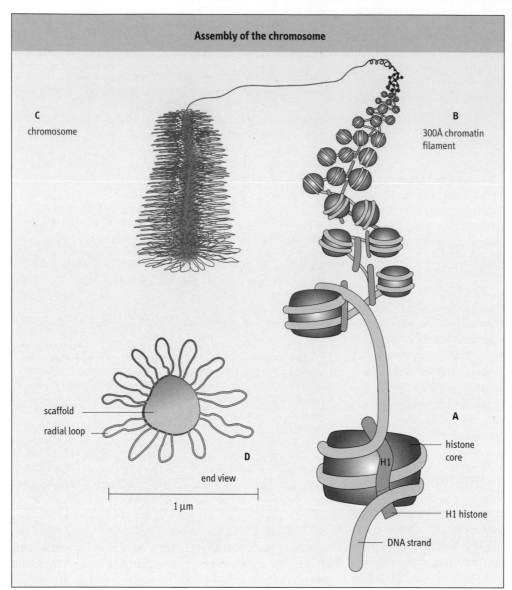

Assembly of the chromosome

C
chromosome

B
300Å chromatin filament

scaffold

radial loop

D

end view

1 μm

A

H1

histone core

H1 histone

DNA strand

Fig. 30.4 **Structures involved in chromosome packaging.** (A) The nucleosome core is composed of two subunits each of H2A, H2B, H3, and H4. The core is twice wrapped with DNA, and the H1 histone binds to the completed complex. (B) The 300 Å chromatin filament is formed by wrapping the nucleosomes into a spring-shaped solenoid. (C) The chromosome is composed of the 300 Å filaments, which bind to a nuclear scaffold, forming large loops of chromatin material. (D) The end view of a chromosome shows the central nuclear scaffold surrounded by the radial loops of chromatin. The diameter of a chromosome is about 1 μm.

Telomeres

The ends of the chromosomes are composed of unique DNA sequences called telomeres. These structures consist of tandem repeats of short, G-rich, species-specific oligonucleotides. In humans, the repeated sequence is TTAGGG. Telomeres can contain as many as 1000 copies of this sequence. During the synthesis of telomeres, the enzyme telomerase adds the preformed hexanucleotide repeats onto the 3′-end of the chromosome. There is no requirement for a DNA template in the elongation of telomeres at chromosome ends.

THE CELL CYCLE

Figure 30.5 shows the various phases of the growth and division of cells, known as the cell cycle. The G1 phase is a period of cell growth that occurs prior to DNA replication. The phase during which DNA is synthesized or replicated is termed the S-phase. A second growth phase, termed G2, occurs after DNA replication, but prior to cell division. The mitosis or M phase is the period of cell division. Following mitosis, the daughter cells either re-enter the G1 phase or enter a quiescent phase termed G0, where growth and replication cease. The passage of cells through the cell cycle is tightly controlled by a variety of proteins termed cyclin-dependent kinases (for details see Chapter 41).

DNA is replicated by separating and copying the strands

For cells to divide, their DNA must be duplicated during the S phase of the cell cycle. The structure of the DNA double helix

Genetic disorders show different modes of inheritance

Chromosomes are inherited according to the tenets of Mendelian genetics. Somatic cells are diploid (2n). They have two copies of each chromosome, and therefore two copies of each gene. During the process of meiosis, chromosome pairs are separated into gamete cells, each having a haploid (1n) chromosome number. The gamete cells, one from each parent, combine to form a daughter cell. Because each gamete has a 50/50 chance of inheriting either parental allele of a gene, inheritance of any particular gene can be statistically predicted.

Some genetic diseases show a dominant phenotype. For example, familial hypercholesterolemia (Chapter 17) is a dominant genetic defect that in the heterozygote results in reduced functional low-density-lipoprotein (LDL) receptors and plasma cholesterol levels that are twice normal. Homozygotes completely lack functional LDL receptors and have a three-to-five-fold higher plasma cholesterol level (see Chapter 17). In contrast, the majority of genetic diseases show a recessive phenotype. Heterozygotes with these recessive diseases are frequently asymptomatic.

A special group of recessive disorders are known as X-linked genetic diseases. These genetic diseases, which include hemophilia, color blindness, Lesch-Nyhan syndrome, and glucose-6-phosphate dehydrogenase deficiency, result from mutations of genes on the X chromosome. Because females have two X chromosomes, these disorders behave like typical recessive disorders in females: one in four are affected. However, in males, with one X chromosome and one Y chromosome, they become X-linked, dominant disorders. With X-linked disorders, females are usually asymptomatic carriers of these diseases and only males are affected.

Many diseases have a genetic component, but several genes may be involved. Examples include hypertension, obesity and type 2 diabetes. Diseases such as cancer, muscular dystrophy, and Xeroderma pigmentosum may also be caused by a range of many different genetic defects.

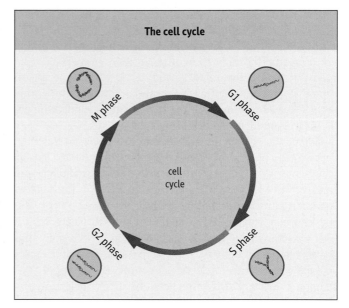

Fig. 30.5 **Stages of the cell cycle.** G1 and G2 are growth phases that occur before and after DNA synthesis respectively. DNA replication occurs during the S phase. Mitosis occurs during the M phase, producing new daughter cells that can re-enter the G1 phase (compare Fig. 41.1).

and its complementarity suggests a mechanism for DNA replication – strand separation followed by strand copying. The separated parent strands serve as templates for the synthesis of the new daughter strands. This method of DNA replication is described as 'semi-conservative' – each replicated duplex, daughter DNA molecule contains one parental strand and one newly synthesized strand.

DNA replication site

The site at which DNA replication is initiated is termed the 'origin of replication'. In prokaryotes, a DNA-binding protein termed DnaA binds to repeated nucleotide sequences located within the origin. Binding of 20–30 DnaA molecules to the origin of replication induces unwinding, which separates the strands in an AT-rich region adjacent to the DnaA-binding sites. Next the hexameric protein DnaB binds to the separated DNA strands. DnaB has helicase activity that catalyzes ATP-mediated unwinding of the DNA helix. DNA gyrase also participates in separation of the strands. As this complex continues unwinding the DNA strands in both directions from the origin of replication, single-stranded-DNA-binding proteins coat the separated strands to inhibit their reassociation.

Once the strands are sufficiently separated, another protein, termed DNA primase, is added, resulting in the formation of a primosome complex at the replication fork. The primosome synthesizes RNA oligonucleotides complementary to each parental DNA strand. These oligonucleotides serve as primers for DNA synthesis. Once each RNA primer has been laid down, two DNA polymerase III complexes are assembled, one at each of the primed sites. Because of the unidirectional synthetic activity of the polymerase and the antiparallel nature of the two strands, the synthesis of DNA along the two strands is different (Fig. 30.6). The two daughter strands being synthesized are termed the leading strand and the lagging strand.

DNA synthesis proceeds along the leading strand in a 5' to 3' direction, producing a single, long, continuous strand. However, because DNA synthesis adds new nucleotides only at the 3'-end of the elongating DNA strand, DNA polymerase III cannot synthesize the lagging strand in one long continuous piece as it does for the leading strand. Instead, the lagging strand is synthesized in small fragments, 1000–5000 base pairs in length, termed Okazaki fragments (Fig. 30.6). The primosome remains associated with the lagging strand and continues periodically to synthesize RNA primers complementary to the separated strand. As DNA polymerase III moves along the parental DNA strand, it initiates the synthesis of Okazaki fragments at the RNA primers, elongating different fragments from each primer.

When the 3′-end of the elongating Okazaki fragment reaches the 5′-end of the previously synthesized Okazaki fragment, DNA polymerase III releases the template and finds another RNA primer further back along the lagging strand, synthesizing another Okazaki fragment. Eventually, the Okazaki fragments are joined by DNA polymerase I. This enzyme, which also has a role in DNA repair, has an exonuclease activity that permits it to remove and replace a stretch of nucleotides as it proceeds along a DNA template. During DNA replication, DNA polymerase I removes the RNA primer and replaces it with DNA. Finally, DNA ligase joins the lagging-strand DNA fragments to form a continuous strand.

Eukaryotes stringently regulate DNA replication

Eukaryotic DNA synthesis is remarkably similar to prokaryotic DNA synthesis. However, eukaryotes have many more origins of replication. These are activated simultaneously during the S-phase of the cell cycle, permitting rapid replication of the entire chromosome. To insure that replicating DNA does not overaccumulate, cells use a protein termed a licensing factor that is present in the nucleus prior to replication. Following one round of replication, this factor is inactivated or destroyed, preventing further replication until more licensing factor is synthesized later in the cell cycle.

Licensing factor is best understood in the yeast. In yeast there is a complex called the origin recognition complex (ORC), composed of six proteins. The ORC marks the origin of replication and remains bound to the origin throughout the cell cycle. It serves as a docking site for the other components that regulate DNA replication. Early events in DNA replication include the binding of several highly unstable proteins to ORC. These proteins include CDC6/18 and CDT1, which facilitate binding of a group of three additional proteins: MCM2, MCM3, and MCM5. Once the MCM proteins bind, the origin exists as a prereplication complex and is 'licensed' to enter S-phase of the cell cycle. The initiation of DNA synthesis is triggered by the action of the CDC7 kinase together with other cyclin-dependent kinases. The activated MCM complex then participates in unwinding the replication origin and is thereby displaced from the origin. Following displacement, the origin forms a postinitiation complex and CDC6 is degraded, thereby preventing the reloading of the origin with additional licensing factor.

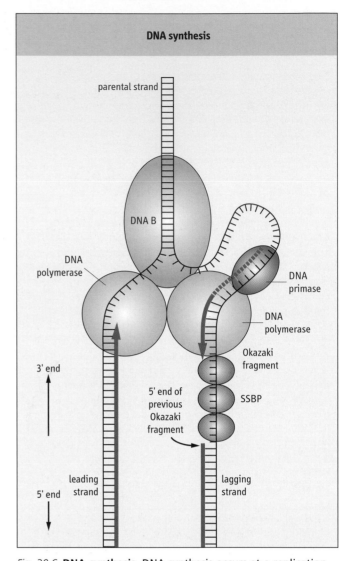

Fig. 30.6 **DNA synthesis.** DNA synthesis occurs at a replication fork producing new strands termed the leading strand and the lagging strand. The 'railroad tracks' represent double-stranded DNA. Some of the enzymes involved in DNA synthesis are shown: DNA B [helicase], DNA primase, DNA polymerase, and single strand DNA binding protein [SSBP]. The leading strand is replicated in a continuous fashion. However, for the lagging strand, RNA primers are periodically added by the DNA primase along the strand. DNA polymerase III elongates these RNA primers to form Okazaki fragments. When the Okazaki fragment is complete, the DNA polymerase III on the lagging strand will shift to the next RNA primer to initiate another Okazaki fragment. The exonuclease activity of DNA polymerase I removes the RNA primers and replaces them with DNA. DNA ligase seals the gaps in the DNA strands to complete synthesis of the lagging strand.

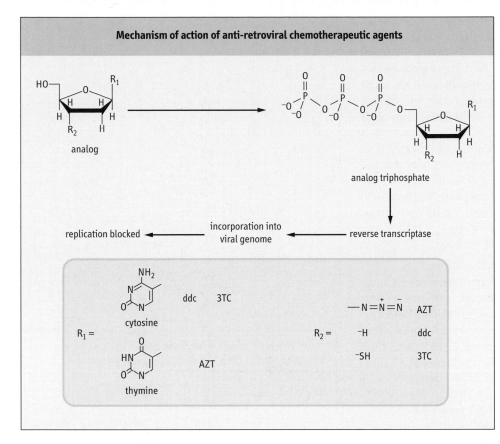

Fig. 30.7 **Mechanism of action of antiretroviral chemotherapeutic agents.** This class of inhibitors includes several compounds with slightly different chemical structures in the nucleobase structure and in substitution at the 3′-carbon of the sugar ring. Structures of some of the most widely used drugs are shown. These compounds are metabolized to the triphosphate form via normal cellular metabolism (see Chapter 29). The triphosphate analogs are then incorporated into the viral genome by reverse transcriptase. This blocks viral DNA synthesis because the modified 3′ end R_2 of the viral DNA molecule is not a substrate for additional rounds of DNA synthesis.

AZT THERAPY FOR HIV INFECTION

Human Immunodeficiency virus (HIV) infection results in a profound weakening of the immune system that leaves the patient vulnerable to a variety of bacterial, fungal, protozoal and viral superinfections. Kaposi's sarcoma may develop and is a cancer-like disease of blood vessels caused by infection with human herpesvirus-8 (HHV-8). AIDS dementia complex may also occur and is one of the few conditions caused by the HIV virus itself.

Effective treatments of the HIV viral infection rely on detailed knowledge of the viral life cycle. For the AIDS virus, the viral genome is RNA. In the infected cell, it is copied into a DNA form by a viral enzyme termed reverse transcriptase. Reverse transcriptase is an error-prone enzyme that does not have the proof-reading capabilities of DNA polymerase III. One therapeutic approach for treatment of AIDS takes advantage

of the enzyme's promiscuity in choice of substrates. Several important antiviral drugs are nucleotide analogs that inhibit reverse transcriptase, including AZT (azido, 2′,3′-dideoxy thymidine; Retrovir, Zidovudine), ddc (2′,3′-dideoxycytidine; Hivid, Zalcitabine), and 3TC (2′,3′-dideoxy-3′-thiacytidine; Epivir, Lamivudine). AZT, for example, is metabolized in the body into the thymine triphosphate (TTP) analog azido-TTP. The HIV reverse transcriptase misincorporates azido-TTP into the reverse-transcribed viral genome. The incorporation of azido-TTP into DNA blocks further chain elongation, because the 3′-azido group cannot form a phosphodiester bond with subsequent nucleoside triphosphates. The inability to synthesize DNA from the viral RNA template results in inhibition of viral replication (Fig. 30.7).

Cells can repair damaged DNA

Because DNA is the reservoir of genetic information within the cell, it is extremely important to maintain the integrity of DNA. Therefore, the cell has developed highly efficient mechanisms for the repair of modified or damaged DNA.

Nature of damage to DNA

DNA is subject to numerous types of endogenous and environmental insults that cause nucleotide deletions, insertions, sequence inversions and transpositions. Some of this damage is secondary to chemical modification of DNA by alkylating agents (including many carcinogens), reactive oxygen species (Chapter 35) and ionizing radiation (ultraviolet or radioactive). Both the sugar and bases of DNA are subject to modification, yielding an estimated 10 000 to 100 000 modifications of DNA per cell per day. The nature of this damage is quite variable, including modification of single bases, single or double-strand breaks, and crosslinking between bases or bases and proteins. Oxidative damage is probably the most common form of DNA damage; it is increased in inflammation, by smoking, in aging and in age-related diseases, including atherosclerosis, diabetes and neurodegenerative diseases (Chapter 42). If not repaired, the accumulated damage will lead to permanent changes in the structure of DNA, setting the stage for loss of cellular functions, cell death, or cancer.

Excision repair

Numerous chemical and environmental agents are known that produce specific chemical modification of the nucleotides in the DNA strand, leading to mismatches during DNA synthesis. After chromosomal replication, the resulting daughter strand contains a different DNA sequence (mutation) from the parent strand. Cells use excision repair to remove alkylated nucleotides and other unusual base analogs, thereby protecting the DNA sequence from mutations. The unmodified strand serves as the template for the repair process.

When short-wavelength ultraviolet (UV) light interacts with DNA, adjacent thymine bases undergo an unusual dimerization, producing a cyclobutylthymine dimer in the DNA strand (Fig. 30.8). The primary mechanism for repair of these intra-strand thymine dimers is an excision repair mechanism. An endonuclease, which appears to be specific for this type of modification, cleaves the dimer-containing strand near the thymine dimer, and a small portion of that strand is removed. DNA polymerase I, the same enzyme that is involved in DNA biosynthesis, then recognizes and fills in the resulting gap. DNA ligase completes the repair by rejoining the DNA strands.

Deamination

Those nucleotides that contain amines, cytosine and adenosine, may spontaneously deaminate to form uracil or hypoxanthine, respectively. When these bases are found in DNA, specific N-glycosylases remove them. This produces base-pair gaps that are recognized by specific apurinic or apyrimidinic endonucleases that cleave the DNA near the site of the defect. An exonuclease then removes the stretch of the DNA strand containing the defect. A repair DNA polymerase replaces the DNA, and, finally, DNA ligase rejoins the DNA strand. This repair mechanism is referred to as excision repair.

Depurination

Single base-pair alterations also include depurination. The purine-N-glycosidic bonds are especially labile, so that an esti-

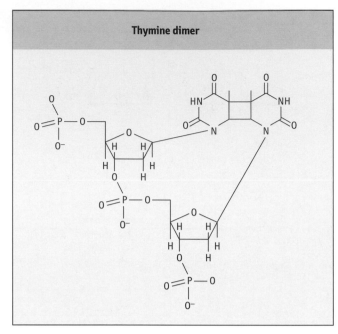

Fig. 30.8 **Thymine dimer.** A thymine dimer consists of a cyclobutane ring joining a pair of adjacent thymine nucleotides.

mated 3–7 purines are removed from DNA per min per cell. Specific enzymes recognize these depurinated sites, and the base is replaced without interruption of the phosphodiester backbone.

Strand breaks

Single-stranded breaks are frequently induced by ionizing radiation. These are repaired by direct ligation or by excision repair mechanisms. Double-stranded breaks are produced by ionizing radiation and some chemotherapeutic agents. Otherwise, double-stranded ends of DNA are rare *in vivo*; they are found at the end of chromosomes and in some specialized complexes involved in gene rearrangement. A specialized enzyme system is designed to recognize and rejoin these ends, but if the ends drift away from one another, the damage is not readily repaired.

Mismatch repair

Errors that escape the proof-reading activity of DNA polymerase III appear in newly synthesized DNA in the form of nucleotide mismatches. While readily repairable, the critical issue is identification of the strand to be repaired: which nucleotide strand is the daughter strand containing the error? In bacterial systems, mismatch repair is accomplished by methylation of DNA at adenine residues in specific sequences spaced along the genome; methylation does not affect base pairing. Newly synthesized strands lack methylated adenine residues, so that the mismatch repair system

Oxidative damage to DNA

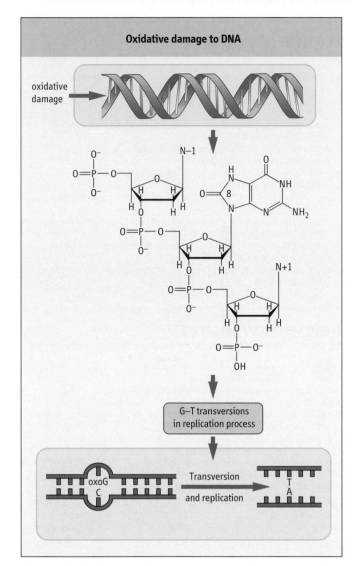

Fig. 30.9 **Oxidative damage to DNA.** 8-Oxo-2′-deoxyguanosine (8-oxoG) is an oxidative modification of DNA that causes mutations in the DNA strand.

enzymes scan the DNA, identify the mismatch, and then repair the unmethylated strand by excision repair. A similar approach is used to correct mismatches occurring during synthesis of mammalian DNA. Defects in mismatch repair are associated with hereditary nonpolyposis colon cancer, an autosomal dominant condition in humans.

8-Oxo-2′-deoxyguanosine

About 20 different oxidative modifications of DNA have been characterized; the most studied is 8-oxo-2′-deoxyguanosine (8-oxoG) (Fig. 30.9). During the process of DNA replication, mismatches between the modified 8-oxoG nucleoside in the template strand and incoming nucleotide triphosphates result in G-to-T transversions, thereby introducing mutations into the DNA strand. Although excision repair mechanisms

 AMES TEST FOR MUTAGENS

Mutagens are chemical compounds that induce changes in the DNA sequence. A large number of natural and man-made chemicals are mutagenic. To evaluate the potential to mutate DNA, the American biochemist Bruce Ames developed a simple test, using special *Salmonella typhimurium* strains that cannot grow in the absence of histidine (His⁻ phenotype). These histidine auxotrophic strains contain nucleotide substitutions or deletions that prevent the production of histidine biosynthetic enzymes.

To test for mutagenesis, about 10^{-9} mutant bacteria are spread on a culture plate lacking histidine. The suspected mutagen is added to the bacteria. The action of the mutagen occasionally results in the reversal of the histidine mutation, yielding a revertant strain that can now synthesize histidine and will grow in its absence. The mutagenicity of a compound is scored by counting the number of colonies that have reverted to the His⁺ phenotype. There is a good correlation between results of the Ames mutagenicity test and direct tests of carcinogenic activity in animals.

Some chemicals (procarcinogens) are not mutagenic *per se*, but are activated to mutagenic compounds during metabolic processes, e.g. during drug detoxification in liver or kidney. Benzopyrene, for example, is not mutagenic, but during its detoxification in liver, it is converted to diolepoxides which are potent mutagens and carcinogens. To provide sensitivity for detecting these compounds, the culture medium is supplemented with an extract of liver microsomes.

are effective, 8-oxoG, like other modified bases, may be re-incorporated into DNA following excision.

Recently a mammalian protein, MTH1, was characterized that specifically degrades 8-oxo-dGTP, thereby preventing misincorporation of this altered nucleotide into DNA. Gene targeting was used to develop an MTH1-knockout mouse. Compared to the wild-type animal, the knockout showed a greater number of tumors in lung, liver, and stomach, illustrating the importance of post-repair protection mechanisms.

In lung cells, inhalation of some particulate materials results in an increase in 8-oxoG levels. The inflammatory process may play a role in asbestos-induced formation of lung tumors. Smoking also induces oxidative damage and increases levels of DNA oxidation products in lungs, blood and urine.

Summary

The genome is composed of DNA, an antiparallel, double-stranded helical polymer of deoxyribonucleotides, stabilized by hydrogen binding between complementary bases. The DNA is packaged in the chromosome in a highly organized, condensed structure. Genetic information is replicated by a semi-conservative mechanism in which the parental strands are separated and both act as templates for daughter DNA. The replication of DNA is a complex, stringently regulated process. DNA is the only polymer in the body that is repaired, rather than degraded, following chemical or biological modification. Repair mechanisms generally involve excision of modified bases and replacement, using the unmodified strand as a template.

ACTIVE LEARNING

1. What are the possible functions of unusual forms of DNA?
2. Discuss the possible roles for middle repetitive and highly repetitive sequences in DNA.
3. Fragile X syndrome is the most common form of inherited mental retardation in humans. What is the role of non-genomic DNA in the pathogenesis of this disease?
4. Hereditary nonpolyposis colon cancer results from a defect in DNA mismatch repair. Why is this condition autosomal dominant?

Further reading

Ahmed A, Tollefsbol T. Telomeres and telomerase: basic science implications for aging. *J Am Geriatr Soc* 2001;**49**:1105–1109.

Cleaver JE, Crowley E. UV damage, DNA repair and skin carcinogenesis. *Front Biosci* 2002;**7**:d1024–d1043.

Norgauer J, Idzko M, Panther E, Hellstern O, Herouy Y. Xeroderma Pigmentosum. *Eur J Dermatol* 2003;**13**:4–9.

Sekiguchi M, Tsuzuki T. Oxidative nucleotide damage: consequences and prevention. *Oncogene* 2002;**21**:8895–8904.

Venter JC, *et al*. (2001) The sequence of the human genome. *Science* 2001;**291**:1304–1351.

Watson JD. A passion for DNA. Genes, genomes and society. (Oxford University Press: Oxford, 2000) 250pp.

Watson JD. The double helix: a personal account of the discovery of the structure of DNA. (Norton: New York, 1980) 298pp.

Wilson III D, Sofinowski T, McNeill D. Repair mechanisms for oxidative DNA damage. Front Biosci 2003;**8**:963–981.

Zannis-Hadjopoulos M, Price GB. Eukaryotic DNA replication. *J Cell Biochem Suppl* 1999;**32/33**:1–14.

Relevant websites

DNA workshop: www.pbs.org/wgbh/aso/tryit/dna

Genetic diseases: www.rarediseases.org

Graphics: www.accessexcellence.org/AB/GG/structure.html

Human Genome Project: www.ornl.gov/TechResources/Human_Genome/

General educational: www.dnaftb.org; www.dnalc.org; www.dnai.org; www.accessexcellence.org/AB/GG/

DNA repair: http://dir.niehs.nih.gov/dirlmg/DNArepair.html

DNA replication: http://dir.niehs.nih.gov/dirlmg/repl.html

Mitochondrial DNA: www.mitomap.org

DNA organization and nucleosomes:
http://medweb4.bham.ac.uk/jspdf/m102pdf/DNA1.pdf
http://medweb4.bham.ac.uk/jspdf/m102pdf/DNA2.pdf

31. Ribonucleic Acid (RNA)

G A Bannon

LEARNING OBJECTIVES

After reading this chapter you should be able to:

- Identify the major types of cellular RNA and the function of each.
- Describe the major steps in transcription of an RNA molecule.
- Explain the function of the different RNA polymerase enzymes.
- Describe the different processing and splicing events that occur during synthesis of eukaryotic mRNAs.

Transcription is defined as the synthesis of a ribonucleic acid (RNA) molecule using deoxyribonucleic acid (DNA) as a template. This rather simple definition describes a series of complicated enzymatic processes that result in the transfer of the genetic information stored in double-stranded DNA into a single-stranded RNA molecule that will be used by the cell to direct the synthesis of its proteins. There are three general classes of RNA molecules found in prokaryotic and eukaryotic cells: ribosomal RNA (rRNA), transfer RNA (tRNA), and messenger RNA (mRNA). Each class has a distinctive size and function (Table 31.1), described by its sedimentation rate in an ultracentrifuge (S, Svedbergs) or its number of bases (nt, nucleotides, or kb, kilobases). Prokaryotes have the same

three general classes of RNA as eukaryotes, but their RNAs differ in size and in some structural features:

- **ribosomal RNA (rRNA)** from prokaryotes consists of three different sizes of RNA, while rRNA from eukaryotes consists of four different sizes of RNA. These RNAs interact with each other, and with proteins, to form a ribosome that provides the basic machinery on which protein synthesis takes place;
- **transfer RNAs (tRNAs)** consist of one size class of RNA that are 65–110 nucleotides in length; they function as adapter molecules that translate the information stored in the mRNA nucleotide sequence to the amino acid sequence of proteins;
- **messenger RNAs (mRNAs)** represent the most heterogeneous class of RNAs found in cells, ranging in size from 500 nt to >6 kb; they are carriers of genetic information, defining the sequence of all proteins in the cell.

In order to understand the complex series of events that lead to the production of these three classes of RNA, this chapter is divided into four parts. The first part deals with the molecular anatomy of the major types of RNA found in prokaryotic and eukaryotic cells; knowing then the chemical nature of the final products of transcription, you will be better prepared to understand the steps involved in generating these molecules. The second part describes the main enzymes involved in transcription, and their specificities. The third part describes the three steps (initiation, elongation, and termination) required to produce an RNA transcript. Finally, in the last section, the modifications that are made to the primary products of transcription (post-transcriptional processing) are described. This information is expanded in Chapter 33: Control of Gene Expression.

MOLECULAR ANATOMY OF RNA MOLECULES

In general, the RNAs produced by prokaryotic and eukaryotic cells are single-stranded molecules that consist of adenine, guanine, cytosine, and uracil nucleotides joined to one another by phosphodiester linkages. The start of an RNA molecule is known as its 5′ end, and the termination of the

General classes of RNA			
RNA	Size and length	Percent of total cellular RNA	Function
rRNA	28s, 18s, 5.8s, 5s (26s, 16s, 5s)*	80	interact to form ribosomes
tRNA	65–110 nt	15	adapter
mRNA	0.5–6 kb	5	direct synthesis of cellular proteins

Table 31.1 **General classes of RNA.** *Size of rRNA in prokaryotic cells. Nt, nucleotides; Kb, kilobases; S, svedbergs.

RNA hairpin loop

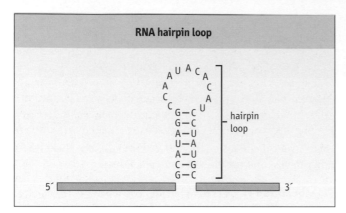

Fig. 31.1 **RNA hairpin loop.** RNA can form secondary structures called hairpin loops. These structures form when complementary bases within an individual RNA share hydrogen bonds and form base pairs. Hairpin loops are known to be important in the regulation of transcription in both eukaryotic and prokaryotic cells.

RNA is known as its 3′end. Even though most RNAs are single stranded, they exhibit extensive secondary structures, including intramolecular double-stranded regions that are important to their function. These secondary structures, one of the most common of which is called a hairpin loop (Fig. 31.1), are the product of intramolecular base pairing that occurs between complementary nucleotides within a single RNA molecule.

rRNAs: formation of the ribosome

The eukaryotic rRNAs are synthesized as a single RNA transcript with a size of 45S and about 13 kb long. This large primary transcript is processed into 28S, 18S, 5.8S, and 5S rRNAs (~3 kb, 1.5 kb, 160 and 120 nt, respectively). The 28S, 5.8S, and 5S rRNAs associate with ribosomal proteins to form what is called the large ribosomal subunit. The 18S rRNA associates with other specific proteins to form the small ribosomal subunit. The large ribosomal subunit with its proteins and RNA has a characteristic size of 60S; the small ribosomal subunit has a size of 40S. These two subunits interact to form a functional ribosome that has a size of 80S (see Chapter 32). Prokaryotic rRNAs interact in a similar fashion to form these ribosomal subunits, but have a slightly smaller size, reflecting the difference in rRNA transcript size that exists between prokaryotic and eukaryotic cells (Table 31.2).

tRNA: the molecular cloverleaf

Prokaryotic and eukaryotic tRNAs are similar in both size and structure. They exhibit extensive secondary structure and contain several ribonucleotides that differ from the usual four by a variety of modifications. All tRNAs have a similar folded

rRNAs and ribosomes

Cell type	rRNA	Subunit	Size	Intact ribosome
prokaryotic	23s, 5s	large	50s	70s
	16s	small	30s	
eukaryotic	28s, 5.8s, 5s	large	60s	80s
	18s	small	40s	

Table 31.2 **rRNAs and ribosomes.** rRNAs interact to form ribosomes.

Structure of tRNA

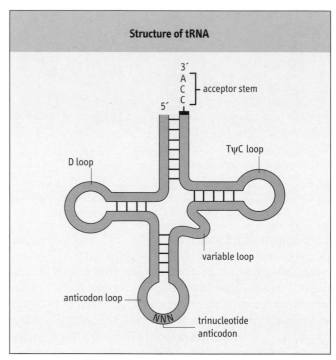

Fig. 31.2 **The structure of a tRNA molecule.** A prototypical tRNA molecule is shown, and the structures important to its function are indicated. The overall structure of the molecule is due to complementary base pairing between nucleotides within a single RNA. All tRNAs have this basic structure.

structure, with four distinctive loops, that has been described as a cloverleaf (Fig. 31.2). The D loop contains several modified bases, including methylated cytosine and dihydrouridine, for which the loop is named. The anticodon loop is the structure responsible for recognition of the complementary codon of an mRNA molecule: specific interaction of an anticodon with the appropriate codon is due to complementary base pairing between these two trinucleotide sequences in tRNA and mRNA. A variable loop, 3–21 bp in length, exists in most tRNAs, but its function is unknown. Finally, there is a TψC loop, which is named for the presence in this loop of the modified base, pseudouridine. Another prominent structure found in all tRNA molecules is the acceptor stem. This structure is formed by base pairing between the nucleotides found at the 5′ and 3′ ends of the tRNA. The last three bases found at the extreme 3′ end remain unpaired, and always have the same sequence: 5′-CCA-3′. The 3′ end of the acceptor stem is the point at which an amino acid is attached via an ester bond between the 3′-hydroxyl group of the adenosine and the carboxyl group of an amino acid.

mRNAs: sorting the prokaryotes from the eukaryotes

mRNAs are the most distinctive class of RNAs when prokaryotic and eukaryotic cells are compared (Fig. 31.3). This is largely because a single prokaryotic mRNA can encode multiple proteins (it is polycistronic), whereas a single eukaryotic mRNA carries the information to encode only a single protein; however, there are also a number of chemical modifications that are unique to eukaryotic mRNAs. For example, the 5′ and 3′ ends of eukaryotic mRNAs are modified, after they have been synthesized, in specific ways that protect them from exonuclease attack. All eukaryotic mRNAs contain a methylated guanine nucleotide 'cap' at their 5′ end, bound in a unique 5′–5′ triphosphate linkage. The 3′ end is even more extensively modified, by the addition of a number of adenine residues – known as a polyA tail. The number of adenine residues added to a particular transcript can vary from as few as 30 to more than 100 residues. Although the vast majority of eukaryotic mRNAs contain a polyA tail, there are notable exceptions to this rule: for example, the mRNAs that encode histone proteins and heat shock proteins do not contain such a tail. While there are many theories, there is little compelling evidence to explain why these particular mRNAs do not contain this structure at their 3′ end.

One of the most striking differences between prokaryotic and eukaryotic mRNAs is that eukaryotic mRNAs are synthesized as large precursors that have to be processed before they are functional. This processing usually involves the removal of portions of the transcript, called introns (**in**travening sequences), and ligation of the remaining sequences, called exons (**ex**pressed sequences), to one another. There is little time for this type of processing to occur in prokaryotic cells, in which the transcript may be partially translated into protein even before transcription is completed; in contrast, simultaneous transcription/translation cannot occur in eukaryotic cells because the nuclear envelope acts as a natural barrier between the process of transcription and translation. The process of removal and ligation of sequences within a primary transcript is called splicing; it is more thoroughly discussed later in this chapter.

RNA POLYMERASES

The enzymes responsible for the synthesis of RNA, using DNA as a template, are called RNA polymerases. All RNAs are synthesized by these enzymes, in a direction that is 5′ to 3′ with respect to their internucleotide linkage. This polarity of synthesis dictates that the DNA strand used as a template is read in the 3′ to 5′ direction (Fig. 31.4). RNA polymerase uses the DNA template strand to synthesize the complementary RNA strand, adding each new nucleotide onto the 3′ end of the growing chain. RNA polymerases have the ability to initiate the synthesis of RNA without the benefit of a free 3′-OH on which to build the new RNA strand. This activity distinguishes them from the DNA polymerases (Chapter 30), which require RNA or DNA primers with a free 3′-OH to begin synthesis.

RNA polymerases are large multimeric enzymes that transcribe defined segments of DNA into RNA with a high degree of selectivity and specificity

The RNA polymerases generally consist of two large-molecular-weight subunits and several smaller subunits, all of which are necessary for accurate transcription to occur. In prokaryotic cells, there is only one type of RNA polymerase, which synthesizes all three of the general classes of RNA. In contrast, eukaryotic cells have three RNA polymerases (I, II, and III), which are distinguished from one another by the class of RNA for which they direct the synthesis. The function of each of the eukaryotic RNA polymerases was determined in part by using a transcription inhibitor, α-amanitin – a toxic compound found in some mushrooms.

- **RNA polymerase I** synthesizes the rRNAs;
- **RNA polymerase II** synthesizes mRNA. It is extremely sensitive to inhibition by α-amanitin;

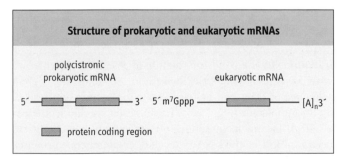

Structure of prokaryotic and eukaryotic mRNAs

polycistronic prokaryotic mRNA

eukaryotic mRNA

5′ ▬□▬□▬ 3′   5′ m⁷Gppp ▬□▬ [A]ₙ3′

□ protein coding region

Fig. 31.3 **Prototypical structures of prokaryotic (polycistronic) and eukaryotic mRNAs.** The boxes indicate those portions of the mRNA that encode a protein. [A]ₙ, polyA tail of adenine residues; m⁷Gppp, 7-methylguanine nucleotide cap.

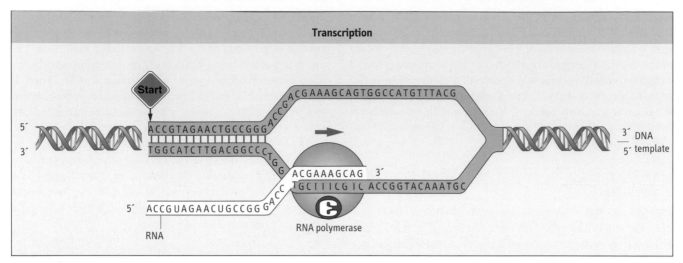

Transcription

Fig. 31.4 **Transcription.** Transcription involves the synthesis of an RNA by RNA polymerase using DNA as a template. The RNA polymerase holoenzyme uses one strand of DNA to direct the synthesis of an RNA molecule that is complementary to this strand.

 PICKING A WRONG MUSHROOM

An otherwise healthy young man presents himself to the emergency room with severe nausea and diarrhea. After his medical history has been taken, he explains that his symptoms came on rather suddenly, about 2–3 hours after he had eaten dinner. The physician suspects some form of food poisoning, and asks the patient to recall everything he has eaten over the past 24 hours. The only suspicious food mentioned were mushrooms that the patient ate for dinner. The mushrooms become prime candidates for the cause of this patient's symptoms when he further relates that they were picked up on a recent hike through the woods. What is the biochemical basis for suspecting that the mushrooms are the cause of this man's illness?

Comment. It is likely that the patient mistakenly picked a member of the family *Amanita phalloides* and ingested them at dinner. The toxin, α-amanitin, binds preferentially to RNA polymerase II and inhibits its function; if a large quantity of the mushrooms had been ingested, even RNA polymerase III could be inhibited. The first cells that encounter the toxin are those of the digestive tract, leading to acute gastrointestinal distress: cells that are incapable of synthesizing new mRNAs and tRNAs would die, causing the diarrhea and nausea that the patient complained of when first examined.

■ **RNA polymerase III** synthesizes the small RNAs, including the tRNAs.

The best-studied RNA polymerase is that of *Eschericha coli*. The core portion of this bacterial polymerase is a tetramer containing two α subunits and a β and β′ subunit, which interact to form what is called the core polymerase. This polymerase is capable of synthesizing RNA, but does so in a nonspecific fashion. It gains specificity and is able to bind and initiate transcription at true initiation sites on DNA when a fifth subunit, the σ-factor, joins the complex. *E. coli* contains a number of different σ-factors that, when joined with the core polymerase, impart specificity for the transcription of certain classes of genes.

THE PROCESS OF TRANSCRIPTION

Transcription is a dynamic process that involves the interaction of enzymes and DNA in specific ways to produce an RNA molecule. In order to understand this process better, it is convenient to divide it into three separate stages:

■ **initiation,**
■ **elongation,**
■ **termination.**

Initiation of transcription

Initiation involves the interaction of the RNA polymerase with DNA in a site-specific fashion, so that the correct sequence of DNA can be used as a template for synthesis of an RNA molecule (Fig. 31.5). The focus on specific sequences of DNA for transcription is an important consideration, because most of the DNA in a cell does not encode proteins. This problem is solved through the interaction of RNA polymerase with specific sites on the DNA, known as promoters. Promoters are characteristic sequences of DNA, usually located in front (upstream) of the gene that is to be transcribed.

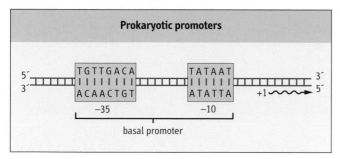

Prokaryotic promoters

Fig. 31.5 **Prokaryotic promoters.** Prokaryotic transcription promoters are located upstream of the gene. DNA sequences that act as transcription promoters are indicated at their respective positions relative to the gene. Position +1 indicates the first nucleotide that will be transcribed into RNA. The TATA box is a common A–T-rich promoter element.

The simplest promoters are found in prokaryotic cells, in which two general types of sequence elements are found in front of most genes: one sequence element is believed to promote initial binding of the RNA polymerase, and the other element usually has a high content of adenine (A) and thymine (T). Because hydrogen bonding is weaker between A–T base pairs than between guanine-cytosine (G–C) base pairs, the increased A–T content helps in the dissociation of the two DNA strands, enabling transcription to begin. These promoter sequences, 6–8 nt in length, are generally located about 35 and 10 bp upstream from the start of transcription of prokaryotic genes. Because these sequence elements are required for any level of transcription to occur, they are called basal promoters. The promoter located at −10 base pair, i.e. 10 bp before the transcription starting site (Fig. 31.5), is known commonly as the TATA or Pribnow box (Chapter 33, Fig. 33.1).

Promoters found in eukaryotic cells are more complicated. In addition to the sequence elements required for basal expression, they have additional sequences that are responsible for regulating the rate of initiation of transcription. These sequence elements are known as either enhancers or silencers, depending on the effect they have on transcription. They can be located at great distances either upstream or downstream of the start of transcription. Promoters with these types of sequence elements exert their effect on transcription by acting as the binding site for a variety of proteins known as trans-acting factors. The type of trans-acting factor that binds to these sequence elements will determine whether the rate of transcription is increased or decreased.

Elongation

Once RNA polymerase has bound to a promoter, it begins the process of selecting the appropriate complementary ribonucleotide and forming phosphodiester bridges between this nucleotide and the nascent chain, in a process called elonga-

THE CASE OF A STUBBORN MICROBE

A patient you were treating for an infected wound last week returns to your clinic, complaining that the infection is worse. You examine the wound and confirm that, indeed, the infection has become worse, even though you had prescribed a high-dose regimen of antibiotics that targeted the bacterial protein synthetic machinery. After questioning the patient to ensure that she was compliant and took the medication, you elect to prescribe rifampicin, a synthetic derivative of the naturally occurring antibiotic, rifamycin. The patient asks you why you think this antibiotic will work.

Comment. Antibiotics work by targeting specific functions in the bacterial cell. In the first round of treatment, you used antibiotics that inhibited the bacterial protein synthetic machinery. In some cases, microbes become resistant to a specific type of antibiotic and it is necessary to target other bacterial functions in order to clear up the infection. Rifampicin inhibits the transcriptional machinery of bacteria, inhibiting the β-subunit of bacterial RNA polymerase. Without the ability to make RNA, the bacterial cell will die.

tion. Elongation can be a very rapid process, occurring at the rate of 40 nt per second. For elongation to occur, the double-stranded DNA must be continually unwound, so that the template strand is accessible to the RNA polymerase; DNA topoisomerases I and II are enzymes associated with the transcription complex that have the ability to separate DNA strands so that they are accessible as templates for RNA synthesis.

Termination

In addition to knowing where to start transcription, RNA polymerase must have a defined site at which to stop RNA synthesis, so that the appropriate size of transcript is produced. The three eukaryotic RNA polymerases employ different mechanisms to terminate transcription. For example, RNA polymerase I uses a specific protein to terminate the transcription of rRNAs, whereas RNA polymerase III uses a specific termination sequence. In contrast, RNA polymerase II is more versatile, utilizing both sequence and protein factors to facilitate pausing of the polymerase and termination of transcription.

Transcription termination in bacterial cells occurs by one of two well-characterized mechanisms (Fig. 31.6). The first mechanism, rho-independent termination, is similar to that described for eukaryotic transcription, except that the secondary structure and sequences involved are much better characterized in bacterial cells. In rho-independent termination, a hairpin loop is formed just before a sequence of six to

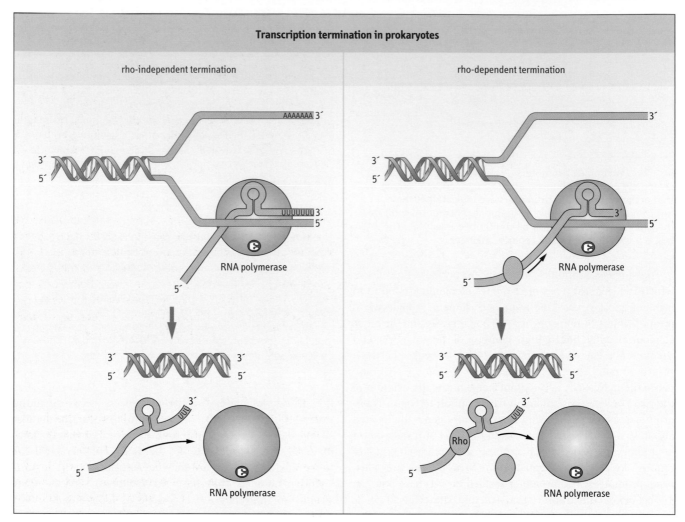

Fig. 31.6 **Transcription termination in prokaryotes.** Two mechanisms of transcription termination in bacterial cells. Rho-independent termination relies on the formation of a secondary structure in the newly transcribed RNA to dislodge the RNA polymerase from the DNA template and stop transcription. Rho-dependent termination requires the action of the rho protein. This protein will move along the newly transcribed RNA, catching up with the RNA polymerase when it pauses at the termination site, and causing the polymerase to leave the DNA template.

eight uridine (U) residues near the 3′ end of the newly synthesized RNA. The formation of this secondary structure dislodges the RNA polymerase from the DNA template, resulting in termination of RNA synthesis in the U stretch. The second mechanism, rho-dependent termination, requires the action of a protein factor called rho, which has an ATP-dependent helicase activity that is required for transcription termination. The rho protein is believed to travel along the newly synthesized RNA, chasing the RNA polymerase. In this mechanism, the formation of a hairpin loop in the RNA structure causes the RNA polymerase to pause, allowing the rho protein to catch up with and displace the RNA polymerase from the template. Transcription termination in eukaryotes resembles the rho-dependent termination in prokaryotes.

POST-TRANSCRIPTIONAL PROCESSING

In eukaryotes, all three classes of RNA (tRNAs, rRNAs, and mRNAs) are synthesized as larger primary transcripts, also known as heterogeneous nuclear (heteronuclear, hn) RNAs. hnRNAs are usually much larger than the RNAs found in the cytoplasm. For any of these transcripts to be functional, they must be processed to a smaller size before leaving the nucleus. Processing may involve either removal of sequences from the primary transcript, or removal and rejoining of segments of the transcript (Fig. 31.7).

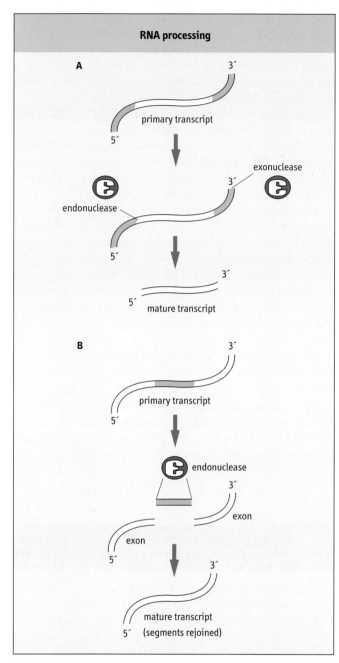

RNA processing

A

3′
primary transcript
5′

endonuclease

exonuclease

3′

5′

3′

5′
mature transcript

B

3′
primary transcript
5′

endonuclease

3′

exon

exon

5′

3′

mature transcript
5′ (segments rejoined)

Fig. 31.7 **RNA processing.** There are two general types of RNA processing events. Processing of an RNA transcript can involve (A) the removal of excess sequences by the action of endonucleases and exonucleases, or (B) the removal of excess sequences and the rejoining of segments of the newly transcribed RNA.

snRNAs and their function in splicing mRNAs		
snRNA	**Size**	**Function**
U1	165 nt	Binds the 5′ exon/intron boundary
U2	185 nt	Binds the branch site on the intron
U4	145 nt	Helps assemble the spliceosome
U5	116 nt	Binds the 3′ intron/exon boundary
U6	106 nt	Helps assemble the spliceosome

Table 31.3 **The function of small nuclear RNAs (snRNAs) in the splicing of mRNAs.**

obtain RNAs of the correct size from the initial transcript, the actions of endoribonucleases and exoribonucleases are required. Endoribonucleases cleave phosphodiester bonds within the primary transcript to release individual RNAs; exoribonucleases remove excess nucleotides from the 5′ and 3′ ends of these RNAs until a molecule of the correct size is produced. After processing, specific nucleotides are modified to give the unusual complement of bases found in most tRNAs.

Processing of eukaryotic mRNAs: 5′ caps and poly(A) tails

Most eukaryotic mRNAs contain specific structures that are added to their 5′ and 3′ ends after transcription has occurred. A 7-methyl guanine residue is added to the 5′ end of eukaryotic mRNAs via a special 5′ to 5′ phosphate linkage by the action of the enzyme guanyl transferase. The function of this structure is two-fold; it is essential for ribosomal binding and it protects the mRNA from attack by 5′ exonucleases. A poly(A) tail of varying length (100–300 residues) is added to the 3′ end of most eukaryotic mRNAs. The A residues are not encoded by the DNA but added by the action of poly(A) polymerase using ATP as a substrate. This structure protects the mRNA from attack by 3′ exonucleases, increasing the half-life of the transcript. Both the 5′ and 3′ ends of eukaryotic mRNAs are modified first, prior to further processing.

Processing of eukaryotic mRNAs: spliceosomes and lariats

In the more complicated post-transcriptional processing of eukaryotic mRNAs, sequences called introns (intravening sequences) are removed from the primary transcript and the remaining segments, termed exons (expressed sequences), are ligated, to form a functional RNA. This process involves a large complex of proteins and auxiliary RNAs called small nuclear RNAs (snRNAs), which interact to form a spliceosome. The function of the five snRNAs (U1, U2, U4, U5, U6) in the spliceosome is to help position reacting groups within the substrate mRNA molecule, so that the introns can be removed and the appropriate exons can be spliced together precisely (Table 31.3). The snRNAs accomplish this task by

Both eukaryotic and prokaryotic tRNAs and rRNAs are subject to processing

As noted above, the rRNAs are initially synthesized as a large precursor RNA that contains the 28S, 18S, 5.8S and 5S RNAs. In some cases, there are tRNAs in addition to the rRNAs contained within this primary transcript. In order to

binding, through base-pairing interactions, with the sites on the mRNA that represent intron/exon boundaries. Accompanying protein factors are responsible for holding the reacting components together to facilitate the reaction.

The removal of an intron and rejoining of two exons can be considered to occur in two steps (Fig. 31.8). The first step involves the breaking of the phosphodiester bond at the exon/intron boundary at the 5′ end of the intron. This is accomplished by a transesterification reaction, which occurs between the 2′-OH of an adenosine nucleotide usually found about 30 nt from the 3′ end of the intron, and the phosphate in the phosphodiester bond of a guanosine residue located at the 5′ end of the intron. This reaction cleaves the nucleotide

chain and produces a branched structure in which the adenine has 2′, 3′, and 5′ phosphate groups. The intron forms a looped structure similar in appearance to that of a cowboy's lariat. The second step in the reaction involves the cleavage of the phosphodiester bond at the 3′ end of the intron, which releases the lariat structure from the complex.

Splicing is completed by the joining of the 3′ end of one exon to the 5′ end of the next exon, through the formation of a regular 5′–3′ phosphodiester bond. Typically, the 3′ end of one exon will be spliced to the 5′ end of the next closest exon, producing a transcript that exhibits all the exons in the order in which they were transcribed. However, depending on cell and tissue type, a single gene can give rise to multiple forms of mature RNA transcripts by a process termed alternative RNA splicing (see Chapter 33). In these instances, some exons may not be represented in the final transcript, yielding an RNA that encodes a different protein. This process represents a major mechanism by which eukaryotic cells control synthesis of different proteins from the same gene transcript in a cell- or tissue-specific manner.

A new light on cellular evolution: self-splicing RNA

The vast majority of transcript processing occurs as described in the preceding paragraphs, but a small percentage of transcripts from a wide variety of organisms undergo splicing reactions without the benefit of protein cofactors. These transcripts are self-splicing and can be classified into two groups,

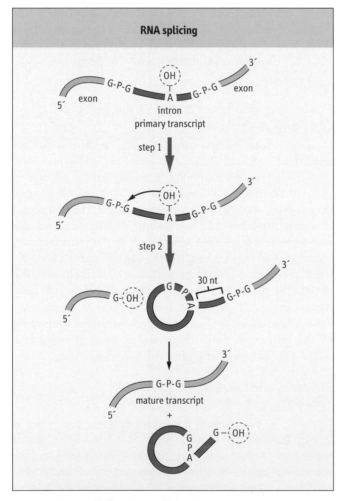

Fig. 31.8 **RNA splicing.** RNA splicing is a two-step process. In the first step, the phosphate bond of a guanosine residue at the 5′ exon/intron boundary is broken and joined to the 2′-OH of an adenine residue located in the middle of the intron. In the second step of the reaction, the phosphate bond at the 3′ intron/exon boundary is first cleaved and then the two exons are spliced together by re-formation of a phosphodiester bond between the nucleotides at either end of the exons.

RIBOZYMES: RNAS THAT ACT LIKE ENZYMES

In some instances, RNAs have a catalytic ability similar to the type of activities previously ascribed only to proteins. These special molecules, known as ribozymes, possess a catalytic activity and a substrate specificity similar to those of proteinaceous enzymes. The substrate specificity of a ribozyme is determined by nucleotide base pairing between complementary sequences contained within the enzyme and the RNA substrate. Just like enzymes that are proteins, the ribozyme will cleave its substrate RNA at a specific site and then release it, without itself being consumed in the reaction. Ribozymes are being considered as possible therapeutic agents for diseases that are caused by the inappropriate expression of an RNA or the expression of a mutated RNA. In these cases, the development of a ribozyme that had specificity for a particular RNA could result in the selective degradation of the substrate, eliminating it from the cell and inhibiting the disease process. Many more years of research on the mechanism of ribozyme activity are required before this type of treatment will be available.

depending on whether a cofactor is required and whether the intron forms a lariat configuration during splicing:

- **group I self-splicing introns**: guanosine acts as a cofactor in the transesterification reaction, which leads to release of the intron without formation of the lariat;
- **group II self-splicing introns**: lariats are formed, and the process is similar to that which occurs in spliceosomes, except that no proteins are required.

The discovery of self-splicing RNA – that is, RNA with an enzymatic activity – has led to new ideas about early cellular evolution, which was originally believed to start with amino acids and proteins. It is now believed that ribonucleotides and RNA may have been the most primitive biopolymers to form on earth, providing for genetic diversity, and that DNA and proteins may have developed later.

Summary

The major products of transcription are the rRNAs, tRNAs, and the mRNAs. These RNAs perform specific functions in the cell. rRNAs interact to form ribosomes, the basic cellular machinery on which protein synthesis occurs. tRNAs function as adapter molecules that translate the information stored in the mRNA nucleotide sequence to the amino acid sequence of proteins. mRNAs carry the genetic information from DNA and direct the synthesis of all proteins in the cell. In eukaryotic cells, each of these classes of RNAs is produced by a specific RNA polymerase (RNA polymerase I, II, or III), while in bacterial cells a single RNA polymerase synthesizes all three classes. The basic structures of rRNAS and tRNAs in eukaryotic and bacterial cells are similar. However, mRNAs from eukaryotic cells have a 5′ (m^7Gppp) cap and a 3′ ($[A]_n$) tail. Prokaryotic cells do not have these modifications on their 5′ and 3′ ends and can be polycistronic. In addition, most eukaryotic mRNAs must undergo a process called splicing to be functional, whereas prokaryotic mRNAs are functional as soon as they are synthesized. Splicing involves the removal of sequences called introns and the joining of other sequences called exons to each other to form a functional mRNA. The process of transcription consists of three parts; initiation, elongation, and termination. Initiation involves the recognition by RNA polymerase of the specific region of DNA that is to be transcribed. To accomplish this, RNA polymerases interact with specific DNA sequences called promoters located upstream (before 5′ end) to the start of transcription. Elongation involves the selection of the appropriate nucleotide, as determined by the DNA strand, and formation of the phosphodiester bridges that exist between each nucleotide in an RNA molecule. Finally, termination involves the dissociation of the RNA polymerase from the DNA template. This can be accomplished by either RNA secondary structure or specific protein factors.

ACTIVE LEARNING

1. Which commonly used antibiotics are directed at inhibition of bacterial RNA polymerase but do not affect the mammalian complex? Why are these drugs less effective against fungal infections?
2. Review the pathogenesis of systemic lupus erythematosus, an autoimmune disease in which antibodies to ribonucleoprotein particles are implicated in the development of chronic inflammation.
3. Review the pathogenesis of the thalassemias, with emphasis on those variants in which gene mutations affect the synthesis, processing and splicing of the RNA for hemoglobin, leading to anemia.

Further reading

Akusjarvi G, Stevenin J. Remodeling of the host cell RNA splicing machinery during an adenovirus infection. *Curr Top Microbiol Immunol* 2003;**272**:253–286.

Herman T, Westhof E. RNA as a drug target: chemical, modeling, and evolutionary tools. *Curr Opin Biotechnol* 1998;**9**:66–73.

Jarad G, Simske JS, Sedor JR, Schelling JR. Nucleic acid-based techniques for post-transcriptional regulation of molecular targets. *Curr Opin Nephrol Hypertens* 2003;**12**:415–421.

Khan AU, Lal SK. Ribozymes: a modern tool in medicine. *J Biomed Sci* 2003 Sep–Oct;**10**:457–467

Raj SM, Liu F. Engineering of RNase P ribozyme for gene-targeting applications. **Gene** 2003 Aug 14;**313**:59–69.

Sassone-Corsi P. Unique chromatin remodeling and transcriptional regulation in spermatogenesis. *Science* 2002;**296**:2176–2178.

Websites

RNA polymerase: www.rcsb.org/pdb/molecules/pdb40_1.html
Spliceosome: www.neuro.wustl.edu/neuromuscular/pathol/spliceosome.htm
Ribozyme: www.ribozyme.no/; highveld.com/pages/ribozyme.html
Thalassemia: www.cooleysanemia.org/; www.ygyh.org/thal/whatisit.htm

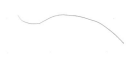

32. Protein Synthesis and Turnover

G A Bannon

LEARNING OBJECTIVES

After reading this chapter you should be able to:

- Describe how the different RNAs involved in protein synthesis interact to produce a polypeptide.
- Outline the structure and redundancy of the genetic code.
- Explain how proteins are targeted to specific subcellular organelles.
- Describe the major steps in synthesis and degradation of a cytosolic protein.

INTRODUCTION

Protein synthesis, also known as translation, represents the culmination of the transfer of genetic information, stored as nucleotide bases in deoxyribonucleic acid (DNA), to protein molecules that are the major structural and functional components of living cells. It is during translation that this information, expressed as a specific nucleotide sequence in a ribonucleic acid (RNA) molecule, is used to direct the synthesis of a protein. The protein then folds into a three-dimensional structure that is defined, in large part, by its amino acid sequence. The interaction between the RNA to be translated and the protein synthetic machinery involves three main components:

- **ribosomes,**
- **messenger RNA (mRNA),**
- **transfer RNA (tRNA).**

The ribosome is the machine on which all proteins are synthesized. mRNA contains the information required to direct the synthesis of the primary sequence of the protein, although only a portion of that information is used to encode the protein. tRNAs carry the amino acids that are to be incorporated into the protein. The ribosome brings together the tRNA molecule and mRNA so that the correct amino acid is incorporated into the protein. In general, the translation of mRNA begins near the 5′ end and moves towards the 3′ end, and proteins are synthesized starting with their amino-terminal ends and progressing toward the carboxy-terminal end; thus the 5′ end of the RNA corresponds to the amino-terminal end of the protein; the 3′ end of the RNA corresponds to the carboxy-terminal end of the protein. In this chapter, we begin our discussion of translation by looking at the general characteristics of the genetic code. Next, we will discuss the structure and function of the ribosome, the macromolecular ribonucleoprotein particle that synchronizes the activity of mRNA and tRNAs to produce a protein. The process of translation (initiation, elongation, and termination of protein synthesis) will be explained, and the mechanism by which proteins are targeted to specific locations in the cell will be discussed. Finally, the many modifications that proteins undergo after synthesis so that they can attain their full activity will be described briefly. During the course of this discussion, we will acknowledge that protein molecules have a defined half-life and address the role of a second macromolecular complex, the proteasome, in protein turnover.

THE GENETIC CODE

The code of life is degenerate, not quite universal, and unpunctuated

When one considers the transfer of information from RNA containing only four different bases (adenine, A; cytosine, C; guanine, G; and uracil, U) to a protein containing 20 different amino acids, it is apparent that there is not a one-to-one correspondence between nucleotide and amino acid sequence. In fact, three nucleotides in the mRNA, known as a codon, are required to specify each amino acid. There is thus a total of 64 possible codons when all combinations of four nucleotides are taken into account three at a time (Table 32.1). Three of these codons (UAA, UAG, UGA) are used as signals to stop the synthesis of a protein, and do not specify an amino acid. This leaves 61 codons to specify 20 amino acids, and illustrates a feature of the genetic code known as degeneracy, i.e. more than one codon can specify a specific amino acid. For example, codons GGU, GGC, GGA, and GGG all code for the amino acid, glycine. Indeed, all the amino acids, with the exception of methionine and tryptophan, have more than one codon. The codon AUG, which specifies only methionine, has a dual role: it encodes methionine anywhere

		The genetic code					
Codon	**Amino acid**	**Codon**	**Amino acid**	**Codon**	**Amino acid**	**Codon**	**Amino acid**
AAA	lysine (Lys)	CAA	glutamine (Gln)	GAA	glutamic acid (Glu)	UAA	Stop
AAG		CAG		GAG		UAG	
AAC	asparagine (Asn)	CAC	histidine (His)	GAC	aspartic acid (Asp)	UAC	tyrosine (Tyr)
AAU		CAU		GAU		UAU	
ACA	threonine (Thr)	CCA	proline (Pro)	GCA	alanine (Ala)	UCA	serine (Ser)
ACC		CCC		GCC		UCC	
ACG		CCG		GCG		UCG	
ACU		CCU		GCU		UCU	
AGA	arginine (Arg)	CGA	arginine (Arg)	GGA	glycine (Gly)	UGA	
AGG		CGC		GGC			
		CGG		GGG		UGG	Stop
AGC	serine (Ser)	CGU		GGU			tryptophan (Trp)
AGU						UGC	cysteine (Cys)
		CUA	leucine (Leu)	GUA	valine (Val)	UGU	
AUG	methionine (Met)	CUC		GUC			
		CUG		GUG		UUA	leucine (Leu)
AUA	isoleucine (Ile)	CUU		GUU		UUG	
AUC							
AUU						UUC	phenylalanine (Phe)
						UUU	

Table 32.1 **Amino acids specified by each of the codons.** Note that the first and second positions of codons that specify the same amino acid are generally the same.

MUTATION OF THE GENETIC CODE

Sickle cell anemia

Sickle cell anemia is an example of a disease in which a single nucleotide change within the coding region of the gene for the β-chain of hemoglobin A, the major form of adult hemoglobin, yields an altered protein that has impaired function. The mutation that causes this disease is a single nucleotide change in a codon that normally specifies glutamate (GAG), and which produces a codon that specifies valine (GUG). Under conditions of low oxygen tension, this single amino acid change causes the protein to polymerize into rod-shaped structures, resulting in deformation and altered rheological properties of red blood cells. This substitution of an acidic for a nonpolar, hydrophobic amino acid is known as a non-conservative mutation. Conservative mutations of one amino acid by another with similar physical and chemical properties usually have less severe consequences.

it occurs in the RNA, and it also marks the start of protein synthesis.

The genetic code as specified by the triplet nucleotides is, for the most part, the same for bacteria and humans, and is referred to as 'universal'. However, there are notable exceptions. In bacteria, if the codons GUG and UUG occur at the beginning of protein synthesis, they can be read as a methionine codon. In addition, the protein synthesis stop-codon, UAA, can encode a tryptophan amino acid in some lower eukaryotic organisms such as *Paramecium* and *Tetrahymena*. There are also minor differences in the genetic code in mitochondria.

Another aspect of the genetic code is that it is translated without punctuation. This means that, once synthesis has started at an AUG codon for methionine, each successive triplet from that start point will be read without interruption until a termination codon is encountered. Thus the 'reading frame' of the mRNA will be dictated by the AUG codon. This means that mutations that cause the addition or deletion of single nucleotides will cause a frame shift, resulting in a protein with a different (nonsense) amino acid sequence after the mutation, or a protein that is prematurely terminated (Table 32.2).

Effect of mutations on protein synthesis													
Normal gene	AUG Met	GCA Ala	UUA Leu	CAG Gln	GUA Val	UUA Leu	CUA Leu	CGA Arg	GGC Gly	ACA Thr	CCU Pro	GAA . . . Glu	functional protein
insertion	AUG Met	GCA Ala	UU**U** Phe	ACA Arg	GGU Gly	AUU Ile	ACU Thr	ACG Thr	AGG Arg	CAC His	ACC Thr	UGA A . . . **Stop**	premature termination
			↓										
deletion	AUG Met	GCA Ala	UAC Tyr	AGG Arg	UAU Tyr	UAC Tyr	UAC Tyr	GAG Glu	GCA Ala	CAC His	CUG Leu	AAA . . . Lys	different protein
altered base	AUG Met	GCA Ala	UUA Leu	CAG Gln	G**A**A Glu	UUA Leu	CUA Leu	CGA Arg	GGC Gly	ACA Thr	CCU Pro	GAA . . . Glu	single amino acid change
altered base	AUG Met	GCA Ala	UUA Leu	CAG Gln	GUA Val	UUA Leu	CU**G** Leu	CGA Arg	GGC Gly	ACA Thr	CCU Pro	GAA . . . Glu	no change

Table 32.2 **Effect of mutations on the primary sequence of the encoded protein.** Note that the location of the mutation will dictate the extent of change observed in the primary sequence. Insertion and deletion mutations cause frame shifts that lead to synthesis of nonsense proteins with either premature or delayed termination.

THE MACHINERY OF PROTEIN SYNTHESIS

Ribosomes consist of a small and a large subunit that, when associated with each other, possess specific sites at which tRNAs bind. These sites are known as the aminoacyl, or A site, and the peptidyl, or P site. The A site is where a tRNA molecule, carrying the appropriate amino acid on its acceptor stem, sits before that amino acid is incorporated into the protein. The P site is the location in the ribosome that contains a tRNA molecule with the amino-terminal polypeptide of the newly synthesized protein still attached to its acceptor stem. It is within these sites that the process of peptide bond formation takes place. This process is catalyzed by peptidyl transferase, an enzyme that forms the peptide bond between the amino group of the amino acid in the A site and the carboxyl terminus of the nascent peptide attached to the tRNA in the P site.

Each amino acid has a specific synthetase that is responsible for attaching it to all the tRNAs that bind it

There is also a distinct tRNA molecule for each of the codons represented in Table 32.1. The amino acid is attached to the acceptor stem of the tRNA by an enzyme called aminoacyl-tRNA synthetase; this enzyme catalyzes the formation of an ester bond linking the 3′ hydroxyl group of the adenosine nucleotide of the tRNA to the carboxyl group of the amino acid (Fig. 32.1). The attachment of an amino acid to a tRNA is a two-step reaction. The carboxyl group of the amino acid is first activated by reaction with adenosine triphosphate

FIDELITY OF TRANSLATION

Aminoacyl-tRNA synthetases have proof-reading ability

To guarantee the accuracy of protein synthesis, mechanisms have evolved to ensure selection of the correct amino acid for acylation and for proof-reading of already charged tRNAs. One such mechanism is found in the enzymes responsible for attaching an amino acid to the correct tRNA. The aminoacyl-tRNA synthetases have the ability not only to discriminate between amino acids before they are attached to the appropriate tRNA, but also to remove amino acids that are attached to the wrong tRNA. This discriminating ability exhibited by the synthetases is accomplished by a series of hydrogen bonding interactions between the enzyme and the amino acid. These two mechanisms combine to ensure accurate transfer of information from RNA to protein.

(ATP) to form an amino-acyladenylate intermediate, which is bound to the synthetase complex. The enzymology of activation of the carboxyl group of amino acids is similar to that for activation of fatty acids by thiokinase, but, rather than transfer of the acyl group to the thiol group of coenzyme A, the aminoacyl group is transferred to the 5′-hydroxyl group of the tRNA – it is now described as a charged tRNA molecule. At this point it is ready to bind to the A site of the ribosome, where it will contribute its amino acid to a growing peptide chain. There is a different synthetase specific for each of the 20 amino acids in protein. This synthetase attaches the

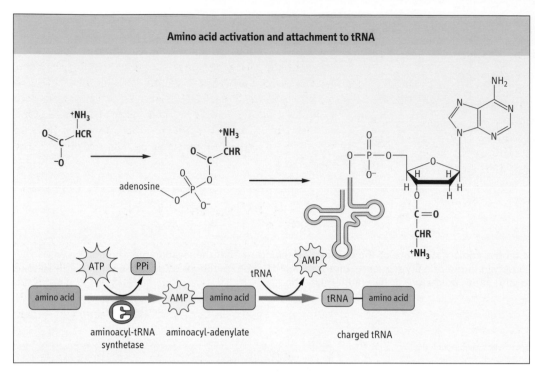

Amino acid activation and attachment to tRNA

Fig. 32.1 **Activation of an amino acid and attachment to its cognate tRNA.** The amino acid must be activated by aminoacyl-tRNA synthetase to form an aminoacyladenylate intermediate, before its attachment to the 3' end of the tRNA. AMP, adenosine monophosphate; PPi, inorganic pyrophosphate.

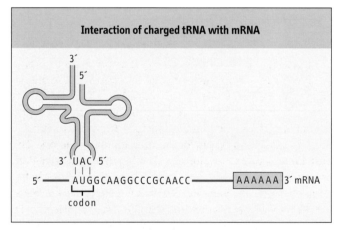

Interaction of charged tRNA with mRNA

Fig. 32.2 **Interaction of charged tRNA with mRNA.** The interaction of a charged tRNA with an mRNA occurs by base pairing of complementary bases in the anticodon loop and the codon of the mRNA.

Codon-anticodon base pairing possibilities

Codon 3' position (mRNA)	Anticodon 5' position (tRNA)
G	C
U	A
A or G	U
C or U	G
A or C or U	I

Table 32.3 **Base pairing possibilities between the 3' nucleotide of the mRNA codon and the 5' nucleotide of the tRNA anticodon.**

appropriate amino acid to all the tRNAs that bind that amino acid.

Some flexibility of base pairing occurs at the 3' base of the mRNA codon

Interaction of the charged tRNA with its cognate codon is accomplished by association of the anticodon loop in tRNA with the codon in mRNA through hydrogen bonding of com-plementary base pairs (Fig. 32.2). The base-pairing rules are the same as those for DNA, except at the 3' base of the codon (see Chapter 30). At this position, non-classical base pairs can form between the last base in tRNA molecule and the 5' base of the anticodon. This observation led to the formulation of the *wobble hypothesis of codon-anticodon pairing.* The basis for this hypothesis lies in the fact that there appears to be less energetic constraint on the type of base pair formed at the 3' position of the codon. For example, if a guanine residue is at the 5' position of the anticodon, it can form a base pair with either a cytidine or a uracil residue in the 3' position of the codon. If the deaminated adenosine residue, inosine, occurs at the 5' position of the anticodon, it can form a base pair with uracil, adenine, or even cytidine at the 3' position of the codon (Table 32.3).

How does the ribosome know where to begin protein synthesis?

The mRNA molecule carries the information that will be used to direct the synthesis of the protein. However, not all of the information carried on the mRNA is used for this purpose. Most eukaryotic mRNAs contain regions both before and after the protein coding region, called 5′ and 3′ flanking sequences or 5′ and 3′ UTRs (untranslated regions). These sequences are involved in regulating the rate of protein synthesis and the stability of the mRNA; however, the fact that, as a consequence of their presence, the protein coding region does not start immediately at the beginning of the mRNA raises the question of how the ribosome knows where to start synthesis. In the case of eukaryotic cells, the ribosome first binds to the 7-methylguanine 'cap' structure at the 5′ end of the mRNA, and then moves down the molecule until it encounters the first AUG codon (Fig. 32.3). This signals the ribosome to begin synthesizing the protein, beginning with a methionine residue, and to continue until it encounters one of the termination codons (UGA, UAA, or UAG).

In the case of bacterial cells, knowing what portion of the mRNA is to be used to synthesize a protein is complicated by the fact that there can be several proteins encoded on a single mRNA, each out of register with one another, so that proteins of different sequence may be obtained from the same ribonucleotide sequence. This problem has been solved by the discovery of a sequence that helps to position the ribosome at the beginning of each protein coding region. This sequence, known as a Shine–Dalgarno sequence, is complementary to a portion of the 16S rRNA in the small bacterial ribosomal subunit. These sequences interact through hydrogen bonding of complementary base pairs, and this interaction helps to target the ribosome to the protein-coding regions of the mRNA.

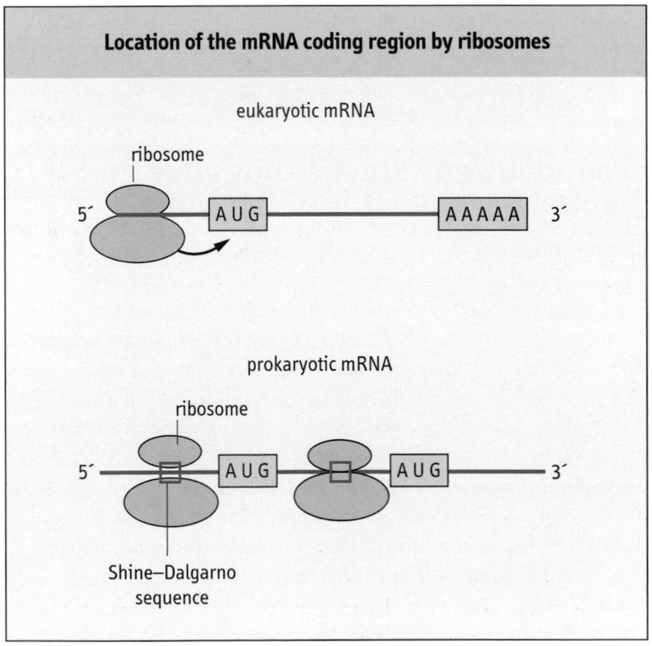

THE PROCESS OF PROTEIN SYNTHESIS

Translation is a dynamic process that involves the interaction of enzymes, tRNAs, ribosomes, and mRNA in specific ways to produce a protein molecule capable of carrying out a specific cellular function. This complex process is normally divided into three steps:

- **initiation,**
- **elongation,**
- **termination.**

Initiation

Initiation of protein synthesis takes place when a ribosome (both large and small subunit) has assembled on the mRNA and the P site is occupied by a methionyl-tRNA (met-tRNA) molecule (Fig. 32.4). This complex is formed by the action of proteins known as initiation factors. In prokaryotic cells, the process (Fig. 32.4) involves three initiation factors. The initiation complex first forms just 5′ to the coding region, as a result of the interaction of the 16S rRNA with the Shine–Dalgarno sequence on the mRNA. *N*-Formyl methionine (fmet) is the first amino acid in all bacterial proteins. In eukaryotic cells, there are at least 12 different initiation factors (eIFs), only a few of which have a known functon. The majority of eIFs help to promote the association of the small ribosomal subunit with the mRNA and a charged met-tRNA. For example, a complex containing the activated initiator, met-tRNA, and eIF-2 first binds to the small ribosomal subunit, which has eIF-3 bound to it. This complex then binds to the 7-methylguanine cap structure of eukaryotic mRNAs by the actions of several factors, including eIF-4F. The small ribosomal subunit moves down the mRNA until the first AUG codon is encountered, at which time the large ribosomal subunit joins the complex and protein synthesis is ready to begin. The assembly of the initiation complex is driven by the hydrolysis of guanosine triphosphate (GTP), and the movement of this complex down the mRNA is driven by the hydrolysis of ATP.

Location of the mRNA coding region by ribosomes

eukaryotic mRNA

ribosome

5′ [AUG] [AAAAA] 3′

prokaryotic mRNA

ribosome

5′ [AUG] [AUG] 3′

Shine–Dalgarno sequence

Fig. 32.3 **Synthesis by multiple ribosomes.** The ribosome binds to the mRNA before locating the protein-coding region. Eukaryotic ribosomes bind to the 5′ end of mRNAs and then move down the mRNA until they encounter the first AUG codon. Bacterial ribosomes bind to complementary sequences in the mRNA –the Shine-Dalgarno sequences – that locate the protein-coding regions on the mRNA.

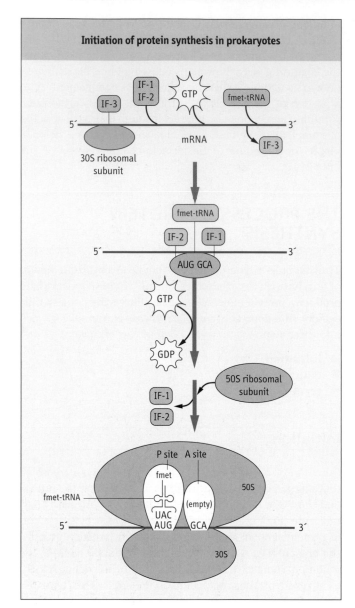

Initiation of protein synthesis in prokaryotes

Fig. 32.4 **Initiation of protein synthesis in bacterial cells.** The 30S ribosomal subunit, mRNA, and formylated met-tRNA (fmet-tRNA) are brought together by the action of initiation factors. Once these components are assembled, the 50S ribosomal subunit completes the initiation complex. Note that, at initiation, the P site is occupied by the initiator tRNA, met-tRNA. GDP, guanosine diphosphate; IF, initiation factor.

Elongation

Factors involved in the elongation stage of protein synthesis are targets of some antibiotics

After initiation is complete, the process of translating the information in mRNA into a functional protein starts. Elongation begins with the binding of a charged tRNA to the

A NONCOMPLIANT PATIENT

A young man you were treating for a sinus infection returns to your clinic after 1 week, still complaining of sinus headaches and stuffiness. He explains that he began to feel better about 3 days after starting to take the antibiotic tetracycline, which you had prescribed. You inquire as to whether he continued to take the full dose of the drug, even after he began to feel better. He reluctantly admits that, as soon as he felt better, he stopped taking the drug. How do you explain to your patient that it is important that he takes the drug for as long as you prescribed it, even if he feels better after only a few days?

Comment. As a physician, you know that tetracycline inhibits the protein synthetic machinery of the bacterial cell by binding to the A site of the ribosome (Table 32.4). You also know that, if the drug is removed, protein synthesis can resume. If the drug is not taken for the entire period recommended, bacteria will begin to grow again, leading to the resurgence of the infection. Further, those bacteria that begin to grow after early termination of treatment are likely to be the most resistant to the drug, either because of selection of more resistant strains, or because of mutation to more resistant strains. The secondary infection is therefore likely to be more difficult to control.

PROTEIN SYNTHESIS: PEPTIDYL TRANSFERASE

Peptidyl transferase is not your typical enzyme. It is a ribozyme

Peptidyl transferase is the enzyme responsible for peptide bond formation during protein synthesis. This enzyme catalyzes the reaction between the amino group of the aminoacyl-tRNA, forming a peptide bond from an ester bond. The enzyme activity is located in the ribosome, but none of the ribosomal proteins has the capacity to catalyze this reaction. In fact, when ribosomes are stripped of all of their associated proteins, the rRNA appears to remain capable of converting an ester bond to a peptide bond. These observations have led investigators to hypothesize that peptidyl transferase activity is contained in the rRNA, rather than in the proteins that associate with ribosomes.

A site of the ribosome. In eukaryotic cells, the charged tRNA molecule is brought to the ribosome by the action of an elongation factor called EF-1α (Fig. 32.5). For EF-1α to be active, it must have a GTP molecule associated with it. If the charged tRNA is the correct one – i.e., one in which the anticodon of

Regeneration of Factor EF-1α

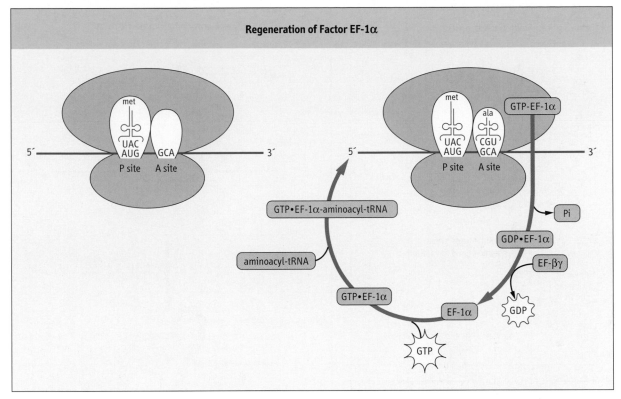

Fig. 32.5 **Recycling of Factor EF-1α.** A charged tRNA molecule is brought to the A site of the initiation complex to begin the process of elongation. Each successive amino acid addition requires that the correctly charged tRNA molecule be brought to the A site of the ribosome. ala, alanine; Pi, inorganic phosphate.

the tRNA forms base pairs with the codon on the mRNA – GTP is hydrolyzed and EF-1α is released. For EF-1α factor to bring another charged molecule to the ribosome, it must be regenerated by an elongation factor called EF-βγ, which will promote the association of EF-1α with GTP so that it may bind to another charged tRNA molecule (Fig. 32.5). Once the correct charged tRNA molecule has been delivered to the A site of the ribosome, peptidyl transferase catalyzes the formation of a peptide bond between the amino acid in the A site and the amino acid at the end of the growing peptide chain in the P site. The tRNA-peptide chain is now transiently bound to the A site. The ribosome is then moved one codon down the mRNA by a factor known as EF-2 and the nascent peptide chain at the A site moves to the P site. The whole process recycles for addition of the next amino acid (Fig. 32.6). This complex process is identical in prokaryotic cells, but the factors are different; this explains the utility of antibiotics that preferentially inhibit protein synthesis in bacteria (Table 32.4).

Antibiotics and their targets

Antibiotic	Target
tetracycline	bacterial ribosome-A site
streptomycin	bacterial 30 S ribosome subunit
erythromycin	bacterial 50 S ribosome subunit
chloramphenicol	bacterial ribosome-peptidyl transferase
cycloheximide	eukaryotic 80 S ribosome
ricin	eukaryotic 60 S ribosome subunit

Table 32.4 **Antibiotics and their targets.** Cycloheximide, and ricin in particular, are potent poisons to humans.

Termination

Termination of protein synthesis in both eukaryotic and bacterial cells is accomplished when the A site of the ribosome reaches one of the stop-codons of the mRNA. Protein factors called releasing factors recognize these codons, and cause the protein that is attached to the last tRNA molecule in the P site to be released (Fig. 32.7). This process is an energy-dependent reaction catalyzed by the hydrolysis of GTP, which transfers a water molecule to the end of the protein, thus releasing it

Peptide bond formation and translocation

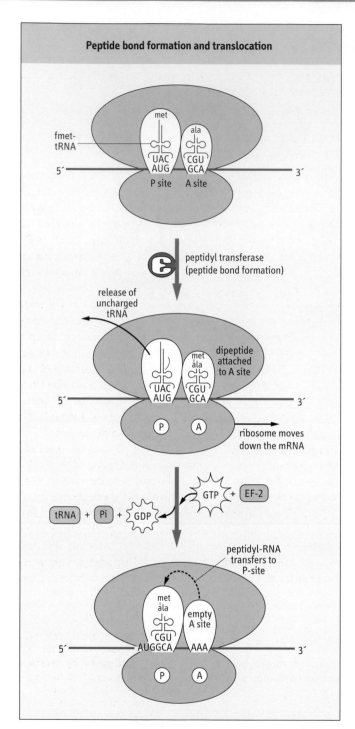

Fig. 32.6 **Peptide bond formation and translocation.** The formation of the peptide bond between each successive amino acid is catalyzed by peptidyl transferase. Once the peptide bond is formed, an elongation factor (EF-2) will move the ribosome down one codon on the mRNA, so that the A site is vacant and ready to receive the next charged tRNA.

Termination of protein synthesis

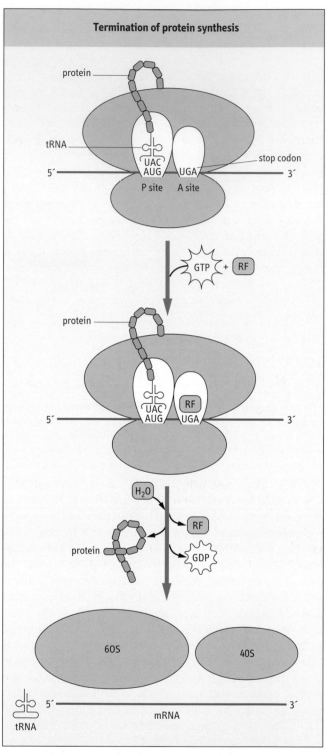

Fig. 32.7 **Termination of protein synthesis.** Termination of protein synthesis occurs when the A site is placed over a termination codon. A releasing factor (RF) will cause the completed protein to be released and the ribosome, mRNA, and tRNA will dissociate from each other.

from the tRNA. After release of the newly synthesized protein, the ribosomal subunits, tRNA, and mRNA dissociate from each other. An initiation factor, such as eIF-2, binds to the small ribosomal subunit, setting the stage for the translation of another mRNA (see Fig. 32.4).

For a newly synthesized protein to become functionally active it must be folded into a unique three-dimensional structure. Newly synthesized proteins achieve their native structures with the help of a class of proteins called chaperones. Chaperones bind to exposed hydrophobic regions of unfolded proteins and prevent their interaction with each other by shielding the interactive surfaces, thereby preventing misfolding of the protein. The chaperones promote the correct folding of newly synthesized proteins by cycles of substrate binding and release regulated by an ATPase activity and by cofactor proteins. The consequences of protein aggregation due to misfolding can be severe. Some forms of Alzheimer's and Huntington's disease are associated with the formation of amyloid, a fibrillar aggregation of mis-folded protein.

PROTEIN TARGETING AND POST-TRANSLATIONAL MODIFICATIONS

Protein targeting

More than one ribosome can translate an mRNA at the same time. An mRNA with several bound ribosomes is known as a polyribosome or polysome (Fig. 32.8). There are two general classes of polysomes found in cells: those that are free in the cytoplasm, and those that are attached to the endoplasmic reticulum. mRNAs encoding proteins destined for the cytoplasm are translated primarily on polysomes free in the cytoplasm, while mRNAs encoding membrane and secre-

tory proteins are translated on polysomes attached to the endoplasmic reticulum. Translation on the endoplasmic reticulum assists in the post-translational modification of proteins and targeting of proteins to specific subcellular compartments.

Cellular fate of proteins is determined by their signal peptide sequences

Proteins that are destined for export, for insertion into membranes, or for specific cellular organelles, must in some way be distinguished from proteins that reside in the cytoplasm. The distinguishing characteristic of all proteins targeted for these locations is that they contain a signal sequence usually comprising the first 20–30 amino acids on the amino-terminal end of the protein. In the case of secretory or membrane proteins, shortly after the signal sequence is synthesized, it is recognized by a ribonucleoprotein complex known as a signal recognition particle (SRP). The SRP binds to the signal sequence and halts translation of the remainder of the protein. This complex then binds to a receptor, known as the SRP docking protein, located on the membrane of the endoplasmic reticulum. After the SRP has delivered the ribosome-bound mRNA with its nascent protein to the endoplasmic reticulum, the signal sequence is inserted through the membrane, the SRP dissociates, and translation continues with the polypeptide chain being moved, as it is synthesized, across the membrane into the interstitial space of the endoplasmic reticulum (Fig. 32.9). The protein is then transferred to the Golgi apparatus, and then to its final destination.

In contrast to secretory and membrane proteins, mitochondrial and nuclear proteins are transported after their translation is complete. In common with membrane and secretory proteins, both mitochondrial and nuclear proteins have signal sequences that mark them to be transported from

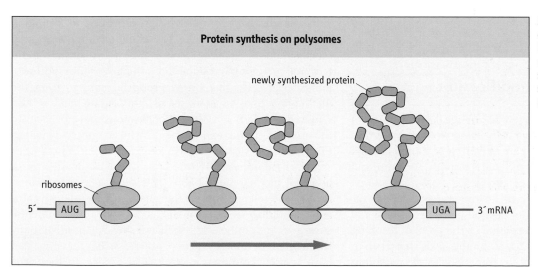

Protein synthesis on polysomes

ribosomes

5′ — AUG — UGA — 3′ mRNA

newly synthesized protein

Fig. 32.8 **Protein synthesis on polysomes.** Protein can be synthesized by several ribosomes bound to the same mRNA, forming a structure known as a polysome.

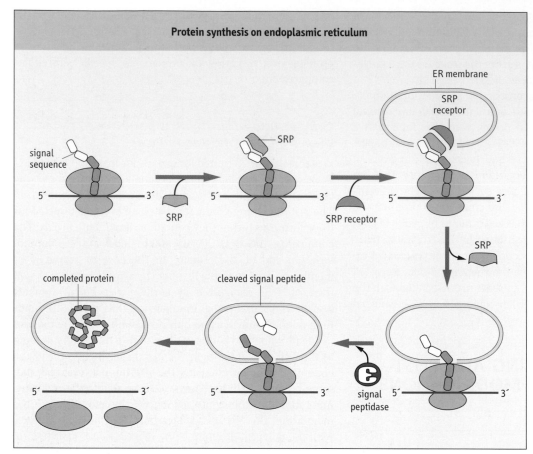

Protein synthesis on endoplasmic reticulum

Fig. 32.9 **Protein synthesis on endoplasmic reticulum.** Proteins can be targeted to specific sites in the cell by recognition of the signal sequence by an SRP. This complex is then recognized by the SRP docking protein (SRP receptor) on the endoplasmic reticulum (ER), where the signal sequence is inserted through the membrane. A signal peptidase removes the signal sequence and translation resumes. Once synthesis of the protein is complete, the protein is delivered to its cellular location.

the endoplasmic reticulum to their respective organelles. In the case of proteins destined for the mitochondrion, they may have two signal sequences on their amino-terminal ends, depending on whether they are destined for the matrix or for the intermembrane space. Mitochondrial proteins must be unfolded before they can be transported; in contrast, nuclear proteins may have nuclear localization signals throughout the entire length of the molecule and do not have to be unfolded before transport. Nuclear pores are very large complexes and apparently accommodate the transport of a protein in its native state.

Post-translational modification

Many proteins must be altered by chemical modification of amino acids before the proteins become biologically active; collectively, these alterations are known as post-translational modifications. It is within the endoplasmic reticulum and Golgi apparatus that two of the major post-translational modifications of proteins occur. In the endoplasmic reticulum, an enzyme called signal peptidase removes the signal sequence from the amino-terminus of the protein, resulting in a mature protein that is 20–30 amino acids shorter than that encoded by the mRNA. In the endoplasmic reticulum

and Golgi apparatus, carbohydrate side chains are added and modified at specific sites on the protein; the specific types of the carbohydrates added are important to the eventual function of the protein. A detailed description of the types of oligosaccharide side chains added to proteins, the mechanism of their addition, and the enzymes involved in this process may be found in Chapter 25.

Post-translational modifications to proteins may also include amino-terminal modification, modification of individual amino acids, proteolytic processing, and formation of disulfide bridges. One of the common amino-terminal modifications of eukaryotic cells is the removal of the amino-terminal methionine residue that initiates protein synthesis; in bacterial cells, the formyl group is removed from the methionine and, in some cases, the amino acid is also removed. In addition to these modifications that can occur to the amino-terminal end of the protein, amino acids within the protein can also be altered: for example, the amino acids serine, threonine, and tyrosine may have phosphate groups attached to their side chains. This type of modification is used by the cell to communicate changes in regulatory pathways resulting from hormone action and environmental stresses. Some amino acids, such as lysine, will be modified by the addition of a methyl group; others, such as cysteine, can have isoprenyl groups or other lipids added to their side chains, to facilitate protein binding to membranes. Cysteine residues also form specific disulfide bridges that are important to the structural integrity of the protein. Finally, many proteins are synthesized as preproteins and proproteins that must be proteolytically cleaved for them to be active. The cleavage of a precursor to its biologically active form is usually accomplished by a specific protease, and is a regulated cellular event.

Proteasomes: Cellular machinery for protein turnover

Protein degradation is a complex process that is critical to cellular regulation. In general, unlike DNA, damaged proteins are not repaired, but degraded, and the amino acids are recycled. In some cases, proteins age passively by gradual denaturation processes at body temperature. Proteins may also be modified by reaction with intracellular carbonyl compounds, such as glycolytic intermediates, or by reaction with products of lipid peroxidation during oxidative stress. Some proteins are induced at specific times in the cell cycle or in response to hormones, and are actively degraded as part of a cell cycle or counter-regulatory response. Some of these proteins have characteristic amino acid sequences or N-terminal residues that promote their turnover. The PEST (ProGluSerThr) sequence marks some proteins for rapid turnover, while proteins with N-terminal arginine residues generally have short half-lives.

Since protein degradation is a destructive process it must be sequestered within specific cellular organelles. Lysosomes, for example, ingest and degrade damaged mitochondria and other membranous organelles. However, most soluble, cytoplasmic proteins are degraded in structures called proteasomes. The 26S proteasome consists of two types of subunits, a 20S multimeric, multicatalytic protease (MCP) and a 19S ATPase. The proteasome is a barrel-shaped structure, formed by a stack of four rings of seven homologous monomers, alpha-type subunits in the outer ends and beta-type subunits on the inner rings of the barrel. The proteolytic activity – three different types of threonine proteases – resides on beta subunits with active sites facing the inside of the barrel, thereby protecting cytoplasmic proteins from random degradation. The ATPase subunits are attached at either end of the barrel and act as gate-keepers, allowing only proteins destined for destruction to enter the barrel. The proteins are unfolded and degraded to small peptides, 6–9 amino acids in length that are released into the cytoplasm for further degradation.

Proteins destined for destruction are directed to the proteasome primarily by covalent modification with a highly conserved, 76 amino acid residue protein called **ubiquitin** which is found in all cells. Ubiquitin must be activated to fulfill its role (Fig. 32.10) and this is accomplished by a ubiquitin-

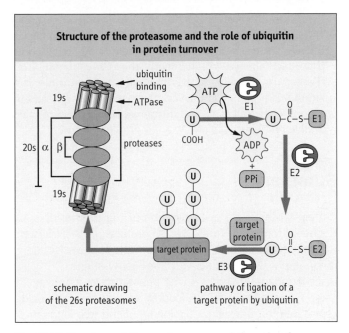

Fig. 32.10 **Structure of the proteasome and the role of ubiquitin (u) in protein turnover.** The proteasome is shown at the left, a barrel-shaped structure. The 20s multicatalytic protease in the middle rings of the barrel has protease activity on their inner face. The 19S caps at the end of the barrel have ubiquitin-binding and release and ATPase activity, and control access of proteins to the inside of the barrel for degradation. The ubiquitin cycle is involved in marking proteins for degradation by the proteasome. Ubiquitin is first activated as a thioester derivative of ubiquitin-activating enzyme E1; it is then transferred to ubiquitin-conjugating enzyme E2, then to a lysine residue on the target protein, catalyzed by ubiquitin-ligase E3. Ubiquitin is frequently co-polymerized on target proteins. The more highly ubiquinated the protein, the more susceptible it is to proteasomal degradation. Note that the drawing is not to scale; the proteasome is a 26S macromolecular complex (>2 000 000 D); target proteins are smaller while ubiquitin molecular weight is less than 10 000 D.

activating enzyme called E1. Activation occurs when E1 is attached via a thioester bond to the C-terminus of ubiquitin via ATP-driven formation of a ubiquitin–adenylate intermediate. The activated ubiquitin is then attached to a ubiquitin carrier protein, known as E2, by a thioester linkage. A ubiquitin protein ligase known as E3 transfers the ubiquitin from E2 to a target protein, forming an isopeptide bond between the carboxyl terminus of ubiquitin and the ε-amino group of a lysine residue on a target protein. Denatured and oxidized proteins are commonly ubiquitinated by this mechanism. The 26S subunit of the proteasome has a ubiquitin binding site that allows proteins with a covalently attached ubiquitin protein to enter the barrel; the ubiquitin is then released by a ubiquitinase activity and recycled to the cytosol. Polymerization of ubiquitin on target proteins (polyubiquitination) enhances degradation of the protein.

The ubiquitin pathway leading to proteasomal degradation of proteins is complex. There are a number of E2 and E3 proteins with differential target specificity, and six different ATPase activities associated with the 19S subunit. The ATPases are thought to be involved in denaturation of ubiquinated proteins. These variations, as well as changes in response to the cell cycle and hormonal stimulation, provide a flexible and regulated pathway for protein turnover.

Summary

Protein synthesis is the culmination of the transfer of genetic information from DNA to proteins. In this transfer, information must be translated from the four-nucleotide-language of DNA and RNA to the twenty-amino acids-language of proteins. The genetic code, in which three nucleotides in mRNA (codon) specify an amino acid, represents the translation dictionary of the two languages. The tRNA molecule is the bridge between these two languages. The tRNA accomplishes this task by virtue of its anticodon loop which interacts with specific codons on the mRNA, and amino acids via its amino acid attachment site located on the 3′ end of the molecule. The process of translation consists of three parts; initiation, elongation, and termination. Initiation involves the assembly of the ribosome and charged tRNA at the initiation codon (AUG) of the mRNA. This assembly process is mediated by initiation factors and requires the expenditure of energy in the form of GTP. Elongation is a stepwise addition of individual amino acids to a growing peptide chain by the action of peptidyl transferase. The charged tRNA molecules are brought to the ribosome by elongation factors at the expense of GTP hydrolysis. Termination of protein synthesis occurs when the ribosome reaches a stop codon and releasing factors catalyze the release of a protein. After release, the newly synthesized protein must be correctly folded with the help of ancillary proteins called chaperones. Many newly synthesized proteins must also be modified, by a variety of chemical and structural changes, before they are biologically active. Once a protein is no longer needed, it is degraded in an equally complex, macromolecular complex called the proteasome.

ACTIVE LEARNING

1. Review the mechanism of action of various drugs that inhibit protein synthesis on the bacterial ribosome.
2. Compare and contrast mechanisms that assure the fidelity of DNA and protein synthesis.
3. Describe the signal sequences that target proteins to the lysosome.
4. Discuss the role of the N-terminal amino acid as a factor regulating the rate of turnover of a cytoplasmic protein.
5. Explain how viruses take control of the cellular protein translation machinery during viral infections to favor the synthesis of viral proteins.

Further reading

Yusupov MM, Yusupova GZ, Baucom A, Lieberman K, Earnest TN, Cate JH, Noller HF. Crystal structure of the ribosome at 5.5 A resolution. Science 2001;**292**:883–896, 2001.

Giasson BI, Lee VM-Y. Are Ubiquitination pathways central to Parkinson's disease? Cell 2003;**114**:1–8.

Gilbert DN, Dworkin RJ, Raber SR, Leggett JE. Outpatient parenteral antimicrobial drug therapy. N Engl J Med 1997;**337**:829–838.

Hartl FU, Hayer-Hartl M. Molecular chaperones in the cytosol: from nascent chain to folded protein. Science 2002;**295**:1852–1858.

Quagliarello VJ, Scheld WM. Treatment of bacterial meningitis. N Engl J Med 1997;**336**:708–716.

Siegel V. A second signal recognition event required for translocation into the endoplasmic reticulum. Cell 1995;**82**:167–170.

Steitz TA, Moore PB. RNA, the first macromolecular catalyst: the ribosome is a ribozyme. Trends Biochem Sci 2003;**28**:411–418.

Zheng N, Gierasch L. Signal sequences: the same yet different. Cell 1996;**86**:849–852.

Websites

Genetic code:
    http://users.rcn.com/jkimball.ma.ultranet/BiologyPages/C/Codons.html
http://www.americanscientist.org/template/AssetDetail/assetid/20831
Ribosome: http://www.rcsb.org/pdb/molecules/pdb10_1.html;
http://info.bio.cmu.edu/Courses/BiochemMols/ribosome/70S.htm
The Proteasome: http://www.ib.amwaw.edu.pl/home/cwojcik/proteas.htm
Ubiquitin:
    http://www.nottingham.ac.uk/biochemcourses/students/ub/ubindex.html

33. Control of Gene Expression

D M Hunt and A Jamieson

LEARNING OBJECTIVES

After reading this chapter you should be able to:

- Describe the general mechanisms of regulation of gene expression, including the role of cis-acting promoters and enhancers and trans-acting transcription factors.
- Describe the many levels at which gene expression may be controlled, using steroid-induced gene expression as a model.
- Explain how alternate splicing, alternate promoters and post-transcriptional editing can modulate expression of a gene.
- Explain how the structure and packaging of chromatin can affect gene expression.
- Explain how genomic imprinting can result in changes in gene expression, depending on whether alleles are maternally or paternally inherited.

INTRODUCTION

The study of genes and the mechanism whereby the information they hold is converted into proteins and enzymes, hormones and intracellular signaling molecules is the realm of molecular biology. One of the most fascinating aspects of this work is the study of the mechanisms that control gene expression, both in time and in place, and the consequences if these control mechanisms are disrupted.

The goal of this chapter is to introduce the basic concepts involved in regulation of protein-coding genes and how these processes are involved in the causation of human disease. The basic mechanism of gene regulation will be described first, followed by a discussion of a specific gene regulation system to highlight various aspects of the basic mechanism. The chapter will end with a discussion of various ways in which the gene regulatory apparatus can be adapted to suit the needs of different tissues and situations.

BASIC MECHANISMS OF GENE EXPRESSION

Gene expression encompasses several different processes

The control of human gene expression occurs principally at the level of transcription. However, transcription is just one step in the conversion of the genetic information encoded by a gene into the final processed gene product, and it has become increasingly clear that post-transcription events occur that may also have an important role in regulating the expression of a gene. The sequence of events involved may be summarized as:

initiation of transcription
→ processing the transcript
→ transport to cytoplasm
→ translation of transcript to protein
→ posttranslational processing of the protein

Gene expression in humans can be regulated in many ways, both at specific phases in development and in differentiated tissues of mature organisms. Clearly, during the growth of a human embryo from a single fertilized ovum to a newborn infant, there must be numerous changes in the regulation of genes, to allow the differentiation of a single cell into many types of cells that develop tissue-specific characteristics. Similarly, at puberty there are changes in the secretion of pituitary hormones that result in the cyclic secretion of ovarian and adrenal hormones in females and the production of secondary sexual characteristics. Such programmed events are common in all cellular organisms, and the production of these phenotypic changes in cells – and thus the whole organism – arises as a result of changes in the expression of key genes. These key genes vary from cell to cell and also in time, but the mechanisms underlying the changes in regulation are less variable. In humans and other eukaryotes, mechanisms that regulate transcription (Table 33.1) are manifold, as are the factors that influence them.

Gene transcription requires key elements to be present in the region of the gene

The key step in the transcription of a protein-coding gene is the conversion of the information held within the DNA of the gene into messenger RNA, which can then be used as a

Regulation of gene expression	
Mechanism	**Example**
Transcriptional level	
transcription by tissue-specific factors	muscle-cell-specific transporter factor (MyoD): in myoblasts
	Ker 1 = keratinocyle differentiation factor – skin cells
	HNF-5 = hepatic nuclear factor-5 – liver cells
	TATA box: binds transcription factor IID (TFIID)
hormone, growth factor, or cellular messenger binding to response element	glucocorticoid response element (GRE): binds glucocorticoid receptor complex
alternative promoters	dystrophin gene
Post-transcriptional level	
tissue-specific RNA processing	alternative splicing, e.g. immunoglobulin genes
	alternative polyadenylation signals, e.g. calcitonin-related gene peptide
RNA editing	editing of apoB mRNA
RNA translation	ferritin and transferrin
RNA stability	transferrin receptor, cyclooxygenase-2

Table 33.1 **Mechanisms involved in the regulation of gene expression in humans.**

template for synthesis of the protein product of the gene. For expression of a gene to take place, the enzyme that catalyzes the formation of mRNA, RNA polymerase II (RNAPol II), must be able to recognize the so-called startpoint for transcription of the gene. RNAPol II uses one strand of the DNA template to create a new, complementary RNA (often called the primary transcript), which is then modified in various ways (commonly including addition of a methylated guanine nucleotide cap, addition of a polyA tail, and splicing out of introns) to form a mature mRNA (Chapter 31). However, RNAPol II cannot initiate transcription alone. This enzyme requires other factors to assist in recognition of critical gene sequences and other proteins in the vicinity of the start point for transcription.

Promoters

Sequences that are relatively close to the startpoint for transcription of a gene (usually within a few hundred or a few thousand nucleotides of the startpoint) and control its expression are collectively known as the promoter. The promoter sequence acts as a basic recognition unit, signaling that there is a gene that can be transcribed and providing the information needed for the RNAPol II to recognize the gene and to correctly initiate RNA synthesis, both at the right place and using the correct strand of DNA as template. The promoter also plays an important role in determining that RNA is synthesized at the right time in the right cell. Most control

regions in the promoter are upstream of the transcription startpoint, and, therefore, are not transcribed into RNA; however, occasionally some elements of the promoter may be downstream of the startpoint for RNA synthesis, and may actually be transcribed into RNA. The structure of promoters varies from gene to gene, but there are a number of key sequence elements that can be identified within the promoter. These elements may be present in varying combinations, some elements being present in one gene but absent in another. Sequences further away from the transcription start site, some of which are known as enhancers, may also have major impact on the transcription of a gene. Enhancers exert their effect independently of their orientation or whether they are upstream or downstream of the start site.

The efficiency and specificity of gene expression is conferred by cis-acting elements

A promoter exerts its effect because it is on the same piece of DNA as the gene being transcribed and is referred to as a *cis*-acting sequence or element to emphasize that it affects only the neighboring gene on the same chromosome. Since the promoter is critical to gene expression, it is often regarded as being part of the gene it controls, since without it the mRNA would not be made.

The nucleotide sequence immediately surrounding the startpoint of a gene varies from gene to gene. However, the first base in mRNA tends to be adenine (A), usually followed by a pyrimidine-rich sequence, termed the initiator (Inr). In general, it has the nucleotide sequence Py_2CAPy_5 (Py = pyrimidine base; C-cytosine, A-adenine) and is found between positions -3 to $+5$ in relation to the startpoint. In addition to Inr, most promoters possess a sequence known as the TATA box. This sequence element is usually approximately 25 bp upstream from the startpoint. The TATA box has an 8 bp consensus sequence that usually consists entirely of adenine-thymine (A–T) base pairs, although very rarely a guanine-cytosine (G–C) pair may be present. This sequence appears to be very important in the process of transcription, as nucleotide substitutions that disrupt the TATA box result in a marked reduction in the efficiency of transcription. The positions of Inr and the TATA box relative to the startpoint are relatively fixed (Fig. 33.1).

In addition to the TATA box, other commonly found *cis*-acting promoter elements have been described. For example, the CAAT box is often found upstream of the TATA box, typically about 80 bp from the startpoint, and may be present and functional in either orientation. As in the case of the TATA box, it may be more important for its ability to increase the strength of the promoter signal rather than in controlling tissue- or time-specific expression of the gene. Another commonly noted promoter element is the GC box. This is a GC rich sequence that can function in either orientation, and multiple copies may be found in a single promoter region.

Figure 33.1 lists some of the common *cis*-acting elements

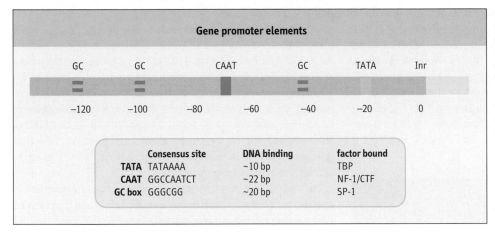

Fig. 33.1 **Idealized version of a promoter comprising various different elements.** Each promoter element has a specific consensus sequence that binds ubiquitous transcription-activating factors. Binding of transcription factors encompasses the consensus site and a variable number of anonymous adjacent nucleotides, depending on the promoter element. CTF, a member of a protein family whose members act as transcription factors; TBP, TATA-binding protein; NF-1, nuclear factor-1; SP-1, ubiquitous transcription factor.

CONSENSUS ELEMENTS

Identifying the function and specificity of nucleotide sequences

Consensus sequences are nucleotide sequences that contain unique core elements that identify the function and specificity of the sequence, for example the TATA box. The sequence of the element may differ by a few nucleotides in different genes, but a core, or consensus, sequence is always present. In general, the differences do not influence the effectiveness of the sequence.

seen within promoters. These promoter elements bind protein factors (transcription factors) that recognize the DNA sequence of each particular element. Some transcription factors stimulate transcription, others suppress it; some are expressed ubiquitously, others are expressed in a tissue- or time-specific fashion. Thus the array of factors bound to a promoter region can vary from cell to cell, tissue to tissue, and be affected by the state of the organism. These factors, bound to promoter sequences, determine how actively the RNApol II copies the DNA into RNA.

Enhancers

Although the promoter is essential for initiation of transcription, it is not necessarily alone in influencing the strength of transcription of a particular gene. Another group of elements, known as enhancers, can regulate the level of transcription of a gene but, unlike promoters, their position may vary widely with respect to the startpoint and their orientation has no effect on their efficiency. Enhancers may lie upstream or downstream of a promoter and may be important in conferring tissue-specific transcription. For instance,

a nonspecific promoter may initiate transcription only in the presence of a tissue-specific enhancer. Alternatively, a tissue-specific promoter may initiate transcription, but with a greatly increased efficiency in the presence of a nearby enhancer that is not tissue-specific. In some genes, for example immunoglobulin genes, enhancers may actually be present downstream of the startpoint of transcription, within an intron of the gene being actively transcribed.

Response elements

Response elements are nucleotide sequences that allow specific stimuli, such as steroid hormones, cyclic AMP, or insulin-like growth factor-1 (IGF-1), to control gene expression. Response elements are often part of promoters or enhancers where they function as binding sites for particular transcription factors. Response elements in promoters are cis-acting sequences that are typically on the order of 6 to 12 bases in length. A single gene may possess any number of different response elements. Multiple genes may possess the same response element, and this facilitates co-induction or co-repression of groups of genes, such as in response to a hormonal stimulus.

Transcription factors

The combination of a promoter and an enhancer linked to a gene is the basic model of a human gene. The transcription of the gene is initiated and regulated by a number of different sequence-specific DNA-binding proteins, known as transcription factors. These factors bind to specific nucleotide sequences and bring about differential expression of the gene, not only during development, but also within tissues of the mature organism (Fig. 33.2). Many transcription factors act positively and promote transcription, while others act negatively and promote gene silencing. The unique pattern of transcription factors present in the cell will determine in large part the different activities of the many genes present in the nucleus. Transcription factors are sometimes referred to as '*trans*-acting' factors, to emphasize that, as soluble proteins, they can diffuse within the nucleus and act on multiple different genes on different chromosomes.

There are other kinds of proteins involved in regulating transcription besides the sequence-specific transcription factors. The so-called general transcription factors form a complex with RNApol II and this complex is necessary for the initiation of transcription. The general transcription factors are needed for the successful use of every promoter; they vary somewhat with the class of gene, being generally different for RNA polymerase I, II, and III. In eukaryotic cells, and mammalian cells in particular, the RNA polymerases cannot recognize promoter sequences themselves. It is the task of the gene-specific factors to create a local environment that can successfully attract the general factors, which in turn, attract the polymerase itself.

In addition, other proteins can bind to the sequence-specific transcription factors and modulate their function by repressing or activating gene expression; these factors are often called co-activators or co-repressors. Thus the overall rate of RNA transcription from a gene is the result of the complex interplay of a multitude of transcription factors, co-activators and co-repressors. Since there are thousands of these factors, there is an almost unimaginably large number of combinations that can occur on any one promoter and thus gene control can be very specific and very subtle.

Initiation of transcription requires binding of transcription factors to DNA

For transcription to occur, transcription factors must bind to DNA. These are trans-acting factors that recognize and bind to short nucleotide sequences in the promoter. For example, a protein known as TATA-binding protein (TBP) binds to the region of the TATA box. TBP is a general transcription factor, associated with the complex of RNApol II and a variable number of other proteins. Binding of TBP to the TATA box directs the positioning of the transcription apparatus at a fixed distance from the startpoint of transcription and thus allows RNApol II to be positioned exactly at the site of initia-

---

WHAT IS A 'GENE'?

Transcription unit versus gene

Exactly what a 'gene' is has become increasingly difficult to define in recent years. The initial notion that a gene was a piece of DNA that gave rise to a single gene product – one gene, one protein – has been challenged. It is now clear that many functional products – different mRNA species or different protein products – may arise from a single region of transcribed DNA, as a result of differences either at the level of transcription or at the post-transcriptional level. Thus there is now a tendency to refer to such 'genes' as transcription units. The transcription units encapsulate, not only those parts of the gene such as the promoters, exons, and introns, classically regarded as the gene unit, but also the molecular events that modify the transcription process from the initiation of transcription to the final post-transcriptional modifications. This is a shift away from the notion of a gene being a single strand of DNA with exons and introns, to one of a gene being a complex structure that directs a dynamic process, giving rise to the final gene product or products at various stages of development of an organism.

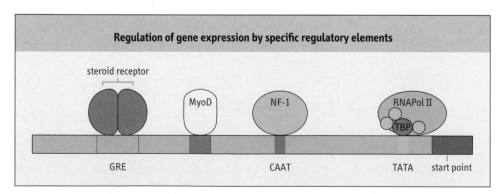

Fig. 33.2 **Regulation of gene expression by specific regulatory elements.** Binding of transcription factors to a steroid response element modulates the rate of transcription of the message. Different elements have varying effects on the level of transcription, some exerting greater effects than others, and may also activate tissue-specific expression. MyoD, muscle-cell-specific transcription factor. GRE, glucocorticoid response element. The proteins are shown in a linear array for convenience, but they interact physically with one another, both because of their size and the folding of DNA.

tion of transcription. Once RNAPol II and a number of other transcription factors have bound to the region of the start-point, transcription can occur. When transcription begins, many of the transcription factors required for binding and alignment of RNAPol II are released, and the polymerase travels along the DNA, forming the primary messenger RNA transcripts (sometimes called pre-mRNA).

Transcription factors have common structures that permit DNA binding

The binding of transcription factors to DNA involves a relatively small area of the transcription factor protein, which comes into close contact with the major and/or minor groove of the DNA double helix to be transcribed. The regions of these proteins that contact the DNA are called DNA-binding domains or motifs, and are highly conserved between species. There are a variety of DNA-binding domains, some of these occur in multiple transcription factors. Four common classes of DNA-binding domain are (Fig. 33.3):

- **helix-turn-helix (HTH) motif:** mediates DNA binding by fitting into the major groove of the DNA helix, allowing precise alignment of the factor in relation to the DNA sequence recognized;

- **helix-loop-helix (HLH) motif:** promotes both DNA binding and protein dimer formation. It is believed that HLH motifs mediate mainly negative influences on gene expression;

- **zinc finger:** loops or fingers of amino acids that have a zinc ion at their core. The adjacent amino acid residues often form α-helices that make contact with the DNA in the major groove;

- **leucine zipper:** enables the protein to form a dimer that grips the DNA double helix like a peg, by inserting into the major groove.

Most sequence-specific transcription factors contain at least one of these DNA-binding motifs. Transcription factors can bind to the DNA in a sequence-specific fashion because the tertiary structure of the DNA-binding site of a transcription factor enables it to interact with the exposed groups of the nucleotide bases in the major or minor groove (see Chapter 30) of the DNA double helix, and the nature of these exposed groups is base-pair specific. Although binding between amino acids and DNA is via weak hydrogen bonds, the average transcription factor has 20 or more sites of contact, which amplifies the strength and specificity of the contact.

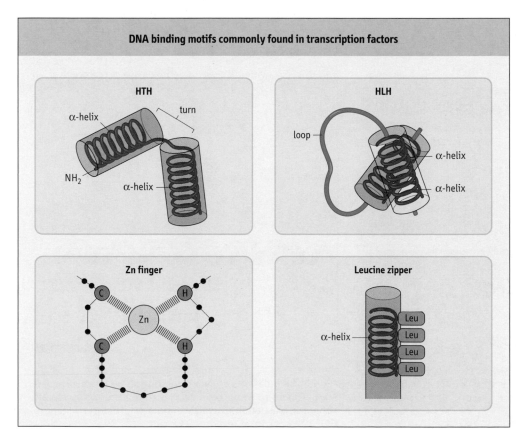

Fig. 33.3 **The four main classes of DNA-binding domains.** Leucine zippers have hydrophobic leucine residues consistently on one face of the helix, which allows two leucine zippers to align with their hydrophobic residues facing each other. HLH, helix-loop-helix; HTH, helix-turn-helix.

In addition to a DNA-binding domain, sequence-specific transcription factors also have a transcription-regulatory domain that is required for their ability to modulate transcription. This domain may function in a variety of ways. It may interact directly with the RNA polymerase-general transcription factor complex, it may have indirect effects via co-activators or co-repressor proteins, or it may be involved in remodeling the chromatin and so alter the ability of the promoter to recruit other transcription factors.

STEROID RECEPTORS

Steroid receptors possess many characteristics of transcription factors and provide a model for the role of zinc finger proteins in DNA binding

Steroid hormones have a broad range of functions in humans and are essential to normal life. They are derived from a common precursor, cholesterol, and thus share a similar structural backbone (Chapter 16). However, differences in hydroxylation of certain carbon atoms and aromatization of the steroid A-ring give rise to marked differences in biological effect. Steroids bring about their biological effects by binding to steroid-specific hormone receptors; these receptors are found in the cell cytoplasm and, on binding steroid molecules, undergo a series of changes that result in the steroid-receptor complex binding to DNA at a specific response element, a so-called steroid response element (SRE). SREs may be found many kilobases upstream or downstream of the startpoint. The steroid-receptor complex functions as a sequence-specific transcription factor and binding of the complex to the SRE results in activation of the promoter and initiation of transcription (Fig. 33.4). As might be expected, because of the large number of steroids found in humans, there is a correspondingly large number of distinct steroid receptor proteins, and each of these recognizes a specific consensus sequence, the SRE, in the region of a promoter.

The zinc finger region

Central to the recognition of the SRE, and to the binding of the receptor to it, is the presence of the so-called zinc finger region in the DNA-binding domain of the receptor molecule. Zinc fingers consist of a peptide loop with a zinc atom at the core of the loop. In the typical zinc finger, each loop comprises two cysteine and two histidine residues in highly conserved positions relative to each other, separated by a fixed number of intervening amino acids. The consensus sequence for a typical zinc finger is:

$$Cys - X_{2-4} - Cys - X_3 - Phe - X_5 - Leu - X_2 - His - X_3 - His$$

where X represents any intervening amino acid (Fig. 33.5).

STEROID RECEPTOR GENE FAMILY

Gene superfamilies: steroid-thyroid-retinoic acid

The steroid receptor gene family, although large, is in fact only a subset of a much larger family of so-called nuclear hormone receptors. All members of this family have the same basic structure as the steroid hormone receptors: a hypervariable N-terminal region, a highly conserved DNA-binding region (49–85% homology), a variable hinge region, and a highly conserved ligand-binding domain (30–87% homology). They are separated into two groups. Type I receptors are a group of receptor proteins that form homodimers and bind specifically to steroid hormone response elements only in the presence of their ligand. Type II receptors form homodimers that can bind to response elements in the absence of their ligand, and may also form heterodimers with other type II receptor subunits, to form active units. The type II receptors include the thyroid hormone, vitamin D, and retinoic acid receptors.

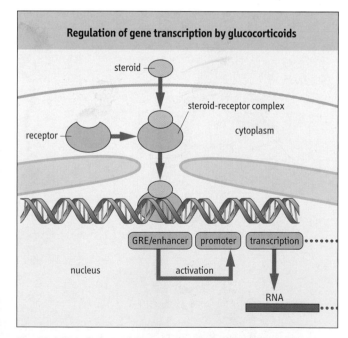

Fig. 33.4 **Regulation of gene transcription by glucocorticoids.** Steroids bind to receptor molecules that, in turn, bind to an enhancer, the action of which stimulates promoter function. GRE, glucocorticoid response element.

This structure holds the zinc atom at the core of a tetrahedron and allows the receptor molecule to sit on the surface of the DNA double helix and interact with a response element, thus enhancing the efficiency of, and conferring specificity to, the promoter. Zinc finger motifs are generally organized as a series of tandem repeat fingers; the number of repeats varies in different transcription factors.

The precise structure of the steroid receptor zinc finger differs from the consensus shown above. Steroid receptor zinc fingers have a simpler structure (Fig. 33.5):

$$Cys - X_2 - Cys - X_{13} - Cys - X_2 - Cys$$

This type of finger recognizes and binds to short palindromic DNA sequences. In the case of steroid receptors, two fingers are found side by side, one binding DNA and the other allowing the receptor to bind to a second steroid receptor molecule of the same type, forming a homodimer.

Organization of the steroid receptor molecule

Steroid receptors are products of a gene family with important similarities

One central feature of all the steroid receptor proteins is the similarity in organization of their receptor molecules. Each receptor has a DNA-binding domain, a transcription-activating domain, a steroid-hormone-binding domain, and a dimerization domain. There are three striking features about the structure of the steroid hormone receptors:

- The DNA-binding region always contains a highly conserved zinc finger region, which, if mutated, results in loss of function of the receptor;
- The DNA-binding regions of all the steroid hormone receptors have a high degree of homology to one another;
- The steroid-binding regions show a high degree of homology to one another.

These common features have identified the steroid receptor proteins as products of a gene family. It would appear that, during the course of evolution, diversification of organisms has resulted in the need for different steroids with varied biological actions and, consequently, a single ancestral gene has undergone duplication and evolutionary change over millions of years, resulting in a group of related, but different receptors (Fig. 33.6).

ALTERNATIVE APPROACHES TO GENE REGULATION IN HUMANS

Promoter access

DNA in the cell nucleus is packaged into nucleosomes and higher order structures in association with histones and other proteins (Chapter 30). Thus, the promoters of some genes may not be readily accessible to transcription factors, even if the transcription factors themselves are present in the nucleus. It has become evident that the degree of packaging

---

A 'standard' and a steroid receptor zinc finger

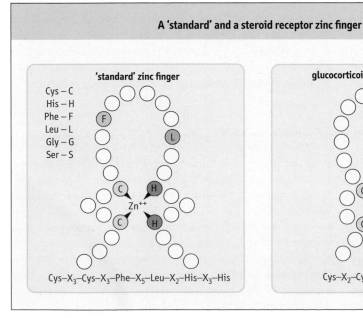

'standard' zinc finger

Cys – C
His – H
Phe – F
Leu – L
Gly – G
Ser – S

Cys–X₃–Cys–X₃–Phe–X₅–Leu–X₂–His–X₃–His

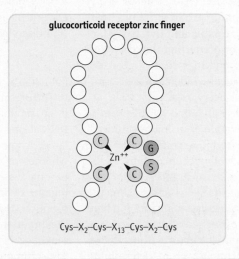

glucocorticoid receptor zinc finger

Cys–X₂–Cys–X₁₃–Cys–X₂–Cys

Fig. 33.5 **A 'standard' zinc finger and a steroid receptor zinc finger.** Zinc fingers are commonly occurring sequences that allow protein binding to double-stranded DNA. X, any intervening amino acid.

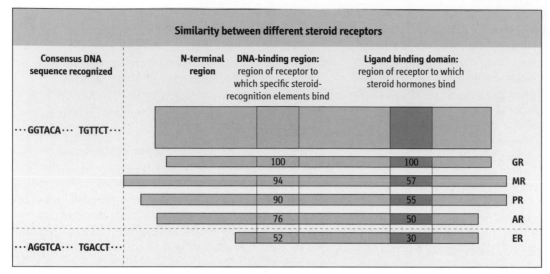

Fig. 33.6 **Similarity between different steroid receptors.** The DNA-binding and hormone-binding regions of steroid receptors share a high degree of homology. The estrogen receptor is less similar to the glucocorticoid receptor than are the others. AR, androgen receptor; ER, estrogen receptor; GR, glucocorticoid receptor; MR, mineralocorticoid receptor; PR, progesterone receptor; nnn, anonymous nucleotides. Numbers denote % homology to sequence in GR.

of a promoter and the presence, absence or precise location of nucleosomes on a promoter can have major effects on the degree of access for both sequence-specific transcription factors and the RNAPol II complex associated with general transcription factors. Condensed chromatin is usually not a good template for transcription and in many cases it is necessary for chromatin remodeling to occur before transcription proceeds. Histone packaging, nucleosome stability and, therefore, the accessibility of DNA is controlled by reversible acetylation and deacetylation of lysine residues in the amino terminal regions of the core histones, particularly histones H3 and H4. Histone acetyl transferases (HAT) transfer acetyl groups from acetyl-CoA to the amino group of lysines, neutralizing the charge on the lysine residue and the strength of histone–DNA interactions, thereby permitting the relaxation of the nucleosome. Conversely, enzymes that remove the acetyl groups and promote the local condensation of chromosomes are known as histone deacetylases.

Reversible acetylation and deacetylation of histones is important in controlling the activation of promoters. Indeed, some transcription factors or transcription co-activators have HAT activity themselves and can remodel chromatin. In the case of some promoters, binding of a transcription factor may result in repositioning of the nucleosomes the next time the DNA replicates, and then other transcription factors can bind and so the gene becomes more expressed after cell division. The dynamic interplay of chromatin structure, transcription factor and cofactor binding is important in determining whether a gene is transcribed and how efficiently the RNA polymerase copies it.

Methylation of DNA regulates gene expression

Certain nucleotides, principally cytosine, can undergo methylation without affecting Watson–Crick pairing of DNA; in mammals, up to 7% of all cytosine residues in DNA are methylated. The methylated cytosine residues are almost always found associated with a guanine, as the dinucleotide CG, and in double-stranded DNA the complementary cytosine is also methylated, giving rise to a palindromic sequence:

$$5' \quad mCpG \quad 3'$$
$$3' \quad GpCm \quad 5'$$

The presence of the methylated cytosine can be examined by susceptibility to restriction enzymes (Chapter 34) that cut DNA at sites containing CG groups only if the CG is unmethylated, compared to other restriction enzymes that cut whether or not the CG is methylated. In this way, it has become clear that methylation is generally associated with regions of DNA that are less active in regulation or transcription. Demethylation of a promoter may be required for the initiation of transcription, and demethylation of a coding sequence of the gene may also be required for efficient transcription.

GENOMIC IMPRINTING

Methylation of DNA is responsible for genomic imprinting

Imprinting is the differential expression of one or other parental allele of a gene. Normally, in Mendelian inheritance, the effect of any particular allele on the offspring would always be expected to be the same, regardless of the parent from which it came. However, if imprinting occurs, the observed phenotype will vary, depending on which parent donated the allele. For imprinting to occur, there must be some event in the passage of the allele through male and female germlines that marks out one allele as maternal and one as paternal. Similarly, there must exist a mechanism whereby the signal can be erased during germ cell formation if necessary. One postulated mechanism is through the methylation and demethylation of DNA.

If, for instance, a gene is expressed in a developing embryo only if derived from the paternal allele, the most likely explanation for this is that the female allele is methylated in the egg but that, in the sperm, the paternal allele is unmethylated. Such is the case for many genes, although the sex of the active allele may be the reverse. Of course, during sperm formation, any maternal imprints need to be erased, and paternal ones need to be imposed. Similarly, during oocyte formation, any paternal imprints need to be erased, and maternal imprints will be imposed. Mechanisms for erasing imprinting do exist in developing spermatocytes and oocytes, and a methylase enzyme also exists that can specifically methylate CG groups during this phase of development.

ALTERNATIVE APPROACHES TO GENE REGULATION IN HUMANS

Tissue-specific expression of a gene

A 17-year-old girl noticed a swelling on the left side of her neck. She was otherwise well, but her mother and maternal uncle have both had adrenal tumors removed. Blood was withdrawn and sent to the laboratory for measurement of calcitonin, which was greatly increased. Pathology of the excised thyroid mass confirms the diagnosis of medullary carcinoma of the thyroid. This family has a genetic mutation causing the condition known as multiple endocrine neoplasia type 2A (MEN 2A). MEN 2A is a Mendelian dominant cancer syndrome of high penetrance caused by a germ line mutation in the RET protooncogene. About 5–10% of cancers result from germline mutations, but additional somatic mutations are required for cancer to develop.

Comment. Expression of the calcitonin gene provides an example of how different mechanisms may regulate gene expression and give rise to tissue-specific gene products. The calcitonin gene consists of five exons and uses two alternative polyadenylation signaling sites. In the thyroid gland, the medullary C cells produce calcitonin by using one polyadenylation signaling site associated with exon 4 to transcribe a pre-mRNA comprising exons 1–4. The associated introns are spliced out and the mRNA is translated to give calcitonin. However, in neural tissue, a second polyadenylation signaling site next to exon 5 is used. This results in a pre-mRNA comprising all five exons and their intervening introns. This larger pre-mRNA is then spliced and, in addition to all the introns, exon 4 is also spliced out, leaving an mRNA comprising exons 1–3 and 5, which is then translated into a neuronal growth factor, calcitonin-related gene peptide (CRGP).

GENE EXPRESSION

Not all gene expression depends on the regulation of transcription

Alternative promoters

Although it is clear that a promoter is essential for gene expression to occur, a single promoter may not possess the tissue specificity or developmental stage specificity to allow it to direct expression of a gene at every correct time and place. Some genes have evolved a series of promoters that confer tissue-specific expression. In addition to the use of different promoters, each of the alternative promoters is often associated with its own first exon and, as a result, each mRNA and subsequent protein has a tissue-specific 5′ or N-terminal sequence. A good example of the use of alternative promoters in humans is the gene for dystrophin, the muscle protein that is deficient in Duchenne muscular dystrophy (see Chapter 19). This gene uses alternate promoters that give rise to brain-, muscle-, and retinal-specific proteins, all with differing N-terminal amino acid structures.

Intron splicing of mRNA

When RNAPol II has completed the transcription of a gene, the initial transcript, the so-called pre-mRNA, has the same organization as the gene. The pre-mRNA then undergoes a process whereby the introns in the RNA are removed, to produce an mRNA molecule that is smaller than the pre-RNA, but contains all the necessary information to allow the gene to be translated into the protein product. This process of RNA or intron splicing relies on the recognition of specific sequences, at the start and finish of introns, which allow specific ribonucleases to cleave the RNA molecule at the exon-intron boundary and re-form the molecules into a single, intron-free, mRNA (see Chapter 31). For many genes, the pre-mRNA can be spliced in several alternate ways. This process, affecting an estimated 30% of human genes, may provide sufficient diversity to explain individual uniqueness, despite similarities in the gene complement of a species. Thus, by alternative splicing, a particular exon or exons may be spliced out on some but not all occasions. Since many genes have a lot of exons, some pre-mRNAs can eventually give rise to many different versions of the mRNA and of the final protein. The proteins may differ by only a few amino acids, or may have major differences; they often have different biological roles. For example, whether an exon is deleted or not may affect where in the cell the protein is localized, whether a protein remains in the cell or is secreted, whether there are specific isoforms in skeletal vs. cardiac muscle. Alternative splicing may also yield a truncated protein that can inhibit the function of the full-length protein. Alternative splicing is regulated, so that certain splice forms may only be seen in certain cells or tissues, or at certain stages of development, or under certain conditions. In the human brain, there is a family of cell surface proteins, the neurexins, which mediate the complex network of interactions between approximately 10^{12} neurons. Thousands of neurexin isoforms are generated from only three genes by alternative promoters and splicing, providing for a diverse range of intercellular communications required for the development of sophisticated neural networks. The neurexins probably have an equally complex set of ligand isoforms, providing tremendous flexibility for reversible cellular interactions during the development of the central nervous system.

Editing of RNA at the post-transcriptional level

RNA editing involves the enzyme-mediated alteration of RNA in the cell nucleus before translation. This process may involve the insertion, deletion, or substitution of nucleotides in the RNA molecule. Like alternative splicing, the substitution of one nucleotide for another can result in tissue-specific differences in transcripts. For example, *APOB*, the gene for human apolipoprotein B (apoB), a component of low-density lipoprotein, encodes a 14.1 kb mRNA transcript in the liver and a 4536-amino-acid protein product, apoB100 (Chapter 17). However, in the small intestine, the mRNA is translated into a protein product, called apoB48, which is 2152 amino acids long, those amino acids being identical to the first 2152 amino acids of apoB100. The difference in transcript size occurs because, in the small intestine, nucleotide 6666 is 'edited' by the deamination of a single cytidine residue, converting it to a uracil residue, and thus generating a premature stop codon in the intestinal mRNA (Fig. 33.7).

IRON STATUS REGULATES TRANSLATION OF AN IRON CARRIER-PROTEIN

A 57-year-old Caucasian male presented to his family doctor with breathlessness and fatigue. He noticed that his skin had become darker. Clinical evaluation indicated cardiac failure with impaired left ventricular function as a result of dilated cardiomyopathy, a low serum concentration of testosterone and an elevated fasting concentration of glucose. Serum ferritin concentration was greatly increased, at >300 µg/L, and the diagnosis of hereditary hemochromatosis was suspected. The man was treated by regular phlebotomy until his serum ferritin was <20 µg/L at which point the phlebotomy interval is increased and maintaining the serum ferritin concentration at <50 µg/L.

Comment. In conditions of iron deficiency, there is an increase in the synthesis of the transferrin receptor protein, which is involved in the uptake of iron, and when there is iron excess, for example in hemochromatosis, there is an increase in the synthesis of ferritin, an iron-binding protein. In both cases, the RNA molecules themselves are unchanged, and there is no increase in the synthesis of the respective mRNAs. However, both the ferritin mRNA and the transferrin receptor mRNA contain a specific sequence known as the iron-response element (IRE). A specific IRE-binding protein can bind to mRNA. In iron deficiency, the IRE-binding protein binds the ferritin mRNA, prevents translation of ferritin, and binds the transferrin receptor mRNA and prevents its degradation. Thus, in iron deficiency, ferritin concentrations are low and transferrin receptor concentrations are high. In states of iron excess, the reverse process occurs and translation of ferritin mRNA increases, whereas transferrin receptor mRNA undergoes degradation, serum ferritin concentrations are high, and transferrin receptor concentrations are low (Fig. 33.8). About 10% of the US population carry the gene for hereditary chromatosis, but only homozygotes are affected with the disease.

Preferential activation of one allele of a gene

The normal complement of human chromosomes comprises 22 pairs of autosomes and two sex chromosomes. Therefore there are 23 pairs of chromosomes, each of which has genes that are present on both chromosomes: they are biallelic. Under normal circumstances, both genes are expressed without preference being given to either allele of the gene – that is, both the paternal and the maternal copies of the gene can be expressed, unless there is a mutation in one allele that prevents this from occurring.

The situation with regard to sex chromosomes is slightly different. Sex chromosomes are of two types, X and Y, the X being substantially larger than the Y. Females have two X

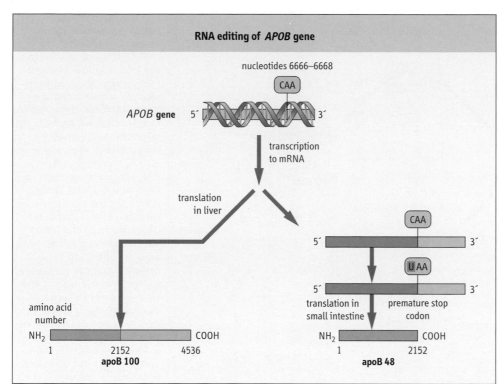

Fig. 33.7 **RNA editing of the APOB gene in man gives rise to tissue-specific transcripts.** In the small intestine, editing of nucleotide 6666 of apoB mRNA, by changing cytosine to uracil, converts a glutamine codon in apoB 100 mRNA to a premature stop codon, and thus produces the truncated product, apoB 48. (See also Chapter 17.)

 ## X CHROMOSOME INACTIVATION

Males have one X chromosome whereas females have two. Thus, genes on the X chromosome are biallelic in females but monoallelic in males. In females, however, one of the X-chromosomes in each cell is inactivated at an early stage of embryogenesis. The inactivated X may be the paternally-derived or the maternally-derived X chromosome, for any particular cell which one is inactivated is random, but the descendants of that cell will have the same X inactivated. The inactivated X chromosome can still express a few genes, however, including XIST (inactive X – Xi – specific transcript) which codes for an RNA which plays an important role in X-chromosome inactivation. The inactivated X-chromosome is reactivated during oogenesis in the female.

Restriction of expression of bi-allelic genes

Genomic imprinting	autosomal genes, Imprinting may be tissue specific – monoallelic expression in some tissues, biallelic in others.
	Examples include insulin-like growth factor 2 (IGF2) and Wilm's tumor susceptibility gene (WT1)
Allelic exclusion	tissue-specific production of a single allele product, for example, synthesis of a single immunoglobulin light or heavy chain in a B cell from one allele only
X chromosome inactivation	some genes on the X chromosome in females. Males exhibit only one allele of the X-linked gene, but females have two, and one is inactivated by switching off the entire X chromosome.
	Examples include XIST, which is expressed only on the inactive X chromosome, and numerous genes on the active X chromosome

Table 33.2 **Examples of types of restriction of biallelic genes in humans.** For some genes, although two alleles exist in any particular cell, only one of these alleles is active. Hence the gene behaves as if it were monoallelic although it is, in fact, biallelic.

chromosomes, whereas males have one X and one Y chromosome. A region of the Y chromosome is identical to a region of the X chromosome, but the X chromosome also contains genes that have no matching partner on the Y chromosome, and some genes on the Y chromosome are specific to the Y chromosome, for example SRY, a sex-determining gene. Such genes are said to be monoallelic; they offer no choice as to which allele of the gene will be expressed.

Thus, apart from the specific cases of sex chromosomes, there would appear to be no reason why both alleles of a gene cannot be expressed. However, in humans, genes have been identified that are biallelic, but only one allele – either maternal or paternal – is preferentially expressed, despite the fact that both alleles are perfectly normal or identical. As a result, only 50% of the gene product is produced, but the product is functionally active. Three different mechanisms have been identified that can restrict the expression of biallelic genes in humans (Table 33.2).

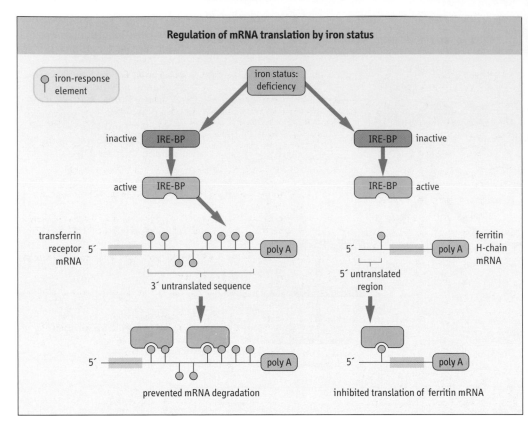

Regulation of mRNA translation by iron status

- iron-response element

iron status: deficiency

inactive — IRE-BP

active — IRE-BP

IRE-BP — inactive

IRE-BP — active

transferrin receptor mRNA 5′ ... poly A

3′ untranslated sequence

ferritin H-chain mRNA 5′ ... poly A

5′ untranslated region

prevented mRNA degradation

inhibited translation of ferritin mRNA

Fig. 33.8 **Regulation of mRNA translation by iron status.** The binding of a specific binding protein to the iron response element (IRE) of the mRNA of iron-responsive genes can alter the translation of the mRNA into functioning proteins in different ways. When iron is deficient, the iron-response element binding protein (IRE-BP) is activated and can bind to the 3′ end of the mRNA for the transferrin receptor. This prevents the degradation of the mRNA, and thus increases the amount of transferrin receptor that can be made (left side of the figure) and thus increases the amount of iron which the receptor can deliver to the cell. However, the IRE-BP also binds to the 5′ end of the ferritin mRNA and prevents its translation (right hand side of the figure). Ferritin is a protein that sequesters and stores iron in the cytoplasm, and less is needed in times of iron deficiency.

THE HUMAN GENOME PROJECT

The objectives of the International Human Genome Project included: construction of a genetic map, identification of all human genes, and sequencing of the entire genome except for a few exceptionally difficult regions such as telomeres and centromeres. Working draft sequences of the human genome were presented by the International Human Genome Project collaboration and Celera Genomics in 2001. The availability of a complete reference sequence for the human genome was announced by the Human Genome Project in April 2003, just a few days prior to the 50th anniversary of the paper by Watson and Crick which first described the double helical structure of DNA. This reference sequence contains approximately 2.9 billion base pairs and represents over 90% of the approximately 3.2 billion base pairs in the human genome. Knowledge of the human genome sequence has been important in many ways,

including identification of gene changes associated with disease. It has also resulted in some surprises; for example, there appear to be fewer genes than originally anticipated. This leads to the question of why the gene number does not increase in more complex organisms by as much as might have been expected. Part of the explanation may be the frequency with which RNA transcripts undergo alternative splicing such that the same gene can give rise to different mRNAs. It has been estimated that more than 30% of human genes may be able to give rise to differentially spliced mRNAs and hence to code for more than one protein per gene. In addition, complex control by hundreds of transcription factors enables cells to express huge numbers of different combinations of genes, and the subtle differences between these combinations can give rise to enormous complexity at the cell and organism level.

Summary

The control of gene expression involves both transcriptional and post-transcriptional events that regulate the expression of a gene in both time and place and in response to numerous developmental, hormonal and stress signals. DNA sequences and DNA binding proteins control gene expression. The DNA sequences include *cis*-acting promoters, such as the TATA box, and enhancer and response elements. The DNA-binding proteins are *trans*-acting transcription factors that bind with high specificity to these sequences, and facilitate the binding and positioning of RNAPol II for synthesis of pre-mRNA. Other factors that affect the conversion of gene to protein include: access of the gene to the transcriptional apparatus, enzymatic modification of histones and nucleotides, and factors that effect alternative intron splicing, post-transcriptional editing of pre-mRNA, and restricted expression of biallelic genes.

ACTIVE LEARNING

1. How are steroid response elements identified in the genome? Discuss the consequences of a mutation in an SRE versus a mutation in the SRE binding protein.
2. What are the biochemical consequences of APOB gene editing in humans? Compare the effects of editing to introduce a substitution, compared to an insertion or deletion, in an mRNA molecule.
3. How many transcription factors are present in a cell? How many are present in all the cells in the body? Compare this number to the total number of genes in the human genome and to the total number of translated proteins in the genome. What is the concentration of an individual transcription factor in the cell, compared to the concentration of a glycolytic enzyme?

Further reading

Cosma MP. Ordered Recruitment: Gene-Specific Mechanism of Transcription Activation. *Molecular Cell* 2002;**10**:227–236.

Howe KJ. RNA polymerase II conducts a symphony of pre-mRNA processing activities. *Biochim Biophys Acta* 2002;**1577**:308–24.

International Human Genome Sequencing Consortium. Initial sequencing and analysis of the human genome. *Nature* 2001;**409**:860–921.

Lee TI, Young RA. Transcription of eukaryotic protein-coding genes. *Annu Rev Genet* 2000;**34**:77–137.

Recillas-Targa F. DNA methylation, chromatin boundaries, and mechanisms of genomic imprinting. *Arch Med Res* 2002;**33**:428–38.

Venter JC, Adams MD, Myers EW et al. The sequence of the human genome. *Science* 2001;**291**:1304–1351.

Yudt MR, Cidlowski JA. The glucocorticoid receptor: coding a diversity of proteins and responses through a single gene. *Mol Endocrinol* 2002;**16**:1719–1726.

Relevant websites

Human Genome Research Institute: www.genome.gov
Human Genome Resources: www.ncbi.nlm.nih.gov/genome/guide/human/
Catalog of Genetic Diseases: www.ncbi.nlm.nih.gov/Omim/
Alternate Splicing: http://hazelton.lbl.gov/~teplitski/alt/
Genomic Imprinting: www.geneimprint.com/

34. Recombinant DNA Technology

W S Kistler and A Jamieson

LEARNING OBJECTIVES

After reading this chapter you should be able to:

- Explain the basis of the molecular attraction that causes nucleic acid hybridization reactions to occur; explain the difference between the probe and target sequences in hybridization assays.
- Describe what is meant by a 'primer pair' used in a PCR assay, and explain how the sequence of these primers determines the product amplified in the PCR process.
- Describe the typical characteristics of restriction endonucleases with regard to their selection of cleavage sites on DNA and the types of fragment ends that are produced.
- Describe the general steps used to perform a Southern blot and the type of information it provides.
- Differentiate between a cDNA and a genomic clone.
- Describe typical features of a bacterial plasmid used for cloning DNA.
- Provide examples of investigations in which it is desirable to carry out hybridization reactions under conditions of either high or low stringency.

INTRODUCTION

There are several key features to all DNA tests

Hand in hand with the development of our understanding of deoxyribonucleic acid (DNA), genes, and their functions has been the explosion of technology for the clinical analysis of DNA and ribonucleic acid (RNA). A full description of all these processes is out of the scope of this chapter but an understanding of the basic principles of the methods and examples of some commonly used applications will become increasingly essential with the shift from experimental DNA analysis to diagnostic services providing genetic analysis in the clinical setting.

There are several key features central to all the DNA methods currently used and these will be discussed prior to outlining some of the commonly used techniques.

HYBRIDIZATION

Hybridization is based on the annealing properties of DNA

Double-stranded DNA exists in life as a double helix, in which the two strands are held together by the hydrogen bonds between complementary bases (A with T, and G with C).

Hybridization is a fundamental feature of DNA technology. It is a process by which a piece of DNA or RNA of known nucleotide sequence, which can range in size from as little as 15 bp to several hundred kilobases, is used to identify a region or fragment of DNA containing complementary sequences. The first piece of DNA or RNA is called a probe. Probe DNA will form complementary base pairings with another strand of DNA, often termed the target, if the two strands are complementary, and a sufficient number of hydrogen bonds is formed.

The principles of molecular hybridization

In molecular hybridization, it is essential that the probe and target are initially single-stranded

Probes can vary in both their size and their nature (Table 34.1). However, one essential feature of any hybridization reaction is that both the probe and the target must be free to base pair with one another. The process of separating the two strands of DNA is called DNA denaturation or melting. Probe DNA is generally denatured by heating. If the target DNA is double-stranded then it too must be denatured, either by heating or treatment with alkali. (NB: alkali is not used to denature RNA because it leads to hydrolysis of the polymer chain.) Once both probe and target DNA are single-stranded, mixing of the two will allow complementary bases to reassociate. This process is called DNA annealing or reassociation.

A single-stranded probe and target can potentially anneal in a variety of ways:

- formation of probe–probe complementary strands (when using a ds probe);
- reannealing of the complementary strands of the target, so-called homoduplexes;
- formation of probe–target heteroduplexes.

Nucleic acid probes used for hybridization studies

Probe type	Origin	Probe characteristics	Labeling method
DNA	cell-based DNA: cloning,	double-stranded	random primer
	polymerase chain reaction (PCR)	cell-based: 0.1–100+ kb PCR-based: 0.1–10 kb	nick translation
RNA	RNA transcription from phage vectors	single stranded: 1–2 kb	run-off transcription
Oligonucleotide	chemical synthesis	single-stranded: 15–50 nucleotides	end-labeling

Table 34.1 **Characteristics of some nucleic acid probes used for hybridization studies.**

Formation of probe-target heteroduplexes is the key to the usefulness of molecular hybridization

The conditions under which DNA hybridization occurs and the reliability and specificity, or stringency, of hybridization are affected by several factors:

- **base composition:** GC pairs have three hydrogen bonds compared with the two in an AT pair. Double-stranded DNA with a high GC content is therefore more resistant to denaturation and melts at a higher temperature;
- **strand length:** the longer a strand of DNA, the greater the number of hydrogen bonds between the two strands. Longer strands require higher temperatures or stronger alkali treatment to denature them; stability varies dramatically with length for very short probes, but above a few hundred base pairs, stability is relatively insensitive to length and is determined primarily by base composition;
- **reaction conditions:** if the sodium concentration of the reaction mix is high, then the formation of double-stranded DNA is favored, whereas substances that disrupt hydrogen bonds in DNA, (e.g. urea or formamide), favor single-stranded DNA.

Thus if a probe is small, e.g. 50 bp, then when stringency is high, i.e. if the probe and template form in the presence of moderate sodium concentration and at high temperature, a single base pair difference may prevent the formation of the probe – target duplex, whereas a larger probe, *e.g.* 500 bp, would still form a stable duplex. The converse may also be true, i.e. if there are substantial differences between the probe and target, annealing of the probe and target may occur even under conditions of low stringency (high sodium and low temperature) (Fig. 34.1).

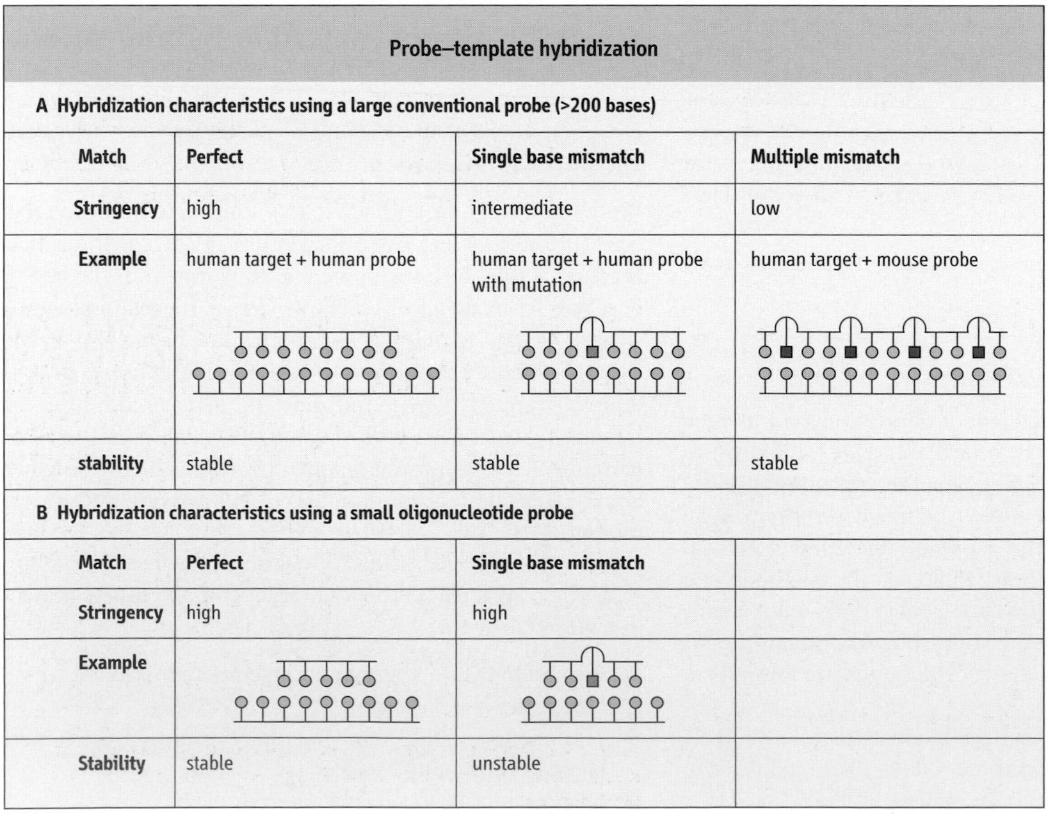

Probe–template hybridization

A Hybridization characteristics using a large conventional probe (>200 bases)

Match	Perfect	Single base mismatch	Multiple mismatch
Stringency	high	intermediate	low
Example	human target + human probe	human target + human probe with mutation	human target + mouse probe
stability	stable	stable	stable

B Hybridization characteristics using a small oligonucleotide probe

Match	Perfect	Single base mismatch	
Stringency	high	high	
Example			
Stability	stable	unstable	

Fig. 34.1 **Probe-template hybridization.** (A) Large probes, e.g. 200 bases or more, can form stable heteroduplexes with the target DNA even if there are a significant number of non-complementary bases in conditions of low stringency. (B) Oligonucleotide probes, in contrast, may discriminate between targets that differ by a single base under stringent conditions.

One means of measuring the stability of a nucleic acid duplex is assessing its melting temperature (Tm)

The melting temperature (Tm) is the temperature, *in vitro*, at which 50% of a double-stranded duplex has dissociated into single-strand form. There are several ways of determining Tm but one simple formula for estimating the melting temperature of moderately sized oligonucleotides, is as follows:

$$Tm\ (°C) = 2\ [\text{number of AT base pairs}] + 4\ [\text{number of base pairs}]$$

This formula emphasizes the importance of the number of hydrogen bonds present between DNA strands and the energy required to disrupt double-stranded DNA. The Tm for human DNA is approximately 87°C under standard conditions and reflects the average GC content – about 40% – of human DNA.

Probes must have a label to be identified

Implicit in the use of probes to identify pieces of complementary DNA is the notion that if hybridization occurs, the heteroduplex can be specifically detected. The probe is labeled so that the probe–target duplex can be identified. There are many ways in which probes can be labeled, but they fall into two categories, either **isotopic**, i.e. involving radioactive atoms, or **nonisotopic**, *e.g.* end-labeling probes with fluorescent tags or small ligand molecules (Table 34.2).

The majority of techniques involving probe hybridization and labeling still involve the use of radioisotopes such as ^{32}P, ^{35}S or ^{3}H and, as such, require a method for detecting and localizing the radioactivity. The most common method involves the process of autoradiography. **Autoradiography** allows information from a solid phase, e.g. as a gel or fixed-tissue samples, to be saved in two-dimensional form as an exposed photographic image.

Methods used in labeling nucleotide probes

Labeling of DNA or RNA probes

Both DNA and RNA can be labeled *in vitro* by several techniques that incorporate a labeled nucleotide (or nucleotides) into the structure of the probe.

There are three general ways in which DNA can be labeled *in vitro*:

- **End-labeling:** this is the addition of a labeled group to one terminus of the probe. Since only single-labeled (or at most a few) groups are added, the specific activity of this type of probe is low, limiting its sensitivity and application. The most common technique of end-labeling involves exchanging a labeled γ-phosphate from adenosine triphosphate (ATP) with a phosphate from the 5′-terminal on single- or double-stranded DNA. The usual substrate is [γ-^{32}P] ATP and the enzyme used to perform the exchange labeling is polynucleotide kinase, which exchanges the unlabelled 5′-phosphate group of the probe DNA for the terminal [γ-^{32}P] of the labeled ATP, resulting in [γ-^{32}P]-labeled probe and unlabelled ATP (Fig. 34.2).
- Polymerase-based labeling: using a DNA polymerase, multiple labeled nucleotides are incorporated into the probe during DNA synthesis. Such a reaction requires deoxyribonucleoside phosphates (dNTPs), and it is customary for one of these to be labeled, e.g. dCTP*. This type of probe has a high specific activity as, on average, up to 25% of the nucleotides

---

 AUTORADIOGRAPHY

The most commonly used imaging technique is direct autoradiography, which involves placing the sample in direct contact with the photographic material, usually an X-ray film. The radioactivity of the bound probe produces a dark image on the developed film. ^{32}P is a commonly used label for nucleic acid probes because of its high specific activity. The beta particle emitted is sufficiently energetic that a substantial fraction passes through ordinary film without exposing it. Therefore it is common to use the same type of intensifying screens used clinically to make film more sensitive to X-rays. Energetic beta particles pass through the film but are absorbed by the intensifying screen, which then emits visible light and exposes the film.

Labels used to prepare probes used for nucleic acid hybridization		
Probe label	**Characteristics**	**Examples**
Radioactive	use radioisotopes emitting β-particles. dNTPs are incorporated into the probe DNA	^{32}P, ^{35}S
Nonradioactive	rely on the coupling of a reporter molecule to a nucleotide precursor, e.g. a dNTP. When the probe hybridizes, another protein with high affinity for the reporter group (an affinity group which has a marker group associated) binds the reporter and the bound complex can be detected	biotin and streptavidin digoxigenin

Table 34.2 **Details of labels used to prepare probes used for nucleic acid hybridization.** dNTP, deoxyribonucleoside triphosphate.

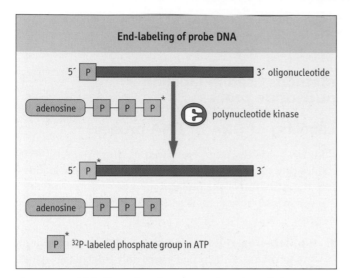

Fig. 34.2 **End-labeling of probe DNA.** Polynucleotide kinase can swap the 5′-terminal phosphate group of the target DNA for the γ-³²P-labeled phosphate group of [γ-³²P]-ATP.

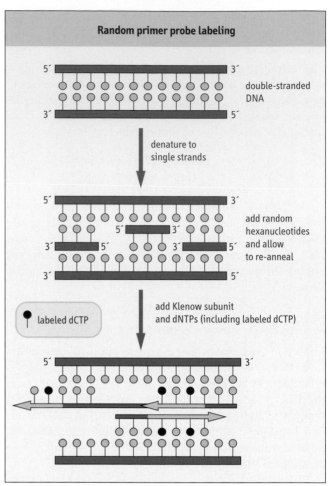

Fig. 34.3 **Random primer labeling of probe DNA.** Random hybridization of hexanucleotides to the template allows the Klenow fragment of *E. coli* DNA polymerase I to fill in the gaps, incorporating radiolabeled dCTP to create radiolabeled complementary strands of DNA.

incorporated are labeled. Random primer labeling is a common technique used to label a defined fragment of DNA for use as a probe. It involves the use of random sequence hexanucleotides, which cover every possible combination of A, T, G, and C. Thus there will always be at least one hexanucleotide that can hybridize to a complementary region in any piece of DNA. The probe to be labeled is denatured to single-stranded DNA and allowed to hybridize with the hexanucleotide mixture. The binding of hexanucleotides to the single-stranded probe provides a starting point for DNA polymerases. The synthesis of DNA is often catalyzed by the Klenow fragment of DNA polymerase I. The full *Escherichia coli* DNA polymerase I enzyme elongates DNA by a repair-like process in which nucleotides ahead of the enzyme are removed and replaced, using a new nucleotide triphosphate from the surrounding medium. The Klenow fragment is a proteolytic digestion product of the *E. coli* DNA polymerase I enzyme, which possesses DNA polymerase activity but lacks the repair-type exonuclease activity. As a result, the enzyme fills in gaps between the hexanucleotides and thus creates a DNA copy of the probe (Fig. 34.3).

■ Nick translation of DNA: nick translation is a sort of 'halfway house' between end-labeling and random priming. When the probe is in its double-stranded form, an endonuclease enzyme such as DNAase I is used to introduce a limited number of random single-stranded breaks in the DNA, leaving exposed 5′-phosphate and 3′-hydroxyl groups. In these nicks, labeled nucleotides can be added at the 3′ hydroxyl terminal and, at the same time, the adjacent nucleotide is excised and replaced by a new labeled nucleotide. This process will proceed in a 5′ to 3′ direction along the 'nicked' DNA strand until the entire strand is replaced. This process is commonly catalyzed by the intact form of *E. coli* DNA polymerase I.

MICROARRAYS

Most of the methods discussed in this chapter enable one to look at one, or a few, genes at one time. However, the ability to obtain a global picture of the genes that a cell is expressing would be a major advantage. Microarray technology makes this possible. Thousands (or tens of thousands) of different DNAs, each corresponding to a fragment of a known gene, are spotted on a slide in an orderly array, such that the position of each DNA is known. A fluorescently-labeled DNA or RNA probe is then made using total RNA extracted from cells of interest. Different fluorophores can be incorporated, so that one could, for example, use a green-labeled probe derived from cancer cells and a red-labeled probe derived from normal cells from the same individual or a red-labeled probe derived from a reference RNA. The two differently colored probes are mixed together, hybridized to the DNA on the slide, and any unhybridized probe is washed away. The slide can then be scanned using an instrument that detects each probe separately. If a gene is expressed only in the tumor RNA, the spot corresponding to that gene will be green. If the gene is expressed only in the reference, the spot will be red. If the gene is expressed equally in both RNAs the spot will be yellow. The results are analyzed and the relative expression in control and reference samples of each spot on the array can be determined. Thus, one can detect differences in the expression of a few genes (out of the thousands on the array) that correlate with a particular disease status or other condition. This is a powerful and rapid way to determine how one cell population, such as diseased cells, differs from other cells at the level of RNA expression.

TISSUE *IN SITU* HYBRIDIZATION

A 37-year-old woman was referred for evaluation of excessive hair growth. Endocrine assessment revealed the presence of an adrenal carcinoma secreting cortisol and testosterone. Imaging of the liver revealed the presence of a 2 cm lesion, which was suspect of metastatic spread. Using ultrasound, a biopsy of the liver lesion was obtained, and the lesion studied by *in situ* hybridization with probes specific to the adrenal cortex. This analysis confirmed that the lesion was a metastasis.

Comment. Labeled riboprobes can be used to detect messenger RNA in tissue sections. The probe is often a single-stranded RNA (cRNA) that is complementary to the transcribed messenger RNA (mRNA) of a gene and will thus hybridize with high efficiency to any mRNA present in the tissue section. A cRNA riboprobe can be prepared by *in vitro* transcription of the gene of interest, which has been cloned into an appropriate plasmid. In order to obtain a complementary RNA to the target, the cloned gene is inserted into the plasmid vector in the reverse orientation relative to a viral promoter. When the gene is transcribed by a viral RNA polymerase, the opposite strand to that normally made *in vivo* is produced and is therefore complementary to the native mRNA.

Hybridization takes place on the microscope slide and the labeled probe will bind to areas of active gene expression. This technique can be also used to study the variation in gene expression in tissues at different times in development, and also tissue-specific gene expression.

RNA PROBES

RNA probes, or **riboprobes**, can be produced by *in vitro* transcription of cloned DNA inserted in a suitable plasmid downstream of a viral promoter. Some bacterial viruses code for their own RNA polymerases, which are highly specific for the viral promoters. Using these enzymes, labeled NTPs, and inserts inserted in both forward and reverse orientations, both sense and antisense riboprobes can be generated from a cloned gene.

Blots used in molecular biology

Blot	Probe	Target
Southern	nucleotide	DNA
Northern	nucleotide	RNA
Western	antibody	protein

Table 34.3 **Types of blots used in molecular biology.** Southern and Northern blots use nucleotide-based probes to hybridize to the DNA or RNA on the membrane. Western blots rely on the ability of a specific antibody to bind to a protein of interest.

DNA storage

Nitrocellulose membranes can store DNA for future use in hybridization studies; Southern blots are the prototype for 'permanent' DNA storage

One of the fundamental steps in the evolution of molecular biology was the discovery that DNA could be transferred from a semisolid gel onto a nitrocellulose membrane in such a way that the membrane could act as a permanent record of the DNA information in the gel and could be used for multiple-probe experiments. The process whereby the DNA is transferred to the membrane was first described by Ed Southern, but subsequent techniques based on the transfer of RNA and proteins have adopted the direction theme and are called Northern and Western blots, respectively (Table 34.3).

Restriction enzymes are crucial in the process of performing Southern blots

Restriction endonucleases comprise a group of enzymes that cleave double stranded DNA. As discussed later, these enzymes are sequence-specific and each enzyme acts at a limited number of sites in DNA called 'recognition' or 'cutting' sites. These enzymes are an element of the bacterial 'immune system'. Bacteria methylate their own DNA, protecting it from their own restriction enzymes, but cleave infecting viral or bacteriophage DNAs at specific sites, thereby inactivating the virus.

If DNA is digested by a restriction enzyme, the resulting digested DNA will be reduced to fragments of varying sizes depending on how many cutting sites for that restriction enzyme are present in the DNA. It is important to note that each enzyme will cut DNA into a unique set of fragments (Fig. 34.5).

Restriction endonucleases

Restriction enzyme	Restriction site	Ends
HaeIII	GG*CC CC*GG	flush
MspI	C*CGG GGC*C	sticky
EcoRV	GAT*ATC CTA*TAG	flush
EcoRI	G*AATTC CTTAA*G	sticky
NotI	GC*GGCCGC CG CCGG*CG	sticky

Table 34.4 **Restriction endonucleases in common use.** Enzymes can cleave DNA to produce 'flush ends' where the DNA is cut 'vertically' leaving two ends that do not have any overhanging nucleotides. However, if the DNA is cleaved 'obliquely', the DNA will have short single stranded overhangs. Such ends are called 'sticky' because they will selectively rejoin (hybridize) to matching overhangs. The sites of cleavage of DNA by restriction enzymes are often described as *palindromic* because of their inverted repeat symmetry – they have identical sequences in opposite directions on the complementary strands.

❋ RESTRICTION ENZYME CUTTING FREQUENCY

Restriction enzymes can cut DNA into fragments at sites determined by the nucleotide sequence of the DNA (Fig. 34.5). The frequency of the cutting sites for various different enzymes varies primarily with the length of the recognition site. Cut sites for an enzymes with a 4-base recognition site, such as *Hae*III, would occur by chance once per 256 base pair sequence. Cut sites for an enzyme with an 8-base recognition site, such as *Not*I, would occur only once in about 65 000 base pairs. As a result of the differing frequencies of cutting sites, there is generally a difference in the size of the cut fragments, frequent cutters generating many small fragments and rare cutters generating fewer and larger fragments. These differences can be exploited when trying to map the location of certain genes to chromosomal locations.

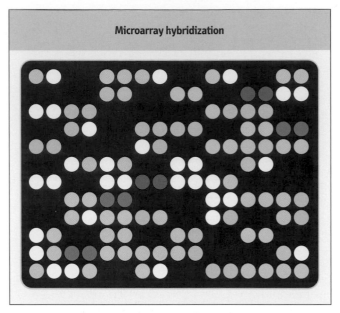

Fig. 34.4 **Microarray hybridization.** Representation of a small region of an array in which each DNA target dot is duplicated. The probe consisted of a mixture of green-tagged cDNA molecules derived from the mRNA of normal cells and red-tagged molecules derived from the mRNA of diseased cells. The color and brightness of the spots indicates the relative prevalence of particular mRNAs in normal as compared with diseased cells. A yellow signal indicates that a particular mRNA was equally common in both normal and diseased cells. No signal indicates genes whose expression is undetectable.

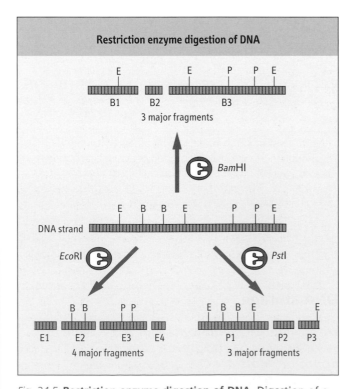

Fig. 34.5 **Restriction enzyme digestion of DNA.** Digestion of a DNA molecule by several different restriction enzymes may result in many different fragments, even though the apparent size of the fragments is similar. For example, fragments E4 and P2 are of similar size but are clearly different pieces of DNA. E, *Eco*RI site; B, *Bam*HI site; P, *Pst*I site.

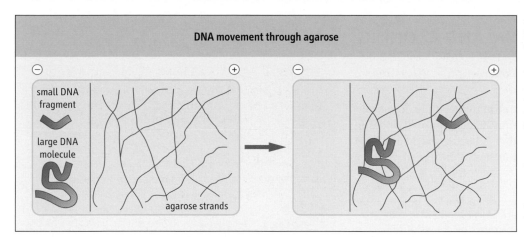

DNA movement through agarose

agarose strands

Fig. 34.6 **Movement of DNA through agarose during electrophoresis.** The molecules must find their way through openings between agarose polymer chains. Small DNA molecules can migrate between the strands with less hindrance. Medium to large DNA molecules take on a random coil geometry and with increasing size have progressively greater difficulty migrating through the polysaccharide network.

Originally the location of cut sites and the number of fragments expected were often unknown. However, with the rapid progress in sequencing the genomes of both mammals and other organisms, cut sites can now often be predicted.

Many restriction enzymes recognize sites that are typically four nucleotides (e.g. *Hae*III), six nucleotides (e.g. *EcoR* I) or eight nucleotides (e.g. *Not*I). Each enzyme recognizes its own site; variation in just one nucleotide within the recognition sequence makes a sequence completely resistant to a particular enzyme.

Southern blotting

Blotting techniques involve transfer of DNA, RNA or proteins in the semisolid phase of a gel to a solid phase that may then be used as a template for exposure to a range of molecular probes

If DNA is digested by a restriction enzyme, the resulting digest can be separated on the basis of size by gel electrophoresis. A solution of digested DNA is placed in a well in an agarose gel and an electric current applied. The rate of migration of DNA fragments depends on their size, with the smallest fragments moving furthest and the largest moving least (Figure 34.6). Agarose gel electrophoresis is used to separate fragments ranging in size from 100 bases to approximately 20 kb in length (above 40 kb, resolution is minimal). Following electrophoresis, the gels are soaked in a strong alkali solution to render the DNA fragments single-stranded. These single-stranded fragments can then be transferred to a nitrocellulose or nylon membrane to which they bind readily and, if preserved properly, permanently. The process of transfer involves the passage of solute through the gel and into the filter, passively carrying the DNA and producing an image of the gel on the filter (Fig. 34.7).

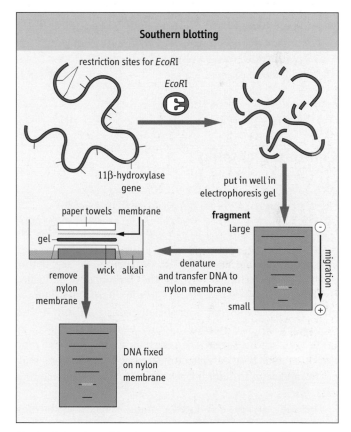

Southern blotting

restriction sites for *EcoRI*

EcoRI

11β-hydroxylase gene

put in well in electrophoresis gel

fragment
large

denature and transfer DNA to nylon membrane

small

migration

paper towels   membrane

gel

remove nylon membrane

wick   alkali

DNA fixed on nylon membrane

Fig. 34.7 **Southern blotting of DNA.** DNA digested with a restriction enzyme is size-fractionated by agarose electrophoresis. The agarose gel is then placed in alkali to denature the DNA. The now single-stranded DNA can pass from the gel to the nylon membrane as buffer solution flows upward by capillary action, forming a permanent record of the digested DNA.

DNA AMPLIFICATION AND CLONING

Two methods exist for mass amplification of DNA in vitro

The amplification of DNA is central to the study of molecular biology and genetics. DNA amplification makes possible an enormous increase in the number of copies of a desired DNA sequence. Two important approaches to the amplification of DNA are:

- **cell-based DNA cloning:** DNA is amplified *in vivo* by a cellular host such that the number of copies of the desired DNA template increases simply due to the exponential increase in number of replicating host cells;
- **enzyme-based DNA cloning (cell-free):** this method is represented by the polymerase chain reaction (PCR) and involves entirely *in vitro* DNA amplification.

Cell-based cloning

The majority of cell-based cloning uses recombinant DNA in replicating bacteria – recombinant human insulin and erythropoietin are prepared by this technique

Cell-based cloning is based on the ability of replicating cells, e.g. bacteria, to sustain the presence of so-called recombinant DNA within them. Recombinant DNA refers to any DNA molecule that is artificially constructed from two pieces of DNA not normally found together. One piece of DNA will be the target DNA that is to be amplified and the other will be the replicating vector or replicon, a molecule capable of initiating DNA replication in a suitable host cell.

The majority of cell-based cloning is performed using bacterial cells. In addition to the bacterial chromosome, bacteria may contain extra-chromosomal double-stranded DNA that can undergo replication. One such example is the bacterial plasmid. Plasmids are circular, double-stranded DNA molecules that undergo intracellular replication and are passed vertically from the parent cell to each daughter cell. However, unlike the bacterial chromosome, plasmids used in these techniques are copied many times during each cell division. Thus, plasmids represent ideal replicons for the amplification of target DNA and methods involving the use of plasmids are widespread throughout molecular biology.

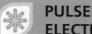

PULSED-FIELD GEL ELECTROPHORESIS

Pulsed-field gel electrophoresis (PFGE) is a technique used to separate large pieces of DNA digested by rare-cutting restriction enzymes. DNA fragments generated by rare cutters can be several hundred kilobases in size and cannot be separated by conventional agarose gel electrophoresis. Conventional gel electrophoresis uses current applied in a single dimension. Very large DNA fragments are thought to orient themselves so that they pass though the gel like a garden hose being drawn through a field thickly overgrown with brush. Once oriented with the voltage field, molecules of different lengths migrate at slow but similar rates. The trick to separating these large fragments is to make them change direction at regular intervals; longer DNAs take longer to orient correctly and so lag behind shorter fragments. Accordingly, in PFGE, an alternating current is applied to the gel, changing the direction of electrophoresis at intervals. The net effect of the time sequence and changes in polarity of the current is to separate large fragments by size in one dimension (Fig. 34.8). Standard agarose gel electrophoresis may take 1–4 hours to complete, whereas PFGE often requires over 24 hours to complete.

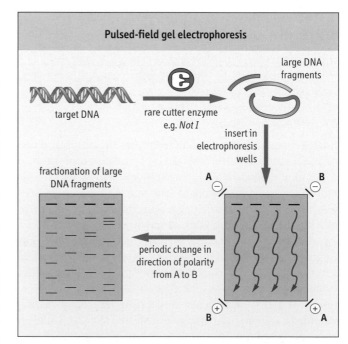

Fig. 34.8 **Pulsed-field gel electrophoresis.** DNA is digested with 'rare-cutting' restriction enzymes to generate large DNA fragments. During electrophoresis, the polarity of the electric field changes direction periodically. Large fragments take longer to re-orient and move in the new direction. The end result is size-fractionated DNA of fragments over 100 kb.

BACTERIAL PLASMIDS ARE BIOENGINEERED TO OPTIMIZE THEIR USE AS VECTORS

Within the circular DNA of a plasmid molecule are several elements that confer specific properties on the plasmid. Naturally occurring plasmids require several modifications to convert them into efficient DNA amplification vectors:

- **a polylinker cloning site:** this is a short sequence of nucleotides that contain unique recognition sites for several common restriction enzymes;
- **an antibiotic resistance gene:** the host bacterial cells used for cloning must be sensitive to an antibiotic, e.g. ampicillin or tetracycline, so that when they are transformed by the plasmid, the host cell acquires resistance to the antibiotic. This then provides a means of selecting out bacteria that contain the plasmid from those that do not. This selection step is important because of the low efficiency of introducing plasmid DNA into bacteria;
- **a recombinant screening system:** it is customary for the plasmid to have an expressible gene within it that can be used to show if foreign DNA is present in the plasmid. This so-called 'marker gene' can be designed to have the polylinker sequence within its reading frame so that, if the plasmid contains the target DNA insert, the normal reading frame is disrupted and the gene becomes nonfunctioning. The most common example is the gene for β-galactosidase. Using chromogenic substrates, bacteria containing this gene can be recognized readily on a culture plate. If there is an insert in the plasmid, the gene product is altered and colonies do not form the colored reaction product (see Fig. 34.9). These colonies are then selected for further study to confirm the presence of the target DNA.

Target DNA is introduced into a replicon by using restriction enzymes to cut target and replicon DNA so that the target DNA and the linearized plasmid DNA will have complementary sticky ends (Fig. 34.9). DNA ligase then covalently joins the target to the ends of the vector to form a closed circular recombinant plasmid.

Once the target DNA is incorporated into the plasmid vector, the next step is to introduce the plasmid into a host cell to allow replication to occur. The cell membrane of bacteria is selectively permeable and prevents the free passage of large molecules such as DNA in and out of the cell. However, the permeability of cells can be altered temporarily by factors such as electric currents (electroporation) and high-solute concentration (osmotic stress), so that the membrane becomes permeable and DNA can enter the cell. Such a process renders the cells competent, i.e. they can take up foreign DNA from the extracellular fluid, a process known as **transformation**. This process is generally inefficient, so that only a small fraction of cells may take up plasmid DNA, and often only a single plasmid per bacterium is introduced during transformation. However, it is this process of cellular uptake of plasmid DNA that forms a critical step in cell-based cloning. Individual recombinant DNAs are easily resolved from one another because they are taken up by separate cells that can be isolated simply by spreading them on an agar surface.

Following transformation, the cells are allowed to replicate, usually on a standard agar plate containing a suitable antibiotic to kill cells that do not harbor a plasmid. Colonies (clones of single cells) are then 'picked' and transferred to tubes for growth in liquid culture and a second phase of exponential increase in cell number. Thus, from a single cell and a single molecule of DNA, an extremely large number of cells containing identical recombinant plasmids can be generated in a relatively small time. (Fig. 34.10). Recovery of the plasmid DNA is easy because it is small, covalently intact circle, and readily separated from the bacterial chromosomal DNA by a variety of techniques.

DNA cloning by the polymerase chain reaction (PCR)

The use of PCR for the amplification of DNA in vitro *has revolutionized molecular biology; it is a method of copying a single template DNA molecule*

PCR is a simple and quick means of generating up to 10^9 copies of a single template DNA molecule within hours. A standard PCR reaction requires the following:

- **DNA template:** DNA containing the sequence to be amplified;
- **amplimers:** small oligonucleotide primers that will hybridize with complementary DNA sequences both upstream and downstream of the desired sequence region and act as a starting point for the synthesis of the newly amplified DNA strands;
- **polymerase enzyme:** typically a heat-stable polymerase that will catalyze the formation of the DNA during the amplification reaction;
- **dNTPs:** these are of course essential for the synthesis of the new DNA strands by the polymerase.

PCR consists of a series of programmed temperature changes that serve to bring about a round of DNA synthesis

Formation of plasmid with target gene

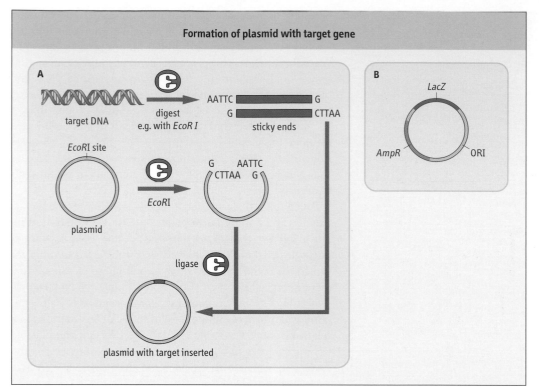

Fig. 34.9 **Formation of a plasmid containing a target gene for cloning.** (A) DNA containing the target gene is digested with a restriction enzyme that will produce 'sticky ends', e.g. *Eco*RI. The plasmid also has a restriction site for *Eco*RI, so that when digested with *Eco*RI it becomes a linear DNA strand with 'sticky ends' complementary to the target. Upon ligation the target and vector form a recombinant molecule. (B) Structure of a typical plasmid. The plasmid contains a gene conferring resistance to the antibiotic ampicillin (AmpR), and a portion of the LacZ gene that encodes the *N*-terminal fragment of the enzyme β-galactosidase. The *E. coli* strain used for this work has a defective β-galactosidase enzyme which is complemented by the plasmid LacZ gene product to form a functional enzyme. Within the plasma LacZ gene segment is a polylinker region containing approximately 10 restriction-enzyme recognition sites, which serve as sites for insertion of target DNA. The plasmid also contains ORI, the site for origin of DNA replication.

VECTOR SYSTEMS FOR CLONING LARGE DNA FRAGMENTS

One critical factor in recombinant DNA manipulations is the size of the target DNA. Conventional bacterial plasmids, although convenient to work with, are limited in the size of insert they can accept; 1–2 kb is the common size of the insert, with an upper limit of 5-10 kb. Some modified plasmid vectors called **cosmids** can accept larger fragments up to 20 kb. Another commonly used vector that has the ability to accept larger DNA fragments is the bacteriophage **lambda** (λ). This viral particle contains a double-stranded DNA genome packaged within a protein coat. The λ–phage can infect *E. coli* cells with high efficiency and introduce its DNA into the bacterium. Infection leads to the replication of viral DNA and the synthesis of new viral particles, which can then lyse the host cell and infect neighboring cells to repeat the process. The viral DNA is then re-isolated to obtain the recombinant DNA.

Larger inserts can be cloned by using modified chromosomes from either **bacteria (bacterial artificial chromosomes, BACs)**, or yeast **(yeast artificial chromosomes, YACs)**. Such vectors can accommodate DNA fragments up to 1–2 Mb. BACs have been particularly important in putting together the sequence of the human genome.

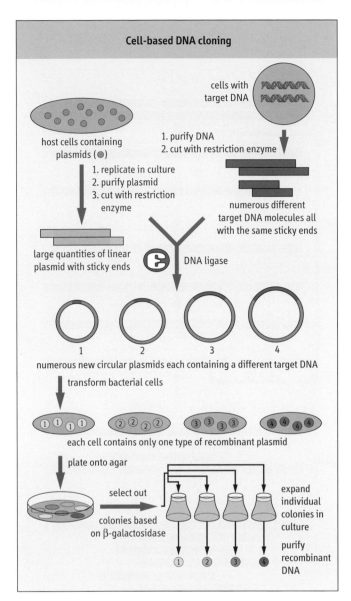

Cell-based DNA cloning

cells with target DNA

host cells containing plasmids (●)

1. purify DNA
2. cut with restriction enzyme

1. replicate in culture
2. purify plasmid
3. cut with restriction enzyme

numerous different target DNA molecules all with the same sticky ends

large quantities of linear plasmid with sticky ends

DNA ligase

1   2   3   4

numerous new circular plasmids each containing a different target DNA

transform bacterial cells

① ① ① ①   ② ② ② ②   ③ ③ ③ ③   ④ ④ ④ ④

each cell contains only one type of recombinant plasmid

plate onto agar

select out

colonies based on β-galactosidase

expand individual colonies in culture

purify recombinant DNA

①   ②   ③   ④

Fig. 34.10 **Cell-based DNA cloning.** An example of cloning genomic DNA using bacterial cells. In general each transformed bacterium will take up only a single plasmid molecule. Therefore individual bacterial colonies will contain many identical copies of just one particular recombinant DNA.

CELL-BASED CLONING IS USED TO PRODUCE CLINICALLY IMPORTANT PROTEINS

A 13-year-old girl was admitted with dehydration, vomiting and weight loss. Her blood glucose level was 19.1 mmol/L (344 mg/dL) and she had ketonuria. A diagnosis of type 1 diabetes mellitus was made. She was started on recombinant human insulin, was rehydrated, and made a prompt recovery.

Comment. Prior to the advent of recombinant DNA technology, insulin therapy involved the use of animal insulins, most commonly pork or beef, which were chemically similar, but not identical, to human insulin. As a result of these differences, animal insulins often led to the development of antibodies, which reduced the efficacy of the insulin and could lead to treatment failures.
Insulin was the first biologically important human molecule to be produced by means of recombinant DNA technology. Following the cloning of the human insulin gene, large-scale production of pure human insulin was possible by inserting the cloned gene into a cell-based amplification system. Large amounts of insulin gene copies were produced, which were then expressed in either bacteria or yeast, and the resulting purified insulin was made available for use in treatment of diabetic patients.
One crucial step in the process is the use of cDNA as a template for transcription and translation of the desired gene. By using insulin mRNA as a template, human insulin cDNA can be generated by reverse transcription (formation of a complementary DNA strand using mRNA as the template) whose product is a DNA molecule that contains all the coding region of the insulin gene without any introns. By this means, human recombinant insulin has almost totally replaced animal insulin in the treatment of diabetes. Other important recombinant human peptides used clinically include growth hormone, erythropoietin and parathyroid hormone.

from the primers (Fig. 34.11). The average PCR involves about 30–35 cycles of reactions, which provide sufficient DNA, as much as a billion copies of the original template, so that it can be visualized following electrophoresis on an agarose gel.

The cycle of the PCR comprises three steps that are repeated continuously by varying temperature in a cyclic fashion:

- **denaturation:** heating of the reaction to approximately 95°C to ensure template and primers are single stranded;
- **annealing:** cooling of the mixture to allow heteroduplexes of primer and template to form. The temperature for this is based on the Tm of the expected duplex (typically in the 50 to 65°C range);
- **elongation:** DNA polymerase elongates the newly synthesized DNA strand from the site of the annealed primer along the template strand (typically about 70°C).

The practical development of PCR was made possible by the discovery of heat-stable DNA polymerases that can withstand the temperature of the denaturation step and still retain enzymatic activity, e.g. *Taq* and *Pfu* polymerases. These enzymes were isolated from organisms that live and reproduce in hot springs and geysers.

The ability of PCR to amplify selectively a single template DNA relies on some prior knowledge of the nucleotide sequences in the regions flanking the target sequence

If the sequences in the regions flanking the target sequence are known, oligonucleotide primers are synthesized that are complementary to:

- the region on the sense (top) strand upstream of the target region; and
- the region on the antisense (lower) strand downstream of the target region (Fig. 34.11).

It is essential that the sequence of the primers be unique to the target DNA being amplified. If, for instance, the downstream primer contains sequences that contain tandem repeats of bases, e.g. TGTGTG, the specificity of the amplification may be reduced as such repetitive sequences occur widely throughout the genome, and the amplified sequence may contain many unwanted products.

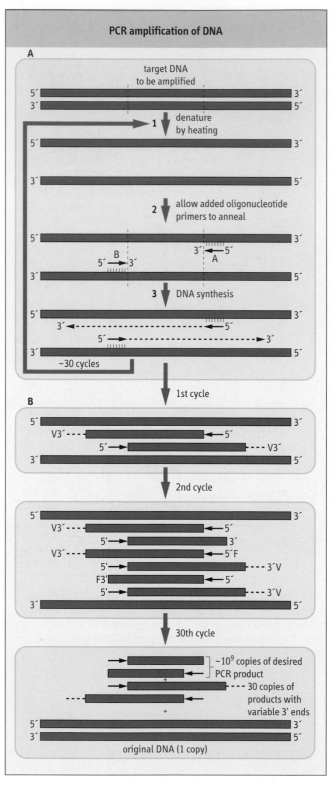

Fig. 34.11 **Polymerase chain reaction (PCR) amplification of DNA.** (A) Cycle 1. The target DNA is heated to 94°C to ensure complete denaturation. The mixture is then cooled to allow the oligonucleotide primers to hybridize to the complementary sequence in the target DNA. Specificity is provided by using two primers that anneal to sequences on opposite strands at opposite ends of the sequence to be amplified. In the presence of dNTPs, *Taq* polymerase catalyzes the elongation, beginning at the 3′end of the primers. Two new duplex DNA molecules: one generated by each primer on its respective template. (B) Subsequent cycles. In the second cycle, products from the first cycle become templates. These templates have primers at their 5′-ends. Accordingly, the DNA made on them stops at the end of the primers used in the first cycle. From now on, molecules will accumulate during each cycle that have both ends defined by the pair of primers used. These accumulate exponentially and soon far outnumber the initial input DNA template. After 30 cycles, the original template and a trivial number of the variable-ended strands copied directly from it remain, but the number of amplified target molecules enclosed by the primers approaches 10^9.

Advantages and disadvantages of PCR cloning

PCR is a quick, simple and robust technique, but prior sequence knowledge is needed, only a relatively small target DNA can be amplified, and DNA replication may be inaccurate

PCR has three principal advantages over cell-based cloning:

■ **time:** by using PCR, a single template strand can be amplified to produce a detectable product very rapidly. Each step takes a few minutes or less, and 30 cycles of this PCR process can be completed in at most a few hours. Cell-based cloning is more expensive and may require days or weeks to produce a similar yield of DNA;

■ **sensitivity:** PCR can amplify a DNA template to usable amounts if only a single copy of the template DNA is present. Indeed, PCR protocols have been developed to allow amplification of target DNA from a single cell. This is why PCR has found such a prominent place in forensic applications and even in paleontology;

■ **robustness:** PCR is able to amplify DNA that is often badly degraded by time or the elements, or is present in previously inaccessible sites, e.g. formalin-fixed tissue. Only a few copies of an unmodified, relatively short sequence to be amplified need to remain intact.

Despite the apparent attraction of PCR, it is not without fault and, depending on the application of the method, it may be an unacceptable means of amplifying DNA. The drawbacks of PCR are as follows:

■ **prior sequence knowledge:** to perform PCR, flanking primers must be synthesized. For this to happen, the sequence of the target DNA, or at least its flanking regions, must be known. This may require prior cell-based cloning to derive the flanking nucleotide information. With the virtual completion of the human genome sequence, this issue is less important than in prior years;

■ **small target DNA amplification:** PCR will reliably amplify target sequences up to about 5 kb, although products of 200–1000 bases are most readily amplified. However, larger products have been amplified recently by so-called 'long PCR' methods, allowing sequences up to 20 kb or more to be amplified;

■ DNA replication may be inaccurate: errors can be introduced during DNA polymerization by *Taq* polymerase since this enzyme lacks proof-reading activity. In a standard PCR reaction, up to 40% of the synthesized products will have some error in the nucleotide sequence introduced by the polymerase enzyme, usually only a single nucleotide substitution. Therefore, the final reaction mixture will contain numerous copies of the target DNA,

which are almost but not quite the same, and the substituted nucleotide may be different in different amplified molecules. Similarly, if there is any contamination of the DNA source by other DNAs that may contain the target sequence (such as with forensic material), unwanted amplification may occur.

Thus, it is safe to say that PCR provides a simple, fast and very efficient means of amplifying DNA that is partly or fully characterized, is of relatively small size and may be present in small amounts or in a poor condition. However, it is a less useful technique if the objective is to amplify DNA accurately without introducing sequence errors or if the target DNA sequence is large.

SPECIFIC METHODS USED IN THE ANALYSIS OF DNA

Hybridization-based methods

There are several ways in which hybridization can be used in the study of DNA, which exploit either the stringency of the hybridization of probe to target or the utility of restriction enzymes for detecting variations in nucleotide sequences.

 OLIGONUCLEOTIDE PRIMER DESIGN

It is the very versatility of PCR that can be its greatest weakness. If the oligonucleotide primers are not sufficiently robust then the reliability of PCR amplification will be significantly reduced. In order to reduce the possibility of unwanted amplification, several simple rules are followed in the design of primers. Primer length should be about 20–30 nucleotides long for amplification of genomic DNA, while amplification of plasmid DNA may be performed with shorter primers. The sequence of the primer should avoid tandem repeats of nucleotides, e.g. CACACACACA, as these are common throughout the genome and will reduce the specificity of the amplification. In addition, it is important to ensure that there is no complementarity between the two primers. If the primers are complementary then they will hybridize to each other rather than the template and amplification will be inefficient.

By analyzing the DNA sequence of the target DNA and paying attention to these simple rules, a large percentage of the PCR amplification problems will be avoided. However, the use of computer software to perform the analysis of suitable sequences is increasingly common, and the software used is becoming extremely sophisticated and almost essential for many large-scale PCR applications.

Restriction fragment length polymorphisms (RFLPs)

Restriction enzymes cleave DNA at specific recognition sites; if these sites are altered by mutation or polymorphism, the size of DNA fragments on a blot will differ

If the recognition sequence is disrupted, either by a pathologic change in the DNA sequence resulting in a disease (a mutation), or a naturally occurring variation in the DNA sequence unaccompanied by disease (a polymorphism), the results of probing a Southern blot of DNA digested by a restriction enzyme may differ. Such differences in DNA sequence may lead to the creation of new restriction sites or the abolition of existing sites, and result in DNA fragments of different lengths – pattern differences known as restriction fragment length polymorphisms (RFLPs) (Fig. 34.12). Such RFLPs can be used either to identify disease-causing mutations, because of a single point mutation creating or abolishing a restriction site, or to study variation in noncoding DNA for use in the study of genetic linkage.

RFLPs can also help detect larger pathologic changes in the DNA sequence, either deletions or duplications. Large deletions of a gene may abolish restriction sites; this leads to the disappearance of a fragment on a Southern blot in homozygous individuals. Alternatively, if a DNA duplication event occurs, a new gene may be formed, which has a different pattern of restriction sites that allow detection of the new gene. This type of hybridization is performed using large probes (0.5–5.0 kb) and is performed under moderate stringency, i.e. it is sufficiently rigid to allow hybridization of probe and target but also to tolerate minor differences, e.g. in introns or flanking, noncoding DNA.

Low stringency hybridization of a probe to a Southern blot of digested DNA may allow genes related to, but not identical to, the starting gene to be identified. Many genes exist in families, or have nonfunctional, nearly identical copies elsewhere in the genome (pseudogenes), and thus hybridization of a probe may identify one or more restriction fragments, corresponding to related genes, which can be identified by other means. Similarly, related genes in different species may be identified by using a single probe that can hybridize at low stringency to complementary sequences in blots of DNA from mouse, rat or other species.

Allele-specific oligonucleotides and dot-blot hybridization

This method uses a small probe to probe the blotted DNA under highly stringent conditions

The other extreme of the RFLP method is to use a small oligonucleotide probe (15–30 nucleotides) and probe the

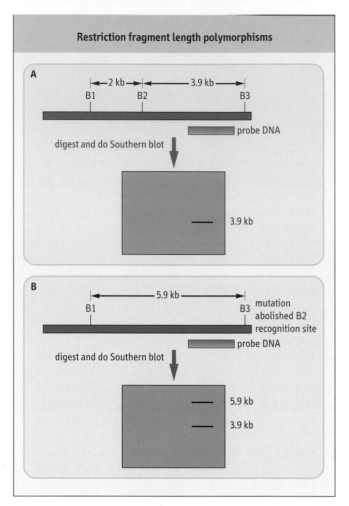

Restriction fragment length polymorphisms

Fig. 34.12 **Restriction fragment length polymorphisms (RFLP).** Variations in the nucleotide sequence of DNA, either due to natural variation in individuals or as a result of a DNA mutation, can abolish the recognition sites for restriction enzymes. This means that when DNA is digested with the enzyme whose site is abolished, the size of the resulting fragments is altered. Southern blotting and probe hybridization can be used to detect this change. Results are shown for (A) homozygous normal and (B) heterozygous mutant individuals. B, *Bam*HI restriction site.

blotted DNA under conditions of high stringency. Careful choice of temperature and solvent ensures that oligonucleotides will only hybridize to complementary sequences where there is a perfect match, down to the single nucleotide level. Mutations that result from a single nucleotide change can be detected by using oligonucleotides that recognize either the mutant or the normal allele of the gene, so-called allele-specific oligonucleotides (ASOs). ASOs can be used to screen DNA for the presence of several mutations, particularly if the template DNA is immobilized on a membrane for dot-blot analysis. Single-stranded DNA is transferred to a membrane as in the case of Southern blotting, but rather

RFLPS CAN BE USED FOR DETECTING PATHOLOGIC MUTATIONS

A 24-year-old Afro-Caribbean woman was referred for prenatal counseling. Her younger brother had sickle-cell anemia, and she had become pregnant. Her partner was known to be a carrier of the sickle-cell mutation (sickle-cell trait) and she wanted to know if her child would develop sickle-cell anemia.

Since the patient is at risk of being a carrier, she opted to have chorionic villus sampling (CVS) performed to detect the presence or absence of the sickle-cell mutation in her child. Analysis of her own DNA revealed that she was a carrier, and the CVS showed that the child was also a carrier and would not develop sickle-cell anemia.

Comment. Occasionally, a mutation will directly abolish or create a restriction site and thus allow the use of a restriction-based method to demonstrate the presence or absence of the mutant allele. One widely examined mutation is the A > T substitution at codon 6 in the sequence for the β-globin gene responsible for sickle-cell disease. This results in a glutamine-valine (Glu-Val) mutation in the amino acid sequence β-globin and also abolishes a recognition site for *Mst*II (CCTN(A > T)GG) in the β-globin gene. Digestion of normal human DNA with *Mst*II and probing the Southern blot with a probe specific for the promoter of the β-globin gene yields a single band of 1.2 kb as the nearest *Mst*II site is 1.2 kb upstream in the 5′ region of the gene. The abolition of the codon 6 restriction site means that the fragment size seen when probing *Mst*II digested DNA is now 1.4 kb, as the next *Mst*II site is located 200 bases downstream in the intron after exon 1. Thus, patients with sickle-cell anemia will show only one band, 1.4 kb, while carriers will have 2 bands, one 1.4 kb and another, 1.2 kb, and unaffected individuals will have a single 1.2 kb band (Figs 34.12 and 34.13).

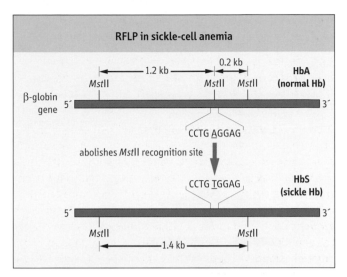

Fig. 34.13 **RFLP analysis in sickle-cell anemia.** An A > T substitution at codon 6 of the β-globin gene abolishes a recognition site for the enzymes, *Mst*II, which can be used to determine the presence or absence of the mutation by studying the RFLP pattern.

Applications of PCR	
Application	
Genetic marker typing	restriction site polymorphisms microsatellite repeats
Detection of point mutations	restriction site polymorphisms amplification refractory mutation systems
Amplification of DNA templates for DNA sequencing	double-stranded DNA single-stranded templates
Genomic DNA cloning	PCR of gene families or genes in different species
Others	genome walking, introduction of mutations *in vitro* to test their effect in biological systems

Table 34.5 **Applications of PCR.**

than transferring size-fractionated digested DNA, total human genomic DNA or PCR-generated fragments are blotted onto the membrane. In this way, ASOs can be hybridized to the membrane under high-stringency conditions and autoradiography performed to determine whether the DNA contains a specific allele. The process can then be repeated for other alleles (Fig. 34.14).

PCR-based methods

PCR is a versatile method applied to a multitude of methods in DNA research (Table 34.5). One of the most widely used clinical applications of PCR is in the identification of genetic mutations within PCR amplified DNA from 'at risk' individuals.

Assay of restriction site polymorphisms

Restriction site polymorphisms (RSPs) are small-scale equivalents of RFLPs

Naturally occurring variations in DNA sequence may abolish or create restriction sites that can be detected conveniently by digesting PCR amplified sequences with the appropriate restriction enzyme.

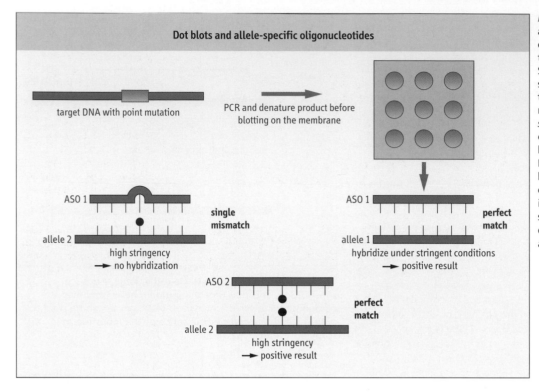

Fig. 34.14 **Dot blots and allele-specific oligonucleotides.** Using a technique similar to Southern blotting, single-stranded PCR products are transferred onto a nylon membrane and fixed *in situ*. Allele-specific oligonucleotides (ASOs) are hybridized to the target DNA under conditions of high stringency. In this case, the ASOs are used to identify a single base substitution, with one detecting the wild type and another the mutant allele.

Detection of microsatellite repeats

This technique detects sets of tandem nucleotide repeats present in mammalian genomes

Tandem microsatellite repeats are sequences that comprise a few nucleotides – between one and four but typically two or three, e.g. CA or CAG, that are repeated in tandem at various locations throughout mammalian genomes, so-called microsatellite repeats. These microsatellites are small blocks of DNA that occur in non-coding regions, either intergenic or within introns of genes. The term 'satellite DNA' has been historically applied to regions of repetitive sequence in which the local base composition may differ from the overall composition of human DNA. One important feature of these microsatellite repeats is that they are highly polymorphic, i.e. the number of tandem repeats in a particular microsatellite may vary from one individual to another. This means that the two copies of a single human microsatellite, one from each chromosome, may be of different lengths and can thus be distinguished in that individual. The number of different alleles of the microsatellite will vary depending on which microsatellite is studied, but may vary from 2–15 or more copies of the repeat per allele (Fig. 34.15). As a result of this high degree of polymorphism, microsatellite repeats are of great value in the study of genetic linkage. This is because a particular microsatellite allele may fortuitously be located in the vicinity of a pathological mutation. Comparison of the DNA of affected families may indicate that a particular microsatellite serves as a marker with which to trace the presence or inheritance of the mutation under study.

Mutation detection by allele-specific PCR

Only mutant DNA will be amplified using this technique

Standard PCR employs two primers to amplify both strands of the DNA and relies on the fact that each primer will reliably amplify the target strand. However, PCR can be performed using allele-specific primers, which will only amplify one allele of a target gene. This means that if a primer contains a sequence that recognizes a mutation, it will only hybridize with the mutant DNA. Thus, only DNA containing the mutation will amplify with this primer. The allele-specific primer has its extreme 3′-nucleotides as the ones that detect the mutation, as the DNA polymerase requires complete hybridization of primer and template at the 3′ end of the primer. This method can be applied to the detection of specific mutations in a single gene, e.g. the gene for cystic fibrosis. This type of PCR is often called an amplification refractory mutation system (ARMS) as PCR amplification will be refractory, *i.e.* will not occur, in the absence of the mutant allele.

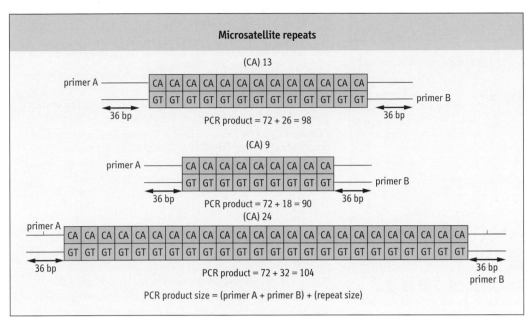

Fig. 34.15 **Microsatellite repeats.** A typical microsatellite contains tandem repeats of a dinucleotide, e.g. CA. The number of repeats can vary from 2 to 20 or more. Amplification of the DNA including the microsatellite repeat is performed by PCR using a radiolabeled primer and the products are then size-fractionated on a polyacrylamide gel to aid resolution. PCR product size = 72 (primer A + primer B) + 26 (13 × 2 for each dinucleotide) = 98. In this instance, three alleles can be identified: $(CA)_{13}$, $(CA)_{9}$, and $(CA)_{24}$.

MICROSATELLITE REPEATS ARE IDEAL MARKERS FOR STUDY OF INHERITANCE

A 7-year-old boy was the subject of disputed paternity. His mother had identified a man as the father and maintained that he should be responsible for the child's financial well-being. All parties consented to DNA testing by means of DNA fingerprinting. Study of the DNA tests revealed that this man was the father and was indeed responsible for the child.

Comment. The most commonly studied microsatellites contain dinucleotide repeats of (CA) or (TG) and may vary in repeat number from one or 2, up to 20 or more. Thus, a standard dinucleotide repeat would be denoted (CA)n, where n is the number of repeats. An ideal microsatellite marker would have a large number of alleles, i.e. n > 100, and each allele would be equally frequent. However, most microsatellites have less than 20, and there is often a preponderance of one or two particular alleles in any population. When microsatellites are typed by PCR amplification and gel electrophoresis, both chromosomes are amplified and thus two possible alleles are generated from each locus for a single individual.
In forensic medicine, simple questions are often asked, e.g. 'Is this man the child's father?' or 'Does this blood stain correspond to blood of the suspect?' By selecting several microsatellite markers, typically six to nine, that are highly polymorphic and have an even spread of allele frequency, i.e. each allele is equally frequent, a series of microsatellite markers can be generated. When an individual's markers are tested, the result is a set of alleles that are virtually unique to an individual, a so-called 'DNA fingerprint'. Thus, by comparing the pattern of microsatellites generated in the subject in question and comparing this with the pathologic sample or the DNA of offspring, the identity of a parent or suspect can be confirmed or refuted with a high degree of certainty.

Microsatellites have also been used to examine the linkage of a disease trait, e.g. type 1 diabetes, to certain regions of the human genome. By studying the inheritance of microsatellite markers in families or the sharing of alleles in affected siblings, a statistical measure of the degree of co-inheritance of a marker can be determined. This approach has been used successfully to identify genetic loci strongly linked to the inheritance of type 1 and type 2 diabetes, and locate the genes causing Huntington's disease, myotonic dystrophy and other single gene disorders (Table 34.6).

Unstable trinucleotide repeats			
Disease	Repeat	Normal Length	Mutation length
Huntington's disease	(CAG)n	A:9–35	37–100
Kennedy disease	(CAG)n	17–24	40–55
Spinocerebellar ataxia I (SCA I)	(CAG)n	19–36	43–81
Dentatopallidoluysian atrophy (DRPLA)	(CAG)n	7–23	49–75+
Machado–Joseph disease (SCA III)	(CAG)n	12–36	69–79+
Fragile X site A (FRAXA)	(CGG)n	6–54	200–1000+
Fragile X site E (FRAXE)	(CCG)n	6–25	>200
Fragile X site F (FRAXF)	(GCC)n	6–29	>500
Fragile 16 site A (FRA16A)	(CCG)n	16–49	1000–2000
Myotonic dystrophy	(CTG)n	5–35	50–4000
Friedreich ataxia	(GAA)n	7–22	>200

Table 34.6 **Unstable trinucleotide repeats.** In all of the cases listed, trinucleotide repeats are present in individuals without clinical disease. However, progressive increase in the number of repeats leads to the onset of clinical signs, although a premutant phase has been described in some disorders, such as FRAXA, where expansions larger than normal are found but with minimal or no clinical features. These premutant states give rise to carriers – females who can subsequently pass on an expanded triplet repeat to their offspring, which may result in the disease.

Detection of deletions in genes causing disease

This is performed using primers that generate PCR products of different sizes

In patients with Duchenne muscular dystrophy, many of the disease-causing mutations are due to deletions of one of relatively few exons in this, one of the largest of human genes. Specific amplification of these exons, using primers that generate PCR products of different sizes for each exon, can be used to screen quickly for the presence of a disease-causing deletion in an affected individual or determine if the fetus of a carrier has the deletion. Such PCR is carried out in a single reaction using a single template and 5–10 different primer pairs, each generating a separate amplification product. This form of PCR is called multiplex PCR.

Other methods for the detection of variation in DNA

Single-strand conformational polymorphism (SSCP)

SSCP is useful for analyzing PCR products of 200 bp and less and is moderately sensitive

Single-stranded DNA has a tendency to form complex structures by folding back on itself, just as tRNA molecules form

TRINUCLEOTIDE REPEATS IN GENES GIVE RISE TO HUMAN DISEASE

A 33-year-old woman has recently been diagnosed as having myotonic dystrophy (MD). MD is characterized by autosomal dominant inheritance, muscular weakness associated with impaired muscular relaxation, frontal balding, endocrine disorders such as diabetes and premature ovarian failure, and premature cataract formation. The patient has muscular problems and frontal balding, whereas her affected father, aged 60 years, has only just developed cataracts. She is concerned about the risk to her own children if she becomes pregnant.

Comment. While the majority of nucleotide repeats are non-coding, several trinucleotide repeats have been described, which are related to human disease. The majority of trinucleotide repeats are clinically silent, but 11 clinical disorders have been identified where trinucleotide repeats appear directly responsible for a disease phenotype (see Fig. 34.16), and where the repeat is said to be unstable. Unstable repeats undergo changes in the size of the repeat during meiotic division and generally undergo expansion of the size of the repeat so that with each successive meiosis, i.e. from generation to generation, the number of repeats will gradually increase. Once trinucleotide expansions reach a critical size they begin to interfere with gene function and then result in the clinical syndrome (Table 34.6). In the case of myotonic dystrophy, with an expansion size of 80 repeats, the patient will exhibit the signs of the disease. Owing to the instability of the triplet repeat during meiosis, offspring of this patient might expect to have a larger expansion and also display features of the disease. Similarly, successive generations may display signs of MD at a younger age. This phenomenon of progressive worsening of the clinical phenotype with successive meioses is known as anticipation and is the result of progressive enlargement of the trinucleotide expansions during meiosis (Fig. 34.17). Interestingly, anticipation may be sex-limited, with the largest expansions only present in eggs, which have larger amounts of cytoplasm than spermatozoa. This observation has been suggested as the explanation for the occurrence of neonatal MD (a life-threatening form of the disease seen in newborn children) only in cases where the mother donates the triplet expansion to the offspring.

hairpin structures. The mobility of single-stranded DNA in an electrophoretic gel depends not only on the length of the DNA but also on its conformation, which is determined by its DNA sequence and folding. Therefore, changes in DNA structure that do not alter the length of the target DNA, i.e. substitutions in contrast to deletions or insertions, can alter the mobility of the fragment in a nondenaturing gel, so-called single-strand conformational polymorphisms (SSCP). SSCP is

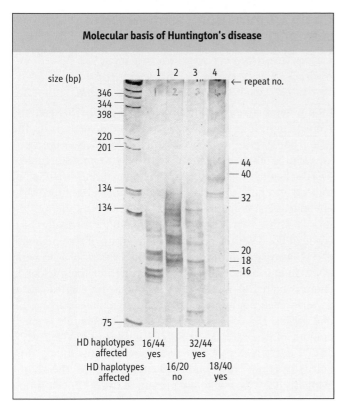

Fig. 34.16 Molecular diagnosis of Huntington's disease. This blot illustrates the use of a PCR-based method to diagnose Huntington's disease (HD). A portion of the HD gene, including the disease-associated triplet expansion region, is amplified by PCR. Each individual has two copies of the gene, one on each chromosome 4, and each PCR generates two PCR products. The PCR products are electrophoresized and compared with a size-specific ladder, which enables the size of the PCR product, and thus the number of triplet repeats in each product, to be assessed accurately. Affected patients will have triplet expansions greater than 35 repeats. HD is inherited as an autosomal-dominant trait, so that the disease is expressed on inheritance of a single copy of the mutant gene.

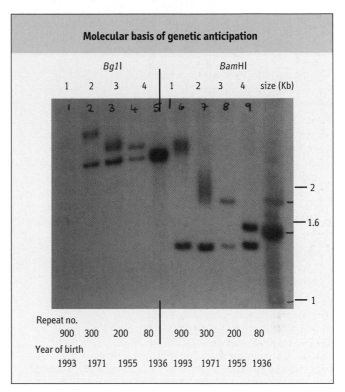

Fig. 34.17 Molecular basis of genetic anticipation. Myotonic dystrophy (MD) exhibits anticipation within families, i.e. the clinical features of the disease become progressively more severe and its age at onset of symptoms is younger with each successive generation. The underlying problem is the presence of an unstable trinucleotide expansion within the MD gene, which progressively expands with each meiosis. This results in the inheritance of larger mutations, which give rise to a more severe clinical picture with the tendency for the features to manifest at an earlier stage. The Southern blot illustrates the progressive increase in size of the trinucleotide expansion in successive generations of a family with MD. The normal allele size is 3.4 kb for the *Bgl*I digest and 1.4 kb for the *Bam*HI digest. It is clear, using both restriction enzymes, that with each generation there is a progressive expansion in the size of the trinucleotide repeat. (This is a good example of an RFLP.)

performed by PCR with a radioactive primer. The reaction products are denatured to render them single-stranded, and diluted to prevent intermolecular hybridization. The DNA is then electrophoresized on non-denaturing polyacrylamide gels. A control sample is also included on the gel to allow identification of the variant from the wild-type allele.

Denaturant-gradient gel electrophoresis (DGGE)

DGGE uses 'melting' of double-stranded DNA

In SSCP, changes in the tertiary structure of single-stranded DNA can result in differing electrophoretic mobilities. However, this type of analysis cannot be used for double-stranded DNA. Nevertheless, if double-stranded DNA under-

goes electrophoresis in a gel that contains a gradient of increasing amounts of denaturant, e.g. urea, double-stranded DNA will then partially denature, to form single-stranded regions and so undergo a marked change in mobility. A single nucleotide change between two alleles of a gene will affect the melting point of the alleles and thus the mobilities of amplified PCR fragments in this kind of denaturing gel.

To perform DGGE, PCR is performed using radiolabeled primers that have a GC clamp at their ends. This is a tail of guanine and cytosine residues added to the PCR primers such that the PCR product will have ends that have artificially created GC ends. These GC ends, or clamps, improve the sensitivity by preventing complete melting of double-stranded

PROTEIN TRUNCATION TESTING IN BREAST CANCER

A hereditary form of breast cancer associated with the coexistence of ovarian cancer is caused by mutations in the *BRCA1* gene. This gene, a tumor suppressor gene, was discovered following the analysis of large pedigrees with breast/ovarian cancer. Analysis of the mutations found in the genes of affected individuals showed that most of the mutations were either nonsense mutations, altered splice sites, or frameshift mutations, which gave rise to abnormally truncated protein products. Following identification of the common mutation types in *BRCA1* (and the subsequently discovered *BRCA2*), a protein truncation test has become a standard procedure for examining both pathologic tissue and blood from individuals at risk for the mutation.

Comment. The translation of mRNA to the final protein product results in a peptide of predictable size. If a gene is disrupted or has an insertion, deletion or a frameshift mutation that produces a premature stop codon, which occurs with 1/64 frequency in a random polynucleotide sequence, then the resulting peptide will be abnormally small. This difference can then be detected by electrophoresis of the protein product in a suitable gel and demonstrating the presence of a truncated protein product.

DNA. PCR products are electrophoresized in the denaturing gel and, following autoradiography, different alleles of the suspect gene are identified (Fig. 34.18). This is particularly useful for rapid scanning of individually amplified exon units from a large gene with many introns.

DNA SEQUENCING

At the heart of many of the foregoing techniques is the notion that at least some of the nucleotide sequence of the DNA being studied is known, particularly when PCR primers are involved. The technologies now used in the sequencing of DNA have become extremely advanced, and automated sequencing of large amounts of DNA is now standard practice in many centers around the world.

Chain termination (Sanger) DNA sequencing

Chain termination sequencing uses a DNA polymerase enzyme, a single-stranded template DNA and a sequencing primer

In this method, originally developed by Fred Sanger, the sequencing primer is designed to be complementary to the region flanking the sequence of interest and acts as the starting point of chain elongation. DNA polymerization requires dNTPs to allow the strand to be elongated but, in addition, radioactive chain-terminating dideoxynucleotides (ddNTPs) are added. These are analogs of the dNTPs but differ in that they lack the 3'-hydroxyl group required for formation of a covalent bond with the 5'-phosphate group of the incoming dNTP. Therefore, during DNA polymerization, if a growing DNA chain incorporates a ddNTP, growth of the nucleotide chain is halted. A total of four reactions are carried out in parallel, each containing the primer, template, polymerase and dNTPs. However, to each of the four reactions, a small amount of one radioactive ddNTP is added (ddATP, ddCTP, ddTTP, ddGTP) so that four separate reactions, the A, T, G, and C reactions, are conducted in parallel. As the chains elongate, ddNTPs, which are present at lower concentration than the natural dNTP, will be incorporated into the chain in place of the corresponding dNTP on a random basis. This means that in any one reaction mixture, there will be many chains of varying lengths, which, when pooled together, represent the total collection of fragments that could terminate at that base. The DNA chains of differing lengths can be separated by electrophoresis on denaturing polyacrylamide gels. These gels allow DNA fragments that differ by only one nucleotide in length to be separated and, if the reaction involves a labeled group, either a dNTP or the primer, then electrophoresis of the four reactions in parallel, with subsequent autoradiography, will allow the sequence of the DNA to be determined (Fig. 34.19). In general, this method can produce sequence data for the 300–500 bases downstream of the sequencing primer, but some protocols permit analysis of much longer sequences.

The chain termination method can be modified by replacing radioactive groups with fluorescence-labeled primers, which then allow sensitive monitoring of each DNA fragment as it reaches the bottom of the gel. This process lends itself to automation (Fig. 34.19).

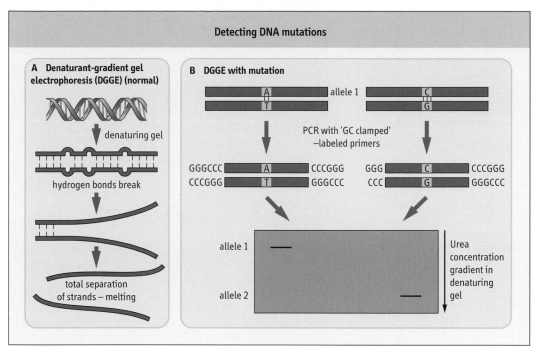

Detecting DNA mutations

A   Denaturant-gradient gel electrophoresis (DGGE) (normal)

denaturing gel

hydrogen bonds break

total separation of strands – melting

B   DGGE with mutation

allele 1

PCR with 'GC clamped' –labeled primers

GGGCCC [A] CCCGGG   GGG [C] CCCGGG
CCCGGG [T] GGGCCC   CCC [G] GGGCCC

allele 1

allele 2

Urea concentration gradient in denaturing gel

Fig. 34.18 **DGGE method to detect DNA mutations.** (A) As double-stranded DNA migrates through a gel containing a gradient of increasing concentration of denaturants, e.g. urea breaks hydrogen bonds between the two strands. At a point unique to that particular DNA, all the hydrogen bonds will be broken and the two strands separate – the so-called melting point. If the nucleotide sequence of a DNA is changed, e.g. by a mutation, the melting point of the DNA will be altered and thus the mobility of the DNA in the gel will be altered, allowing the change to be detected by autoradiography. (B) DGGE with mutation. In this case, a single A > C substitution has occurred. This increases the number of hydrogen bonds between the two strands and alters the mobility in the denaturant gradient. The difference in mobility through the gel only highlights the difference in the two strands' nucleotide sequence – it does not say what or where the difference is.

 ## REVERSE TRANSCRIPTASE-PCR

From whole blood, or pathologic tissue, cDNA for a gene can be prepared by the process of reverse transcription. Reverse transcription uses a reverse transcriptase enzyme to polymerize a DNA molecule complementary to the mRNA molecule, using a single poly T primer, which binds to the mRNA at its 3′ poly A tail. The reverse transcriptase proceeds along the mRNA to manufacture a complementary strand, cDNA. The resulting cDNA is then used as a template for PCR where the entire cDNA can be amplified to produce a DNA molecule containing the entire coding sequence of a gene. Clearly in some cases, gene expression is tissue-specific and one would not expect some mRNAs to be present in blood, e.g. dystrophin from muscle. However, ectopic transcription of genes occurs in white blood cells at a low level and allows analysis of transcripts of genes not normally expressed. This can be useful if the desired transcript is derived from a tissue that is not easily accessible or if study of the cDNA can give definitive information about the presence of a mutation.

The cDNA can then be incorporated into a cell-based cloning vector for further amplification or can be introduced into a cellular expression system to produce the gene product *in vitro*. Such methods are used increasingly in the study of the functional aspects of mutant gene products.

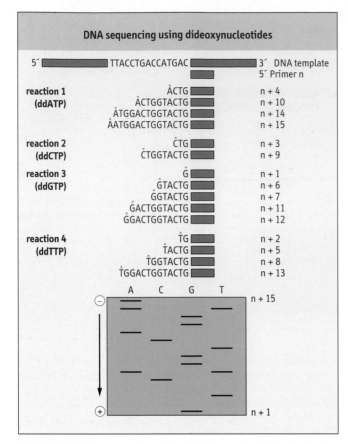

Fig. 34.19 **DNA sequencing using dideoxynucleotides.** A single reaction involving the DNA template and primer will proceed until a ddNTP is incorporated into the chain at random. This halts the reaction and that particular chain can grow no longer. Four reactions are performed in parallel, and each reaction is identical other than the ddNTP that is included, ddATP, ddCTP, ddGTP, and ddNTP. Each reaction generates hundreds of different reaction products with the same 5′ end, the sequencing primer, but differing 3′ ends. The length of the 3′ end will vary from 1 to over 300 bases depending on when a ddNTP was incorporated into the chain. In order to visualize the sequence a radiolabeled dNTP is added to all four reactions to facilitate autoradiography. Once completed, the four reactions are electrophoresized simultaneously on a polyacrylamide gel and the resultant autoradiograph is read and the sequence determined.

REAL-TIME PCR

It is sometimes necessary to quantify amounts of RNA or DNA in a clinical sample. For example, in cases of human immunodeficiency virus (HIV) infection, knowledge of the amount of viral RNA in the bloodstream can be a valuable guide to prognosis and treatment. In standard PCR reactions, one usually examines the DNA produced after 30 or more cycles, when it has been amplified 1 000 000 000 times or more. This is a useful qualitative test, but is not good for quantification. For example, the amount of PCR products approximately doubles each cycle so small differences in efficiency at earlier cycles result in large differences at later cycles. In addition, all reactions eventually reach a plateau phase due to many reasons, including the accumulation of end-products that inhibit the reaction, and many reactions will have reached plateau phase before 30 cycles. To circumvent many of these problems, real-time PCR machines have been developed which measure how much product is formed at very early stages in the reaction when it is proceeding at the maximal rate. If there is more target DNA in a particular sample, fewer cycles will be needed to make a defined amount of product, so the number of cycles needed to make a defined amount of product is a measure of how much of that DNA sequence was present at the beginning of the PCR. In real-time PCR, the formation of product is followed either by using a dye which fluoresces brightly when bound to double-stranded DNA, or by using some form of fluorescently-labeled hybridization probe. The amount of product is measured continuously at the end of every PCR cycle, e.g. by measuring fluorescence, using a probe that intercalates into double-stranded DNA and changes or increases its fluorescence on binding. Sensitive optics and powerful electronics are used so that very small amounts of product can be detected at early cycles and the process can easily be automated. This is a convenient way to quantify accurately, sensitively and quickly small amounts of DNA or RNA (which must first be transcribed to cDNA) and the technology is rapidly moving from research laboratories to clinical applications.

Summary

There are a myriad of DNA techniques available for the analysis of every aspect of DNA metabolism and function. However, regardless of the complexity of the methods, they all rely on the basic principles of hybridization and polymerization by appropriate enzymes. There is no doubt that the most significant recent advance in the study of DNA has been the discovery and automation of PCR. PCR is now used widely in all aspects of biomedical research, in particular, the study of human genetics. Whether in the diagnostic laboratory, or in the search for new disease genes, analysis has been totally transformed by PCR. There are now many hundreds of human genetic diseases whose diagnosis can be made by a single PCR-based method on DNA from a single blood sample. In many cases the PCR-based diagnosis has replaced complex biochemical tests or allowed a definitive diagnostic test to be available for the first time, e.g. in Huntington's disease. As a result of the expansion of the use of PCR and the versatility of PCR-based techniques, the use of Southern blotting and RFLPs has decreased. However, the basic principles of Southern blotting are at the center of all protocols that require radioactive labels to identify the reaction products, and an understanding of the principle of probe–target hybridization is essential.

The virtual completion of the Human Genome Project, within just 50 years of the discovery of the three dimensional structure of DNA, stands as one of mankind's great achievements. Of course this vastly simplifies the study of both normal and mutant genes, since the information to design PCR primers and to predict restriction enzyme cut-sites is now available for all genes. Recombinant DNA technology has replaced complex biochemical assays as the major biological scientific technology in most laboratories. The subject is continually evolving, but at its center are several key principles that are modified to fit the application of a particular method. Understanding these key steps is the key to grasping the seemingly abstract nature of some of the newer techniques.

ACTIVE LEARNING

1. A 14-year-old female patient appeared to be undergoing normal sexual development, except for rather scant body hair. Her complaint was that she has never had a menstrual period. Physical examination indicated a very short vagina ending in a blind pouch. How could you use the human genome sequence to design primer pairs that would amplify exons of the androgen receptor to check for possible mutations that could account for androgen insensitivity syndrome?
2. New human pathogenic viruses appear with some regularity. If you were in charge of a large research group, how could you apply cell-based cloning techniques to establish the sequence of a new viral DNA and then suggest possible viral proteins that could be expressed to use in a recombinant vaccine?
3. An unsorted collection of clones derived from the DNA of an organism is called a genomic library. Similarly, an unsorted collection of clones derived from the mRNA of a particular tissue is termed a cDNA library. Why are cDNA libraries most useful if the goal is to express a specific human pituitary protein in yeast cells, but a genomic library would be required if the aim was to characterize binding sites for transcription factors in the promoter of the same gene?

Further reading

Braude P, Pickering S, Flinter F, Ogilvie CM. Preimplantation genetic diagnosis. *Nat Rev Genet* 2002;**3**:941–953.

Chance RE, Frank BH. Research, development, production, and safety of biosynthetic human insulin. *Diabetes Care* 1993;**16** Suppl 3:133–142.

Cockerill FR. Application of rapid-cycle real-time polymerase chain reaction for diagnostic testing in the clinical microbiology laboratory. *Arch Pathol Lab Med* 2003;**127**:1112–1120.

Copland JA, Davies PJ, Shipley GL, Wood CG, Luxon BA, Urban RJ. The use of DNA microarrays to assess clinical samples: the transition from bedside to bench to bedside. *Recent Prog Horm Res* 2003;**58**:25–53.

Guo, OM. DNA microarray and cancer. *Curr Opin Oncol* 2003;**5**:36–43.

Ivnitski D, O'Neil DJ, Gattuso A, Schlicht R, Calidonna M, Fisher R. Nucleic acid approaches for detection and identification of biological warfare and infectious disease agents. *Biotechniques* 2003;**35**:862–869.

Primrose SB, Twyman, R. Principles of Genome Analysis and Genomics. Oxford: Blackwell, 2002.

Tuzmen S, Schlechter AN. Genetic diseases of hemoglobin: diagnostic methods for elucidating beta-thalassemia mutations. *Blood Rev* 2001;**15**:19–29.

Relevant websites

http://www.ncbi.nlm.nih.gov National Center for Biotechnology Information: an entry site that leads to full genome sequences for human and mouse as well as much other sequence-related information.

http://www.ensembl.org Sanger Center for Genome Analysis: An alternative presentation of data from human and mouse genomes.

http://health.nih.gov US National Institutes of Health: a portal to health related information. Look under "Genetics/Birth defects."

Institutional websites for Recombinant DNA:
  web.mit.edu/esgbio/www/rdna/rdnadir.html;
  www.genome.ou.edu/protocol_book/protocol_index.html;
  http://www.blc.arizona.edu/INTERACTIVE/recombinant3.dna/recombinant.html

35. Oxygen and Life

J W Baynes

LEARNING OBJECTIVES

After reading this chapter you should be able to:

- Explain the nature of reactive oxygen species (ROS), and identify the cellular sources of major ROS.
- Identify targets of reactive oxygen damage and describe the effects of ROS on biomolecules.
- Identify the major antioxidant enzymes, vitamins, and biomolecules that provide protection against ROS damage.
- Describe the role of reactive oxygen in regulatory biology and immunological defenses.
- Explain the role of ROS in development of chronic and inflammatory diseases.

IRON OVERLOAD INCREASES RISK FOR DIABETES AND CARDIOMYOPATHY

Patient with hematologic disorders such as hereditary hemochromatosis, thalassemias and sickle cell disease, or who receive frequent blood transfusions, gradually develop iron overload, a condition that increases the risk for development of cardiomyopathy and diabetes. The heart and β-cells are iron-rich in the mitochondria. The development of secondary disease in iron overload is considered the result of iron-mediated enhancement of mitochondrial ROS production in these tissues. Mutations in the mitochondrial genome may lead to progressive mitochondrial dysfunction.

INTRODUCTION

The element oxygen (O_2) is essential for the life of aerobic organisms. Although it is highly reactive in combustion reactions at high temperature, oxygen is relatively inert at body temperature; it has a high activation energy for oxidation reactions. This is fortunate, otherwise we might spontaneously combust. About 90% of our O_2 usage is committed to oxidative phosphorylation. Enzymes that use O_2 for hydroxylation and oxygenation reactions use another fraction of about 10%. A residual fraction, about 1%, is converted to reactive oxygen species (ROS), such as superoxide and hydrogen peroxide, which are inherently toxic, reactive forms of oxygen. ROS are important in metabolism – some enzymes use H_2O_2 as a substrate – and they play a role in regulation of metabolism and in immunological defenses against infection. However, ROS are also a source of chronic damage to tissue biomolecules. One of the risks of harnessing O_2 as a substrate for energy metabolism is that we may, and do, get burned. For this reason, we have a range of antioxidant defenses that protect us against ROS. This chapter will deal with the biochemistry of reactive oxygen, the mechanisms of formation and detoxification of ROS, and their role in human biology.

THE INERTNESS OF OXYGEN

In most textbooks, oxygen is shown as a diatomic molecule with two bonds between the oxygen atoms. This is an attractive presentation, from the viewpoint of the electron dot structures and electron pairing to form chemical bonds, but it is incorrect. In fact, at body temperature, O_2 is a biradical, a molecule with two unpaired electrons (Fig. 35.1). These electrons have parallel spins and are unpaired. Since most organic oxidation reactions, e.g. the oxidation of an alkane to an alcohol or an aldehyde to an acid, are two-electron oxidation reactions, O_2 is generally not very reactive. In fact, O_2 is completely stable in the presence of H_2, a strong reducing agent, until enough heat is provided to flip an O_2 electron and initiate the combustion reaction. Once it is started, the combustion provides the heat needed to propagate the reaction, sometimes explosively.

Metabolic reactions are conducted at body temperature, far below the temperature required to activate free oxygen. In biological redox reactions involving O_2, the oxygen is activated by redox active metal ions, such as iron and copper. All enzymes that use O_2 *in vivo* are metalloenzymes and, in fact, even the oxygen transport proteins, hemoglobin and myoglobin, contain iron in the form of heme. These metal ions provide one electron at a time to oxygen, activating O_2 for

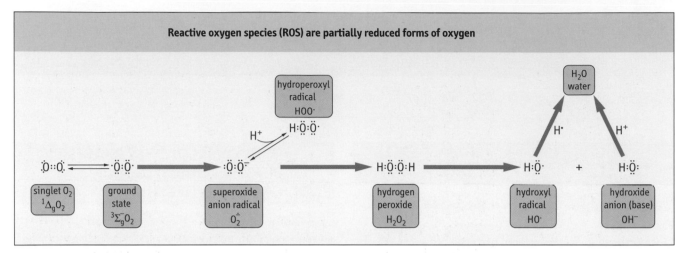

Reactive oxygen species (ROS) are partially reduced forms of oxygen

Fig. 35.1 **Structure of oxygen and reactive oxygen species (ROS).** Oxygen is shown at the far left as the incorrect double-bonded diatomic form. This form, known as singlet oxygen, exists to a significant extent only at high temperature or in response to irradiation. The diradical is the natural, ground-state form of O_2 at body temperature. ROS are partially reduced, reactive forms of oxygen. The first product is the anion radical, superoxide ($O_2^•$), which is in equilibrium with the weak acid, hydroperoxyl radical (pKa ≈ 4.5). Reduction of superoxide yields hydroperoxide O_2^{-2}, in the form of H_2O_2. Reduction of H_2O_2 causes a hemolytic cleavage reaction that releases hydroxyl radical ($OH^•$) and hydroxide ion (OH^-). Water is the end product of complete reduction of O_2.

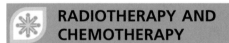 ## RADIOTHERAPY AND CHEMOTHERAPY

Applications of reactive oxygen

Exposure to radiation from nuclear explosions or accidents, or breathing or ingestion of radioactive elements, such as Strontium-90 or radon gas, produces a flux of ROS in the body, causing mutations in DNA. Radiation therapy uses a focused beam of high-energy electrons or γ-rays from an X-ray or Cobalt-60 source to destroy tumor tissue. The radiation produces a flux of hydroxyl radicals (from water) and organic radicals at the site of the tumor, oxidizing and destroying the DNA of the tumor cell. Irradiation of food is also used as a method of sterilization to destroy bacterial and viral contaminants or destroy insect infestations in order preserve food products during long-term storage.

 ## ISCHEMIA/REPERFUSION INJURY

A patient suffered a severe myocardial infarction, which was treated with tissue plasminogen activator, a clot-dissolving (thrombolytic) enzyme. During the days following hospitalization, the patient experienced palpitations, irregular rapid heartbeat, associated with weakness and faintness. The patient was treated with anti-arrhythmic agents.

Comment. Ischemia, meaning limited blood flow, is a condition in which a tissue is deprived of oxygen and nutrients. There is growing evidence that damage to heart tissue occurs not during the hypoxic or ischemic phase, but during reoxygenation of the tissue. This type of damage occurs following coronary occlusion, transplantation, and cardiovascular surgery. It is generally accepted that ROS play a major role in reperfusion injury. When cells are deprived of oxygen, they must rely on anaerobic glycolysis and glycogen stores for ATP synthesis. NADH and lactate accumulate, and all of the components of the mitochondrial electron transport system are saturated with electrons, because they cannot be transferred to oxygen. The mitochondrial membrane potential is increased, and when oxygen is reintroduced, great quantities of ROS are rapidly produced, overwhelming the scavenging mechanisms. ROS flood throughout the cell, damaging membrane lipids, DNA and other vital cellular constituents, leading to necrosis. There is considerable research on the evaluation of antioxidant supplements to protect tissues prior to transplantation, during surgery and during recovery from ischemia.

metabolism. Because iron and copper, and sometimes manganese and other ions, activate oxygen, these redox-active metal ions are present at very low (sub-micromolar) free concentrations *in vivo*. Normally, they are tightly sequestered in inactive form in storage or transport proteins, and they are locally activated at the active sites of enzymes where oxidation chemistry can be contained and focused on a specific substrate. Free redox-active metal ions are dangerous in biological systems because, in free form, they activate O_2.

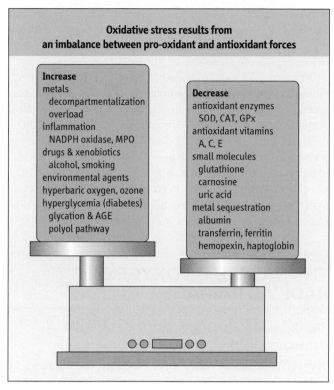

Fig. 35.2 **Oxidative stress: an imbalance between pro-oxidant and antioxidant systems.** As described in this chapter, numerous factors contribute to the enhancement and inhibition of oxidative stress. AGE, advanced glycation end-product; CAT, catalase; GPx, glutathione peroxidase; MPO, myeloperoxidase.

 TOXICITY OF HYPEROXIA

Supplemental oxygen therapy may be used for treatment of patients with hypoxemia, respiratory distress, or following exposure to poisons, such as carbon monoxide. Under normobaric conditions, the fraction of oxygen in air can be increased to nearly 100% using a facial mask or nasal cannula. However, patients develop chest pain, cough and alveolar damage within a few hours of exposure to 100% oxygen. Edema gradually develops and compromises pulmonary function, leading eventually to pulmonary fibrosis. The damage results from production of ROS in the lung. Rats can be protected from oxygen toxicity by gradually increasing the oxygen tension over a period of days. During this time, superoxide dismutase in lung tissue is induced and provides increased protection against oxygen toxicity.

The lung is not the only tissue affected by hyperoxia. Premature infants, especially those with acute respiratory distress syndrome (Chapter 26), often require supplemental oxygen for survival. During the 1950s, it was recognized that the high oxygen concentration used in incubators for premature infants increased the risk for blindness, resulting from retinopathy of prematurity (retrolental fibroplasia).

REACTIVE OXYGEN SPECIES (ROS) AND OXIDATIVE STRESS (OxS)

ROS are reactive, strongly oxidizing forms of oxygen (Fig. 35.1)

Oxidative stress (OxS) is defined as a condition in which the rate of generation of ROS exceeds our ability to protect ourselves against them, resulting in an increase in oxidative damage to biomolecules (Fig. 35.2). OxS is a characteristic feature of inflammatory diseases in which cells of the immune system produce ROS in response to challenge. OxS may be localized, for instance in the joints in arthritis or in the vascular wall in atherosclerosis (see Boxes), or can be systemic, e.g. in systemic lupus erythematosus (SLE), and possibly diabetes.

Among the ROS, OH• is the most reactive and damaging species; its half-life, measured in nanoseconds, is diffusion-limited, i.e. determined by the time to collision with a target biomolecule. The hydroperoxy radical (HOO•) and H_2O_2 are small, uncharged molecules that readily penetrate membranes. At physiological pH, HOO• represents only a small fraction of total $O_2^{\bullet}$ (about 0.1%), but this radical is intermediate in reactivity, between $O_2^{\bullet}$ and OH•. Myeloperoxidase in the macrophage catalyzes the reaction of H_2O_2 with Cl⁻ to produce another ROS, hypochlorous acid (HOCl).

ROS are formed by three major mechanisms *in vivo*: by reaction of oxygen with 'decompartmentalized' metal ions (Fig. 35.3); as a side reaction of electron transport (Fig. 35.4); or by normal enzymatic reactions, e.g. by the monoamine oxidase involved in dopamine metabolism (Chapter 18) and fatty acid oxidases in the peroxisome (Chapter 14).

REACTIVE NITROGEN SPECIES (RNS)

Nitric oxide synthases catalyze the production of the free radical, nitric oxide (NO•) from the amino acid L-arginine. NO•, known as the endothelium derived relaxation factor (EDRF), is an important signaling molecule with neurotransmitter activity. It has a role in the regulation of vascular tone (Chapter 17, p. 236), and is now thought to be an important regulator of the electron transport system. NO• competes with O_2 for cytochrome c oxidase (complex IV), and decreases the membrane potential by inhibiting proton pumping and ATP production. At high levels of NO•, complex IV is strongly inhibited, and ROS production is increased.

NO• reacts with $O_2^{\bullet}$ to form the strong oxidant, peroxynitrite (ONOO⁻), an RNS which has many of the strong

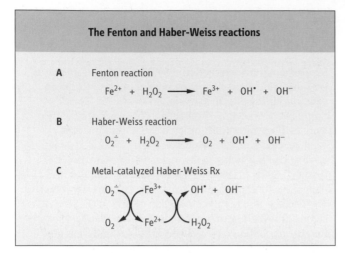

The Fenton and Haber-Weiss reactions

A   Fenton reaction

$$Fe^{2+} + H_2O_2 \longrightarrow Fe^{3+} + OH^{\bullet} + OH^{-}$$

B   Haber-Weiss reaction

$$O_2^{\cdot -} + H_2O_2 \longrightarrow O_2 + OH^{\bullet} + OH^{-}$$

C   Metal-catalyzed Haber-Weiss Rx

Fig. 35.3 **Formation of ROS by the Fenton and Haber-Weiss reactions.** (A) Fenton first described the oxidizing power of solutions of Fe^{2+} and H_2O_2. This reaction generates the strong oxidant $OH^{\bullet}$. Cu^{+} catalyzes the same reaction. (B) The Haber–Weiss reaction describes the production of $OH^{\bullet}$ from $O_2^{\cdot}$ and H_2O_2. (C) Under physiological conditions, the Haber–Weiss reaction is catalyzed by redox-active metal ions.

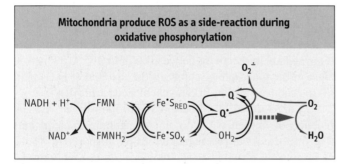

Mitochondria produce ROS as a side-reaction during oxidative phosphorylation

Fig. 35.4 **Formation of superoxide by mitochondria.** After the oxidation of NADH, the electron transport chain catalyzes single-electron redox reactions. The semiquinone radical, an intermediate in the reduction of Q to QH₂ by Complex I or II, is sensitive to oxidation by molecular oxygen and is considered a major source of superoxide radicals in the cell. This reaction is enhanced at high oxygen tension and also at high membrane potentials, when the electron transport chain is saturated with electrons, e.g. at low oxygen tension during ischemia-reperfusion injury (see Box).

oxidizing properties of $OH^{\bullet}$, but has a longer biological half-life. $ONOO^{-}$ is a potent nitrating agent, and there is some evidence that $ONOOH$ degrades, in part, by homolytic cleavage to produce two reactive species, $OH^{\bullet}$ and $NO_2^{\bullet}$. Simultaneous production of $NO^{\bullet}$ and $O_2^{\bullet}$, with the concomitant increase in $ONOO^{-}$ and a decrease in $NO^{\bullet}$, is thought to limit vasodilatation and cause inflammation of the vascular wall during

ischemia-reperfusion injury, setting the stage for vascular disease. $NO_2^{\bullet}$, another RNS with strong oxidizing and nitrating activity, is formed by eosinophil peroxidase or myeloperoxidase catalyzed oxidation of $NO^{\bullet}$ by H_2O_2.

ROS and RNS induce oxidative, chemical (nonenzymatic) damage to biomolecules. Damage to proteins is often site-specific, occurring at sites of metal binding to proteins, suggesting that metal-oxo complexes participate in ROS-mediated damage *in vivo*. As described later in this chapter, we have a range of antioxidant defenses against ROS, involving chelation of metal ions, enzymatic inactivation of ROS, trapping or degrading of ROS and intermediate reactive oxidation products by small molecules, vitamins and enzymes, and, in some cases, repair processes.

THE NATURE OF OXYGEN RADICAL DAMAGE

The hydroxyl radical is, by far, the most damaging ROS

The hydoxyl radical reacts with biomolecules primarily by hydrogen abstraction and addition reactions. Characteristic products, described as biomarkers of oxidative stress, are formed in these reactions. One of the most sensitive sites of free radical damage is the cell membrane, which is rich in readily oxidized polyunsaturated fatty acids (PUFA). Peroxidative damage to cell membranes affects the integrity and function of the membrane, compromising the cell's ability to maintain ion gradients and membrane phospholipid asymmetry.

As shown in Fig. 35.5, $OH^{\bullet}$ abstracts a hydrogen atom from a PUFA, setting off a chain of lipid peroxidation reactions. Lipid peroxides formed in this reaction degrade to form characteristic products, such as malondialdehyde (MDA) and hydroxynonenal (HNE). These compounds react with proteins to form adducts and crosslinks, known as advanced lipoxidation end-products (ALE). MDA and HNE adducts to lysine residues have been measured in lipoproteins in the vascular wall in atherosclerosis (Chapter 17) and in neuronal plaque in Alzheimer's disease (Chapter 42), implicating oxidative stress and damage in the pathogenesis of these diseases.

Hydroxyl radicals also react by addition to phenylalanine, tyrosine and nucleic acids to form characteristic hydroxylated derivatives and crosslinks (Fig. 35.6). Other ROS and RNS leave tell-tale tracks, such as nitro- and chloro-tyrosine, formed from ONOOH and HOCl, respectively, and methionine sulfoxide, formed by reaction of H_2O_2 or HOCl with methionine residues in proteins (Fig. 35.6). Nitrotyrosine, like ALEs, is increased in atherosclerotic and Alzheimer's plaques.

ROS also react with carbohydrates to form dicarbonyl compounds that react with protein to form crosslinks and

Pathway of lipid peroxidation

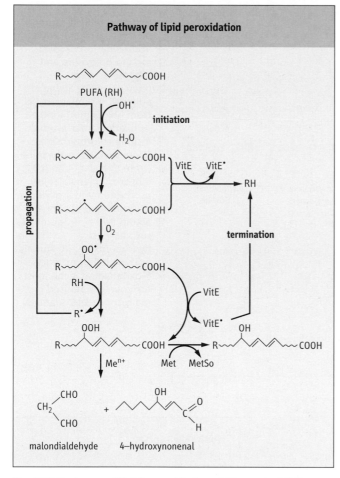

Fig. 35.5 **Pathway of lipid peroxidation.** OH• attacks PUFA, forming a carbon-centered lipid radical. The radical rearranges to form a conjugated dienyl radical. This radical reacts with ambient O₂, forming a hydroperoxyl radical, which then abstracts a hydrogen from a neighboring lipid, forming a lipid peroxide and starting a chain reaction. This reaction continues until the supply of PUFA is exhausted, unless a termination reaction occurs. Vitamin E (discussed below) is the major chain-terminating antioxidant in membranes; it reduces both the conjugated dienyl and hydroperoxyl radicals, quenching the chain or cycle of lipid peroxidation reactions. Lipid peroxides may also be reduced by methionine residues in lipoproteins, forming methionine sulfoxide and lipid alcohols. Otherwise, they decompose to form a range of 'reactive carbonyl species' such as malondialdehyde and hydroxynonenal, which react with protein to form advanced lipoxidation end-products (ALE), which are biomarkers of oxidative stress. The reaction scheme shown here for PUFA also occurs with intact phospholipids and cholesterol esters in lipoproteins and cell membranes.

adducts, known as glycoxidation products or advanced glycation end-products (AGE). AGE are increased in tissue proteins in diabetes as a result of hyperglycemia and oxidative stress, and the increase in chemical modification of proteins by AGE and ALE is implicated in the development of diabetic vascular, renal, and retinal complications (see also Chapter 42).

 ## SENTINEL FUNCTION OF METHIONINE

Methionine (Met) residues are located on the surface of proteins and are easily oxidized to methionine sulfoxide (MetSO) by H_2O_2 or HOCl. Met is generally on the surface of proteins and rarely has a role in the active site mechanism of action of enzymes. However, there is evidence that Met serves as an 'antioxidant pawn', protecting the active site of enzymes. Half of the Met residues of glutamine synthetase could be oxidized without affecting the enzyme's specific activity. These residues were physically arranged in an array that guarded the entrance to the active site. MetSO can be reduced back to methionine by the enzyme methionine sulfoxide reductase, providing a catalytic amplification of the antioxidant potential of each methionine residue. In addition to its scavenging role, there is evidence that oxidation of Met may be involved in the regulation of enzyme activity and targeting enzymes for proteolytic degradation.

 ## GLUTATHIONYLATION OF PROTEIN

S-glutathionylation or S-glutathiolation of proteins describes the formation of a disulfide bond between GSH and an –SH group on a target protein. S-thiolation of proteins is induced by both ROS and RNS and is thought to have a dual role in protecting cysteine against irreversible oxidation during oxidative stress and in modulating cellular metabolism (redox regulation). Target proteins include a wide range of regulatory enzymes with active site –SH groups, such as protein kinases and transcription factors. S-thiolation also appears to protect proteins against ubiquitin-mediated proteasomal degradation. It is reversed by nonenzymatic reduction by GSH or by enzymes using thiol protein cofactors (thioredoxin, glutaredoxin).

ANTIOXIDANT DEFENSES

There are several levels of protection against oxidative damage

ROS damage to lipids and proteins is addressed largely by degradation and re-synthesis. Oxidized proteins, for example, are preferred targets for proteasomal degradation (Chapter 32, Fig. 32.10), and damaged DNA is repaired by a number of excision–repair mechanisms (Chapter 30). The process is not perfect. Some proteins, such as collagens and crystallins, turn over slowly, so that damage accumulates and function may be impaired, *e.g.* age-dependent browning of lens proteins,

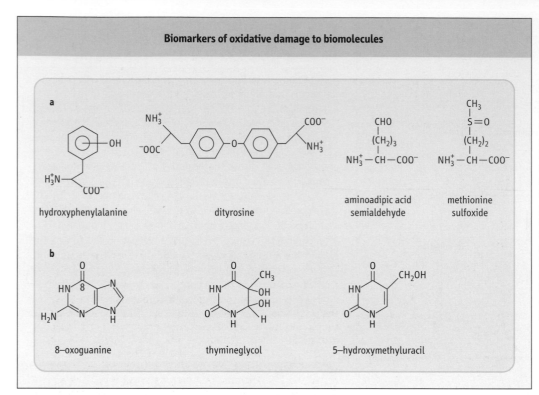

Biomarkers of oxidative damage to biomolecules

a

hydroxyphenylalanine   dityrosine   aminoadipic acid
semialdehyde   methionine
sulfoxide

b

8–oxoguanine   thymineglycol   5–hydroxymethyluracil

Fig. 35.6 **Products of hydroxyl radical damage to biomolecules.** (A) Amino acid oxidation products: *o*-, *m*- and *p*-tyrosine and dityrosine from phenylalanine; amino adipic acid semialdehyde from lysine; methionine sulfoxide. Other products include chlorotyrosine (from HOCl), nitrotyrosine (from ONOO-•— and NO_2•, dihydroxyphenylalanine produced by hydroxylation of tyrosine, and aliphatic amino acid hydroperoxides, such as leucine hydroperoxide. (B) Nucleic acid oxidation products: 8-oxoguanine is the most commonly measured indicator of DNA damage.

crosslinking of collagen and elastin, and loss of elasticity or changes in permeability of the vascular wall and renal basement membrane (see Chapter 42). The association between chronic inflammation and cancer also indicates that ROS cause some residual damage to the genome in the form of mutations in DNA.

Our first line of defense against oxidative damage is sequestration or chelation of redox-active metal ions

These chelators include a number of metal-binding proteins that sequester iron and copper in inactive form, such as transferrin and ferritin, the transport and storage forms of iron. Hemopexin binds heme, a lipid-soluble form of iron, which catalyzes ROS formation in lipid environments; it delivers the heme to the liver for catabolism. Haptoglobin binds to hemoglobin and decreases the pro-oxidant activity of hemoglobin and delivers the intact hemoglobin molecule to the liver for catabolism. Albumin, the major plasma protein, has a strong binding site for copper and effectively inhibits copper-catalyzed oxidation reactions in plasma. Carnosine (β-alanyl-L-histidine) and related peptides are present in muscle and brain at millimolar concentrations; they are potent copper chelators and may have a role in intracellular antioxidant protection.

Despite efficient chelation of metals, ROS are formed in the body and do cause chemical damage. In these cases, there are a group of enzymes that act to detoxify the precursors of

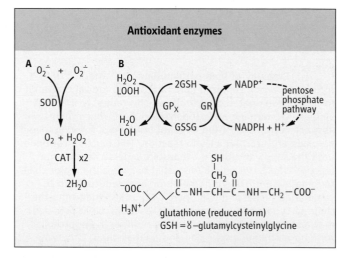

Antioxidant enzymes

Fig. 35.7 **Enzymatic defenses against ROS.** (A) SOD and CAT are dismutases, catalyzing oxidation and reduction of separate substrate molecules; both are highly specific for their substrates, O_2• and H_2O_2, respectively. (B) GPx reduces H_2O_2 and lipid peroxides (LOOH), using GSH as a co-substrate. The GSH is recycled by glutathione reductase (GR) using NADPH from the pentose phosphate pathway. (C) Structure of GSH.

hydroxyl radicals. These include superoxide dismutase (SOD), catalase (CAT), and glutathione peroxidase (GPx) (Fig 35.7). CAT, which inactivates H_2O_2, is found largely in peroxisomes, the major site of H_2O_2 generation in the cell. SOD converts O_2• to the less toxic H_2O_2. There are two classes of SOD, an

ANTIOXIDANT DEFENSES IN THE RED BLOOD CELL (RBC)

The RBC does not use oxygen for metabolism, nor is it involved in phagocytosis. However, because of the high O_2 tension in arterial blood and heme iron content, ROS are formed continuously in the RBC. Hb spontaneously produces superoxide ($O_2^•$) in a side reaction associated with binding of O_2. The occasional reduction of O_2 to $O_2^•$ is accompanied by oxidation of Hb to methemoglobin (ferrihemoglobin), a rust-brown protein that does not bind or transport O_2. Methemoglobin may release heme, which reacts with $O_2^•$ and H_2O_2 to produce hydroxyl radical ($OH^•$) and reactive iron–oxo species. These ROS initiate lipid peroxidation reactions which can lead to loss of membrane integrity and cell death. The RBC is well-fortified with antioxidant defenses to protect itself against oxidative stress. These include catalase (CAT), superoxide dismutase (SOD) and glutathione peroxidase (GPx), as well as a methemoglobin reductase activity that reduces methemoglobin back to normal ferrohemoglobin. Normally, less than 1% of Hb is present as methemoglobin. Persons with congenital methemoglobinemia, resulting from methemoglobin reductase deficiency, typically have a dark and cyanotic appearance. Treatment with large doses of ascorbate (vitamin C) is used to reduce their methemoglobin to functional hemoglobin.

GSH, present at a concentration of approximately 2 mmol/L in the RBC, not only supports antioxidant defenses, but is also an important sulfhydryl buffer, maintaining –SH groups in hemoglobin and enzymes in the reduced state. Under normal circumstances, when proteins are exposed to O_2, their sulfhydryl groups gradually oxidize to form disulfides, either intramolecularly or intermolecularly with other proteins. GSH nonenzymatically reverses these reactions, leading to regeneration of the sulfhydryl group.

MnSOD isozyme which is found in mitochondria, and CuZnSOD isozyme which is widely distributed throughout the cell. An extracellular, secreted glycoprotein isoform of CuZnSOD (EC-SOD) binds to proteoglycans in the vascular wall and is thought to protect against $O_2^•$ and $ONOO^−$ injury.

GPx is widely distributed in the cytosol and in the mitochondria and the nucleus. It reduces both H_2O_2 and lipid hydroperoxides to water and a lipid alcohol, respectively. It requires reduced glutathione (GSH) as a co-substrate. GSH is a tripeptide (Chapter 2) that is present at 1–5 mM concentration in all cells. The GSH is recycled by an NADPH-dependent enzyme GSH reductase. The NADPH, provided by the pentose phosphate pathway, maintains a $\approx100:1$ ratio of GSH:GSSG in the cell. GPx is actually a family of selenium-containing isozymes; a phospholipid hydroperoxide glutathione peroxidase will reduce lipid hydroperoxides in phospholipids in lipoproteins and membranes, while other

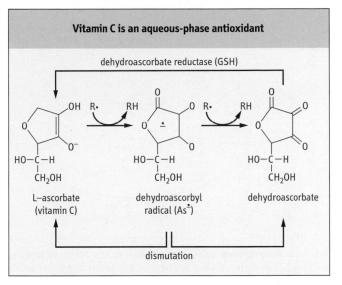

Fig. 35.8 **Antioxidant activity of ascorbate.** Vitamin C exists as the enolate anion at physiological pH. The enolate anion spontaneously reduces superoxide, organic ($R^•$) and vitamin E radicals, forming a dehydroascorbyl radical ($As^•$). Dehydroascorbate, formed by a second reduction reaction or by a dismutation reaction, is recycled by dehydroascorbate reductase, a GSH-dependent enzyme present in all cells. Dehydroascorbyl radical may also dismutate to ascorbate and dehydroascorbate.

PEROXIDASE ACTIVITY FOR DETECTION OF OCCULT BLOOD

Peroxidases, such as the glutathione peroxidase (GPx), are enzymes that catalyze the oxidation of a substrate using H_2O_2. Hemoglobin and heme have a pseudo-peroxidase activity *in vitro*. In a test for occult blood, hemoglobin in a stool specimen oxidizes phenolic compounds in guaiac acid to quinones. A positive test is indicated by a blue stain along the edge of the fecal smear. Hemoglobin and myoglobin from animal meat will cause false positives as will many vegetables containing plant peroxidases. To eliminate false positives, the assay should be confirmed by retesting 48 hours later. Similar peroxidase-dependent assays are used to identify bloodstains at crime scenes.

isozymes require the free fatty acid or cholesterol ester hydroperoxide. There is also an isoform of GPx in intestinal epithelial cells, which is thought to have a role in detoxification of dietary hydroperoxides.

Three antioxidant vitamins, A, C, and E provide the third line of defense against oxidative damage. These vitamins, primarily vitamin C (ascorbate) (Fig. 35.8) in the aqueous phase and vitamin E (α- and γ-tocopherol; Fig. 35.9) in the lipid phase act as chain-breaking antioxidants (Fig. 35.5).

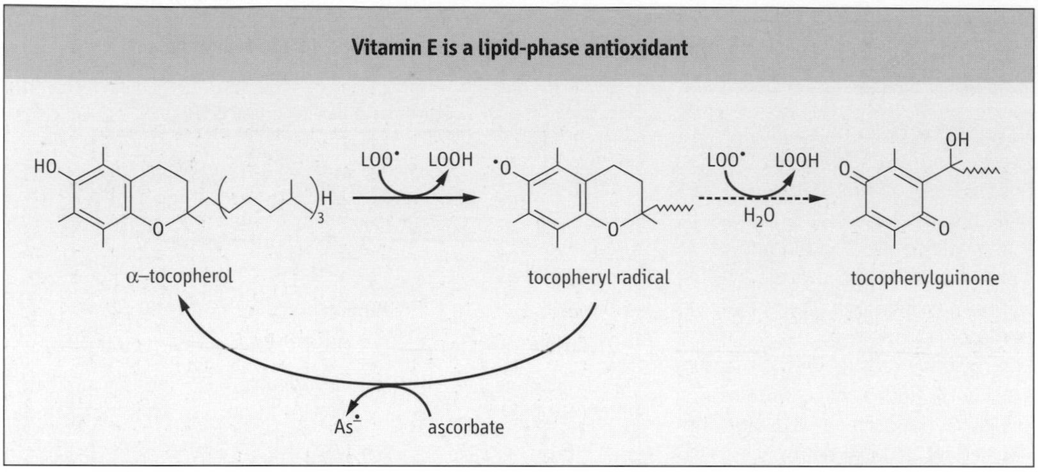

Fig. 35.9 **Antioxidant activity of vitamin E.** The term, vitamin E, refers to a family of related tocopherol and tocotrienol isomers with potent lipophilic antioxidant and membrane stabilizing activity (see Fig. 10.3). Tocopherols reduce lipid hydroperoxyl radicals and also inactivate singlet oxygen. α-tocopherol is the most effective form in humans and the major form of vitamin E in the diet. It consists of a chromanol ring structure with a polyisoprenoid side chain; the isoprene units are unsaturated in the tocatrienols. α, β, γ, and δ differ in the pattern of methyl groups at R_1, R_2 and R_3 (see Fig. 10.3). The major commercial form of vitamin E is α-tocopherol acetate, which is more stable than free tocopherol during storage. The tocopheryl radical, the major product formed during antioxidant action of vitamin E, is recycled by ascorbate. Tocopheryl quinone is also formed in small quantities.

✳ CELLULAR RESPONSE TO ROS

Cells adapt to oxidative stress by induction of antioxidant enzymes. Many of these are controlled by the antioxidant response elements (ARE), also known as the electrophilic responsive elements. The central regulator of the ARE-response is the transcription factor Nrf2, which on stimulation dissociates from its cytoplasmic inhibitor Keap1, translocates to the nucleus and transactivates ARE-dependent genes. Electrophilic lipid peroxidation products, such as hydroxynonenal and acrolein, are potent activators of ARE through modification of Keap1 thiol residues. Keap1 is also activated in response to electrophilic carcinogens that alkylate DNA. ARE-dependent enzymes include CAT and SOD, and other enzymes that catalyze the oxidation and conjugation of carcinogens and oxidants for excretion.

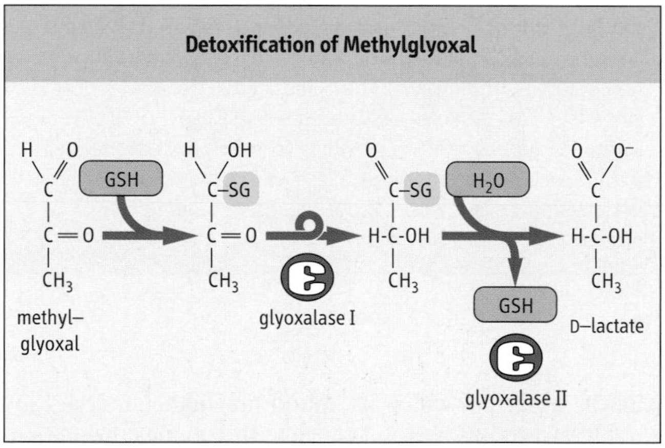

Fig. 35.10 **The glyoxalase system.** Glyoxalase I catalyzes the formation of a thiohemiacetal adduct between GSH and MGO and its rearrangement to a thioester. Glyoxalase II catalyzes the hydrolysis of the thioester forming D-lactate and regenerating GSH. Unlike GPx, this pathway does not consume GSH. MGO, methylglyoxal.

These vitamins are reducing agents; they donate a hydrogen atom ($H^\bullet$) to radical intermediates formed by reaction of ROS with biomolecules. The vitamin C and E radicals produced in this reaction are resonance-stabilized species; they do not propagate radical damage and are recycled, e.g. by dehydroascorbate reductase. Vitamin C reduces superoxide and lipid peroxyl radicals, but also has a special role in reduction and recycling of vitamin E. These antioxidants work together to inhibit lipid peroxidation reactions in plasma lipoproteins and membranes. In response to severe oxidative stress, vitamin E is maintained at constant concentration in the lipid phase until all of the vitamin C is consumed. Vitamin A (carotene; see Fig. 10.1) is a lipophilic antioxidant. Although best understood for its role in vision, it is a potent singlet oxygen scavenger and protects against damage from sunlight in the retina and skin.

THE GLYOXALASE PATHWAY: A SPECIAL ROLE FOR GLUTATHIONE

A small fraction of triose phosphates produced during metabolism spontaneously degrades to methylglyoxal (MGO), a reactive dicarbonyl sugar. MGO is also formed during metabolism of glycine and threonine, and as a product of nonenzymatic oxidation of carbohydrates and lipids; as such it is a significant precursor of advanced glycation and lipoxidation end-products (AGE/ALEs) (see Chapter 42). MGO reacts with amino, guanidino, imidazole, and sulfhydryl groups in proteins, leading to enzyme inactivation and protein crosslinking.

MGO is inactivated by enzymes of the glyoxalase pathway, a GSH-dependent system found in all cells in the body. The glyoxalase pathway (Fig. 35.10) consists of two enzymes that catalyze an internal redox reaction in which carbon-1 of MGO is oxidized from an aldehyde to a carboxylic acid group and carbon-2 is reduced from a ketone to a secondary alcohol. The end product, D-lactate, does not react with proteins (D-lactate is distinct from L-lactate, the product of glycolysis, but may be converted into L-lactate, for further metabolism). Levels of MGO and D-lactate are increased in blood of diabetic patients, because levels of glucose and glycolytic intermediates, including triose phosphates, are increased intracellularly in diabetes. The glyoxalase system also inactivates glyoxal, and is reactive with other dicarbonyl sugars produced by nonenzymatic oxidation of carbohydrates and lipids.

THE BENEFICIAL EFFECTS OF REACTIVE OXYGEN

As outlined in Fig. 35.11, the macrophage initiates a sequence of ROS producing reactions during a burst of oxygen consumption accompanying phagocytosis. NADPH oxidase in the macrophage plasma membrane is activated to produce $O_2^{\bullet}$ which is then converted to H_2O_2 by superoxide dismutase. The H_2O_2 is used by another macrophage enzyme, myeloperoxidase (MPO), to oxidize chloride ion, ubiquitous in body fluids, to hypochlorous acid (HOCl). H_2O_2 and HOCl mediate bactericidal activity by oxidative degradation of microbial lipids, proteins, and DNA. The macrophage has a high intracellular concentration of antioxidants, especially ascorbate, to protect itself during ROS production.

The consumption of O_2 by NADPH oxidase is responsible for the 'respiratory burst', the sharp increase in O_2 consumption for production of ROS, which accompanies phagocytosis. The end product of this reaction sequence, HOCl, is also the active oxidizer in chlorine-containing laundry bleaches. Before the advent of penicillin and other antibiotics, intravenous infusion of dilute HOCl solutions was actually used for treatment of bacterial sepsis in battlefield hospitals during World War I.

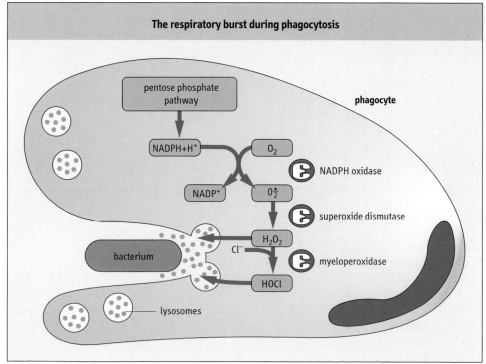

Fig. 35.11 **Generation and release of ROS during phagocytosis.** A cascade of reactions generating ROS is initiated during phagocytosis to kill invading organisms. Hydrolytic enzymes are also released from lysosomes to assist in degradation of microbial debris.

Summary

Reactive oxygen species (ROS) are the sparks of the oxidative metabolism. Oxidative stress is the price we pay for using oxygen. ROS and reactive nitrogen species (RNS), such as superoxide, peroxide, hydroxyl radical, and peroxynitrite, are reactive and toxic, sometimes difficult to contain, but their production is important for regulation of metabolism, turnover of biomolecules and protection against microbial infection. ROS and RNS cause oxidative damage to all classes of biomolecules: proteins, lipids and DNA. There are a number of protective antioxidant mechanisms, including sequestration of redox-active metal ions, enzymatic inactivation of major ROS, inactivation of organic radicals by small molecules, such as GSH and vitamins, and, when all else fails, repair or turnover. Biomarkers of oxidative stress are readily detected in tissues in inflammation, and oxidative stress is increasingly implicated in the pathogenesis of chronic disease.

ACTIVE LEARNING

1. Review the evidence that atherosclerosis is an inflammatory disease initiated by production of ROS in the vascular wall.
2. Discuss the evidence that hyperglycemia in diabetes induces a state of oxidative stress that leads to renal and vascular complications.
3. Review the data on use of antioxidants in therapy for atherosclerosis and diabetes. Based on these studies, how strong is the evidence that these diseases are the result of increased oxidative stress? What are the limitations of these studies?
4. Discuss recent advances in the use of antioxidants for tissue protection during cardiac surgery and transplantation.

Further reading

Aliev G, Smith MA, Seyidov D et al. The role of oxidative stress in the pathophysiology of cerebrovascular lesions in Alzheimer's disease. *Brain Pathol* 2002;**12**:21–35.

Baynes JW, Thorpe SR. Glycoxidation and lipoxidation in atherogenesis. *Free Radic Biol Med* 2000;**28**:1708–1716.

Cracowski JL, Durand T, Bessard G. Isoprostanes as a biomarker of lipid peroxidation in humans: physiology, pharmacology and clinical implications. *Trends Pharmacol Sci* 2002;**23**:360–666.

Janero DR. Ischemic heart disease and antioxidants: mechanistic aspects of oxidative injury and its prevention. *Crit Rev Food Sci Nutr* 1995 Jan;**35**(1–2):65–81.

Jollow DJ, McMillan DC. Oxidative stress, glucose-6-phosphate dehydrogenase and the red cell. *Adv Exp Med Biol* 2001;**500**:595–605.

Koutsilieri E, Scheller C, Grunblatt E, Nara K, Li J, Riederer P. Free radicals in Parkinson's disease. *J Neurol* 2002;**249** Suppl 2:1–5.

Kuroki T, Isshiki K, King GL. Oxidative stress: the lead or supporting actor in the pathogenesis of diabetic complications. *J Am Soc Nephrol* 2003;**14**(Suppl 3):S216–220.

Meagher EA. Treatment of atherosclerosis in the new millennium: is there a role for vitamin E? *Prev Cardiol* 2003;**6**:85–90.

Nedeljkovic ZS, Gokce N, Loscalzo J. Mechanisms of oxidative stress and vascular dysfunction. *Postgrad Med J* 2003;**79**:195–199.

Roberts LJ 2nd, Morrow JD. Products of the isoprostane pathway: unique bioactive compounds and markers of lipid peroxidation. *Cell Mol Life Sci* 2002;**59**:808–820.

Relevant websites

Antioxidants: http://www.nlm.nih.gov/medlineplus/antioxidants.html

Oxidative Stress and Aging Association: http://www.o2sa.org/O2SAHomepage/HomePage.htm

Reactive oxygen species and antioxidant vitamins: http://lpi.oregonstate.edu/f-w97/reactive.html

Society for Free Radical Biology and Medicine: http://www.sfrbm.org/

Virtual Free Radical School: http://www.medicine.uiowa.edu/FRRB/VirtualSchool/Virtual.html#S

The Immune Response

A Farrell

LEARNING OBJECTIVES

After reading this chapter you should be able to:

- Discuss, compare and contrast the nonspecific and the specific immune response.
- Describe the activation of the complement system.
- Outline the functions of cytokines and chemokines.
- Characterize the cellular and humoral elements of nonspecific and specific immune response.
- Describe the basis for antibody diversity.
- Define autoimmune response.

INTRODUCTION

The immune system consists of the tissues, cells and molecules, and genes involved in the recognition, reaction with, and elimination of, foreign and nonself substances (antigens) that may disturb the homeostasis of the body. Immunity can be categorized as being either nonspecific or innate, and specific and adaptive.

THE NONSPECIFIC IMMUNE RESPONSE

Nonspecific immunity is the body's first line of defense

Nonspecific immunity uses physicochemical barriers, such as the skin and mucosal epithelia, and their associated secreted products, e.g. sweat, mucus and acid. It also involves inflammatory response. Inflammation is the body's response to injury or tissue damage. Its purpose is to limit, and then repair, the damage brought about by any injurious agent. It involves the interaction of the microvasculature, circulating blood cells, other cells in the tissues, and their secreted products. The cells that line blood vessels, endothelium, play a major role in the vascular effects, such as increased permeability and vasodilatation. The cellular effects involve phagocytic and secretory responses of cells that usually circulate in the blood as well as of some that are tissue-based (Table 36.1).

Inflammatory mediators contribute to the immune response

All the cells involved can synthesize and secrete a wide variety of different types of soluble chemical substances termed inflammatory mediators. Since some of these mediators are present in the blood, they are also known as humoral components and include acute-phase reactants such as C-reactive protein (CRP) (see Chapter 3) and components of the complement system.

The complement system

Complement is activated in a series of sequential steps

The complement system consists of a series of proteins that are normally present in the inactive form. The components of the system are sequentially activated, in a cascade, after contact with surfaces or particles that have a specific molecular composition or configuration. Please refer to Figure 36.1 throughout the following explanation of complement activation:

- The activation of the first component leads to the unlocking of serine protease activity;
- The activation of the next component in the sequence is achieved by it being cleaved by the first component into two unequally sized fragments;
- The larger of the resulting fragments exhibits serine protease activity and attaches to the activating surface, while the smaller fragment has distinctive biologic activities, which include the facilitation of phagocytosis (termed opsonization), the attraction of cells (chemotaxis), and the stimulating degranulation of mast cells (anaphylatoxin activity);
- This series of activation events is then repeated with further early components, thereby creating a cascade effect;
- By activating the next component, the large enzymatically active fragment of the previous component is itself inactivated. When components further down the sequence – the so-called 'late' components of the pathway – are activated, instead of demonstrating enzyme activity they show the ability to coalesce with each other and with subsequently activated components, to form a multimolecular

Cells involved in inflammation		
Circulating		**Tissue based**
Polymorphonuclear leukocytes	neutrophil	
	eosinophil	
	basophil	
		mast cell
Mononuclear phagocytes	monocyte	macrophage
Lymphocytes		
Platelets		
Endothelial cells		

Table 36.1 **Cells involved in inflammation.**

complex that can breach the integrity of the bacterial surface that bears the molecular complex – which had activated the complement cascade in the first place.

Cytokines

Cytokines have several characteristics in common

Cytokines are soluble mediators of the inflammatory and immune response. They are produced by a variety of cells and tissues, are peptides or glycoproteins in nature, and are active at concentrations between 10^{-9}–10^{-15} molar. They act by interacting with receptors on the surfaces of their target cells. The majority act within short distances of the site of their production (paracrine action) or on the cells that produced them (autocrine action). A few, however, are capable of acting on cells distant to their site of production. They show significant overlap in their functions (redundancy) and they may act on multiple cell types (pleiotropy); they also have potential for interaction via the effects they mediate (for cytokine signaling, see Chapter 38).

Cytokines may be classified into families or by their principal effect

Cytokines can be grouped into families:

■ **interferons (IFNs):** while IFN-α and IFN-β have a role in protection against viral replication, IFN-g plays a significant part in regulating the specific immune response (SIR);

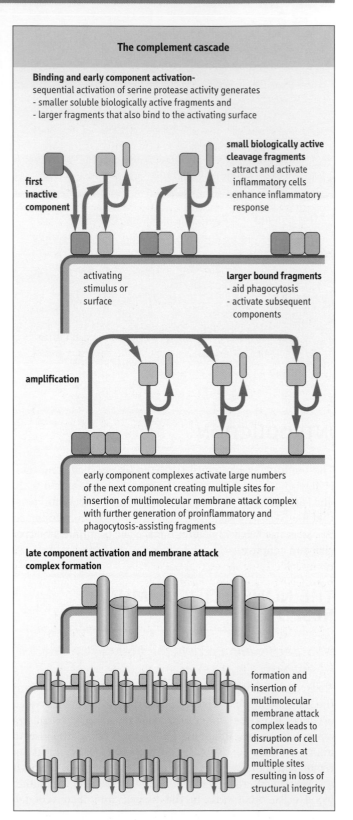

The complement cascade

Binding and early component activation- sequential activation of serine protease activity generates
- smaller soluble biologically active fragments and
- larger fragments that also bind to the activating surface

first inactive component

small biologically active cleavage fragments
- attract and activate inflammatory cells
- enhance inflammatory response

activating stimulus or surface

larger bound fragments
- aid phagocytosis
- activate subsequent components

amplification

early component complexes activate large numbers of the next component creating multiple sites for insertion of multimolecular membrane attack complex with further generation of proinflammatory and phagocytosis-assisting fragments

late component activation and membrane attack complex formation

formation and insertion of multimolecular membrane attack complex leads to disruption of cell membranes at multiple sites resulting in loss of structural integrity

Fig. 36.1 **The complement cascade.** Activating stimuli bear surfaces that trigger complement activation, and to which the activated component can attach itself. The late components of the cascade do not show enzymatic activity. Instead, they coalesce to form a polymeric macromolecule (the membrane attack complex), which can insert itself into the activating surface (the cell wall in the case of bacteria), breach its integrity and cause osmotic lysis.

- **interleukins (ILs):** currently there are in excess of 20 interleukins recognized, all of which participate in regulating the cells involved in both nonspecific and specific immune responses;
- **chemokines:** these are a family of cytokines that bring about chemokinesis – movement in response to chemical stimuli. Interest has increased dramatically in the receptors for these mediators since some appear to act as coreceptors for infection, in particular HIV infection of lymphocytes. Some overlap in activity with cytokines can be seen with IL-8 which demonstrates chemokine properties. In general cytokines are more practically grouped by their principal effects or roles, examples of which are shown below:
- **proinflammatory cytokines:** tumor necrosis factor (TNF)-α, IL-1, IL-6, IL-8 and other chemokines, IL-12 and IL-15;
- **anti-inflammatory:** transforming growth factor (TGF)-β and IL-10;
- **immunostimulatory:** for cellular responses IL-2 and IFN-γ; for humoral, including allergic, responses: IL-4, IL-13, TGF-b, and IL-10.

As will be seen later, the specific immune response is driven by direct cell interactions together with the effects of cytokines. Cells and soluble mediators of the nonspecific immune response participate in the initiation of these responses and then help to deal with the antigen.

Arachidonic acid metabolites

The prostaglandins (PGs) and leukotrienes (LTs) form another group of inflammatory mediators. On each stimulation, the nonspecific immune response follows the same sequence of nonspecific and stereotypical events.

THE SPECIFIC IMMUNE RESPONSE

The specificity of the immune response is achieved through special receptors that recognize antigen

The specific immune response is brought into play if the nonspecific defenses are unsuccessful, e.g. due to the persistence of the triggering agent. The specific response focuses on the individual antigen by using specific receptors that can be viewed as being individually tailored to the stimulating element. The antigen and receptors can be considered to have a 'hand-in-glove' relationship, fitting together in a unique three-dimensional manner. A prerequisite for such response is the ability of the system to distinguish between self and nonself. This is achieved by thymic education and self-tolerance.

ALLERGY TO BEE VENOM

A young man was brought into the emergency room in a state of shock with stridor and widespread urticaria. A companion told the admitting medic that the patient had just been stung by a bee. A diagnosis of anaphylaxis was made. An intramuscular injection of epinephrine was given promptly and also treatment with intravenous antihistamine, corticosteroid, and cardiorespiratory support. The man recovered.

Comment. While the physiologic role of the IgE response is considered to be protection against parasite infestation, this response is seen to be subverted in those who experience atopic diseases and anaphylaxis. The atopic diseases include allergic rhinitis, allergic conjunctivitis and asthma. The major fraction of IgE is bound via receptors to mast cells in the tissues. When antigen binds and crosslinks its specific IgE on the mast cells, it triggers the degranulation of the cells and release of preformed mediators (principally histamine), as well as the synthesis of other mediators, including arachidonic acid metabolites. The clinical effects depend on the location and/or extent of mast cell degranulation. When localized to one site, such as the nasal or bronchial mucosa, it usually gives rise to only localized reactions in the form of allergic rhinitis and asthma, respectively. If the degree of sensitization with the antigen-specific IgE and/or the antigenic burden is much greater, systemic degranulation can occur, with consequent anaphylactic shock. This is primarily due to the effects of the released mediators on vessels and vascular integrity. Significant vasodilation takes place, reducing the blood pressure. This is accompanied by large increases in vessel wall permeability, leading to shifts of fluid from the intravascular to the extracellular compartment and substantial swelling of any tissues with the capacity, which particularly affects the skin and other loose connective tissue such as those in the larynx. Smooth muscle spasm also occurs, leading to bronchoconstriction and contraction of the gut wall, with consequent marked respiratory difficulty and wheezing. These features are accompanied by increased secretory activity of seromucous glands in the respiratory and gastrointestinal tract as well as itching of the skin.

When a specific immune response is initiated, relatively few components are likely to be available that could react specifically with any chosen antigenic substance. There is a delay or lag period while these components increase to a level at which they can ensure elimination of the antigen, or at least reduce it to such a level that would be manageable by the nonspecific immune response. This delay can have disastrous consequences for the organism and its survival.

In addition to generating specificity, the specific immune response also employs a mechanism to remember a specific encounter so that if the same foreign or nonself substance is encountered again, it can be dealt with more quickly and effectively. Thus, in comparison to the nonspecific immune response, the specific immune response shows both the specificity for the foreign or nonself substance – the memory of the event.

Similarly to the nonspecific response, specific immune response is mediated by cellular and humoral elements. The cells primarily responsible are the lymphocytes that reside in the lymphoid tissues; there are two major types:

- **T cells** which are responsible for cellular specific immunity,
- **B cells** which are responsible for humoral specific immunity.

The terms 'cellular' and 'humoral' have a slightly different meaning than when used in the context of nonspecific response. 'Cellular' refers to those aspects which are driven by T cells and 'humoral' to the aspects mediated by antibodies (which are the products of the other major lymphocyte type: the B cell).

LYMPHOID TISSUES AND TRAFFIC BETWEEN THEM

The lymphoid tissues are classified as being primary or secondary.

Primary lymphoid tissues

Primary lymphoid tissues include the fetal yolk sac, the embryonic liver; the fetal and adult bone marrow and the thymus

Lymphocytes originate in primary lymphoid tissue and undergo early development and differentiation there. Their location alters during gestation: in the early embryo the main site of lymphocyte production is the fetal yolk sac but later in embryonic life this shifts to the liver. Later there is yet another shift to the bone marrow and the thymus, the sites at which it will remain throughout the rest of the individual's life. Within the bone marrow, pluripotential stem cells become committed to the lymphoid lineage. Those that remain within the bone marrow for the rest of their maturation become B cells. In T-cell development, the primitive lymphocytes have to travel to the thymus. It is still uncertain at which point in their development lymphocytes become committed to a T-cell lineage.

The thymus has epithelial and mesenchymal (supporting) components in addition to the lymphoid tissue. The thymus is a two-lobed lobulated structure found in the anterior chest or mediastinum. At the microscopic level, there is an outer cortex and an inner medullary area within each lobule. In the thymus, T-cell development progresses further as the imma-

ture T cells migrate from the cortex to the medulla. During this time, the early T cells interact with nonlymphoid elements, including thymic epithelia and dendritic cells. These cells are thought to be responsible for the important processes of positive and negative selection that take place as part of the 'thymic education of T cells'. During this process the T cells are assessed for their ability to discriminate between what is and is not 'self'. During early development and differentiation, the T and B cells demonstrate changes in expression of surface molecules that would determine their future role and functional capabilities. The development of both early T and B cells in the primary lymphoid tissues is independent of extrinsic antigen stimulation.

Secondary lymphoid tissues

The secondary lymphoid tissues comprise lymph nodes, spleen, and mucosa-associated lymphoid tissues (MALT)

These tissues are functionally organized to enable the interaction of lymphocytes with other cells and the antigen, and it is at these sites that immune reactions actually develop. Common to them all is a degree of compartmentalization, with specific areas for T cells and B cells and areas of overlap where they interact.

Within the lymph node, the T-cell area is the paracortex and the B-cell area the follicular areas of the medulla. Here follicular structures of two types can be found: the unstimulated primary follicle; and stimulated secondary follicles, characterized by the presence of germinal centers. The spleen contains nonlymphoid tissue (the red pulp) as well as lymphoid areas – termed the white pulp. The white pulp surrounds the splenic arterioles and is called the periarteriolar lymphoid sheath. Within the white pulp, follicular B-cell areas are evident, and the T-cell areas lie between them in the interfollicular space. MALT comprises the lymphoid elements found adjacent to the mucosal surfaces lining the internal body surfaces; they are found at the entrance to the respiratory tract and gut, and include the tonsils and adenoids. Further down the digestive tract, unencapsulated aggregates of lymphoid cells referred to as Peyer's patches are found, overlain by specialized areas of epithelium for sampling the antigenic environment. Solitary lymphocytes are also found throughout the mucosal epithelium.

Traffic between the secondary lymphoid tissues is via the lymphatics and blood vessels

The site of antigen localization in the lymphoid tissues after antigens gain access to the body depends upon the route of exposure. Entry via the circulation leads to localization in marginal zone lymphatics of the spleen. Entry via the gut and dome epithelia leads to localization in the MALT. With entry via the skin, the antigen may pass directly to the local lymph node via the lymphatics, or it can be taken up by the epidermal Langerhans cells, which then pass via lymphatics to the interdigitating cell-rich area of the paracortex of the local lymph node. Entry via other sites/tissues leads to the local lymph node.

LYMPHOCYTES

Lymphocyte circulation

The regulation of lymphocyte circulation depends on the expression of markers of location and activation by the cells and tissues involved

The entry of antigen into the lymphoid tissues has several effects on lymphocyte traffic into and out of these tissues, especially the lymph nodes. These effects occur in four phases:

- within hours, increased blood flow leads to increased lymphocyte entry. In the case of some antigens this is also accompanied by decreased lymphocyte outflow;
- by 1–2 days, there is an increased outflow of small, antigen-nonspecific lymphocytes; this represents the antigen-specific nonmigratory phase. Expansion of primed antigen-reactive B cells leads to the formation of primary follicle, in which the antigen-reactive B cells are located, to become a secondary follicle later;
- at 4 days, activated lymphocytes that have undergone blast transformation (blast cells) emigrate from the lymph node and home in with increased affinity on the high endothelial venule (HEV) to reach site of their first antigen contact, using adhesion molecules and their respective receptors;
- in the final phase, blast cell output falls and memory cells are generated.

Adhesion molecules

Adhesion molecules mediate adhesion between cells

The whole process of the immune response is dependent on the expression of the molecules and ligands that mediate adhesion between cells and the connective tissue elements such as fibronectin or collagen (Chapter 27). These are termed 'adhesion molecules' (see Fig. 25.14). They are found on a wide variety of cell types and they play important roles in interactions between the lymphocytes and the endothelium lining the small blood vessels. A major determinant of their expression is the prevailing cytokine environment and the surrounding connective tissue matrix.

Adhesion molecules are grouped into the following families:

- integrins;
- immunoglobulin supergene family adhesion molecules;
- selectins.

T and B lymphocytes

Distinction between T and B cells is most easily made with reference to the cells' antigen-specific receptors

The cells primarily involved in the immune response are the lymphocytes. In total, lymphocytes are present in the peripheral blood at between 1.5×109 and $3.5 \times 109/L$. Of these, approximately 50–70% are T cells and 10–20% are B cells. A third population termed 'natural killer' (NK) cells make up the remainder. NK cells are so called because they demonstrate the ability to kill neoplastic cells without prior exposure or sensitization. Despite their different function it is not possible to discern any morphologic features that could be used to distinguish between these lymphocyte populations. Instead, their identification is based on immunophenotypic or functional studies.

Each of the major populations of lymphocytes carry particular collections of markers that can assist in assigning their lineage. The distinction between T and B cells is most easily made with reference to their antigen receptors (Figs 36.2 and 36.3). In the B cell, the receptor is a surface immunoglobulin termed 'sIg'; it is an integral part of the cell membrane. On binding to its antigen, it brings about the cell's activation and subsequent proliferation and differentiation. In addition to sIg, B cells express several other markers, the best characterized of which include CD19, CD20 and the major histocompatibility complex (MHC) class II DR molecules. The T cell antigen receptor is termed the T-cell receptor (TCR) and it is complexed with CD3. Two other CD markers whose expression appears to be mutually exclusive on T cells are the CD4 and CD8, and they are useful in further categorizing the T cell function. NK cells are currently identified by the expression of the combination of CD16 and CD56. These markers are used in flow cytometric technology to identify cell types.

MOLECULES INVOLVED IN ANTIGEN RECOGNITION

T and B cells are involved in antigen recognition

The specificity of the immune response is made possible through the recognition of the antigen by specific receptors

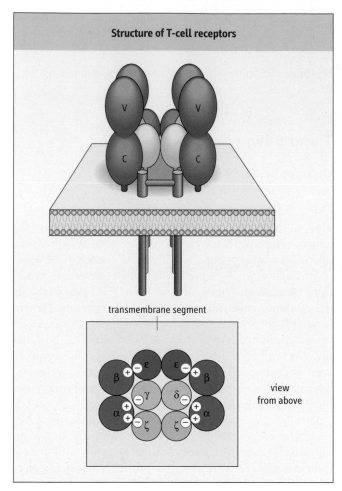

Fig. 36.2 **Structure of the α/β, γ/δ T-cell receptors.** V and C refer to the variable and constant sequence domains, respectively, of each of the α, β, γ and δ chains. Modified from Roitt IM *et al*. *Immunology*, 5th edn. London: Mosby, 1998.

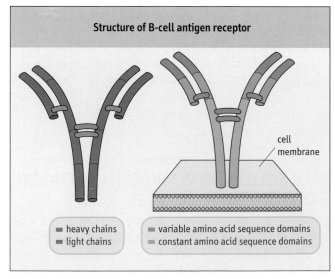

Fig. 36.3 **Structure of B-cell antigen receptor.**

on T and B cells. The ability to recognize the enormous number of possible antigenic configurations is achieved by differences in amino acid sequence of these receptors, which gives rise to differences in protein shape or conformation. As mentioned earlier, the antigen and its specific receptor have a 'hand-in-glove' relationship. Both T- and B-cell antigen receptors show marked variability in the sequence of amino acids that come into contact with the antigenic element, while other parts of these molecules are relatively constant with regard to their amino acid sequences.

T-cell antigen receptors

The T-cell antigen receptor (TCR) is made up of two nonidentical polypeptide chains: TCRαβ or TCRγδ.

The TCR is a heterodimer made up of two nonidentical polypeptide chains (Fig. 36.2). These chains are termed the TcRα, β, γ and δ, and the only functional combinations are αβ and γδ. The structure is based on the immunoglobulin domain (see Chapter 3). Each chain comprises two domains – one constant and one variable amino acid sequence. The antigen-binding site of the TCR is in the cleft formed by the adjoining single *N*-terminal variable domains of the constituent alpha (Vα), beta (Vβ), gamma (Vγ), or delta (Vδ) chains. The effector function of the constant domain in each of the antigen receptor chains is signal transduction. The two chains come into close contact via the covalent bonds between the variable domains and noncovalent hydrophobic interactions between the opposing faces of the constant domains.

The B-cell antigen receptor

The B-cell antigen receptor is merely the membrane form of the immunoglobulin found circulating in serum. Immunoglobulins are Y-shaped molecules made up of four polypeptide chains (Fig. 36.3; see also Chapter 3) – a pair of heavy chains each of approximate molecular weight 150 kDa and a pair of light chains each of approximate molecular weight 23 kDa. The arms interact with antigen and their structure is based on immunoglobulin domains with constant and variable sequences of amino acids in both the heavy and the light chains. It is the variably sequenced amino (NH_2) terminal domains of both the heavy (VH – variable heavy) and the light (VL – variable light) chains that form a pocket that constitutes the antigen binding site – the 'fragment antigen binding' (Fab) portion sits at the end of the arms. The remaining relatively constant amino acid sequence domains of the chains are termed constant heavy (CH) or constant light (CL) and form the stem that provides transduction effects (Fig. 36.4)

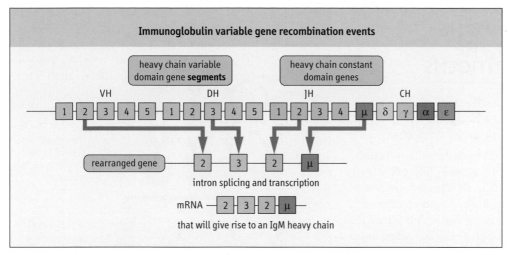

Fig. 36.4 **Immunoglobulin variable gene recombination events.** The apparent requirement for a huge number of genes required for antibody diversity is resolved by using a gene rearrangement strategy. The variable domains of both the heavy (H) and light (L) chains are encoded by a number of gene segments, two for the L chain (Variable L [VL] and Junctional L [JL]) and three for the H chain (Variable H [VH], Diversity H [DH], and Junctional H [JH]). The constant domains that make up the majority of the heavy chain molecules and half the light chain molecules are coded for by single gene segments, CH and CL, respectively.

IMMUNOGLOBULIN VARIABLE GENE RECOMBINATION EVENTS

The ability to generate molecules of variable amino acid sequence, using a basic template onto which some variation is superimposed provides the capability to generate as many different shapes as there are sequences. This is made possible by the organization of the genes that give rise to the T- and B-cell antigen receptors. They both undergo similar rearrangements and recombinations to generate a vast repertoire of antigen recognition units. This is illustrated by the idealized representation of the organization of a hypothetical immunoglobulin heavy-chain gene (see Fig. 36.4).

One gene from each of the variable domain gene segments combines with one gene from each of the other segments to produce a whole rearranged variable domain gene. This then associates with the gene coding for the constant domains of the particular heavy chain class being produced. In the case of a light chain, only two segments are involved in the production of a variable domain gene and this is then associated with the gene coding, whichever of the light chain types is going to be produced. The whole rearranged gene can be transcribed and subsequently translated. Thus multiple gene segments contribute to the formation of each individual variable domain gene and, together with the gene encoding, the constant domains complete light- and heavy-chain genes.

In the example shown in Figure 36.4, the number of genes available in each segment has been limited for simplicity. In reality, the actual numbers available at the three segments are 65, 10 and 6, giving rise to a huge number of possible permutations for the variable domain of just the heavy chain derived from one chromosome alone. Therefore there is an enormous potential for variation in the translated amino acid sequence and thus shape of the variable domains of both light and heavy chains; these chains, when combined, are capable of fitting with the huge variety of antigenic conformations likely to be encountered. By concentrating diversity to the variable domain genes, the amount of DNA required is also conserved.

Thus several similarities and differences between the TCR and the B-cell antigen receptor are evident. The TCR is described as a member of the immunoglobulin supergene family and is structurally similar to the B-cell antigen receptor with regard to the immunoglobulin domains and folding. Whereas there are two types of TCR, there are five classes of immunoglobulin that can be found on the B cell. Unlike B cells, no secretory version of the TCR is made. The most important is that the TCR needs to interact with antigen that has been 'processed' and which is presented against a background of self-molecules (in the form of MHC or human leukocyte antigen (HLA) molecules).

THE REACTION WITH, THE RESPONSE TO, AND THE ELIMINATION OF, ANTIGENS

On binding to the antigen, the cell divides and then differentiates into progeny with an effector function or a memory function

On successful antigen binding, accompanied with a requisite number of so-called costimulatory signals, the cell is activated to enter the cell cycle leading to repeated division or proliferation. This results in multiple daughter cells or a clone. This is followed by differentiation which alters the functional capabilities of the cell, and it may be accompanied by a change in the cell's appearance. Differentiation can either lead to the development of an effector function or the generation of memory. The aim is to create clones of cells that have precisely the same specificity for antigen and the process is termed the clonal selection. Antigen therefore determines the specific lymphocyte that will undergo activation. This outcome is assisted by the structural organization of the lymphoid tissues, together with the lymphoid traffic between them. This ensures that antigen is inspected by many lymphocytes and can select for proliferation and differentiation the cell that bears a specific and reciprocal antigen receptor.

Clonal selection (Fig. 36.5) ensures not only an adequate number of effector cells to deal with the threat at the time of initial stimulation, but also a suitable number of part-primed memory cells that will be able to complete their activation more rapidly on subsequent exposure.

Memory is one of the components that distinguish the specific immune response from the nonspecific response

How memory is generated is still the subject of continuing research: it has been suggested that the partial triggering of lymphocytes is an important mechanism. The partially triggered cells fail to undergo complete differentiation to the effector cell state and appear to return to a resting state. On subsequent exposure to the same antigen that partially triggered them previously, the time to complete proliferation and activation is significantly shortened, thus leading to a quicker and more effective response.

Specific immune response is responsible for the elimination of antigens that are intracellular or integral to the cell surface

As indicated above, specific immune response is mediated by cellular and humoral elements. The specific immune response has been classically described as having cellular and humoral arms, T cells being considered responsible for cellular immunity and B cells for humoral immunity. It is now established that the role of cellular, or T-cell mediated, immunity is dealing

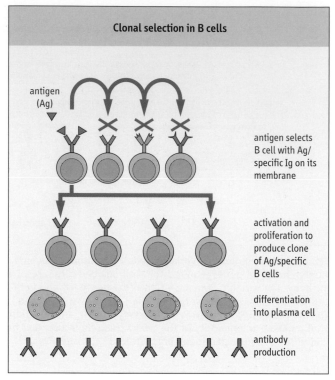

Fig. 36.5 **Clonal selection in B cells.** Antigen-specific (Ag-specific) secretory immunoglobulin (sIg) on the B-cell membrane has a shape reciprocal to the antigen. Antigen-immunoglobulin binding leads to activation and proliferation to produce a clone of antigen-specific B cells. Each member of the specifically activated clone then undergoes differentiation into a plasma cell, which produces large quantities of a single homogeneous immunoglobulin with identical specificity to the sIg that triggered the response in the first instance.

with chronic intracellular infections, mediating the immune response to tumors, the rejection of transplanted tissue and contact hypersensitivity. Chronic intracellular infections may be bacterial (e.g. tuberculosis), viral, fungal or parasitic,

T cells are responsible for the regulation of the activities of the other arms of the immune response

These functions include:

- increasing the numbers of cells capable of responding to the particular antigen;
- preventing the antigen gaining access to so far unaffected cells;
- limiting damage, i.e. assisting already altered cells to rid themselves of antigens by enhancing the capacity the affected cells have for self-cure and destroying those cells that do not have such capacity;
- making sure that any antigenic material released will be mopped up by other elements of the immune response, (both specific and nonspecific), clearing the damage and generating memory of the process.

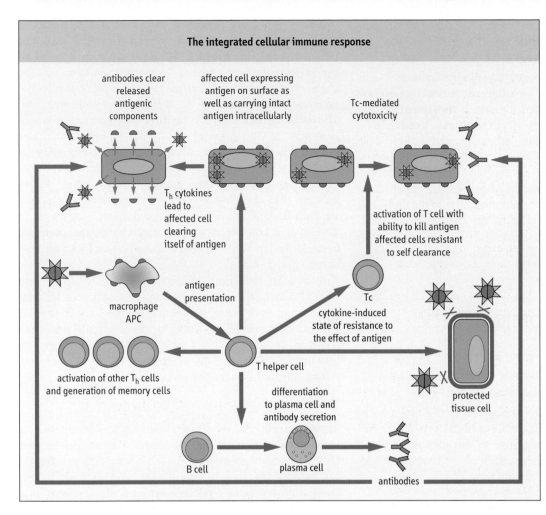

The integrated cellular immune response

antibodies clear released antigenic components

affected cell expressing antigen on surface as well as carrying intact antigen intracellularly

Tc-mediated cytotoxicity

T_h cytokines lead to affected cell clearing itself of antigen

activation of T cell with ability to kill antigen affected cells resistant to self clearance

macrophage APC

antigen presentation

Tc

cytokine-induced state of resistance to the effect of antigen

activation of other T_h cells and generation of memory cells

T helper cell

differentiation to plasma cell and antibody secretion

protected tissue cell

B cell

plasma cell

antibodies

Fig. 36.6 **The integrated cellular immune response.** T-helper cells (Th cells) are involved in many aspects of the cellular immune response. Cytokine and direct Th cell-mediated activation of B cells leads to differentiation to plasma cells, which secrete antibody. AG:AB, antigen–antibody; APC, antigen presenting cell; Tc, cytotoxic T cell; Th, T helper cell.

All of these other functions can be achieved either by direct cell–cell contact or by the secretion of soluble mediators that interact with the relevant cells, be they other T cells, B cells, NK cells, cells involved in the nonspecific immune response, or cells of other tissues. The responsibilities for providing all these functions, with the exception of killing cells, resides in a subpopulation of T cells. Not surprisingly, as they have the role of assisting the rest of the immune response and host response, these cells have been termed T-helper cells (Fig. 36.6).

This population of T cells achieves its goals for the elimination of intracellular antigen by the secretion of cytokines and direct interaction with the B cells responsible for antibody-mediated immunity, other T cells, and macrophages

These cells can be identified phenotypically by its expression of CD4, together with its nonexpression of CD8. The term CD4 T cell is synonymous with T-helper cell.

T-helper cells can also differentiate into those that drive a proinflammatory response and those that drive an anti-inflammatory response

It is now recognized that T-helper cells can be further divided into helper cells that drive the immune response towards a proinflammatory or antibody-based response and helper cells that drive the response towards an antagonistic anti-inflammatory or cell-orientated response. This differentiation is made on the basis of the profiles of secreted cytokines.

The lymphocyte-derived cytokines perform the following actions:

- augment further the nonspecific immune response;
- determine the form of the specific immune response to be used;
- assist the relevant cellular components in mediating it.

Other cells are cytotoxic and kill cells that carry a 'recognizable' antigen, i.e. the antigen for which the killer cells carry a receptor

The other major T cell subpopulation are the cytotoxic T cells (Tc) specifically responsible for killing those cells that express on their surface the antigen for which the Tc carries the appropriate TCR. Like T-helper cells, cytotoxic T cells can be identified phenotypically and are CD8+, CD4−. These cells employ a mechanism of killing that is similar to that used by the complement system (see earlier) but requires direct cellular interaction between the Tc and the target cell. A polymeric macromolecule termed perforin is inserted into the target cell wall, breaching its integrity. Unlike the complement system, reliance is not placed on this alone and enzymes (granzymes) from the Tc cell are introduced into the target cell, to hasten cell death.

MAJOR HISTOCOMPATIBILITY COMPLEX (MHC)

The MHC is responsible for how T cells 'see' an antigen against a background of self

For the TCR to interact with antigen there must be a background of self-molecules in the form of MHC or HLA molecules. For an immune response to be initiated, antigen cannot simply bind to the nearest T cell, but must be 'formally' presented to the immune system which acts as a means of regulating input and stimulation.

The MHC complex of genes is found on the short arm of chromosome 6 and is grouped into three regions termed class I, II and III with the same nomenclature being applied to the respective polypeptide products (Fig. 36.7). Class I and II molecules are directly involved with immune recognition and cellular interactions, whereas class III molecules are involved in the inflammatory response by coding for soluble mediators, including complement components and TNF.

Class I genes are organized into several loci, the most important of which are those termed HLA-A, HLA-B and HLA-Cw. Alleles are transmitted and expressed in Mendelian codominant fashion. Owing to their closeness on the chromosome, they are inherited *en-bloc* as parts of a haplotype and are expressed on the surface of all nucleated cells. The α-chains they encode have three domains, one of which is similar to those found in immunoglobulin molecules but the other two show significant differences. The α-chains combine with β2-microglobulin to give rise to a functional class I molecule (Fig. 36.8). Crystallographic studies indicate that the chains combine to produce a molecule which is designed to offer processed antigenic fragments to T cells in a cup-like structure, the sides of the molecule being formed by two α-helices and the bottom by a β-pleated sheet.

In contrast, the class II subregion genes are organized into α- and β-loci, giving rise to α- and β-polypeptide chains, respectively. Both are of approximately the same molecular weight and combine to form a heterodimer with a tertiary structure similar to a class I molecule, with a peptide groove into which the processed antigenic fragment is inserted during intracellular antigen processing.

The HLA system is intensely polymorphic

Many (currently in excess of 1000) allelic variants can be identified in each of the loci associated with antigen presentation. There are six major loci each having between 10 and 60 functionally recognizable alleles, and as each parent passes on one set or haplotype on each chromosome, it is easy to appreciate that the likelihood of another individual in the same species having an identical set is remote.

The genetic polymorphism is predominantly in exon 2 of the β-chain of class II molecules and α-chain of class I molecules. These encode amino acids on the floor and sides of the peptide grooves and thus have a significant bearing on the capacity to bind differing antigenic fragments. The combination of the antigenic fragment with the edge of the peptide groove of the MHC molecule is then recognized by the

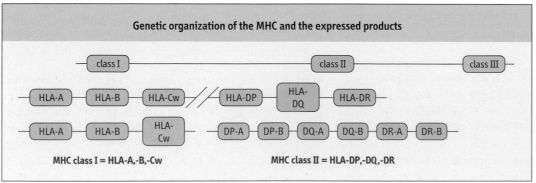

Fig. 36.7 **Genetic organization of the MHC and expressed products.** Genes of the MHC in humans are located on chromosome 6. The gene products are the human leukocyte antigens (HLA).

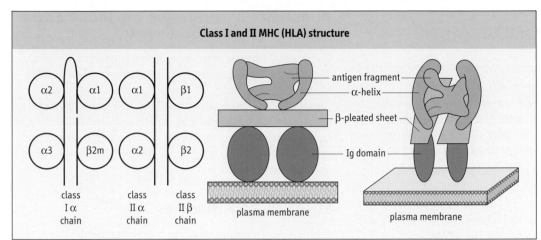

Class I and II MHC (HLA) structure

Fig. 36.8 **Class I and II MHC (HLA) structure.** On the left there are class I and class II MHC molecules. In class I molecules β2-microglobulin (β2m) provides the fourth domain. On the right, this is related to the types of protein conformation in the MHC molecules.

relevant T cell. This is another mechanism that ensures appropriate stimulation. It limits the possibility of a single microorganism being able to subvert or circumvent the immune response of an entire species, as there is a huge potential for binding to at least some component of a microbe, together with a similarly high potential for a T cell to be able to recognize the antigen in combination with an element that says 'self + antigen'. At the same time, it prevents any single pathogen from infecting the entire population – either by using the system as a back-door receptor into cells of every member of the species, or avoiding detection and elimination by mimicking one particular HLA allele.

MHC EXPRESSION PATTERNS AND MHC RESTRICTED STIMULATION

MHC molecules can restrict stimulation to a limited number of cell types through differing properties of class I and class II molecules

Class I molecules are expressed on all nucleated cells of the body, whereas class II molecules are expressed on only a limited variety of cells. The latter includes cells whose primary role is to present antigen (antigen-presenting cells, APCs), including macrophages and the cortical cells of the lymph nodes, as well as B cells and activated T cells. In this way, the MHC molecules can restrict stimulation to a limited number of cell types but at the same time, using similar mechanisms, permit appropriate targeting of any cell in the body. Without such a control, the immune system could be triggered repeatedly for no good reason.

As well as restricting input, the class I and II molecules also provide a differential mechanism for processing antigens that originate from within cells, e.g. viruses, and those that arise

RECURRENT INFECTION IN AN IMMUNOCOMPROMISED PATIENT

A 2-year-old child presented with a history of recurrent *Candida albicans* and chest infections. Investigations reveal decreased number of neutrophils, IgG and IgA. Assessments of lymphocyte proliferative response show decreased expression of CD40 on T cells. A diagnosis of X-linked hyper IgM was made and a treatment with intravenous immunoglobulin was commenced.

Comment. T cell help is required for effective B-cell responses. Particular interactions are required for the switch of isotype from the IgM response that is typical of a primary antibody response, to the more mature IgG and or IgA isotypes seen in secondary antibody responses produced to subsequent challenges. CD40L on the T cell is required to interact with the CD40 on B cells to achieve this. In its absence, antibody production is limited to IgM and the affected individual is immunocompromised owing to the lack of the other important isotypes so critical to the integrity of the immune response. The problem of infection more typically associated with cellular problems suggests the T-cell defect has functional consequences for this arm of the immune response.

from the extracellular environment, e.g. bacterial antigens. The different class MHC molecules also lead such antigens through different pathways to interact with the immune system, in particular with the T cells, on the basis that each will be better dealt with by differing effector systems: class I leads to CD^{8+} T-cytotoxic responses, and class II leads to antibody-mediated responses via CD^{4+} T- helper pathways.

HUMORAL SPECIFIC IMMUNE RESPONSE

Humoral- or antibody-mediated specific immunity is directed at extracellular infection, especially by bacteria and their products, and also at the extracellular phase of viral infection and individual cell transplantation

Humorally mediated immune reactions require a soluble and cell-free antigen receptor to match the soluble and cell-free nature of the antigens. The act of antibody binding to antigen may go some way to counter the antigen's potential for causing harm, by blocking the adhesion of bacteria or viruses, or the effect of bacterial toxins on the hosts cells – a process termed neutralization. However, simple binding, in most situations, will not guarantee elimination of the antigen. These two issues are dealt with by generating secreted forms of the B cell receptor – recognized as immunoglobulin – and giving it an additional effector function. This is provided by the nonantigen binding (Fc) part of the molecule and it is capable of recruiting components of the nonspecific immune response. The secreted immunoglobulins have effector functions encoded in the nonantigen-binding fragment of the molecule. This is achieved by genetic recombinations of the heavy chain genes, additional to those present to generate diversity and specificity of the antigen-binding component. Thus the original antigen specificity is preserved whilst effector functions can alter.

As with T cells, B cell subsets are operative in the humoral immune response

However, unlike the T cell subsets which are categorized on a functional basis, B cell subsets are defined by the timing of their participation in the humoral response. The B1 subset is responsible for the production of antibody that appears during the earliest stages of development of the organism. This subset and the antibodies it produces persist as a carry-over from this period. Although these cells possess a lesser degree of specificity than the antibodies produced later by the more mature B2 cells, they form a relatively effective first line of defense against a broad spectrum of antigens. Similar to T cell subsets, it is possible to distinguish these subsets on the basis of their phenotypic properties: B1 cells express CD5 in addition to CD19 and CD20 found in the B2 population. It may be this population of B cells, that is responsible for the production of autoantibodies when dysregulated – this is but one of many theories of the pathogenesis of autoimmune reactions. As noted earlier, T cells, particularly Th cells interact with B cells both directly and indirectly via cytokines. This happens to such a degree that effective B cell responses are described as being T cell-dependent.

Antibodies illustrate the capability of the immune system for diversity

The normal human immune system is apparently capable of producing a limitless number of antibodies with the ability of recognizing any and all nonself elements it comes into contact with. Antibodies therefore represent an excellent demonstration of the diversity of the immune response with regard to its ability to recognize antigen and its methods for antigen elimination. The terms antibody, gamma globulin and immunoglobulin are synonymous.

Structure of antibodies

Five classes of immunoglobulin are recognized: IgG, IgA, IgM, IgD, and IgE, with subclasses being recognized for IgG (IgG1, 2, 3, and 4) and for IgA (1 and 2). When studied at the individual molecular level, no other proteins show such amino acid sequence variation between individual members of the same class or subclass. This is most evident in the NH_2-terminal domains of both heavy and light chains. As mentioned earlier, antibodies are capable of discriminating between the molecules that characterize the outer capsular coverings of differing bacterial species and may vary by a single amino acid or a monosaccharide residue. This is a consequence of the dimensions of the area recognized by the antibody molecule being 10×20 Å (10^{-10} m) and thus being significantly influenced by the alteration in three-dimensional conformation brought about by the change of a single residue.

Functions of antibodies

Antibodies are also good examples of how function is intimately related to structure. They are Y-shaped molecules. The arms interact with antigen and the stem provides additional or effector functionality. This secondary or effector function endows the antibody with an ability to not only recognize the antigen but also to help eliminate it.

The activation of the complement system (a component of nonspecific immune response, discussed above) is one of the most important antibody effector functions of the specific immune response

This is achieved by using a set of components termed the 'classical activation pathways', which comprise C1q, C1r, C1s, C4, and C-2. Sequential activation of these components leads to the activation of the pivotal and critically important C-3 component, which is an absolute requirement for full complement activation. Once this is achieved, the terminal membrane attack complex, which comprises the components C5, C6, C7, C8, and C9, is activated. This complex eventually generates the polymeric ring structure that inserts into the

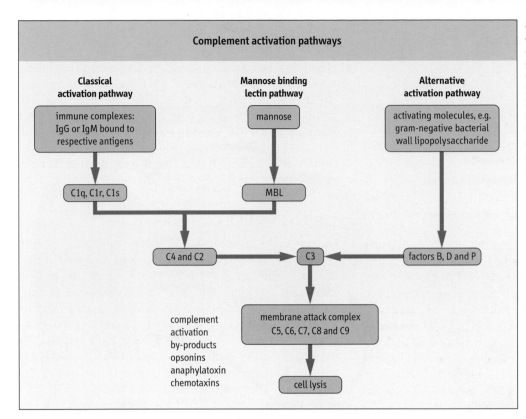

Fig. 36.9 **Complement activation pathways.** There are three possible pathways of complement activation. Only the classical pathway is triggered by the specific immune response. The mannose binding ligand (MBL) pathway and the alternative activation pathway are triggered directly by microbes and their products.

cell membrane of bacteria and is responsible for cell lysis. This classical pathway is triggered by C1q binding IgG or IgM that is already bound to its specific antigen (Fig. 36.9).

Two other pathways of activation exist, both constituting parts of the nonspecific immune response; they are probably older in evolutionary terms. These are the alternative pathway, which can be activated by lipopolysaccharide such as is found in Gram-negative bacterial walls, and the mannose binding ligand (MBL) pathway, which can be activated by mannose and other particular carbohydrates found in the cell wall of fungi, bacteria and viruses. The effector functions of antibodies are summarized in Table 36.2.

THE CELLULAR AND MOLECULAR ELEMENTS OF THE INTEGRATED IMMUNE RESPONSE

Vaccination depends on the integrated specific immune response

Probably the single most beneficial application of the basic function of the immune response, as we have now described it, has been the vaccination. The process of vaccination illustrates well the interactions of the humoral and cellular

Effector functions of antibodies

Type	Functions	Concentration in peripheral blood
IgG	neutralisation	5.0–16.0 g/L
	opsonization for neutrophils and macrophages	
	passive immunity for foetus via transplacental passage	
	complement activation via classical pathway	
	antibody – dependent, cell – mediated cytotoxicity	
	natural killer – cell killing of antibody bound cells achieved by FcRs (receptors for the Fc portion)	
	major isotype used in a secondary antibody response	
IgA	defence of mucosal surfaces as the most predominant immunoglobulin produced by MALT, neutralisation	0.5–4.0 g/L
IgM	neutralisation	0.5–2.0 g/L
	most effective classical complement pathway activator,	
	predominant isotype in primary antibody responses	
IgD	possible role in signal transduction and B cell maturation,	0.03 g/L
	significance of circulating IgD is undefined	
IgE	major role is defence of mucosal surfaces against multicellular microorganisms	<120 kU/L

Table 36.2 **Effector functions of antibodies.**

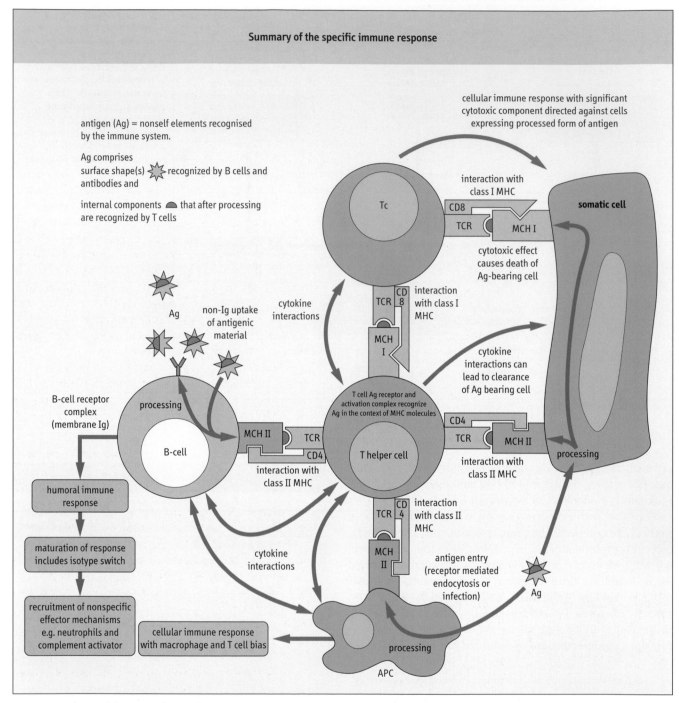

Summary of the specific immune response

cellular immune response with significant cytotoxic component directed against cells expressing processed form of antigen

antigen (Ag) = nonself elements recognised by the immune system.

Ag comprises surface shape(s) recognized by B cells and antibodies and

internal components that after processing are recognized by T cells

interaction with class I MHC

Tc

CD8

TCR   MCH I

somatic cell

cytotoxic effect causes death of Ag-bearing cell

Ag

non-Ig uptake of antigenic material

cytokine interactions

TCR CD 8 interaction with class I MHC

MCH I

cytokine interactions can lead to clearance of Ag bearing cell

B-cell receptor complex (membrane Ig)

processing

MCH II   TCR

B-cell   CD4

interaction with class II MHC

T cell Ag receptor and activation complex recognize Ag in the context of MHC molecules

T helper cell

CD4

TCR   MCH II

interaction with class II MHC

processing

humoral immune response

maturation of response includes isotype switch

recruitment of nonspecific effector mechanisms e.g. neutrophils and complement activator

cytokine interactions

TCR CD 4 interaction with class II MHC

MCH II

antigen entry (receptor mediated endocytosis or infection)

Ag

cellular immune response with macrophage and T cell bias

processing

APC

Fig. 36.10 **Summary of the specific immune response.** Interrelationships between cellular and humoral components of the specific immune response. APC, antigen presenting cell; Th, T-helper cell; Tc, cytotoxic T cell; MHC, major histocompatibility complex; TCR, T-cell receptor.

arms of the specific immune response and the features that characterize it best – specificity and memory. On first encounter with antigen, the immune system and antigen interact to select lymphocytes with the receptors specific for that antigen. These undergo activation, proliferation and dif-

ferentiation into effector memory cells, a process that may take up to 14 days to complete (Fig. 36.10). However, the process of memory cell generation, now leaves a body of cells semi-primed for that specific antigen. On subsequent exposure, the response is more rapid in view of the partly activated state of the memory cells, and more effective as a consequence of a degree of maturation of the response, due to the differentiation of the lymphocytes that has already taken place.

With reference to antibody responses, the primary challenge elicits a predominantly IgM response. On subsequent challenge, the lymphocytes undergo further maturation and differentiation and isotype switching more rapidly to produce a predominantly IgG response. This provides additional effector functions to that obtained with just IgM. It is this heightened and more specific response that can reduce both the severity and the duration of any damage sustained by the offending antigen; this may be critical to the survival of the organism.

IMMUNOLOGIC DYSFUNCTION

Autoimmunity is normally avoided by thymic education; a breakdown in the processes involved leads to autoimmune disease

While the immune system's activities are mostly beneficial, there are several situations in which they can have deleterious effects. These are best considered as aberrations of the quality, quantity or direction of the response (Table 36.3).

One particular aspect of these immunodysregulatory disorders, that of autoimmunity (self-reactivity), is avoided by the processes of thymic education. This is achieved via positive and negative selection and tolerance, which includes the processes of clonal deletion, clonal abortion and energy. These terms refer to the processes whereby self-reactive clones are eliminated or rendered impotent. These mechanisms can be seen as a multilayered fail-safe strategy. Should

these processes breakdown or be circumvented, the resulting state of self-reactivity and the resulting inflammatory damage constitute autoimmune disease. The form of disease is determined by the target antigen and the form of the immune response. At its simplest, reactions against ubiquitous antigens lead to what are termed nonorgan-specific autoimmune diseases, whereas reactions to unique components of individual tissues, organs or systems lead to organ-specific disease. The former are best exemplified by systemic lupus erythematosus (SLE), in which the apparent target antigens are components common to all nuclei. Damage is seen in several tissues, including the skin, joints, kidneys, and nervous system. The latter are exemplified by autoimmune thyroiditis, where the apparent target is thyroid peroxidase enzyme. The use of the word 'apparent' should be noted here, as on more detailed investigation it becomes clear that these particular antigen systems, while acting as markers or indicators of autoimmune disease, are not pathogenically responsible for the damage being inflicted. The methods used to detect such autoantibodies include indirect and direct immunofluorescence, particle agglutination, electroimmunodiffusion and enzyme immunoassay.

These diseases, and the others mentioned in Table 36.3, are the focus of the discipline of clinical immunology and immunopathology. More information can be found by reading the books cited in the Further Reading list below.

Summary

- Integrated immune response to non-self or altered-self elements (antigen(s)) is made up of a number of components. Some of these show unique specificity for the particular stimulating antigen(s) and comprise the specific or adaptive immune response, whilst others do not and comprise the nonspecific or innate immune response.
- The nonspecific response represents the first line response and can be considered cruder and more primitive. The cells and soluble mediators involved are primarily those associated with the processes of acute inflammation and endothelial cell activation.
- The specific response is more refined and usually invoked only in the face of either failure/continued stimulation of the nonspecific response. The cells responsible for the specific immune response are the lymphocytes; T, B and NK. The specificity they show for the inciting antigen is achieved via the use of specific antigen receptors, T cell and B cell receptors, expressed on cell surface.
- T cells recognize processed antigen via the TcR interacting with antigen presented by MHC-bearing

Disorders of immune regulation		
Antigen source **Level of response**	**Polyclonal response** **Exogenous**	**Monoclonal response** **Endogenous**
Decreased response	immunodeficiency primary and secondary	
Increased response	tuberculosis, leprosy, immune complex disease	lymphoproliferative disease
Inappropriate response	allergic disease – IgE	
Increased and inappropriate response	allergic disease – EAA	autoimmune disease

Table 36.3 **Disorders of immune regulation.**

cells, leading to the secretion of additional cytokines and the generation of effector functions such as T cell help and T cell-mediated cytotoxicity brought about by the T-helper and T-cytotoxic subsets respectively. Historically, T cell responses have been termed the cellular immune response.

- B cells recognize native antigen and secrete soluble forms of the individual B cell antigen receptors which we recognize as antibodies. Historically, B cells and their antibody products have been termed the humoral immune response. Both T and B cells and their products are able to recruit and utilize components of the nonspecific response in a more effective and targeted manner, with the aim of eliminating or eradicating the antigen.

- In addition to demonstrating specificity, the specific immune response also demonstrates another critically important characteristic not seen with the nonspecific response – the memory for its encounter with all types of antigen. The benefit of this is that, on subsequent contact with the same antigen, the antigen can be eliminated more quickly and effectively, and with less tissue damage, than on the previous occasion.

ACTIVE LEARNING

1. Compare T and B lymphocytes.
2. What are adhesion molecules and what is their role in the immune response?
3. Can one distinguish T and B lymphocytes under a microscope?
4. What is the role of the Fc fragment of an immunoglobulin?
5. What is the role of the thymus in the immune response?

Further reading

Roitt IM. *Immunology*, 5th edn. London: Mosby, 1998.

Janeway C, Traver P, Hunt S, Walport M. *Immunobiology*, 5th edn. London: Garland, 2002.

Chapel H, Heaney M, Misbah S, Snowden N. *Essentials of Clinical Immunology*, 4th edn. Oxford: Blackwell; 1999.

Parkin J, Cohen B. An overview of the immune system. *Lancet* 2001;**357**:1777–1789.

LEARNING OBJECTIVES

After reading this chapter you should be able to:

■ Describe the pathway and regulatory processes controlling the biosynthesis of thyroid hormones and the mechanism of their transport to and action on target tissues.

■ Describe the pathway and mechanisms regulating synthesis and activity of glucocorticoids, from the hypothalamus to target organs.

■ Outline the pathway and mechanisms regulating the synthesis and activity of sex steroid hormones and their role in regulation of male and female reproduction.

■ Describe the direct and indirect actions of growth hormone, including the role of IGF-I.

■ Outline the role of prolactin in reproduction.

■ Describe the many and variable consequences of deficiencies and excesses of hormones regulated by the hypothalamo–pituitary axis.

INTRODUCTION

The endocrine system provides communication between cells, tissues and organs. In higher species, such as humans, sophisticated control mechanisms are required to ensure optimal communication between cells, tissues, and organs. Along with the nervous system, the endocrine system provides this communication and is responsible for the regulation of a wide range of functions including growth, development, reproduction, homeostasis, and the response to external stimuli and stress. Failures in this communication channels are common and lead to many diseases of the endocrine system.

Several organs secrete hormones

Many organs in the body secrete biologically active compounds called endocrine hormones, which are transported via the bloodstream to other tissues or organs where they exert a biological effect. Some hormones, termed paracrine hormones, are made and act locally, affecting the tissue that synthesizes them. Others, termed autocrine hormones act on the cell that synthesized them or on neighboring cells

of the same type. All of these hormones act by binding to specific receptors, either on the cell surface or within the target cell (see Chapter 38). It is this hormone–receptor interaction that triggers and coordinates a wide range of biological effects.

Negative feedback regulation is important for homeostatic control

In order to ensure tight homeostatic control, the final output of hormone action involves a complex feedback loop that regulates either further hormone synthesis or secretion, or hormone sensitivity (Fig. 37.1).

Several hormones may control one process, or one hormone may control several processes

While it may be convenient to think of the endocrine system as being compartmentalized so that one hormone has control over one process, this is rarely the case. For example, at least four different hormones are involved in the regulation of plasma glucose concentration (see Chapter 20). Conversely, single hormones such as testosterone influence a range of metabolic processes.

HORMONES

Types of hormones

Hormones may be simple or complex, and may have very different chemical structures

Many different types of molecules function as hormones (Table 37.1). At the simplest level, modified amino acids, such as epinephrine (adrenaline), have hormonal activity. Other hormones are polypeptides, synthesized on the ribosome, and vary in size from a tripeptide (e.g. thyrotropin releasing hormones, TRH) up to complex glycoproteins (e.g. luteinizing hormone, LH). The smaller peptide hormones are synthesized as larger polypeptide or protein pre- or pro-hormones, then are cleaved by specific proteolytic enzymes to release the active hormone from the endocrine gland. Other hormones are derived by modification of simple lipids such as cholesterol or fatty acids. Some of these molecules require further metabolism within their target cell before they can exert their full biological effect (e.g. the conversion of circulating testosterone to its active form dihydrotestosterone).

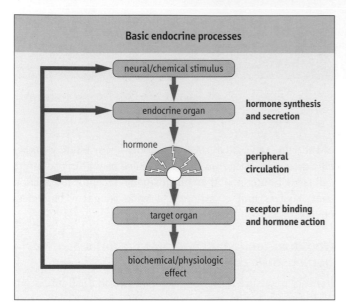

Fig. 37.1 **Basic endocrine processes.** The feedback regulation of hormone action is a classical example of self-regulation.

Chemical derivation of hormones

Derived from amino acids	
Amino acid derivatives	catecholamines, serotonin, thyroxine
Tripeptides	TRH
Small peptides	VP (ADH), somatostatin
Intermediate-size peptides	insulin, parathyroid hormone
Complex polypeptides and glycoproteins	gonadotropins, TSH
Derived from lipid precursors	
Cholesterol derivatives	cortisol, testosterone, estradiol, vitamin D
Fatty acid derivatives	prostaglandins, leukotrienes
Phospholipid derivative	platelet-activating factor
Derived from other chemicals	
Purines	adenosine
Gases	nitric oxide

Table 37.1 **The chemical derivation of hormones.** AVP/ADH, arginine vasopressin or antidiuretic hormone; TRH, thyrotropin releasing hormone; TSH, thyroid stimulating hormone.

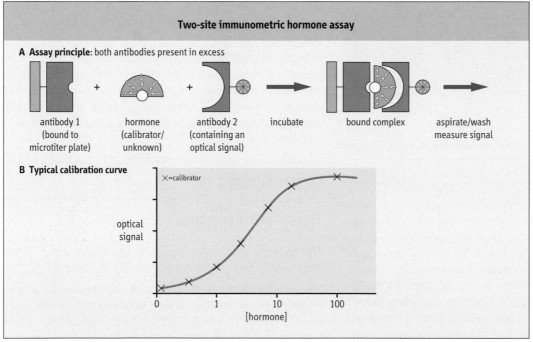

Fig. 37.2 **The sandwich design for enzyme–linked immunosorbent assay (ELISA) for the measurement of hormone concentration.** The amount of signal present on the microplate after washing of the serum/reagents is a measure of the concentration of a hormone.

Circulation, action, and inactivation of hormones

Many hormones are transported to their site of action by carrier proteins, where they exert their action and are then inactivated by further metabolism

Within the circulation, small or hydrophobic hormones are transported bound to carrier proteins. For example, thyroxine and cortisol are transported on specific plasma binding globulins such as thyroid-binding globulin (TBG) and cortisol-binding globulins (CBG). The transport proteins extend the biological half-life and increase the plasma concentration of the smaller hormones, which would otherwise be eliminated rapidly in the liver or kidney. The rate of clearance of different hormones varies enormously, from a few minutes (insulin), to hours (steroids), to days (thyroxine). At the cellular level, hormones exert their actions through a wide range of signal transduction mechanisms (Chapter 38). Hormone inactivation usually occurs by further metabolism (e.g. proteolysis, hydroxylation, and conjugation), followed by

HORMONE IMMUNOASSAY – A BILLION DOLLAR BUSINESS

Immunoassay is the most widely applied technique for measuring hormones in biological samples. Antibodies are produced that bind to antigenic sites on the hormone. Ideally, this antibody should possess both high specificity and affinity for the hormone of interest, e.g. the β-subunit of glycoprotein hormones.

In the first immunoassays, the antibodies were produced in the serum of animal species (e.g. rabbit or sheep) that had been immunized with human hormone preparations. Such antisera contained a range of different antibodies (polyclonal) capable of binding to different sites on the hormone antigen. However, antibody specificity and titer varied with the animal and duration of the immune response. Today most immunoassays employ monoclonal antibodies, which are produced by fusion of spleen cells from an immunized mouse with a mouse myeloma cell line. Hybridoma cells may be cloned to produce a cell line that secretes a single antibody species for an indefinite period of time.

Many commercial producers have designed proprietary methods for quantifying the hormone-antibody interaction. One of the most widely used formats is the two-site (sandwich) immunometric or ELISA assay assay outlined in Figure 37.2. This assay employs two antibodies binding to different epitopes on the hormone, one of which is modified to be capable of generating an optical signal. Spectrophotometric, fluorometric, luminescence and radiochemical reporter systems are in common use.

 ## HORMONE MEASUREMENT – A MATTER OF TIMING

Since hormones are involved with homeostatic mechanisms, their secretion is not constant. In response to a specific stimulus, most hormones are released in bursts ranging from single spikes (e.g. growth hormone, GH) to sustained release (e.g. insulin). Hormone secretion often conforms to strict biological rhythms, which may be at intervals of 1–2 hours (LH), 24 hours (cortisol) or 28 days (progesterone). For these reasons, it is always necessary to standardize the time and status of the patient before sampling, and it is often necessary to perform multiple sampling or dynamic testing.

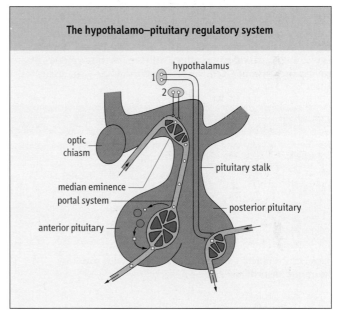

Fig. 37.3 **The hypothalamo–anterior pituitary regulatory system.** Hormones of the posterior pituitary are synthesized and packaged in the supraoptic and paraventricular nuclei of the hypothalamus (1), transported along axons and stored in the posterior pituitary prior to release into the circulation. The anterior pituitary releasing or release-inhibiting hormones are synthesized in various hypothalamic nuclei (2) and transported to the median eminence. From there they travel to the anterior pituitary via a portal venous system.

excretion of the metabolites. Measurement of urinary concentrations of hormone metabolites can be used to diagnose pregnancy or disease.

THE HYPOTHALAMO–PITUITARY REGULATORY SYSTEM

Hormones of the posterior pituitary gland are distinct from those of the anterior pituitary

The pituitary gland is an oval organ weighing about 0.6 g, encased in a bony cavity of the skull (*sella turcica*) below the brain. It communicates with the hypothalamus via the pituitary stalk, which contains a complex array of axons and portal blood vessels (Fig. 37.3). The pituitary gland is divided into two lobes. The anterior lobe (adenohypophysis), accounting for ~80% of the gland, may be seen as a target organ for endocrine hormones released from hypothalamic nuclei and transported via the median eminence and the portal circulation. The hormones of the posterior pituitary (neurohypophysis) are actually synthesized and packaged in the supraoptic and paraventricular nuclei of the hypothalamus and transported in granules along axons to the pituitary.

Hormones of the posterior pituitary gland

The posterior pituitary gland secretes two hormones into the circulation. Oxytocin is a small peptide hormone that stimulates smooth muscle contraction in the uterus and breast; it functions in parturition and lactation. Vasopressin (VP), also known as antidiuretic hormone (ADH), is a nine-amino-acid cyclic peptide with functions linked to the control of water metabolism, as described in Chapter 22.

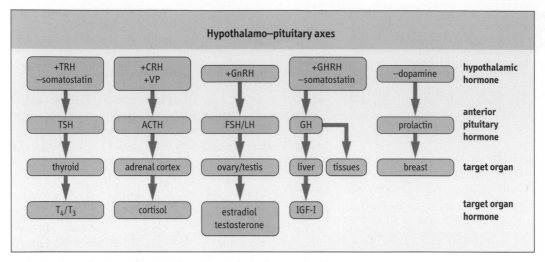

Fig. 37.4 **Hypothalamo–anterior pituitary regulatory target organ axes.** The hypothalamo-anterior pituitary regulatory system comprises five parallel endocrine axes, regulating the biosynthesis and release of: (1) thyroid hormone; (2) glucocorticoids; (3) sex steroids; (4) growth hormone; and (5) prolactin. T_4, thyroxine; T_3, triiodothyronine; GHRH, growth-hormone-releasing hormone; GnRH, gonadotropin-releasing hormone; IGF_1, insulin growth factor-1. (+) indicates stimulatory action and (–) inhibitory action.

Pituitary hormone disorders		
Hormone	**Deficiency**	**Excess**
TSH	hypothyroidism	thyrotoxicosis
ACTH	hypoadrenalism	Cushing's disease
FSH/LH	hypogonadism	precocious puberty
GH	short stature	gigantism/acromegaly
prolactin	none	galactorrhea/infertility

Table 37.2 **Clinical conditions associated with pituitary hormone disorders.**

Hormones of the hypothalamo–anterior pituitary regulatory system

There are five separate endocrine axes within this system (Fig. 37.4). Three of these are part of a complex three-level endocrine axis in which the hormones of the pituitary gland (thyroid stimulating hormone (TSH), adrenocorticotropic hormone (ACTH), follicle-stimulating hormone (FSH) and luteinizing hormone (LH) may be regarded solely as tropic hormones for other target organs (i.e. thyroid, adrenals, gonads). In these axes, sophisticated control is exercised via a cascade in which each endocrine organ in the axis amplifies both the amount of hormone secreted and the biological half-life of its hormone product compared with the previous organ. The fourth endocrine axis is a hybrid: growth hormone (GH) is both a tropic hormone and has actions in its own right. The fifth endocrine axis mediates the secretion of prolactin, unique in that it is not a tropic hormone. With one exception, there are distinct endocrine disorders associated with both deficiency and excess secretion by the anterior pituitary hormones (Table 37.2).

THE HYPOTHALAMO–PITUITARY-THYROID AXIS

Thyrotropin-releasing hormone (TRH)

TRH is manufactured in the hypothalamus and transported via the portal circulation to the pituitary where it ultimately leads to secretion of TSH

TRH is a modified tripeptide synthesized as a 26 kDa prohormone by peptidergic hypothalamic nuclei and transported, after processing, to the anterior pituitary by the portal circulation. It is secreted in pulsatile fashion. TRH stimulates TSH synthesis and secretion by binding to receptors on the pituitary thyrotroph cell membrane that are linked to phospholipase C. The resulting phosphoinositides stimulate the release of calcium from intracellular storage sites and so lead to secretion of TSH. More chronic actions of TRH include stimulation of TSH subunit biosynthesis and TSH glycosylation. The number of TRH receptors on the thyrotrophs is downregulated both by the concentration of TRH itself and by thyroid hormones.

Thyroid-stimulating hormone

TSH (also known as thyrotropin) is a 28 kDa glycoprotein synthesized by the pituitary thyrotroph. It consists of two noncovalently linked subunits and contains about 15% carbohydrate. The α-chain is identical to that found in other pituitary glycoprotein hormones and so the specificity is determined by the β-chain and the three-dimensional configuration. The synthesis of each subunit is directed by separate messenger ribonucleic acids (mRNAs) encoded by separate genes on different chromosomes. The carbohydrate side chains are complex mixtures of unmodified, acetylated, and sulfated sugars.

TSH is secreted in a pattern that is both pulsatile and circadian. The plasma half-life of TSH is about 65 minutes. The normal plasma reference concentration is approximately 0.4–4.0 mU/L although logarithmic transformation is required to give it a Gaussian distribution (Fig. 37.5).

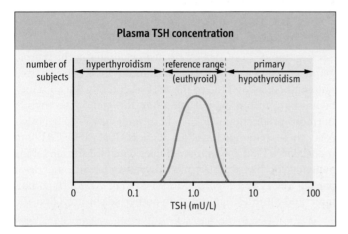

Fig. 37.5 **Distribution of plasma TSH concentrations.** The reference range is 0.4–4.0 mU/L.

TSH acts on the thyroid gland and influences virtually every aspect of thyroid hormone biosynthesis and secretion

TSH acts via a specific transmembrane receptor on the target cell of the thyroid gland. Binding of TSH to the receptor activates adenylate cyclase; cAMP-dependent protein kinases control virtually every aspect of thyroid hormone biosynthesis and secretion, including iodide transport, iodothyronine formation, thyroglobulin proteolysis, and thyroxine deiodination. TSH also stimulates growth of the thyroid gland.

Negative feedback by thyroid hormones occurs at both hypothalamic and pituitary levels. At the pituitary level, thyroxine (T_4) and tri-iodothyronine (T_3) inhibit TSH secretion by decreasing both the biosynthesis and release of TSH through regulation of gene transcription and TSH glycosylation. T_3, the biologically active form of the hormone, is a more potent feedback inhibitor than T_4.

Thyroxine and tri-iodothyronine

T_4 is produced exclusively in the thyroid gland and is more abundant than T_3, which is the biologically active form

T_4 (also known as tetra-iodothyronine) and T_3 are structurally simple molecules, being iodinated thyronines produced by the coupling of a phenyl group detached from one tyrosine to the phenyl group of a second intact tyrosine (Fig. 37.6). The biosynthesis of T_4 and T_3 occurs within thyroglobulin, a large (660 kDa) glycoprotein that accounts for about 75% of the protein content of the thyroid gland. Iodination of thyroglobulin occurs late after it has been secreted

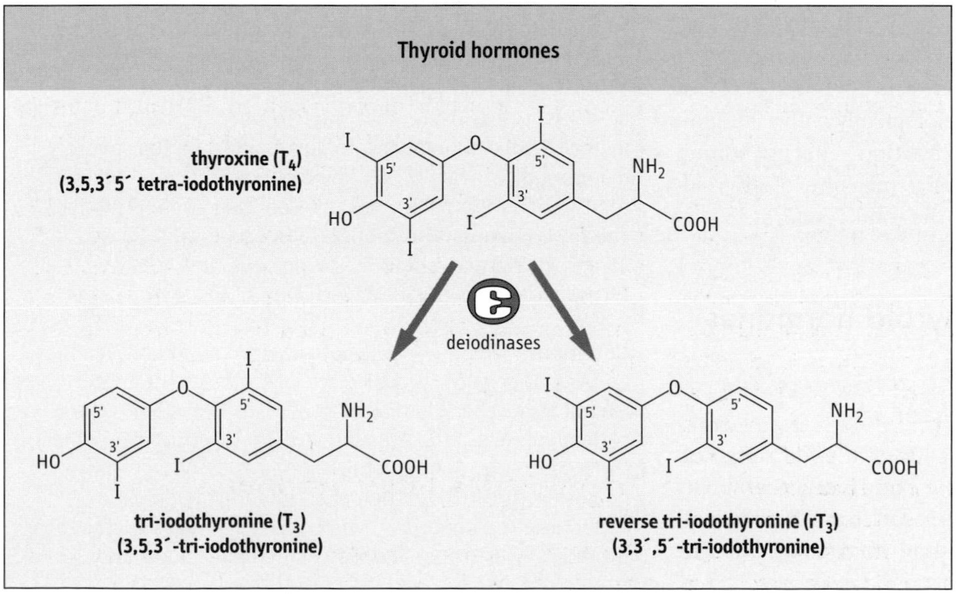

Fig. 37.6 **Structures of the thyroid hormones T_4, T_3, and rT_3.**

Thyroid hormones

thyroxine (T_4)
(3,5,3´5´ tetra-iodothyronine)

deiodinases

tri-iodothyronine (T_3)
(3,5,3´-tri-iodothyronine)

reverse tri-iodothyronine (rT_3)
(3,3´,5´-tri-iodothyronine)

into the follicular lumen. The secretion of T_4 and T_3 requires enzymatic hydrolysis of thyroglobulin, which is located in the follicular colloid. During hydrolysis and subsequent deiodination, the released iodide is conserved and reutilized. About 25 mg of thyroglobulin are hydrolyzed daily for production of ~100 µg of T_4.

Thyroid hormone bioactivity is regulated by controlling the conversion of T_4 into T_3 by deiodination; this is mediated by three deiodinase enzymes

T_4 is quantitatively the most important thyroid hormone and it is produced exclusively by the thyroid gland. T_3 is the biologically active form of thyroid hormone produced by 5'- deiodination of T_4. This process may occur in the thyroid gland, in target tissues, or in other peripheral tissues, and is accomplished by iodothyronine deiodinases I and II. The type I enzyme regulates plasma T_3 levels, while the type II enzyme controls nuclear T_3 levels. The type III enzyme is the major catabolic enzyme; it catalyzes the removal of an iodide from the 5- rather than 5'-position, resulting in reverse T_3, which is inactive. Thus, control of the deiodination of T_4 is one method of controlling thyroid hormone bioactivity (see Fig. 37.6). About 80% of T_4 is metabolized by deiodination with about equal amounts of T_3 and rT_3 being produced. The remaining T_4 is conjugated with sulfate or glucuronic acid and deactivated by deamidation or decarboxylation.

The biologically active fraction of T_3 and T_4 in plasma (free T_3 or free T_4 i.e. a fraction which is not bound to protein) represents, in each case, less than 1% of the total concentration of the hormone

The daily production of T_4 is approximately 10% of the extrathyroidal pool, much of which is bound to TBG or albumin in plasma. Approximately 80% of this T_4 is converted to T_3 by extrathyroidal deiodination. The turnover of T_3 is much greater than that of T_4. The biologically active component of T_4 and T_3 in plasma is the free fraction – that not bound to proteins. This fraction, which is a measure of thyroid hormone status, represents <1% of the total T_4 and T_3.

Biochemical actions of thyroid hormones

The thyroid hormones may be considered the accelerator pedal of metabolism

T_3 and T_4 increase the metabolic rate of a wide range of tissues and thereby affect the whole body, basal metabolic rate. Most, if not all, of these actions result from altered transcription brought about by the binding of T_3 to its nuclear receptor (see Chapter 38).

Thyroid hormones augment thermogenesis by increasing mitochondrial oxidative metabolism driven by the increase in ATP utilization that occurs as a result of increased sodium-potassium (Na^+/K^+)-dependent ATPase activity. Lipolysis is stimulated by cAMP-dependent activation of hormone sensitive lipase, thus producing fatty acids that can be oxidized to generate the ATP used for thermogenesis. Increase in both glycogenolysis and gluconeogenesis occurs to balance the increased use of glucose as a fuel for thermogenesis. The rate of synthesis of many structural proteins, enzymes, and other hormones is also affected as a result of thyroid hormone action.

Clinical disorders of thyroid function

Thyroid disease is common, affecting almost 3% of the population; nine times as many women as men are affected

Greater than 95% of thyroid disease originates in the thyroid gland and much of this is autoimmune in origin. Thyroid autoantibodies can bind to the TSH receptor. If the autoantibodies bind to but do not stimulate the gland, the thyroid hormone production will fall and the patient will be hypothyroid; these patients have an increased plasma TSH and reduced free T_4. If the autoantibodies bind and stimulate, the patient will be hyperthyroid (thyrotoxic) with increased plasma free T_4 and suppressed TSH (see Fig. 37.5). Hypothalamic and pituitary causes of hypothyroidism are often the

 HYPOTHYROIDISM

The symptoms of hypothyroidism are nonspecific and easily missed. A 60-year-old woman comes to the outpatient clinic and complains of weight gain, intolerance of cold, and tiredness. She also says that she has recently become less alert mentally, but attributes this to aging. She says that two members of her family had 'thyroid trouble'. On examination, she is moderately obese, has dry, cool skin and a puffy face. The thyroid gland is not palpable. Her thyroxine (T_4) was 15 nmol/L (normal range: 55–144 nmol/L) and TSH was 25 mU/L (range 0.4–4 mU/L) (see Fig. 37.5).

Comment. Symptoms of hypothyroidism at an early stage can be fairly non-specific, as they are in this case. The best laboratory test for the diagnosis of hypothyroidism is the plasma TSH level. The elevated level of TSH suggests primary thyroid disorder. Subsequently this lady's blood was shown to be positive for the microsomal and antithyroglobulin antibodies. A diagnosis of lymphocytic thyroiditis (Hashimoto's thyroiditis) was made. She was treated with thyroxine.

result of impaired TSH secretion secondary to pressure from an adjacent tumor. Pituitary TSH-secreting tumors are an extremely rare cause of hyperthyroidism.

THE HYPOTHALAMO–PITUITARY-ADRENAL AXIS

Two hypothalamic peptides are the principal regulators of pituitary ACTH release, corticotropin-releasing hormone (CRH) and vasopressin

Two hypothalamic peptides, CRH and VP/ADH, are the principal but not the sole regulators of pituitary ACTH synthesis and release. They act independently and synergistically. CRH is a 41-amino-acid peptide secreted by the paraventricular nucleus; it acts via the cAMP second messenger system. VP/ADH is a nine-amino-acid peptide synthesized by both the supraoptic and paraventricular nuclei; it acts by altering intracellular calcium ion channels. Negative feedback by cortisol inhibits the stimulation of the pituitary by both CRH and VP/ADH.

Adrenocorticotropic hormone (ACTH)

ACTH is synthesized as a 241-amino-acid precursor molecule pro-opiomelanocortin (POMC). POMC is cleaved at multiple sites to release several hormonally active peptides, including the endorphins and melanocyte stimulating hormones. In addition to the pituitary, POMC may also be produced in large quantities by certain malignancies giving rise to ectopic ACTH syndrome.

   ACTH itself is comprised of 39 amino acids with the biological activity residing in the N-terminal 24 moieties. It is secreted in stress-related bursts superimposed on a marked diurnal rhythm that shows a peak at 05.00 h. It is transported unbound in plasma and has a half-life of about 10 minutes. ACTH stimulates the synthesis and release of glucocorticoid hormones by interacting with cell-surface receptors on the adrenal cortex that stimulate the production of intracellular cAMP. Acute increases in the adrenal synthesis of cortisol occur within 3 minutes, principally by stimulating the activity of cholesterol esterase. Chronic effects of ACTH include induction of transcription of the genes that encode steroidogenic enzymes.

   Negative feedback by cortisol occurs within two time frames, acting at both the hypothalamic and pituitary levels. Fast feedback alters the release of hypothalamic CRH and the CRH-mediated secretion of ACTH. Slow feedback results from reduced synthesis of CRH and AVP/ADH plus suppression of POMC gene transcription, which results in reduced ACTH synthesis.

HYPERTHYROIDISM

A 35-year-old woman came to her physician complaining of palpitations, difficulty climbing stairs and general fatigue. She also said that she had lost 4 kg of weight recently despite a good appetite and no attempt at dieting. She reported occasional diarrhea.

Comment. On examination her skin was warm and moist and she had a fine tremor of outstretched hands. There was mild weakness of the thigh muscles. She had tachycardia (110/min). She also has a mild thyroid enlargement (goiter) and a bruit over the gland. Thyroid function tests show suppressed TSH level (<0.05; range 0.4–4 mU/L) (see Fig. 37.5) and increased thyroxine ($T_4 = 220$; range: 55–144 nmol/L) and tri-iodothyronine ($T_3 = 4.0$; range 0.9–2.8 nmol/L). Thyroid receptor antibodies were detected. In hyperthyroidism, the TSH level tends to be suppressed by high circulating thyroid hormones. The low TSH level and high thyroid hormone concentrations suggest hyperthyroidism. The presence of thyroid receptor antibodies confirms that the cause is Graves disease, an autoimmune thyroid disorder. The antireceptor antibodies bind to the TSH receptors in the thyroid gland and mimic the effect of TSH, producing thyroid over-secretion.

Biosynthesis of cortisol

Cortisol is the major glucocorticoid synthesized in man in the adrenal cortex and is under the direct control of pituitary ACTH

A simplified scheme of steroid biosynthesis is shown in Figure 37.7 (see also Fig. 16.7, p. 219). Cholesterol is the precursor for all steroid hormones. Cleavage of the cholesterol side chain liberates the C-21 corticosteroids; further side chain cleavage yields the C-19 androgens, and aromatization of the A ring results in the C-18 estrogens. The structures of the key steroid hormones are shown in Chapter 16. Several of the steroidogenic enzymes are members of the cytochrome P450 superfamily of oxidases.

   The plasma concentration of cortisol shows a pronounced diurnal rhythm, being some 10 times higher at 08.00 h than at 24.00 h. This parallels the marked diurnal rhythm of secretion of ACTH. Approximately 95% of cortisol in plasma is bound to proteins, mainly CBG. As cortisol concentration rises, the percentage of free cortisol also rises, indicating that CBG binding is saturable. Cortisol has a half-life in plasma of about 100 minutes. It is metabolized in the liver and other organs by a combination of reduction, side chain cleavage, and conjugation to produce a wide range of inactive metabolites that are excreted in urine.

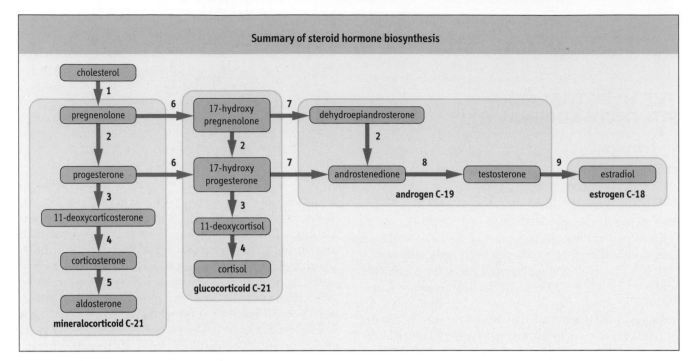

Fig. 37.7 **Summary of steroid hormone biosynthesis. 1**, cholesterol 20,22-desmolase; **2**,3β-hydroxysteroid dehydrogenase$\Delta\alpha^{4,5}$-oxosteroid isomerase; **3**, 21-hydroxylase; **4**, 11-hydroxylase; **5**, aldosterone synthase; **6**, 17α-hydroxylase; **7**, 17,20-lyase/desmolase; **8**, 17β-hydroxysteroid dehydrogenase; **9**, aromatase. These enzymes are part of the cytochrome P450-dependent superfamily of NADPH-dependent mono-oxygenases (see also Chapter 16).

Cortisol has a major influence on gluconeogenesis

As the name glucocorticoid suggests, cortisol has a major influence on glucose homeostasis. It is a counter-regulatory hormone, like glucagon but slower acting, working through nuclear receptors to induce the biosynthesis of gluconeogenic enzymes. At the same time, cortisol has a diabetogenic effect, inhibiting glucose uptake and metabolism in peripheral tissues. Glycogen synthesis and deposition are increased, and lipolysis is stimulated. Protein and RNA synthesis are stimulated in the liver, but inhibited in peripheral tissues (muscle); proteolysis in muscle produces the amino acid substrates for hepatic gluconeogenesis. In this role, cortisol is working in tandem with several other hormones including insulin and GH.

Excess cortisol has a wide range of effects on the immune system, inhibiting the immune response and inflammation. Cortisone, a related glucocorticoid, is used as a topical anti-inflammatory agent. Cortisol also influences the heart, vasculature, blood pressure, water excretion, and electrolyte balance. It influences bone turnover through a variety of mechanisms, and osteoporosis is a recognized consequence of sustained cortisol excess.

Clinical disorders of cortisol secretion

Hyposecretion of cortisol may occur as a result of hypothalamic, pituitary, or adrenal failure

The diagnosis of the cause of cortisol hyposecretion relies on the clinical presentation, measurement of cortisol and ACTH, and the extent of the cortisol response to synthetic ACTH (Synacthen).

Deficiencies of CRH and ACTH are often accompanied by deficiencies of other hypothalamic or pituitary hormones. Addison's disease is a primary adrenal failure in which secretion of all adrenal hormones is decreased, usually because of autoimmune disease or infection. Biochemically, it is characterized by hyponatremia, an impaired cortisol response to Synacthen, and an elevated plasma ACTH. Cortisol replacement, usually with a mineralocorticoid, is an effective treatment for this life-threatening condition.

Rarely, cortisol hyposecretion results from a genetic disorder in the steroid biosynthetic pathway: congenital adrenal hyperplasia. The most frequently affected enzyme is the steroid 21-hydroxylase (see Fig. 37.7). Hyponatremia develops in neonates and may be accompanied by ambiguous

PRIMARY ADRENAL INSUFFICIENCY – AN ENDOCRINE EMERGENCY

A 40-year-old woman was admitted as a medical emergency after collapsing at home 2 days after contracting influenza. For 1 year she had been complaining of chronic weakness and fatigue, and lately of abdominal pain, nausea, vomiting, anorexia and confusion. She was dehydrated and hypotensive with pigmentation of the palmar creases and buccal mucosa. Biochemical analysis revealed Na$^+$ 115 mmol/L (135–145 mmol/L); K$^+$ 5.9 mmol/l (3.5–5.0 mmol/L); urea 12 mmol/L (2.5–6.5 mmol/L) and glucose 2.9 mmol/L (4.0–6.0 mmol/L). Baseline serum cortisol was 95 nmol/L rising to 110 nmol/L 30 minutes after administration of synthetic ACTH (Synacthen).

Comment. This is an acute presentation of Addison's disease resulting from progressive autoimmune destruction of the adrenal cortex. The nonspecific symptoms of cortisol deficiency became critical after the stress of a minor illness. The hypotension and electrolyte imbalance result from mineralocorticoid deficiency. The pigmentation is due to elevated ACTH and other POMC peptides (notably melanocyte stimulating hormone). The diagnosis is made by the impaired cortisol response to synthetic ACTH (normal increment >200 nmol/L). Treatment is rehydration with intravenous saline, plus a bolus of intravenous hydrocortisone followed by daily maintenance therapy with hydrocortisone and a mineralocorticoid.

CUSHING'S SYNDROME – A DIAGNOSTIC DILEMMA

A 65-year-old man presented with a history of rapid weight gain, central obesity, a plethoric face (full, moon-shape) and abdominal bruising. He was mildly hypertensive. Urinary cortisol was 1000 nmol/24 h (normal <250 nmol/24 h); serum cortisol was 500 nmol/L at 24.00 h (normal <50 nmol/L) and his 08.00 h cortisol was 550 nmol/L after 1 mg of dexamethasone (a potent synthetic glucocorticoid) (normal <50 nmol/L). Plasma ACTH was 100 ng/L (normal <80 ng/L).

Comment. This man has hypercortisolism, known as Cushing's syndrome. The elevated urine cortisol, elevated evening serum cortisol and failure to suppress following dexamethasone administration support the diagnosis. The ACTH result indicates that the cause is either a pituitary tumor or ectopic ACTH secretion from an occult tumor (probably carcinoid). In this case magnetic resonance imaging (MRI) of the pituitary revealed a clear tumor of 0.5 cm diameter; the differential diagnosis is not often this easy. Pituitary surgery is the appropriate treatment in this case.

genitalia resulting from the metabolism of accumulated 17-hydroxyprogesterone into androgens. A milder form presents in teenage girls where the androgen excess results in hirsutism and menstrual irregularity. A clinical example of this condition is given in Chapter 16 (clinical box on p. 218).

Hypersecretion of cortisol results in Cushing's syndrome – easily the most challenging of all endocrine disorders

Exogenous glucocorticoids, commonly used to suppress the immune system in a range of gastrointestinal or dermatologic disorders, may cause clinical Cushing's syndrome. However, Cushing's syndrome may also result from a disorder of the hypothalamus, pituitary, or adrenal gland; or it may be the consequence of ectopic ACTH syndrome. The symptoms are often nonspecific and cyclical, but there is general deposition of fat in the face and trunk, wasting of skeletal muscle, and development of glucose intolerance. Once cortisol excess is demonstrated, the diagnosis can be made using ACTH measurements, dexamethasone (a synthetic glucocorticoid) suppressibility tests, and selective venous catheterization of the pituitary or the adrenal glands. Treatment is usually surgical and should be targeted at the primary cause of the condition.

THE HYPOTHALAMO–PITUITARY– GONADAL AXIS

Gonadotropin-releasing hormone (GnRH)

GnRH is essential for the secretion of intact FSH and LH

The hypothalamus has a major role in the control of gonadal function in both males and females. The secretion of GnRH is the first stage in the onset of puberty. GnRH, in turn, influences the relative secretion of pituitary FSH and LH. GnRH is a decapeptide synthesized as a 92-amino-acid precursor by various hypothalamic nuclei and transported to the pituitary via the portal system. It is secreted in a pulsatile fashion and induces the synthesis and secretion of both FSH and LH from the same gonadotroph cell type. GnRH acts through its cell surface receptor to increase intracellular calcium, hydrolyze phosphoinositides, and activate protein kinase C. Through feedback loops, estrogens increase and androgens decrease the number of GnRH receptors. Long-acting GnRH agonists can also cause down-regulation of GnRH receptors and reduced FSH and LH secretion. Such agonists are now used to treat prostate cancer and to prepare infertile women for assisted-conception programs.

BIOCHEMICAL CONFIRMATION OF PREGNANCY

Biochemical confirmation of pregnancy is now achieved by means of a simple and sensitive test that can give reliable results within 2 weeks of fertilization (i.e. before the next menstrual period). Pregnancy tests may be performed by doctors, nurses, or even the patients themselves since they are readily purchased from pharmacies.

Pregnancy tests are immunoassays that measure the production of human chorionic gonadotropin (HCG). A specific two-site immunoassay is employed (see Fig. 37.2). One antibody recognizes the α-subunit of HCG, while the other only binds to the 32-amino-acid segment of the β-subunit that is unique to HCG (see Fig. 37.8). Since nonpregnant women do not normally produce HCG, the detection of even low levels from the first stages of placental development is sufficient to confirm pregnancy.

Follicle-stimulating hormone and luteinizing hormone

Although FSH and LH have been given their names on the basis of their function in the female, it is now clear that identical hormones are secreted and function in the male

Both FSH and LH are secreted in the male and female and appear to be under the influence of the same stimulus (GnRH). There is growing evidence that alterations in the GnRH pulse frequency and amplitude can influence the relative amounts of FSH and LH secreted by the gonadotroph. Inhibin, as a selective feedback inhibitor of FSH, also affects the relative output of FSH and LH from the cell.

FSH and LH are both glycoproteins with molecular weights of approximately 28 kDa. Each contains an identical α-subunit (shared with TSH) and a specific β-subunit. The gene for LH has recently undergone duplication to produce HCG, a gonadotropin secreted by embryonic tissues (Fig. 37.8).

Although GnRH is essential for the secretion of intact FSH and LH, feedback from estradiol and testosterone plus gonadal peptides such as inhibin have a secondary effect. Feedback by estradiol is especially interesting because it may have either negative or positive effects on gonadotropins depending on the stage of the menstrual cycle. An outline of the control of the hypothalamo-pituitary-gonadal axes, both for adult men and women, is shown in Figure 37.9.

The production rate of LH in men and ovulating women is about 200 IU/day; the corresponding figure for FSH is around 50 IU/day. These production rates are greatly increased in postmenopausal women in whom there is no negative feedback from ovarian steroids. The half-life of LH in plasma is approximately 50 minutes, FSH has a longer half-life of about

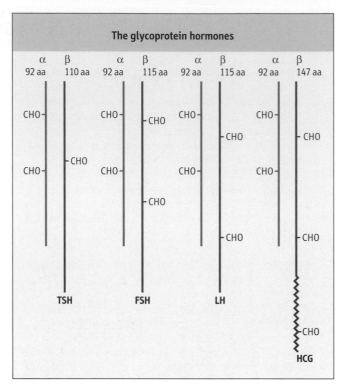

Fig. 37.8 **Relative structures of glycoprotein hormones.** The three pituitary glycoprotein hormones (TSH, FSH, LH) and the placental glycoprotein (HCG) share a common α–subunit. Hormone specificity is conveyed by the β-subunit and the resulting three-dimensional protein structure. CHO indicates the approximate location of carbohydrate side chains. HCG differs from LH solely by having an additional 32 amino acids in its β-subunit. aa, amino acids.

4 hours. Both FSH and LH concentrations vary considerably depending on age and sex (Fig. 37.10).

Actions of FSH and LH on the testes

FSH and LH influence spermatogenesis

In the male, testosterone biosynthesis occurs in the Leydig cells of the testes under the primary influence of LH (see Fig. 37.9). The LH receptor is a member of the G-protein coupled superfamily, which includes the receptors for TSH and FSH among many others (see Chapter 38). These receptors, with seven transmembrane spanning units, mediate the activation of adenylate cyclase, leading to regulation of the steroidogenic enzymes shown in Figure 37.7.

Among other functions, testosterone facilitates the effects of FSH on spermatogenesis in the spermatic tubule. FSH binds to its specific receptor on the Sertoli cell of the testes and, by a mechanism similar to LH, induces increased synthesis of several proteins, including androgen-binding protein (ABP) and inhibin. ABP is secreted into the seminiferous tubular lumen where it binds testosterone (or its active form dihydrotestosterone). This ensures a high local androgen

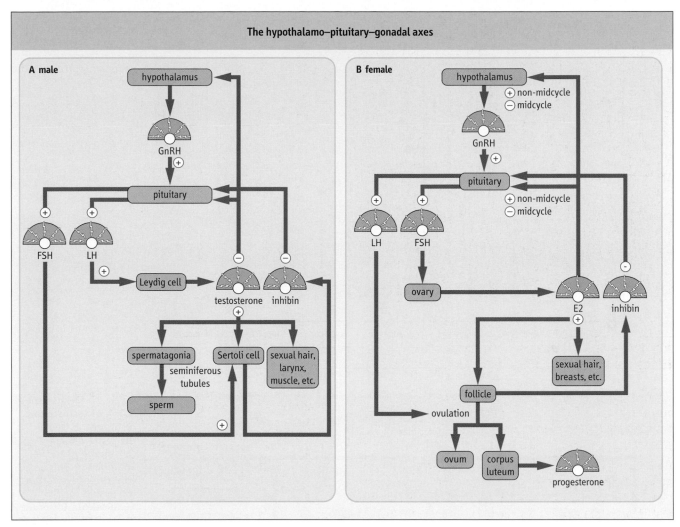

Fig. 37.9 **Control of the hypothalamo-pituitary-gonadal axes.** (A) In men, testosterone is produced from cholesterol in the Leydig cell under LH stimulation. Testosterone and FSH support spermatogenesis. (B) In women, estradiol (E_2) is produced by the granulosa cell and the developing follicle after feedback stimulation. E_2 feedback is mainly negative but, in midcycle, there is a positive E_2 feedback resulting in the surge of LH that causes ovulation. Progesterone (P) is secreted by the resultant corpus luteum.

concentration that, together with FSH, brings about the meiotic divisions that are necessary for spermatogenesis. Inhibin has a role in the FSH negative feedback loop (see Fig. 37.9).

Biochemical actions of testosterone in the male

Testosterone not only influences gonadotropin regulation and spermatogenesis, but is also a natural anabolic steroid

The testes secrete about 7 mg of testosterone each day into the peripheral circulation. A further 500 μg of testos-terone originates from the adrenal gland. More than 97% of the circulating testosterone is bound to protein, with equal amounts bound to albumin and to the specific sex hormone-binding globulin (SHBG), which is similar in structure to ABP. Testosterone is further metabolized to dihydrotestosterone (DHT) via 5-α reduction; this modification more than doubles its affinity for the nuclear androgen receptor. In addition to effects on gonadotropin regulation and spermatogenesis, androgens induce the development of the reproductive tract from the Wolffian ducts during male sexual differentiation. They also have anabolic effects, stimulating protein synthesis and an increase in muscle mass (Fig. 37.11).

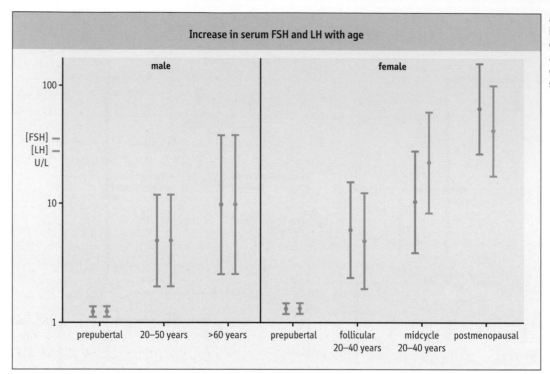

Fig. 37.10 **Variations in serum FSH and LH during life.** Serum FSH and LH levels vary depending on age and sex.

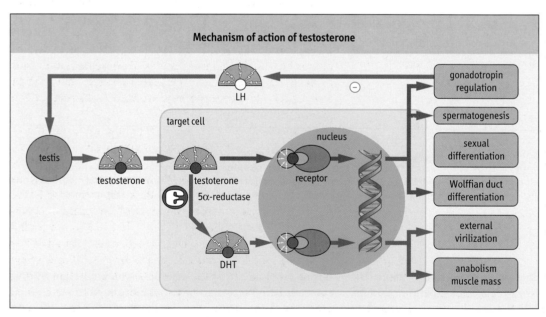

Fig. 37.11 **Mechanism of action of testosterone.** Testosterone from the testis enters a target cell and binds to the androgen receptor, either directly or after conversion to 5α-dihydrotestosterone (DHT). DHT binds more tightly than testosterone, and the DHT-receptor complex binds more efficiently to chromatin. Actions mediated by testosterone are shown by purple lines, those mediated by DHT are shown by blue lines.

Clinical disorders of testosterone secretion in males

Testosterone deficiency may originate from a wide range of disorders of the hypothalamus, pituitary or testes

A genetic hypothalamic disorder in children (Kallmann's syndrome) results in deficient GnRH production; affected individuals present with delayed puberty and subnormal FSH, LH, and testosterone. A genetic testicular disorder of the seminiferous tubules (Klinefelter's syndrome, karyotype 47XXY) presents with gynecomastia (abnormal increase in size of the male breast), eunuchoidism, and varying degrees of hypogonadism. Serum FSH is elevated, and LH is usually elevated, but testosterone may be subnormal. The external effects of hypogonadism may be corrected by androgen administration but these patients are sterile. Androgen deficiency in older men may have a specific cause (e.g. a pituitary tumor or mumps orchitis, which is an infection of the testes) or it may be part of the natural aging process. Muscle and fat distribution also change,

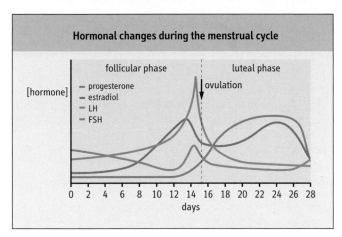

Hormonal changes during the menstrual cycle

Fig. 37.12 **Changes in hormone secretion during the normal menstrual cycle.** LH, luteinizing hormone; FSH, follicle stimulating hormone.

and these may be corrected, to some extent, by androgen administration.

Androgen excess in males is only seen in precocious puberty

Precocious puberty is a rare condition that may result either from early maturation of the normal hypothalamo–pituitary–gonadal axis, gain-of-function mutations in the LH receptor, or as a result of a tumor that is secreting either androgen or HCG.

Actions of FSH and LH on the ovary

In the female, FSH promotes estradiol synthesis leading to follicular maturation, while LH leads to follicle rupture and oocyte release

In the mature female the GnRH pulse generator is responsible for the control of all the hormonal changes seen in the normal menstrual cycle (Figs. 37.9 and 37.12). The initiation of follicular growth begins in the last few days of the preceding menstrual cycle and terminates at the time of ovulation. FSH is the dominant hormone acting through its receptors on the ovarian granulosa cells. Rising FSH concentrations stimulate estradiol synthesis through induction of the aromatase and other enzymes (see Fig. 37.7). As estradiol is secreted so FSH falls, and this combination leads to the selection of a dominant follicle for further development. Follicular maturation continues under the influence of rising estradiol concentrations. At midcycle there is a further estradiol surge, which causes positive feedback at the pituitary to initiate the LH surge. This LH binds to its receptors on the dominant follicle and, in tandem with steroid hormones and other factors such as prostaglandins, results some 36 hours later in rupture of the follicle and release of the oocyte, i.e. ovulation. At this time there is a sharp fall in plasma estradiol, followed

by a fall in LH. The ruptured follicle transforms into the corpus luteum, which secretes progesterone and lesser amounts of estradiol both to sustain the oocyte and to prepare the estrogen primed uterine endometrium for implantation of a fertilized ovum and the establishment of early pregnancy. In the absence of fertilization, corpus luteum function declines, and progesterone and estradiol secretion fall. This brings about vascular changes in the endometrium leading to tissue death and menstruation. The decline in steroid secretion stimulates FSH secretion, setting the stage for initiation of the next cycle.

Actions of steroid hormones in the female

In a woman with a normal menstrual cycle, it is the progesterone level that is of diagnostic significance

The concentrations of FSH, LH, estradiol, and progesterone vary considerably during the menstrual cycle. In a normally cycling woman it is only progesterone that is of diagnostic significance: a serum concentration of more than 20 nmol/L in the luteal phase is consistent with ovulation. The production rate of estradiol is 80 µg/day early in the cycle rising 10-fold during the follicular phase. In contrast the production rate of progesterone is 2 mg/day in the follicular phase and 10-fold greater in the luteal phase. Estradiol binds to SHBG in plasma, although with a lower affinity than testosterone. Progesterone binds to CBG in plasma with a lower affinity than cortisol.

Aside from their roles in the menstrual cycle and reproduction, both estradiol and progesterone have other effects, acting via their specific nuclear receptors in target cells. Estradiol, working in tandem with other hormones such as insulin-like growth factor-I (IGF-I), is responsible for linear growth, breast development and maturation of the urogenital tract and the female habitus. In adult life, both estradiol and progesterone support breast function, and estradiol has an important role in influencing bone turnover. Progesterone is responsible for the rise in basal body temperature during the luteal phase of the menstrual cycle and decreases in progesterone secretion may contribute to changes in mood as seen in premenstrual tension.

Disorders of steroid secretion in the female

Just as in the male, endocrine disorders of subnormal sex steroid secretion in the female may result from a wide range of disorders in the hypothalamus, pituitary, or ovary

Kallmann's syndrome is seen in females as well as males, but the most common genetic disorder affecting the ovary is

POLYCYSTIC OVARY SYNDROME – A COMMON CAUSE OF INFERTILITY

A 24-year-old woman presented with a 2-year history of oligomenorrhea (infrequent menstruation) and infertility. She was obese with facial acne and mild hirsutism. Basal hormone studies showed normal FSH, LH prolactin and estradiol, but she has a serum testosterone of 4.5 nmol/L (0.9–3.2 nmol/L).

Comment. This woman's polycystic ovary syndrome (PCOS) was confirmed by ultrasound of the ovaries showing enlargement with the characteristic cysts that secrete testosterone (and other androgens). The androgen is the cause of the hirsutism and its interference with the normal estrogen feedback at the pituitary causes the oligomenorrhea and infertility. The cause of the syndrome is unclear but hyperinsulinaemia secondary to peripheral insulin resistance has been implicated. Insulin and insulin growth factor stimulate the ovaries to secrete androgens.

HORMONE REPLACEMENT THERAPY (HRT)

Women normally reach menopause at 45–55 years of age. The absence of ovarian follicles leads to an absence of estrogen and inhibin secretion resulting in a marked rise in pituitary FSH. There are vasomotor symptoms of estrogen deficiency (flushing) associated with menopause. Long-term postmenopausal estrogen deficiency is known to increase the rate of bone loss, leading to osteoporosis, and also alters lipoprotein metabolism in a way that increases the risk of cardiovascular disease.
HRT with an estrogen preparation was standard practice in most developed countries both to relieve the acute symptoms and to provide prophylaxis against the long-term risks. However, recent studies have shown that HRT increases a woman's risk for breast cancer, cardiovascular disease, stroke, and pulmonary embolism. Although HRT did have a modest effect on preventing osteoporosis, there are newer drugs, the bisphosphonates, that are just as effective. The current recommendations are that HRT should only be used as short-term therapy for vasomotor symptoms that do not respond to other treatment.

Turner's syndrome (karyotype 45X), which has characteristic somatic features and an elevated plasma FSH and prepubertal estradiol pattern. In the mature female there are various endocrine causes of infertility, which is beyond the scope of this text. Although reduced estradiol secretion is a natural consequence of menopause, hormone replacement therapy (HRT) can no longer be routinely recommended because of the numerous undesirable side-effects (box).

Syndromes of excess ovarian steroid secretion lead to precocious puberty in children and infertility and/or hirsutism in the adult

Precocious puberty may arise from early maturation of the normal axis, an estradiol- or androgen-secreting cyst or tumor of the ovary or the adrenal gland, or congenital adrenal hyperplasia. In the mature female, hypersecretion of androgen in the polycystic ovary syndrome (PCOS) may result both in infertility and/or hirsutism (growth of male type and distribution of hair in women).

THE GROWTH HORMONE AXIS

Growth hormone-releasing hormone (GHRH) and somatostatin

GHRH is a 44-amino-acid peptide belonging to the secretin–vasointestinal peptide-glucagon family of hormones, and is synthesized as part of a 108-amino-acid prohormone. Immunohistochemical studies have located GHRH in the arcuate and ventromedial nuclei of the hypothalamus and in the median eminence. GHRH binds to its receptor on the pituitary somatotroph cell and triggers both the adeny-late cyclase and intracellular calcium-calmodulin systems to stimulate GH transcription and secretion from the anterior pituitary. Negative feedback from GH and IGF-I results in both a decrease in GHRH synthesis and secretion and an increase in somatostatin synthesis and secretion.

Somatostatin is found in two forms with 14 and 28 amino acids, both of which are produced from the same 116-amino-acid gene product. Somatostatin and its receptors are found throughout the brain and also in other organs, notably the gut. Binding of somatostatin to its receptor is coupled to adenylate cyclase by an inhibitory guanine nucleotide-binding protein, resulting in a decrease in intracellular cAMP. In the context of growth, somatostatin inhibits the secretion of GH. GHRH and somatostatin are released in separate bursts to provide a very fine level of control of GH release. Somatostatin also inhibits basal and stimulated TSH release. Long-acting analogs of somatostatin are effective in the management of GH excess and tumors secreting a wide range of other hormones including TSH, insulin, and glucagon.

Growth hormone

The greatest secretion of GH occurs in children and young adults; it occurs chiefly during sleep

Although GH can exist in variant forms, the major species is a 22 kDa protein. Nearly two-thirds of GH in the circulation is associated with a 29 kDa binding protein that is identical to the extracellular domain of the GH receptor. This binding protein prolongs the half-life of GH in plasma, about 20 minutes.

The normal human pituitary contains approximately 10 mg of GH; less than 5% of this is released each day. GH is released in bursts with a periodicity of 3-4 hours and greatest secretory activity occurs during sleep. At the peak of a secretory burst, the plasma GH concentration may be 100-fold greater than baseline; this means that no meaningful reference interval can be derived for this hormone. Secretory bursts occur most frequently in children and young adults.

Control of GH secretion

GH has a wide range of actions in regulating growth and intermediary metabolism

It is not surprising, in view of the wide range of actions of GH, that several factors other than GHRH and somatostatin can influence GH secretion. These include other hormones (estradiol) and metabolic fuels (glucose). Several pharmacologic agents are also known to influence GH secretion. These factors act at the higher centers and the hypothalamus to alter the pattern of GHRH and somatostatin secretion.

Biochemical actions of GH

Binding of GH to its receptor precipitates a complex series of intracellular events that lead to the transcription of many enzymes, hormones and growth factors, including IGF-I

The diversity of action of GH makes it difficult to understand or integrate all of its functions; thus it is convenient to think in two distinct phases (Fig. 37.13). The direct actions of GH are on lipid, carbohydrate, and protein metabolism. During hypoglycemia, GH stimulates lipolysis and induces peripheral resistance to insulin. These effects stimulate the use of fatty acids in peripheral tissues, sparing glucose for use in the brain. Previously, GH therapy was used only for treatment of GH-deficiency in children in order to stimulate

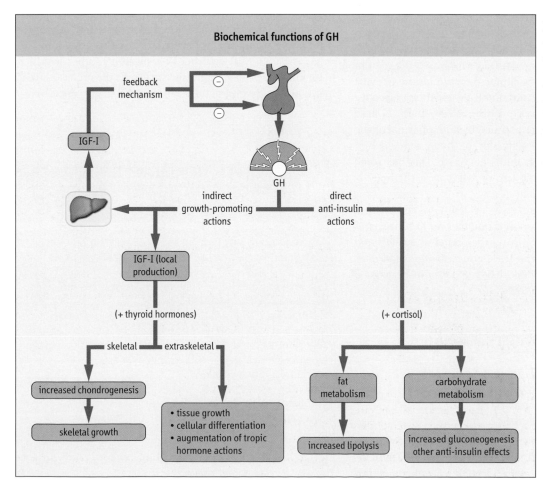

Fig. 37.13 **Biochemical functions of GH.** These can be divided conveniently into direct actions on lipid and carbohydrate metabolism and indirect actions on protein synthesis and cell proliferation.

growth; however treatment is now often extended into adulthood because untreated individuals are susceptible to hypoglycemia. This change in treatment strategy illustrates the complex effects of GH on metabolism. During growth, GH stimulates the uptake of amino acids and their incorporation into protein, especially in muscle. The indirect actions of GH are mediated by IGF-I. These actions promote the proliferation of chondrocytes and the synthesis of cartilage matrix in skeletal tissues. Although GH is most often associated with its role in stimulating linear growth, it clearly has other roles in influencing the relative amount and distribution of fat and muscle tissue.

Insulin-like growth factor I

IGF-I is the most GH-dependent of a series of growth factors

IGF-I is a 70-amino-acid single-chain basic peptide; it has considerable homology with proinsulin. In response to tropic hormones like GH, IGF-I is produced in many tissues, whose growth is then stimulated; that is, IGF-I acts as a parahormone. The liver is the major source of circulating IGF-I, whose function is primarily feedback inhibition of GH secretion. In plasma and other extracellular fluids, IGF-I is complexed to a series of IGF-binding proteins (IGFBPs) of which IGFBP-3 is the most abundant. IGF-I works through the type 1 IGF receptor, which is structurally similar to the insulin receptor and linked to intracellular tyrosine kinase activity. The relative affinities of insulin and IGF-I for their respective receptors mean that, in normal physiology, there is little cross-binding, although in pathologic and pharmacologic situations it is possible for insulin to have some action through the IGF-I receptor, and vice versa. This has some implications for the possible use of IGF-I as a therapeutic agent in type 2 diabetes mellitus.

The plasma reference interval for IGF-I in adults aged 20–60 years is fairly constant. It is much lower in young children but rises dramatically during the period of growth and progression through puberty. IGF-I concentrations fall after the sixth decade of life. Thus, IGF-I appears to be a good marker of integrated GH activity.

Clinical disorders of GH secretion

GH deficiency in children is one of several causes of short stature, while GH excess in children leads to gigantism and, in adults, acromegaly

The absence of a plasma reference range for GH means that GH deficiency may only be diagnosed by studying the dynamics of GH secretion, either during sleep or following a stimulation test. Basal IGF-I or IGFBP-3 measurements may serve

as a preliminary screening test. Treatment is by regular injection of recombinant human GH. Adults with a definite cause of GH deficiency (hypopituitarism) are also candidates for GH replacement therapy. A rare genetic cause of short stature is Laron dwarfism in which GH levels are elevated but IGF-I levels are subnormal – a GH receptor defect is responsible.

In most cases, GH excess is caused by a pituitary tumor

GH excess is almost always due to a GH-secreting pituitary tumor, although GHRH-secreting tumors in the hypothalamus and ectopic GHRH production from pancreatic tumors have been described. In children, GH excess manifests itself as gigantism. In adults, the epiphyses of the long bones have closed and so further linear growth is not possible. Therefore, the adult form, acromegaly, is characterized by a thickening of tissues and overgrowth of the bones in the hands, feet and face. Enlarged lips and tongue with mandibular overgrowth give rise to a classic facial appearance. Excessive sweating and arthritis are also common symptoms. Unfortunately, the progression of acromegaly is so slow that an average of 9 years elapses between the onset of symptoms and diagnosis. Classically, the diagnosis of GH excess has relied on showing inadequate GH suppression during a standard 75 g oral glucose tolerance test and on elevated IGF-I levels. However, pubescent patients may have paradoxical responses to glucose, and IGF-I levels are normally elevated during this developmental stage. As such, MRI evidence of a pituitary tumor is critical in making the proper diagnosis. Surgery is the preferred treatment, although long-acting somatostatin is also effective.

GROWTH HORMONE RESISTANCE (LARON SYNDROME) – INCIDENCE ~1 PER 1–2 MILLION

A 5-year-old boy was brought to his GP because his mother was concerned that he had been the smallest in his class, and of the same size as his 3-year-old brother. Both parents were of average height. He was referred to hospital. His measured height was well below the 0.3 centile.

He underwent an insulin tolerance tests to assess his GH reserve and high levels were found throughout (GH >30 iU/l). The endocrinologist asked for the measurement of the insulin growth factor-I (IGF-I) to be performed. The IGF-I concentration was very low.

Comment. The high circulating levels of GH with the corresponding failure to produce IGF-I in the liver are diagnostic of the Laron syndrome. This is a defect in the GH receptors inherited in an autosomal recessive pattern. Without treatment the final height is likely to be 120–130 cm. GH is ineffective and specific treatment with IGF-I is required.

THE PROLACTIN AXIS

Dopamine

Dopamine is an inhibitor of prolactin secretion

Prolactin is unique among the pituitary hormones in that it is under predominantly inhibitory control from the hypothalamus (see Fig. 37.4). Furthermore, the controlling agent is the very simple molecule dopamine, which is produced by tuberoinfundibular dopamine neurons. Dopamine works by stimulating the pituitary lactotroph D2 receptor to inhibit adenylate cyclase and consequently inhibits both prolactin synthesis and secretion. Several neuropeptides, including TRH, have prolactin-releasing properties, but there is little evidence for a physiologic role.

Prolactin

Prolactin may assist breast growth and milk formation in association with other pregnancy-related hormones

Prolactin is a 23 kDa protein, which is homologous to GH. The primary role for prolactin in humans occurs during pregnancy when prolactin binds to its receptor in mammary tissue and stimulates the synthesis of several milk proteins, including lactalbumin (see Chapter 25). In other animals, prolactin also has gonadotropic, immunological, and hematological effects: it is required for maintenance of pregnancy in rodents, is mitogenic for some immune cells, and it ameliorates some forms of anemia. Prolactin exerts its effects on female reproductive function by blocking the action of FSH on follicular estrogen secretion and by enhancing progesterone levels by inhibiting steroid-metabolizing enzymes.

Clinical disorders of prolactin secretion

There are no known prolactin deficiency syndromes but hyperprolactinemia is very common

Hyperprolactinemia may result from a prolactin-secreting pituitary tumor (prolactinoma), a deficient supply of dopamine from the hypothalamus, or the use of any of a wide range of antidopaminergic drugs. In women, the presenting features of hyperprolactinemia include menstrual irregularity and galactorrhea (discharge of milk from the breast). A grossly elevated serum prolactin is usually diagnostic of a prolactinoma. For subjects with modest hyperprolactinemia, who are not taking antidopaminergic drugs, the differential diagnosis is difficult; pituitary imaging and/or dynamic tests of prolactin secretion will assist the diagnosis of a microprolactinoma. Treatment options include long-acting dopamine agonist drugs or surgery. In men, hyperprolactinemia can cause impotence and prostatic hyperplasia. However, because other conditions more commonly produce these symptoms, the diagnosis of hyperprolactinemia is often missed until prolactinomas become very large and present as hypopituitarism with visual field defects. The latter symptoms arise when the tumor expands out of the pituitary fossa and impinges on the optic chiasm. Such tumors often shrink with dopamine agonist therapy.

Summary

The endocrine system produces hormones, a structurally diverse group of chemical messengers that regulate and coordinate whole body metabolism, growth, reproduction, and responses to external stimuli. The hypothalamic–anterior pituitary axis controls the synthesis and action of several major hormones: thyroid hormone, glucocorticoids, sex steroids, growth hormone, and prolactin. The hypothalamic–posterior pituitary axis controls the production and release of oxytocin and AVP/ADH. The action of these hormones on cells is controlled by receptors located either on cell membranes or intracellularly. Feedback mechanisms are important in controlling the endocrine systems. Both over-activity and under-activity of a hormone produce distinct clinical syndromes. Laboratory diagnosis of endocrine disorders relies heavily on the measurements of hormones in blood and also on function tests that check the integrity of endocrine regulatory systems.

The human body contains several other endocrine systems not considered in this chapter. Some of these are considered in other chapters as part of the physiologic function that they control. Thus the reader is referred to Chapter 20 for carbohydrate homeostasis, Chapter 24 for calcium homeostasis and Chapter 22 for water and electrolyte homeostasis and the control of blood pressure. The intracellular signaling systems through which hormones exert their effects are described in the next chapter.

ACTIVE LEARNING

1. Trace the flow of information from the hypothalamus to the ovum early in the menstrual cycle.
2. How do GH, cortisol, and insulin interact to regulate lipid and carbohydrate metabolism?
3. Because dietary iodide can vary greatly, thyroid hormones need to be synthesized and stored when iodide is available; but thyroid hormones are hydrophobic and cannot be contained within membrane vesicles. How does the thyroid gland solve this problem?

Further reading

Buffet NC, Bouchard P. The neuroendocrine regulation of the human ovarian cycle. *Chronobiol Int* 2001;**18**:893–919.

Hasinski S. Assessment of adrenal glucocorticoid function. Which tests are appropriate for screening? *Postgrad Med* 1998;**104**:6–4, 69–72.

Merza Z. Modern treatment of acromegaly. *Postgrad Med J* 2003;79:189–194.

Monzavi R, Cohen P. IGFs and IGFBPs: role in health and disease. *Best Pract Res Clin Endocrinol Metab* 2002;**16**:433–447.

Niewoehner CB, Niewoehner DE. Steroid-induced osteoporosis. Are your asthmatic patients at risk? *Postgrad Med* 1999;**105**:79–83, 87–8, 91.

Ribela MT, Gout PW, Bartolini P. Synthesis and chromatographic purification of recombinant human pituitary hormones. *J Chromatogr B Analyt Technol Biomed Life Sci* 2003;**790**:285–316.

Yen PM. Physiological and molecular basis of thyroid hormone action. *Physiol Rev* 2001;**81**:1097–1142.

Relevant websites

Endotext: www.endotext.org

Cushing's Syndrome: www.medstudents.com.br/endoc/endoc7.htm

www.cushings-help.com/HPA_axis.htm

Thyroid hormone: www.thyroidmanager.org

Glucocorticoids: www.uspharmacist.com/NewLook/CE/glucocort/lesson.htm

38. Membrane Receptors and Signal Transduction

M M Harnett and H S Goodridge

After reading this chapter you should be able to:

- Distinguish between steroid and polypeptide hormones, and outline their mechanisms of action.
- Describe G-protein-coupled receptors.
- Outline the activation of downstream intracellular signaling cascades by heterotrimeric G-proteins.
- Discuss the generation of second messengers such as cyclic AMP, IP_3, DAG and Ca^{2+}, and explain how they activate key protein kinases.
- Explain how phospholipases generate a diverse array of lipid second messengers.
- Discuss how the generation of a variety of second messengers can amplify hormone signals and lead to the generation of specific biological responses.

INTRODUCTION

Cells sense, respond to, and integrate a multiplicity of signals from their environment. Although some of these signals may be mediated by cell–cell contact, in multicellular organisms many signal molecules, such as hormones, originate in organs distant from their site of action and must be carried in the blood to their target effector cells. Likewise, immune cells such as phagocytes are recruited from the blood to sites of inflammation by migrating along chemo-attractant gradients. Signals generated in these ways are sensed and processed by cellular signal transduction cassettes that comprise specific cell-surface membrane receptors, effector signaling elements, and regulatory proteins. These signaling cassettes serve to detect, amplify, and integrate diverse external signals to generate the appropriate cellular response (Fig. 38.1). In this chapter, we first discuss how cell-surface receptors sense and transduce their specific hormone signal by transmembrane coupling to effector enzyme systems, generating low-molecular-weight molecules termed second messengers. We then discuss the diversity of these second messengers and how they influence the activity of a range of key protein kinases with distinct substrates that ultimately determine the type of obtained biological response.

HORMONE RECEPTORS

Hormones are biochemical messengers that act to orchestrate the responses of different cells within a multicellular organism (Chapter 37). They are generally synthesized by specific tissues and secreted directly into the blood, which transports them to their target responsive organs. Hormones can broadly be subdivided into two major classes:

- steroid hormones
- polypeptide hormones

These hormones achieve their biological effects by interacting with specific receptors to induce intracellular signaling cascades.

Intracellular receptors: steroid hormone receptors

Steroid hormones traverse cell membranes

Because of the cholesterol-based nature of their structure, steroid hormones, such as cortisol (made in the cortex of the adrenal gland), sex hormones, and vitamin D, can directly traverse the plasma membrane of cells to initiate their responses via cytoplasmically located receptors called steroid hormone receptors (see Fig. 38.1). These receptors belong to a superfamily of cytoplasmic receptors called the intracellular receptor superfamily, which also transduce signals from other small hydrophobic signaling molecules such as the tyrosine-derived thyroid hormones (e.g. thyroxine) and the vitamin A-derived retinoids (e.g. retinoic acid).

Intracellular receptors are transcription factors

The intracellular receptors for these steroid and thyroid hormones and retinoids are transcription factors; they bind to regulatory regions of the DNA of genes that are responsive to the particular steroid/thyroid hormone. Such 'ligand binding' (ligation) induces a conformational change in the

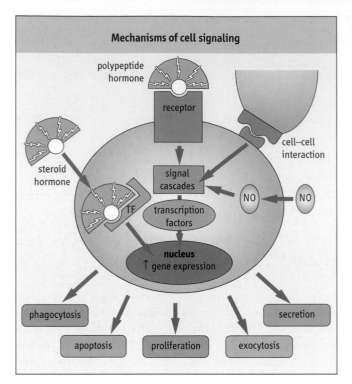

Fig. 38.1 **Mechanisms of cell signaling.** NO, nitric oxide; TF, transcription factor.

transcription factor that allows it to activate, or repress, gene induction. Although all the target cells have specific receptors for the individual hormones, they express distinct combinations of cell-type-specific regulatory proteins that cooperate with the intracellular hormone receptor to dictate the precise repertoire of genes that are induced. Hence the hormones induce distinct sets of responses in different target cells.

Cell–surface receptors: polypeptide hormone receptors

Polypeptide hormones act through membrane receptors

In contrast to the steroid hormones, polypeptide hormones cannot cross cell membranes and must initiate their effects on their target cells via specific cell surface receptors (see Fig. 38.1). As they do not themselves enter the target cell, they are termed 'first messengers' and their intracellular effects are mediated by low-molecular-weight signaling molecules, such as cyclic adenosine monophosphate (cAMP) or calcium, which are called 'second messengers'. In fact, the term 'polypeptide hormones' encompasses a wide range of families of hormones, growth factors, and cytokines that use transmembrane signal transduction cassettes to elicit their biological effects.

Receptor-independent signaling mechanisms

Some low-molecular-weight signaling molecules traverse the cell membrane

Although most extracellular signals mediate their effects via receptor ligation of either cell surface or cytoplasmic receptors, some low-molecular-weight signaling molecules are able to traverse the plasma membrane and directly modulate the activity of the catalytic domains of transmembrane receptors or cytoplasmic signal transducing enzymes (see Fig. 38.1). For example, nitric oxide (NO), which has been postulated to have a variety of functions including signaling the relaxation of smooth muscle cells in blood vessels, can stimulate guanylate cyclase, leading to the generation of the second messenger, cGMP. Patients with angina are treated with glyceryl trinitrate, which is converted to NO, resulting in relaxation of the blood vessels. The consequent improvement in oxygen delivery to the heart muscle eases the pain that was caused by inadequate blood flow to the heart.

RECEPTOR COUPLING TO INTRACELLULAR SIGNAL TRANSDUCTION

Some sensory systems use receptor-coupled signaling

In addition to hormone receptors, sensory systems such as vision (Chapter 39, Fig. 39.4), taste and smell use similar mechanisms of cell-surface membrane receptor-coupled signal transduction (see Table 38.1). Some of these receptors, for example the β-adrenergic receptors (see Fig. 38.2) or the antigen receptors on lymphocytes, have no intrinsic catalytic activity and serve simply as specific recognition units. These receptors use a variety of mechanisms, including adaptor molecules or catalytically active regulatory molecules such as G-proteins (guanosine triphosphatases, GTPases, which hydrolyze GTP), to couple them to their effector signaling elements, which are generally enzymes (often called signaling enzymes or signal transducers) or ion channels (Fig. 38.3). In contrast, other receptors – such as the intrinsic tyrosine kinase receptors for growth factors (e.g. platelet-derived growth factor, PDGF) or the intrinsic serine kinase receptors for molecules like transforming growth factor-β (TGF-β) – have extracellular ligand-binding domains and cytoplasmic catalytic domains. Thus, after receptor-ligand interactions (receptor ligation), these receptors can directly initiate their signaling cascades by phosphorylating and modulating the activities of target signal-transducing molecules (downstream signaling enzymes). These in turn propagate the growth factor signal by modulating the activity of further

Membrane receptors				
Receptor class	**Transmembrane-spanning domains**	**Intrinsic catalytic activity**	**Accessory coupling/regulatory molecules**	**Examples of receptor subclasses**
G-protein-coupled receptors (serpentine receptors)	multipass (seven transmembrane α-helices)	none	G-proteins	β-adrenergic α-adrenergic muscarinic chemokines (IL-8) rhodopsin (vision)
Ion-channel receptors (ligand-gated receptors)	multipass; generally form multimeric complexes	none	none	neurotransmitters ions nucleotides inositol trisphosphate (IP$_3$)
Intrinsic receptor tyrosine kinases	single-pass transmembrane domain, but may be multimeric (e.g. insulin receptor)	tyrosine kinase	none	epidermal growth factor (EGF) nerve growth factor (NGF) platelet-derived growth factor (PDGF) fibroblast growth factor (FGF) insulin
Tyrosine kinase-associated receptors	single-pass transmembrane domain, but generally form multimeric receptors	none	some require ITAM/ITIM-containing proteins	antigen receptors (ITAM–Src-related kinases) FcγR (ITIM–Src-related kinases) hemopoietin cytokine receptors (Janus kinases)
Intrinsic tyrosine phosphatase receptors	single-pass transmembrane domain	tyrosine phosphatase	none	CD45-phosphatase receptor
Intrinsic serine–threonine receptor kinases	single-pass transmembrane domain	serine–threonine kinase	none	tumor growth factor β (TGF-β)
Intrinsic guanylate cyclase receptors	single-pass transmembrane domain	guanylate cyclase (generates cGMP)	none	atrial natriuretic peptide (ANP) receptors
Death-domain receptors	single-pass transmembrane domain	none	death-domain accessory proteins (TRADD, FADD, RIP, TRAFs)	tumor necrosis factor (TNF-α) Fas

Table 38.1 **Classification of membrane receptors.** cGMP, cyclic guanosine monophosphate; FADD, fas-associated death domain; FcγR, Fc-γ receptor (receptor for immunoglobulin G); IL, interleukin; ITAM/ITIM, immunoreceptor tyrosine activation/inhibition motif; RIP, receptor-interacting protein; Src, Src-tyrosine kinase; TRADD, TNF-receptor-associated death domain; TRAFs, TNF-receptor-associated factors.

specific signal transducers or transcription factors, leading to gene induction (see Chapter 41).

G-protein-coupled receptors

G-protein-coupled receptors comprise a superfamily of structurally related receptors for hormones, neurotransmitters, inflammatory mediators, proteinases, taste and odorant molecules, and light photons. A classic example of this class of receptors is the β-adrenergic receptor (for which the ligand is epinephrine); its structure-function properties have been extensively studied with respect to its activation of signal transduction cascades (see Fig. 38.2). G-protein-coupled receptors are integral membrane proteins characterized by the seven transmembrane-spanning helices within their

structure. They generally comprise an extracellular N-terminus, seven transmembrane-spanning α-helices (20–28 hydrophobic amino acids each), three extracellular and intracellular loops, and an intracellular C-terminal tail. Ligands, such as epinephrine, typically bind to the G-protein-coupled receptor by sitting in a pocket formed by the seven transmembrane helices. G-protein-coupled receptors have no intrinsic catalytic domains; they therefore recruit guanine nucleotide-binding proteins (G-proteins), via their third cytoplasmic loop, to couple to their signal transduction elements.

G-proteins

G-proteins constitute a group of regulatory molecules that are involved in the regulation of a diverse range of biological processes, including signal transduction, protein synthesis,

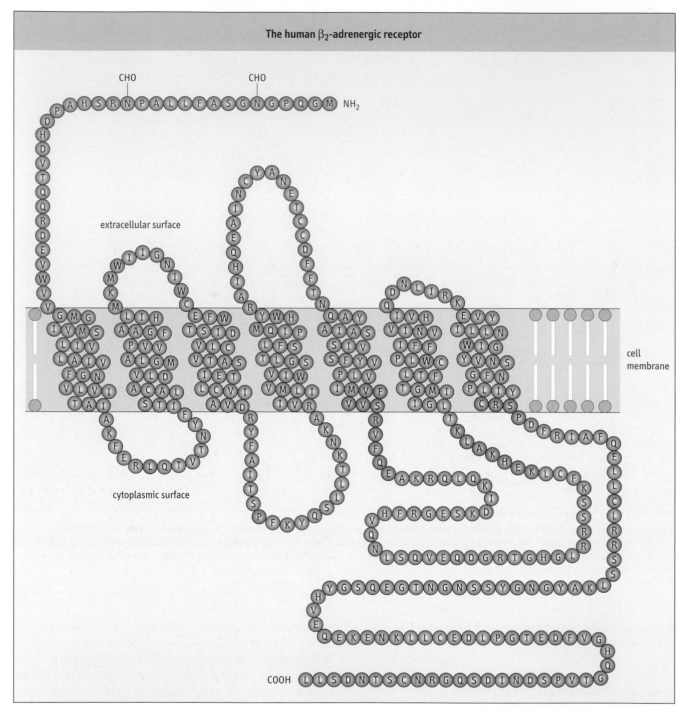

Fig. 38.2 **The human β-adrenergic receptor.** The sequence of this receptor is organized about the plasma membrane according to the seven membrane-spanning helices model. The ligand-binding site is deep within the plane of the membrane and is formed by amino acids from several of the transmembrane helices. Residues shown in blue in the third cytoplasmic loop and at the beginning of the cytoplasmic tail represent regions that, when deleted or substituted, prevent coupling of the mutated receptor to adenylyl cyclase. The blue residues in the first and second cytoplasmic loops (Leu[64] and Pro[138]) and the carboxyl tail (Cys[341]) are conserved in many G-protein-coupled receptors and, when mutated, are found to affect markedly both the expression and the functionality of the receptor (see also Chapter 39).

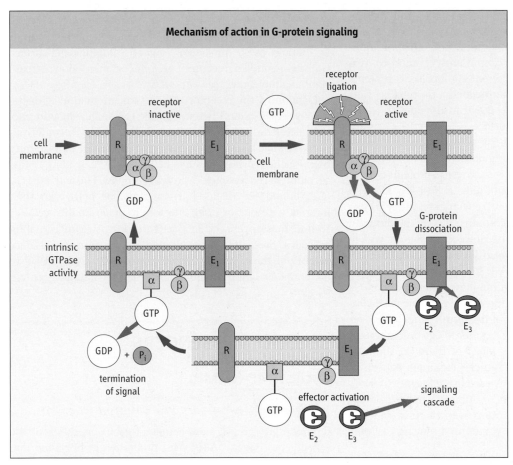

Mechanism of action in G-protein signaling

Fig. 38.3 **Mechanism of G-protein signaling.** In the inactive state, G-proteins exist as heterotrimers with GDP bound tightly to the α-subunit. None of the subunits are integral membrane proteins; however, the G-protein is anchored to the plasma membrane by lipid modification of the γ-subunits (prenylation) and some of the α-subunits (myristoylation of the $G_{i\alpha}$ family). Ligation of the receptor (R) drives exchange of GDP for GTP and induces a conformational change in Gα, which results in a decrease in its affinity both for the receptor and for the βγ-subunits, leading to dissociation of the receptor-G-protein complex. The activated Gα (GTP-bound) or the released βγ-subunits, or both, can then interact with one or more effectors, to generate intracellular second messengers that activate downstream signaling cascades. Signaling is terminated by the intrinsic GTPase activity of the α-subunit, which hydrolyzes GTP to GDP to allow re-association of the inactive, heterotrimeric G-protein, Gαβγ. (See also Fig. 39.4.)

 ## BACTERIAL TOXINS WHICH TARGET G-PROTEINS CAUSE A RANGE OF DISEASES

A variety of bacterial toxins exert their toxic effects by covalently modifying G-proteins and hence irreversibly modulating their function. For example, cholera toxin (choleragen) from *Vibrio cholerae* contains an enzyme (subunit A) that catalyzes the transfer of ADP-ribose from intracellular NAD to the α-subunit of G_s; this modification prevents the hydrolysis of G_s-bound GTP, resulting in a constitutively (permanently) active form of the G-protein. The resulting prolonged increase in cAMP concentrations within the intestinal epithelial cells leads to phosphokinase A-mediated phosphorylation of Cl^- channels, causing a large efflux of electrolytes and water into the gut, which is responsible for the severe diarrhea that is characteristic of cholera. Enterotoxin action is initiated by specific binding of the B (binding) subunits of choleragen (AB_5) to the oligosaccharide moiety of the monosialoganglioside, GM_1, on epithelial cells. A similar molecular mechanism has been attributed to the action of the heat-labile enterotoxin, labile toxin, secreted by several strains of *Escherichia coli* responsible for 'traveler's diarrhea'. In contrast, pertussis toxin (another AB_5 toxin) from *Bordetella pertussis*, the causative agent of whooping cough, catalyzes the ADP-ribosylation of G_i, which prevents G_i from interacting with activated receptors. Hence, the G-protein is inactivated and cannot act to inhibit adenylyl cyclase, activate PLA_2 or PLC, open K^+ channels, or open and close Ca^{2+} channels, causing a generalized uncoupling of hormone receptors from their signaling cascades. For example, the α2-adrenergic receptor mediates inhibition of insulin secretion from pancreatic islet cells by inhibiting adenylyl cyclase in a G_i-dependent manner.

intracellular trafficking (targeted delivery to the plasma membrane or intracellular organelles) and exocytosis, as well as cell movement, growth, proliferation and differentiation. The G-protein superfamily predominantly comprises two major subfamilies: the small, monomeric *Ras*-like G-proteins (see Chapter 41) and the heterotrimeric G-proteins. Heterotrimeric G-proteins regulate the transduction of transmembrane signals from cell–surface receptors to a variety of intracellular effectors, such as adenylyl cyclase, phospholipase C (PLC), cGMP-phosphodiesterase (PDE) and ion-channel effector systems (Fig. 38.3). These G-proteins consist of three distinct classes of subunits: α (39–46 kDa), β (37 kDa), and γ (8 kDa). In general, effector specificity is conferred by the α-subunit, which contains the GTP-binding site and an intrinsic GTPase activity. However, it is now widely accepted that $\beta\gamma$ complexes can also directly regulate effectors such as phospholipase A_2 (PLA_2), PLC-β isoforms, adenylyl cyclase and ion channels in mammalian systems, as well as cellular responses such as mating-factor receptor pathways in yeast. Four major subfamilies of α-subunit genes have been identified on the basis of their cDNA homology and function: G_s, G_i, G_q, and G_{12} (Table 38.2). Many of these Gα subunits have been shown to exhibit a rather ubiquitous pattern of expression in mammalian systems, at least at the mRNA level, but it is also clear that certain α-subunits have a tissue-restricted profile of expression. Moreover, there is evidence of differential expression of α-subunits during cellular development.

G-proteins act as molecular switches

Heterotrimeric G-proteins regulate transmembrane signals by acting as a molecular switch, linking cell-surface G-protein-coupled receptors to one or more downstream signaling molecules (see Fig. 38.3).

Ligation of the receptor initiates an interaction with the inactive, GDP-bound heterotrimeric G-protein. This interaction drives exchange of GDP for GTP, inducing a conformational change in Gα, which results in a decrease in its affinity both for the receptor and for the $\beta\gamma$-subunits, leading to dissociation of the receptor-G-protein complex. The activated Gα (GTP-bound) or released $\beta\gamma$-subunits, or both, can then interact with one or more effectors to generate intracellular second messengers, which activate downstream signaling cascades. Signaling is terminated by the intrinsic GTPase activity of the α-subunit, which hydrolyses GTP to GDP to allow reassociation of the inactive heterotrimeric G-protein (G$\alpha\beta\gamma$).

SECOND MESSENGERS

Cyclic AMP (cAMP)

β-adrenergic receptors are coupled to cAMP

β-adrenergic receptors are coupled to the generation of the second messenger, cAMP. The β-adrenergic hormone epi-

Properties of mammalian G-proteins					
G-protein subfamily	**α subunits**	**Molecular mass (kDa)**	**Toxin substrate**	**Tissue distribution**	**Effector**
G_i	G_z	41	none	brain, adrenal medulla, platelets	inhibits adenylate cyclase
	G_i	40	pertussis toxin	nearly ubiquitous	G_i α-subunits activate
	G_0	40	pertussis toxin	brain, neural systems	PLC and PLA_2 and K^+ channels, and inhibit adenylate cyclase and Ca^{2+} channels
	G_t	40	pertussis/cholera toxin	retinal rods and cones	activates cGMP-phosphodiesterase
	G_{gust}	40	pertussis toxin	taste buds	activates phosphodiesterase
G_s	G_s	44–46	cholera toxin	ubiquitous	G_s activates adenylate cyclase and Ca^{2+} channels
	G_{oll}	45	cholera toxin	olfactory neuroepithelium	activates adenylate cyclase
G_{12}	G_{12}	44	none	ubiquitous	$G_{12/13}$ subunits regulate
	G_{13}	44	none	ubiquitous	Na^+/H^+ exchange, voltage-dependent Ca^{2+} channels, and eicosanoid signaling
G_q	G_q	42	none	nearly ubiquitous	PLC
	G_{11}	42	none	nearly ubiquitous	
	G_{14}	42	none	lung, kidney, liver, spleen, testis	
	G_{15}	43	none	hemopoietic cells	
	G_{16}	44	none	hemopoietic cells	

Table 38.2 **Properties of the four main classes of mammalian G-protein α-subunits.** Some G-proteins can be characterized using different bacterial toxin substrates. PDE, phosphodiesterase; cGMP, cyclic guanosine monophosphate; PLC, phospholipase C; PLA_2, phospholipase A_2.

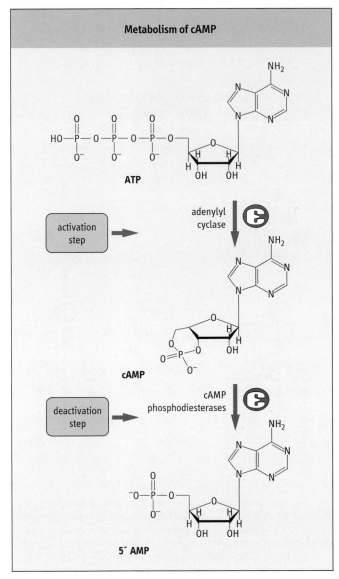

Fig. 38.4 Metabolism of cyclic AMP. Adenylyl cyclase catalyzes a cyclization reaction to produce the active cAMP, which is then deactivated by cAMP-phosphodiesterases. cAMP, cyclic adenosine monophosphate.

nephrine induces the breakdown of glycogen to glucose in muscle and, to a lesser extent, in the liver. In the latter organ, the breakdown of glycogen is predominantly stimulated by the polypeptide hormone glucagon, which is secreted by the pancreas when blood sugar is low (Chapters 12 and 20). One of the earliest signaling events after binding of these hormones to their receptors is the generation of cAMP, a small molecule that has a key role in the regulation of intracellular signal transduction, leading to the conversion of glycogen to glucose. cAMP is derived from ATP by the catalytic action of the signaling enzyme, adenylyl cyclase (Fig. 38.4). This

cyclization reaction involves the intramolecular attack of the 3′-OH group of the ribose unit on the α-phosphoryl group of ATP to form a phosphodiester bond; this is driven by the subsequent hydrolysis of the released pyrophosphate. The activity of cAMP is terminated by the hydrolysis of cAMP to 5′-AMP by specific cAMP-phosphodiesterases. The importance of cAMP in regulating glycogen breakdown was demonstrated by a series of experiments showing not only that hormones that activate adenylyl cyclase activity in fat cells also stimulate glycogen breakdown, but also that cell-permeant analogs of cAMP, such as dibutyryl cAMP, can mimic the effects of these hormones in inducing glycogen breakdown.

Adenylyl cyclase is activated by a G-protein

The β-adrenergic receptor is coupled to adenylyl cyclase activation by the action of the α-subunit of the stimulatory G-protein, called G_s. Because each molecule of bound hormone can stimulate many G_s α-subunits, this form of transmembrane signaling amplifies the original hormone signal. Although hydrolysis of GTP by the intrinsic GTPase of the G_s α-subunit acts to switch off adenylyl cyclase activation, the hormone–receptor complex must also be deactivated to return the cell to its resting, unstimulated state. This receptor desensitization, which occurs after prolonged exposure to the hormone, involves phosphorylation of the C-terminal tail of the hormone-occupied β-adrenergic receptor by a kinase known as β-adrenergic receptor kinase. G-protein-coupled receptors, such as α-adrenergic receptors, which act to inhibit cAMP generation, are coupled to the inhibition of adenylyl cyclase via the inhibitory, G_i-, G-protein.

Protein kinase A

Protein kinase A binds cAMP and phosphorylates other enzymes

cAMP transduces its effects on glycogen–glucose interconversion by regulating a key signaling enzyme, protein kinase A (PKA), which phosphorylates target proteins on serine and threonine residues. PKA is a multimeric enzyme comprising two regulatory (R) subunits and two catalytic (C) subunits: the R_2C_2 tetrameric form of PKA is inactive, but binding of four molecules of cAMP to the R subunits leads to the release of catalytically active C-subunits, which can then phosphorylate and modulate the activity of two key enzymes, phosphorylase kinase and glycogen synthase (see Fig. 38.5), which are involved in regulation of glycogen metabolism (see Chapter 12). Involvement of such a multilayered signal transduction cascade leads to substantial amplification of the original signal at each stage of the cascade (Fig. 38.6), ensuring that binding of only a few hormone molecules leads to release of a large number of sugar molecules.

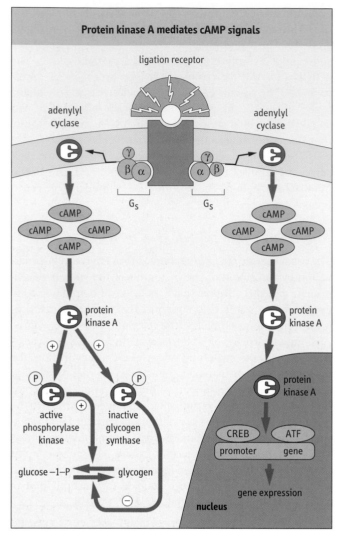

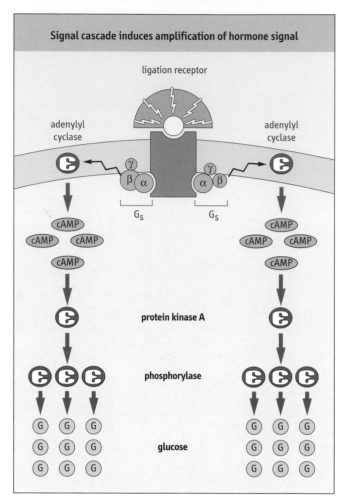

Fig. 38.5 **Protein kinase A (PKA) acts as a signaling enzyme for the second messenger, cAMP.** Binding of a stimulatory G-protein (Gs) to the hormone-receptor complex activates adenylyl cyclase, which catalyses the production of cAMP. Protein kinase A is activated by binding four molecules of cAMP. Translocation of PKA into the nucleus modulates activity of transcription factors – for example CREB and ATF (see text) – leading to induction or repression of gene expression.

Fig. 38.6 **Signal cascade induces amplification of hormone signal.** Each activated hormone-receptor complex can stimulate multiple Gs molecules. Each adenylyl cyclase can catalyze the generation of many cAMP molecules, and each protein kinase A can activate many phosphorylase molecules, leading to the release of a large number of glucose molecules (G) as a result of glycogen degradation.

Many other cellular responses can be mediated by the cAMP–PKA signaling cassette

PKA-mediated phosphorylation can regulate the activity of a number of ion channels, such as K^+, Cl^- and Ca^{2+} channels, and that of phosphatases involved in the regulation of cell signaling. In addition, translocation of PKA into the nucleus allows modulation of the activity of transcription factors such as the cAMP-responsive-element-binding protein (CREB) or the activation transcription factor (ATF) families, leading to either the induction or the repression of expression of specific genes (see Fig. 38.5 and Chapter 33).

Transcription requires binding of RNA polymerase (RNApol) to non-transcribed regions of the gene, called promoters, which are located upstream (5′) of the start site. Transcription factors are activators or repressors of gene expression that act by altering the rate of formation of the basal transcriptional complex on the promoter (Chapter 32). Transcription factors binding to regulatory sites on DNA can therefore be regarded as passwords that cooperatively open multiple locks to give RNA polymerase access to specific genes. It should be noted that binding of multiple transcription factors might be required for the induction of a single gene; hence, activation of different combinations of transcription factors provides the specificity for the switching on of particular genes in response to different hormones or growth factors.

The amplification of a hormonal signal involving G-proteins, adenylyl cyclase, protein kinase A and phosphorylase is illustrated in Fig. 38.6 (compare Fig. 12.4).

Phosphodiesterases

Phosphodiesterases terminate the cAMP signal

Phosphodiesterases (PDEs) terminate the cAMP signal by converting cAMP to its 5′AMP metabolite (see Fig. 38.4); thus they have the potential to play key roles in the regulation of various physiologic responses in many different cells and tissues. Indeed, they have been postulated to regulate platelet activation, vascular relaxation, cardiac muscle contraction, and inflammation, making them attractive targets for the development of selective inhibitors as potential therapeutic agents. For example, one group of compounds, the methylxanthines – which include theophylline and isobutylmethylxanthine – have been used as bronchodilators in the treatment of asthma, and are also able to exert positive inotropic responses in the heart. Moreover, drugs selective for the PDE_3 class of enzymes – such as milrinone – are cardiotonic and increase the force of contraction of the heart, presumably by increasing the concentrations of cAMP and stimulating PKA, leading to phosphorylation of cardiac calcium channels and a subsequent increase in intracellular calcium concentration.

Calcium Ion

Calcium ion (Ca^{2+}) is a ubiquitous messenger and has an important role in the transduction of signals leading to cellular responses such as cell motility changes, egg fertilization, neurotransmission and protein secretion, as well as cell fusion, differentiation and proliferation.

Cells expend a considerable amount of energy maintaining a steep extracellular/intracellular Ca^{2+} concentration gradient: for example, the intracellular Ca^{2+} concentration in resting, unstimulated cells is of the order of 10^{-7} mol/L (100 nM), whereas the extracellular Ca^{2+} concentration is typically 10^{-3} mol/L (1 mM). This steep gradient allows for rapid, abrupt, transient changes in Ca^{2+} concentration: ligation of a wide range of hormone receptors, for example, leads to a rapid (within seconds) and transient increase in intracellular Ca^{2+} concentration to the micromolar range. The rapid raising and lowering of Ca^{2+} concentrations is very tightly regulated and utilizes a variety of mechanisms involving cell compartmentalization. For example, intracellular Ca^{2+} concentrations can be lowered by sequestration of Ca^{2+} into the endoplasmic reticulum by Ca^{2+}-ATPases, or into the mitochondria using the energy-driven electrochemical gradient. Alternatively, free Ca^{2+} can be chelated by Ca^{2+}-binding proteins such as calsequestrin.

Calmodulin

Many downstream signaling events mediated by Ca^{2+} are modulated by a Ca^{2+}-sensing and binding protein, calmodulin

Calmodulin is a 17-kDa protein found in all animal and plant cells (comprising up to 1% of cellular protein). It belongs to a family of proteins characterized by one or more copies of a Ca^{2+}-binding structural motif called an EF hand motif (Fig. 38.7). Calmodulin is comprised of two similar globular domains joined by a long (6.5 nm; 65 Å) α-helix, each globular lobe having two EF hand motifs/Ca^{2+}-binding sites, 1.1 nm (11 Å) apart. Binding of three to four calcium ions (which occurs when the intracellular calcium ion concentration is increased to about 500 nmol/L) induces a major conformational change that allows calmodulin to bind to and modify target proteins such as cAMP-PDE. Binding of several calcium ions allows cooperativity in the activation of calmodulin, such that small changes in Ca^{2+} concentration cause large changes in the concentration of an active Ca^{2+}-calmodulin (Ca^{2+}/CAM) complex, providing amplification of the original hormone signal.

Calmodulin has a wide range of target effectors, including Ca^{2+}/CAM-dependent protein kinases, which phosphorylate serine-threonine residues on proteins to regulate a variety of processes. For example, the broad-specificity kinase, Ca^{2+}/CAM-kinase II, is involved in the regulation of fuel metabolism, ion permeability, neurotransmitter biology, and myosin light-chain kinase and phosphorylase kinase activity. Interestingly, calmodulin serves as a permanent regulatory subunit of phosphorylase kinase and may also regulate non-kinase effectors such as certain adenylyl cyclase isoforms and also cAMP-PDEs, indicating 'cross-talk' between cAMP- and Ca^{2+}-dependent signaling pathways. Moreover, mice defective in the calmodulin-dependent adenylyl cyclase are deficient in spatial memory, showing that this signal transduction system is important for learning and memory in vertebrates.

Phosphatidylinositol 4,5-bisphosphate (PIP₂)

Hydrolysis of a membrane phospholipid phosphatidylinositol 4,5-bisphosphate generates two second messengers

The major breakthrough in the search for the second messenger responsible for calcium mobilization came in the early 1980s, when it was found that stimulation of receptors that were known to increase the intracellular free Ca^{2+} concentration could activate the prior phospholipase C (PLC)-mediated hydrolysis of a minor phospholipid species, phosphatidylinositol 4,5-bisphosphate (PIP₂). PIP₂, which typically represents about 0.4% of total phospholipids in membranes,

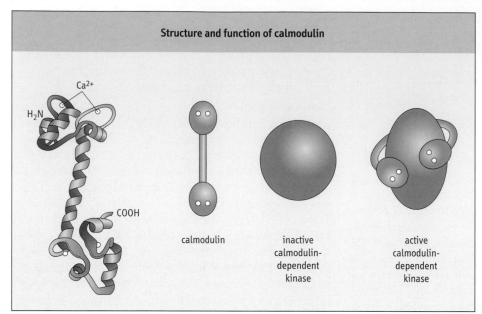

Structure and function of calmodulin

calmodulin

inactive calmodulin-dependent kinase

active calmodulin-dependent kinase

Fig. 38.7 **Structure and function of calmodulin.** Binding of calcium induces a conformational change, allowing calmodulin to bind to and modify the activity of target signaling enzymes.

is generated from phosphatidylinositol by two kinases, phosphatidylinositol-4-kinase (PI-4-K or PI kinase) and phosphatidylinositol-5-kinase (PI-5-K or PIP kinase), both of which are found in the plasma membrane (Fig. 38.8A). PIP_2 is hydrolyzed (Fig. 38.8B) by a PIP_2-specific PLC, to generate two-second messengers: inositol trisphosphate (I-1,4,5-P_3 or IP_3) and diacylglycerol (DAG). IP_3 is a water-soluble product, which is released into the cytosol and has been shown to mobilize intracellular stores of calcium. DAG is a lipid second messenger, which is anchored in the plasma membrane by virtue of its hydrophobic fatty-acid side chains and activates a key family of signaling enzymes known as protein kinase C (PKC) (Fig. 38.8B).

Inositol 1,4,5-trisphosphate (IP_3)

IP_3 is important in intracellular calcium mobilization

The rapid production (<1 second) and removal ($t\frac{1}{2} = 4$ seconds in liver) of IP_3 that precedes an increase in intracellular Ca^{2+} concentration implied that it could be a second messenger signaling calcium mobilization. Two types of experiment confirmed that IP_3 is indeed a second messenger:

- **microinjection of IP_3 into cells**, or simply including IP_3 in incubations of cells in which detergent treatment had induced the formation of holes or pores in the plasma membrane (permeabilized cells), mobilized calcium in the absence of hormone stimulation;
- **structure-function analyses** of a variety of inositol phosphate molecules suggested that calcium mobilization was dependent on specific IP_3 receptors.

IP_3 receptors that exhibit IP_3 binding and calcium release have now been cloned. These receptors are expressed on the endoplasmic reticulum of all cells as a family of related glycoproteins (molecular mass 250 kDa) comprising six transmembrane-spanning domains. The active receptor is expressed as a multimer of four IP_3 receptor molecules; this tetrameric structure gives rise to cooperativity in Ca^{2+}-channel activity. It has been estimated that stimulated IP_3 (typically 2–3 mmol/L) releases 20–30 calcium ions. This calculation reveals the amplification inherent in this signaling cascade because, typically, only nanomolar concentrations of growth factor are required to elicit millimolar concentrations of this second messenger. Consistent with the transient nature of the release of intracellular calcium that is observed after hormone receptor ligation, cellular concentrations of IP_3 are rapidly returned to resting values (0.1 mmol/L) by more than one route of degradation (Fig. 38.9).

Diacylglycerol (DAG)

DAG activates protein kinase C

DAG fulfils its second messenger role by activating the key signaling enzyme, protein kinase C (PKC), which phosphorylates a wide range of target signal-transduction proteins on serine or threonine. PKC was originally identified as a calcium- and lipid (phosphatidylserine)-dependent kinase important in the regulation of cell proliferation. However, in recent years it has become clear that PKC is, in reality, a generic name for a superfamily of related kinases that have different tissue distribution and activation requirements (Table 38.3). Nevertheless, all these enzymes share some conserved features;

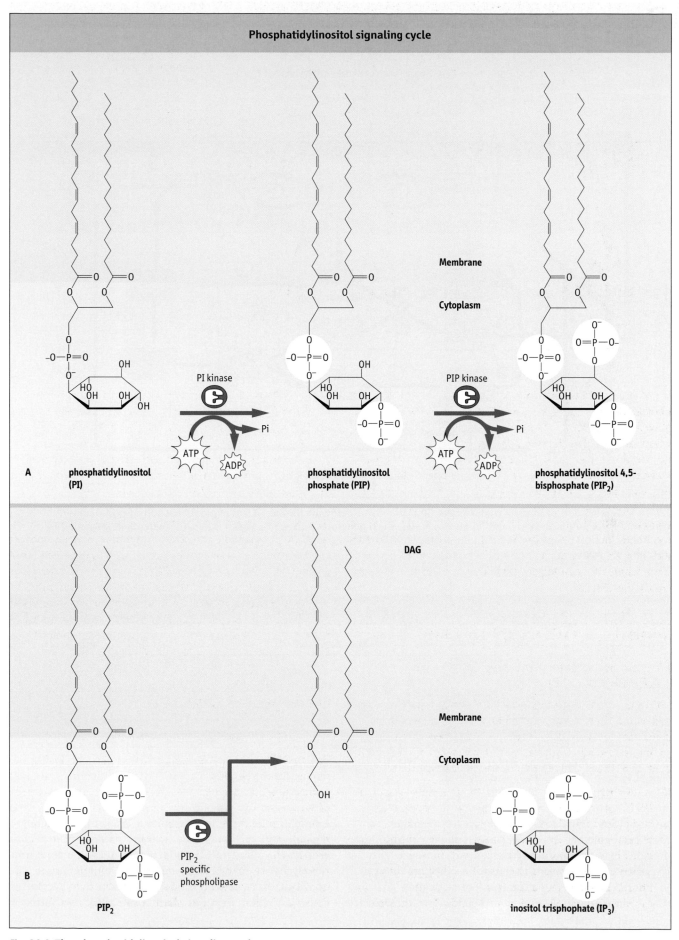

Fig. 38.8 **The phosphatidylinositol signaling cycle.**

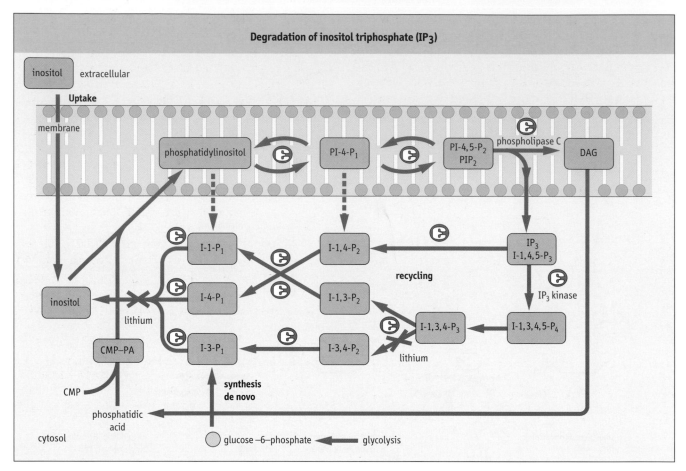

Fig. 38.9 **Degradation of inositol triphosphate (IP₃).** The major pathways involve (i) the sequential action of phosphatases converting I-1,4,5-P₃ to inositol, and (ii) an IP₃ kinase, which generates I-1,3,4,5-P₄, which is in turn sequentially degraded to inositol by inositol phosphate-specific phosphatases. DAG, diacylglycerol; PA, phosphatidic acid; CMP-PA, cytosine monophosphate-phosphatidic acid.

	Classical PKCs				Novel PKCs					Atypical PKCs	
PKC designation	α	β1	β2	γ	δ	ε/ε′	η	θ	μ	ι/λ	ζ
molecular mass (kDA)	82	80	80	80	78	90	80	79	115	74	72
activators											
[Ca²⁺]	yes	yes	yes	yes	no	no	no	no		no	no
DAG	yes	yes	yes	yes	yes	yes	yes	yes		no	no
tissue distribution	all	some	many	neural	all	neural	many	muscle, skin		ovary, testis	all

Protein kinase C superfamily (table header)

Table 38.3 **The protein kinase C (PKC) superfamily.** This is a multigene family, except for β1, β2 and ε/ε′, which are alternatively spliced forms of β and ε. DAG, diacylglycerol.

most notably they comprise two major domains: an N-terminal regulatory domain and a C-terminal catalytic kinase domain. The regulatory domain contains a pseudosubstrate sequence that resembles the consensus phosphorylation site in PKC substrates. In the absence of activating cofactors (Ca²⁺, phospholipid, DAG), this pseudosubstrate sequence interacts with the substrate-binding pocket in the catalytic domain and represses PKC activity; binding of cofactors reduces the affinity of this interaction, induces a conformational change in the PKC, and allows stimulation of PKC activity. Consistent with the fact that the activator/cofactor, DAG, is anchored in the membranes, PKC activation is generally associated with translocation from the cytosol to the plasma or nuclear membranes. Although PKC is generally considered to be a serine kinase, it can phosphorylate threonine, but never tyrosine, residues. Interestingly, PKC can phosphorylate the same protein targets as PKA but, whereas PKC generally phosphorylates the protein at serine residues, PKA usually phosphorylates threonine residues.

Phospholipases

Phospholipases hydrolyse phosphatidylcholine or phosphatidylethanolamine generating lipid second messengers

In many hormone systems, although receptor-stimulated hydrolysis of PIP_2 is transient and rapidly switched off (desensitized), generation of DAG is sustained. Together with the recent emergence of the multiple isoforms of PKC, some of which do not require Ca^{2+} or DAG for activation (Table 38.3), these findings led to the discovery of additional receptor-coupled lipid-signaling pathways involving hydrolysis of phosphatidylcholine or phosphatidylethanolamine (Fig. 38.10), which can give rise to DAG and other biologically active lipids (Fig. 38.11) in response to a wide range of growth factors and mitogens. Phosphatidylcholine comprises about 40% of total cellular phospholipids. It can be hydrolyzed by distinct phospholipases, generating a diversity of lipid second messengers, including arachidonic acid (generated by PLA_2) as well as different species of DAG (generated by PLC) and phosphatidic acid (generated by PLD). In addition, hormone-stimulated phosphatidylethanolamine-PLD activities have also been reported.

Some hormones or growth factors can stimulate only one or other of these phospholipases, but other ligands can stimulate all these pathways after binding to their specific receptors. There is therefore the potential to generate multiple distinct species of DAG and phosphatidic acid, reflecting

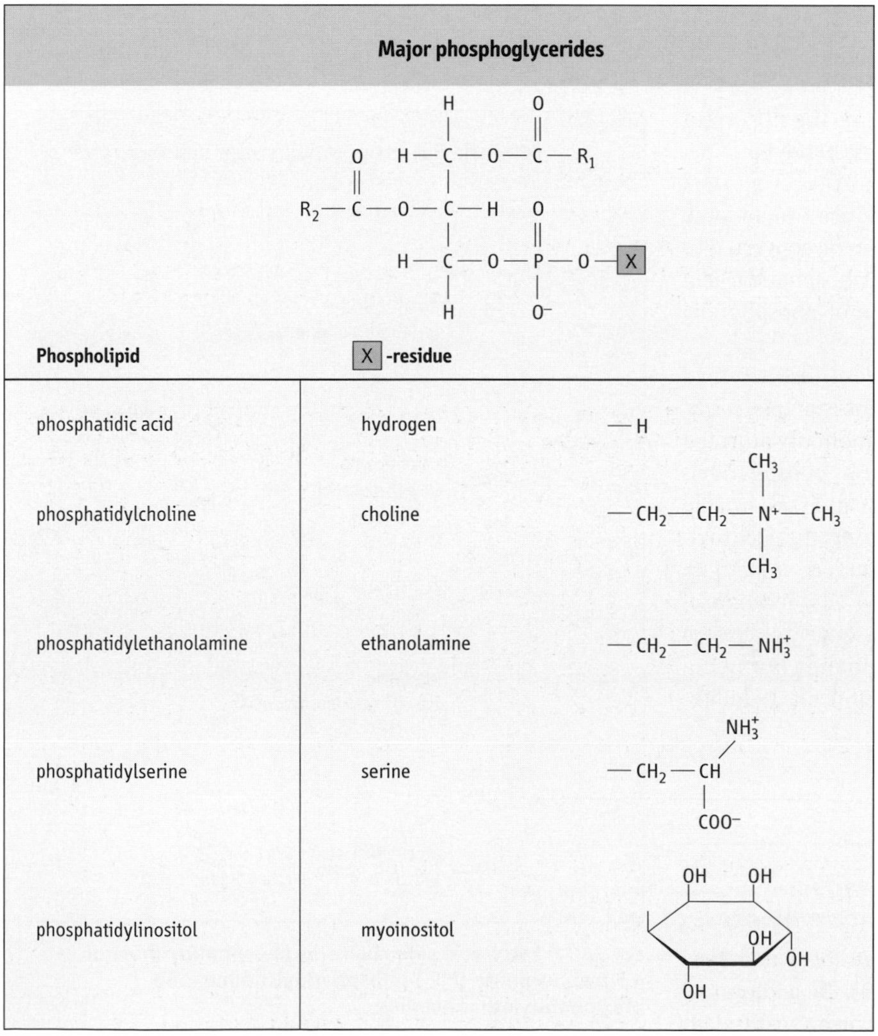

Fig. 38.10 **Potential lipid second messengers: phosphoglycerides.** R1/R2, fatty acid side chains.

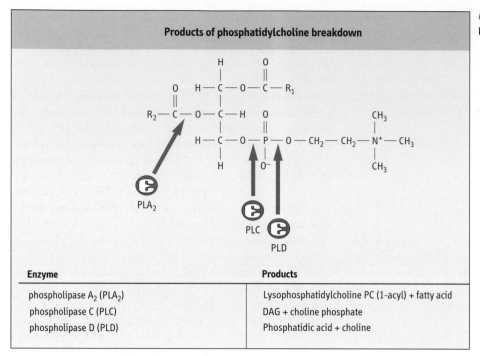

Products of phosphatidylcholine breakdown

Enzyme	Products
phospholipase A$_2$ (PLA$_2$)	Lysophosphatidylcholine PC (1-acyl) + fatty acid
phospholipase C (PLC)	DAG + choline phosphate
phospholipase D (PLD)	Phosphatidic acid + choline

Fig. 38.11 **Products of phosphatidylcholine breakdown.**

different fatty-acid side chains (Fig. 38.12) of the PIP$_2$ (predominantly stearate/arachidonate) and phosphatidylcholine, and phosphatidylethanolamine substrates. Moreover, DAG species can be further metabolized to produce arachidonic acid via DAG lipase or, alternatively, DAG can be converted to phosphatidic acid via DAG kinase. Likewise, phosphatidic acid can be interconverted to DAG by the action of phosphatidic acid phosphohydrolase.

There is growing evidence that all these distinct lipid second messengers have different targets. For example, it has recently been suggested that the saturated/monounsaturated fatty-acid-containing DAGs derived from phosphatidylcholine-specific phospholipase D (PLD) activation are unable to activate PKC isoforms, and that it is only the stearoyl-arachidonyl–phosphatidic acid species that can modulate activity of the GTPase *Ras* (see Chapter 41). Generation of these diverse, but related, lipid second messengers therefore provides a mechanism for initiating or terminating hormone-specific responses via particular signal transducers, including differential activation of PKC isoforms.

Arachidonic acid

Arachidonic acid is a second messenger regulating phospholipases and protein kinases

Arachidonic acid is a C20 polyunsaturated fatty acid containing four double bonds (see Fig. 38.12). In addition to being implicated as a lipid second messenger involved in

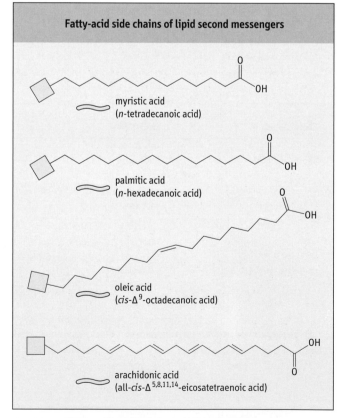

Fatty-acid side chains of lipid second messengers

myristic acid
(*n*-tetradecanoic acid)

palmitic acid
(*n*-hexadecanoic acid)

oleic acid
(*cis*-Δ^9-octadecanoic acid)

arachidonic acid
(all-*cis*-$\Delta^{5,8,11,14}$-eicosatetraenoic acid)

Fig. 38.12 **Fatty acid side chains in phosphatidylinositol 4,5-bisphosphate (PIP$_2$) phosphatidylcholine, and phosphatidylethanolamine.**

ANTI-INFLAMMATORY DRUGS TARGET PROSTAGLANDIN SYNTHESIS

Non-steroid anti-inflammatory drugs (NSAIDs) such as aspirin and ibruprofen decrease inflammation, pain, and fever through inhibition of the synthesis of prostaglandins, by blocking the first stage whereby arachidonic acid is converted to the common prostaglandin precursor, PGG_2 by a cyclo-oxygenase enzyme. There are two forms of the enzyme. Cyclo-oxygenase 1 (COX-1) is mainly constitutive and found in platelets, stomach, and kidney. Cyclo-oxygenase 2 (COX-2) is mainly inducible and responsible for synthesis of inflammatory prostaglandins. Aspirin (acetylsalicylate) covalently modifies and irreversibly inactivates both forms of the enzyme by acetylation. Because abrogation of cyclo-oxygenase activity will also block production of the potent vasoconstrictor and aggregator of blood platelets, thromboxane A_2 (TXA_2, also derived from the common precursor, PGG_2), aspirin can also be used as a prophylactic agent, to prevent the excessive blood clotting that can lead to heart attacks and stroke. The Antiplatelet Trialists Collaboration meta-analysis of aspirin in secondary prevention showed that the reduction in risk of recurrent stroke was about 15%. The combination of aspirin with dipyridamole, which reduces platelet aggregation by increasing cAMP concentrations may further reduce risk. Other effective antiplatelet drugs are the thienopyridines, ticlopicline and clopidogrel which block ADP-induced platelet aggregation. Selective inhibitors of COX-2 such as celecoxib are also effective treatments for inflammatory conditions such as rheumatoid arthritis and their effectiveness and tolerability are being compared with conventional NSAIDs. Corticosteroid hormones, such as cortisone, are also anti-inflammatory drugs that target prostaglandin synthesis; in this case, however, such reagents do not affect cyclo-oxygenase but, rather, appear to inhibit activation of the PLA_2 activity that generates the key intermediate, arachidonic acid. Such drugs are therefore useful for treating inflammatory responses involving leukocyte recruitment or asthma, as targeting arachidonic acid production will, in addition to blocking synthesis of prostaglandin, also abrogate the production of leukotriene.

Comment. Prostaglandins orchestrate a myriad of physiologic responses: they stimulate inflammation, regulate blood flow to organs such as the kidney, control ion transport across membranes, modulate synaptic transmission, and induce sleep. Prostaglandins are generally derived from the key inflammatory mediator, arachidonic acid, which in turn can be produced by PLA_2-mediated hydrolysis of various phospholipids such as phosphatidylcholine.

the regulation of signaling enzymes, such as PLC-γ, PLC-δ and PKC-α, -β and -γ isoforms, arachidonic acid is a key inflammatory intermediate. However, the arachidonic acid involved in these disparate functions appears to be generated by two distinct PLA_2 routes. Arachidonic acid generated for signaling purposes appears to be derived by the action of a phosphatidylcholine-specific cytosolic phospholipase A_2 ($cPLA_2$), which has a molecular mass of 85 kDa and is regulated by phosphorylation of key serine residues. In contrast, inflammatory arachidonic acid is generated by the action of a family of low-molecular-weight secretory PLA_2 ($sPLA_2$) proteins (14–18 kDa), which appear to be ubiquitous and are found in high concentrations in snake venom and pancreatic juices. In addition, arachidonic acid can be generated by DAG lipase.

Eicosanoids

Arachidonic acid is the precursor of eicosanoids, which encompass prostaglandins, prostacyclins, thromboxanes, and leukotrienes

As a key inflammatory mediator, arachidonic acid (see Chapter 15) is the major precursor of the group of molecules termed eicosanoids, which encompass prostaglandins, prostacyclins, thromboxanes, and leukotrienes. Eicosanoids (Fig. 38.13) act like hormones and signal via G-protein-coupled receptors. They have a wide variety of biological activities, including modulating smooth muscle contraction (vascular tone), platelet aggregation, gastric acid secretion, and salt and water balance, as well as mediating pain and inflammatory responses. Moreover, knockout mice defective in prostaglandin production have shown that prostaglandins have wider roles than was previously realized, being involved in the control of complex processes such as pregnancy, and tumor spread and metastasis in colon cancer (see Chapter 41).

Prostaglandins are synthesized in membranes from arachidonic acid

The first stage in the conversion of arachidonic acid to prostaglandins involves the cyclo-oxygenase component of prostaglandin synthase, which induces the formation of a cyclopentane ring and the introduction of four oxygen atoms to generate the intermediate, prostaglandin G_2 (PGG_2). PGG_2 is then subject to a hydroperoxidase reaction that catalyzes the two-electron reduction of the 15-hydroperoxy group to a 15-hydroxyl group and generates the highly unstable intermediate, PGH_2, which can then be converted into other prostaglandins, prostacylin and thromboxane.

Two distinct isoforms of cyclo-oxygenase, termed COX-1 and COX-2, have been identified. Whereas COX-1 is constitutively expressed, COX-2 is made only in response to

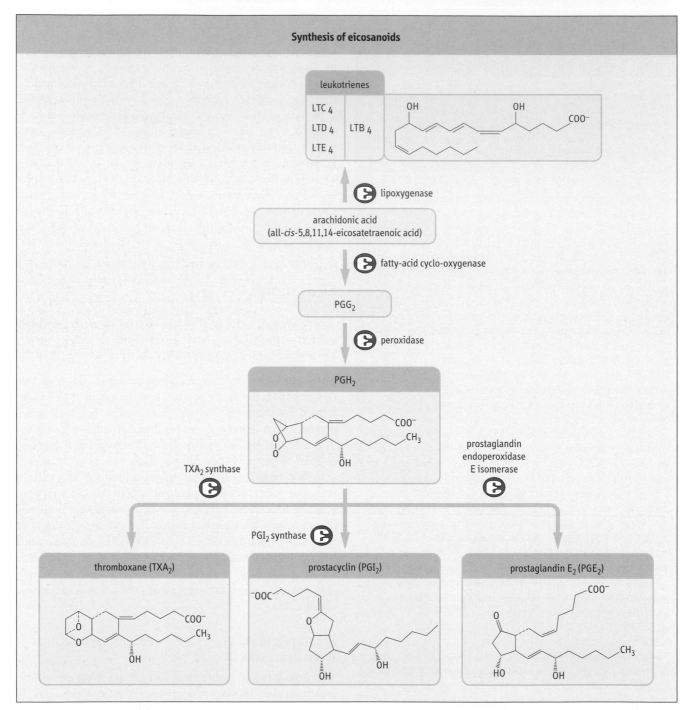

Fig. 38.13 **Synthesis of eicosanoids.** Eicosanoids are primarily derived from arachidonic acid. Leukotrienes (LT) are synthesized via a lipoxygenase-dependent pathway, whereas prostaglandins (PG), prostacyclins and thromboxanes (TX) arise from cyclo-oxygenase-dependent routes.

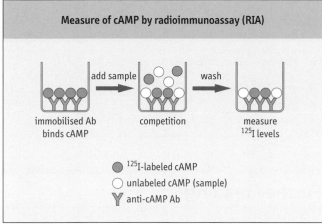

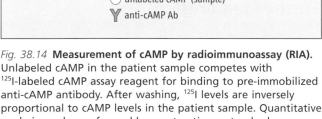

Fig. 38.14 **Measurement of cAMP by radioimmunoassay (RIA).** Unlabeled cAMP in the patient sample competes with ^{125}I-labeled cAMP assay reagent for binding to pre-immobilized anti-cAMP antibody. After washing, ^{125}I levels are inversely proportional to cAMP levels in the patient sample. Quantitative analysis can be performed by constructing a standard curve. Compare the immunoradiometric sandwich assay for hormones (Fig. 37.2).

 cAMP RADIO-IMMUNOASSAY (RIA)

The action of parathyroid hormone (PTH) on the renal tubule results in release of cAMP into the urine (see Chapter 23). The clinical assessment of cAMP levels is a useful indicator of parathyroid function. 90% of patients with hyperparathyroidism have increased levels of nephrogenous cAMP (urinary cAMP minus plasma cAMP filtered but not reabsorbed in the kidney). Furthermore, infusion with PTH causes a dramatic increase in urinary cAMP concentrations in patients with idiopathic hypoparathyroidism but not type I pseudohypoparathyroidism patients, who have a mutation in $G_s\alpha$ and thus exhibit a defective renal tubular response to PTH, resulting in reduced cAMP secretion.

cAMP levels can be analyzed by radio-immunoassay (RIA), which measures the competition for binding to an immobilized cAMP-specific antibody between ^{125}I-labeled cAMP assay reagent and unlabeled cAMP in the patient sample (Fig. 38.14). Quantitative measurement of cAMP levels can be performed using known concentrations of unlabeled cAMP assay reagent to construct a standard curve.

 McCUNE–ALBRIGHT SYNDROME (INCIDENCE 1 IN 25 000)

A 3-year-old girl was brought to hospital because her mum had been concerned about apparent breast development over the last 6 months, and a spot of blood on her pants last week. On examination, she had Tanner Stage 3 breast development. On her trunk she had three areas of brown skin pigmentation with ragged edges.

Comment. This child is suffering from McCune–Albright Syndrome. She is likely to develop polyostotic fibrous dysplasia, with areas of thinning and sclerosis in her long bones which may fracture. Other endocrinopathies include thyrotoxicosis, GH hypersecretion, Cushing's syndrome (cortisol excess) and hyperparathyroidism. The cause is an activating missense mutation in the gene encoding the $G_{s\alpha}$ subunit of the G protein that stimulates cyclic AMP formation. The problem presents following a somatic cell mutation with clinical features dependent on a mosaic distribution of aberrant cells.

inflammatory mediators such as cytokines. Cyclo-oxygenase inhibitors, the non-steroidal anti-inflammatory drugs (NSAIDs) such as aspirin and ibuprofen, act to reduce inflammation and provide pain relief by blocking this first step in the production of prostaglandins. Although the currently marketed drugs preferentially block COX-1, a number of COX-2-selective drugs are under development because it is believed that COX-2, being induced under conditions of inflammation, may have a more important role than COX-1 in mediating inflammatory responses. Moreover, the major side effects of blocking COX-1 are bleeding and the inflammation of gastric mucosa, and the use of inhibitors selective for COX-2 may make it possible to target inflammatory activity and thus avoid most of the sequelae associated with the use of COX-1 inhibitors.

Leukotrienes

Arachidonic acid is also converted into other inflammatory and vasoactive mediators, called leukotrienes, by the action of a variety of structurally related lipoxygenases (see Fig. 38.13). For example, 5-lipoxygenase comprises both a dioxygenase activity that converts arachidonate to 5-hydroperoxyeicosatetraenoic acid (5-HPETE), and a dehydrase activity that transforms 5-HPETE to leukotriene A_4 (LTA_4). Natural deficiencies in lipoxygenases have been associated with human disease: for example, in one study, 40% of patients with myeloproliferative disorders were found to have reduced platelet lipoxygenase activity and increased synthesis of thromboxane. In addition, mice deficient in 5-lipoxygenase exhibit defects in the responses of their neutrophils to immune complexes and platelet-activating factor, supporting the idea that leukotrienes have important roles in inflammatory responses.

Summary

■ Cells specifically respond to a multiplicity of signals from their environment via signal transduction cassettes, which comprise specific cell–surface membrane receptors, effector signaling systems (e.g. adenylyl cyclase, phospholipases, or ion channels) and regulatory proteins (e.g. G-proteins or tyrosine kinases).

■ These signal transduction cassettes serve to detect, amplify and integrate diverse external signals to generate the appropriate cellular response.

■ The variety of families of cell-surface receptors sense and transduce their specific hormone signal by transmembrane coupling to different effector systems to generate low-molecular-weight molecules, termed second messengers, such as cAMP, IP_3, DAG, and Ca^{2+}, which mediate their signaling functions by activating key protein kinases.

■ The specificity of a particular hormone response can be further heightened by the variety of available phospholipase-signaling activities (PLC, PLD and PLA_2). Taking into account their range of potential lipid substrates (e.g. PIP_2, phosphatidylcholine, and phosphatidylethanolamine) and products (e.g. DAG, phosphatidic acid and arachidonic acid), the phospholipases can generate a diverse array of lipid second messengers to influence differentially the activity of the key protein kinases. Because, for example, many of the members of the PKC family appear to have distinct substrate repertoire of downstream signal transducers, differential activation of particular PKC isoforms can ultimately determine the specific type of biological response obtained.

ACTIVE LEARNING

1. How are appropriate cellular responses triggered by specific hormones?
2. How do second messengers propagate intracellular signals?
3. How do NSAIDs such as aspirin and ibuprofen work?

Further reading

Hur EM, Kim KT. G protein-coupled receptor signaling and cross-talk: achieving rapidity and specificity. *Cell Signal* 2002;**14**:397–405.

Kohout TA, Lefkowitz RJ. Regulation of G protein-coupled receptor kinases and arrestins during receptor desensitization. *Mol Pharmacol* 2003;**63**:91–8.

Perez J et al. Abnormalities of cAMP signaling in affective disorders: implication for pathophysiology and treatment. *Bipolar Disord* 2000;**2**:27–36.

Pierce KL, Premont RT, Lefkowitz RJ. Seven-transmembrane receptors. *Nat Rev Biol Mol Cell* 2002;**3**:639–50.

Rockman HA, Koch WJ, Lefkowitz RJ. Seven-transmembrane-spanning receptors and heart function. *Nature* 2002;**415**:206–12.

Relevant websites

Science Magazine's Signal Transduction Knowledge Environment
www.stke.org
Kimball's Biology Pages
www.biology-pages.info/C/CellSignaling
The Biology Project (University of Arizona)
www.biology.arizona.edu/cell_bio/problem_sets/signaling
BioCarta's Cell Signaling Pathways
www.biocarta.com/genes/CellSignaling.asp

39. Neurochemistry

E J Thompson

LEARNING OBJECTIVES

After reading this chapter you should be able to:

- Describe the cellular components of the central nervous system.
- Discuss the function of the blood–brain barrier in health and disease.
- Describe the basic principles of neuronal signaling and receptors.
- Describe adrenergic and cholinergic transmission.
- Describe the role of ion channels in nerve transmission.
- Comment on the role of sodium, potassium and calcium ions in nerve transmission.
- Discuss the process of vision as an example of chemical process underlying neuronal function.

GUILLAIN–BARRÉ SYNDROME

Three weeks after an acute diarrheal illness, a 65-year-old man presented with progressive ascending weakness of the limbs followed by respiratory muscle weakness requiring assisted ventilation. On examination, he was hypotonic and areflexic, with profound general weakness. Isoelectric focusing of CSF and parallel serum samples showed a similar abnormal pattern of oligoclonal bands in both.

Comment. This predominantly motor neuropathy is Guillain–Barré syndrome and the patient has antibodies developed as a result of infection with the bacterium *Campylobacter jejuni*. The organism contains the antigen ganglioside sugar GM1, which is shared with a ganglioside on peripheral nerves. Antibodies bind to peripheral motor nerves and cause the neuropathy. It is an example of molecular mimicry.

INTRODUCTION

The brain is, in many ways, a chemist's delight. This is so because it illustrates various general principles of biology applied to a highly specialized tissue that ultimately regulates all the other tissues of the body. This chapter highlights the differences between the central nervous system – that is, the brain and spinal cord – and the peripheral nervous system, which is outside the dura (the thick fibrous covering that contains the cerebrospinal fluid [CSF]).

BRAIN AND PERIPHERAL NERVE

The distinction between brain and peripheral nerve essentially reflects the division between the central nervous system (CNS) and the peripheral nervous system (PNS): a convenient dividing line being the confines of the dura, within which watertight compartment is the CSF, partially produced (about one-third of the total volume) through the action of the blood–brain barrier. Myelin insulates the axons of nerves; the chemical composition of CNS myelin is quite distinct from that of PNS myelin, not least because the two forms are produced by two different types of cells: the oligodendrocyte within the CNS, and the Schwann cell within the PNS. The distinction between the separate functions of the CNS and those of the PNS is fundamental to differential diagnosis in neurology, and many tests exist to discriminate between the two. A typical example is the difference between the demyelination of the CNS that occurs in multiple sclerosis, and the demyelination of the PNS that occurs in Guillain–Barré syndrome.

The blood–brain barrier

The term blood–brain 'barrier' is a slight misnomer, in that the barrier is not absolute, but relative: its permeability depends on the size of the molecule in question

Initially, experiments based upon use of a dye (Evans' Blue) bound to albumin showed that, over a period of hours, an animal progressively turned blue in all tissues, with the notable exception of the brain, which remained white. It subsequently became clear that 1 molecule in 200 of serum albumin passed normally into the CSF, which is analogous to lymph. It also became obvious that, for any given protein, the ratio of its concentrations in CSF and serum was a linear function of the molecular radius of the molecules in solution.

There are a total of six sources of the CSF which contain different 'barriers'. Under normal and pathologic conditions, proteins pass from these cellular or tissue sources into the

CSF, and their degrees of filtration or rates of local synthesis, or both, vary.

The total quantity of the CSF therefore constitutes the algebraic summation of these six sources (Fig. 39.1):

- **the blood–brain barrier** (the parenchymal capillaries) gives rise to about one-third of the volume of CSF, and has been termed the interstitial fluid source;
- **the blood–CSF barrier** provides the bulk of CSF (almost all of the remaining two-thirds), termed choroidal fluid, as it is principally provided by the choroid plexi (capillary tufts) situated in the lateral ventricles and, to a lesser degree, the plexi situated in the third and fourth ventricles;
- **the dorsal root ganglia** contain capillaries that have a much greater degree of permeability. In the animal experiments with the Evans' blue referred to above, although the brain was otherwise white, the dorsal roots took up the blue color reflecting their greater permeability to albumin;
- **the brain parenchyma of the CNS** produces a number of brain-specific proteins. These include prostaglandin synthase (formerly called β-trace protein), which shows an 11-fold increase from the choroid plexus to the lumbar sac, and transthyretin (a protein formerly called prealbumin which is produced locally by the choroid plexi), for which the reverse is found: it has a much greater relative concentration in ventricular than in lumbar CSF;
- **CSF circulating cells**, mainly lymphocytes within the CNS, synthesize local antibodies; however, in the CNS there is strong presence of immune suppressor cells. Because of this, in brain infections such as meningitis, steroids are given in addition to antibiotics, to suppress the potentially devastating effects, within this confined space, of inflammation associated with the intrathecal immune response;
- **the meninges** represent a sixth source of CSF under pathologic conditions; they can give rise to dramatic increase in the concentrations of CSF proteins.

CELLS OF THE NERVOUS SYSTEM

Fewer than 10% of the cells of the nervous system are large neurons. The three major cell types in the nervous system (which each constitute about 30%) are:

- **astrocytes**, which also make up part of the blood/brain barrier;
- **oligodendrocytes**, which are principally composed of fat, and serve to insulate the axons;
- **microglia**, which are essentially resident macrophages (scavengers).

These different cell types are associated with predominant protein molecules that are important in various brain pathologies (Table 39.1). Other minor constituents of the

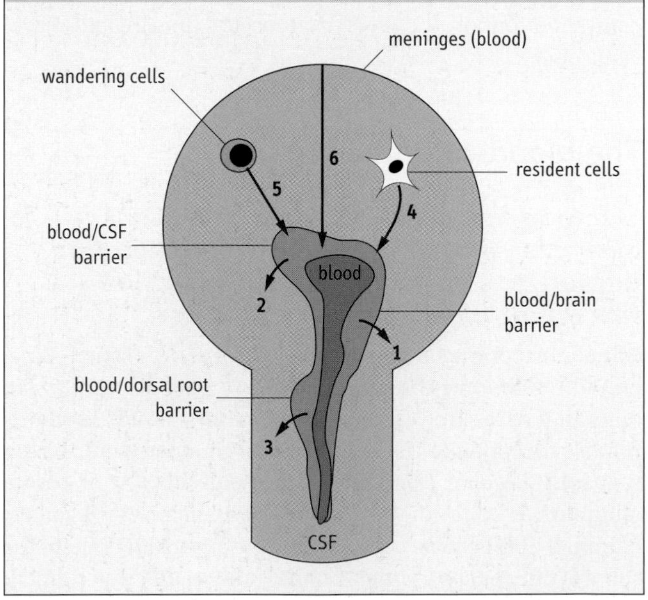

Fig. 39.1 **The six main sources of cerebrospinal fluid (CSF).** The involved processes comprise passage across barriers (from the blood, i.e. 1,2,3) and direct sources of local production (CNS cells, i.e. 4,5,6).

REGIONAL FLUIDS WITHIN THE BRAIN

CSF leak

It is essential, on clinical grounds, to distinguish CSF rhinorrhea from local nasal secretions caused by, say, influenza infection. The ENT surgeon must know whether the fluid present is CSF, as any leak must be surgically repaired lest it remain a chronic potential source of meningitis as a result of the migration of nasal flora into the subarachnoid space. One characteristic and useful marker protein in the CSF is asialotransferrin, which is transferrin lacking sialic acid. In the systemic circulation, this absence of sialic acid gives a molecular signal for the protein to be recycled, and it is thus immediately removed from the systemic circulation by all reticuloendothelial cells. The brain has no true reticuloendothelial cells along the path of CSF flow, and hence asialotransferrin is present in quite high concentrations. The aqueous humor of the anterior chamber of the eye also produces the characteristic asialotransferrin, and the same asialotransferrin can also be found in the perilymph of the semicircular canals.

nervous system include the ependymal cells, which are ciliated cells secreting brain-specific proteins such as prostaglandin synthase. The brain endothelial cells also merit special comment because, unlike other tissue capillaries, these contiguous cells have tight junctions that bind them together; this feature is believed also to contribute to the blood/brain barrier, although it is the basement membrane which is the major source of molecular sieving of the different-sized proteins.

Neurons

The significant features of neurons are their length, their many interconnections, and the fact that they do not divide post-partum

There is an archetypal notion of the electrical activity of the nervous system – in particular, of the electrical activity of

CNS cells and markers for brain pathology		
Cell	Protein	Pathology
neuron	neuron-specific enolase	brain death
astrocyte	GFAP	plaque (or scar)
oligodendrocyte	myelin basic protein	de/remyelination
microglia	ferritin	stroke
choroid plexi	asialotransferrin	CSF leak (rhinorrhea)

Table 39.1 **The different cells of the CNS, and their protein markers indicating brain pathologies.** GFAP, glial fibrillary acidic protein.

neurons. However, three other biological features of neurons are particularly worthy of note: their length, their prolific interconnections, and the fact that they do not divide *postpartum*. Further to the last of these features – many embryonic neurons are destined to die (through apoptosis), as they have no postembryonic target organ. The existence of cervical and lumbar swellings of the spinal cord, reflecting segmental neurons for which, respectively, the target organs were the hands and feet, is evidence for reduced diameter of the cord due to neuronal death. The capacity for memory and learning similarly indicates the importance of the plasticity of the synaptic system afforded by the extensive interconnections of and between neurons.

Because of their great length, neurons depend upon an efficient system of axonal transport

Neurons can typically be 1 m long; thus the nucleus, the source of information for the synthesis of neurotransmitters, is typically quite remote from the synaptic terminal, the site of release of those transmitters. Because of this extensive length – a crucial requirement is the neuron's ability to transport material both from the nucleus towards the synapse (anterograde transport) and from the synapse to the nucleus (retrograde transport). Neurons have evolved special characteristics to deal with this separation of their two functional sites, and to maintain electrical activity at the nodes of Ranvier (the remainder of the axon is electrically quiet during the saltatory process of electrical conduction (Fig. 39.2).

The normal 'resting' movement within the axon is mediated by separate molecular 'motors' (motile proteins): kinesin in the case of anterograde transport, and dynein in retrograde transport. The materials being transported in each direction are also rather different, and the different components of axonal structure shown in Figure 39.2 possess the

IRON IN THE CNS

During normal maturation of the oligodendrocytes that form the myelin sheath, iron appears to be important, as there are increased local concentrations of this cation and of the transferrin protein that is required to bind it (including the asialo form). An apparent discrepancy between the amounts of iron and those of transferrin is readily explained by the local synthesis of the latter, particularly of the asialo form; large amounts of mRNA are found in oligodendrocytes and in the choroid plexus.

There is also local synthesis of ferritin by the normal CNS. Free iron can have a particularly toxic effect on the CNS and, by binding to it, ferritin provides a store for it. This is clearly evident in the event of cerebrovascular accidents, after which there is a further dramatic increase in the local synthesis of ferritin, to bind the iron that has been released by the destruction of red cells.

CSF CIRCULATING CELLS

'Regional' immunology

As mentioned in the text, the brain is essentially an immunologically 'quiet' place. There is an almost 10-fold difference between the ratio of helper cells (CD_4) to suppressor cells (CD_8) in the CSF, where the ratio is 3:6, and that in the brain parenchyma, where the ratio is 0:4, reflecting a preponderance of suppressor cells within the CNS (see also Chapter 36). Approximately one-third of CNS cells are resident macrophages; within the CSF, two-thirds of the cells are lymphocytes and the remaining one-third are macrophages. There are very few lymphatic vessels within the brain itself, and CSF itself can be thought of as being analogous to lymph.

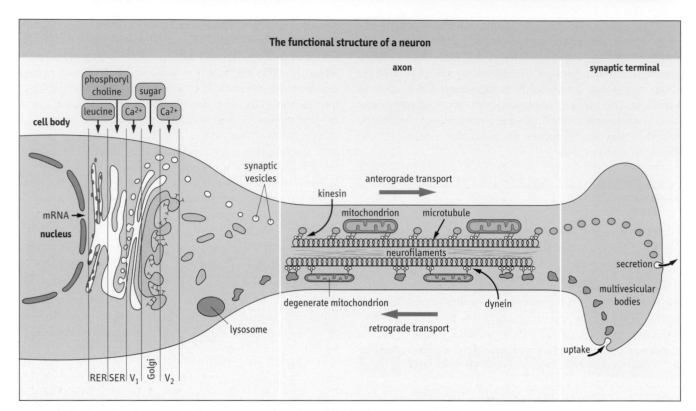

The functional structure of a neuron

Fig. 39.2 **The functional structure of a neuron.** Within the cell body, there is specialized movement through the Golgi stack by the components required to form synaptic vesicles (V_1, V_2). In the axon, there is fast axonal transport along microtubules via the motile proteins, kinesin (in anterograde transport) or dynein (in retrograde transport). RER, rough endoplasmic reticulum; SER, smooth endoplasmic reticulum.

Differing speeds of axonal transport

Component	Rate (mm/day)	Structure and composition of transported substances
Fast transport		
anterograde	200–400	small vesicles, neurotransmitters, membrane proteins, lipids
mitochondria	50–100	mitochondria
retrograde	200–300	lysosomal vesicles, enzymes
Slow transport		
slow component a	2–8	microfilaments, metabolic enzymes, clathrin complex
slow component b	0.2–1	neurofilaments, microtubules

Table 39.2 **Differing speeds of axonal transport.**

capacity for different speeds of transportation (Table 39.2). During growth, a separate form of transport (toward the synapse) occurs that takes place at the rate of about 1 mm/day; this flow constitutes bulk movement of the building blocks such as the filamentous proteins.

Neuroglial structures

Essentially, the astrocytes and the oligodendrocytes comprise the neuroglial structures

In the cortex, or gray matter, one typically finds a protoplasmic astrocyte with one set of processes surrounding the endothelial cells, thereby helping to 'filter' materials from the blood, and a separate set of processes surrounding the neurons, which are thereby being 'fed' selected substances that have been extracted from the blood for passage to the neurons. In the white matter, the astrocytes have a rather more fibrous appearance, and have more of a structural role. Under pathologic conditions in which there is injury to the CNS, astrocytes can play a major part in the reaction, synthesizing large amounts of the glial fibrillary acid protein (GFAP). This is the cellular equivalent of scar tissue, and is found in diseases such as multiple sclerosis, in which it is the major constituent of the characteristic plaques. Astrocytes are not found in the PNS.

The oligodendrocytes of the CNS can wrap round as many as 20 axons, forming the myelin sheath that insulates these neuronal processes from one another, and stops cross-talk between neurons. There is also intense oligodendrocyte mitochondrial activity at the nodes of Ranvier, which are parallel to the sites of depolarization within the underlying axon. In the PNS, the Schwann cells form the myelin and, typically, wrap round only a single axon. As noted previously, the chemical constituents of the myelin sheath are different when produced by Schwann cells rather than by oligodendrocytes.

SYNAPTIC TRANSMISSION

One of the unique chemical characteristics of the brain is the massively high density of synapses between different neurons, at which a locally acting neurohormone is released by one axon onto many other cell bodies. On the receiving end, a given cell body will typically receive a myriad of cellular products via its profusely branched dendritic tree: each branch can be smothered in synapses. The first chemical messenger or 'neurotransmitter' to traverse the synaptic cleft is the neurohormone, which is released by the axon of the first cell onto the dendrite of the second cell. This action is mediated by a neurotransmitter receptor on the respondent cell. There is usually a second messenger such as a cyclic nucleotide, which may also lead to a third messenger such as a phosphorylated protein. Typically, G-proteins are found just under the neurotransmitter receptor protein spanning the cell membrane, where they act to 'couple' the first messenger (e.g. norepinephrine) to a second messenger (e.g. cyclic AMP [cAMP]) (see also Chapter 38).

Neurotransmitters are normally inactivated after their postsynaptic actions on the target cell, hydrolysis being a major mechanism by which this is achieved. The best studied example is that of the enzyme, acetylcholinesterase. There can also be blockade at the level of the second messenger, such as cAMP, which is broken down by the enzyme phosphodiesterase. This enzyme is inhibited by methylxanthines and caffeine, and thereby mimics many of the effects of adrenergic neurotransmission.

Synaptic transmission also involves the recycling of membrane components

In addition to release of a specific neurohormone, there is also an extensive system for recycling of membrane constituents associated with this process. The synaptic vesicles contain a very high concentration of the relevant neurotransmitter, which is bounded by a membrane (see Chapter 40). During synaptic release of the transmitter, there is fusion of the synaptic vesicle membrane (containing the neurotransmitter) with the presynaptic membrane. This increase in total membrane mass is redressed by invagination of the lateral aspects of the nerve terminals, where an inward puckering movement of the membrane is effected by contractile movements of the protein, clathrin. There then follows a form of pinocytosis of the excess membrane, which is transported in retrograde fashion toward the nucleus, to be digested in lysosomes.

Types of synapse

Because of the multitude of different synaptic inputs to a given neuron, the final algebraic summation results in a

---

 AMYLOIDOSIS

A 75-year-old woman complained of postural dizziness, dry mouth, intermittent diarrhea, and numbness in both her feet. On examination, there was a marked decrease in blood pressure on assuming the upright posture. A chest radiogram revealed lytic lesions in the sternum. Her urine contained Bence–Jones protein. A bone marrow examination demonstrated increased numbers of plasma cells (see also Chapter 3).

Comment. Her neurological condition was caused by amyloidosis in which the free light-chain component of myeloma globulin produced by tumor of plasma cells in the bone marrow, accumulates in peripheral nerves. The light chains adopt the configuration of a β-pleated sheet, with multiple copies that are intercalated and resistant to normal proteolysis.

 MULTIPLE SCLEROSIS

It is essential to make a diagnosis of a disease which relapses and remits since the patient may show no abnormalities at the time of physical examination by the clinician. Lumbar puncture therefore plays a major role with the demonstration of oligoclonal bands in CSF which are absent from the parallel serum specimen. This means that there is an intrathecal rather than a systemic immune response. The converse is seen in, e.g. neurosarcoidosis, in which the systemically synthesized immunoglobulins are transferred passively into the spinal fluid, giving rise to a so-called 'mirror' pattern, where the oligoclonal bands are the same in both CSF and serum. The test involves isoelectric focusing of CSF with a parallel serum sample. The separated immunoglobulins are exposed to anti-IgG to identify bands which are present in CSF but absent from the corresponding serum. Such patterns indicate local synthesis of IgG within the brain.

'decision' at the level of the axon hillock (the site of origin of the axon from the cell body) as to whether or not to transmit an action potential down the axon as an all-or-none phenomenon. However, even before this decision is made, the input of a particular neurotransmitter can essentially be classified as excitatory or inhibitory.

In addition to the relatively short-term decisions concerning action potentials (Chapter 40), there is a longer-term modulation of the resting membrane potential, moving it either closer to (excitation) or further from (inhibition) the critical membrane potential, which is the level at which the resting membrane potential will finally trigger an action potential at the axon hillock. Many drugs have a longer-term effect on modulation, in addition to the short-term effect, which partially explains their addictive effect; this can be seen with alcohol or the opioid drugs. There are also long-term effects during treatment with various drugs – for example those used to treat endogenous depression – such that it may be weeks before any beneficial effects are seen.

Cholinergic transmission

Acetylcholine (Ach) is the neurotransmitter that has been best studied. As a model system, this transmitter can have two rather different effects, depending upon its site of origin within the nervous system (i.e. central or peripheral): those effects originally demonstrated by experiments with nicotine are characteristic of the nicotinic receptor, whereas those demonstrated with muscarine characterize the muscarinic receptor. Modern developments in pharmacology and DNA technology have produced a complex picture of the agonists and antagonists associated with the regional actions of ACh (Fig. 39.3). The classical antagonist of the muscarinic effect

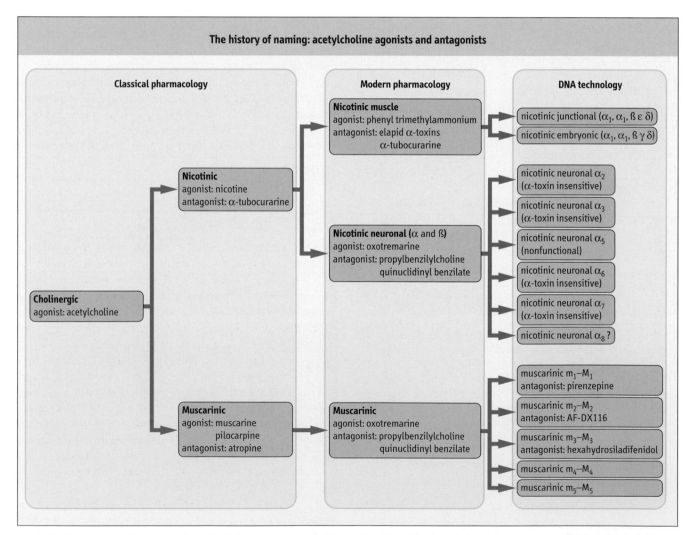

Fig. 39.3 **The history of naming: acetylcholine agonists and antagonist.** The changes in nomenclature, from early to modern terms, for the agonists and antagonists of the different central (neuronal) versus peripheral (muscle) regional actions of acetylcholine (ACh).

ION CHANNELS

Defects of sodium channels

Different molecular lesions at various sites of the sodium channel pores can give rise to hyperkalemic periodic paralysis. As this name suggests, the patient has intermittent muscle weakness, during which time the serum potassium concentration is increased. This is caused by an imbalance of cationic movements in which sodium enters the cell and potassium leaves it. For these patients, the abnormal flux of sodium into the muscle is not correctly regulated with its counterflux of potassium ions.

 ## CHANNELOPATHIES

An 18-year-old male awoke in the night with intense weakness of the proximal muscles of his arms and legs. Before retiring he had consumed a meal of pasta and cake. His brother and father had previously been similarly affected. He was taken to the emergency room of the local hospital where the weak limbs were noted to be hypotonic with depressed tendon reflexes. Serum concentration of potassium was mildly reduced at 2.9 mmol/L (normal 3.5–5.5). By the next day he had fully recovered and serum potassium had risen spontaneously to normal levels. A further attack of paralysis was induced by an infusion of intravenous glucose thereby confirming a diagnosis of familial periodic paralysis.

Comment. Hypokalaemic periodic paralysis is inherited as a Mendelian dominant and results from a mutation in the gene encoding the L-type calcium channel. Genetic diseases that affect ion channel function are called channelopathies. (See also Chapter 7.)

is atropine, and the best-studied blocker for the nicotinic receptor is the poisonous snake venom, α-bungarotoxin.

In myasthenia gravis, autoantibodies are formed against the nicotinic receptor for ACh. However, by blocking the hydrolysis of ACh, for example by means of the drug edrophonium (which inhibits the hydrolytic enzyme, acetylcholinesterase), the concentration of ACh can be effectively increased (see Chapter 40).

Adrenergic transmission

After ACh, epinephrine and norepinephrine are the neurotransmitters that have received most study. Again, they have two separate receptors:

- α-**adrenergic receptor**, blocked by phentolamine;
- β-**adrenergic receptor**, blocked by propranolol (see Fig. 38.2).

The latter drug used to be commonly used by cardiologists (many other β-blockers the mainstay of treatment in coronary heart disease), but neurologists also use it as part of the treatment of Parkinson's disease. This disease results from a deficiency of dopamine, the precursor of epinephrine and norepinephrine. Many adrenergic effects are promoted by cAMP, but other neurotransmitters have either excitatory or inhibitory effects (Fig. 39.3) (see Chapter 40).

Ion channels

Even at rest, the neuron is working to pump ions along ionic gradients

The 'resting' neuron is, nevertheless, continually pumping sodium out of the cell and potassium in, through ion channels. During an action potential, there is a momentary reversal of these ionic movements, such that sodium enters the cell and potassium then leaves, effectively repolarizing the resting

membrane. Mutations of sodium channels can occur at different sites and give rise to hyperkalemic periodic paralysis. The negative ion, chloride, moves through separate channels, which are implicated in specific pathologic states such as myotonia.

Calcium ions have an important role in the synchronization of neuronal activity

The movement of calcium ions within cells often provides a 'trigger' for the cells to synchronize an activity such as synaptic release of neurotransmitter; this synchronization of movement is also seen to have a prominent role in the sarcoplasmic reticulum of muscle (see Chapter 19). Within the central nervous system, the Lambert–Eaton syndrome is a disease that affects predominantly the P/Q subtype of calcium channels, in an example of molecular mimicry. The patient may have a primary oat–cell carcinoma of the lung; the immune system responds by making antibodies against these malignant cells. However, the malignancy and the calcium channels possess a common epitope, the effect of which is that the immune response causes the release of neurotransmitter to be blocked at the presynaptic site. This is analogous to, but nevertheless can be clearly distinguished from, the condition in myasthenia gravis, in which the block is postsynaptic.

It is also worth noting that blockade of the presynaptic release of neurotransmitter may be usefully exploited by therapeutic application of botulinus toxin (a protein derived from anerobic bacteria), which contains enzymes to hydrolyze the presynaptic proteins involved in release of neurotransmitters.

This toxin is used in special cases of spasticity such as torticollis, in which the patient can be relieved of the excessive contractures of the neck muscles, which turn the head chronically to one side and thus cause pain and distraction if untreated.

THE MECHANISM OF VISION

The mechanism by which the human eye can detect a single photon of light provides a marvelous example of the chemical processes underlying neuronal function. It involves both trapping of photons and the transducer effect, whereby the energy of light is converted into a chemical form, which is then ultimately transmuted into an action potential by a retinal ganglion neuron. A number of the intermediates are as yet not precisely known, but the underlying hypothesis is that the receptor protein, rhodopsin, is coupled to the G-protein. There are several sequence homologies of rhodopsin with the adrenergic β-receptor and with the muscarinic ACh receptor. The main steps take place in the following order (Fig. 39.4):

- *Cis*-retinal is converted to *trans*-retinal,
- Rhodopsin becomes activated,
- The level of cGMP decreases,
- Na$^+$ entry is blocked,
- The rod cell hyperpolarizes,
- There is release of glutamate (or aspartate),
- An action potential depolarizes the adjacent bipolar cell,
- This depolarizes the associated ganglion neuron, to send an action potential out of the eye.

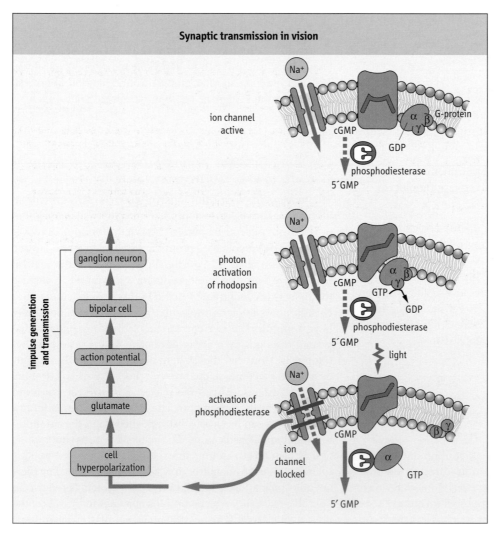

Fig. 39.4 **Neurochemistry of synaptic transmission in the mechanism of vision.** The figure shows the consequences of photon activation of rhodopsin via G-protein coupling in a rod cell. Phosphodiesterase is activated and hydrolyzes the second messenger, cGMP, thereby blocking the entry of sodium and causing hyperpolarization of the cell. Currently, the steps through which neurotransmission subsequently proceeds to produce the final ganglion neuron action potential are not known in detail. Compare G-protein-coupled receptor (Fig. 38.3).

BOTULISM

Twenty-four hours after eating home-preserved vegetables, a healthy young woman experienced progressive onset of blurred vision, severe vomiting, dysphagia, and advancing limb weakness starting in the shoulders. Her doctor admitted her to hospital, and electrophysiological studies confirmed the clinical diagnosis of botulism. Trivalent antiserum, made from inactivated toxin is administered immediately and, with the help of assisted ventilation, the patient recovers within a few weeks.

Comment. The vegetables contained the exotoxin of the anerobe, *Clostridium botulinum*, which had not been destroyed during the preservation process. The toxin hydrolyzes the presynaptic proteins involved in the release of neurotransmitter, and thus the blockade is similar to the functional lesion in Lambert–Eaton myasthenic syndrome; however, in botulism the blockade can be lethal, especially at the level of the phrenic nerve which is essential for appropriate respiratory lung movement.

ACTIVE LEARNING

1. G-proteins are widely used throughout the body as 'coupling' agents between the first extracellular messenger and the second intracellular messenger. Discuss some of the different roles for which the G-protein has been adapted amongst various cell types.
2. Mitochondria play an important role in providing for the metabolic requirements of electrical activity at the notes of Ranvier along the considerable length of the axon. Discuss the role of the two molecular motors in recycling the mitochondria required to support his function.
3. Chloride is an important anion which forms part of the complex movements with other cations such as sodium and potassium during depolarization. Discuss how congenital abnormalities in this anion transported can give rise to abnormal activities dependent upon action potentials.
4. Discuss how the brain can produce a 'gradient' for different proteins along the rostro–caudal axis.
5. Describe the reactions in vision which illustrate how light is converted into changes in ion flux.
6. Give an example of molecular mimicry.

Summary

- The nervous system contains a number of distinct cells, each of which synthesizes its own individual proteins.
- The specialized functions of the nervous system mean that these proteins are effectively compartmentalized in different loci.
- In order to facilitate communication within the brain there are two specialized methods of moving cells, organelles and proteins, i.e. the cerebrospinal fluid and axonal transport.
- The blood–brain barrier is diverse in anatomic origin and is not absolute, but it is relative (specifically based on molecular size).
- The synthesis of antibodies within the CSF, but not in parallel serum is unequivocal evidence for the brain as the source of antigenic stimulation.

Further reading

Cohen BA. Clinical applications of new cerebrospinal fluid analytic techniques for the diagnosis and treatment of central nervous system infections. *Curr Neurol Neurosci Rep* 2001;**1**:518–525.

Streilein JW, Ohta K, Mo JS, Taylor AW. Ocular immune privilege and the impact of intraocular inflammation. *DNA Cell Biol* 2002;**21**:453–459.

Brown A. Axonal transport of membranous and nonmembranous cargoes: a unified perspective. *J Cell Biol* 2003;**160**:817–821.

Bashir ZI. On long-term depression induced by activation of G-protein coupled receptors. *Neurosci Res* 2003;**45**:363–367.

Kleopa KA, Barchi RL. Genetic disorders of neuromuscular ion channels. *Muscle Nerve* 2002;**26**:299–325.

40. Neurotransmitters

S Heales

LEARNING OBJECTIVES

After reading this chapter you should be able to:

- Outline the criteria that need to be met before a molecule can be classified as a neurotransmitter.
- Identify the major neurotransmitter types and be aware that some molecules have neurotransmitter properties but cannot in the strictest sense be classified as neurotransmitters.
- Explain generation of action potentials, appreciate how neurotransmitters can be excitatory or inhibitory and summarize the process whereby a neurotransmitter is released from the presynaptic cell.
- Describe the different neurotransmitter receptors and their general mode of action.
- Describe the major biochemical pathways for neurotransmitter synthesis and degradation.
- Identify some clinical disorders that can arise as a result of disruption of neurotransmitter metabolism.

INTRODUCTION

Neurotransmitters are molecules that act as chemical signals between nerve cells

Nerve cells communicate with each other and with target tissues by secreting chemical messengers, called neurotransmitters. This chapter describes the various classes of neurotransmitters and how they interact with their target cells. It will discuss their effects on the body, how alterations in their signaling may cause disease, and how pharmacologic manipulation of their concentrations may be used therapeutically.

DEFINITION OF A NEUROTRANSMITTER

Traditionally, for a molecule to be labeled as a neurotransmitter a number of criteria have to be met. These include:

1. Synthesis of the molecule must occur within the neurone, i.e. all biosynthetic enzymes, substrates, cofactors, etc., are present for *de novo* synthesis.

2. Storage of the molecule occurs within the nerve ending prior to release, e.g. in synaptic vesicles.

3. Release of the molecule from the presynaptic ending occurs in response to an appropriate stimulus such as action potential.

4. There is binding and recognition of the putative neurotransmitter molecule on the postsynaptic target cell.

5. Mechanisms exist for the inactivation and termination of the biological activity of the neurotransmitter.

Rigorous adherence to the above criteria means that some molecules that are involved in the crosstalk between neurons are not in the strict sense classified as neurotransmitters. Thus, nitric oxide (NO), adenosine, neurosteroids, polyamines, etc., are often termed neuromodulators rather than neurotransmitters.

CLASSIFICATION OF NEUROTRANSMITTERS

A classification of neurotransmitters based on chemical composition is shown in Table 40.1. Many are derived from simple compounds, such as amino acids (Table 40.2), but peptides are also now known to be extremely important. The principal transmitters in the peripheral nervous system are norepinephrine and acetylcholine (Ach) (Fig. 40.1).

Several transmitters may be found in one nerve

An early dogma of nerve function held that one nerve contained one transmitter. However, this is now known to be an oversimplification and combinations of transmitters are the rule. The pattern of cellular transmitters may characterize a particular functional role, but details of this also remain unclear. A major low-molecular-weight transmitter such as an amine is often present, along with several peptides, an amino acid, and a purine. Sometimes, there may even be more than one possible transmitter in a particular vesicle, as is believed to be the case for adenosine triphosphate (ATP) and norepinephrine in sympathetic nerves. In some cases, the intensity of stimulation may control which transmitter is released, peptides often requiring greater levels of stimulus. Furthermore, different transmitters may have a different timescale of action. Sympathetic nerves are good examples of nerves for which this is the case: it is believed that ATP causes their rapid excitation, whereas norepinephrine and the

Classification of neurotransmitters

Group	Examples
	acetylcholine (ACh)
amines	norepinephrine, epinephrine, dopamine, 5-HT
amino acids	glutamate, GABA
purines	ATP, adenosine
gases	nitric oxide
peptides	endorphins, tachykinins, many others

Table 40.1 **Classification of neurotransmitters.**
Neurotransmitters can be classified in several ways. The scheme shown relies on chemical similarities. All except the peptides are synthesized at the nerve ending and packaged into vesicles there; peptides are synthesized in the cell body and transported down the axon. 5-HT, 5-hydroxytryptamine; GABA, γ-amino butyric acid.

Neurotransmitters of low molecular weight

Compound	Source	Site of production
Amino acids		
glutamate		central nervous system (CNS)
aspartate		CNS
glycine		spinal cord
Amino acid derivatives		
GABA	glutamate	CNS
histamine	histidine	hypothalamus
norepinephrine	tyrosine	sympathetic nerves, CNS
epinephrine	tyrosine	adrenal medulla, a few CNS nerves
dopamine	tyrosine	CNS
5-HT	tryptophan	CNS, enterochromaffin gut cells, enteric nerves
Purines		
ATP		sensory, enteric, sympathetic nerves
adenosine	ATP	CNS, peripheral nerves
Gas		
nitric oxide	arginine	genitourinary tract, CNS
Miscellaneous		
ACh	choline	parasympathetic nerves, CNS

Table 40.2 **Neurotransmitters of low molecular weight.** Many neurotransmitters are of low molecular weight, and are simple compounds, often derived from common amino acids.

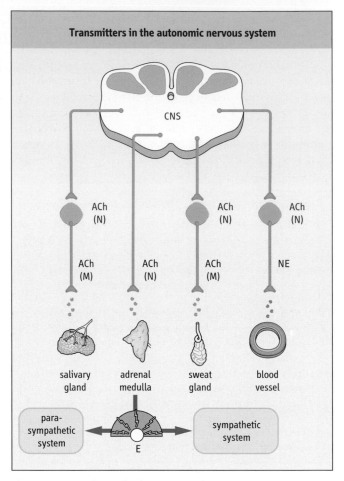

Fig. 40.1 **Transmitters in the autonomic nervous system.** Catecholamines and acetylcholine are transmitters in the sympathetic and parasympathetic nervous systems. Preganglionic nerves all release ACh, which binds to nicotinic (N) receptors. Most postganglionic sympathetic nerves release norepinephrine (NE), whereas postganglionic parasympathetic nerves release ACh, which acts at muscarinic (M) receptors. Motor neurons release ACh, which acts at distinct nicotinic receptors. E, epinephrine.

neuromodulator, neuropeptide Y (NPY), cause a slower phase of action. In some tissues, NPY on its own may be able to produce a very slow excitation.

NEUROTRANSMISSION

Action potentials are caused by changes in ion flows across cell membranes

The signal carried by a nerve cell reflects an abrupt change in the voltage potential difference across the cell membrane. The normal resting potential difference is a few millivolts, with the inside of the cell being negative, and is caused by an imbalance of ions across the plasma membrane: the concentration of K⁺ ions is much greater inside cells than outside, whereas the opposite is true for Na⁺ ions. This difference is maintained by the action of the Na⁺/K⁺-ATPase (see Chapter 39). Only those ions to which the membrane is permeable can affect the potential, as they can come to an electrochemical steady state under the combined influence of concentration and voltage differences. Because the membrane in all resting cells is comparatively permeable to K⁺ as a result of the presence of voltage-independent (leakage) K⁺ channels, this ion largely controls the resting potential.

A change in voltage which tends to drive this resting potential towards zero from the normal negative voltage is known as a depolarization, whereas a process that increases the negative potential is called hyperpolarizing

So far, this picture is common to all cells. However, nerve cells contain voltage-dependent sodium channels that open very rapidly when a depolarizing change in voltage is applied. When they open, they allow the inward passage of huge numbers of Na⁺ ions from the extracellular fluid (Fig. 40.2), which swamps the resting voltage and drives the membrane potential to positive values. This reversal of voltage is the

action potential. Almost immediately afterwards, the sodium channels close and so-called delayed potassium channels open. These restore the normal resting balance of ions across the membrane and, after a short refractory period, the cell can conduct another action potential. Meanwhile, the action potential has spread by electrical conductance to the next segment of nerve membrane, and the entire cycle starts again.

Neurotransmitters alter the activity of various ion channels to cause changes in the membrane potential

Excitatory neurotransmitters cause a depolarizing change in voltage, in which case an action potential is more likely to occur. In contrast, inhibitory transmitters hyperpolarize the membrane, and an action potential is then less likely to occur.

Neurotransmitters act at synapses

Neurotransmitters are released into the space between cells at a specialized area known as a synapse (Fig. 40.3). In the

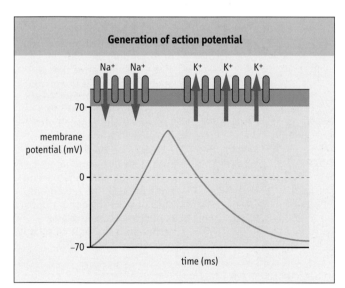

Fig. 40.2 **Generation of action potential.** Action potential is formed as follows. At the start of an action potential, the membrane is at its resting potential of about −70 mV; this is maintained by voltage-independent K⁺ channels. When an impulse is initiated by a signal from a neurotransmitter, voltage-dependent Na⁺ channels open. These allow inflow of Na⁺ ions, which alter the membrane potential to positive values. The Na⁺ channels then close, and K⁺ channels, called delayed rectifier channels, open to restore the initial balance of ions and the negative membrane potential.

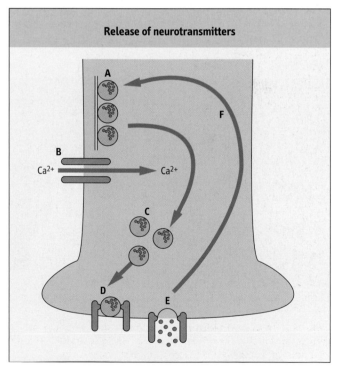

Fig. 40.3 **Release of neurotransmitters.** Neurotransmitters are released from vesicles at the synaptic membrane. (A) In the resting state, vesicles are attached to microtubules. (B) When an action potential is received, calcium channels open. (C) Vesicles move to the plasma membrane, and (D) bind to a complex of docking proteins. (E) Neurotransmitter is released, and (F) vesicles are recycled.

simplest case, they diffuse from the presynaptic membrane, across the synaptic space or cleft, and bind to receptors at the postsynaptic membrane. However, many neurons, particularly those containing amines, have several varicosities along the axon, containing transmitter. These varicosities may not be close to any neighboring cell, so transmitter released from them has the possibility of affecting many neurons. Nerves innervating smooth muscle are commonly of this kind.

When the action potential arrives at the end of the axon, the change in voltage opens calcium channels. Calcium entry is essential for mobilization of vesicles containing transmitter, and for their eventual fusion with the synaptic membrane and release through it.

Because transmitters are released from vesicles, impulses arrive at the postsynaptic cell in individual packets, or quanta. At the neuromuscular junction between nerves and skeletal muscle cells, a large number of vesicles are discharged at a time, and a single impulse may therefore be enough to stimulate contraction of the muscle cell. The number of vesicles released at synapses between neurons, however, is much smaller; consequently, the recipient cell will be stimulated only if the total algebraic sum of the various positive and negative stimuli exceeds its threshold. As each cell in the brain receives input from a huge number of neurons, this implies that there is a far greater capability for the fine control of responses in the central nervous system (CNS) than there is at the neuromuscular junction.

Receptors

Neurotransmitters act by binding to specific receptors and opening or closing ion channels

There are several mechanisms by which receptors for excitatory neurotransmitters can cause the propagation of an action potential in a postsynaptic neuron. Directly or indirectly, they cause changes in ion flow across the membrane, until the potential reaches the critical point, or threshold, for initiation of an action potential. Receptors that directly control the opening of an ion channel are called ionotropic, whereas metabotropic receptors cause changes in second messenger systems, which, in turn, alter the function of channels that are separate from the receptor.

Ionotropic receptors (ion channels)

Ionotropic receptors contain an ion channel within their structure (Fig. 40.4; see also Chapter 38). Examples include the nicotinic ACh receptor and some glutamate and γ-amino butyric acid (GABA) receptors. These are transmembrane proteins, with several subunits, usually five, surrounding a pore through the membrane. Each subunit has four transmembrane regions. When the ligand binds, there is a change in the three-dimensional structure of the complex, which allows the flow of ions through it. The effect on membrane

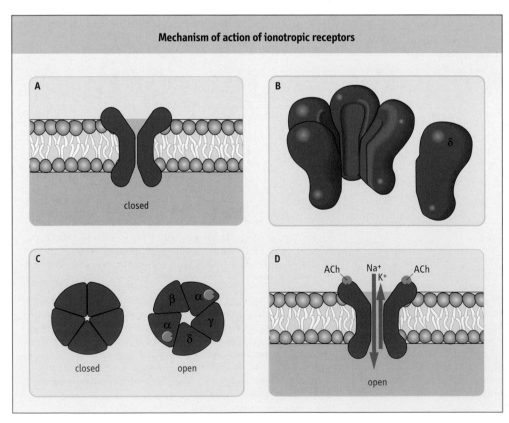

Fig. 40.4 **Mechanism of action of ionotropic receptors.** Ionotropic receptors directly open ion channels (ionotropic receptors are themselves ion channels). The best-studied example is the nicotinic ACh receptor. This is a transmembrane protein (A) consisting of five nonidentical subunits (B), each one passing right through the membrane. The subunits surround a pore (C) that selectively allows certain ions through when it is opened by a ligand (D).

potential depends on the particular ions that are allowed to pass: the nicotinic ACh receptor is comparatively nonspecific towards sodium and potassium, and causes depolarization, whereas the GABA$_A$ receptor is a chloride channel, and causes hyperpolarization.

Metabotropic receptors

All known metatropic receptors are coupled to G-proteins

Metabotropic receptors are coupled to second messenger pathways and act more slowly than ionotropic receptors. All known metabotropic receptors are coupled to G-proteins (see Chapter 38) and, like hormone receptors, have seven transmembrane regions. Typically, they couple either to adenylate cyclase, altering the production of cyclic adenosine monophosphate (cAMP), or to the phosphatidyl inositol pathway, which alters calcium fluxes. Ion channels that are separate from the receptor are then usually modified by phosphorylation. For instance, the β-adrenergic receptor, which responds to norepinephrine and epinephrine, causes an increase in cAMP, which stimulates a kinase to phosphorylate and activate a calcium channel. Some of the muscarinic class of ACh receptors have similar effects on K$^+$ channels.

Regulation of neurotransmitters

The action of transmitters must be halted by their removal from the synaptic cleft

When transmitters have served their function, they must be removed from the synaptic space. Simple diffusion is probably the major mechanism of removal of neuropeptides. Enzymes such as acetylcholinesterase, which cleaves ACh, may destroy any remaining transmitter. Surplus transmitters may also be taken back up into the presynaptic neuron for reuse, and this is a major route of removal for catecholamines and amino acids. Interference with uptake causes an increase in the concentration of transmitter in the synaptic space; this often has useful therapeutic consequences.

Concentrations of neurotransmitters may be manipulated

The effects of neurotransmitters can be altered by changing their effective concentrations or the number of receptors. Concentrations can be altered by:

- **changing the rate of synthesis**,
- **altering the rate of release at the synapse**,
- **blocking reuptake**,
- **blocking degradation**.

Changes in the number of receptors may be involved in long-term adaptations to the administration of drugs.

VARIOUS CLASSES OF NEUROTRANSMITTERS

Amino acids

It has been particularly difficult to prove that amino acids are true neurotransmitters; they are present in high concentrations because of their other metabolic roles, and therefore simple measurement of their concentrations did not provide conclusive evidence. Pharmacologic studies of responses to different analogs and the cloning of specific receptors finally provided the proof.

Glutamate

Glutamate is the most important excitatory transmitter in the CNS

It acts on both ionotropic and metabotropic receptors. Clinically, the receptor characterized *in vitro* by N-methyl-D-aspartate (NMDA) binding is particularly important (Fig. 40.5).

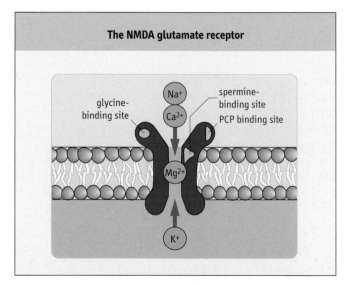

Fig. 40.5 **The NMDA glutamate receptor.** The glutamate receptor that binds *N*-methyl-L-aspartate (NMDA) is complex. This receptor is clinically important because it may cause damage to neurons after stroke (excitotoxicity, see following page). It contains several modulatory binding sites, so it may be possible to develop drugs that could alter its function. Glycine is an obligatory cofactor, as are polyamines such as spermine. Magnesium physiologically blocks the channel at the resting potential, so the channel can open only when the cell has been partially depolarized by a separate stimulus. It therefore causes a prolongation of the excitation. This receptor also binds phencyclidine (PCP). Because this drug of abuse can cause psychotic symptoms, it is possible that dysfunction of pathways involving NMDA receptors causes some of the symptoms of schizophrenia.

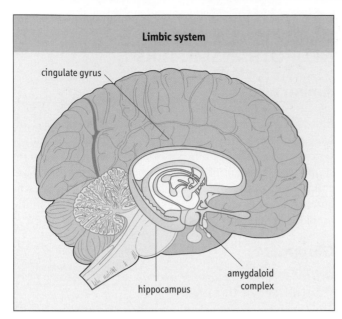

Fig. 40.6 **Limbic system.** The limbic system of the brain is involved in emotions and memory. It consists of various areas surrounding the upper brain stem, including the hippocampus, the amygdaloid body, and the cingulate gyrus. Removal of the hippocampus prevents the laying down of short-term memory, whereas intact amygdaloid function is required for the emotion of fear.

The hippocampus (Fig. 40.6) is an area of the limbic system of the brain that is involved in emotion and memory. Certain synaptic pathways there become more active when chronically stimulated – a phenomenon known as long-term potentiation. This represents a possible model of how memory is laid down, and it requires activation of the NMDA receptor and the consequent influx of calcium.

Glutamate is recycled by high-affinity transporters into both neurons and glial cells. The glial cells convert it into glutamine, which then diffuses back into the neuron. Mitochondrial glutaminase in the neuron regenerates glutamate for reuse.

Glutamate and Excitotoxicity

Extracellular glutamate concentration is increased after trauma and stroke, during severe convulsions, and in some organic brain diseases such as Huntington's chorea, AIDS-related dementia, and Parkinson's disease, because of release of glutamate from damaged cells and damage to the glutamate uptake pathways.

Excess glutamate is toxic to nerve cells

The NMDA receptor is activated, which allows calcium entry into cells. This activates various proteases, which in turn initiate the pathway of programmed cell death, or apoptosis (see also Chapter 29). There may, in addition, be changes in other ionotropic glutamate receptors that also cause aberrant calcium uptake. Uptake of sodium ions is also implicated, and causes swelling of cells. Activation of NMDA receptors also increases the production of nitric oxide, which may in itself be toxic. Cell death in some models of excitotoxicity can be prevented by inhibitors of nitric oxide production, but the mechanism of toxicity is not clear.

Attempts are being made to develop drugs to inhibit NMDA activation and suppress excitotoxicity. The hope is that damage caused by stroke can be limited or even reversed. Unfortunately, many of the drugs have side effects because they bind to the phencyclidine-binding site and have unpleasant psychologic effects such as paranoia and delusions.

γ-Amino butyric acid (GABA)

GABA is synthesized from glutamate by the enzyme glutamate decarboxylase (Fig. 40.7)

It is the major inhibitory transmitter in the brain. There are two known GABA receptors: the $GABA_A$ receptor is ionotropic, and the $GABA_B$ receptor is metabotropic. The $GABA_A$ receptor consists of five subunits that arise from several gene families, giving an enormous number of potential receptors with different binding affinities. This receptor is the target for several useful therapeutic drugs. Benzodiazepines bind to it and cause a potentiation of the response to endogenous GABA; these drugs reduce anxiety and also cause muscle relaxation. Barbiturates also bind to the GABA receptor and stimulate it directly in the absence of GABA; because of this lack of dependence on endogenous ligand, they are more likely to cause toxic side effects in overdose.

Glycine

Glycine is primarily found in inhibitory interneurons in the spinal cord, where it blocks impulses traveling down the cord in motor neurons to stimulate skeletal muscle. The glycine receptor on motor neurons is ionotropic and is blocked by strychnine; motor impulses can then be passed without negative control, which accounts for the rigidity and convulsions caused by this toxin.

Catecholamines

Norepinephrine, epinephrine, and dopamine, known as catecholamines, are all derived from the amino acid tyrosine (see Fig. 40.7). In common with other compounds containing amino groups, such as serotonin, they are also known as biogenic amines. Nerves that release catecholamines have varicosities along the axon, instead of a single area of release at the end. Transmitter is released from the varicosities, and diffuses through the extracellular space until it meets a receptor. This allows it to affect a wide area of tissue, and these compounds are believed to have a general modulatory effect on overall brain functions such as mood and arousal.

Synthesis of neurotransmitters

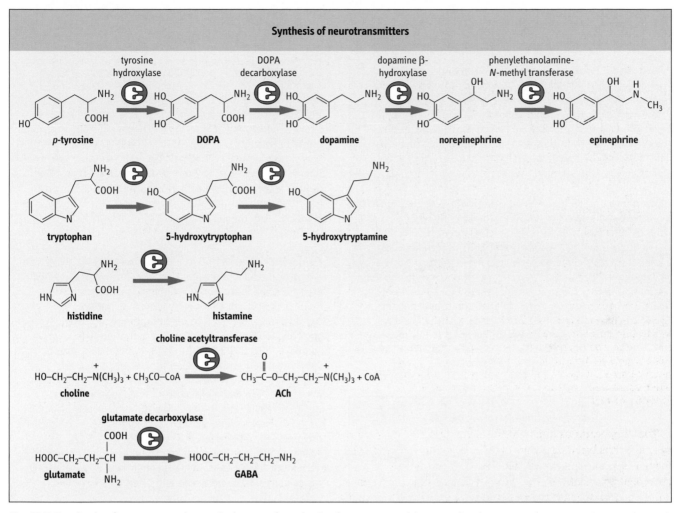

Fig. 40.7 **Synthesis of neurotransmitters.** Pathways of synthesis of neurotransmitters are simple.

 DISORDERS OF NEUROTRANSMISSION

Depression as a disease of amine neurotransmitters

Monoamine oxidase (MAO) inhibitors prevent the catabolism of catecholamines and serotonin. They therefore increase the concentrations of these compounds at the synapse and increase the action of the transmitters. Compounds with this property are antidepressants. Reserpine, an antihypertensive drug that depletes catecholamines, caused depression and is no longer in use. These dual findings gave rise to the 'amine theory of depression': this states that depression is caused by a relative deficiency of amine neurotransmitters at central synapses, and predicts that drugs which increase amine concentrations should improve symptoms of the condition.

In support of this theory, tricyclic antidepressants inhibit transport of both norepinephrine and serotonin into neurons, thereby increasing the concentration of amines in the synaptic cleft. Specific serotonin reuptake inhibitors (SSRIs), such as fluoxetine (Prozac), are also highly effective antidepressants. However, as the symptoms of depression do not resolve for several days after treatment is started, it is likely that long-term adaptations of concentrations of transmitters and their receptors are at least as important as acute changes in amine concentrations in the synaptic cleft.

This role of monoamines in depression is undoubtedly an oversimplification. Thus, cocaine is also an effective reuptake inhibitor, but is not an antidepressant, and amphetamines both block reuptake and cause release of catecholamines from nerve terminals, but cause mania rather than relief of depression.

AN UNUSUAL REACTION TO CHEESE

A 50-year-old man had been suffering from depression for some years. His condition was treated with tranylcypromine, an inhibitor of monoamine oxidase types A and B. He developed a severe, throbbing headache and his blood pressure was found to be 200/110 mmHg. The only unusual occurrence had been that he had attended a cocktail party the previous evening at which he ate cheese snacks and drank several glasses of red wine.

Comment. The patient was experiencing a hypertensive crisis caused by an interaction between the food he had eaten and the drug he was treated with – a MAO inhibitor. This drug inhibits the main enzyme that catabolizes catecholamines. Several foods, including cheese, pickled herring, and red wine, contain an amine called tyramine, which is similar in structure to natural amine transmitters and is also broken down by MAO. If this enzyme is not functional, the concentrations of tyramine increase and it starts to act as a neurotransmitter. This can cause a hypertensive crisis, as it did in this patient.

A NEUROTRANSMITTER CAUSE OF HYPERTENSION

A 56-year-old woman presented with severe hypertension. She suffered from attacks of sweating, headaches, and palpitations. Her high blood pressure had not responded to treatment with an angiotensin converting enzyme inhibitor and a diuretic. A sample of urine was taken for measurement of catecholamines and metabolites. The rate of excretion of norepinephrine was 1500 nmol/24 h (253 mg/24 h); (reference range <900 nmol/24 h [<152 mg/24 h]), that of epinephrine 620 nmol/24 h (113 mg/24 h); (reference range <230 nmol/24 h [<42 mg/24 h]) and that of vanillylmandelic acid 60 mmol/24 h (11.9 mg/24 h); (reference range <35.5 mmol/24 h [<7.0 mg/24 h]).

Comment. The patient had a pheochromocytoma which is a tumor of the adrenal medulla that secretes catecholamines. Both norepinephrine and epinephrine may be secreted: norepinephrine causes hypertension by activating α-1-adrenoceptors on vascular smooth muscle, and epinephrine increases heart rate by activating β-1-adrenoceptors on the heart muscle. Hypertension may be paroxysmal and severe, leading to stroke or heart failure. Diagnosis is made by measuring catecholamines in plasma or urine, or their metabolites, such as metanephrines and vanillylmandelic acid, in urine. The tumor is usually localized by radiological techniques such as magnetic resonance (MR) or computed tomography (CT) scanning.
Although this is a rare cause of hypertension, comprising only about 1% of cases, it is very important to remember it, as the condition is dangerous and often amenable to surgical cure.

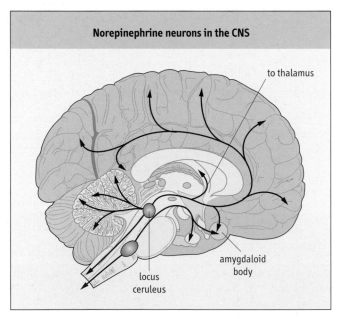

Norepinephrine neurons in the CNS

to thalamus

amygdaloid body

locus ceruleus

Fig. 40.8 **Norepinephrine neurons in the CNS.** Norepinephrine-containing neurons arise in the locus ceruleus in the brain stem and are distributed throughout the cortex.

Norepinephrine and epinephrine

Norepinephrine (also known as noradrenaline) is a major transmitter in the sympathetic nervous system. Sympathetic nerves arise in the spinal cord and run to ganglia situated close to the cord, from which postganglionic nerves run to the target tissues. Norepinephrine is the transmitter for these postganglionic nerves, whereas the transmitter at the intermediate ganglia is ACh. Stimulation of these nerves is responsible for various features of the 'fight or flight' response, such as stimulation of the heart rate, sweating, vasoconstriction in the skin, and bronchodilation.

There are also norepinephrine-containing neurons in the CNS, largely in the brain stem (Fig. 40.8). Their axons extend in a wide network throughout the cortex, and alter the overall state of alertness or attention. The stimulatory effects of amphetamines are caused by their close chemical similarity to catecholamines.

Epinephrine (also known as adrenaline) is produced by the adrenal medulla under the influence of ACh-containing nerves analogous to the sympathetic preganglionic nerves. It is more active than norepinephrine on the heart and lungs, causes redirection of blood from the skin to skeletal muscle, and has important stimulatory effects on glycogen meta-

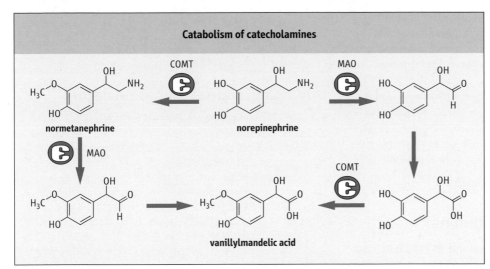

Catabolism of catecholamines

normetanephrine

norepinephrine

vanillylmandelic acid

Fig. 40.9 **Catabolism of catecholamines.** Catecholamines are degraded by oxidation of the amino group by the enzyme monoamine oxidase (MAO), and by methylation by catecholamine-*O*-methyl transferase (COMT). The pathway shown is for norepinephrine, but the pathways for epinephrine, dopamine, and 5-HT are analogous.

bolism in the liver. In response to epinephrine, a sudden extra supply of glucose is delivered to muscle, the heart and lungs work harder to pump oxygen round the circulation, and the body is then prepared to run or to defend itself (see Chapter 20). Epinephrine is not essential for life, however, as it is possible to remove the adrenal medulla without serious consequences.

The receptors for norepinephrine and epinephrine are called adrenoceptors. They are divided into α- and β-receptor classes and subclasses on the basis of their pharmacology. Epinephrine acts on all classes of the receptors, but norepinephrine is more specific for α-receptors. β-Blockers, such as atenolol, are used to treat hypertension and chest pain (angina) in ischemic heart disease because they antagonize the stimulatory effects of catecholamines on the heart. Nonspecific α-blockers have limited use, although the more specific α_1-blockers such as prazosin, and α_2-blockers such as clonidine, can be used to treat hypertension. Certain subclasses of β-receptors are found in particular tissues; for instance, the β_2-receptor is present in lung, and β_2-receptor agonists such as salbutamol are therefore used to produce bronchial dilatation in asthma without stimulating the β_1-receptor in the heart.

Norepinephrine is taken up into cells by a high-affinity transporter and catabolized by the enzyme monoamine oxidase (MAO). Further oxidation and methylation by catecholamine-*O*-methyl transferase (COMT) convert the products to metanephrines and vanillylmandelic acid (4-hydroxy-3-methoxymandelic acid) (Fig. 40.9), which can be measured in the urine as indices of the function of the adrenal medulla. They are particularly increased in patients who have the tumor of the adrenal medulla known as pheochromocytoma. This tumor causes hypertension because of the vasoconstrictor action of the catecholamines it produces.

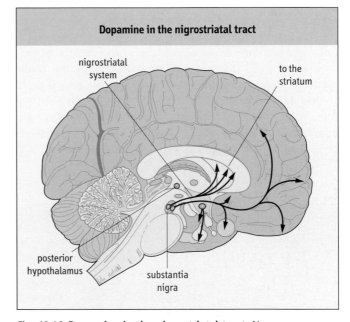

Dopamine in the nigrostriatal tract

nigrostriatal system

to the striatum

posterior hypothalamus

substantia nigra

Fig. 40.10 **Dopamine in the nigrostriatal tract.** Nerves containing dopamine run in well-defined tracts. One of the most important tracts, the nigrostriatal, connects the substantia nigra in the mid brain with the basal ganglia below the cortex. Damage to this causes Parkinson's disease, with loss of fine control of movement.

Dopamine

Dopamine is both an intermediate in the synthesis of norepinephrine and a neurotransmitter. It is a major transmitter in nerves that interconnect the nuclei of the basal ganglia in the brain and control voluntary movement (Fig. 40.10). Damage to these nerves causes Parkinson's disease, which is characterized by tremor and difficulties in initiating and controlling movement. Dopamine is also found in pathways affecting the limbic systems of the brain, which are involved in emotional responses and memory. Defects in dopaminergic systems are implicated in schizophrenia, because many antipsychotic drugs used to treat this disease have been found to bind to dopamine receptors.

In the periphery, dopamine causes vasodilatation, and it is therefore used clinically to stimulate renal blood flow, and is important in the treatment of renal failure (Chapter 22). The catabolism of dopamine is comparable to norepinephrine. However, the major metabolite formed is homovanillic acid (HVA).

Serotonin (5-hydroxytryptamine)

Serotonin, also called 5-hydroxytryptamine (5-HT), is derived from tryptophan (see Fig. 40.7). In addition, serotonin biosynthesis has a number of biochemical similarities to dopamine synthesis. Thus, tryptophan hydroxylase like tyrosine hydroxylase displays a cofactor requirement for tetrahydrobiopterin (BH_4) (see below). Furthermore, 5-hydroxytryptophan is converted to serotonin by dopa decarboxylase (also known as aromatic amino acid decarboxylase).

Serotoninergic neurons are concentrated in the raphe nuclei in the upper brain stem (Fig. 40.11), but project up to the cerebral cortex and down to the spinal cord. They are more active when subjects are awake than when they are asleep, and serotonin may control the degree of responsiveness of motor neurons in the spinal cord. In addition, it is

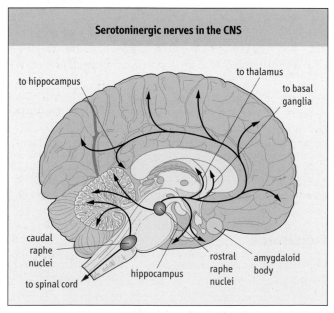

Fig. 40.11 **Serotoninergic nerves in the CNS.** Serotonin-containing nerves arise in the raphe nuclei, part of the reticular formation in the upper brain stem. In common with those containing norepinephrine, they are distributed widely.

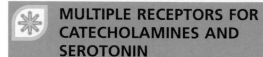

MULTIPLE RECEPTORS FOR CATECHOLAMINES AND SEROTONIN

Dopamine and serotonin receptors

Multiple receptors have been isolated for dopamine and serotonin. Not all those that have been cloned have yet been shown to be functional, but the possible relevance in terms of drug development is obvious. In some cases, specific actions on particular receptors can be exploited therapeutically.

There are five known dopamine receptors, falling into two main groups – D_1-like (D_1 and D_5) and D_2-like (D_2, D_3, and D_4) – that differ in their signaling pathways. D_1 receptors increase the production of cAMP, whereas D_2 receptors inhibit it. Antipsychotic drugs such as phenothiazines and haloperidol tend to inhibit D_2-like receptors, suggesting that excessive dopamine activity may be important in causing the symptoms of schizophrenia.

The D_2 receptor is a major receptor in the nerves that interconnect the basal ganglia. As it is known that destruction of these nerves causes Parkinson's disease, it is not surprising that antipsychotic drugs that inhibit the D_2 receptor tend to have the side effect of causing abnormal movements. Drugs, such as clozapine, that bind preferentially to the D_4 receptor appear to be free of such side effects, although that particular drug also binds to several other receptors.

More than a dozen serotonin (5-HT) receptors have been isolated using molecular biological techniques. They have been divided into classes and subclasses on the basis of their pharmacologic properties and their structures. Most are metabotropic, although the $5-HT_3$ receptor is ionotropic and mediates a fast signal in the enteric nervous system. The $5-HT_{1A}$ receptor is found on many presynaptic neurons, where it acts as an autoreceptor to inhibit the release of 5-HT.

In general, increasing the brain concentration of 5-HT appears to increase anxiety, whereas reducing its concentration is helpful in treating the condition. The antidepressant, buspirone, acts as an agonist at $5-HT_{1A}$ receptors, and presumably causes a decrease in production of 5-HT. In addition to its effects on the D_4 dopamine receptor, clozapine binds strongly to the $5-HT_{2A}$ receptor, and it may be that a combination of a high level of $5-HT_{2a}$ antagonism and low D_2-binding activity is desirable for drugs that can be used to treat schizophrenia with the minimum frequency of side effects. The $5-HT_3$ blocker, ondansetron, is an anti-emetic, extensively used to prevent vomiting during chemotherapy. Migraine can be treated with sumatriptan, a $5-HT_{1D}$ agonist. The central role of 5-HT in controlling brain function and the huge number of associated receptors suggest that it may possible to tailor a large number of drugs to treat specific disorders, and that pharmacological manipulation of the function of the nervous system is probably still in its infancy.

ANALYSIS OF CEREBROSPINAL FLUID FOR THE DETECTION OF DISORDERS OF DOPAMINE AND SEROTONIN METABOLISM

Cerebrospinal fluid (CSF) flows around the major structures of the brain and spinal cord (see also Chapter 39). During circulation, molecules reflecting cellular metabolism diffuse into the CSF. Included in this range of metabolites are the dopamine and serotonin degradation products, homovanillic acid (HVA) and 5-hydroxyindoleacetic acid (5-HIAA). Furthermore, tetrahydrobiopterin (BH$_4$) precursors, metabolites and BH$_4$ itself are also released into the CSF. Thus, determination of such molecules in CSF provides a powerful indicator of the integrity of dopamine and serotonin metabolism within the central nervous system. Such analyses have identified a number of inborn errors of metabolism affecting dopamine and/or serotonin availability, e.g. disorders of BH$_4$ metabolism, pyridoxal phosphate metabolism, tyrosine hydroxylase deficiency and aromatic amino acid decarboxylase (dopa decarboxylase) deficiency. Quantification of the above metabolites is usually achieved by high-performance liquid chromatography (HPLC). For the above molecules, there is a concentration gradient in the CSF, known as the rostral-caudal gradient. Thus, CSF fractions taken from closer to the brain have a high concentration of these metabolites. Furthermore, for many of these metabolites, their concentration declines with age. Consequently, in view of these factors, specialist laboratories providing a diagnostic service require that the same fraction of CSF is provided for analysis. In addition, appropriate age-related reference ranges must be available for correct interpretation of the results generated.

FLUSHING ATTACKS CAUSED BY A TUMOR

A 60-year-old man complained of attacks of flushing, associated with an increased heart rate. He also had troublesome diarrhea and abdominal pain, and had lost weight. The symptoms suggested a diagnosis of carcinoid syndrome caused by excessive secretion of serotonin and other metabolically active compounds from a tumor. To confirm this, a urine sample was taken for measurement of 5-hydroxyindoleacetic acid (5-HIAA), the major metabolite of 5-HT; the concentration was found to be 120 mmol/24 h (23 mg/24 h); (reference range 10–52 mmol/24 h [3–14 mg/24 h]).

Comment. The patient had the carcinoid syndrome, which is caused by tumors of enterochromaffin cells usually originating in the ileum which have metastasized to the liver. These cells are related to the catecholamine-producing chromaffin cells in the adrenal medulla and convert tryptophan to serotonin (5-HT). Serotonin itself is believed to cause diarrhea, but other mediators, such as histamine and bradykinin, may be more important in the flushing attacks. The urinary concentration of 5-HIAA provides a useful diagnostic test and can be used to monitor the response of the cancer to treatment.

Acetylcholine

Acetylcholine (ACh) is the transmitter of the parasympathetic autonomic nervous system and of the sympathetic ganglia. Stimulation of the parasympathetic system produces effects that are broadly opposite to those of the sympathetic system, such as slowing of the heart rate, bronchoconstriction, and stimulation of intestinal smooth muscle. ACh also acts at neuromuscular junctions, where motor nerves contact skeletal muscle cells and cause them to contract. Apart from these roles, ACh may be involved in learning and memory, as neurons containing this transmitter also exist in the brain.

ACh is synthesized from choline by the enzyme choline acetyl transferase. After it is secreted into the synaptic cleft, it is largely broken down by acetylcholinesterase. The remainder is taken back up into the nerve cell by transporters similar to those for amines.

There are two main classes of ACh receptors: nicotinic and muscarinic (see Chapter 39, Fig. 39.3). Both respond to ACh, but can be distinguished by their associated agonists and antagonists; they are quite different structurally and differ in their mechanisms of action:

■ **Nicotinic receptors are ionotropic**. They bind nicotine and are found on ganglia and at the neuromuscular junction. When ACh or nicotine binds, a pore opens, which allows both Na$^+$ and K$^+$ to pass

implicated in so-called vegetative behaviors such as feeding, sexual behavior, and temperature control.

Serotonin has effects on mood. Reuptake inhibitors, which increase its concentration at the synapse, relieve depression. An excess of serotonin may cause panic attacks; these can be controlled by 5-HT$_{1A}$-receptor agonists, which are believed to act on autoreceptors to reduce the production of serotonin.

Serotonin also has substantial effects on the peripheral nervous system and enteric neurons. It is a powerful vasoconstrictor, and increases motility of the gastrointestinal tract. Some of the serotonin in the gut arises not from neurons, but from enterochromaffin cells, which are similar to the chromaffin cells in the adrenal medulla that produce epinephrine.

The degradation pathway of serotonin is similar to that of catecholamines, resulting in the formation of 5-hydroxyindoleacetic acid (5-HIAA). This is a useful marker of excessive production or deficiency of serotonin.

through. Because the action of the ligand on the channel is direct, action is rapid;

- **Muscarinic receptors, responding to the fungal toxin, muscarine, are metabotropic.** They are much more widespread in the brain than are nicotinic receptors, and are also the major receptors found on smooth muscle and glands innervated by parasympathetic nerves. Atropine specifically inhibits these receptors. There are several separate muscarinic receptors, differing in their tissue distribution and signaling pathways. As yet, no clear pattern has emerged as to their specific functions.

Clinically, ACh agonists, in common with acetylcholinesterase inhibitors, are used to treat glaucoma, an eye disease characterized by high intra-ocular pressure, by increasing the tone of the muscles of accommodation of the eye, and to stimulate intestinal function after surgery. On the other hand, when acetylcholinesterase is inhibited by organophosphate insecticides or nerve gases, a toxic syndrome is caused by the resulting excess of ACh. There may be diarrhea, increased secretory activity of several glands, and bronchoconstriction. This syndrome can be antagonized by atropine, although longer-term treatment involves the use of drugs that can remove the insecticide from the enzyme, such as pralidoxime.

Nitric oxide gas

In autonomic and enteric nerves, nitric oxide (NO) is produced from arginine by the tetrahydrobiopterin-dependent nitric oxide synthases. NO has a number of attributed physiological functions including relaxation of both vascular and intestinal smooth muscle and the possible regulation of mitochondrial energy production. Furthermore, within the brain, NO may have a role in memory formation. However, excessive NO formation has been implicated in the neurodegenerative process associated with Parkinson's and Alzheimer's disease. Whilst the exact mechanism whereby excessive NO causes neuronal death is not known, a growing body of evidence suggests that irreversible damage to the mitochondrial electron transport chain may be an important factor.

NO is a gas it is not stored in vesicles, but released directly into the extracellular space. Consequently, NO does not, in the strictest sense, meet all the current criteria to be labeled as a neurotransmitter. NO itself diffuses comparatively easily between cells and binds directly to heme groups in the enzyme guanylate cyclase, stimulating the production of cyclic guanosine monophosphate. (See also Chapter 17, p. 236.)

TETRAHYDROBIOPTERIN IS AN ESSENTIAL COFACTOR FOR DOPAMINE AND SEROTONIN SYNTHESIS

Tetrahydrobiopterin (BH_4) is a member of the group of chemicals known as the pterins. Normally, BH_4 is synthesized, via a number of enzymatic steps, from the precursor guanosine triphosphate. With regards to the central nervous system an adequate supply of BH_4 is essential for tyrosine and tryptophan hydroxylase activities. When acting as a cofactor, BH_4 is oxidized to quinonoid dihydrobiopterin (qBH_2). BH_4, under normal conditions, is regenerated from qBH_2 by the enzyme, dihydropteridine reductase (DHPR). Several inborn errors of BH_4 metabolism are now known. These can arise as a result of a failure of *de novo* BH_4 synthesis or recycling by DHPR. If untreated, these patients have a number of severe neurological problems which include mental retardation, epilepsy and a movement disorder similar to that seen in Parkinson's disease. Following diagnosis, patients are treated by L-DOPA and 5-hydroxytryptophan, to bypass the metabolic block created by the BH_4 deficiency. Following initiation of treatment, there is usually clinical improvement, resulting from the correction of dopamine and serotonin metabolism. However, BH_4 is also the cofactor for all isoforms of nitric oxide synthase. There is now evidence to suggest that patients with BH_4 deficiency also have an impaired ability to generate NO. Thus, research is now in progress to develop means to correct this impairment of the NO signaling pathway as well, for instance by gene therapy targeting the deficient enzyme of BH_4 metabolism. Such an approach has the advantage of correcting the primary defect, i.e. the BH_4 deficiency.

Other small molecules

ATP and other purines derived from it are now known to have transmitter functions. ATP is present in synaptic vesicles of sympathetic nerves, along with norepinephrine, and is responsible for rapid excitatory potentials in smooth muscle. Adenosine receptors are widespread in the brain and in vascular tissue. Adenosine is largely inhibitory in the CNS, and inhibition of adenosine receptors is believed to underlie the stimulatory effects of caffeine.

Study of histamine in nerves is complicated by the large amounts that are present in mast cells. Histamine is found in a small number of neurons, mainly in the hypothalamus, although their projections are widespread throughout the brain. It has been shown to control the release of pituitary hormones, arousal, and food intake. Antihistamines designed to control allergies caused by release from mast cells act on the H_1 receptor and tend to be sedative, suggesting that other central functions also probably exist. The histamine receptor

A DISEASE CAUSING MUSCLE WEAKNESS

A 35-year-old woman noticed that she had difficulty in keeping her eyes open. She also had periods of double vision when her voice was indistinct and nasal and she had difficulty swallowing. Her physician suspected myasthenia, a disease of nerve–muscle conduction. The serum titer of anti-acetylcholine receptor antibodies, was measured and found to be elevated.

Comment. The patient was suffering from myasthenia gravis. This is a disease that manifests itself as weakness of voluntary muscles and is corrected by treatment with acetylcholinesterase inhibitors. It is caused by autoantibodies directed against the nicotinic acetylcholine receptor, which circulate in serum. Because of these autoantibodies, transmission of nerve impulses to muscle is much less efficient than normal.
Drugs that inhibit acetylcholinesterase increase the concentration of acetylcholine in the synaptic space, which compensates for the reduced number of receptors. Improvement in nerve–muscle conduction in response to endrophonium can be used as a diagnostic test but requires several precautions, and long-acting acetylcholinesterase inhibitors such as pyridostigmine can be used to treat the disease but corticosteroids are often effective.

in the stomach is of the H_2 class, therefore the H_2 inhibitors, such as cimetidine and ranitidine, that are used to treat peptic ulcers have no effect on allergy.

Peptides

Many peptides act as neurotransmitters

It is an open question whether all of the peptides that have been described are really true neurotransmitters. Nevertheless, more than 50 small peptides have now been shown to influence neural function. All known peptide receptors are metabotropic and coupled to G-proteins (see Chapter 38), and so act comparatively slowly. There are no specific uptake pathways or degradative enzymes, and the main route of disposal is simple diffusion followed by cleavage by a number of peptidases in the extracellular fluid. This allows a peptide to affect a number of neurons before it is finally degraded.

Vasoactive intestinal peptide (VIP) is one of many peptides that affect the function of the intestine through the enteric nervous system. It was originally described as a gut hormone that affected blood flow and fluid secretion, but it is now known to be an important enteric neuropeptide, inhibiting smooth muscle contraction. It also causes vasodilatation in several secretory glands, and potentiates stimulation by ACh.

Many neuropeptides belong to multigene families

The opioid peptides (receptors) provide a good example of a multigene family. They are the endogenous ligands for opiate analgesics such as morphine and codeine. The control of pain is complex, and opioid peptides and receptors are found both in the spinal cord and in the brain itself. There are at least three genes that code for these peptides, and each contains the sequences for several active molecules:

- **pro-opiomelanocortin** contains β-endorphin, which binds to opiate μ-receptors, and also adrenocorticotropic hormone (ACTH) and the melanocyte-stimulating hormones (MSH), which are pituitary hormones (see Chapter 37);
- **proenkephalin A** contains the sequences for Met- and Leu-enkephalins, which bind to δ-receptors and are involved in pain regulation at local levels in the brain and spinal cord;
- **prodynorphin** contains sequences for dynorphin and several other peptides, which bind to the κ class of receptors.

Opiates also affect pleasure pathways in the brain, which explains their euphoriant effects, and they also have side effects, such as respiratory depression, that limit their use. In excess, they cause contraction of the muscles of the eye, resulting in 'pinpoint' pupils. It has been shown that endorphins are released after strenuous exercise, giving the so-called 'jogger's high'. It is hoped that increased knowledge of the specific opioid receptors and neural opioid pathways will allow the development of analgesics with fewer side effects and less likelihood of abuse.

Substance P is another example of a member of a multigene family, known as the tachykinin family. It is present in afferent fibers of sensory nerves and transmits signals in response to pain. It is also involved in so-called neurogenic inflammation stimulated by nerve impulses, and is an important neurotransmitter in the intestine.

Neuropeptides can act as neuromodulators

Some peptides do act as true neurotransmitters, but they have many other actions in addition. They often alter the action of other transmitters, acting as neuromodulators but having no action of their own. For instance, VIP enhances the effect of ACh on salivary gland secretion in cat submandibular glands (glands located under the jawbone) by causing vasodilatation and potentiating the cholinergic component. NPY causes inhibition of the release of norepinephrine at autonomic nerve terminals, acting at presynaptic autoreceptors, and potentiates the action of norepinephrine in certain arteries while having only weak actions itself. Opioid peptides also are capable of modulating neurotransmitter release.

Summary

Neurons communicate at synapses by means of neurotransmitters. A large number of compounds, whether of low molecular weight, such as the biogenic amines, or larger peptides, can act as neurotransmitters. They act on specific receptors, and there is normally more than one receptor for each neurotransmitter. The presence of several transmitters in the same nerves and the identification of multiple receptors suggest that there is a high degree of flexibility and complexity in the signals that can be produced in the nervous system.

ACTIVE LEARNING

1. Does nitric oxide meet all the criteria to be defined as a true neurotransmitter?
2. Explain how a neurotransmitter such as serotonin can have so many diverse effects within the central nervous system.
3. Explain how neurotransmitters can be excitatory or inhibitory.
4. What neurotransmitter types are likely to become deficient in the brain of a patient with an inborn error of tetrahydrobiopterin metabolism?
5. Discuss the factors that need to considered when establishing a diagnostic method for disorders of dopamine and serotonin metabolism.
6. Explain the concept of ionotropic and metabotropic receptors.

Further reading

Clayton PT, Surtees RA, DeVile C, Hyland K, Heales SJ. Neonatal epileptic encephalopathy. *Lancet* 2003;**361**,1614.

Cooper JR, Bloom FE, Roth RH. *The biochemical basis of neuropharmacology*, 8th ed. Oxford: Oxford University Press; 2002.

Siegel GJ, Agranoff BW, Albers RW, Fisher SK, Uhler MD. *Basic Neurochemistry*, 6th ed. New York: Lippincott-Raven; 1998.

Stewart VC, Heales SJ. Nitric oxide-induced mitochondrial dysfunction: implications for neurodegeneration. *Free Radic Biol Med* 2003;**34**:287–303.

Relevant websites

http://www.indstate.edu/thcme/mwking/nerves.html
http://www.bh4.org

41. Cell Growth, Differentiation, and Cancer

M M Harnett and H S Goodridge

LEARNING OBJECTIVES

After reading this chapter you should be able to:

- Define the stages of the mammalian cell cycle.
- Describe how growth factors regulate cell proliferation.
- Outline the regulation of cell cycle progression by cyclins and cyclin-dependent kinases.
- Discuss the regulation of apoptosis by caspases and Bcl-2 family members.
- Explain how deregulation of growth control leads to the development of tumors.
- Distinguish between oncogenes and tumor suppressor genes, and describe the roles they play in tumor progression.

INTRODUCTION

In unicellular organisms such as bacteria, natural selection favors those cells that are most efficient at growing and dividing and, generally, proliferation is simply limited by the availability of nutrients. In contrast, in multicellular organisms such as human beings, there are elaborate controls on the proliferation of individual cell types to maintain the overall integrity of the organism both in terms of the number of individual cell types and also with respect to their spatial organization. Indeed, in adults, despite a plentiful supply of nutrients, the vast majority of cells are not dividing; furthermore, deregulation of growth control leads to the development of tumors and cancer. However, under certain conditions such as tissue repair and senescence, regulated growth and proliferation is promoted. Thus, as cells die, either by senescence or as a result of tissue damage, they must be replaced in a strictly regulated manner.

Cellular homeostasis maintains organ integrity through controlled cell survival, proliferation and cell death (by apoptosis) to ensure that normal cells, unlike cancerous (transformed) cells, generally stop dividing when they contact neighboring cells.

Much of what we now know about the control of normal cell growth and division has arisen from cancer research; analysis of the genetic alterations in cancer cells has revealed mutations in a large number of genes involved in the control of normal cell proliferation. These genes can be classified as proliferative or antiproliferative.

Mutated proliferative genes are called oncogenes (cancer-causing genes), the normal cellular counterparts of which are called proto-oncogenes

Proto-oncogenes are predominantly signal transducers that act to promote normal cell growth and division; aberrant regulation of these processes leads to cellular transformation.

In contrast, the antiproliferative genes or tumor suppressor genes normally act to suppress cell proliferation

Mutations that inactivate or lead to loss of expression of tumor suppressor genes therefore also lead to uncontrolled proliferation. Thus, whereas the mutant phenotype of tumor suppressor genes is usually recessive and generally requires loss or inactivation of both alleles for its expression, a mutation in only one allele of a proto-oncogene is required to bring about cell transformation (dominant mutant phenotype).

THE CELL CYCLE

Cells reproduce by duplicating their contents and then dividing in two; this is a closely regulated and complex process that is termed the cell cycle. In recent years a number of key control points in the cell cycle have been elucidated. In mammals, the duration of the cell cycle varies greatly from one cell type to another, ranging from minutes to years. However, cultured immortalized mammalian cells, which are studied in experimental systems, are, typically, relatively rapidly dividing cells with a cell cycle division time of approximately 24 hours.

Traditionally, the cell cycle is divided into several phases (Fig. 41.1). Mitosis (M-phase) is the stage of cell division; in most cells this takes only about an hour. The remainder of the cell cycle, during which cell growth and deoxyribonucleic acid (DNA) synthesis occur, is known as interphase. Replication of the nuclear DNA occurs during the synthesis (S) phase of interphase. The interval between the M- and S-phases is called the G1-phase, and the interval between the S- and M-phases is called G2. The G1- and G2-phases afford time, not only for cell growth, but also to provide checkpoints at which the progress of the cell cycle may be controlled, and

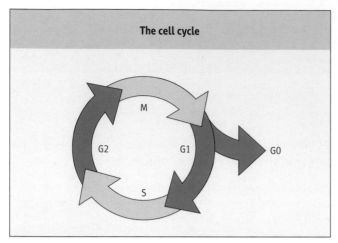

The cell cycle

Fig. 41.1 **The phases of the cell cycle.** The mitosis (M) phase is the stage of cell division, and takes about an hour in most cells. The G1, S, and G2 phases comprise the remaining interphase, during which cell growth and DNA synthesis occur. The restriction point is of significance in mitogenesis (see later in text). S, the synthesis phase of interphase, during which replication of nuclear DNA occurs; G1, the interval between M- and S-phases; G2, the interval between S- and M-phases.

the incorporation of DNA damage prevented, before cell division. As mentioned above, individual cell cycle times vary enormously and it is during G1-phase that most of this variability occurs. This is because cells in G1-phase, which are not committed to DNA replication, can enter a specialized resting state, called G0-phase, until they receive appropriate signals allowing them to progress further through the cell cycle. In mammals, the time required for a cell to progress from the beginning of S-phase through mitosis is typically 12–24 hours irrespective of the duration of the G1-phase. Thus, almost all the variation in proliferation rates between cell types is attributable to the amount of time spent in this G0/G1 state. Furthermore, in conditions that favor cell growth, the total ribonucleic acid (RNA) and protein content of the cell increases continuously, except in M-phase, when the chromosomes are too condensed to allow transcription.

GROWTH FACTORS

Regulation of cell proliferation

Cells of a multicellular organism have to receive specific positive signals in order to grow and divide. Many of these signals are in the form of polypeptide hormones (e.g. insulin), growth factors (e.g. platelet-derived growth factor, PDGF) or cytokines (e.g. interleukins, designated IL-1 to IL-29). These growth factors bind to specific cell–surface receptors and initiate intracellular signaling cascades that ultimately act to counter those negative controls in resting cells that prevent growth and block cell cycle progression. Proliferation of most cell types generally requires signaling via a specific combina-

tion of growth factors, rather than stimulation by a single growth factor; thus a relatively small number of growth factors can selectively regulate the proliferation of many cell types. Moreover, although most factors that stimulate cell growth also stimulate cell proliferation, some factors will induce cell growth but not division. This reflects the reality that, within an organism, individual cell types vary enormously in size. Indeed, some cells, such as neurons (in the G0-phase), grow very large without ever dividing. Furthermore, although proliferating cells stop growing when they are deprived of growth factors, they continue to progress through the cell cycle until they reach the point in the G1-phase at which they can enter the G0-phase or resting state.

Growth factors bind to specific cell-surface receptors, which are generally transmembrane proteins with cytoplasmic protein tyrosine kinase domains (see also chapter 38). There are now about 50 known growth factors; PDGF was one of the first to be identified. The growth and proliferative responses to PDGF have proved to be prototypic of many other growth factors and include:

- **immediate increase in intracellular Ca²⁺**, indicative of initiation of transmembrane signaling (see Chapter 38);
- **reorganization of actin stress fibers**, which is necessary for the anchorage-dependence of cell attachment that is required for cell cycle progression;
- **activation, nuclear translocation, or both, of transcription factors** (see Chapter 33) that bind to regulatory regions of the DNA of genes that are responsive to the particular growth factor. These transcription factors regulate the transcription of early response genes, which often encode additional transcription factors that are necessary for the induction of components of the cell cycle machinery such as cyclin proteins and, ultimately:
- **DNA synthesis and cell division**.

Growth factors activate distinct combinations of signal transducers (see Chapter 38) and transcription factors to dictate the precise repertoire of genes that is induced, thereby enabling the initiation of characteristic differential classes of responses.

Growth factor binding generally induces receptor dimerization and activation of the tyrosine kinase intrinsic to the receptor, causing phosphorylation of the dimerized receptor at specific sites on its cytoplasmic domains (transphosphorylation; Fig. 41.2). This tyrosine phosphorylation of the receptor creates 'docking sites' that allow protein-protein interactions, leading to recruitment and activation of signaling enzymes or 'adapter molecules', which are signal transducers that serve as enzyme modulators for signaling enzymes. Transphosphorylation of receptor cytoplasmic domains thus allows recruitment and activation of a scaffold

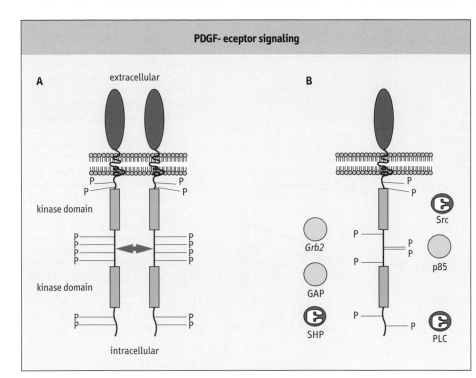

Fig. 41.2 **Recruitment of the downstream signaling element scaffold to the activated PDGF receptor.** Growth factor ligation of the receptor induces dimerization and activation of the tyrosine kinase intrinsic to the receptor cytoplasmic domains, leading to tyrosine phosphorylation (transphosphorylation, P) of the dimerized receptor at specific sites on the cytoplasmic domains (A). Docking sites thus created (B) enable protein-protein interactions that lead to recruitment and activation of downstream signaling enzymes, for example phospholipase C (PLC), GTPase-activating protein (GAP), protein tyrosine kinases (PTKs) such as *Src*, phosphotyrosine phosphatases such as SHP (SH2 domain-containing phosphatase), and adapter molecules such as Grb2 (which recruits Ras).

THE ROLE OF PROTEIN TYROSINE KINASES IN SIGNAL TRANSDUCTION

Protein tyrosine kinase (PTK)-dependent interactions in cell signaling

PTKs are enzymes that transfer the γ-phosphate group of ATP to tyrosine residues on target substrate proteins. The term 'protein tyrosine kinase' is a generic term for a large superfamily of enzymes comprising both transmembrane-spanning receptors with an intrinsic tyrosine kinase activity in their cytoplasmic domains and a wide range of subfamilies of cytoplasmic tyrosine kinases such as the *Src*, *Abl* or Janus kinase (JAK) families. Tyrosine phosphorylation, which is a covalent modification of proteins, provides a rapid and reversible (by the action of protein tyrosine phosphatases) mechanism of modifying the enzymic activity of target proteins. In addition, it can modify their ability to act as adapter molecules to recruit other signaling molecules to the protein networks involved in transmembrane cell signaling. For example, the tyrosine phosphorylation of receptors or signaling molecules creates 'docking sites' that allow protein-protein interactions leading to recruitment of downstream signal transducers. Signal transducers are recruited to these phosphorylated tyrosines by virtue of protein-protein interaction domains, called SH2 domains, contained within the sequence of many signal transducers. SH2 stands for *Src*-homology region 2, from the cytoplasmic *Src* tyrosine kinase, a signal transducing element in which this protein domain was first characterized. SH2 domains comprise approximately 100 amino acids and specifically recognize a phosphotyrosine plus the three amino acids immediately C-terminal to that phosphotyrosine.

of signal transduction elements (see Fig. 41.2) such as phospholipase C-γ (PLC-γ), GTPase-activating protein (GAP), protein tyrosine kinases (PTKs) such as *Src*, *Fyn* and *Abl*, phosphotyrosine phosphatases (PTPases) and adapter molecules such as *Shc* or *Grb2*, which we will discuss in more detail below.

PDGF-receptor signaling

PDGF signals through the phosphatidylinositol and Ras-MAPK cascades

Ligation of the PDGF-receptor (PDGF-R) leads to the recruitment and activation of phospholipase C-γ (PLC-γ), which catalyzes the hydrolysis of phosphatidylinositol 4,5-bisphosphate (PIP$_2$) to generate the intracellular second messengers, inositol 1,4,5-trisphosphate (IP$_3$) and diacylglycerol (DAG) (see Chapter 38). IP$_3$ stimulates release of Ca^{2+} from intracellular stores and DAG activates an important signal transducer family, protein kinase C (PKC). Ligation of the PDGF-R also leads to recruitment of another lipid signaling enzyme, phosphoinositide-3-kinase (PI-3-kinase). This enzyme phosphorylates PIP$_2$ yielding the lipid second messenger, phosphatidylinositol 3,4,5-trisphosphate (PIP$_3$), which can also activate certain members of the PKC family. In addition, PIP$_3$ can activate another kinase called PIP$_3$-dependent kinase.

Thirty percent of all tumors have constitutively active mutants of a signaling element called *Ras*, which acts as a molecular switch for a key signal transduction pathway in the control of growth and differentiation.

Ras is a GTPase, which cycles between an inactive *Ras*-GDP form and an active *Ras*-GTP form (Fig. 41.3). GTP/GDP

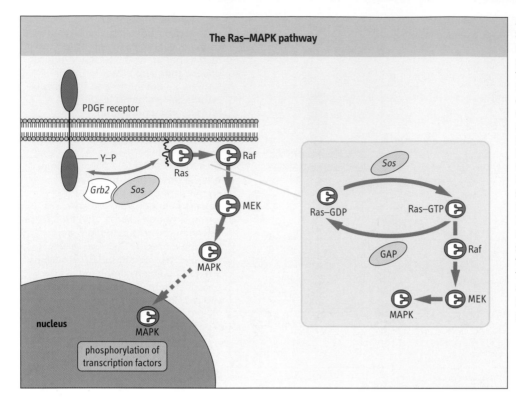

Fig. 41.3 **Recruitment and activation of Ras by the PDGF receptor.** Ras is anchored in the plasma membrane and recruited to the activated PDGF-R via interaction with the Grb2—Sos complex. Receptor-stimulated GTP/GDP exchange, and hence activation of Ras, is promoted by Sos, whereas GAP inactivates Ras by stimulating its intrinsic GTPase activity. Ras couples the PDGF-R to MAPK activation via stimulation of the intermediary kinases, Raf and MEK kinase. MAPK translocates to the nucleus and phosphorylates (on serine and threonine) key transcription factors involved in the regulation of DNA synthesis and cell division.
MAPK: mitogen-activated protein kinase

exchange is promoted by a guanine nucleotide exchange factor, called *Sos*, and the GTPase-activating protein (GAP) inactivates *Ras* by stimulating its intrinsic GTPase activity (as does the intrinsic GTPase of the α-subunit of heterotrimeric G-proteins; see Chapter 38). *Ras* is constitutively targeted to the plasma membrane by a post-translational modification involving the addition of a lipophilic farnesyl group (Chapter 16) and is then recruited to the activated PDGF-R by interaction with an adapter protein called *Grb2*.

One of the main effector functions of *Ras* is to regulate the mitogen-activated protein kinase (MAPK) cascade. MAPK is a serine–threonine kinase that is itself activated by phosphorylation by a dual specificity (tyrosine/threonine) MAPK kinase called MEK. MAPK has two major isoforms, extracellular regulated kinases (ERK) 1 and 2, which translocate to the nucleus and phosphorylate (on serine and threonine) key transcription factors involved in the regulation of DNA synthesis and cell division.

Cytokine receptor signaling

Cytokines are growth factors that specifically act to orchestrate the development of hemopoietic cells and the immune response

However, they can also have multiple effects on non-hemopoietic cell types (see Chapter 36). In common with growth

X-SCID: INTERLEUKIN COMMON γ-CHAIN DEFICIENCY

X-linked severe combined immunodeficiency (X-SCID) is a disorder causing very severe immunodeficiency. It is characterized by profoundly defective cellular and humoral immunity resulting in greatly increased susceptibility to infection, and is uniformly fatal by the time the patient is 1–2 years of age unless treated by bone-marrow transplantation. X-SCID males typically have profoundly defective cell-mediated and humoral immunity, with low numbers of T cells, or none at all, but normal numbers of B cells.

Comment. The gene responsible for X-SCID was initially reported to code for the γ-chain of the IL-2 receptor. The extracellular domain of this γ-chain has been implicated in the high-affinity binding of IL-2 to its receptor and its intracellular domain associates with the signal transducer, JAK3, leading to gene induction, and cell growth and proliferation. However, the recent finding that the γ-chain is shared with the receptors for IL-4, IL-7, IL-9, IL-13, and IL-15 suggests that the severe immunodeficiency in X-SCID must be due to the patient's inability to respond to a number of or all these cytokines. (See also Chapter 36.)

SIGNALING CASCADES

Mitogen-activated protein kinase (MAPK) signaling cascades

The MAPK cascade was originally elucidated by genetic studies in yeast, but the pathway has proved to be evolutionarily very highly conserved from yeast to mammals, allowing the mammalian elements to be identified by homology cloning. It has emerged in recent years that MAPKs are key components of an interacting network of sequential protein kinase cascades (MAPK cassettes) that serve to link early receptor-transduced signals with growth and differentiation-related transcriptional events in the nucleus. 'MAPK' is the generic name for a superfamily of signal transducing kinases that, to date, encompasses three major subfamilies, termed the extracellular regulated kinase (ERK; e.g. *p44*ERK1 and *p42*ERK2), stress activated protein kinase (SAPK) or *Jun* N-terminal kinase (JNK), and *p38*-reactivating kinase (*p38*RK) MAPK cassettes. These MAPK cassettes can phosphorylate transcription factors implicated in immediate early gene induction, such as AP-1 (*Jun* and *Fos*), ELK-1, and SAP1. Furthermore, whereas activation of the SAPKs and *p38*RKs can selectively induce apoptosis, under certain conditions, ERK1 and ERK2 generally act to promote cell survival and proliferation.

ATAXIA TELANGIECTASIA

Ataxia telangiectasia is a rare autosomal recessive disease caused by mutations in the ataxia telangiectasia-mutated (*ATM*) gene. Symptoms and signs include an unsteady gait, telangiectasia, skin pigmentation, infertility, immune deficiencies, and an increased incidence of cancer, especially lymphoreticular tumors.

Comment. ATM belongs to a protein kinase family that regulates the induction of DNA damage responses in reaction to ionizing radiation, anticancer treatment, or programmed DNA breaks during meiosis. Patients with ataxia telangiectasia show a large increase in cancer susceptibility and increased sensitivity to ionizing radiation. Ataxia telangiectasia cells show chromosomal instability, hypersensitivity to reagents that induce DNA-strand breaks, and defects in the G1/G2-phases, and altered regulation of the expression of *p53* and *p21* WAF1. *ATM* protein is constitutively expressed during the cell cycle and has been assigned a checkpoint function in monitoring DNA damage and determining whether *p53*-mediated growth arrest and DNA repair or *p53*-dependent apoptosis occurs in response to severe DNA damage. In ataxia telangiectasia, cells with mutated *ATM* fail to adequately activate *p53*, and hence to induce growth arrest or apoptosis in response to ionizing radiation. Moreover, when *p53* is also mutated, the cell cycle is deregulated and the risk of tumor formation is enhanced as a result of the accumulation of mutations.

factors, they mediate their effects via specific cell-surface receptors; although there are several major classes of receptors, most cytokine receptors belong to the receptor superfamily called the hemopoietic receptors. These receptors are transmembrane glycoprotein receptors characterized by their conserved extracellular domains, which contain characteristic cysteine pairs and a pentapeptide WSXWS (tryptophan-serine–any–tryptophan-serine) motif. The receptors have no intrinsic catalytic activity, and many are multisubunit receptors, although not all of the chains necessarily belong to this receptor superfamily. These multisubunit receptors are generally characterized by a unique ligand-binding subunit that confers specificity, and a common signal transducer subunit that is often shared by several related cytokines and is the basis of the subdivison of the receptors into a number of distinct subfamilies. The sharing of common signal transducer subunits serves to explain the severe immunodeficiencies that result from naturally arising defects in these receptors.

As stated above, the hemopoietic receptors express no intrinsic catalytic activity; however, after ligation, these receptors stimulate tyrosine kinase activity and most cytokines, in common with the classical growth factors, signal through PLC, PI-3-K, and *Ras*-MAPK pathways (Fig. 41.4). However, a family of cytosolic protein tyrosine kinases (PTKs) has a crucial role in hemopoietic receptor signaling;

these kinases, called Janus kinases (JAKs), couple hemopoietic receptors to a novel transduction pathway that provides a direct link between receptor activation and gene transcription. Like the *Src* kinases, the JAKs are cytosolic tyrosine kinases. They associate with the hemopoietic receptors at conserved regions near the transmembrane domain and are activated and phosphorylated after cytokine binding and oligomerization of hemopoietic receptors.

The major breakthrough in identifying the role of these kinases was obtained when the downstream targets of JAKs were identified as transcription factors called signal transducers and activators of transcription (STATs). STATs are found in a monomeric latent form in the cytoplasm of unstimulated cells. Cytokine stimulation leads to JAK-mediated phosphorylation and dimerization of STATs. STATs translocate to the nucleus, where they bind specific DNA sequences in the promoters of target genes and thus directly modulate gene induction (see Fig. 41.4). Recently, growth factors such as epidermal growth factor (EGF) and PDGF have also been shown to activate JAK/STAT pathways; thus this novel signaling cascade may provide a universal mechanism by which growth factors mediate gene induction and cellular responses.

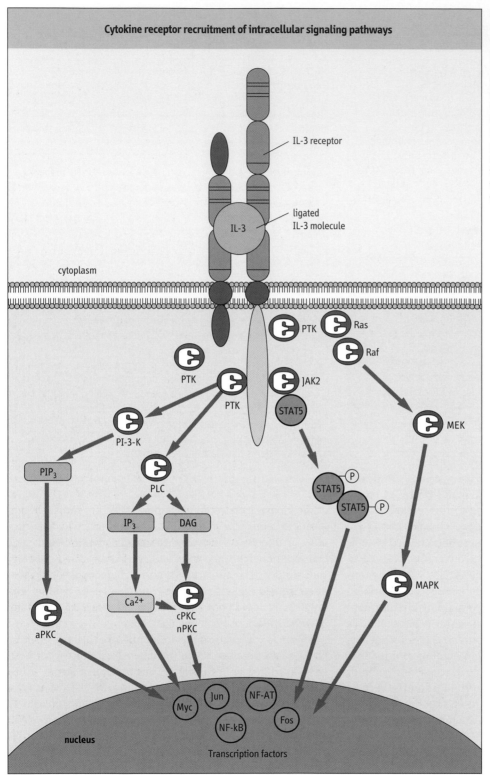

Cytokine receptor recruitment of intracellular signaling pathways

Fig. 41.4 **Cytokine receptor recruitment of JAK, STAT, and other intracellular signaling pathways.** *Fos*, *Jun*, *Myc*, NF-kB, NF-AT transcription factors; GAS, gamma activation sequence; PKC: protein kinase C. cPKC, nPKC, aPKC: classical, novel, and atypical forms of protein kinase C (PKC); PLC, phospholipidase C; DAG, diacylglycerol; PIP_3, inositol-3,4,5-trisphosphate; IP_3, inositol-1,4,5-trisphosphate; PTK, protein tyrosine kinase; JAK, janus kinase.

REGULATION OF THE CELL CYCLE

Growth factor stimulation results in the induction of proteins involved in regulating the cell cycle, such as the cyclin-dependent kinases (CDKs) and cyclins.

Cyclins were originally defined as proteins that were specifically degraded at every mitosis

CDKs are kinases that must to bind to a cyclin in order to be active. This cyclin-dependent activation of CDKs regulates key steps in cell cycle progression (Fig. 41.5).

The activity of the cyclins is modulated by changes in their levels of expression at both the mRNA and the protein level (transcriptional and translational control). In contrast, the CDKs are expressed in relatively constant amounts and their activities are modulated by their phosphorylation status. Moreover, a further level of control has been revealed by the recent identification of CDK inhibitors (CDKIs), which bind CDKs and act as inhibitory subunits to block their catalytic activity.

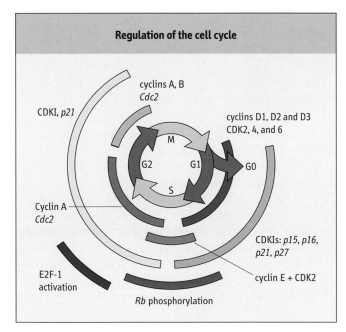

Fig. 41.5 **Regulation of the cell cycle.** Stimulation of growth factors leads to cyclin-dependent activation of the regulation of key steps in the cell cycle by CDKs and their inhibitors. The cyclins and their respective CDK partners acting at the different stages of cell cycle progression are shown. CDK, cyclin-dependent kinase; CDKI, CDK inhibitor; E2F-1, a transcription factor; *Rb*, retinoblastoma protein.

Mitogenesis

Mitogenic growth factors exert their effects between the onset of G1-phase and a point in late G1-phase called the restriction point

Once the cell has passed through the restriction point, the remaining phases of the cell cycle through to M-phase are virtually unaffected by extracellular signals and are committed to progress rather than to quiesce. The retinoblastoma protein, *Rb*, controls the expression of genes that commit cells that are at the restriction point late in G1-phase to enter S-phase (DNA synthesis phase) of the cell cycle. Thus, in early G1-phase, hypophosphorylated *Rb* represses advance of the cell cycle by binding to, and preventing the DNA-binding activity of, a family of transcription factors, called *E2F*, which have key roles in the G1/S-phase transition. In contrast, close to the restriction point, growth factor stimulation induces the cyclin D-CDK4 and 6 complexes and then the cyclin E-CDK2 complex to hyperphosphorylate *Rb*. The resulting release of inhibition of *E2F* allows activation of genes, the products of which are important for entry into S-phase (see Fig. 41.5).

Monitoring for DNA damage

The tumor suppressor protein, *p53*, is a predominantly DNA-damage-sensing protein by which the cell monitors DNA damage throughout the cell cycle. It can halt cell cycle progression to allow DNA repair, by induction of the *p21* CDKI, (WAF1), which prevents the CDK-dependent phosphorylation and inactivation of *Rb*. As WAF1 can affect a variety of cyclin-CDK complexes, it appears that growth arrest can occur at any point in the cell cycle. However, although minimal repairable damage induces *p53*-mediated growth arrest to allow DNA repair and avoid accumulation of mutations by preventing replication of the damaged DNA in the S-phase, serious, irreparable damage triggers *p53*-dependent programmed cell death by apoptosis.

The link between growth factor receptor signaling and cell cycle progression can be seen by examining two important examples. First, the growth factor, transforming growth factor – β (TGF-β), which negatively regulates growth in many cell types, mediates many of its effects by inhibition of the cyclin D-CDK4 and 6 complexes that promote cell cycle progression. Indeed, in some tumors, transformation appears to result from deletion or functional inactivation of TGF-β receptors or associated downstream signal-transducing elements. Second, the key signaling element, *Ras*, which has been found to be mutated to a constitutively activated form in approximately 30% of all tumors, similarly appears to exert many, if not all, of its effects ultimately by upregulating concentrations of cyclin D and, hence, by stimulating cell cycle progression. This upregulation of cyclin D expression results from stimulation of the MAPK cascade by *Ras* and the induction of the transcription factor, AP-1, which regulates induction of cyclin D expression (Fig. 41.6).

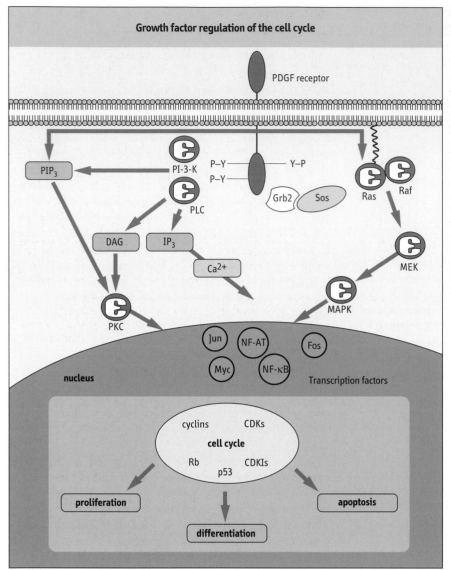

Growth factor regulation of the cell cycle

Fig. 41.6 **Growth factor regulation of the cell cycle.** Growth factor signals generated at the plasma membrane can transduce gene induction, cell cycle progression, and proliferation, differentiation, or apoptosis. Growth factor receptor signaling leads to activation of transcription factors such *Jun* and *Fos* (which dimerize to form AP-1), *Myc*, NF-AT, and NF-κB. These regulate the induction of components of the cell cycle machinery that monitor and direct cell cycle progression, cell growth arrest and cell differentiation. Induction of DNA damage that would result in the accumulation of mutations leads to cell cycle arrest and DNA repair. Alternatively if the DNA damage is too great, cell death occurs by apoptosis. DAG, diacylglycerol; IP$_3$, inositol-1,4,5-trisphosphate; PI-3K, phosphoinositide-3-kinase; PIP$_3$, inositol-3,4,5-trisphosphate; PKC, protein kinase C; PLC, phospholipidase C.

APOPTOSIS

Apoptosis, a form of programmed cell death, occurs during normal cellular development

It is a fundamentally important biological process that is required to maintain the integrity and homeostasis of multicellular organisms. Whereas inappropriate apoptosis can lead to degenerative conditions, such as neurodegenerative disorders, subversion and disruption of the apoptosis machinery can result in cancer (Table 41.1) or autoimmune disease. Cells that die from damage typically swell and burst (necrosis), but apoptosis is characterized by dramatic morphologic changes in the cell, including shrinkage, chromatin condensation, cleavage, and disassembly into membrane-enclosed vesicles called apoptotic bodies that undergo rapid phagocytosis by neighboring cells. It is the accumulation of sterols in

the plasma membrane and translocation of phosphatidylserine to the outer leaflet of the plasma membrane that serve to flag the apoptotic cell for elimination via phagocytosis by neighboring cells or macrophages.

Recent research has elucidated many of the biochemical signals that regulate apoptosis, and has identified two key families of proteins that appear to be central to the regulation of mammalian cell death by apoptosis. These are the family of cysteine proteases called caspases, and the B cell lymphoma protein 2 (*Bcl-2*)-related family members, which serve to modulate cell survival by regulating caspase activity.

Caspases

Caspases are involved in apoptosis

The caspases act by cleaving key target proteins, resulting in the systematic disassembly of the apoptotic cell by:

Cancer and the cell cycle

Cancer	Cell cycle element	Outcome: status of the retinoblastoma protein (Rb)
breast cancer, leukemia testicular carcinomas breast tumors	cyclin expression increased as a result of gene amplification or chromosomal translocation cyclin D1 cyclin D2 cyclin E	hyperphosphorylation and inactivation of retinoblastoma protein (Rb), leading to deregulated malignant cell proliferation
retinoblastomas small-cell lung carcinomas osteosarcomas	mutational inactivation of Rb genes	loss of Rb control of cell cycle, leading to deregulated malignant cell proliferation
cervical carcinomas	sequestration of Rb by the human papilloma virus E7 protein	loss of Rb control of cell cycle
variety of tumor cells	deletion of CDKI genes, $p14$, $p15$	loss of inhibition of cyclin D-CDK4/6 complexes, resulting in inappropriate hyperphosphorylation and inactivation of Rb
melanomas	mutant CDK4 demonstrating resistance to CDKI gene products, $p14$, $p15$	loss of inhibition of cyclin D-CDK4/6 complexes, resulting in loss of Rb control of cell cycle

Table 41.1 **Relationship between various cancers and stages of the cell cycle.** Some degree of disruption of the cell cycle machinery is likely to occur in every type of cancer cell (Table 41.2). As most proliferative decisions are made at the restriction point in late G1-phase, the key target for cellular transformation appears to be the retinoblastoma protein, *Rb*. Indeed, it is now clear that the signal transduction events leading to *Rb* phosphorylation and functional inactivation are disrupted in many cancer cells, suggesting that *Rb* inactivation may be crucial to deregulated, malignant cell proliferation.

 # APOPTOSIS

Disruption of the apoptotic machinery in B cell leukemias

During lymphopoiesis, B (75%) and T (95%) cell progenitors that fail to rearrange their antigen receptor genes in a productive, non-self manner are programmed to die by apoptosis. The finding that the cell survival gene, *Bcl-2*, was subject to a chromosomal translocation in human follicular lymphomas suggested that subversion of apoptotic pathways may have a key role in malignant transformation. Thus, by deregulating the key antiapoptotic protein, *Bcl-2*, this translocation promotes the survival of cells that would otherwise die, and which then acquire the additional mutations required for malignant transformation.

Bcl-2 has now been shown to belong to a family of proteins that modulate caspase activity and hence are intimately involved in the regulation of selection of the alternative pathways of cell survival or apoptosis. Thus, whereas family members such as *Bcl-2* and *Bcl-x$_L$* inhibit apoptosis, their cell survival activities can be antagonized by *Bcl-x$_S$* (a lower-molecular-weight splice variant of *Bcl-x$_L$*), Bak, Bax, and Bad. The antagonistic actions of these proteins can be illustrated by studies showing that, whereas loss of Bax promotes tumor formation in mice, overexpression of Bax can suppress cellular transformation *in vitro*. Similarly, a number of viruses (e.g. adenovirus, Epstein–Barr virus, African swine fever virus, herpes virus Saimiri, and human herpes virus 8) enhance their replication by encoding viral homologs of *Bcl-2* to promote survival of the host cell. Finally, the tumor suppressor, *p53*, appears to activate apoptosis, at least in part, by downregulating the expression of *Bcl-2* and upregulating that of Bax; this provides an additional rationale for *p53* being the most commonly mutated gene in human cancer.

- **halting cell cycle progression;**
- **disabling homeostatic and repair mechanisms;**
- **initiating the detachment of the cell** from its surrounding tissue structures;
- **dismantling structural components** such as the cytoskeleton;
- **flagging the dying cell for phagocytosis.**

Overexpression of active caspases is sufficient to cause cellular apoptosis.

Caspases are expressed as inactive procaspases, and it is likely that caspase activation occurs in a cascade fashion, with the initial activation of a regulatory caspase serving to activate downstream effector caspases by proteolysis. Cell death

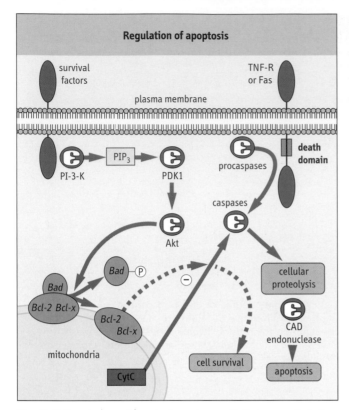

Fig. 41.7 **Regulation of apotosis and growth factor-mediated cell rescue.** Cell death receptors, such as TNF receptor (TNF-R) or *Fas*, recruit procaspases such as caspase 8 to their 'death domain' transducing molecules (FADD, TRADD, RIP, and RAIDD), thereby inducing the proteolytic caspase activation cascade of apoptotic cell death. In contrast, the *Bcl-2* family-regulated cascade may be modulated by survival factors coupled to phosphoinositide-3-kinase (PI-3-K), leading to rescue of cells from apoptosis and promotion of cell survival. PI-3-K catalyses the production of phosphatidylinositol 3,4,5-trisphosphate (PIP₃), which stimulates a PIP₃-dependent kinase (PDK), resulting in phosphorylation and activation of the protein kinase, *Akt*. In turn, *Akt* phosphorylates the proapoptotic *Bcl-2* family member, Bad, inducing dissociation of Bad from heterodimeric complexes with *Bcl-2* or *Bcl-x*$_L$ and allowing *Bcl-2/Bcl-x*$_L$ to antagonize cell death by preventing release of cytochrome c (Cyt c) and caspase activation. CAD, caspase-dependent endonuclase.

ANALYSIS OF CELL CYCLE PROGRESSION AND APOPTOTIC CELLS

The DNA content of cells varies through the cell cycle, increasing during S phase from diploid chromosomal DNA in G0/G1 to tetraploid at G2/M, before returning to diploid again after M phase. Furthermore, subdiploid DNA content is an indicator of apoptosis. The cell cycle status of cells can therefore be assessed in the laboratory by measuring DNA content. Flow cytometry, which measures the fluorescence of individual cells, can be combined with a variety of fluorescent staining techniques to assess the proportions of cells in a population that are at the different stages of the cell cycle or undergoing apoptosis.

For example, staining with propidium iodide (PI), which intercalates into the DNA helix, measures the total DNA content of cells; 4'-6'-diamidino-phenylindole-2HCl (DAPI) works in a similar manner by preferentially binding to A–T base pairs. Incorporation of bromodeoxyuridine (*BrdU*), an analog of the DNA precursor thymidine, into the newly synthesised DNA of cells progressing through S phase can also be detected by flow cytometry using anti-*BrdU* antibodies conjugated to fluorescent dyes.

Non-fluorescent carboxy-fluoresceindiacetate succinimidyl ester (CFDA SE), which is converted to fluorescent CFSE by the action of cytoplasmic esterases, is a very effective reagent for studying the division of proliferating cells. When CFSE-stained cells divide, CFSE is uniformly distributed between daughter cells; each division reduces the CFSE fluorescence intensity of daughter cells by approximately half. Flow cytometric analysis therefore reveals discrete frequency distributions of cells with progressively reduced fluorescence levels (histogram peaks), representing successive generations of cells (Fig. 41.8).

Multi-color staining using fluorescent dyes with different emission spectra can also be performed to yield extra information about cell subpopulations. For example, antibodies against cell-specific markers conjugated to other fluorescent dyes can be employed to establish whether an agent causes all cells or an individual cell type within a mixed cell population to proceed through the cell cycle, arrest in G0 phase, or undergo apoptosis.

receptors, such as tumor necrosis factor (TNF)-R and *Fas* (also known as CD95 or APO-1), mediate apoptotic cell death pathways in a number of cell types but particularly in cells of the immune system. They initiate apoptosis by directly recruiting procaspases, such as caspase 8, to their accessory 'death domain' transducing molecules thereby inducing the proteolytic caspase activation cascade (Fig. 41.7). These death domain molecules include *Fas*-associated death domain protein (FADD), TNF-receptor associated death domain protein (TRADD), receptor interacting protein (RIP), and RIP-associated ICE-like protease with a death domain (RAIDD). The precise molecular mechanisms of effector caspase activation are as yet unknown. However, it has recently

emerged that proteolysis and activation of effector caspases is facilitated by binding to cytochrome c, which is released from the mitochondria during the process of apoptosis.

The *Bcl-2* gene family

Bcl-2 is a key antiapoptotic protein

The *Bcl-2* gene family comprises structurally related proteins that form homo- or heterodimers and act either to

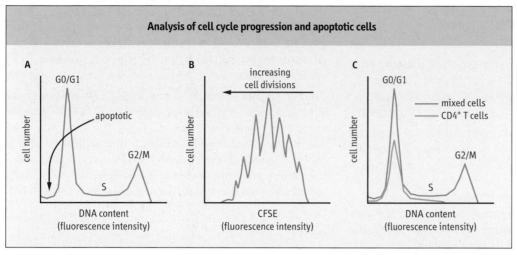

Fig. 41.8 **Analysis of cell cycle progression and apoptotic cells.** (A) Measurement of DNA content in PI- or DAPI-stained cells by flow cytometry allows assessment of the cell cycle status of individual cells in a population. Tetraploid = G2/M, diploid = G0/G1, intermediate = S phase; subdiploid DNA content indicates cells undergoing apoptosis. (B) When CFSE-stained cells divide, CFSE is shared equally between daughter cells, reducing the fluorescence intensity of daughter cells by half with each division. Flow cytometry reveals discrete cell subpopulations representing successive generations of cells. (C) Surface staining of cells with a fluorescent antibody specific for the T helper cell marker CD4 suggests that CD4⁺ T cells in this mixed population of cells are arrested in G0.

GENETIC MUTATIONS UNDERLYING DEVELOPMENT OF A COLORECTAL CANCER

Screening of colorectal cancer cells with DNA probes specific for known proto-oncogenes and tumor suppressor genes showed that 50% of these tumors had an activating point mutation in a *Ras* oncogene, and 75% of these cancers had an inactivating mutation in *p53*. Moreover, studies of familial adenomatous polyposis (FAP; see below) have shown that more than 70% of colon cancers have a mutation in the adenomatous polyposis coli (APC) gene. Indeed, it now seems clear that mutations inactivating APC may represent an early stage in the development of a colon cancer cell, because APC mutations can be detected at the same frequency in small benign polyps as in large malignant tumors. These APC mutations appear to promote the transformation of normal epithelium through a stage of hyperproliferative epithelium to early adenoma. The next stage seems to involve the activating mutation of *Ras* (rarely found in small polyps, but common in large polyps), which induces changes in cell differentiation typical of cell transformation (intermediate adenoma) and which allow the cells to grow in an anchorage-independent manner in culture. These changes are followed by a mutation in a tumor suppressor gene called 'deleted in colon carcinoma' (DCC), to generate a late adenoma that is converted to an adenocarcinoma by the subsequent loss of *p53*. Loss of the DNA-damage sensing function of *p53* allows the cells to accumulate, at a rapid rate, the further mutations required for metastasis.

Comment. Although these mutations appear to be the rate-limiting steps in a large number of colorectal cancers, it should be noted that other sequences of mutations can also generate this disease. Indeed, in about 15% of cases, patients with a hereditary syndrome called hereditary nonpolyposis colorectal cancer (HNPCC) have a mutation of the HNPCC gene that normally acts to repair mismatches in the nucleotide sequences of the DNA double helix. Thus, in such patients, the likelihood of the development of colorectal cancer is enhanced, as the HNPCC mutation decreases the fidelity of DNA replication and hence increases the tendency of the cells to undergo mutation.

promote or to antagonize apoptosis by modulating caspase activation.

Bcl-2 was initially discovered as a chromosomal transloca-tion in a follicular B cell lymphoma, which was found to con-tribute to neoplastic growth by inhibiting normal B cell apoptosis. The molecular mechanisms underlying *Bcl-2-* mediated survival signals are as yet poorly defined, but it appears that *Bcl-2*, which is located on the outer mitochon-drial membrane, may act by preventing leakage of cytochrome C from the mitochondria and, hence, activation of effector caspases (see Fig. 41.7).

CANCER

Cells that undergo mutation(s) that disrupt the regulation of cell division will divide without regard to the overall needs of the organism and become apparent as a tumor or neoplasm

As long as the neoplastic cells remain as an intact tumor, the tumor is said to be benign, and can be removed surgically. However, if further mutations allow such tumor cells to invade and colonize other tissues, creating widespread secondary tumors or metastases, the tumor is described as malignant, and classified as a cancer. Each cancer is derived from a single cell that has undergone some heritable mutation that allows it to outgrow its surrounding cells: by the time they are first detected, tumors typically contain a billion cells. Cancers are classified according to the tissue and cell type that they are derived from: those from epithelial cells are carcinomas, those from connective tissue or muscle cells are termed sarcomas, and those from the hemopoietic system are called leukemias. About 90% of human cancers are carcinomas, the five most common being those of the lung, stomach, breast, colon/rectum, and uterine cervix.

A single mutation is not sufficient to convert a healthy cell to a cancer cell; several rare mutations have to occur together

Mutations in DNA occur spontaneously at a rate of 10^{-6} mutations per gene per cell division (even more in the presence of mutagens). Thus, since approximately 10^{16} cell divisions occur in the human body over an average lifetime, every human gene is likely to undergo mutation on about 10^{10} occasions. Clearly then, a single mutation is not sufficient to convert a healthy cell to a cancer cell; several rare mutations have to occur together, as demonstrated by epidemiologic studies showing that, for any given cancer, the incidence increases exponentially with age. Indeed, it has been estimated that three to seven independent mutations are usually required, leukemias apparently needing the fewest mutations and carcinomas the most.

Tumor progression can be observed when initial minor disruptions of cell regulation escalate into a full cancer. For example, chronic myelogeneous leukemia (CML) is initially characterized by the overproduction of white blood cells, as a result of chromosomal translocation. This chronic stage of the disease remains stable for several years before transforming into the acute, rapidly progressing phase of the disease, in which the cells have accumulated several other mutations that cause them to proliferate more rapidly. Alternatively, mutations may have arisen such that committed progenitors of the cells continue to divide indefinitely, rather than terminally differentiating and dying after a strictly regulated number of cell divisions as happens to their normal counterparts.

Mutations that block the normal development of cells towards an end-differentiated, non-dividing cell, or a cell that would normally be programmed to die by apoptosis, have been shown to play an essential part in many cancers

Thus drugs that promote cell maturation may turn out to be at least as useful as those targeted to prevent cell proliferation (cytotoxic drugs).

In order to metastasize, cells in a tumor must be able to escape their adhesion to neighboring cells, invade surrounding tissues, enter the blood or lymph systems, and, finally, invade and colonize a new tissue. The mechanisms involved

THE PAPANICOLAOU OR 'PAP SMEAR' TEST OF THE UTERINE CERVIX

The epithelium of the uterine cervix resembles the epidermis of the skin, and comprises a proliferating basal layer that generates cells that differentiate into flat, keratin-rich cells that are eventually shed from the surface. Cancers of the uterine cervix are strongly associated with infection by human papilloma virus types 16 and 18 and arise from mutations in the basal epithelial cells, which are no longer then confined to the basal layer but invade the area normally occupied by the differentiated keratin-rich cells (dysplasia). These proliferating cells are shed at a less mature stage of differentiation than normal. Whereas the differentiated cells are characterized by their large size and highly condensed nuclei, the mutant cells have relatively large nuclei and little cytoplasm so that dysplasia can be identified in the Pap smear test, which simply involves microscopic examination of the morphology of a sample of cells scraped from the cervix. Dysplasia often remains stable or even spontaneously regresses. However, it may progress to a more serious lesion, called carcinoma *in situ*, in which the epithelium is entirely made up of undifferentiated proliferating cells with nuclei of variable size and shape. This lesion can be completely cured by surgery; however, in 20–30% of cases carcinoma *in situ* progresses over several years into a malignant cervical carcinoma.

Comment. Abnormal nuclear morphology is a key diagnostic tool of pathologists for identifying cancer, and correlates with the destabilization of karyotypes of cancer cells when they are cultured. These unstable karyotypes exhibit genes that become amplified or deleted, and chromosomes that are highly susceptible to loss, duplication, or translocation. These findings suggest that the cells have developed one or more mutations in the mechanisms regulating chromosomal replication, repair, recombination, or segregation, thereby facilitating the accumulation of the multiple mutations required for development of cancer.

are as yet poorly understood, but it appears that, in epithelia, loss of expression of the adhesion molecule, E-cadherin, has a key role in the ability of the cell to leave its parent tumor. Moreover, in order to bind to and traverse the basal lamina, the cells must express specific integrins to bind laminin, and type IV collagenase to digest the lamina.

Oncogenes: mutant signal transducers

As mentioned above, mutations that lead to the uncontrolled proliferation of cancer cells can result either from disruption of the control of normal cell division or, alternatively, from a reduction in the normal processes of terminal differentiation or apoptosis.

This distinction is reflected by the two main groups of genes targeted for mutation: oncogenes and tumor suppressor genes (Table 41.2).

Oncogene, transcription factors, and tumor suppressor genes (antioncogenes)	
Oncogene	**Intracellular signaling role**
overexpressed growth factors	*v-Sis* encodes a sequence almost identical to the active PDGF-β
	Int-2 and k-Fgf-hst are related to fibroblast growth factor (FGF)
overexpressed and/or constitutively active growth factor receptors	v-ErbB is analogous to the activated cytoplasmic domain of EGF-receptor (EGF-R)
	v-Fms is related to macrophage colony stimulating factor receptor (M-CSF-R)
	v-kit is related to PDGF-R
	Mas is related to the G-protein-coupled angiotensin receptor also, overexpression of normal receptors can lead to transformation
G-proteins	mutated Gs (*gsp*) in pituitary/thyroid tumors
	mutated Gi (*gip2*) in adrenocortical/ovarian tumors
	Ras: mutated in 30% of human tumors
kinases	Src, Abl: protein tyrosine kinases
	Raf: serine-threonine kinase
oncomodulin	calcium-binding protein similar to calmodulin, found only in cancer cells
growth regulation genes	*Jun* and *Fos*: transcription factors
	Myc: a transcription factor regulating Cdc25 protein tyrosine phosphatase
	Myb and *Mos*: regulate Gi/S-phase transition
	Cdc2: regulation of S/M-phase transition
	Bcl-2 family: cell survival
tumor suppressor genes	*p53*: most frequently mutated gene in human cancer; cell cycle and apoptosis regulator
	Rb gene; cell cycle regulator
	neurofibromatosis gene – analogous to *Ras* GTP-ase activating protein (GAP)

Table 41.2 **Factors involved in the uncontrolled proliferation of cancer cells.**

Oncogenes were first identified as viral genes that infect normal cells and transform them into tumor cells

For example, the Rous sarcoma virus, which is a retrovirus that causes connective tissue tumors in chickens, will infect and transform fibroblast cells grown in cell culture. The transformed cells outgrow the normal cells and exhibit a number of growth abnormalities, such as a loss of cell contact-mediated inhibition of growth and loss of anchorage-dependence of growth. In addition, the cells have a rounded appearance and can proliferate in the absence of growth factors. Moreover, the cells are immortal, do not senesce, and can induce tumor formation when injected into a suitable animal host.

The key to understanding cell transformation lay in the mutation of a normal cellular gene that controls cell growth. The use of mutant Rous sarcoma viruses that, despite multiplying normally, have lost the ability to transform host cells showed that it was the *Src* gene that was responsible for such cell transformation. The breakthrough in our understanding of how this single gene could transform cells in culture came when it became apparent that the viral oncogene was a mutated homolog of a normal cellular gene. This gene is now called the *c-Src* proto-oncogene and has been identified as a protein tyrosine kinase signal transducer involved in the normal control of cell growth. As expression of this gene is not essential to the survival of the retrovirus, it is likely that *Src* was accidentally incorporated by the virus from a previous host genome and was somehow mutated in the process. In the case of the Rous sarcoma virus, the introns normally present in c-*Src* are spliced out and, in addition, there are a number of mutations causing amino acid substitutions, resulting in a constitutively active enzyme.

Cell transformation can, however, also result from overexpression of an oncogene in an abnormally high number of copies, as a consequence of the gene being under the control of powerful promoters or enhancers in the viral genome. Alternatively, for retroviruses, DNA copies of the viral RNA inserted into the host genome at or near sites of proto-oncogenes (insertional mutation) can cause abnormal activation of these proto-oncogenes. In this situation, the altered genome is inherited by all progeny of the original host cell.

Most human tumors are nonviral in origin, and arise from spontaneous or induced mutations. Approximately 85% of human tumors arise as a result of point or deletion mutations, rather than through viral involvement. The mutations may be spontaneous, or induced by carcinogens or radiation, resulting in overexpression or hyperactivity of the proto-oncogenes. In addition, karyotyping of tumor cells has shown, for example, that the conversion of the *Abl* (tyrosine kinase) proto-oncogene into an oncogene in CML results from a chromosomal translocation between chromosomes 9 and 22, with breakpoints in the *Abl* and *Bcr* genes, respectively, leading to the generation of a chromosome called the

Philadelphia chromosome. This translocation results in the generation of a fusion protein comprising the N-terminus of *Bcr* and the C-terminus of *Abl*. The *Abl* kinase domain of this fusion protein is hyperactive and drives the abnormal proliferation of a clone of hemopoietic progenitors in the bone marrow. In other cases, the translocation brings the oncogene under the control of an inappropriate promoter. For example, in Burkitt's lymphoma, overexpression of the *Myc* gene occurs through its translocation into the vicinity of one of the Ig loci. Because *Myc* normally acts as a nuclear proliferative signal, overexpression of *Myc* induces the cell to divide, even under conditions that would normally dictate growth arrest.

Oncogene actions are dominant and mutation in only one allele is therefore sufficient to transform culture cells

However, studies in transgenic mice overexpressing mutiple oncogenes have illustrated the point, made above, that human cancers are usually generated after the accumulation of mutations over several years. For example, transgenic mice overexpressing either the *Myc* or *Ras* oncogenes typically exhibit some tissues that are abnormally large. Occasionally, with age, some of these mice develop a few tumors, in a manner that is consistent with the expression of an inherited oncogene that increases the risk of accumulating further mutations and, hence, of initiating cancers. However, the vast majority of these transgenic cells do not develop any cancers. In contrast, double transgenic mice overexpressing both the *Myc* and the *Ras* oncogenes develop cancers at a much greater rate – a phe-

nomenon known as oncogene collaboration. An example of such synergistic action in human cancers is provided by B cell lymphoma, which relies on cooperation between overexpressed *Myc* (to drive inappropriate cell division) and *Bcl-2* (to inhibit apoptosis and promote B cell survival).

Tumor suppressor genes

Subversion of the cell cycle

Mutations in tumor suppressor genes are recessive and, thus, mutations in both copies of the gene are usually required for transformation. As it is very difficult to identify the loss of function of a single gene in a cell, much of the initial information relating to tumor suppressor genes was obtained by studying a range of inherited cancer syndromes (Table 41.3).

The retinoblastoma (Rb) gene

The rare human cancer, retinoblastoma, affords a good example of a cancer syndrome that has been an important source of information on tumor suppressor genes. In this cancer, neural progenitor cells in the immature retina are transformed by an unusually low number of mutations. Retinoblastoma occurs in childhood, with an incidence of about 1 in 20 000. In the hereditary form of the disease, multiple tumors occur, affecting both eyes, whereas in the (very rare) nonhereditary form, only one eye is affected by a single tumor. Sufferers of both forms of the disease were found to

Selected inherited cancer syndromes		
Syndrome	**Cancer**	**Gene product**
familial retinoblastoma	retinoblastoma	Rb 1: cell cycle and transcriptional regulation
	osteosarcoma	
Li-Fraumeni	sarcomas, adrenocortical carcinomas	p53: transcription factor
	carcinomas of breast, lung, larynx, and colon	DNA damage and stress
	brain tumors	
	leukemia	
Familial adenomatous polyposis (FAP)	colorectal cancer: colorectal adenomas, duodenal and gastric tumors, jaw osteomas, and desmoid tumors (Gardner syndrome), medulloblastoma (Turcot syndrome)	APC: regulation of β-catenin, microtubule binding
Wiedmann-Beckwith syndrome	Wilm's tumor, organomegaly, hemihypertrophy, hepatoblastoma, adrenocortical cancer	p57/KIP2: cell cycle regulator
neurofibromatosis type 1 (NF1)	neurofibrosarcoma AML brain tumors	GTP-ase activating protein (GAP) for *p21*Ras
hereditary papillary renal cancer	renal cancer	Met
		HGF-receptor
familial melanoma	melanoma	*p16* (CDK): inhibitor of cyclin-dependent kinase (CDK4/6)
	pancreatic cancer	
	dysplastic nevi	
	atypical moles	cyclin-dependent kinase (CDK4)

Table 41.3 **Selected inherited cancer syndromes.** AML, acute myelogenous leukemia; HGF, hepatocyte growth factor; KIP2, 57KDa inhibitor of cyclin-CDK complexes.

have a deletion of a specific band on chromosome 13; analysis of this genetic defect in individual patients showed that patients with the hereditary disease had a deletion or loss-of-function mutation of the *Rb* gene in every cell. This mutation predisposed these cells to become cancerous, because a single somatic mutation to knock out the remaining copy of *Rb* gene was sufficient to initiate a cancer. In fact, in approximately 70% of cases, the second *Rb* gene and its flanking regions on the chromosome are either completely deleted, or replaced with the corresponding regions of the defective chromosome by a process of mitotic recombination (loss of heterozygosity). In contrast, although patients with the non-hereditary disease show no mutations in either copy of their *Rb* genes in noncancerous cells, both copies are defective in

their cancer cells. This explains the rarity of the nonhereditary disease, because somatic mutations in both copies of *Rb* in a single retinal cell are required for transformation. Given the key role of the retinoblastoma protein, *Rb*, in the negative regulation of cell cycle progression (see above), it is perhaps not surprising that loss of *Rb* function plays such a major part in tumor progression. Thus, although retinoblastoma is a rare disease, mutations of *Rb* are not, and occur in many of the most common cancers such as lung, breast, and bladder carcinomas.

p53

p53 is a cell cycle regulator that has a key role, not only in regulating G1/S-phase cell cycle progression, but also in monitoring DNA damage

Individuals with only one functional copy of the *p53* gene are predisposed to develop a wide range of tumors, including sarcomas, carcinomas of the lung, breast, larynx and colon, brain tumors and leukemias. In common with retinoblastoma, this syndrome, called Li–Fraumeni syndrome, is rare and tumor cells in affected patients have defects in both copies of *p53*. Again like retinoblastoma, although the Li–Fraumeni syndrome is rare, the incidence of *p53* mutations in common cancers is extremely high. Deletion of *p53*, in addition to allowing uncontrolled cell cycle progression, also permits replication of damaged DNA, leading to further carcinogenic mutations or gene amplification; it is perhaps not surprising therefore, that the most common genetic lesion in cancer is found in *p53*.

FAMILIAL ADENOMATOUS POLYPOSIS (FAP) AND COLON CANCER

Investigation of inherited cancer genes has advanced our understanding of somatic mutations in sporadic cancers and the function of these signaling elements in the normal regulation of cell growth. FAP, a rare condition affecting 1 in 7000 in the USA, is characterized by inactivating germline mutations in the *APC* gene. Although germline mutations in *APC* are infrequent, somatic mutations in APC are present in more than 70% of adenomatous polyps and carcinomas of the colon and rectum. *APC* acts to promote degradation of the protein, β-catenin, in normal cells; β-catenin, through its interactions with transcription factors, drives transcriptional activation. Thus, in APC-mutated cells, β-catenin accumulates and binds and activates transcription factors, resulting in deregulated growth control and cancer. Additional evidence for a key role for β-catenin signaling in cancer development has been provided by cancer cells bearing β-catenin mutations that render β-catenin insensitive to APC-mediated degradation and repression of transcriptional activation.

Comment. Studies of the use of aspirin in humans have suggested that inhibitors of cyclo-oxygenase (COX: enzymes that have a key role in the conversion of the inflammatory mediator, arachidonic acid, to various prostaglandins; see Chapter 38) can alter the natural history of colon cancer. A randomized, double blind trial showed that aspirin prevented adenomas from arising in patients with previous colorectal cancer. Indeed, not only does the risk of the disease appear to be reduced in regular users of aspirin, but also the risk of fatal or metastatic colon cancer appears to be reduced by up to 50% in chronic users of the drug. This effect of aspirin appears to result from inhibition of COX-2, which is expressed at high levels in most colon tumors, and reflects the important roles that prostaglandins have in the pathogenesis of cancer as a result of their modulation of a wide range of cellular responses such as mitogenesis, cellular adhesion, immune surveillance, and apoptosis.

Summary

- Most proto-oncogenes and tumor suppressor genes that have been identified, function in signal transduction to mimic the effects of persistent mitogenic stimulation, thereby uncoupling cells from normal external controls.
- These signaling pathways converge on the machinery that controls passage of the cell through the G1-phase and prevent cell cycle exit.
- In addition, other genes, many of which are targeted by cancer-specific chromosomal translocations, lead to aberrant lineage-specific differentiation and developmental decisions that would normally induce apoptosis. The two tumor suppressor proteins, p53 and Rb, which have key roles in determining cell cycle progression and apoptosis, and the genes coding for these proteins are most frequently disrupted in cancer cells.

ACTIVE LEARNING

Test your new knowledge:

1. How is progression through the cell cycle regulated?
2. What roles do caspases and *Bcl-2* family members play in the regulation of apoptosis?
3. How do mutations in the *Rb* or *p53* genes contribute to tumor progression?

Further Reading

O'Connor L, Huang DCS, O'Reilly LA, Strasser A. Apoptosis and cell division. *Curr Op Cell Biol* 2000;**12**:257–263.

Zhu L, Skoultchu AI. Coordinating cell proliferation and differentiation. *Curr Op Genet Dev* 2001;**11**:91–97.

Harbour JW, Dean DC. Rb function in cell cycle regulation and apoptosis. *Nature Cell Biol* 2000;**2**:E65–67.

Hengartner MO. The biochemistry of apoptosis. *Nature* 2000;**407**:770–776.

Vogelstein B, Lane D, Levine AJ. Surfing the p53 network. *Nature* 2000;**408**:307–310.

Evan GI, Vousden KH. Proliferation, cell cycle and apoptosis in cancer. *Nature* 2001; **411**:342–348.

Relevant Websites

The WWW Virtual Library of Cell Biology (cell cycle, apoptosis etc.)
www.vlib.org/Science/Cell_Biology
Kimball's Biology Pages
www.biology-pages.info
Nature's Encyclopedia of Life Sciences
www.els.net
The Genetics of Cancer Resource Center
www.intouchlive.com/cancergenetics

LEARNING OBJECTIVES

After reading this chapter you should be able to:

- Describe the relationship between aging and disease.
- Explain the Gompertz plot and how it describes the rate of aging of different species.
- Differentiate between biological and chemical theories of aging.
- Explain the precepts of the free radical theory of aging, including identification of characteristic oxidation products that accumulate in long-lived proteins with age.
- Outline the evidence that the rate of mutation of DNA is an important determinant of the rate of aging.
- Explain the evidence in support of mitochondrial theories of aging and describe how this theory interfaces with the free radical theory of aging.
- Describe the etiology and pathology characteristic of several diseases of accelerated aging.
- Describe the effects of caloric restriction on the rate of aging of rodents.

INTRODUCTION

Aging may be defined as the time-dependent deterioration in function of an organism. While it has broad-based physiological effects, aging is fundamentally the result of changes in cellular structure and function, biochemistry and metabolism (Table 42.1). The result of aging, even healthy aging, is increased susceptibility to disease and increased probability of death – the end-point of aging. However, aging is not a disease. Diseases affect a fraction of the population; aging affects all of us, whether it is programmed or stochastic.

With the aging of the population, gerontology and geriatric medicine are becoming increasingly important in the practice of medicine. This chapter focuses on the biochemical changes associated with aging and addresses them from the viewpoint of chemical theories of aging, with emphasis on the free radical theory of aging. General factors affecting longevity and the impact of interventions on aging and longevity are discussed, including discussion of the aging of specific organ systems.

Aging of complex systems

Excluding genetic defects, childhood disease and accidents, humans survive until about age 50 with limited maintenance requirements or risk of death, then we become increasingly frail and our death rate increases, reaching a maximum at about age 76. Our lifespan is affected by our genetics and our environmental exposure, and our death is usually attributable to failure of a critical system (cardiovascular, renal, pulmonary, etc.). The capacity of these inter-dependent physiological systems usually declines as a linear function of age, leading to an exponential increase in our age-specific death rate (Fig. 42.1). Historically, improvements in health care and environment have resulted in rectangularization of the survival curve – the mean lifespan is increased without an increase in the maximum lifespan potential.

THE HAYFLICK LIMIT – REPLICATIVE SENESCENCE

Differentiated cells from higher animals undergo only a limited number of cell divisions (population doublings) in tissue culture, unless they become transformed or are infected with certain viruses. The number of potential cell divisions is greater in longer-lived animals, suggesting a relationship between cell division potential and longevity. Human neonatal fibroblasts will divide about 60 times, then enter a non-dividing state. Cells from younger donors have greater replicative capacity, a greater number of cell divisions in cell culture, but with each generation, the number of dividing cells decreases. This limited doubling capacity, described by Dr Leonard Hayflick, is known as the Hayflick limit. The relevance of the Hayflick limit to human aging is still debated – certainly human cells retain some replicative capacity, even at advanced age, and major tissues, such as muscle and nerve, are largely post-mitotic, *i.e.* not actively dividing. However, changes in the metabolism and morphology of senescent cells, their responsiveness to hormones and their synthetic and degradative capacity, e.g. in the immunological and endothelial systems, may affect our adaptability and susceptibility to age-related diseases, placing limits on our lifespan.

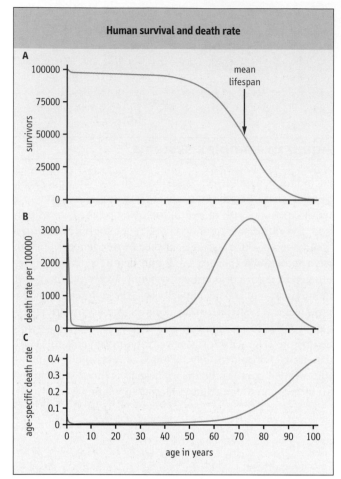

Fig. 42.1 **Survival curve and death rate.** (A) Mean lifespan is defined as the age at which 50% of a population survives (or has died). The negative slope of the survival curve reaches a maximum at the mean lifespan of a species. (B) The death rate reaches a maximum at the mean lifespan. (C) The age-specific death rate, defined as the number of deaths per time at a given age, e.g. deaths per 100 000 persons of a specific age per year, increases exponentially with age. The lifespan or maximum lifespan potential (MLSP) is defined as the maximum age attainable by a member of the population, which is 120 years for humans.

Changes in biochemistry and physiology during aging

Biochemical	Physiological
Basal metabolic rate	Lung expansion volume
Protein turnover	Renal filtration capacity (glomerular)
Glucose tolerance	Renal concentration capacity (tubular)
Reproductive capacity	Cardiovascular performance
Telomere shortening	Musculoskeletal system
Oxidative phosphorylation	Nerve conduction velocity
	Endocrine and exocrine systems
	Reproductive and immunological systems
	Sensory systems (vision, audition)

Table 42.1 **Decline in biochemical and physiological systems with age.**

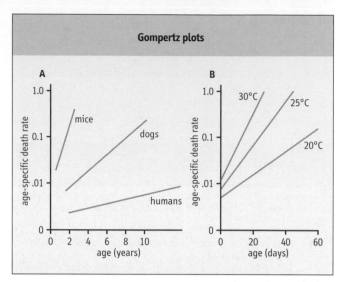

Fig. 42.2 **Gompertz plots for humans and other species.** (A) Humans and other vertebrates; (B) Flies raised at various temperatures (adapted from work of Prof RS Sohal).

Mathematical models of aging

In the early 19th century, Gompertz observed that the age-specific death rate of humans increased exponentially after 35 years of age, and that human survival curves could be modeled by what is now known as the Gompertz equation:

$$m(t) = Ae^{\alpha t}$$

where: m is the age specific death rate at age t;
A is the intercept (death rate at birth); and
α is a slope constant (the effect of time on the death rate).

The Gompertz–Makeham equation: $m(t) = Ae^{\alpha t} + B$, adds a constant, B, to correct for the age-independent death rate, e.g. as a result of infant mortality or accidents, and provides a better fit to actuarial data.

The Gompertz plots in Fig. 42.2 illustrate the time-dependent changes in death rate for three different species of vertebrates and for flies raised at different temperatures. Shorter-lived mammals have a greater age-adjusted rate of death (α), while the death rate for poikilotherms varies with ambient temperature – flies live longer when grown at lower temperatures. This observation has been interpreted as evidence for 'rate of living' or 'wear and tear' theories of aging. Flies, being more active at higher temperature, consume more energy and die more rapidly. Flies that are restrained, e.g. in a matchbox, rather than a large carboy, also live longer; wingless flies live longer; and male flies, segregated from females, also live longer. In each case, in small enclosures, without wings and in the absence of the opposite sex, male flies are less active, have lower basal metabolic rates, and have longer mean and maximum lifespans.

THEORIES OF AGING

Theories of aging can be divided into two general categories: biological and chemical

Biological theories treat aging as a genetically controlled event, determined by the programmed expression or repression of genetic information. Aging and death are seen as the orchestrated end-stage of birth, growth, maturation and

PROGERIAS – DISEASES OF ACCELERATED AGING CAUSED BY DEFECTS IN DNA REPAIR

Certain genetic diseases are considered models of accelerated aging (progeria). These monogenic diseases display many, but never all, of the features of normal aging. Few progeric patients develop dementia or age-related pathologies, such as Alzheimer's disease. The progerias are sometimes described as caricatures of aging, but are useful models for understanding the aging process. Werner's and Bloom's syndromes are autosomal recessive diseases caused by mutation of distinct DNA helicase genes which are thought to have a role in replication and repair of damaged DNA. Patients with Werner's syndrome appear normal during childhood, but stop growing in their teens. They gradually show many symptoms of premature aging, including graying and loss of hair, thinning of skin, development of early cataracts, impaired glucose tolerance and diabetes, atherosclerosis and osteoporosis, and increased rates of cancer. Death usually occurs in the mid-40s from cardiovascular disease. Fibroblasts from Werner's patients divide only about 20 times in cell culture and have higher levels of protein-bound carbonyl groups, an indicator of increased oxidative stress. Bloom's Syndrome is also characterized by increased frequency of chromosomal breaks, dwarfism, photosensitivity and increased frequency of cancer and leukemia; death occurs typically in the mid-20s. Ataxia-telangiectasia, or fragile chromosome syndrome, is associated with increased loss of telomeres with cell division and deficiency in repair of double-strand DNA breaks. It is caused by a defect in a protein kinase involved in signal transduction, cell cycle control and DNA repair.
Hutchinson–Gilford syndrome is a severe, pediatric form of progeria. Patients have many of the symptoms of Werner's syndrome, but the symptoms appear at an earlier age and death usually occurs by the mid-20s. This syndrome is caused by a defect in a gene for lamin, a component of the nuclear lamina, which together with nuclear membranes and pore complexes comprise the nuclear envelope. Hutchinson-Gilford is one of several distinct syndromes associated with lamin mutations. The progeric mutation appears to increase nuclear fragility and aberrant mRNA splicing; as in Werner's syndrome, cultured fibroblasts become prematurely senescent. These progeric diseases suggest that efficient repair of DNA is essential for prevention of cancer and for normal aging.

reproduction. Apoptosis (programmed cell death) and thymic involution are examples of genetically programmed events at the level of cells and organs, and the decline in the immunological, neuroendocrine and reproductive systems may be seen, in a broader context, as evidence for action of a biological clock affecting the integrated functions of an organism. Biological theories attribute differences in lifespan to interspecies differences in genetics, but also provide an explanation for the observation that there is a genetic component to longevity within a species, e.g. in families with a history of longevity. Differences in lifespan among species are also closely correlated with the efficiency of DNA repair mechanisms. Longer-lived species have more efficient DNA repair processes (Fig. 42.3). Numerous diseases of accelerated aging (progeria) also illustrate the importance of genetics and maintenance of the integrity of the genome during aging.

Chemical theories of aging treat aging as a somatic process resulting from cumulative damage to biomolecules. At one extreme, the error–catastrophe theory proposes that aging is the result of cumulative errors in the machinery for replication, repair, transcription, and translation of genetic information. Eventually, errors in critical enzymes, such as DNA

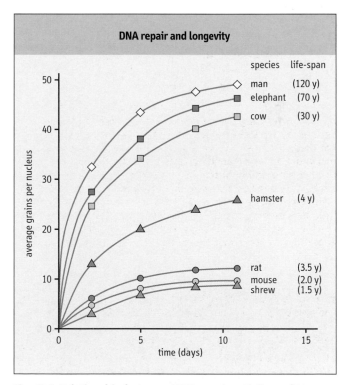

Fig. 42.3 **Relationship between DNA repair activity and longevity.** Fibroblasts from various species were irradiated briefly, forming thymine dimers and thymine glycol (Chapter 30). The oxidized bases are removed and replaced by excision repair. DNA repair was assessed by the rate of incorporation of a [³H]thymidine tracer into DNA by autoradiography (adapted from Hart RW, Setlow RB: Correlation between deoxyribonucleic acid excision-repair and life-span in a number of mammalian species. *Proc Natl Acad Sci USA*. 1974;**71**:2169–2173.)

and RNA polymerases or enzymes involved in the synthesis and turnover of proteins, gradually affect the fidelity of expression of genetic information and permit the accumulation of altered proteins. The propagation of errors and resultant accumulation of dysfunctional macromolecules leads eventually to the collapse of the system. Consistent with this theory, increasing amounts of immunologically detectable, but denatured or modified, functionally inactive, enzymes accumulate in cells as a function of age.

More general chemical theories treat aging as the result of chronic, cumulative chemical (non-enzymatic) modification, insults, or damage to all biomolecules (Table 42.2). Like rust, erosion, or corrosion, the accumulation of damage with age gradually affects function. This damage is most apparent in long-lived tissue proteins, such as lens crystallins and extracellular collagens, which accumulate chemical modifications with age. A brown color commonly results from formation of a wide range of conjugated compounds with absorbance in the yellow–red region of the spectrum (Fig. 42.4). Chemical damage to the integrity of the genome also occurs, but is more difficult to quantify because of the efficiency of repair processes that excise and repair modified nucleotides. As noted in Table 42.2, there are a number of silent consequences of DNA damage. This damage is primarily

Chemistry and aging

Protein modification	DNA modification and mutation	Other
crosslinking	oxidation	lipofuscin
oxidation	depurination	inactive enzymes
deamidation	substitutions	
D-aspartate	insertions and deletions	
protein carbonyls	inversions and transpositions	
glycoxidation		
lipoxidation		

Table 42.2 **Age-dependent chemical changes in biomolecules.** Long-lived proteins, such as lens crystallins and tissue collagens accumulate damage with age. Modification and crosslinking of proteins occurs as a result of non-oxidative (deamidation, racemization) or oxidative (protein carbonyls) mechanisms or by reactions of proteins with products of carbohydrate or lipid peroxidation (glycoxidation, lipoxidation). Damage to DNA is often silent, i.e. modified forms of nucleotides may not accumulate, but the damage increases in the form of mutations resulting from errors in repair.

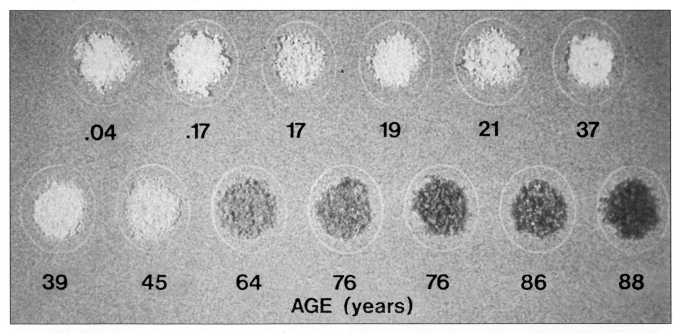

Fig. 42.4 **Changes in lens protein and costal cartilage with age.** Browning is a characteristic feature of the aging of proteins, not just in the lens, which is exposed to sunlight, but also in tissue collagens throughout the body. Crosslinking of proteins also increases with browning. Crosslinking contributes to the gradual insolubilization of lens protein with age. Aggregates of lens protein disperse light, contributing to the development of 'senile' cataracts. Crosslinking of articular and vascular collagens decreases the resilience of vertebral disks and compliance of the vascular wall with age. These changes in extracellular proteins, shown here for costal collagen, are similar to changes induced by reaction of carbohydrates and lipids with protein during the cooking of foods, a process known as the Maillard or browning reaction. At one level, humans have been described as low temperature ovens, operating at 37°C, with long cooking cycles (~75 years). Many of the Maillard reaction products detected in the crust of bread and pretzels have been identified in human crystallins and collagens, and increase with age. (See also discussion of diabetic complications in Chapter 20.)

endogenous, but is enhanced by xenobiotic and environmental agents.

Organ system theories of aging incorporate various aspects of the above theories. These theories attribute aging to the failure of integrative systems, such as the immunological, neurological, endocrine, or circulatory system. While they do not assign a specific cause, these theories integrate biological and chemical theories, acknowledging both genetic and environmental contributions to aging.

The free radical theory of aging

The most widely accepted chemical theory of aging is the free radical theory of aging (FRTA). This theory treats aging as the result of cumulative oxidative damage to biomolecules: DNA, RNA, protein, lipids, and glycoconjugates. From the viewpoint of the FRTA, longer-lived organisms have lower rates of production of reactive oxygen species (ROS; Chapter 35), better antioxidant defenses, and more efficient repair or turnover processes. While generally considered a chemical theory, the FRTA does not ignore the importance of genetics and biology in limiting the production of ROS, and in antioxidant and repair mechanisms. It also interfaces with other theories of aging, such as the rate of living theory because the rate of generation of ROS is considered a function of the overall rate and/or extent of oxygen consumption, and the crosslinkage theory because some products of ROS damage crosslink protein. Finally, as a chemical hypothesis, the FRTA does not exclude cumulative chemical damage, independent of ROS, such as racemization, deamidation and alkylation reactions, but focuses on ROS as the primary source of damage and the fundamental cause of aging.

The FRTA is supported by the inverse correlation between basal metabolic rate (rate of oxygen consumption per unit weight) and maximum lifespan of mammals, and by evidence of increased oxidative damage to proteins with age. Protein carbonyl groups, such as glutamic and aminoadipic acid semialdehyde, formed by oxidative deamination of arginine and lysine, respectively, are formed in proteins exposed to ROS. The steady-state level of protein carbonyls in intracellular proteins increases logarithmically with age and at a rate inversely proportional to the lifespan of species. Protein carbonyls are also much higher in fibroblasts from patients with Werner's or Hutchinson–Gilford syndromes, compared to age-matched subjects. Similar concentrations of protein carbonyls are also present in tissues of old rats and elderly humans, arguing that similar changes occur at old age in a range of organisms, regardless of the difference in their lifespans.

Figure 42.5 illustrates the accumulation of two relatively stable amino acid oxidation products in human skin collagen: methionine sulfoxide and *ortho*-tyrosine. These compounds are formed by different mechanisms involving different ROS

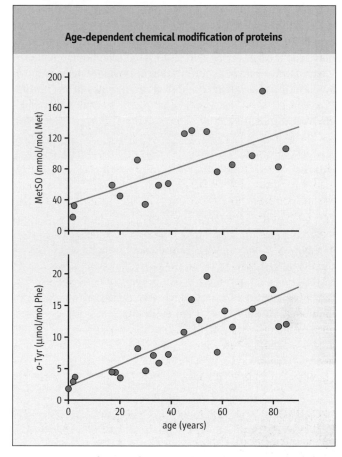

Age-dependent chemical modification of proteins

Fig. 42.5 **Accumulation of amino acid oxidation products in human skin collagen with age.** Methionine is oxidized to methionine sulfoxide (MetSO) by HOCl or H_2O_2; *ortho*-tyrosine is a product of hydroxyl radical addition to phenylalanine. Despite a 100-fold difference in their rate of accumulation in collagen, levels of MetSO and *o*-tyrosine correlate strongly with one another, indicating that multiple ROS contribute to oxidative damage to proteins (adapted from Wells-Knecht MC, *et al.*: Age-dependent accumulation of *ortho*-tyrosine and methionine sulfoxide in human skin collagen is not increased in diabetes: evidence against a generalized increase in oxidative stress in diabetes. *J Clin Invest* 1997;**100**:839–846.)

(Chapter 35) and are present at significantly different concentrations in skin collagen, but increase in concert with age. Other amino acid modifications that accumulate in skin collagen with age include advanced glycoxidation and lipoxidation end-products (AGE/ALEs), such as carboxymethyllysine and pentosidine (Fig. 42.6), and D-aspartate. The rate of accumulation of these modifications depends on the rate of turnover of the collagens (Fig. 42.7) and is accelerated in diabetes and hyperlipidemia. The increase in AGE/ALEs in collagen is thought to impair the normal turnover and contribute to the thickening of basement membranes with age. Increased age-adjusted levels of AGE/ALEs in collagen are implicated in the pathogenesis of complications of diabetes and atherosclerosis.

D-aspartate is a non-oxidative modification of protein that is formed by spontaneous, age-dependent racemization of L-aspartate, the natural form of the amino acid in protein. The more rapid turnover of skin, compared to articular, collagen yields a lower rate of accumulation of D-aspartate in skin collagen and also explains the difference in rates of accumulation of AGE/ALEs in skin versus articular collagen. AGE/ALEs are even higher in lens crystallins, which have the slowest rate of turnover among proteins in the body. Deamidation of asparagine and glutamine is another non-oxidative chemical modification that increases with age in proteins; it has been described primarily in intracellular proteins.

AGE/ALEs: BIOMARKERS OF OXIDATIVE STRESS AND AGING

Advanced glycoxidation and lipoxidation end-products (AGE/ALEs) are carbohydrate- and lipid-derived chemical (nonenzymatic) modifications and crosslinks in protein. They are formed by reaction of proteins with products of oxidation of carbohydrates and lipids (Fig. 42.6). Some compounds, such as N^ε-(carboxymethyl)lysine (CML), may be formed from either carbohydrates or lipids; others, such as pentosidine, are formed only from carbohydrates, and others, such as the malondialdehyde adduct to lysine, are formed exclusively from lipids. Carbohydrate sources of AGEs include glucose, ascorbate, and glycolytic intermediates; polyunsaturated fatty acids in phospholipids are considered the primary source of ALEs. Lysine, histidine and cysteine residues are the major sites of AGE/ALE formation in protein. Over 20 different AGE/ALEs have been detected in tissue proteins, and many of these are known to increase with age. AGE/ALEs are useful biomarkers of the aging of proteins and their exposure to oxidative stress.

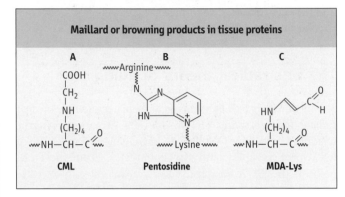

Fig. 42.6 **Structure of major advanced glycoxidation and lipoxidation end-products (AGE/ALEs).** (A) the AGE/ALE, N^ε-(carboxymethyl)lysine (CML), which is formed during both carbohydrate and lipid peroxidation reactions; (B) the AGE pentosidine, a fluorescent crosslink in proteins; (C) the ALE, malondialdehyde-lysine (MDA-Lys), a reactive ALE that may proceed to form aminoenimine (RNHCH=CHCH=NR) crosslinks in proteins.

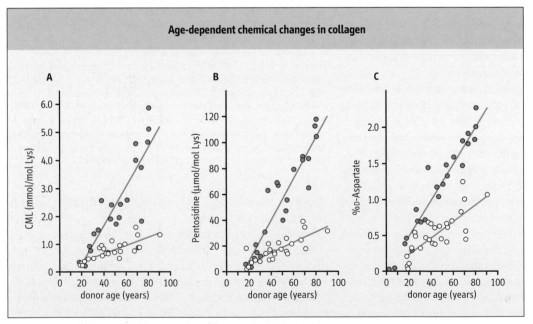

Fig. 42.7 **Accumulation of advanced glycoxidation and lipoxidation end-products (AGE/ALEs) and D-aspartate in collagens with age.** N^ε-(carboxymethyl)lysine (CML) is formed by oxidative mechanisms from glycated proteins or reaction of glucose, ascorbate or lipid peroxidation products with protein. The fluorescent crosslink pentosidine is formed by oxidative reaction of glucose or ascorbate with proteins. D-Aspartate is formed non-oxidatively by racemization of L-aspartate residues in protein. Differences in rate of accumulation of both oxidative and non-oxidative biomarkers are attributable to differences in rates of turnover of collagens. (adapted from Verzijl N, *et al.*: Effect of collagen turnover on the accumulation of advanced glycation endproducts. *J Biol Chem* 2000;**275**:39027–39031.)

AGING OF THE CIRCULATORY SYSTEM

The extracellular matrix of the aorta and major arteries becomes thicker and more highly crosslinked with age, contributing to both the decrease in elasticity and the capacity of the endothelium to dilate blood vessels in response to physical and chemical stimuli. These changes occur naturally with age, independent of pathology, but may account for the increase in cardiovascular risk in the elderly. AGEs and ALEs are implicated in the crosslinking of the vascular extracellular matrix, explaining the increase in arterial crosslinking in diabetes and dyslipidemia. A new class of drugs, known as AGE-breakers, is being evaluated clinically for reversal of increased vascular stiffness in aging and disease.

The fluorescent age-pigment lipofuscin is considered the accumulated debris of reactions between lipid peroxides and proteins. Lipofuscin accumulates in granular form, possibly residual bodies derived from lysosomes, in the cytoplasm of post-mitotic cells at a rate that is inversely related to species lifespan. It may account for 10–15% of the volume of cardiac muscle and neuronal cells at advanced age, and its rate of deposition in cardiac myocytes in cell culture is accelerated by growth under hyperoxic conditions. In flies, the rate of accumulation of lipofuscin varies directly with ambient temperature and activity, and inversely with lifespan.

Overall, there are a number of chemical modifications, both oxidative and non-oxidative, that accumulate in proteins with age. While much of the research in this area has focused on slow, cumulative chemical modification of long-lived extracellular proteins, there is growing evidence that these reactions also proceed inside the cell where ROS are formed from mitochondria and from reactive metabolic intermediates, such as glyceraldehyde-3-phosphate and methylglyoxal (Chapter 35). The generation of these compounds is also accelerated under pathological conditions, for example, in plaque deposits in the vascular wall in atherosclerosis and in neurodegenerative diseases (see Box).

Mitochondrial theories of aging

Mitochondrial theories of aging are a blend of biological and chemical theories, treating aging as the result of chemical damage to mitochondrial DNA (mtDNA). Mitochondria contain proteins specified by both nuclear and mitochondrial DNA, however only 13 mitochondrial proteins are encoded by mitochondrial DNA. While this may seem trivial, these include essential subunits of the three proton pumps and ATP synthase. MtDNA is especially sensitive to mutations: mitochondria are the major site of ROS production in the cell,

mtDNA is not protected by a sheath of histones, and mitochondria have limited capacity for DNA repair.

Mitochondrial diseases commonly involve defects of energy metabolism, including the pyruvate dehydrogenase complex, pyruvate carboxylase, complexes I, II, III, and IV, cytochrome c, ATP synthase (complex V), and biosynthesis of ubiquinone. These defects can be caused by mutations in both nuclear and mitochondrial DNA, but mtDNA suffers many more mutations than nuclear DNA. Such defects often result in the accumulation of lactic acid because of impaired oxidative phosphorylation, and may cause cell death, especially in skeletal (myopathies) and cardiac muscles (cardiomyopathies) and nerve (encephalopathies) tissues, which are heavily dependent on oxidative metabolism (Chapters 8 and 13). The number of mitochondria and multiple copies of the mitochondrial genome in the cell may provide some protection against mitochondrial dysfunction as a result of mutation.

TELOMERES – A CLOCK OF AGING

Telomeres are the repetitive sequences at the ends of chromosomal DNA, typically thousands of copies of short, highly redundant, repetitive DNA, TTAGGG in humans (Chapter 30). DNA polymerase requires a double-stranded template for DNA biosynthesis. During normal DNA replication, RNA primers at the 5′ end of the template serve to initiate DNA synthesis. However, at the extreme ends of the chromosomes, DNA synthesis is restricted, because there are no sequences further upstream for DNA primase engagement. Therefore, each round of chromosome replication results in chromosome shortening. The enzyme telomerase is a reverse transcriptase containing an RNA with a sequence complementary to the telomere DNA. It functions to maintain the length of telomeres at the 3′-end of chromosomes. Telomerase is found in fetal tissues, adult germ cells and in tumor cells, but the somatic cells of multicellular organisms lack telomerase activity. This has led to the hypothesis that shortening of the telomere may contribute to the Hayflick limit and is involved in aging of multicellular organisms. Increased expression of telomerase in human cells results in elongated telomeres and an increase in the longevity of those cells by at least 20 cell doublings. Cells from individuals with premature aging diseases (progeria) also have short telomeres. In contrast, cancer cells, which are immortal, express an active telomerase activity. All of these observations suggest that the decrease in telomere length is associated with cellular senescence and aging. Knockout mice, in which the telomerase gene has been deleted, have chromosomes lacking detectable telomeres. These mice have high frequencies of aneuploidy and chromosomal abnormalities. The disease, autosomal *dyskeratosis congenital,* features a mutation in the telomerase locus, with inability of somatic cells to reconstitute their telomeres, and hence loss of epidermis and hematopoietic marrow. This disease has many of the characteristics of accelerated aging.

AGING OF MUSCLE – DAMAGE TO MITOCHONDRIAL DNA

Old age is characterized by a general decrease in skeletal muscle mass (sarcopenia) and strength, as a result of a decrease in both the number of motoneurons and the number and size of myofibers. The fiber loss is accompanied by an increase in interstitial, fibrous connective tissue, and a reduction in capillary density, which limits the blood supply. The decrease in muscle mass and strength contributes to frailty and the increased risk of mortality. The loss in skeletal muscle mass may also contribute to glucose intolerance in the elderly as a result of the decreasing mass of tissue available to take up glucose from blood.

One of the major changes in muscle biochemistry with age in an increase in the number of muscle cells with mitochondria deficient in cytochrome oxidase, which limits the muscle's ability to do work. As mitochondria become less efficient in oxidizing NADH, they become more reduced, and the accumulation of partially reduced ubiquinone (semiquinone) promotes the reduction of molecular oxygen, leading to increased superoxide production in older mitochondria. Under these conditions, when oxidative phosphorylation is impaired, cells appear to generate ATP primarily by glycolysis. NADH is oxidized extramitochondrially, primarily by NADH oxidases in the plasma membrane, which produce hydrogen peroxide, but no ATP. NADH oxidase:

$$NADH + H^+ + O_2 \rightarrow NAD^+ + H_2O_2.$$

These changes are observed in both cardiac and skeletal muscle and appear to result from major, random deletions in mitochondrial DNA (25–75% of total mtDNA), which are then amplified by clonal expansion, leading to fiber atrophy and breakage. The muscle fiber is only as strong as its weakest link, so that small regions of fiber loss affect overall muscle capacity. Fortunately, sarcopenia can be delayed and partially reversed by resistance exercise, thus the emphasis on regular exercise among the elderly.

INTERVENTIONS TO DELAY AGING – WHAT WORKS AND WHAT DOESN'T

Antioxidant supplements

Based on the FRTA, it seems reasonable to speculate that antioxidant supplementation should have an effect on longevity. In fact, however, there is no rigorous, reproducible experimental evidence that antioxidant supplements have any effect on maximum lifespan of humans or other vertebrates. At the same time, antioxidant supplements, most of which include vitamins, may improve health, particularly in those subjects with vitamin deficiencies. Thus, effects of antioxidant

therapy on mean (and healthy) lifespan are not unexpected. Failure to affect maximum lifespan may result from the fact that there are so many mechanisms for production and control of free radicals and inhibiting or reversing damage to biomolecules. Many of these processes depend on the activity of enzymes that detoxify ROS or regenerate endogenous antioxidants. These enzymes, such as superoxide dismutase and glutathione peroxidase (Chapter 37), are induced in response to oxidative stress, and may also be repressed during times of low oxidative stress. Thus, the body may respond to maintain a homeostatic balance between pro-oxidant and antioxidant forces (see Fig. 37.1), countering efforts to enhance antioxidant defenses. This response may be essential, for example, to maintain effective bactericidal activity during the respiratory burst accompanying phagocytosis.

Calorie restriction

Calorie restriction (CR) is the only intervention that consistently extends maximum lifespan in a variety of species, including mammals, fish, flies, worms, and yeast. Reduction in total caloric intake appears to be the essential feature of this intervention, i.e. the beneficial, life-extending effects are observed whenever CR is applied and regardless of dietary composition, although early and prolonged intervention has more impressive effects. As shown in Figure 42.8, CR leads to a significant increase in the maximum lifespan of laboratory rats, equivalent to extending human lifespan to about 180 years. The extension in maximum lifespan is accompanied by an overall improvement in the health of the animal. Control experiments have established that the effects of CR are not attributable to toxins in the animal chow.

Based on analysis of gene expression, CR appears to limit chemical damage to DNA to and to promote the turnover of tissue proteins. Calorie-restricted rats had fewer muscle fibers lacking in cytochrome oxidase and decreased levels of deletions in muscle mitochondrial DNA. CR mice also have lower levels of inducible genes for hepatic detoxification, DNA repair and response to oxidative stress (heat shock proteins), suggesting a lower rate of chemical damage to proteins and DNA during CR. In CR experiments, it has been difficult to differentiate between the effects of dietary restriction on energy consumption versus the reduction in body weight that accompanies dietary restriction. However, recent experiments in a mouse model with knock-out of the adipose tissue insulin receptor gene, suggest that adiposity may be more important than caloric consumption *per se*. Compared to normal littermates, the knock-out mice were leaner, with a 50% decrease in fat mass, but consumed identical amounts of food per day (actually more than the control animals when normalized to their body weight). The 20% increase in lifespan of the knock-out mice, compared to controls, suggests that energy utilization and storage is more important than total caloric intake in determining maximum lifespan potential.

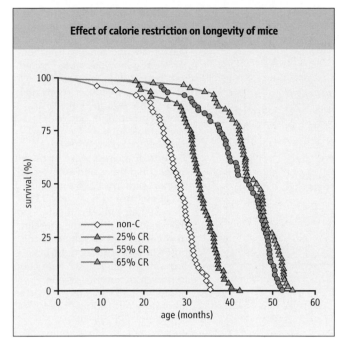

Fig. 42.8 Calorie restriction extends longevity of mice. The Non-CR group received food *ad libitum*. Other groups were restricted by 25, 55 and 65% of the *ad lib* diet, starting at 1 month of age: (◇) *ad libitum* fed mice; (▲) 25% CR; (●) 55% CR; (▲) 65% CR (adapted from Weindruch R, *et al.*: Retardation of aging in mice by dietary restriction. *J Nutr* 1986;**116**:651–654).

GENETIC MODELS OF AGING

There is increasing interest in development of mammalian genetic models with increased lifespan. If genetic manipulation of the lifespan of mice can be achieved, then it may be possible to translate this knowledge to treatment of human aging. Ames and Snell dwarf mice have separate, homozygous defects in growth hormone, thyroid hormone and prolactin production in the pituitary and a 40% increase in both mean and maximum lifespan, compared to long-lived progenitor strains. Their skin collagen is less crosslinked and they are less susceptible to some age-related diseases and declines in organ function, but they are infertile and have poor thermoregulation. In contrast to CR-mice, these mice are obese, although their body weight and food intake are decreased, compared to normal mice. Studies on these mice suggest that the onset of multiple, late-life functional declines and diseases may be decelerated in parallel by a few, underlying, unifying control mechanisms.

Studies in longer-lived primate species have been underway since the late 1980s, and there is clear evidence of health benefits of CR in primates, although effects on maximum lifespan are not yet available. Even if CR can be shown to extend human lifespan, it is unlikely that humans will be able to adopt the strict dietary control required for this regimen. There are also some risks associated with caloric restriction, e.g. sterility and possibly increased susceptibility to environmental stress and microbial infection. However, understanding the biological mechanisms of the effects of CR may lead to alternative strategies that mimic CR and extend lifespan. In this context, it is important to emphasize that CR contributes to overall health and extends the healthy lifespan, not just total lifespan. CR delays the onset of a wide range of age-related diseases, including cancer (Fig. 42.9), and is, in fact, the most potent, broad-acting cancer-prevention regimen in experimental animals. While CR has not been tested in humans, obesity is recognized as a risk factor for cancer in humans. It is argued that the extension of maximum lifespan by CR is achieved by delaying the onset of cancer. Long-lived animals are more efficient in protecting their genome and

ALZHEIMER'S DISEASE – A ROLE FOR OXIDATIVE STRESS IN NEURODEGENERATIVE DISEASE?

Alzheimer's disease (AD) is the most common form of progressive cognitive deterioration in the elderly. It is characterized microscopically by the appearance of neurofibrillary tangles and senile plaques in cortical regions of the brain. The tangles are localized inside neurons, and are rich in τ (tau) protein, which is derived from microtubules; it is hyperphosphorylated and poly-ubiquitinated. Plaques are extracellular aggregates, localized around amyloid deposits, formed from insoluble peptides derived from a family of amyloid precursor proteins. AD affects primarily cholinergic neurons, and drugs that inhibit the degradation of acetylcholine within synapses are the mainstay of therapy. A similar approach is used for preservation of dopamine in dopaminergic neurons in Parkinson's disease, i.e. by inhibiting the degradative enzyme, monoamine oxidase.

Several studies have shown that both AGEs and ALEs are increased in tangles and plaques in brain of AD patients, compared with age-matched controls. Other indicators of generalized oxidative stress in the AD brain include increased levels of protein carbonyls, nitrotyrosine and 8-OH-deoxyguanosine, all detected by immunohistochemical methods. The amyloid protein is toxic to neurons in cell culture and appears to provoke inflammatory responses in glial cells. Significant quantities of decompartmentalized, redox-active iron are also detectable histologically in the AD brain and can be removed reversibly (*in vitro*) by treatment with chelators, such as desferrioxamine. Based on these data, oxidative stress is strongly implicated in the development and/or progression of AD, and chelators are being evaluated clinically for treatment of AD. Epidemiological studies also indicate that long-term treatment with non-steroidal anti-inflammatory drugs, such as ibuprofen and Tylenol, reduces the risk of AD and may delay its onset or slow its progression. Anti-inflammatory drugs are now being tested for treatment of AD.

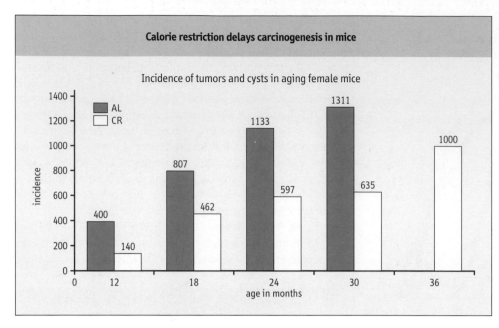

Incidence of tumors and cysts in aging female mice

Calorie restriction delays carcinogenesis in mice

Fig. 42.9 **Effect of calorie restriction (CR) on development of tumors in mice.** Over 1000 mice, 50:50 male and female, from four different genotypes were divided into two groups, one fed *ad libitum* (AL), the other receiving 60% of the caloric intake of the control group (CR), but with comparable intake of vitamins, minerals and micronutrients. Cohorts of animals were sacrificed at specified times and total lesions (tumors plus cysts) were measured. At 24 months, 51% AL and 13% CR mice had tumors. CR extended the mean and maximum lifespan of the mice and also delayed the onset of cancer (adapted from Bronson RT, Lipman RD: Reduction in rate of occurrence of age related lesions in dietary restricted laboratory mice. *Growth Dev Aging* 1991;**55**:169–184).

thereby delaying carcinogenesis. Lifespan depends on preservation of the integrity of the genome.

Summary

Aging is characterized by a gradual decline in the capacity of physiological systems, leading eventually to failure of a critical system, then death. At the biochemical level, aging is considered the result of chronic chemical modification of all classes of biomolecules. According to the free radical theory of aging, ROS are the primary culprits, causing alterations in the sequence of DNA (mutations) and structure of proteins. Longevity is achieved by developing efficient systems to limit and/or repair chemical damage. Caloric restriction is, at present, the only widely applicable mechanism for delaying aging and extending the mean, healthy, and maximum lifespan of species. CR appears to work, in part, by inhibiting the production of ROS and limiting damage to biomolecules, delaying many of the characteristic features of aging, including cancer.

Further reading

Barja G. Endogenous oxidative stress: relationship to aging, longevity and caloric restriction. *Ageing Res Rev* 2002 Jun;**1**(3):397–411.

Baynes JW. From life to death – the struggle between chemistry and biology during aging. *Biogerontology* 2000;**1**(3):235–246.

Butler RN *et al.* Is there an anti-aging medicine? *J Gerontol A Biol Sci Med Sci* 2002 Sep;**57**(9):B333–338.

Chomyn A, Attardi G. MtDNA mutations in aging and apoptosis. *Biochem Biophys Res Commun* 2003;**304**(3):519–29.

Knight JA. The biochemistry of aging. *Adv Clin Chem* 2000;**35**:1–62.

ACTIVE LEARNING

1. Discuss the evidence that caloric restriction increases the mean and maximum lifespan of primates.
2. Review recent literature on mouse genetic models of mammalian aging and discuss the relationship between growth rate, obesity, calorie restriction and aging in the mouse.
3. Describe the basis for the decline in renal glomerular and tubular function during aging.
4. Discuss the nature of protein carbonyls and lipofuscin and their relevance to aging.
5. Discuss the relative importance of chemical damage to protein and DNA during aging.

Martin GM, Oshima J. Lessons from human progeroid syndromes. *Nature* 2000 Nov 9;**408**(6809):263–266.

Olshansky SJ *et al.* Position statement on human aging. *J Gerontol A Biol Sci Med Sci* 2002 Aug;**57**(8):B292–297.

Levine RL, Stadtman ER. Oxidative modification of proteins during aging. *Exp Gerontol* 2001;**36**:1495–1502.

Szweda PA *et al.* Proteolysis, free radicals, and aging. *Free Radic Biol Med* 2002 Jul 1;**33**(1):29–36.

Relevant websites

Aging research: http://www.innovitaresearch.org/index.html

Caloric restriction: www.calorierestriction.org

Lecture notes on gerontology:
http://family.georgetown.edu/geriatrics/syllabus/Physio.htm
http://www.pathguy.com/lectures/aging.htm
www.benbest.com/lifeext/aging.html

Progeria: http://www.progeriaresearch.org/index.asp; http://www.hgps.net/

Telomeres: www.medslides.com/member/Oncology/Basic_Science/telomerase.ppt

Reference values and clinical decision limits for laboratory tests
M H Dominiczak

Reference values (also, less accurately, called the normal values) are values of a given substance (analyte) obtained in a reference population, which is usually a group of healthy individuals. If such values demonstrate normal (Gaussian) distribution, the range used as reference is the population mean ± 2 standard deviations (this constitutes the central 95% interval of the distribution). When a non-Gaussian distribution is observed in a population, mathematically transformed (for instance log-transformed) values are used to obtain a normal distribution. The interpretation of results from laboratory tests is based on comparing them with reference values. If the value falls outside the reference interval, it tells one that the result varies from that seen in the reference population. Note that it is not necessarily abnormal: by definition, 5% of individuals in a reference population will have results outwith the reference range. However, the further the result is from the reference range, the greater is the probability that it is associated with a pathology.

In some cases (such as with glucose, lipids, or cardiac troponin measurements), instead of reference values, we use clinical decision limits: these are usually derived from epidemiological studies linking the levels of a particular analyte with either the presence, or the risk of, a particular disease.

Below we have listed reference intervals of more commonly used laboratory tests. Note that reference ranges may be age- and sex-dependent. They also may differ for the arterial and venous blood, and may be affected by posture, fast-feed cycle, and specific diets. The detailed discussion of factors which affect the test results is beyond the scope of this appendix: the reader should refer to the specialist clinical chemistry texts.

The reference values given here are either those used in North Glasgow University Hospitals, Glasgow, UK, or are quoted from publications listed in Further Reading below. These values are given for guidance only: it is good practice to always check the reference ranges used by the laboratory which provided the result. On the other hand, the clinical decision limits for glucose and lipids are laboratory-independent, provided these measurements are performed using standardized methods and appropriate quality control.

REFERENCE VALUES FOR SELECTED LABORATORY TESTS

(Reference ranges are given for serum, unless otherwise stated.)

Selected serum proteins

Total serum protein: 63–86 g/L
Conversion to SI units: g/l = g/dl × 10
Albumin: 35–45 g/L
Urinary protein excretion: <0.15 g/24 h
Microalbuminuria – albumin excretion: >30 μg/24 h or >30 mg/mg creatinine.
C-reactive protein: <10 mg/L
C-reactive protein by a high sensitivity method (quantitation below 10 mg/dL) is used to assess cardiovascular risk
Transthyretin (prealbumin): 0.2–0.5 g/L

Blood gases

Arterial blood hydrogen ion concentration: 36–43 nmol/L (pH 7.37–7.44)
pCO_2: 4.6–6.0 kPa (34–45 mm Hg)
pO_2: 10.5–13.5 kPa (79–101 mm Hg)
Conversion to SI units: kPA × 7.5 = mm Hg
See also Table 23.2 on p. 337.

Calcium and phosphate

Total serum calcium: 2.2–2.60 mmol/L (8.8–10.4 mg/dL)
Conversion to SI units: mmol/l = mg/dL × 0.25
Adjusted calcium: 2.2–2.6 mmol/L (8.8–10.4 mg/dL)
Ionized calcium: 1.1–1.3 mmol/L (4.4–5.2 mg/dL)
Phosphate: 0.7–1.4 mmol/L [2.2-5.6 mg/dL]),
Conversion to SI units: mmol/L = mg/dL × 0.323
Parathyroid hormone PTH (intact PTH): 1.1–6.9 pmol/L (11–69 mg/mL)

Cerebrospinal fluid (CSF)

Ratio of CSF glucose to blood glucose: 0.65
CSF lactate: <2.2 mmol/L (<20 mg/dL)
Conversion to SI units: mmol/L = mg/dL × 0.111

Coagulation tests

Platelet count in blood: 150–400 × 190/L
Activated partial thromboplastin time (APTT): 30–50 seconds
Prothrombin time (PT): 10–15 seconds
Thrombin time: 10–15 seconds
Fibrin D-dimer: <0.25 g/L

Electrolytes (the urea and electrolytes) profile

Sodium: 135–145 mmol/L
Potassium: 3.5–5.0 mmol/L
Bicarbonate: 20–25 mmol/L
Urea: 2.5–6.5 mmol/L (16.2–39 mg/dL)
Conversion to SI units: mmol/L × 6.02 = mg/dL
Blood urea nitrogen: 3–6.4 mmol/L (8-18) mg/dL
Conversion to SI units: mmol/L = mg/dL × 0.357
Creatinine: 20–80 μmol/L (0.23–0.90 mg/dL)
Conversion to SI units: μmol/L × 0.0113 = mg/dL
Anion gap: upper limit 5–15 mmol
Osmolality: 285–295 mmol/L
Magnesium: 0.7–1.0 mmol/L (1.7–2.4 mg/dL)
Conversion to SI units: mmol/L = mg/dL × 0.411

Selected endocrine tests

Thyroid function tests:
TSH range 0.4–4 mU/L
Conversion to SI units: mU/L = μU/dL
Thyroxine (T4) 55–144 nmol/L (4.2–11 μg/dL)
Conversion to SI units: nmol/l = μg/dL × 12.87
Tri-iodothyronine (T3) (0.9–2.8 nmol/L) (0.6–1.8 ng/mL).
Conversion to SI units: nmol/L = ng/mL × 1.54
Cortisol
Cortisol at 08.00 h: 190–690 nmol/L (7–25 μg/dL)
Cortisol at 24.00 h: <50 nmol/L <2 μg/dL
Urinary free cortisol: <250 nmol/24 h;
Conversion to SI units: nmol/L = μg/dL × 27.59
ACTH: <80 ng/L

Conversion to SI units: ng/L = pg/ml
17-hydroxyprogesterone: <50 nmol/L (< 16 pg/L)
Conversion to SI units: nmol/l = 3.026 × pg/L
Aldosterone: supine 83–277 pmol/L (3–10 ng/dL); upright 139–832 pmol/L (5–30 ng/dL)
Conversion to SI units: pmol/L = 27.74 × ng/dL
Dietary salt affects results

Full blood count

Hematocrit: 0.41–0.46
Hemoglobin: men g/L 13–18 g/dL; women 12–16 g/dl
g/l = g/dL × 10
Erythrocyte count: men 4.4–5.9 × 10^6/μL; women 3.8–5.2 × 10^6/mm^3
Mean corpuscular volume: (normal 80–100 fL).
White blood cell count: 4–11 × 103/mm^3
Platelet count: 150–400 × 103/mm^3
Note: mm^3 = μL
Carboxyhemoglobin fraction of total Hb: (normal = 0.5–1.0%).
See also Table 4.2 on p. 48.

Glucose and glycated hemoglobin

Plasma glucose normal range: 4.0–6.0 mmol/L (72–109 mg/dL)
Conversion to SI units: mmol/L × 18 = mg/dL
Fasting (no caloric intake for approx 10 h): below 6.1 mmol/L (<110 mg/dL).
Impaired fasting glucose (IFG): above 6.1 mmol/L but below 7.0 mmol/L (126 mg/dL)
Diabetes: 7.0 mmol/L (126 mg/dL) or above.

Oral glucose tolerance test (OGTT) plasma glucose rises to a peak concentration after approximately 60 min and returns to a near-fasting concentration within 120 min. If it remains above 11.1 mmol/L (200 mg/dL/min) in the 120-min sample, the patient has diabetes, even if the fasting blood glucose is normal. If fasting blood glucose is normal but post-load glucose is between 6.1 and 7.8 mmol/L (= 100 mg/dL and = 140 mg/dL), the condition is classified as impaired glucose tolerance (IGT).

HbA1c: 4–6% of total HbA. Levels below 7% indicate acceptable control of diabetes. Higher levels suggest poor control

See also Table 20.5 on p. 287.

Lipids

Total cholesterol desirable; <5 mmol/L (190 mg/dL)
LDL-cholesterol: optimal <2.6 mmol/L (<100 mg/dL)
HDL-cholesterol: low <1 mmol/L (40 mg/dL);
    high >1.6 mmol/L (60 mg/dL)
Conversion to SI units: mmol/L = mg/dL × 02586

Triglycerides (triacylglycerols)
Desirable: below 1.7 mmol/L (150 mg/dL)
Conversion to SI units: mmol/L = mg/dL × 0.01129

Liver function tests

Bilirubin: <17 mmol/L (<1.0 mg/dL)
Conversion to SI units: mmol/L = mg/dl × 17.1
Aspartate transaminase AST: 5–45 U/L
Alanine transaminase ALT: 5–40 U/L
Alkaline phosphatase (ALP): 50–260 U/L; (ALP is
    physiologically elevated in children and adolescents).
Gamma-glutamyl transpeptidase (GGT): men <90U/L,
    women <50 U/L
These are given in the legend to Table 28.2, p. 409.

Key metabolites

Ammonia: 15–88 μmol/L (25–150 μg/dL)
Conversion to SI units: μmol/l × 1.7 = μg/dl
Lactate: 0.7–1.8 mmol/L (6–16 mg/dL)
Conversion to SI units: mmol/L = mg/dL × 0.111
Porphobilinogen, urine: <9 μmol/24h (<2 mg/24h)
Conversion to SI units: umoL/24 h = mg/24 h × 4.42
Pyruvate, arterial: 02–08 mmol/L (0.2–0.7 mg/dL)
Conversion to SI units: –0.10 (0.3–0.9 mg/dL)
Conversion to SI units: mmol/L = mg/dL × 0.114
Urate: 0.20–0.5 mmol/L (3.5–8.0 mg/dL) men; 0.1–
    0.4 mmol/L (2.5–6.2 mg/dL) women;
Conversion to SI units: mmol/l = mg/dL × 0.0595

Diagnosis of myocardial infarction

Cardiac troponins (note that clinical decision limits for
    cardiac troponins may vary in different laboratories)
Troponin T: >0.1 ng/ng/mL
Troponin I: >2.5 ng/mL
Creatine kinase CK: <210 U/L
Creatine kinase MB fraction CK-MB CK/CK-MB: = <6%

Neurotransmitters and their metabolites

Norepinephrine: 1094–1625 pmol/L (185–275 ng/L)
Urine norepinephrine: <900 nmol/24 h (<152 mg/24 h)
Conversion to SI units: pmol/L = ng/L × 5.9
Epinephrine: 164–464 pmol/L (30–85 ng/L)
Conversion to SI units: pmol/L = ng/L × 5.5
Urine epinephrine: <230 nmol/24 h (<42 mg/24 h)
Urine vanillylmandelic acid reference range: <35.5
    mmol/24 h (<7.0 mg/24 h)
Conversion to SI units: umol/24 h = mg/24h × 5.05
Urine 5-hydroxy indoleacetic acid (5-HIAA), the major
    metabolite of 5-HT; reference range: 10–52 mmol/24 h
    (3–14 mg/24 h)
Conversion to SI units: mmol/24 h = mg/24 h × 5.24

Marker of pancreatitis

Amylase: 0–100 U

Trace metals and metal-binding proteins

Copper: 12–25 μmol/L (80–160 μg/dL)
Conversion to SI units: umol/l = μg/dL × 0.157
Urinary copper excretion: 0.2–1.6 μmol/24 h
    (6–10 mg/24h)
Conversion to SI units: mmol/24 = μg/24h × 0.0157
Ceruloplasmin: 200–450 mg/L (20–45 mg/dL)
Iron: 10–30 μmol/L (56–167 mg/dL)
Conversion to SI units: mmol/l = μg/dl × 0.179
Ferritin: 30–280 mg/L. Conversion to SI units: mg/L =
    ng/mL
Selenium: 0.8–2.0 μmol/L (6-16 mg/dL)
Conversion to SI units: mmol/L = mg/dL × 7.9
Zinc: 9–20 μmol/L (60–130 μg/dl)
Conversion to SI units: mmol/l = mg/dL × 0.1530
Transferrin: 2.2–4.0 g/L

VITAMINS

Vitamin A: 1.05–2.8 µmol/L (300–800 µg/dL)
Conversion to SI units: mmol/L= mg/dL × 0.0349
Vitamin B_6 pyridoxal phosphate: 5–50 µg/L deficiency <3 µg/L
Vitamin B_{12}: 148–590 pmol/L (200–800 pg/mL)
Conversion to SI units: pmol/L = pg/ml × 0.7378
Vitamin C plasma: 0.6–2.0 mg/dL acceptable level plasma 0.30 mg/dL; leukocytes >15 mg/dL. Conversion to SI units: mmol/l = mg/dL × 56.8
Vitamin D25-OHD$_3$: Winter 35–104 pmol/L (14–42 ng/mL); Summer 37–197 pmol/L (15–80 ng/mL)
Conversion to SI units: pmol/L = ng/ml × 2.469
Vitamin E: 11.6–37.1 µmol/L (0.5–1.6 mg/dL)
Conversion to SI units: µmol/L = ug/dL × 23.22
Folate: ≥7 nmol/L (3 ng/mL)
Conversion to SI units: nmol/l = ng/ml × 2.27
Red blood cell folate: 362–1586 nmol/L (160–700 ng/mL)
Conversion to SI units: nmol/L = ng/mL × 2.266

Further reading

Bakerman, S (revised by Bakerman P and Strausbauch P). *Bakerman's ABC's of interpretive laboratory data.* 4th edn. Scottsdale AZ: Interpretive Laboratory Data; 2002: pp 580.

Dominiczak MH (Ed.) *Seminars in Clinical Biochemistry.* Glasgow: University of Glasgow; 1997: pp 415.

Jakob M. *Normal values pocket.* Hermosa Beach CA: Borm Bruckmeier; 2002: pp 220.

Burtis C, Ashwood ER. *Tietz textbook of clinical chemistry.* 3rd Edn., Philadelphia PA, USA: Saunders; 1999: pp 1917.

Note: Every effort has been made to ensure the accuracy of data given in this appendix. However, you should always verify normal ranges used by the local laboratory, particularly when treatment is to be based on laboratory results.

Multiple Choice Questions (MCQs)

Chapter 2

1. What is the approximate isoelectric point (pI) of (i) glycine? (ii) glutamine? (iii) glutamate? (iv) lysine?
(a) 6, the average of the pKa of the amino and carboxyl groups.
(b) 6, the average of the pKa of the amino and carboxyl groups.
(c) 4; the mean of the pKa of the carboxyl groups.
(d) 9, the mean of the pKa of the amino groups.

2. In which direction will the tetrapeptide, Gly-Lys-Glu-Ala, migrate during electrophoresis at (i) pH 4? (ii) pH 7? (iii) pH 9?
(a) Toward the cathode; the peptide has a positive charge at acidic pH.
(b) Neither; the peptide has no net charge at neutral pH.
(c) Toward the anode; the peptide has a negative charge at basic pH.
(d) Neither; the peptide will have no net charge.

3. Which of the following does not contribute to the tertiary structure of a protein?
(a) Hydrogen bonds between side chains of amino acids.
(b) Hydrogen bonds between amine and carbonyl groups in the peptide backbone.
(c) Disulfide bonds between cysteine residues.
(d) Hydrophobic interactions between side chains of amino acids.
(e) Salt bridges between ionized groups in side chains of amino acids.

4. Which of the following proteins does not have a significant quaternary structure?
(a) Collagen.
(b) Hemoglobin.
(c) Superoxide dismutase.
(d) Carbonic anhydrase.

5. Gel filtration chromatography is a method for fractionation of proteins on the basis of:
(a) Size.
(b) Charge.
(c) Hydrophobicity.
(d) Isoelectric point.
(e) Posttranslational modifications.

6. Which of the following methods is commonly used to estimate the size of the subunits of a protein?
(a) Isoelectric focusing.
(b) Sodium dodecylsulfate polyacrylamide gel electrophoresis.
(c) Amino acid analysis.
(d) Ion exchange chromatography.
(e) Salting out from solution.

Chapter 3

7. Which of the following is not a function of albumin?
(a) Transport of hormones.
(b) Osmoregulation.
(c) Solubilization of glucose.
(d) Transport of bilirubin.

8. Transferrin is involved in the following (indicate true or false):
(a) Transport of iron.
(b) Utilization of iron.
(c) Hormone metabolism.
(d) Diagnosis of Wilson's disease.

9. The principal plasma protein responsible for exerting colloid osmotic pressure is:
(a) Hemoglobin.
(b) Albumin.
(c) Haptoglobin.
(d) CRP.

10. Which of the following does not increase as part of the acute phase response?
(a) CRP.
(b) α_1-antitrypsin.
(c) Albumin.
(d) Fibrinogen.

11. Which of the following statements about paraproteins are correct (indicate true or false)?
(a) Paraprotein bands usually consist of structurally identical immunoglobulins.
(b) Paraproteins derive from plasma cells resulting from a single B-cell clone.
(c) Paraproteins are exclusively seen with malignant disease.

(d) Bence Jones proteins are seen only in the presence of serum paraproteins.

(e) IgE is the most common paraprotein.

Chapter 4

12. The primary form in which oxygen is transported in blood is:

(a) In solution in plasma as dissolved oxygen.

(b) In the red cell bound to hemoglobin.

(c) In plasma bound to myoglobin.

(d) In solution in ionized form as bicarbonate.

13. Which of the following elements is not normally involved in coordination to iron in hemoglobin?

(a) Iron.

(b) Nitrogen.

(c) Oxygen.

(d) Sulfur.

14. Which protein has the strongest affinity for oxygen?

(a) Albumin.

(b) Myoglobin.

(c) Hemoglobin A.

(d) Hemoglobin F.

15. Which of the following changes increases the oxygen affinity of hemoglobin?

(a) Shifting the equilibrium toward the R-state.

(b) Decreasing the pH of the solution.

(c) Increasing the concentration of CO_2.

(d) Increasing the concentration of 2,3-bisphosphoglycerate.

16. The Bohr Effect refers to:

(a) The right shift in the oxygen saturation curve of hemoglobin at lower pH.

(b) The binding of H^+ concomitant with binding of oxygen to hemoglobin.

(c) The decrease in P_{50} for oxygen binding at lower pH.

(d) The decrease in oxygen affinity of hemoglobin on binding of CO_2.

17. Which of the following substitutions at Glutamate[6] would cause a decrease in the pI of hemoglobin?

(a) Glutamine.

(b) Lysine.

(c) Aspartate.

(d) Glycine.

(e) None of the above.

Chapter 5

18. Enzymes increase reaction rates by:

(a) Altering the change in free energy of the reaction.

(b) Inhibiting the rate of reverse reactions.

(c) Changing the equilibrium constant of the reaction.

(d) Decreasing the energy of activation.

(e) Selectively enhancing the rate of the forward reaction.

19. An example of irreversible regulation of enzyme activities is:

(a) Phosphorylation by protein kinases.

(b) Allosteric regulation by substrates.

(c) Dissociation of subunit into oligomeric enzymes.

(d) Inhibition by competitive inhibitors.

(e) Proteolytic conversion of digestive enzymes.

20. The Michaelis constant (K_m) is:

(a) Not changed by the presence of a noncompetitive inhibitor.

(b) The substrate concentration at $v = \frac{1}{2}V_{max}$.

(c) The intercept on the $1/v$ axis of a Lineweaver–Burk plot.

(d) Equal to $\frac{1}{2}V_{max}$.

(e) The equilibrium constant for the dissociation of ES to E + P.

21. Captopril, a competitive inhibitor for angiotensin converting enzyme, can be used as a therapeutic agent for hypertension. Competitive inhibitors change:

(a) The V_{max} of the reaction.

(b) The K_m of the reaction.

(c) Both the V_{max} and K_m of the reaction.

(d) The substrate specificity of the enzyme.

(e) None of the above.

22. Choose the correct description of an enzymatic reaction.

(a) An enzyme that catalyzes $A + B \rightarrow C + D$ accelerates the reaction velocity of $A + B \rightarrow C + D$, but does not accelerate the reaction velocity of $C + D \rightarrow A + B$.

(b) Enzymes decrease the activation energy of reactions, but do not affect the free-energy change, ΔG.

(c) Enzymes can change the reaction velocity without directly interacting with substrates.

(d) Enzymes mainly consist of proteins. Coenzymes are small compounds that support the structure of the enzyme, but are not involved in the reaction.

(e) Since enzymes catalyze chemical reactions in much the same manner as inorganic catalysts, the higher the reaction temperature, the higher the reaction velocity becomes.

23. Which of the following amino acids would **not** be involved in the catalytic triad in the active site of a serine protease?
(a) Aspartate.
(b) Histidine.
(c) Leucine.
(d) Serine.

Chapter 6

24. Which, if any, of the following compounds are inhibitors of platelet aggregation?
(a) Adenosine diphosphate.
(b) Aspirin.
(c) Thromboxane A_2.
(d) Clopidogrel.
(e) Prostacyclin.

25. Which, if any, of the following statements is/are true of classical hemophilia (factor VIII deficiency)?
(a) Autosomal dominant inheritance.
(b) Prolonged prothrombin time.
(c) Prolonged activated partial thromboplastin time.
(d) Aspirin administration is safe.
(e) Prolonged skin bleeding time.

26. Which, if any, of the following statements is/are true of von Willebrand's disease (vWF deficiency)?
(a) Autosomal dominant inheritance.
(b) Prolonged prothrombin time.
(c) Prolonged activated partial thromboplastin time.
(d) Aspirin administration is safe.
(e) Prolonged skin bleeding time.

27. Which, if any, of the following statements is/are true of warfarin?
(a) Competitive antagonist of vitamin K.
(b) Co-administration of aspirin is safe.
(c) Prolonged prothrombin time.
(d) Reduces synthesis of coagulation factor VIII.
(e) Reduces synthesis of coagulation factor VII.

28. Which, if any, of the following statements is/are true of tissue-type plasminogen activator (t-PA)?
(a) Used in treatment of acute myocardial infarction.
(b) Inhibited by α_2 antiplasmin.
(c) Synthesized by vascular endothelial cells.
(d) Activity is stimulated by fibrin.
(e) High therapeutic doses can cause excessive bleeding.

29. Which, if any, of the following statements is/are true of antithrombin?
(a) Cofactor for the anticoagulant drug, warfarin.
(b) Inactivates coagulation factor VIII.

(c) Inactivates coagulation factor X.
(d) Congenital deficiency causes excessive bleeding.
(e) Inheritance of deficiency is autosomal dominant.

30. Which, if any, of the following statements is/are true of thrombin?
(a) It stimulates platelet aggregation.
(b) Its formation is reduced by warfarin.
(c) Its formation is reduced in patients with protein C deficiency.
(d) It promotes activation of protein C.
(e) It promotes crosslinking of fibrin strands.

31. Which, if any, of the following statements is/are true of vitamin K?
(a) Deficiency reduces prothrombin levels.
(b) Deficiency reduces antithrombin levels.
(c) It can be given to treat excessive warfarin activity.
(d) Deficiency reduces protein C levels.
(e) Low levels are observed in patients with liver disease.

32. Which, if any, of the following statements is/are true of plasma fibrinogen?
(a) Low levels prolong the skin bleeding time.
(b) Low levels prolong the thrombin time.
(c) Binds to the platelet receptor Gp Ib/IX.
(d) Low levels follow thrombolytic therapy.
(e) High levels are associated with thrombosis.

Chapter 7

33. Which of the following statements about membrane lipids is/are true?
(a) Membrane structure can be modeled by phospholipid bilayers or liposomes.
(b) Phospholipids are amphipathic compounds.
(c) Flip-flop movement of phospholipids is catalyzed by an energy-dependent enzyme called flippase.
(d) Compared with unsaturated fatty acids, saturated fatty acids have lower melting points and are more fluid.

34. Of the following characteristics of biomembranes, which is/are true?
(a) They act as a barrier to gases such as CO_2 and O_2.
(b) Ion gradients are formed across membranes.
(c) They are composed of phospholipids and proteins.
(d) They are freely permeable to ionic compounds.

35. Which of the following statements about transporters is/are true?
(a) Transporters use only ATP for driving chemical gradients.
(b) Facilitated diffusion is a passive transport process.

(c) Transporters are distributed in various cell-surface and intracellular membranes.

(d) Transporters are intrinsic transmembrane proteins.

36. Which of the following statements about protein-mediated transport kinetics is/are true?

(a) K_m for transport corresponds to the substrate concentration which gives the half-maximal transport rate.

(b) Glucose transporters with greater K_m values respond to increases in glucose concentration upon food intake.

(c) The transport rate is directly proportional to the substrate concentration.

(d) Glucose transport is stereospecific.

37. Which of the following statements about the glucose transporter is/are true?

(a) The GLUT family of transporters transport glucose by facilitated diffusion.

(b) The Na^+-coupled SGLT family of transporters transport glucose against a concentration gradient.

(c) In insulin-sensitive cells, GLUT-4 sequestered in the cytoplasmic vesicle is translocated to the plasma membrane in response to insulin stimulation.

(d) Sulfonylureas bind to the glucose transporter on pancreatic β-cells.

38. Which of the following statements about Ca^{2+} mobilization in muscle cells is/are true?

(a) Cytoplasmic Ca^{2+} is sequestered within the sarcoplasmic reticulum.

(b) Ca^{2+}-ATPase increases cytoplasmic Ca^{2+} concentration upon muscle contraction.

(c) Ca^{2+}-ATPase is a primary active transporter.

(d) Relaxation of muscle is associated with the decrease of cytoplasmic Ca^{2+} concentration.

Chapter 8

39. Succinate is added to a suspension of freshly isolated mitochondria in phosphate buffer. Respiration starts when ADP is added at point (A), stops on addition of unknown compound at point (B), but begins again when DNP is added at point (C). What is the most likely identity of the compound added at (B)?

(a) Oligomycin.
(b) Cyanide.
(c) Rotenone.
(d) Antimycin A.
(e) Malate.

40. Which of the following does not contribute to the chemiosmotic force required for ATP synthesis?

(a) The pH gradient across the inner mitochondrial membrane.

(b) The voltage gradient across the inner mitochondrial membrane.

(c) The hydrogen ion gradient across the inner mitochondrial membrane.

(d) The pumping of protons by the several electron transport complexes in the inner mitochondrial membrane.

(e) The phosphate concentration gradient across the inner mitochondrial membrane.

41. Which one of the following reduces oxygen to water?

(a) Q-cytochrome c reductase.
(b) ATP synthase.
(c) TCA cycle.
(d) Cytochrome c oxidase.
(e) Glycerol-3-P dehydrogenase.

42. All of the following are true regarding mitochondrial cytochromes, except:

(a) They all contain heme groups.

(b) Iron must remain in the ferrous state for them to function in electron transport.

(c) All are bound to protein components.

(d) They are found in complex III, IV, and cytochrome c, but not complex I and II.

(e) They accept or donate one electron at a time.

43. Which of the following compounds or complexes would exist in the most oxidized state in mitochondria treated with antimycin?

(a) $FAD/FADH_2$
(b) $NAD^+/NADH$
(c) Complex I (NADH-Q reductase)
(d) Complex II (Succinate-Q reductase)
(e) Complex IV (cytochrome oxidase complex)

44. Which of the following changes would **not** occur on treatment of respiring mitochondria with dinitrophenol?

(a) Decrease in the rate of ATP synthesis.
(b) Increase in the P:O ratio.
(c) Increase in the rate of fuel consumption.
(d) Increase in the rate of oxygen consumption.
(e) Increase in heat production.

Chapter 9

45. The digestion of carbohydrates is:
(a) Associated with increased uptake of glycerol by the intestinal epithelial cell.
(b) Associated with increased osmolality of the gut lumen fluid.
(c) Associated with decreased osmolality of the gut lumen fluid.
(d) Initiated by enzymes secreted by the gastric mucosa.

46. Lactase produced at the intestinal brush border:
(a) Is an inducible enzyme dependent on the amount of lactose in the diet.
(b) Produces equivalent amounts of galactose and fructose.
(c) Produces equivalent amounts of glucose and galactose.
(d) Is associated with delivery of gut digest to the lacteals.

47. Which of the following enzymes are involved in the digestion and absorption of protein?
(a) Trypsinogen.
(b) Amylase.
(c) Phospholipase A_2.
(d) Pepsin.

48. Di- and tripeptides are absorbed by the intestinal epithelial cell by a process of:
(a) Passive diffusion.
(b) Na^+-dependent carrier-mediated system.
(c) H^+-dependent carrier-mediated system.
(d) Surface membrane-directed hydrolysis and absorption of amino acids.

49. Which of the following is associated with the process of fat digestion?
(a) Increased production of surfactants.
(b) Stimulation of carbohydrate digestive enzymes.
(c) Hydrolysis of triglycerides to 1-monoacylglycerol.
(d) Increased acid production and change in blood pH.

50. Micelles:
(a) Are the same as emulsion droplets in terms of size and composition.
(b) Formation is independent of bile salt concentrations.
(c) Are not involved in increasing lipid absorption.
(d) Are equilibrium structures dependent on bile salt concentrations.

Chapter 10

51. Eating no animal products may lead to deficiencies of:
(a) Vit B_{12}.
(b) Vit C.
(c) Iron.
(d) Calcium.
(e) Potassium.

Chapter 11

52. Which of the following compounds inhibits ATP production during glycolysis in a manner most analogous to the effect of Dinitrophenol during oxidative phosphorylation?
(a) Fluoride.
(b) ATP.
(c) AMP.
(d) Iodoacetamide
(e) Arsenate.

53. Enzymes that catalyze the equilibrium between aldoses and ketoses are known as:
(a) Mutases.
(b) Isomerases.
(c) Aldolases.
(d) Epimerases.
(e) Reductases.

54. Which two of the following enzymes produce a product used for synthesis of ATP by substrate-level phosphorylation?
(a) Phosphofructokinase-1.
(b) Aldolase.
(c) Glyceraldehyde-3-phosphate dehydrogenase.
(d) 1,3-bisphosphoglycerate mutase.
(e) Enolase.

55. The raison *d'être* for lactate dehydrogenase in the red blood cell is:
(a) To produce lactate from pyruvate so that it can be excreted from the cell.
(b) To produce lactate from pyruvate, providing additional negative free energy for driving glycolysis.
(c) To recycle NADH to NAD^+ for use in glycolysis.
(d) To convert the unstable metabolite, pyruvate, into the stable product, lactate.
(e) To produce NADPH for antioxidant protection.

56. 2,3-bisphosphoglycerate is:
(a) A high-energy substrate used for substrate-level phosphorylation.
(b) An intermediate in the *interconversion* stage of the pentose phosphate pathway.

(c) A product of the phosphoglycerate kinase reaction.
(d) An allosteric effector that decreases the O_2 affinity of Hb.
(e) The product of the glyceraldehyde 3-phosphate dehydrogenase reaction.

57. Which of the following is the primary function of the pentose phosphate pathway in the red cell?
(a) Provision of ribose for synthesis of ribonucleic acid.
(b) Provision of deoxyribose for synthesis of deoxyribonucleic acid.
(c) Synthesis of NADPH for electron transport.
(d) Synthesis of NADPH for maintenance of antioxidant defenses
(e) Synthesis of NADPH for biosynthesis of fatty acids and cholesterol

Chapter 12

58. Why is muscle glycogen not available for maintenance of blood glucose concentration?
(a) There is insufficient glycogen in muscle for maintenance of blood glucose concentration.
(b) Muscle lacks glycogenolytic enzymes required for response to blood glucagon.
(c) Muscle lacks glucagon receptors, so it does not respond to blood glucose concentration.
(d) Muscle lacks Glc-6-Pase activity, so it cannot form free glucose from glycogen.
(e) The muscle glucose transporter, GLUT-4, is internalized when blood insulin is low.

59. Which of the following mechanisms does **not** contribute to the increase in glycolysis in muscle during prolonged exercise?
(a) Activation of phosphorylase by phosphorylation in response to epinephrine.
(b) Activation of phosphorylase in response to the increase in muscle cytoplasmic Ca^{2+}.
(c) Activation of PFK-1 by Fru-2,6-BP.
(d) Activation of phosphorylase in response to an increase in cAMP.
(e) Activation of phosphorylase in response to the gradual increase in blood glucagon concentration during exercise.

60. What controls the rate of glucose entry into muscle and adipose tissue for energy storage?
(a) The rate of phosphorylation of glucose by glucokinase.
(b) The concentration of glucose in blood.
(c) The rate of perfusion of the tissue by blood.
(d) The intracellular ratio of cAMP to ATP concentrations.
(e) The concentration of GLUT-4 in muscle or adipocyte plasma membranes.

61. During the early stages of dieting, it is relatively easy to lose a few pounds rapidly, but then the rate of weight loss slows down to less than 250 g/day. Why?
(a) People are generally less committed to their weight-losing diet after the first few days.
(b) The initial weight loss is the result of loss of water from blood and extravascular fluids.
(c) The initial weight loss results from rapid consumption of liver and muscle glycogen.
(d) The body switches from glucose to protein as its major source of energy.

62. What is primary the metabolic fate of lactate released from muscle during intense exercise?
(a) Excretion in urine as sodium lactate.
(b) Gluconeogenesis in liver for replenishment of blood glucose.
(c) Conversion into pyruvate for aerobic metabolism in liver and other tissues.
(d) Gradual reuptake in muscle for metabolism during the recovery phase following exercise.

63. What is the major mechanism for inhibition of glycolysis in liver during gluconeogenesis?
(a) GK is inhibited by the high concentration of Glc-6-P.
(b) Phosphorylation of PFK-2/Fru-2,6-BPase leads to decreased levels of Fru-2,6-BP, which is an allosteric activator of PFK-1.
(c) Increased hepatic acetyl-CoA inhibits the activity of PDH.
(d) Hydrolysis of Glc-6-P to glucose decreases the availability of Glc-6-P for glycolysis.

64. Which one of the following will yield a net synthesis of glucose?
(a) Acetoacetic acid.
(b) Leucine.
(c) Palmitic acid.
(d) Acetic acid.
(e) Glutamic acid.

Chapter 13

65. Malonate is:
(a) A competitive inhibitor of malate dehydrogenase.
(b) An allosteric inhibitor of the TCA cycle.
(c) An alternative substrate for succinate dehydrogenase.
(d) A reversible inhibitor of succinate dehydrogenase.
(e) A suicide substrate for succinate thiokinase.

66. Which one of the following statements is most true of the TCA cycle?
(a) It participates in the synthesis of glucose from pyruvic acid.
(b) Some of the enzymes are located in the cytoplasm.
(c) It is an endergonic series of reactions.
(d) Two NADH are produced per turn.
(e) It requires the coenzymes biotin, FAD, NAD^+, and Coenzyme A.

67. Starting with one mole of succinic acid and ending with one mole of oxaloacetic acid, how many maximum moles of ATP could the TCA cycle produce when coupled to the electron transport system and ATP synthase?
(a) 2.
(b) 3.
(c) 4.
(d) 5.
(e) 6.

68. All of the following are true of the TCA cycle except which one?
(a) It begins with the condensation of acetyl-CoA and oxaloacetic acid.
(b) If the cycle begins with one mole of oxaloacetic acid and one mole of acetyl-CoA, one mole of oxaloacetic acid will be regenerated.
(c) The cycle requires molecular oxygen (O_2) in one of its enzymatic reactions.
(d) The cleavage of two thioester linkages helps drive the cycle to make it exergonic.
(e) GTP is produced by a substrate-level phosphorylation in the cycle.

69. Which of the following compounds is both an inhibitor of pyruvate dehydrogenase and an activator of pyruvate carboxylase?
(a) NADH.
(b) $FADH_2$.
(c) ATP.
(d) AMP.
(e) Acetyl-CoA

70. Which of the following statements about regulation of pyruvate dehydrogenase is correct?
(a) PDH is activated by increasing NADH concentration in the mitochondrion.
(b) PDH is activated by phosphorylation by PDH kinase.
(c) PDH is activated allosterically by ATP.
(d) PDH is inactivated by phosphorylation by cAMP-dependent protein kinase.
(e) PDH and pyruvate carboxylase are reciprocally regulated by acetyl CoA.

71. A major function of the tricarboxylic acid cycle is:
(a) Generation of CO_2 from energy substrates.
(b) Oxidation of acetate to oxaloacetate.
(c) Disposal of acetic acid generated during oxidation of energy substrates.
(d) Oxidation of acetate and reduction of nucleotide coenzymes.
(e) Generation of heat from redox reactions to maintain body temperature.

72. Which of the following vitamins or coenzymes does not participate in the oxidative decarboxylation of pyruvate?
(a) Lipoic acid.
(b) Thiamin.
(c) Biotin.
(d) Niacin.
(e) Riboflavin.

73. Which of the following reactions does not catalyze a decarboxylation reaction?
(a) Pyruvate dehydrogenase.
(b) Isocitrate dehydrogenase.
(c) α-ketoglutarate dehydrogenase.
(d) PEP carboxykinase.
(e) Pyruvate carboxylase.

Chapter 14

74. β-oxidation of fatty acids in liver:
(a) Requires fatty acids with an even number of carbon atoms.
(b) Produces only acetyl-CoA.
(c) Requires the citric acid cycle for ATP production.
(d) Degrades fatty acids to CO_2 and H_2O.
(e) Occurs primarily in the mitochondrial matrix.

75. Which of the following intermediates in the oxidation of odd-chain fatty acids is likely to appear in the urine in vitamin B_{12} deficiency?
(a) Formic acid.
(b) Methylmalonic acid.
(c) Pentanoic acid.
(d) Propionic acid.
(e) Succinic acid.

76. Which of the following fatty acids would yield the highest level of gluconeogenic precursors?
(a) C-16:0 (palmitic acid).
(b) C-17:0 (heptadecanoic acid).
(c) C-18:0 (stearic acid).
(d) C-20:5 (arachidonic acid).
(e) C-20 polyisoprenoid (phytanic acid).

77. Carnitine has an active role:
(a) In transport of fatty acids across the plasma membrane into the cytosol.
(b) In activation of fatty acids in the cytosol.
(c) As an allosteric regulator of acyl-CoA dehydrogenase.
(d) In transport of fatty acids across the mitochondrial inner membrane.
(e) As a carrier of acetate during conversion of acetyl-CoA to ketone bodies.

78. Most of the redox nucleotides produced in liver during oxidation of fatty acids are produced:
(a) By the carnitine cycle.
(b) During β-oxidation.
(c) In the TCA cycle.
(d) During ketogenesis.
(e) In peroxisomes.

79. Which of the following statements about ketogenesis is false?
(a) Ketone bodies appear in urine during fasting and starvation.
(b) Ketone bodies are produced during times when the liver is gluconeogenic.
(c) Ketogenesis is a mechanism for regeneration of CoA in the mitochondrion.
(d) Ketone bodies have more caloric value per gram than glucose.
(e) Ketone bodies are a major source of energy in the liver during fasting and starvation.

Chapter 15

80. Which one of the following statements is correct?
(a) Fatty acid biosynthesis is a series of oxidation reactions.
(b) Fatty acid biosynthesis requires NAD^+ as a cofactor.
(c) Fatty acid biosynthesis requires NADPH as a cofactor.
(d) Fatty acid biosynthesis is a mitochondrial function.

81. The role of the citrate in fatty acid biosynthesis is:
(a) To activate fatty acid synthetase.
(b) To activate acetyl-CoA carboxylase.
(c) To act as a precursor for addition of carbon.
(d) To inhibit oxidation of fatty acids.

82. Which of the following is not a property of the fatty acid synthase complex?
(a) A multienzyme complex.
(b) Requires pantothenic acid as a cofactor.
(c) Requires biotin as a cofactor.
(d) Is found within the cytosol.

83. Which of the following is true in fatty acid elongation?
(a) It is a requirement in the provision of essential fatty acids.
(b) It is a single chemical reaction.
(c) It is a mitochondrial and not a cytoplasmic function.
(d) It is a series of reactions requiring CoA and NADPH.

84. Which of the following is true for synthesis of TAG in the liver?
(a) It is usually accompanied by increased glycolysis.
(b) It is associated with gluconeogenesis.
(c) It occurs in the mitochondria.
(d) It requires cytochrome b_5.

85. Which of the following statements is true of lipoprotein lipase?
(a) It is an extracellular enzyme.
(b) It is important in the release of fatty acids from adipose tissue.
(c) Is induced and activated by insulin.
(d) Is transported from the liver bound to VLDL.

Chapter 16

86. Which of the following enzymes is the rate-limiting enzyme in the biosynthesis of cholesterol?
(a) HMG-CoA synthase.
(b) HMG-CoA reductase.
(c) Mevalonate kinase.
(d) cis-Prenyl transferase.
(e) Squalene synthase.

87. Which of the following statements about the structure of cholesterol are true?
(a) It contains 27 carbon atoms.
(b) It contains only carbon, hydrogen, and one oxygen atom.
(c) It is saturated (no double bonds).
(d) It contains four hexane rings fused together.

88. Which of the following are biologically active steroid hormones?
(a) Cortisol.
(b) Aldosterone.
(c) Testosterone.
(d) Cholesterol.
(e) Estradiol.

89. Which of the following statements is true?
(a) Membranes contain equal amounts of protein and carbohydrate.
(b) Phospholipids are amphipathic.
(c) Cholesterol-rich regions increase membrane fluidity.

(d) Membrane rigidity is reduced by saturated fatty acids.
(e) Cholesterol is almost absent from plasma membranes.

90. Which of the following is the biologically active form of vitamin D?
(a) Cholecalciferol.
(b) 24-hydroxycholecalciferol.
(c) 25-hydroxycholecalciferol.
(d) 1,25-dihydroxycholecalciferol.
(e) 24,25-dihydroxycholecalciferol.

91. Which of the following is a primary bile acid?
(a) Glycocholic acid.
(b) Glycochenodeoxycholic acid.
(c) Deoxycholic acid.
(d) Taurocholic acid.
(e) Taurochenodeoxycholic acid.

92. Individual variation in cholesterol is genetically determined in:
(a) 10%.
(b) 20%.
(c) 30%.
(d) 50%.
(e) 80%.

Chapter 17

93. Apoprotein B48 is:
(a) The main apoprotein of LDL.
(b) The N-terminal fragment of apoB100.
(c) The apoprotein of Lp(a).
(d) The oxidized form of apoB.

94. LDL:
(a) Delivers cholesterol to cells.
(b) Contains only one apoprotein.
(c) Is a marker for cardiovascular risk.
(d) Contains apoB48.

95. Free fatty acids are transported in plasma:
(a) As a component of VLDL.
(b) As a component of chylomicron remnants.
(c) As a part of Lp(a).
(d) As a ligand bound to albumin.

96. The concentration of the following is inversely related to the risk of cardiovascular disease:
(a) VLDL.
(b) IDL.
(c) LDL.
(d) HDL.

97. The following apolipoprotein may play a role in the development of Alzheimer's disease:
(a) ApoB48.
(b) ApoB100.
(c) ApoE.
(d) ApoC.

Chapter 18

98. The principal mechanism for the removal of amino groups from most amino acids before their catabolism is:
(a) Oxidative deamination.
(b) Transamination.
(c) The action of a dehydratase enzyme.
(d) The action of glutamine synthase.

99. The primary nitrogenous excretion product in human urine is:
(a) Ammonium ion.
(b) Uric acid.
(c) Creatinine.
(d) Urea.

100. A compound common to the urea cycle and the tricarboxylic acid cycle is:
(a) Lactate.
(b) Fumarate.
(c) Pyruvate.
(d) α-ketoglutarate.

101. Which of the following amino acids has an important role in the transport of amino groups from peripheral tissues to the liver?
(a) Serine.
(b) Methionine.
(c) Glutamine.
(d) Arginine.

102. Which of the following amino acids is not classified as glucogenic?
(a) Leucine.
(b) Tryptophan.
(c) Serine.
(d) Aspartate.

103. Which of the following amino acids is required in the diet of a healthy adult?
(a) Aspartate.
(b) Serine.
(c) Tryptophan.
(d) Glutamine.

Chapter 19

104. Which compound is the storage form of high energy phosphate in muscle?
(a) Carnitine phosphate.
(b) Creatine phosphate.
(c) Creatinine phosphate.
(d) Cyclic AMP
(e) Carnosine phosphate

105. Which allosteric activator of phosphofructokinase in muscle is analogous in function to fructose-2,6-bisphosphate in liver?
(a) ATP.
(b) ADP.
(c) AMP.
(d) Cyclic AMP.
(e) Citrate.

106. Which component of the sarcomere has ATPase activity?
(a) Myosin.
(b) Actin.
(c) Tropomyosin.
(d) Troponin.
(e) Dystrophin

107. The region of overlap of actin and myosin in the sarcomere, which shortens during contraction, is known as:
(a) Z-line.
(b) M-line.
(c) I-band.
(d) A-band.
(e) H-zone.

108. Which cardiac isozyme is commonly measured to confirm the diagnosis of myocardial infarction?
(a) Cardiac myoglobin.
(b) Creatine phosphokinase CK-MB.
(c) Creatine phosphokinase CK-MM.
(d) Creatine phosphokinase CK-BB.
(e) Lactate dehydrogenase M_4.

109. What is the major source of energy in muscle during long-term endurance exercise?
(a) Blood glucose.
(b) Blood fatty acids.
(c) Muscle glycogen.
(d) Creatine phosphate.
(e) Lactate.

Chapter 20

110. After a meal the following occurs:
(a) Stimulation of gluconeogenesis.
(b) Stimulation of glycogen synthesis.
(c) Inhibition of lipolysis.
(d) Stimulation of glycolysis.

111. The principal source of glucose after an overnight fast is:
(a) Glycolysis.
(b) Gluconeogenesis.
(c) Glycogenolysis.
(d) Lactate.

112. Which of the following cannot take place in the human body?
(a) Transformation of lactate into glucose.
(b) Transformation of acetate into glucose.
(c) Transformation of glycerol into glucose.
(d) Transformation of alanine into pyruvate.

113. The differences between type 1 and type 2 diabetes are:
(a) Insulin secretion is preserved in type 2 but not in type 1 diabetes.
(b) Type 2 diabetic patients do not develop ketoacidosis.
(c) Type 2 diabetes normally develops later in life than type 1.
(d) Insulin resistance is important in the development of type 2 diabetes.

Chapter 21

114. Which factors determine the nutritional state?
(a) Level of exercise.
(b) The presence of disease.
(c) The phase of the life cycle.
(d) Sex.
(e) Genetic background.

115. Obesity is concordant in dizygotic twins in:
(a) 32%.
(b) 54%.
(c) 15%.
(d) 25%.
(e) 85%.

116. Refined carbohydrates include:
(a) Sucrose.
(b) Beta-glucan.
(c) Starch.
(d) Potatoes.
(e) Cellulose.

117. Saturated fatty acids are:
(a) Palmitic acid.
(b) Arachidonic acid.
(c) Myristic acid.
(d) Linoleic acid.
(e) Docahexanoic acid.

Chapter 22

118. The dominant cation in the intracellular fluid is:
(a) Sodium.
(b) Potassium.
(c) Calcium.
(d) Magnesium.

119. An increased anion gap is consistent with:
(a) An increase in plasma concentration of acetoacetic and β-hydroxybutyric acids.
(b) An increase in plasma chloride.
(c) An increase in plasma bicarbonate.
(d) A decrease in plasma sodium.

120. A decreased oncotic pressure will result in:
(a) The movement of water from ECF to ICF.
(b) The movement of sodium from ICF to ECF.
(c) The movement of fluid out of capillaries into the interstitial space.
(d) The movement of proteins into capillaries.

121. Transport of sodium in the renal tubules involves:
(a) Na^+/K^+-ATPase located on the luminal membrane.
(b) Na^+/K^+-ATPase located on the basolateral membrane.
(c) Entry of sodium into tubular cells by active transport.
(d) cAMP.

122. Excess of aldosterone causes:
(a) Sodium and water retention.
(b) An increase in urinary sodium concentration.
(c) Hyperkalemia.
(d) A decrease in renal blood flow.

123. A diuretic acting on the ascending part of the loop of Henle:
(a) Inhibits the action of aldosterone.
(b) Promotes potassium reabsorption.
(c) Inhibits ACE.
(d) Decreases sodium reabsorption.

124. Potassium:
(a) Is the main extracellular ion.
(b) Hyperkalemia may lead to cardiac arrest.
(c) Hypokalemia never leads to arrhythmias.
(d) Potassium intake needs to be restricted in renal disease.
(e) Potassium is mainly excreted in feces.

Chapter 23

125. The kidney contributes to acid-base balance by:
(a) Secretion of ammonia.
(b) Reabsorption of bicarbonate.
(c) Increased ketogenesis.
(d) Decreased CO_2 uptake.

126. pKa:
(a) Indicates the strength of an acid.
(b) Reflects the pH of a solution.
(c) Points to an effective range of a buffer solution.
(d) Is a measure of buffer capacity.

127. Respiratory acidosis may occur when:
(a) Chest wall expansion is impaired.
(b) A patient hyperventilates.
(c) There is anemia.
(d) A fluid accumulates in pulmonary alveoli.

128. Carbon dioxide:
(a) Is more soluble in water than oxygen.
(b) Does not bind to hemoglobin.
(c) Cannot diffuse through cell membranes.
(d) Has a decreased partial pressure in blood in respiratory acidosis.

Chapter 24

129. Which of the following is true of PTH?
(a) It is synthesized in the chief cells of the parathyroid gland.
(b) It promotes renal gluconeogenesis.
(c) It is secreted as 139-, 141-, and 173-amino acid isoforms.
(d) It stimulates renal excretion of phosphate.

130. With which of the following is hypocalcemia associated?
(a) Muscle twitching and cramp.
(b) Vitamin D deficiency.
(c) Hypomagnesemia.
(d) Decreased osteoid formation.

131. Osteoporosis is commonly caused by:
(a) Hypogonadism.
(b) Excessive weight.
(c) HRT.
(d) Consumption of dairy products.

Chapter 25

132. Galactosemia may be treated most practically by:
(a) Adopting a high-carbohydrate diet.
(b) Eliminating all sugar from the diet.
(c) Eliminating all dairy products from the diet.
(d) Adopting a high-protein diet.
(e) Avoiding the use of sucrose.

133. In I-cell disease, lysosomal enzymes are found in plasma rather than in the lysosomes, because they lack:
(a) High-mannose oligosaccharides.
(b) O-linked oligosaccharides.
(c) Specific protein epitopes.
(d) Glucose 6-phosphate.
(e) Mannose 6-phosphate.

134. Biosynthesis of N-linked oligosaccharides involves:
(a) Sequential addition of sugars to the polypeptide chain.
(b) Activation of sugars to nucleoside diphosphate sugars and transfer to cytoplasmic proteins.
(c) Addition of galactose to hydroxylysine and then transfer of other sugars.
(d) Assembly of oligosaccharide chains on Dolichol-PP and transfer to the growing polypeptide chain.
(e) Assembly of oligosaccharide in cytoplasm and processing in the ER.

135. Carbohydrate-deficient glycoprotein syndromes are a family of diseases in which:
(a) Individuals lack the ability to make glycoproteins.
(b) Formation of O-linked oligosaccharides is defective.
(c) Individuals cannot secrete glycoproteins normally.
(d) N-linked oligosaccharides are not synthesized or processed normally.
(e) The protein portion of the glycoproteins does not contain the amino acids necessary for attaching sugars.

136. Which of the following amino acids is **not** involved in the linkage of carbohydrates to proteins:
(a) Asparagine.
(b) Hydroxylysine.
(c) Serine.
(d) Threonine.
(e) Glutamate

137. Which of the following sugars is commonly found at the non-reducing terminus of oligosaccharides on plasma glycoproteins and mucins?
(a) Glucose.
(b) Sialic acid.
(c) Mannose.
(d) N-acetylglucosamine.
(e) Fructose.

Chapter 26

138. GPI anchors are composed of:
(a) Phosphatidylcholine attached to cholesterol and fatty acids.
(b) Phosphatidylinositol, a glycan, and ethanolamine.
(c) A hydrophobic region of amino acids interacting with various phospholipids.
(d) Phosphatidylglycerol or phosphatidylinositol linked to an *N*-linked oligosaccharide of a glycoprotein.
(e) Plasmalogen and a hydrophilic core region.

139. Cytidine nucleotides are involved in phospholipid synthesis because:
(a) They provide the energy to convert phosphatidylethanolamine to phosphatidylcholine.
(b) They are involved in the phosphorylation of choline and ethanolamine.
(c) They are involved in the activation of choline, ethanolamine, and DAG.
(d) They are recognition molecules for phospholipid transferases.
(e) They are important in signal transduction.

140. Which of the following activities are associated with gangliosides in cell membranes?
(a) They are binding sites for toxins.
(b) They are energy-yielding molecules for nerve cells.
(c) They are hydrolyzed to inositol triphosphate for signaling.
(d) They can give rise to fatty acids for acylation reactions.
(e) They are receptors for epinephrine and insulin.

141. Tay-Sachs disease is characterized by a(n):
(a) Inability to synthesize gangliosides.
(b) Lesion in the conversion of globoside to ganglioside.
(c) Absence of the enzymes that remove fatty acids from cerebrosides.
(d) Inability to degrade gangliosides completely because of absence of a lysosomal glycosidase.
(e) Inability to move gangliosides into the lysosome.

142. Synthesis of ceramide involves which of the following?
(a) Choline and sphingosine.
(b) Palmitoyl-CoA, serine, reducing agents and fatty acyl CoA.
(c) Serine, NADP$^+$, FAD, and CDP-fatty acids.
(d) UDP-glucose, sphingosine, and FAD.
(e) Sphingosine produced from sphingomyelin.

143. Platelet activating factor is a form of:
(a) Sphingomyelin.
(b) Phosphatidylcholine.
(c) Ganglioside.
(d) Plasmalogen.
(e) Glycosylphosphatidylinositol anchor.

Chapter 27

144. Which of the following is the most abundant amino acid in collagens?
(a) Alanine.
(b) Glycine.
(c) Hydroxyproline.
(d) Hydroxylysine.
(e) Proline.

145. Which of the following (types of) crosslinks is unique to elastins in the ECM?
(a) Allysine.
(b) Desmosine.
(c) Glycyl glycine.
(d) Lysinonorleucine.
(e) Schiff base (imine) crosslinks.

146. The RGD sequence in proteins is:
(a) A characteristic repeating tri-peptide sequence of collagen.
(b) A site for cleavage of collagen by procollagen proteinases.
(c) An interrupt sequence in the collagen triple helix.
(d) A tripeptide sequence contributing to the elasticity of elastin.
(e) A binding site for integrins in the plasma membrane.

147. Which of the following proteins is not found in the extracellular matrix?
(a) Fibronectin.
(b) Laminin.
(c) Elastin.
(d) Collagen.
(e) Integrin.

148. Glycosaminoglycan chains are bound to serine and threonine residues in core protein by:
(a) Glucuronic acid.
(b) N-acetylgalactosamine.
(c) N-acetylglucosamine.
(d) Xylose.
(e) Galactose.

149. Which of the following statements about proteoglycans is false?
(a) Their repeating disaccharides typically consists of a uronic acid and a hexosamine residue.
(b) The majority of the carbohydrates are found in long, unbranched glycan chains, attached at multiple sites to a core protein.
(c) Proteoglycans are typically strongly anionic in nature.
(d) Proteoglycans are degraded in lysosomes by acid exoglycosidases.
(e) Defects in glycosyl transferases involved in their synthesis result in mucopolysaccharidoses.

Chapter 28

150. Which one of the following is not synthesized by hepatocytes?
(a) Prothrombin.
(b) Ceruloplasmin.
(c) Immunoglobulin.
(d) Ferritin.

151. In the hepatic metabolism of ethanol, which one of the following is false?
(a) Hepatic oxidation of lactate is inhibited.
(b) Gluconeogenesis is impaired.
(c) The NADH/NAD$^+$ ratio increases.
(d) Alcohol dehydrogenase is a P450 cytochrome.

152. In bilirubin metabolism, which one of the following is true?
(a) Hepatocytes oxidize heme to biliverdin.
(b) Conjugated bilirubin is colorless.
(c) Unconjugated bilirubin is soluble in water.
(d) Feces normally contain urobilin.

153. In cholestatic jaundice, which one of the following is false?
(a) Urine bilirubin is conjugated.
(b) Plasma alkaline phosphatase activity indicates the site of obstruction.
(c) Malabsorption of fat is common.
(d) Plasma bile acid concentrations are increased.

154. Which of the following statements is incorrect?
(a) Neonatal jaundice is common after 48 hours.
(b) In neonatal jaundice, conjugated hyperbilirubinemia requires investigation.
(c) In neonatal jaundice, conjugated bilirubin causes kernicterus.
(d) Neonatal jaundice in the first 24 hours may indicate hemolytic disease.

155. In acetaminophen overdose, which one of the following is false?
(a) Alcoholics are at increased risk of hepatotoxicity.
(b) Sulfation of acetaminophen becomes the major route of detoxification.
(c) The prothrombin time is prolonged.
(d) The plasma creatinine concentration is related to prognosis.

156. Major illness is associated with changes in hepatic protein synthesis of:
(a) CRP.
(b) Collagen.
(c) Haptoglobin.
(d) α1-acid glycoprotein.
(e) Apoprotein B.

Chapter 29

157. Which of the following types of amino acids are involved as precursors for synthesis of nucleic acids?
(a) Nonessential amino acids.
(b) Basic amino acids.
(c) Aromatic amino acids.
(d) Aliphatic hydrophobic amino acids.

158. Which of the following statements about ribonucleotide reductase (RNR) is false?
(a) RNR is specific for nucleoside diphosphates.
(b) RNR reduces ADP to dADP during purine biosynthesis.
(c) RNR reduces TDP to dTDP during pyrimidine biosynthesis.
(d) RNR is part of both de novo and salvage pathways of nucleotide biosynthesis.

159. Which of the following is an intermediate in the *de novo* biosynthesis of dATP?
(a) Adenine.
(b) Adenosine.
(c) dAMP.
(d) AMP.

160. Which of the following is an inhibitor of xanthine oxidase, used for the treatment of Gout?
(a) Hypoxanthine.
(b) Orotic acid.
(c) Allopurinol.
(d) Thioredoxin.
(e) Fluorodeoxyuridylate.

161. Which of the following inhibitors of thymidylate synthase is used as a chemotherapeutic agent?
(a) Allopurinol.
(b) Methotrexate.
(c) Aminopterin.
(d) Trimethoprim.
(e) Fluorouridine.

162. Which of the following enzymes in the purine salvage pathway is deficient in Severe Combined Immunodeficiency Syndrome?
(a) Ribonucleotide reductase.
(b) Aspartate transcarbamoylase.
(c) Xanthine oxidase.
(d) Hypoxanthine/Guanine Phosphoribosyltransferase.
(e) Adenosine deaminase.

163. Fluorocytosine is an effective antimicrobial compound, but is nontoxic to humans because:
(a) Microbes have cytosine deaminase but mammals do not.
(b) Fluorocytosine blocks salvage pathways for pyrimidines.
(c) Bacterial thymidylate synthase is inhibited by fluorocytosine.
(d) Its metabolite, 5-fluorouracil, is a potent inhibitor of microbial, but not mammalian, thymidylate synthase.

164. Which of the following compounds would be useful as a chemotherapeutic agent designed to inhibit synthesis of purine nucleotides?
(a) Allopurinol.
(b) 5-fluorouracil.
(c) Methotrexate.
(d) Sulfanilamide.

Chapter 30

165. The therapeutic rationale for using AZT for treatment of AIDS is based on the fact that:
(a) AZT is incorporated into DNA, but forms a base-pair mismatch.
(b) AZT is incorporated into DNA, but inhibits the movement of DNA polymerase during replication.
(c) AZT is incorporated into DNA, but blocks the elongation of viral DNA by reverse transcriptase.
(d) AZT is incorporated into viral RNA, causing nonsense mutations in the viral genome.
(e) AZT is incorporated into viral RNA, yielding mutant proteins that cannot support virus assembly.

166. Which of the following tests is commonly used to test for mutagenic activity of a compound?
(a) Evaluation of the effect of the compound on the activity of DNA polymerase.
(b) Evaluation of the effect of the compound on the melting temperature of DNA.
(c) Evaluation of the effect of the compound on the rate of mutation of Salmonella typhimurium.

(d) Evaluation of the effect of the compounds on the size of Okazaki fragments.

(e) Evaluation of the effect of the compound on the rate of repair of DNA.

167. Which of the following enzymes is **not** involved in the synthesis of DNA along the lagging strand during replication?
(a) DNA ligase.
(b) DNA polymerase I.
(c) DNA polymerase III.
(d) DNA gyrase.
(e) Telomerase.

168. Which of the following compounds is a classical biomarker of oxidative damage to DNA?
(a) 8-oxo-2′-deoxyguanosine.
(b) Thymine dimers.
(c) Okazaki fragments.
(d) Satellite DNA.
(e) Telomeres.

169. Which of the following sequences of DNA would form a duplex with a complementary sequence to yield the highest melting point?
(a) AAAAAAAAA
(b) ATATATATA
(c) AGTAGTAGT
(d) GCGCGCGCG
(e) AGAGAGAGA

170. Which nucleotide in DNA forms dimers on exposure to ultraviolet light?
(a) Adenine.
(b) Guanine.
(c) Cytosine.
(d) Thymin.
(e) Uracil.

171. The Ames test is used:
(a) For paternity testing.
(b) For prenatal diagnosis of disease.
(c) To differentiate between single and double stranded DNA.
(d) For identification of mutagens.
(e) To determine the sex of the fetus.

Chapter 31

172. Which of the following best describes the role of σ-factor in RNA synthesis?
(a) Sigma factor is essential for elongation.
(b) Sigma factor is responsible for the recognition of specific initiation sites on a DNA template.

(c) Sigma factor is responsible for separation of DNA strands
(d) Sigma factor is responsible for releasing the completed chain.

173. All of the following are true for DNA polymerases and RNA polymerases except which one?
(a) Both require a template.
(b) Both reactions produce pyrophosphate as a product.
(c) Both add 5′ nucleotides to 3′ hydroxyl groups.
(d) Both utilize 5′-nucleoside triphosphate as substrate.
(e) Both require a primer.

174. If the DNA strand that is complementary to the strand of DNA that is transcribed into RNA has the base sequence 5′-AGCTCACTG-3′ the RNA transcribed would have which of the following sequences?
(a) CAGUGAGCU.
(b) AGCUCACUG.
(c) AGCTCACTG.
(d) CAGTGAGCU.
(e) None of the above.

175. Synthesis and maturation of mRNA in eukaryotic cells can involve:
(a) Post-transcriptional addition of polyA to the 3′ termini of RNA molecules.
(b) Nucleic acid sequences that are separated from one another in DNA and next to one another in mRNA.
(c) Giant precursor molecules that are largely destroyed.
(d) Addition of the cap structure to the 5′ termini of mRNA.

176. During nuclear processing of an hnRNA in a eukaryotic cell, the portions that are discarded are referred to as:
(a) Exons.
(b) Introns.
(c) Duplicate genes.
(d) PolyA chains.

177. Which of the following statements about eukaryotic RNA polymerase promoters is/are true?
(a) They all lie relatively close to the transcription start site in untranscribed regions outside genes.
(b) RNA polymerase II promoters contain conserved nucleotide sequences that may determine the exact start site and efficiency of transcription.
(c) Precursors of mRNA are transcribed by RNA polymerase II.
(d) None of the above.

Chapter 32

178. Codons on mRNA can be described by which of the following statements?
(a) They are read in a non-overlapping fashion.
(b) The same codon may specify more than one amino acid.
(c) They are recognized by complementary base pairs on tRNA.
(d) They may specify start and stop sites for protein synthesis.

179. Methionine initiates protein synthesis and
(a) Is removed from most eukaryotic proteins.
(b) Every eukaryotic protein has this amino acid on its carboxy-terminal end.
(c) Every mature eukaryotic protein has this amino acid on its amino-terminal end.
(d) Also terminates protein synthesis.

180. Charging of a tRNA molecule with the correct amino acid is dependent on:
(a) The anticodon loop.
(b) The variable loop.
(c) The codon of the mRNA.
(d) An aminoacyl synthetase specific for that tRNA.

181. Translation requires:
(a) A methionyl initiator tRNA molecule.
(b) Elongation factors for translocation of ribosomes along the mRNA.
(c) GTP for energy.
(d) Initiation factors for bringing mRNA, ribosomes, and tRNA together.

182. An amino acid is attached to the tRNA via:
(a) Hydrogen bonds.
(b) Ester bonds.
(c) Amide bonds.
(d) Glycosidic bonds.
(e) Ether bonds.

183. During protein synthesis, the newly synthesized peptide
(a) Is covalently bound to DNA.
(b) Is covalently bound to the 5' end of mRNA.
(c) Is covalently bound to the small rRNA subunit.
(d) Is covalently bound to the end of tRNA.

Chapter 33

184. Which of the following is/are essential for gene transcription?
(a) RNA polymerase.
(b) DNA methylase.

(c) A CAAT box.
(d) A promoter region.
(e) Glucocorticoids.

185. Which of the following is/are true of promoter elements in genes?
(a) Share common elements.
(b) Always confer tissue specificity.
(c) Act as sites for upregulation of transcription.
(d) May contain consensus sequences.
(e) If mutated, may diminish the efficiency of gene expression.

186. Which of the following is/are true of steroid receptors?
(a) Contain manganese atoms that confer biological activity.
(b) Have a high degree of similarity at their DNA-binding site.
(c) Bind to a wide range of DNA sequences.
(d) Are similar to thyroid hormone receptors.
(e) In humans are very different from those in nonprimate mammals.

187. Which of the following is/are true of gene expression?
(a) Only involves transcription-related processes.
(b) May be influenced by the sex of the individual.
(c) Is always regulated by glucocorticoids.
(d) Regulation of the expression of a single gene may involve two different processes.
(e) Is never influenced by age.

188. Which of the following mechanisms is/are involved in gene expression?
(a) Methylation of cytosine nucleotides.
(b) Intron splicing.
(c) Use of alternative promoters.
(d) Mutation of consensus sequences.
(e) Binding of transcription factors to RNA.

189. Which of the following methods of regulating gene expression is/are common?
(a) Use of alternative promoters.
(b) Post-translational cleavage.
(c) RNA editing.
(d) Alternative splicing of DNA.
(e) Multigenic transcription units.

Chapter 34

190. Human insulin, produced by recombinant DNA technology, is made primarily by:
(a) *In vitro* synthesis by the polymerase chain reaction.
(b) Cell-based cloning using a bacterial host.

(c) Cell-based cloning using an insect host.

(d) Cell-based cloning using an immortalized mouse β-cell line.

(e) Cell-based cloning using a transformed human β-cell line.

191. Single base mutations (substitutions) in DNA may be detected by all of the following **except**:

(a) Change in DNA fragment sizes on a Southern blot.

(b) Change in Southern blot analysis of DNA under high stringency conditions.

(c) Change in Southern blot analysis of DNA under low stringency conditions.

(d) Change in sensitivity to cleavage by a restriction enzyme.

(e) Change in DNA migration on denaturant-gradient gel electrophoresis.

192. Which reagent in a DNA sequencing procedure leads to production of DNA fragments that are used for sequencing?

(a) DNA ligase

(b) DNA endonuclease (Nickase)

(c) Deoxynucleotide triphosphates.

(d) Ribonucleotide triphosphates.

(e) Dideoxynucleotide triphosphates.

193. During the polymerase chain reaction, the double stranded DNA is dissociated by:

(a) DNA gyrase.

(b) DNA helicase.

(c) Heat.

(d) Urea.

(e) Addition of amplimers.

194. Which of the following reagents is **not** needed for the polymerase chain reaction?

(a) *Taq* polymerase.

(b) DNA template.

(c) Amplimers.

(d) Deoxynucleotide triphosphates.

(e) RNA primers.

195. Which method is commonly used to evaluate the full range of changes in gene expression in response to environmental stresses?

(a) Measurement of restriction fragment length polymorphism.

(b) Microarray technology.

(c) Tissue *in situ* hybridization.

(d) 2-D Polyacrylamide gel electrophoresis.

(e) Pulsed-field gel electrophoresis.

Chapter 35

196. Which is the most reactive of reactive oxygen species?

(a) Molecular oxygen.

(b) Superoxide anion radical.

(c) Hydrogen peroxide.

(d) Hypochlorous acid.

(e) Hydroxyl radical.

197. Which is the most reduced form of oxygen?

(a) Water (H_2O).

(b) Superoxide anion radical ($O_2^{\cdot-}$).

(c) Hydroperoxy radical ($HOO^\bullet$).

(d) Hydroxyl radical ($OH^\bullet$).

(e) Peroxynitrite ($ONOO^-$)

198. Which of the following is considered an important source of hydroxyl radicals in the cell?

(a) The Haber-Weiss reaction.

(b) Superoxide dismutase.

(c) Redox cycling of ubiquinone.

(d) The Fenton reaction.

(e) Catalase.

199. Which of the following enzymes does not participate in the defense against oxidative stress?

(a) Catalase.

(b) Superoxide dismutase.

(c) Myeloperoxidase.

(d) Glutathione peroxidase.

(e) Glucose-6-phosphate dehydrogenase.

200. Which of the following biomolecules are most susceptible to oxidative damage?

(a) Nuclear DNA.

(b) Carbohydrates on glycoconjugates.

(c) Sphingosine in sphingolipids.

(d) Polyunsaturated fatty acids in phospholipids.

(e) Side chains of hydrophobic amino acids.

201. Which of the following antioxidants has the primary role as a chain-breaking antioxidant in the lipid phase of plasma membranes?

(a) Ascorbic Acid.

(b) Vitamin E.

(c) Ubiquinone

(d) Glutathione.

(e) Nitric oxide.

202. Which tripeptide has a major role in protection against reactive oxygen?

(a) Insulin.

(b) Glutathione.

(c) Carnitine.
(d) Creatine.
(e) Methionine.

203. Which of the following enzymes does not participate in bactericidal activity during phagocytosis?
(a) Superoxide dismutase.
(b) Glutathione peroxidase.
(c) Myeloperoxidase.
(d) NADPH oxidase.

Chapter 36

204. Which of the following statements are true of the nonspecific immune responses? (Choose more than one.)
(a) Lymphocytes are central to these responses.
(b) CRP is an acute-phase reactant.
(c) The humoral mediators include components of the classical pathway of complement.
(d) Interleukins are products of arachidonic acid metabolism.
(e) Epithelial barriers are integral components

205. Which of the following is true of antigens? (Choose more than one.)
(a) Can only be polysaccharide in nature.
(b) Are usually of less than 10 kD in molecular weight.
(c) Alone are always capable of stimulating specific immune responses.
(d) Are processed prior to recognition by T cells.
(e) In the native state are recognized by B cells.

206. Which of the following is not true of B cells? (Choose more than one.)
(a) Characteristically express the CD3 molecule.
(b) Are responsible for the cellular arm of the specific immune response.
(c) When activated may differentiate into a morphologically different cell type.
(d) Are responsible for the humoral specific immune responses.
(e) Are typically found in the lymph node paracortex.

207. Which of the following is not true of CD4-positive lymphocytes? (Choose more than one.)
(a) Can interact with B cells.
(b) May typically show cytotoxic effector function.
(c) Are MHC class 2-restricted.
(d) Are depleted in HIV infection.
(e) Secrete monokines.

208. Which of the following is true of the major histocompatibility complex of genes? (Choose more than one.)
(a) Include the genes responsible for kappa chains
(b) Are located on the short arm of chromosome 5.
(c) Are genetically transmitted as part of a haplotype.
(d) Are described as producing three classes of protein products.
(e) Are responsible for the molecules that have the greatest influence on the rejection of grafted tissue

209. Which of the following is not true of immunoglobulin molecules? (Choose more than one.)
(a) Are composed of alpha and beta chains.
(b) Show marked variability in the sequence of their C terminal amino acids.
(c) In the monomeric form have two antigen binding sites.
(d) Of the IgG class are the isotype responsible for protection of mucosal surfaces.
(e) Of the IgE isotype can be responsible for life-threatening anaphylaxis.

Chapter 37

210. Hormone concentrations in plasma are usually measured by:
(a) Colorimetric assays for specific functional groups.
(b) High performance liquid chromatography.
(c) Liquid chromatography – mass spectrometry.
(d) Functional assays in animal model systems.
(e) Specific immunoassays.

211. Which of the following hormones has the primary role in regulation of thyroid status in the body?
(a) Thyroglobulin.
(b) Triiodothyronine (T_3).
(c) Thyroxine (T_4).
(d) Thyroid releasing hormone (TSH).
(e) Thyrotropin releasing hormone (TRH).

212. Which of the following is **not** a characteristic feature of Addison's disease?
(a) Hyponatremia.
(b) Hypercortisolemia.
(c) Elevated plasma ACTH.
(d) Impaired cortisol response to synthetic ACTH agonists.
(e) Positive response to therapy with cortisol.

213. Which of the following abnormalities is **not** associated with Cushing's syndrome?
(a) Weight loss.
(b) Hypertension.
(c) Diabetes.
(d) High plasma cortisol concentration.
(e) High plasma ACTH concentration.

214. Which of the following hormones is commonly measured in urine for diagnosis of pregnancy?
(a) Human chorionic gonadotropin (HCG).
(b) Follicle stimulating hormone (FSH).
(c) Luteinizing hormone (LH).
(d) Progesterone.
(e) Gonadotropin releasing hormone (GnRH).

215. Growth hormone exerts its growth promoting effects primarily through the action of:
(a) Insulin.
(b) Cortisol.
(c) Testosterone.
(d) Insulin-like growth factor-1 (IGF-1).
(e) Prolactin.

Chapter 38

216. The intrinsic enzyme activity associated with the a-subunit of regulatory G-proteins is:
(a) A kinase that transfers the γ-phosphate of GTP to serine residues of proteins.
(b) A GTPase that hydrolyzes GTP to GDP.
(c) A guanylate cyclase that converts GTP to cGMP.
(d) A cGMP-dependent kinase.

217. G-protein-coupled receptors have:
(a) Single-pass transmembrane domains.
(b) Seven transmembrane-spanning domains.
(c) Seven subunits.
(d) Seven single-pass transmembrane domains.

218. β-adrenergic receptors are coupled to:
(a) G_s-stimulated adenylate cyclase activity.
(b) G_i-mediated inhibition of adenylate cyclase.
(c) G_s-stimulated guanylate cyclase activity.
(d) G_i-stimulated adenylate cyclase activity.

219. The PIP_2-derived second messenger that mobilizes intracellular calcium is:
(a) PIP_3.
(b) $I-1,4,5-P_3$.
(c) Phosphatidic acid.
(d) DAG.

220. Diacyl glycerol is converted to phosphatidic acid by:
(a) Phosphatidic acid phosphohydrolase.
(b) DAG lipase.
(c) DAG kinase.
(d) PLA_2.

221. Increasing cAMP concentrations is found to alleviate the symptoms of asthma; should you therefore design drugs to:
(a) Inhibit adenylyl cyclase?
(b) Inhibit cAMP PDEs?
(c) Inhibit PKA?

222. How do the increased concentrations of cAMP resulting from cholera toxin-mediated activation of adenylyl cyclase result in the efflux of water and electrolytes into the gut that is responsible for the severe diarrhea that is characteristic of cholera?
(a) PKA phosphorylates and modulates the activity of plasma membrane Cl^- channels.
(b) PKA phosphorylates and modulates the activity of plasma membrane Ca^{2+} channels.
(c) PKA phosphorylates and modulates IP3 receptors on the endoplasmic reticulum.

223. Aspirin is a pain-relieving and anti-inflammatory mediator because it inhibits prostaglandin synthesis by:
(a) Inhibiting fatty-acid-specific lipoxygenase activity.
(b) Inhibiting fatty-acid-specific cyclo-oxygenase activity.
(c) Inhibiting fatty-acid-specific hydroperoxidase activity.

Chapter 39

224. In the diagnosis of multiple sclerosis, which of the following is the most common abnormal pattern of CSF and serum?
(a) No bands in CSF or serum.
(b) Bands in both CSF and serum.
(c) Different bands in CSF and serum.
(d) Bands in CSF but not serum.
(e) Monoclonal pattern in CSF and serum.

225. The most useful test for the definitive diagnosis of myasthenia gravis is:
(a) Antibodies against calcium channels.
(b) Administration of edrophonium.
(c) Antibodies against double-stranded DNA.
(d) Antibodies against the acetylcholine receptor.
(e) Serum manganese concentration.

226. The most common fate of neurons during embryogenesis is:
(a) Connection to muscle cells.
(b) Connection to glandular organs.
(c) Connection to other neurons in the CNS.
(d) Connection to other neurons in the PNS.
(e) Cell death.

227. The rate at which axons will regrow after a nerve is severed in a limb is:
(a) 0.1 mm/day.
(b) 0.3 mm/day.
(c) 1 mm/day.
(d) 3 mm/day.
(e) 6 mm/day.

228. The brain contains approximately what percentage of fat?
(a) 10%.
(b) 20%.
(c) 30%.
(d) 40%.
(e) 50%.

229. CSF rhinorrhea is best diagnosed by measuring which of the following analytes?
(a) Total protein.
(b) Glucose.
(c) Chloride.
(d) Asialotransferrin.
(e) Sodium.

Chapter 40

230. Examples of excitatory neurotransmitters in the CNS are:
(a) Glutamate.
(b) Dopamine.
(c) Aspartate.
(d) Glycine.

231. Which of the following processes is/are important in the removal of neuropeptides?
(a) Specific degradation.
(b) Diffusion.
(c) Uptake into neurons.
(d) Metabolism in the urea cycle.

232. An ionotropic receptor:
(a) Allows ions to pass through a membrane pore.
(b) Is connected to G-proteins.
(c) Responds only to excitatory amino acids.
(d) Produces a rapid response to stimulation.

233. Catecholamines:
(a) Are derived from tryptophan.
(b) Are released from varicosities along the nerve.
(c) Cause hypertension when present in excess.
(d) Inhibit glycogen metabolism.

234. Opiate peptides:
(a) Stimulate breathing.
(b) Are coded by several genes.
(c) Increase painful stimuli.
(d) Act on receptors in the spinal cord.

235. In the sympathetic nervous system:
(a) Nerves run directly from the brain to the target organs.
(b) Norepinephrine is the major postganglionic transmitter.
(c) Stimulation causes bronchoconstriction.
(d) Stress is an important stimulus.

Chapter 42

236. The age at which 50% of a population of humans has deceased is known as:
(a) The mean lifespan of the population.
(b) The half-life of the population.
(c) The Hayflick Limit for the population.
(d) The maximum lifespan of the population.

237. Which of the following **do not** contribute to lengthening of the maximum lifespan of animals?
(a) Caloric restriction.
(b) Reduced energy expenditure.
(c) Improved health care.
(d) Genetic manipulation.

238. Which form of DNA is most susceptible to oxidative damage in eukaryotic cells?
(a) Nuclear DNA.
(b) Mitochondrial DNA.
(c) Satellite DNA.
(d) Telomeric DNA.
(e) Nucleosomal DNA.

239. Which of the following types of posttranslational, chemical modifications of protein **does not** accumulate in tissues with age?
(a) Glycoxidation products.
(b) Amino acid oxidation products.
(c) Phosphorylated amino acids.
(d) Lipofuscin.
(e) Racemized amino acids.

240. Which factor does not contribute to the loss of oxidative metabolic capacity in aged muscle?
(a) Decrease in total skeletal muscle mass.
(b) Decreased efficiency of perfusion of muscle tissue.
(c) Decrease in cytochrome oxidase in muscle mitochondria.
(d) Decrease in number of functional mitochondria per muscle cell.
(e) Decrease in glycolytic activity in muscle.

241. Which of the following is **not** a characteristic of animals whose lifespan is extended by calorie restriction?
(a) Increased fertility.
(b) Decreased rate of oncogenesis.
(c) Extension of mean lifespan.
(d) Extension of maximum lifespan.
(e) Decreased rate of development of age-related, chronic diseases.

Patient Oriented Problems (POPs)

Note: Normal values for laboratory lests are shown in parentheses. Alternative units of measurement are shown in square brackets.

---

1. A young woman, while hyperventilating (frequent, deep, sighing respirations to sustained, obvious, rapid, deep breathing) fell unconscious to the floor. An attending physician diagnosed her condition as 'hyperventilation syndrome' caused by her anxiety and mental stress. He successfully treated her by rebreathing expired CO_2 from a paper bag and she completely recovered. What happened to the acid-base balance in her body? Describe the rationale for the treatment.

---

2. A 20-year-old African-American complaining of severe back pain was hospitalized and sickle cell anemia was diagnosed. In patients with sickle cell anemia abnormal hemoglobin called hemoglobin-S is observed. Hemoglobin consists of two α chains and two β-chains. The sickle cell mutation causes the substitution of valine at the 6th position of normal hemoglobin (Hb-A) β chain to glutamic acid and the mutated hemoglobin is called Hb-S. The estimated frequency of sickle cell anemia in Afro-Americans is 1:655 and in some parts of Africa over 45% of the population are carriers for the sickle cell gene. When you analyze the hemolysate of the patient on electrophoresis, how does Hb-S migrate on an electrophoresis at pH 8.6? What will happen in the case of the other mutation called Hb-C that causes mutation of glutamic acid to lysine in the 6th amino acid residue of the β-chain?

---

3. A 3-year-old boy was admitted to hospital with a red, scaly rash on the exposed areas of his body. The symptoms were characteristic of pellagra, a dermatitis often accompanied by motor dysfunction and mental retardation or psychosis, resulting from niacin (nicotinamide) deficiency. After exhaustive evaluation, the patient was shown to have high levels of amino acids in urine, a hyperamino-aciduria characterized by excessive excretion of neutral amino acids. He was diagnosed as having Hartnup disease. Hartnup disorder is an autosomal recessive impairment of neutral amino acid transport limited to the kidneys and small intestine. The characteristic biochemical feature in urine is specific aminoaciduria that is caused by a diminished capacity for renal reabsorption of a group of mono amino-mono carboxylic amino acids except glycine, proline and sulfur-containing amino acids. These free amino acids are sometimes excreted in the amount of five to 20 times normal. The symptoms of the disease appear to result from deficiencies in the metabolism or transport of tryptophan which is a precursor to both niacin and the neurotransmitter, serotonin. The incidence of the disorder is approximately 1:300,000. Name the amino acids that are excreted in excess in this disorder.

---

4. After a traffic accident, a 34-year-old lady was admitted to the intensive care unit for treatment. Her biochemical profile on the second day of admission showed:

Albumin 30 g/L (35–45 g/L)
CRP 68 mg/L (<10 mg/dL)
Transferrin 1.8 g/L (2.2–4.0 g/L)

These results are consistent with:
(a) Acute nutritional deficiency.
(b) Acute phase response to injury.
(c) Severe infection.
(d) Nephrotic syndrome.

---

5. A 70-year-old man was seen at the outpatient clinic. He had experienced generalized bone pain and severe back pain. A fractured thoracic vertebra was apparent on a radiograph of his spine. The bones were thin, with multiple lytic (radiolucent) areas throughout the spine and ribs. Investigations that would help make a diagnosis are:
(a) Measurement of CRP.
(b) Measurement of albumin.
(c) Serum and urine protein electrophoresis.
(d) Immunoglobulin quantitation.
(e) All the above.

---

6. A 10-year-old boy is admitted to hospital with hepatic failure. Which of the following are consistent with a diagnosis of Wilson's disease?
(a) Increased ceruloplasmin.
(b) Low serum concentrations of copper.
(c) Low serum concentrations of transferrin.
(d) Markedly increased concentrations of copper in the liver.
(e) Normal concentrations of copper in the urine.

7.   A 3-year-old female, of nonconsanguineous parents from southern Italy, first presented with jaundice and splenomegaly; her Hb level was 6.5 g/dL (12–16 g/dL). In the next year she lost 0.5 kg, and her weight and height fell to the 5th percentile. Because of persistent pallor and jaundice, she was transfused and underwent a splenectomy. A regular transfusion regimen was initiated at age 7 years. Hb analysis showed no abnormalities in the structure of the α- or β-globin polypeptides. Genetic analysis, however, revealed mutations in the β-globin gene cluster. What is a likely explanation for the severe β-thalassemia phenotype?

8.   Patients with chronic pulmonary disease or congenital heart defects often have decreased arterial saturation of Hb (78–85%; normal > 96%) and elevated erythrocyte 2,3-BPG levels (5.3–7.0 mmol/L [1.4–1.9 g/L] cells; normal = 4.1 ± 0.5 mmol/L [1.1 ± 0.1g/L]). What do these observations tell you about the properties of Hb in this group of individuals?

9.   A 65-year-old man shows elevation of plasma levels of LDH1 and creatine phosphokinase. This patient is likely to have (indicate the correct answer):
(a)   Bone disease.
(b)   Myocardial infarction.
(c)   Malignant tumor.
(d)   Acute hepatitis.
(e)   Colitis.

10.   A 48-year-old man was exposed to a toxic dose of organic fluorophosphate, and was treated with atropine sulfate immediately. The reaction mechanism for organic fluorophosphate is (indicate the correct answer):
(a)   Blocking the binding of acetylcholine to an acetylcholine receptor.
(b)   Inactivation of acetylcholine by direct binding.
(c)   Acceleration of acetylcholine excretion into urine.
(d)   Activation of acetylcholinesterase.
(e)   Irreversible inhibition of acetylcholinesterase.

11.   Parents who have a good reason such as a family history, commonly request testing for cystic fibrosis. Social agencies also request testing for cystic fibrosis before adoption. In these cases, what laboratory test would you try?
(a)   Genotyping, which can detect 70 mutations among 500 reported, 90% of the mutated genes being detectable.
(b)   Sweat testing, which measures the concentration of chloride in sweat. If the chloride concentration is ≥80 mmol/L [284 mg/dL], the test result is strongly positive.

12.   The patient was the 10th child of consanguineous Saudi Arabian parents, whose third child was affected with PHHI. She was born at term after normal gestation, weighed 4.25 kg [9.35 lb], but had features of hyperinsulinism *in utero*. Glucose was undetectable in a capillary blood sample after delivery. Simultaneous intravenous infusions of glucose and glucagon were required to maintain normoglycemia. Because of the excessive requirement for glucose and lack of response to medical treatment, 95% of the patient's pancreas was removed 17 days after her birth. After surgery, the patient had recurrent hypoglycemia. A second resection of the pancreas (99%), performed 2 weeks later, resulted in hyperglycemia, necessitating insulin replacement treatment. The child is now 18 months old and continues to require insulin replacement treatment. Genetic analysis of the patient demonstrated the presence of a homozygotic mutation in the *SUR1* gene. What medical treatment was probably used for management of this patient before pancreatic resection?

13.   Patients with gastric or duodenal ulcer, or both, often experience chronic recurrence. In these cases, what treatment would you choose?

14.   A 23-year-old man, who works in the wood preservative division of a local sawmill, comes to his physician because of unremitting fever and weakness. He has severe chloracne and is complaining of gastrointestinal symptoms as well. Could this patient be suffering from effects of occupational exposure to a toxic substance? If so, how would you explain his fever?

15.   A 1-month-old infant is brought to her pediatrician because of hypotonia, vomiting, spasticity and ataxia. The most remarkable finding in blood is very high levels of pyruvic and lactic acids. How would you explain the high levels of pyruvic and lactate, and how could this relate to the symptoms displayed?

16.   A patient complains of abdominal bloating and diarrhea after eating some brands of ice-cream. Lactose (50 g) dissolved in 200 ml of lemon-flavored water was administered after an overnight fast, and the following blood glucose results were obtained:

Time (min)	Blood glucose
0	4.6 mmol/l [83 mg/dl]
30	4.7 mmol/l [85 mg/dl]
60	4.9 mmol/l [88 mg/dl]
90	4.6 mmol/l [83 mg/dl]
120	4.5 mmol/l [81 mg/dl]

These results indicate:
(a) Normal lactose tolerance.
(b) Impairment of galactose absorption.
(c) Lactase deficiency.

17. A 64-year-old patient presents with a history of increasing frequency of passage of feces. On questioning, he tells you that the stools are pale in colour, are passed in copious amounts, are foul-smelling, and difficult to flush away. Does this suggest:
(a) Dissacharidase deficiency?
(b) Malabsorption of fat?
(c) The absence of secreted HCl in the stomach?

18. A 45-year-old man is admitted to the emergency room because of complications of chronic alcoholism. It is determined that he is severely malnourished, and his water-soluble B-vitamin levels are very low in blood. In addition, it is found that he has several organic acids in his urine, particularly pyruvic acid and α-ketoglutaric acid. These are not normally found in urine. Why would chronic alcoholism result in malnutrition? Why would this man's water-soluble vitamins be so low? How would a vitamin deficiency result in the excretion of pyruvate and α-ketoglutaric acid?

19. A 13-year-old boy is brought to his family pediatrician, because he is urinating frequently throughout the day and night, and he is continually thirsty. His breath has a 'fruity' odor, and he is on the verge of becoming comatose. It is quickly determined that he has a high concentration of blood glucose. Clearly, this young man most likely has insulin-dependent diabetes mellitus (Type I diabetes). Which one of the following mitochondrial enzymes, that is essential in the net conversion of alanine to glucose, would be most active. Why?
(a) Citrate synthase.
(b) Isocitrate dehydrogenase.
(c) Pyruvate carboxylase.
(d) Pyruvate dehydrogenase.
(e) Fumarase.

20. A 56-year-old man presented with an enlarged liver that felt lumpy on examination. He admitted to drinking 1–2 bottles of vodka per day. A blood sample taken on his admission to hospital was excessively turbid and resembled a strawberry milkshake. This increase in turbidity was most probably due to:
(a) Increase in total cholesterol alone.
(b) Increase in VLDL and thus triglyceride.
(c) Increase in circulating denatured proteins.

21. Two brothers from a family with a high degree of consanguinity presented at ages 8 and 10 years with gross obesity and marked hyperphagia. All previous behavioral therapy had failed. Attempts to measure circulating concentrations of leptin revealed its absence in both children. To which of the following would you attribute their obesity?
(a) Lack of leptin receptors in the hypothalamus.
(b) Failure by adipose tissue to produce leptin.
(c) High circulating concentrations of insulin and stimulation of lipoprotein lipase.

22. A 17-year-old woman presents with oligomenorrhea and hirsutism. All her endocrine biochemistry is 'normal' except: testosterone 4.5 nmol/L (0.9–3.2 nmol/L) 17–hydroxyprogesterone 80 nmol/L (<50 nmol/L)
(a) What is the most likely diagnosis in this woman?
(b) Where is the excess androgen coming from?
(c) What is the appropriate form of therapy?
(d) Can this condition present in a different patient population?

23. An 80-year-old woman falls and fractures her femur. During her subsequent management, the serum biochemistry profile reveals the following results:

calcium 1.85 mmol/L (2.20–2.60 mmol/L)
albumin 40 g/L (35–45 g/L)
alkaline phosphatase 600 U/L (50–260 U/L)
creatinine 55 µmol/L (20–80 µmol/L)
parathyroid hormone 19 pmol/L (1.1–6.9 pmol/L)

These results indicate the likelihood of:
(a) Uncomplicated osteoporosis.
(b) Osteomalacia.
(c) Primary hyperparathyroidism?.

On questioning, she confirms that she has been housebound for the last 5 years and that she is a strict vegetarian. Which test would you perform to confirm your diagnosis? What would be the appropriate therapy for this woman?

24. A 15-year-old boy collapses while playing football. A week earlier he had finished a course of high-dose glucocorticoids as treatment for severe eczema. The most notable findings in his biochemical profile are:

cortisol <30 nmol/L (160–690 nmol/L)
ACTH <3 ng/L (<80 ng/L)

The most likely cause of his subnormal cortisol is:
(a) Primary adrenal failure (Addison's disease).
(b) A defect in one of the enzymes making cortisol (congenital adrenal hyperplasia).
(c) Suppression of pituitary ACTH by exogenous steroid.

Why do you think that the boy collapsed when he did?

25. A 34-year-old man comes to the outpatient clinic. He is asymptomatic. His cholesterol is 8 mmol/L [308 mg/dL] and his triglycerides are 15 mmol/L [1363 mg/dL]. On inspection his serum is white and cream-like.
(a) Which lipoproteins are likely to be increased?
(b) What is the risk associated with very high triglyceride concentration?
(c) Which enzyme activity is likely to be impaired?

26. A 9-year-old girl is brought to the outpatient clinic by her mother. The mother requests cholesterol testing because the girl's father died of myocardial infarction at the age of 42. Cholesterol is 8 mmol/L [308 mg/dL] and triglycerides are 1 mmol/L [91 mg/dL].
(a) Can this be simply diet related?
(b) Which lipid tests would you request from the laboratory?
(c) Which of the lipid metabolic disorders would you suspect here?

27. An obese 45-year-old man who smokes 20 cigarettes a day is referred to the lipid clinic. Triglycerides are 3.5 mmol/L [318 mg/dL], cholesterol is 6.7 mmol/L [258 mg/dL], and HDL is 0.85 mmol/L [33 mg/dL]. His blood pressure is 160/100 mmHg (the desirable level is below 140/90 mmHg), and the fasting plasma glucose is 7.5 mmol/L [135 mg/dL].
(a) How do you rate the cardiovascular risk of this man?
(b) What lifestyle changes would you advise to improve his health?
(c) Does he have an abnormality of carbohydrate metabolism?

28. A 3-month-old girl has been admitted to hospital for evaluation of periodic epileptic seizures. The child had light pigmentation and eczema on her arms and legs. She appeared to be detached, and somewhat unresponsive to her surroundings. No abnormalities were evident on an electroencephalogram or on magnetic resonance imaging of the brain. However, the blood phenylalanine level was high. A diagnosis of phenylketonuria is made, and the child is placed on a low-phenylalanine diet. While a noticeable improvement is noted in the hyperphenylalaninemia, no improvement is observed in the child's development or neurologic problems. Can you speculate as to what the metabolic defect may be in this infant and why no neurologic improvement is observed?

29. A 35-year-old male patient is admitted to hospital after several episodes of bizarre behavior and a finding of ammonia toxicity. The patient's history indicates a long-standing problem with alcoholism, and laboratory findings are consistent with acute hepatitis. Which of the following would it be helpful to administer to this patient in order to reduce the toxic concentrations of ammonia in his blood? Why?
(a) Sodium benzoate.
(b) Arginine.
(c) Lysine.
(d) Glutamine.

30. Growing children and patients recovering from surgery, burns, or other trauma require more high-quality protein (protein rich in essential amino acids) than normal, healthy adults. In addition, they excrete less nitrogen than they consume (negative nitrogen balance). Can you explain why this is the case and illustrate your answer with some specific examples from amino acid metabolism?

31. During his first week of military basic training, a young man in relatively poor physical condition collapsed at the end of a day of strenuous exercise. He failed to respond to a dousing with cold water and was admitted to the emergency room. Serum electrolytes were unremarkable, except that sodium was 130 mM (135–145 mM), and potassium was 5.0 mM (3.5–5.0 mM). The patient was acidotic as a result of excessive serum lactic acid build-up (15 mM, normal <2 mM), BUN (urea) was increased (150 mg/dL, 8× upper limit of normal), as was serum creatinine, 10× upper limit of normal). Serum levels of creatine phosphokinase were 4000 IU/mL (<100 IU/mL). Isozyme analysis indicated that the CPK was primarily the MM isoform. Urine was red-brown in color, pH 6.2, but free of erythrocytes. Urine flow was limited (<10 ml/hour), even following hydration. Myoglobin was detected in serum and urine at 1 and 25 mg/dL, respectively (normal <10 mg/dL), indicating severe muscle injury. How does muscle injury (rhabdomyolysis) lead to renal failure?

32. These are the results of an OGTT performed on a 53-year-old woman:

Time (min)	Plasma glucose concentration
0	4.5 mmol/L [81 mg/dL]
30	8.6 mmol/L [155 mg/dL]
60	9.8 mmol/L [176 mg/dL]
90	9.5 mmol/L [171 mg/dL]
120	8.5 mmol/L [153 mg/dL]

These results indicate:
(a) Normal glucose tolerance.
(b) Impaired glucose tolerance.
(c) Diabetes mellitus.

33. A 14-year-old boy comes to the outpatient clinic complaining of increased thirst and tiredness. His random blood glucose level is 13.0 mmol/L [234 mg/dL]. Would you:
(a) Repeat the random plasma glucose measurement?
(b) Perform the fasting plasma glucose measurement?
(c) Perform the OGTT?
(d) Measure urine ketones?
(e) Do all of the above?

34. A 24-year-old man has a blood glucose concentration of 12 mmol/L [216 mg/dL], HbA1c 8%, urine ketones (++). Urine protein excretion is 3 g/24 h. What do these results tell you about:
(a) The present state of his fuel metabolism?
(b) The history?
(c) The possible complications of diabetes?

35. A 65-year-old diabetic man is admitted to hospital with signs and symptoms of dehydration. His blood glucose is high, 20 mmol/L [360 mg/dL]; normal less than 6 mmol/L [108 mg/dL]. Only a small volume of urine is available for testing, but it shows a high (++++) sugar level. The likely cause of dehydration is:
(a) The patient is unable to drink.
(b) The concentration of glucose exceeded the capacity of the renal transport system and, by passing into the urine, the glucose contributed to osmotic diuresis.
(c) Independent of diabetes.

36. A 59-year-old woman underwent abdominal surgery. In the postoperative period, she received standard intravenous fluid treatment. On the fourth day, her plasma sodium concentration was 125 mmol/L (135–145 mmol/L). On examination, she was found to have edema of the hands and ankles. The most probable explanation of her reduced plasma sodium concentration is:
(a) Loss of sodium in the urine.
(b) Water retention as a result of excess secretion of ADH in the postoperative period.
(c) Undiagnosed diabetes insipidus.
(d) Increased insensible water loss.

37. A 49-year-old woman is admitted to hospital with a history of glomerulonephritis. Her creatinine concentration is 200 mmol/L [2.26 mg/dL] (20–80 mmol/L) [0.28-0.90 mg/dL]. The most probable interpretation of these findings is:
(a) Her renal function is normal.
(b) Approximately 50% of her nephrons are not functioning.
(c) None of her nephrons is functioning.
(d) There is an overproduction of phosphocreatine.

38. A 46-year-old woman comes to the outpatient clinic with high urea and creatinine concentrations indicating renal damage. The expected acid-base disorder will be:
(a) Respiratory acidosis caused by CO_2 retention.
(b) Acidosis caused by overproduction of nonvolatile acids.
(c) Metabolic acidosis caused by impaired excretion of nonvolatile acids.

39. A 56-year-old smoker comes to the hospital having difficulty breathing. His pO_2 is 6 kPa [45 mmHg], his pCO_2 5 kPa [37.5 mmHg], and his pH 7.40 (hydrogen ion concentration 40 nmol/L). This patient:
(a) Does not have a significant respiratory problem.
(b) Is likely to have respiratory acidosis.
(c) Has hypoxia, but is unlikely to have acidosis.

40. The patient with diabetic acidosis as a result of the accumulation of acetoacetic and hydroxybutyric acids in plasma is likely:
(a) To breathe at a normal rate.
(b) To hyperventilate as a compensation for the present metabolic acidosis.
(c) To hyperventilate to prevent the increase in CO_2 caused by acidosis.

41. An 18-year-old student presents in the casualty department with a rapid ventilatory rate, marked tetany of hands and feet, and in significant distress. You would expect to find:
(a) Decreased total calcium.
(b) Decreased ionized calcium.
(c) Increased serum albumin.
(d) Respiratory acidosis.

42. A young child was developing normally until he began to make the transition from breast feeding to infant foods. During this time he had frequent but intermittent bouts of vomiting and intestinal distress, and slept poorly at night. He was brought to the doctor's office one afternoon about an hour following a severe reaction to his food, a simple lunch of pureed vegetables and grape juice. His blood sugar was 2 mM [40 mg/dL], blood lactate was 4 mM (<1 mM), and serum phosphate was 2 mg/dL [0.6 mM] (4–7 mg/dL), [1.3–2.3 mM]. He was sweaty and lethargic, and there was evidence of mild jaundice and hepatomegaly. What metabolic abnormality might cause these problems? What analyses should be done to confirm your diagnosis?

43. The following results are obtained from investigation of a jaundiced patient: AST 300 IU/L, ALP 175 IU/L; urine bilirubin and urobilin both present. The cause of jaundice is:
(a) Hemolytic.
(b) Hepatocellular.
(c) Cholestatic.

44. A 1-day-old baby becomes jaundiced, but results of liver function tests are normal. Which course of action would you take initially?
(a) Attribute this to physiologic jaundice.
(b) Investigate for an inborn error of metabolism.
(c) Investigate for hemolytic disease and infection.

45. An asymptomatic, 55-year-old man is found to have an increased transaminase concentration, with otherwise unremarkable liver function tests. Which one of the following tests is not relevant to the differential diagnosis?
(a) Direct and indirect bilirubin.
(b) Autoimmune antibody screen.
(c) A differential blood cell count and film.
(d) Plasma ceruloplasmin.

46. A university president, on a speaking engagement to Miami Beach, noticed a dull ache in her right hip. During her return trip home, the pain increased to such a level that while on layover in Atlanta, she cancelled her remaining flight and went instead to the hospital where she was admitted. On admission the patient had a temperature of 101°C and a pulse rate of 90. Physical examination was unremarkable. X-ray examination of the abdomen and pelvis showed no distinct abnormalities. Urinalysis revealed cloudy, acidic urine, along with protein in the urine. After centrifugation, the sediment revealed a fine crystalline material. Analysis of this material showed that it was uric acid. What is your diagnosis? Discuss with your patient the biochemical basis for allopurinol treatment.

47. A baby boy was admitted to the hospital at 5 months of age with extreme lethargy, a persistent cough, nasal discharge, and loose, foul-smelling stools. He was found to be severely anemic. His urine contained a crystalline sediment, which was later identified as orotic acid. The patient was given large doses (150 mg/kg body weight) of uridine, which resulted in decreased excretion of orotic acid along with a return to normal hematocrit levels. With continued treatment, he gained weight and became active.
Explain the biochemical basis for the improved response of the patient when treated with uridine.

48. Humans cannot synthesize folic acid. Instead they obtain it through their diet. Compare the structure of sulfanilamide, a common sulfonamide antibiotic, and tetrahydrofolic acid.
Propose a mechanism of action for the sulfonamide antibiotics. Identify those steps in purine and pyrimidine biosynthesis that are blocked by sulfonamide antibiotics. Why are these drugs toxic to micro-organisms, but not to humans?

49. A frustrated couple brought their 5-year-old daughter to your office with complaints about excessive skin eruptions and blistering on the face, neck, hands, and arms. The parents noted that the young girl showed excessive freckling and blistering with only minimal sun exposure. The girl shows diminished stature and also shows some hearing and movement impairment. Lymphocytes were isolated from the patient, and an analysis of sensitivity to UV irradiation demonstrated a level of nucleotide excision repair that was 30–40% that of normal cells. What is your diagnosis of this child and what are your recommendations to her parents?

50. One of your patients, a young married woman of middle-Eastern origin, is pregnant with her first child. Ultrasound demonstrates that the child is a boy. Her father has a severe form of β-thalassemia. Her husband is apparently healthy; however, his maternal grandfather was a hemophiliac. Explain to the young couple the nature of the modes of inheritance of these diseases and evaluate the likelihood that her baby will be normal. How would your advice differ if ultrasound demonstrated that the baby were a girl?

51. You are treating a young man who has been diagnosed as carrying HIV (Human Immunodeficiency Virus), the primary cause of AIDS (Acquired Immune Deficiency Syndrome). One of the drugs the patient is taking is AZT (3'-azido-3'-deoxythymidine), a pyrimidine analog. Your patient asks you to explain why he is taking this drug when he has no symptoms of AIDS and how this drug is working.

52. A young mother brings her first child into your office to begin an immunization injection schedule which will provide the child protection against diptheria, pertussis, and tetanus. The young woman wants to ensure that her baby is well cared for but cannot see the need for immunization against diptheria since she has never heard of a child having this illness and the seriousness of the disease. How do you explain to the young mother the importance of protecting her child against this often fatal disease?

53. A 17-year-old man presents with hypertension. His blood pressure is increased: 210/110 mmHg; his urine sediment is clear. Examination of the optic fundi reveals grade II changes of established hypertension, and left ventricular hypertrophy is demonstrated by echocardiography. Examinations reveal hypokalemia, increased plasma aldosterone, and suppressed plasma renin activity, suggesting primary aldosterone excess from the adrenal glands. Computed tomography (CT) scanning of the adrenal glands reveals no adrenal tumor. The patient is given oral dexamethasone, a potent glucocorticoid drug that has no mineralocorticoid activity, and his hypertension and the biochemical abnormalities resolve.

This patient had a genetic disorder called glucocorticoid-suppressible hyperaldosteronism. This is an uncommon form of human hypertension caused by the inheritance of a chimeric gene that possesses aldosterone synthetic activity. How might dexamethasone have brought about resolution of the clinical abnormalities – hypertension and hypokalemia?

54. Thalassemias are common world-wide causes of anemia. Often, however, DNA sequencing of the exons of the β-globin genes reveals no abnormal nucleotides, but the β-globin mRNA is smaller than expected, and the hemoglobin produced is defective. How might genetic mutations cause such abnormal gene expression?

55. It is often observed in clinic that the response of individuals to steroid treatment varies. How might the effect of steroids on gene expression explain this variation?

56. A 27-year-old woman has a brother with Duchenne muscular dystrophy (DMD). Her affected brother is now dead, and his work-up was performed overseas but you know that he was said to have 'a deletion of his DNA'. The woman wishes to become pregnant but would wish to know if her child is likely to be affected by DMD. What strategy would you use to determine whether she and her child have a DMD-causing mutation?

57. A 25-year-old man with type II neurofibromatosis (NF-II) has a maternal cousin who has also developed deafness. Her MRI of the brain has a suspicious appearance, suggestive of a vestibular neurinoma (a tumor of the 8th cranial nerve highly associated with NF-II). Knowing that the gene for NF-II is large, how would you attempt to define a diagnostic method to determine whether or not the cousin has NF-II using DNA technology?

58. A 3-year-old boy is referred for investigation of learning difficulties. There is a strong family history of learning difficulties, particularly his maternal cousins, and his mother and her sister both attended special schools, yet his mother's brother did not. Screening investigations have found the mutation in the FMR-1 gene causing Fragile X syndrome (FRAXA). How can you explain the pattern of inheritance of the learning difficulties based on your knowledge of the DNA methods used to diagnose FRAXA?

59. A 27-year-old woman complains of 'walking on pillows'. Lumbar puncture shows oligoclonal bands in CSF, but not in serum. What is the most likely diagnosis?
(a) Neurosarcoidosis.
(b) Multiple sclerosis.
(c) Myasthenia gravis.
(d) Guillain-Barré syndrome.

60. A 48-year-old man has difficulty in keeping his eyes open. An edrophonium test dramatically alters this. What test would you perform next?
(a) Lumbar puncture.
(b) Serum theobromine.
(c) Acetylcholine receptor antibodies.
(d) Nerve conduction studies.

61. Calcium channel antibodies are positive in a 53-year-old male smoker. What would you see on a chest film?
(a) Bilateral basal fluid.
(b) Hilar lymphadenopathy.
(c) Lytic lesions in the sternum.
(d) Apical bronchiectasis.

62. A 67-year-old man's hands shake uncontrollably. He finds it difficult to start walking and, once he has managed to start, he cannot stop easily. His facial expression is blank and fixed. The patient has:
(a) Depression.
(b) Parkinson's disease.
(c) Cushing's syndrome.
(d) Organophosphate toxicity.

63. A 19-year-old man presents collapsed, with a slow ventilation rate. He has pin-point pupils. His symptoms are caused by:
(a) Myasthenia gravis.
(b) Diabetes mellitus.
(c) Opiate overdose.
(d) A stroke.

Short Answer Questions (SAQs)

1. The interactions between different parts of a protein play important roles in protein structure. These interactions are weak because they compete for interaction with water. Boiling water denatures proteins. Which types of interactions may be destroyed by boiling water?

2. A certain protein was purified from human erythrocytes, and in order to obtain the molecular mass of the protein, a purified sample was subjected to SDS–PAGE. In the absence of 2-mercaptoethanol, the molecular mass of 60 000 Da was observed, whereas in the presence of 2-mercaptoethanol, the value was 30 000 Da. Explain the data obtained in the presence or absence of 2-mercaptoethanol.

3. Plasma H_2CO_3 concentration is approximately 0.00125 mol/L. Calculate the level of HCO_3^- in plasma according to the Henderson-Hassebalch equation when pH of plasma is 7.4. The pKa of H_2CO_3 in blood is 6.1.

4. Which peptide(s) is produced on digestion of the peptide Gly-Val-Arg-His-Met-Trp-Lys-His-Ala-Met-Gly-Gly by trypsin? How could trypsin and cyanogen bromide (CNBr) be used together to determine the complete sequence of this peptide?

5. In the laboratory, after separating HbA into its globin subunits, you determine the O_2 saturation behavior of the intact HbA tetramer and the isolated α-globin monomer. Draw the O_2-binding curves for the two proteins. Give the approximate Hill coefficient for each protein.

6. Describe the molecular basis of the higher O_2 affinity of HbF compared with maternal HbA. Explain why this adaptation is necessary.

7. In the laboratory analysis of abnormal Hb, explain the difference in mobility on isoelectric focusing between normal and sickle cell Hb (HbA vs HbS).

8. What determines the substrate specificity and reaction specificity of an enzyme? Use serine proteases as an example.

9. Explain why high temperatures decrease enzymatic activity.

10. What biological benefit derives from the allosteric regulation of enzymes?

11. The optimum pH of pepsin is 1.5–2.0, and that of trypsin is 7.8. Explain the physiologic meaning of the difference in pH optima of these enzymes.

12. Explain in terms of K_m of enzymatic reactions why treatment with ethanol is useful for methanol poisoning.

13. A serine protease has histidine and aspartate at the catalytic center and is markedly inactivated at both lower pH (< 3) or higher pH (> 8). What type of ionic state do the side chains of these amino acids have when the enzyme is active?

14. Describe the major features of the currently accepted model for the structure of biomembranes.

15. Describe the relationship between Michaelis–Menten (enzyme) kinetics and those of facilitated diffusion.

16. Describe the essential features, and provide examples, of uniport, symport, and antiport systems.

17. Outline the mechanism of glucose absorption from the intestine.

18. Outline the mechanism of gastric acidification, describing multiple transport systems involved in this process.

19. Describe the two main types of ionophores and their mechanism of action.

20. Iron is an important constituent of the diet, and some people become iron deficient. One of the symptoms of iron deficiency anemia is fatigue. How could you explain this symptom in biochemical terms?

21. Some physicians are recommending that people taking inhibitors of HMG CoA reductase should supplement their diets with ubiquinone. What is the rationale for this recommendation?

22. Inhibitors of the electron transport system target specific components such that all of the components above the point of inhibition are reduced and those below it are oxidized. How would one go about monitoring this phenomenon?

23. Indicate how the process of digestion of protein is stimulated by gastric activity and how this affects activation of pancreatic peptidases.

24. Discuss the enzymic steps and intermediates formed during the process of complete digestion of glycogen to glucose.

25. Illustrate the mechanism by which glucose is absorbed into the intestinal epithelial cell and transported to the portal blood.

26. Describe the mechanisms available for the absorption of protein digests into the enterocyte.

27. Illustrate the role of micelle formation in the digestion and absorption of fat.

28. Indicate the different fates of a medium-chain and long-chain fatty acid on sn-3 carbon of a triacylglycerol.

29. Outline the role of vitamin A in the visual process, paying attention to both light/dark adaptation and the development of total blindness.

30. Vitamin D should be reclassified as a hormone – discuss.

31. Explain why folate and B_{12} deficiency present with some hematological abnormalities.

32. Outline those vitamins with an antioxidant function, indicating their differing roles in this process.

33. Outline methods for assessing zinc status in man.

34. Discuss the biological roles of copper.

35. What are the likely consequences of defects in glycolytic enzymes in the red blood cell? Consider enzymes that are thermolabile and have shorter than normal half-lives, or enzymes that have altered substrate affinities. Consider effects of enzyme defects on ATP production and explain why defects in both hexokinase and pyruvate kinase cause peripheral hypoxia.

36. The measurement of blood glucose in the clinical laboratory is carried out by enzymes in which phosphorylation of glucose is coupled enzymatically to the reduction or oxidation of NAD(P)(H). In this case the change or rate of change in absorbance at 340 nm, the λ_{max} for NAD(P)H, is used to estimate the glucose concentration in the sample. Outline two possible NAD(P)H-linked enzymatic assays for blood glucose using enzymes in glycolysis and/or the pentose phosphate pathway.

37. How could you estimate the relative distribution of glucose 6-phosphate metabolism between glycolysis and the pentose phosphate pathway? Consider the measurement of end-products of the two pathways. Consider the use of isotopically labeled $[^{14}C]$glucose, with ^{14}C labeling at various positions in the glucose molecule.

38. How does regulation of glycogenolysis differ between liver and muscle?

39. PKA works directly on glycogen synthase, but phosphorylase kinase is interposed between PKA and glycogen phosphorylase in both liver and muscle. Can you explain?

40. Discuss the rationale for 'carbohydrate loading' prior to a marathon run, including effects on both liver and muscle glycogen? Assuming that marathon runners metabolize about 500 kcal/h (500 Cal equals approximately 2000 kJ) how long would muscle glycogen reserves last during a marathon run?

41. Consider that one of the TCA cycle enzymes is defective, and its maximal activity is 60% of the normal enzyme. How would this affect metabolism and function in various tissues?

42. Suppose that a person is recuperating after a massive hemorrhage. How would this affect the TCA cycle?

43. Dietary citric acid can enter mitochondria and be oxidized in the TCA cycle. Explain how citric acid constitutes an anaplerotic compound.

44. Lipolysis in adipose tissue produces both glycerol and fatty acids. Describe the metabolic fate of the glycerol component of triglycerides.

45. Predict the biochemical and clinical consequences of a deficiency in an enzyme involved in carnitine biosynthesis in liver and kidney. Is this disease likely to be life threatening? Under what conditions? How would it be treated?

46. There is a old dictum that 'fats burn in the flame of carbohydrates'. Explain this, and discuss the requirement for glycolysis in order for fat catabolism to proceed efficiently in muscle.

47. Why does ketogenesis occur during fasting and starvation?

48. What is the rationale for the 'ketogenic diet', in which calories are restricted until the appearance of ketone bodies in urine. What does the appearance of urinary ketone bodies signify?

49. Ketone bodies are often described as 'water-soluble fats'. Compare the ATP yield per gram and per mole of acetoacetate and glucose, respectively, oxidized in cardiac muscle.

50. Outline the mechanisms by which long-chain fatty acids are synthesized from malonyl CoA.

51. Discuss the control mechanisms involved in the activation of acetyl-CoA carboxylase.

52. Fatty acid biosynthesis is an inducible, food-linked process. Discuss.

53. Outline the pathway for long-term storage of fat.

54. Explain why linoleic and linolenic acids are essential for humans.

55. How is cholesterol entry into the hepatocyte regulated?

56. Explain the importance of cytochrome P450 mono-oxygenase enzymes in the synthesis of estradiol from cholesterol.

57. Why is the enterohepatic circulation important in bile acid metabolism?

58. How is it possible to have a high serum cholesterol on a low-cholesterol diet?

59. Why is the concentration of cholesterol in plasma 1000 times greater than the solubility of cholesterol in water?

60. Outline the basic principles of the sliding filament model of muscle contraction.

61. Identify the major sites or mechanisms of regulation of the TCA cycle and explain their *raison d'être*.

62. Identify the sources of ATP (or ATP equivalents) in the TCA cycle and compare the efficiency of ATP production from glucose by glycolysis and by oxidative metabolism.

63. Compare the structure and activities of the pyruvate and α-ketoglutarate dehydrogenase complexes.

64. Explain how observations on malonate inhibition of succinate dehydrogenase contributed to the description of the TCA cycle.

65. Yeast are facultative anaerobes. They have mitochondria but will grow under anerobic conditions. The Pasteur effect is observed when a suspension of yeast is transferred from anaerobic to aerobic conditions. The yeast respond by:
(a) Decreasing their consumption of glucose;
(b) Decreasing their rate of evolution of CO_2. Explain.

66. Discuss the mechanisms involved in calcification of bone.

67. Outline the normal physiological responses observed when serum ionized calcium decreases acutely.

68. Explain how the bone remodeling cycle maintains bone mass, and indicate how this may be disturbed in patients with osteoporosis.

69. Outline the general pathways by which galactose and fructose enter glycolysis.

70. Describe some of the functions of the N-linked oligosaccharides.

71. Differentiate between the mechanism of biosynthesis of the *N*-linked and *O*-linked oligosaccharides on glycoproteins.

72. How are sugars activated for polymerization reactions and why is that necessary?

73. What is I-cell disease and what is its relation to protein targeting?

74. Where in the cell are *N*-linked and *O*-linked oligosaccharides synthesized?

75. What is the role of phosphatidic acid in the biosynthesis of triglycerides and phospholipids?

76. Describe two alternative routes for synthesis of phosphatidylcholine (PC), phosphatidylethanolamine (PE), and phosphatidylserine (PS).

77. What is the role of phospholipids in respiratory distress syndrome?

78. Discuss how phosphatidylinositol is involved in cell signaling.

79. Why are glycosphingolipids more likely than glycerophospholipids to have a role in intercellular recognition and signaling?

80. Discuss the pathogenesis of glycosphingolipidosis.

81. Explain how glycolipids mediate blood incompatibility reactions.

82. Describe the structural basis for formation of the collagen triple helix and the reason for the banded pattern of fibrillar collagens seen with the electron microscope.

83. Explain the effects of interrupting nonhelical segments on the structure of collagen domains.

84. How does collagen differ from elastin?

85. What are the principal noncollagenous glycoproteins in connective tissue? Discuss their interaction with ECM components and with integrins in plasma membranes.

86. Distinguish proteoglycans from glycoproteins.

87. How does the structure and composition of proteoglycans contribute to their function in the ECM?

88. When and why is the measurement of direct and indirect bilirubin of clinical value?

89. Why are low protein diets used for patients with severe liver disease?

90. Why may the effects of therapeutic drugs be altered by liver disease?

91. List the laboratory tests which are useful in an adult with jaundice, and explain why they are helpful.

92. When is neonatal jaundice of clinical concern?

93. Outline the *de novo* and salvage pathways for synthesis of GTP and TTP.

94. Describe the biochemical basis for chemotherapeutic treatment with fluorodeoxyuridylate (FdUMP).

95. Discuss the benefits of substrate channelling in multifunctional enzymes.

96. Describe the biochemical basis for the elevated purine levels in Lesch–Nyhan patients.

97. Imagine that you are attempting to identify a gene that you have mapped to a specific location on human chromosome 15. You have narrowed the region on this chromosome that contains this gene to a contiguous DNA fragment of about 450 kb. The 450-kb fragment is sequenced and you can now begin to identify the genes contained on this fragment. What are the types of sequence elements that will help you identify these regions?

98. The rho protein is involved in what stage of RNA transcription? What enzymatic activity does rho have, and why is this activity required for it to perform its function in transcription?

99. If you were developing a new antibiotic that specifically targeted bacterial protein synthesis as its mode of action, what specific enzymes, structures, or molecules would be likely targets?

100. Assume that you are studying a new anti-microbial drug that resulted in the termination of protein synthesis shortly after the initiation complex had formed. What is a good possibility for the target of the drug?

101. Describe the key features of a transcription unit.

102. If you were designing a gene for red hair, what regulatory features would you include?

103. List five ways of altering gene transcription.

104. Does genomic imprinting matter in man?

105. Compare and contrast the benefits and limitations of PCR versus cell-based DNA amplification.

106. One method of looking for genetic mutations is to screen entire genes for variations in their nucleotide sequence. How would you design a PCR experiment to detect mutations in a gene with eight exons, three of which are almost identical in size?

107. Describe the characteristics of an ideal PCR reaction, and contrast this with the reality of PCR using Taq polymerase.

108. Many genetic disorders can be detected *in utero* by analysis of fetal DNA. What limitations on the yield of target DNA would such prenatal diagnosis present, and how would this limit the methods used to detect any mutation?

109. Some times PCR can yield either no products or many products (not necessarily including the one you want!). Why may this occur and what simple steps can you take to prevent this from happening?

110. Paternity testing is becoming increasingly common. Describe the features that are essential for paternity testing to be successful using microsatellite repeats.

111. Explain why a single GH measurement may not provide optimal clinical information in a child being investigated for possible GH deficiency.

112. Explain the cellular basis of autoimmune primary hypothyroidism.

113. Give three reasons why the hypothalamo-prolactin axis is different from any of the other hypothalamo-pituitary axes.

114. Explain how a deficiency of the enzyme steroid 21-hydroxylase can lead to an increase in androgen production.

115. Suggest reasons why it is possible to use a two-site immunoassay for measurement of FSH but not estradiol.

116. Explain why some hormones are transported in plasma in association with specific binding proteins.

MCQ Answers

1. (i) (a), (ii) (b), (iii) (c), (iv) (d)
2. (i) (a), (ii) (b), (iii) (c)
3. (b)
4. (d)
5. (a)
6. (b)
7. (c)
8. (a) T, (b) T; (c) F; (d) F
9. (b)
10. (c)
11. (a) T, (b) T, (c) F, (d) F, (e) F
12. (b)
13. (d)
14. (d)
15. (a)
16. (a)
17. (e)
18. (d)
19. (e)
20. (b)
21. (b)
22. (b)
23. (c)
24. (b), (d), (e)
25. (c)
26. (a), (c), (e)
27. (a), (e)
28. (a), (c), (d), (e)
29. (c), (e)
30. (a), (b), (d), (e)
31. (a), (c), (d)
32. (a), (b), (d), (e)
33. (a), (b), (c)
34. (b), (c)
35. (b), (c), (d)
36. (a), (b), (d)
37. (a), (b), (c)
38. (a), (c), (d)
39. (a)
40. (e)
41. (d)
42. (b)
43. (e)
44. (b)

45. (b)
46. (c)
47. (d)
48. (c)
49. (a)
50. (d)
51. (a), (c), (d)
52. (e)
53. (b)
54. (c), (e)
55. (c)
56. (d)
57. (d)
58. (d)
59. (e)
60. (e)
61. (c)
62. (b)
63. (b)
64. (e)
65. (d)
66. (a)
67. (d)
68. (c)
69. (e)
70. (e)
71. (d)
72. (c)
73. (e)
74. (e)
75. (b)
76. (e)
77. (d)
78. (b)
79. (e)
80. (c)
81. (b)
82. (c)
83. (d)
84. (a)
85. (a)
86. (b)
87. (a), (b)
88. (a), (b), (c), (e)
89. (b)
90. (d)

91. (a), (b), (d), (e)
92. (d)
93. (b)
94. (a), (b), (c)
95. (d)
96. (d)
97. (c)
98. (b)
99. (d)
100. (b)
101. (c)
102. (a)
103. (c)
104. (b)
105. (c)
106. (a)
107. (d)
108. (b)
109. (b)
110. (a)
111. (b)
112. (b)
113. (a), (c), (d)
114. (a), (b), (c), (e)
115. (a)
116. (a)
117. (a), (c)
118. (b)
119. (a)
120. (c)
121. (b)
122. (a)
123. (d)
124. (b), (d)
125. (a), (b)
126. (a), (c)
127. (a), (d)
128. (a)
129. (d)
130. (a), (b), (c), (d)
131. (a)
132. (c)
133. (e)
134. (d)
135. (d)
136. (e)

137. (b)
138. (b)
139. (c)
140. (a)
141. (d)
142. (b)
143. (b)
144. (b)
145. (b)
146. (e)
147. (e)
148. (d)
149. (e)
150. (c)
151. (d)
152. (d)
153. (b)
154. (c)
155. (b)
156. (a), (c), (d)
157. (a)
158. (c)
159. (d)
160. (c)
161. (e)
162. (e)
163. (a)
164. (c)
165. (c)
166. (c)
167. (e)
168. (a)
169. (d)
170. (d)
171. (d)
172. (b)
173. (e)
174. (b)
175. (a), (b), (c), (d)
176. (b)
177. (b), (c)
178. (a), (c), (d)
179. (a)
180. (d)
181. (a) ,(b), (c), (d)
182. (b)

183. (d)
184. (a), (d)
185. (a), (c), (d), (e)
186. (d)
187. (b), (d)
188. (a), (b), (c), (e)
189. (a), (d)
190. (b)
191. (c)
192. (e)
193. (c)
194. (e)
195. (b)
196. (e)
197. (a)

198. (d)
199. (c)
200. (d)
201. (b)
202. (b)
203. (b)
204. (b)
205. (d), (e)
206. (a), (b), (e)
207. (b), (e)
208. (c), (d), (e)
209. (a), (b), (d)
210. (e)
211. (e)
212. (b)

213. (a)
214. (a)
215. (d)
216. (b)
217. (b)
218. (a)
219. (b)
220. (c)
221. (b)
222. (a)
223. (b)
224. (d)
225. (d)
226. (e)
227. (c)

228. (c)
229. (d)
230. (a), (c)
231. (b)
232. (a), (d)
233. (b), (c)
234. (b), (d)
235. (b), (d)
236. (a)
237. (c)
238. (b)
239. (c)
240. (e)
241. (a)

Patient-Oriented Problem Answers

1. Increased rate of respiration due to hyperventilation causes the lungs to remove more CO_2 from the blood than normal and then this will decrease pCO_2 and increase blood pH. This is because, in plasma, CO_2 is considered an acid and HCO_3^- its conjugate base. The decrease in acid relative to the level of its conjugate base causes an increase in pH, which is an example of respiratory alkalosis. Rebreathing from the paper bag in which CO_2 is accumulated will normalize the pCO_2 and reduce the blood pH to normal or near normal levels.

2. The sickle cell mutation results in the loss of two negative charges in the Hb tetramer at pH 8.6. Hb-C has an additional two positive charges because of glutamic acid to lysine and migrates more rapidly toward the cathode (negative pole) than Hb-S or Hb-A.

3. Alanine, serine, threonine, valine, leucine, isoleucine, phenylalanine, tyrosine, tryptophan, histidine. Actually monoamine dicaboxylic amino acids such as glutamine and aspargine are also excreted.

4. (b).

5. (c), (d).

6. (b), (d) for multiple myeloma.

7. This individual cannot synthesize a sufficient level of β-globin, leading directly to the profound anemia and requirement for transfusion therapy. The homozygous β-thalaessemia genotype arises from different mutations to each of the two alleles that encode β-globin. One of her β-globin gene alleles includes an RNA translation defect that terminates prematurely; the other contains a processing defect that limits the production of normal β-globin mRNA. Together, these mutations result in the synthesis of a fraction of the amount of normal β-globin polypeptide.

8. The concentration of 2,3-BPG should shift the O_2 saturation curve further to the right. The compensatory benefit of this shift is to facilitate O_2 delivery to peripheral tissues. But the physiologic cost is a somewhat diminished re-oxygenation of Hb in the pulmonary alveoli.

9. (b).

10. (e).

11. Option (a) provides a definitive diagnosis, but (b) is a reliable screening test and is appropriate for the first testing. The diagnosis can be confirmed by (a).

12. To reduce the secretion of insulin from β-cells, drugs that activate the K^+-ATP channel, such as diazoxide, and/or those that inhibit VDDC, such as nifedipine, would be given.

13. Consider maintenance treatment using a proton pump inihibor, or aggressive antibiotic therapy to eradicate *Helicobacter pylori*, if that organism is detected.

14. Pentachlorophenol has been used as a wood preservative and an insecticide. Workers exposed to it and people living in log homes, where the wood is preserved with pentachlorophenol, may suffer from exposure, because it has a significant vapor pressure. One of the symptoms of pentachlorophenol exposure is chloracne, which is a type of acne caused by exposure to chlorinated hydrocarbons. Pentachlorophenol is also known to act as an uncoupler of the mitochondrial electron transport system, and it stimulates respiration and wastes metabolic energy by dissipating the proton gradient across the inner mitochondrial membrane, generating larger quantities of heat and causing fever.

15. Clearly there is something metabolically wrong with the central nervous system. The high levels of pyruvate and lactate indicate that pyruvate is not being metabolized as a fuel. Defects could be in any of the enzymes leading to the TCA cycle, in the TCA cycle, in the electron transport system or ATP synthase. Such disorders fall under the category of Leigh's syndrome.

16. (c).

17. (b).

18. Distilled spirits are said to be empty calories, because they supply plenty of energy, but they are devoid of essential nutrients like vitamins and minerals, proteins and their essential amino acids, and essential fatty acids. Of the water-soluble vitamins, humans require more thiamin than any of the others, and its deficiency will be expressed first. Since thiamin is required by both pyruvate dehydrogenase and by α-ketoglutarate dehydrogenase, pyruvate and α-ketoglutarate metabolism will be impaired and they will accumulate in plasma to such an extent that they will be excreted by the kidneys.

19. (c) Pyruvate carboxylase converts pyruvate to oxaloacetic acid, a key reaction during the net synthesis of glucose from alanine.

20. (b).

21. (b).

22. (a) Partial steroid 21-hydroxylase deficiency.
(b) The adrenal gland.
(c) Glucocorticoid replacement therapy (e.g. hydrocortisone).
(d) Yes, in neonates who present with hyponatremia and/or ambiguous genitalia

23. (b) Osteomalacia. 25-hydroxycholecaferol, vitamin D therapy plus a calcium enriched diet.

24. (c) Suppression of pituitary ACTH by exogenous steroid. He was unable to produce cortisol during a time of exercise-related stress.

25. (a) Chylomicrons.
(b) Very high triglyceride concentration is associated with the risk of pancreatitis.
(c) Lipoprotein lipase.

26. (a) Taking into account the level of cholesterol and the family history, it is unlikely that dyslipidaemia in this child is diet related.
(b) Fasting lipid profile including total cholesterol, triglycerides and HDL cholesterol to confirm the previous results.
(c) Familial hypercholesterolemia.

27. (a) This cardiovascular risk is high on account of a moderate increase in cholesterol level, low HDL cholesterol, smoking, hypertension, and probably diabetes. High glucose level will have to be confirmed.
(b) Weight reduction, low cholesterol diet, smoking cessation, and mild regular exercise.

(c) This level of fasting glucose is consistent with diabetes mellitus. It needs to be confirmed as the diagnosis cannot be made on the basis of a single measurement.

28. The key to this child's problems is likely to stem from abnormal neurotransmitter generation. This may be due to a poor supply of tyrosine (although it is presumed that the low phenylalanine diet provided to the child was supplemented with tyrosine). It is more likely that this child may suffer an abnormality in biopterin cofactor metabolism since this same cofactor is required for tyrosine hydroxylase, a prerequisite step for catecholamine neurotransmitter biosynthesis and tryptophan hydroxylase, a prerequisite step for serotonin biosynthesis.

29. The useful compound from this list would clearly be sodium benzoate. This compound will form hippuric acid after conjugation with the glycine molecule. The hippuric acid is excreted in the urine, carrying nitrogen out of the body and relieving some of the ammonia load, since glycine biosynthesis from non-nitrogen containing precursors can utilize ammonia. Phenylacetate, which conjugates with glutamine, is also used in a similar approach aimed at removing amino groups and lowering free ammonia in patients suffering from ammonia toxicity. The ultimate solution in all cases is to define the cause of the elevated ammonia levels and when possible address the problem directly. These agents are stop-gap measures.

30. In both cases (rapid growth or tissue regeneration from trauma), there is an increased requirement for all amino acids in new protein synthesis. This will result in a higher portion of dietary essential amino acids, as well as non-essential amino acids being incorporated into new protein, rather than being channelled into energy metabolism, etc., with the loss of nitrogen. Thus, the amount of nitrogen excreted is less than that consumed and they are considered to be in positive nitrogen balance. Certain amino acids, like lysine and histidine, are required in higher amounts in the diet under these circumstances, because our ability to synthesize them is limited.

31. Diagnosis. This patient experienced severe muscle trauma during prolonged, strenuous exercise, as indicated by the release of muscle potassium, enzymes, and myoglobin into serum. Myoglobin is a low molecular weight protein which is filtered through the glomerulus and partially resorbed in renal tubules. Under acidic conditions, the heme group of myoglobin induces oxidative stress and renal tubular damage. Alkalinization of urine by administration of an antacid ($NaHCO_3$) with simultaneous dialysis therapy reduces renal injury and may lead to complete recovery. Other causes of rhabdomyolysis and subsequent renal failure include crush injuries, electrocution, severe hyperthermia, metabolic diseases (e.g. McArdle's disease) and drugs.

32. (b).

33. (b), (d).

34. (a) The patient is hyperglycaemic and the increased ketones indicate increased lipolysis and ketogenesis.
(b) Hemoglobin A_{1c} level suggests that he has been hyperglycemic for the last 3–6 weeks.
(c) Urine protein level suggests diabetic nephropathy.

35. (b).

36. (b).

37. (b).

38. (c).

39. (c).

40. (b).

41. (b)
Results consistent with overbreathing. Tetany as a result of respiratory alkalosis lowering ionized calcium.

42. This child shows symptoms of hereditary fructose intolerance, resulting from aldolase B deficiency. The disorder appears when children begin to consume fruit products and juices rich in fructose or sucrose. The liver is the primary site of fructose metabolism. Fructose 1-phosphate accumulates because of aldolase B deficiency. The resulting hypophosphatemia inhibits glycogenolysis by limiting the action of glycogen phosphorylase. Lactate accumulates in blood because fructose 1-phosphate also inhibits aldolase A, limiting gluconeogenesis.

43. (b).

44. (c).

45. (a).

46. Gout. See Figure 29.4

47. Uridine provides a source of UMP by the salvage pathway, reducing the need for de novo synthesis.

48. Bacteria synthesize folic acid *de novo*. They use sulfonamide, instead of *p*-aminobenzoic acid, forming an inactive folate analog, which inhibits bacterial nucleic acid

metabolism and causes cell death. Humans are protected because they cannot synthesize the vitamin, folic acid. Sulfonamides block tetrahydrofolate-dependent steps in purine synthesis (Fig. 29.2) and thymidylate synthase in pyrimidine (Fig. 29.6) biosynthesis.

49. Diagnosis of xeroderma pigmentosum can be confirmed by analysis of DNA repair activity in cultured fibroblasts. Recommendations include avoidance of sunlight, use of sunscreen, and frequent checks for skin cancer, plus genetic counseling.

50. β-Thalassemia is an autosomal recessive disease. Hemophilia is an X-linked recessive disease. Because her father had β-thalassemia, there is a 50% chance that she carries one copy of the β-thalassemia gene. Based on the frequency of β-thalassemia in the population, her husband has about 10% probability of carrying the same gene, so their son is unlikely (<5%) to suffer from β-thalassemia. Her husband does not suffer from hemophilia, so their child will be normal in this respect. Despite the genetic background of the family there is every reason to be optimistic. The advice would be the same for a female child.

51. You explain to the young man that AZT, once it is phosphorylated by the cell, acts like the nucleotide thymidine used for DNA synthesis. However, once AZT is incorporated into a newly synthesized DNA strand, no other nucleotides can be added because it lacks a 3'-OH necessary for strand elongation. This prevents the virus from replicating, helping to keep the virus in check. It is effective against the AIDS virus because the AIDS virus DNA polymerase is about 100 times more sensitive to the drug than the cellular enzyme.

52. You could start by explaining to her that diptheria is caused by a bacterium called *Corynebacterium diptheriae* and that the disease is highly contagious. You go on to explain that this bacterium produces a toxin that attacks the protein synthetic machinery of her child's cells leading to cell death. The toxin is so specific that it only targets a eukaryotic elongation factor (EF-2) and ignores the bacterial protein synthetic machinery. Since the toxin is covalently attached to the elongation factor it is impossible to rescue cells once they are affected, thus the importance of having preventive immunity against this deadly microbe.

53. Dexamethasone inhibits pituitary ACTH secretion. This results in a down regulation in the activity of ACTH-response genes. ACTH acts via generation of cAMP which binds to a cAMP response element on transcribable genes. In this case the chimeric gene is ACTH responsive and thus dexamethasone will suppress ACTH secretion which in turn switches off the chimeric gene and thus aldosterone secretion falls. This fall in aldosterone concentration leads to resolution of the clinical abnormalities.

54. In some cases of β-thalassemia there is a mutation of one or other end of an intron at the cervical splice donor or acceptor site. This means that when the ribonuclease enzyme performing the splicing reaches the mutation, it is unable to splice one exon to the next. The result is often a non-functional peptide due to the loss of a group of important amino acids. If the sequence of the exons alone is examined, the intron boundaries will be missed but the mRNA transcribed will be abnormally small.

55. The mechanism of action of steroid hormones is very complex. Although in theory the formation of a steroid-receptor-response element-complex would appear to be at the heart of their mode of action, there are many other steroid-related effects which are subject to natural variation. The affinity of the steroid for the receptor, the binding of the steroid-receptor complex, and the effectiveness of transcription can all vary from one person to another and thus the effect of steroids on human disease will vary accordingly.

56. As the majority of deletions causing Duchenne muscular dystrophy occur within a limited number of exons, then PCR-based approaches to the detection of deleted exons would be the first step. The use of multiplex PCR is particularly useful in this case. If such a deletion was detected in the patient then testing of a pregnancy by multiplex PCR or exon-specifi PCR of DNA obtained by chorionic villous sampling would the be investigation of choice.

57. As the NF-II gene is large, it would be impossible to sequence the gene quickly to detect a point mutation or some other small mutation responsible for the condition. It may therefore be easier to employ methods that can detect variation between normal alleles and mutant alleles without necessarily defining the nature of the mutation. This could involve RFLP analysis of the affected man with a normal individual and then comparing his RFLP patterns with his cousin. Similar strategies employing SSCP or DGGE analysis of PCR amplified regtion of the gene are also potentially useful.

58. Fragile X syndrome (FRAXA) is due to the inheritance of an unstable trinucleotide repeat in the FMR-1 gene on the X chromosome. As the trinucleotide expansion increases in size, the ability for it to cause the FRAXA phenotype increases. Small expansions may not give rise to clinical manifestations, but can act as 'pre-mutations' which if inherited can be passed on and result in a larger disease causing expansion. FRAXA can be diagnosed by using Southern blots of digested DNA to show increasing fragment sizes in those individuals with normal, premutant and mutant alleles. In this case the boy has inherited a trinucleotide repeat sufficient to cause FRAXA from his mother. She has a smaller expansion that has caused milder learning difficulties that are also present in her sister. Both these women must have inherited the mutation from a carrier of a 'premutation', either mother or father, whereas their brother has inherited a non-FRAXA X chromosome from the parent with the FRAXA 'premutation'.

59. (b).

60. (a).

61. (b).

62. (b).

63. (c).

Short Answers

1. Hydrogen bonds.

2. This is because the protein consists of two subunits with molecular mass of 30,000 Da.

3. 25 mM.

4. Digestion by trypsin yields Gly-Val-Arg, His-Met-Trp-Lys and His-Ala. These three peptides are isolated and then sequenced by Edman degradation. CNBr treatment cleaves the peptides at Met residue into two peptides. Following isolation, they are also subjected to sequencing. N-terminal amino acid sequence is obtained when the peptide is sequenced without cleavage. By these sequence data, you can determine the complete sequence.

5. HbA has a sigmoid curve with n = 2.7. The isolated globin monomer has a hyperbolic curve with n =1, identical to that of Mb because of the loss of subunit cooperativity.

6. A mutational loss of a positively charged amino acid side chain in γ-globin.

7. HbS differs from HbA at residue 6 of β-globin: Glu in the normal; Val in the mutant. With the loss of a negative charge on each of the subunits, HbS migrates more slowly toward the positive electrode (anode) than HbA. Homozygotes exhibit a single band representing the $\alpha_2\beta^s_2$ tetramer. A mixture of two tetrameric structures, $\alpha_2\beta_2$ (60% of total) and $\alpha_2\beta^s_2$ (40% of total), is present in heterozygotes; the proportion of the mixed tetramer $\alpha_2\beta\beta^s$ is too slow to be detected readily.

8. Active site of enzymes is composed of catalytic site and substrate binding site. In enzyme reactions, ionizable amino acids, such as histidine and cysteine, often participate in catalytic reaction. Specific serine, histidine, and aspartate residues form a 'catalytic triad' in serine proteases. Chymotrypsin, trypsin, and elastase, three serine proteases, are similar in many respects. However, their substrate specificities are quite different because structures and charges of the binding sites are different from each other.

9. In the case of an inorganic catalyst, the reaction rate increases with the temperature of the system. The tertiary (three-dimensional) structure of a protein involves weak bonds such as hydrogen bonds, which can be disrupted by high temperature. Thus, enzymes function at body temperature 37°C, but also many of them display a temperature optimum at this range.

10. Allosteric enzymes undergo conformational changes in response to surrounding conditions such as substrates, products, and other regulatory factors. For example, an allosteric enzyme can become more active in the presence of positive, allosteric effectors and produce products more efficiently than an isosteric enzyme.

11. Pepsin works in the stomach where the pH is extremely low (1.5–2.0) due to gastric juice, while trypsin exists in the intestinal tract where the pH is about neutral (7–8). Thus these enzymes have ideal characteristics for working where they are found.

12. In methanol poisoning, toxic compounds are produced by metabolic conversion of methanol. Both methanol and ethanol are metabolized by alcohol dehydrogenase. This enzyme, however, has much lower Km, i.e. higher affinity, for ethanol than for methanol. Thus, ethanol can competitively inhibit conversion of methanol to toxic metabolites.

13. Histidine is protonated and aspartate is ionized between pH 3 and pH 8 when the enzyme is active.

14. See Figure 7.2. Biomembranes are composed of proteins and lipids. As proposed by Singer & Nicolson, the phospholipid bilayer is a basic structure of biomembrane into which globular proteins are embedded. Polar head groups of phospholipids are located in the membrane surface and their fatty acyl chains face inside the membranes. Variations in the size and degree of unsaturation of fatty acids in the phospholipids affect the fluidity of biomembranes. While membrane lipids and proteins easily move on the membrane surface (lateral diffusion), the 'flip-flop' movement of lipids between outer and inner bilayer leaflets rarely occurs. Membrane proteins are classified into integral transmembrane proteins and peripheral membrane proteins. The former proteins are deeply embedded into lipid bilayer and some of them traverse the membrane several times. Peripheral membrane proteins are bound to the membrane lipids and proteins by electrostatic interaction.

15. See Figure 7.5. In a fashion similar to enzymic reactions, proteins participate in facilitated diffusion. The kinetics of facilitated transport of substrate can be described by the same equation that is used for enzyme catalysis (the Michaelis–Menten equation). Facilitated diffusion is a saturable process, having a maximum transport rate (V_{max}). When the concentration of extracellular transport substrate becomes very high, the V_{max} value is achieved, as a result of saturation of the protein with substrate. K_m is the dissociation constant of substrate and transporter, and equal to the concentration that gives the half-maximal transport rate.

16. See Table 7.3. Transport substrates move in the same direction during symport, whereas they move in opposite directions in antiport systems. The movement of one substrate against its concentration gradient is driven by movement of another substrate (usually cations such as Na^+ and H^+) down a gradient. Charged substrates are electrophoretically driven by membrane potential in uniport. Examples: uniporter, glucose transporter (GLUT); symporter, Na^+-coupled glucose transporter (SGLT) in kidney and intestine; antiporter, Na^+/Ca^{2+} antiporter in heart muscle and Cl^-/HCO_3^- antiporter in gastric parietal cells.

17. See Table 7.4. Dietary glucose is transported into intestinal epithelial cells against a concentration gradient. The Na^+-coupled glucose symporter (SGLT) functions in this process. The Na^+ ions symported into the cell are pumped out by an Na^+/K^+-ATPase. The intracellular glucose concentration increases and glucose is transported across the membrane to the blood by facilitated diffusion, using the GLUT family of glucose transporters.

18. See Figure 7.8. The lumen of the stomach is highly acidic (pH≈1) because of the presence of a proton pump (H^+/K^+-ATPase) that is specifically expressed in gastric parietal cells. The pump protein is localized intracellularly in vesicles in the resting state. Stimuli such as histamine induce fusion of the vesicles with the plasma membrane. The pump antiports two cytoplasmic hydrogen ions and two extracellular potassium ions, coupled with hydrolysis of a molecule of ATP. Cl^- is secreted through a Cl^- channel, producing HCl (gastric acid) in the lumen. The cytoplasmic K^+ is secreted by a K^+ channel. The CO_2 gas transported by simple diffusion into the parietal cells is hydrated immediately, producing H^+ and HCO_3^-. The HCO_3^- is exchanged with extracytoplasmic Cl^- by a Cl^-/HCO_3^- antiporter. Thus HCl is supplied in the parietal cell.

19. There are two classes of ionophores: mobile ion carriers (or caged carrier) and channel formers. Valinomycin is a typical example of a mobile ion carrier. K^+ binds to the center of the peptide ring structure at the aqueous interface of membrane. The complex diffuses across the hydrophobic membrane to the distal aqueous interface, where the ion is released. Gramicidin A is a linear peptide with 15 amino acid residues. A β-helical gramicidin A molecule forms a pore. The head-to-head dimer formation makes a transmembrane channel that allows movement of monovalent cations (H^+, Na^+, and K^+). (Figure 7.4)

20. Hemoglobin and myoglobin clearly require iron for oxygen transport. Mitochondrial cytochromes also require iron. Iron deficiency could affect all of these components. Both oxygen transport and energy production would be impaired, causing fatigue.

21. Ubiquinone is synthesized from the same isoprenoid precursors as cholesterol. HMG CoA reductase catalyzes a reaction that leads to these intermediates, so its inhibition will result in less synthesis of both cholesterol and ubiquinone, which functions both as a component of the respiratory chain and as an antioxidant. Its antioxidant function may by important in the prevention of atherosclerosis caused by oxidized LDL.

22. Many of the respiratory chain components have unique absorption spectra and can be identified spectrophotometrically. The absorption spectrum of each also shifts when reduced or oxidized. The point of inhibition is known as the crossover point and can be determined spectrophotometrically by monitoring the absorption spectrum of each respiratory chain component.

23. The low pH of gastric fluid denatures dietary protein. Pepsinogen is secreted by gastric chief cells and is spontaneously and autocatalytically activated to pepsin at acid pH, beginning the digestive process. The peptide digest stimulates cholecystokinin release in the duodenum, which then stimulates secretion of pancreatic enzymes.

24. Carbohydrate digestion begins with salivary amylase, continues with pancreatic amylase, yielding dextrins, which are degraded to glucose by intestinal brush border glucosidases.

25.   Glucose is absorbed from the lumen primarily by an active transport process involving cotransport with Na^+. High luminal Na^+ is maintained by a Na^+,K^+-ATPase. Thus glucose uptake occurs by an indirect, active transport process. Glucose moves from the enterocyte into blood by passive transport involving GLUT-5.

26.   Amino acids and di- and tri-peptides are absorbed from the gut. Amino acids are absorbed by a family of Na^+ symporters with broad specificity for similar types of amino acids (aromatic, basic, acidic, etc.). Di- and tri-peptides are cotransported with H^+ ions; digestion to amino acids is completed in the enterocyte.

27.   Bile salts, with some assistance from dietary lipids and lipid digestion products (fatty acids), disperse fats into small micelles with large surface areas, facilitating degradation by pancreatic lipase. Water-soluble products (fatty acids, 2-monoacylglycerols) are absorbed by intestinal epithelial cells.

28.   Fatty acids at the sn-3 position of triglycerides are released by pancreatic lipase. Very long-chain, water-insoluble fatty acids are largely unabsorbed. Long-chain fatty acids are absorbed into the enterocyte, reassembled into tryglycerides and secreted into the lymphatic circulation. Medium- and short-chain fatty acids are absorbed directly into the portal circulation.

29.   Vitamin A is a precursor of the visual pigment, rhodopsin, which is essential for function of rod cells. Deficiency of vitamin A leads to poor vision at low light levels (night blindness), and may lead to complete blindness as a result of abnormalities in growth and development of corneal epithelia.

30.   Vitamin D is a steroid derivative. Following activation in liver and kidney, it binds to transport proteins in target cells and affects gene expression. Its mechanism of action is identical to that of steroid hormones.

31.   Folate and cobalamin are required for 1-carbon transfer reactions in nucleic acid synthesis and methionine metabolism. Deficiencies in these vitamins affect cell division, particularly the production and development of red cell precursors (reticulocytes in the bone marrow) leading to anemia.

32.   Vitamins A and E are fat soluble vitamins, providing antioxidant protection in membrane environments. Vitamin C is a water-soluble vitamin and provides protection in aqueous compartments.

33.   Zinc status was originally evaluated by measurement of serum zinc concentration. Because many dietary, health, and environmental factors affect serum zinc concentration, measurements of red cell levels of the zinc-containing protein, metallothioneine, have proven more useful for assessing zinc status.

34.   Copper is a cofactor for oxygenases and oxidases which use molecular oxygen for metabolism, and for proteins and enzymes involved in antioxidant defenses and scavenging of reactive oxygen species (ceruloplasmin and superoxide dismutase).

35.   Hemolytic anemia is a common consequence of defects in glycolytic enzymes, leading to low hematocrit and inadequate oxygen transport.

36.   (A) hexokinase + Glc-6-P dehydrogenase, yielding increase in NADPH. (B) hexokinase, pyruvate kinase, lactate dehydrogenase, yielding decrease in NADH.

37.   [1-^{13}C]-glucose is used to assess the activity of the pentose phosphate pathway by measuring the rate of release of $^{13}CO_2$. Release of $^{13}CO_2$ from [6-^{13}C]-glucose provides a measure of the relative rate of other pathways of glucose metabolism.

38.   Glucagon response in liver, response to neural stimulation in muscle.

39.   Phosphorylase kinase provides an additional site for regulation of glycogenolysis.

40.   Carbohydrate loading builds up both hepatic and muscle glycogen. Storage of 500 grams of glycogen would provide sufficient energy for 4 hours of intense exercise; however, after a short duration of exercise, fatty acids become the major energy source in muscle.

41.   Since one of the major precursors to acetyl-CoA is pyruvate, it would probably accumulate producing excess lactic acid, which could lead to lactic acidosis. TCA cycle defects are very rare, because when they occur, the organism probably dies before the fetal stage and aborts. Since the nervous system generally has the highest metabolic rate in the body, it would probably be severely impaired and cell death would occur, resulting in encephalopathy.

42.   Heme and proteins would be synthesized at a rapid rate because of the loss of blood. The TCA cycle activity would be accelerated to produce heme, because the synthesis of heme starts with succinyl-CoA supplied by the

TCA cycle. A source of carbons would be required to make up for the deficit created by the loss of succinyl CoA. For example, glutamate could undergo trasamination to α-ketoglutarate, an anaplerotic reaction. In addition, the cycle would supply reductive power in the form of reduced nucleotide coenzymes for the production of mitochondrial ATP, which would be needed for biosynthetic reactions.

43. Citric acid increases the net carbons in the cycle and will result in the net synthesis of oxaloacetic acid, as well as other intermediates.

44. Conversion to glycerol phosphate, then dihydroxyacetone phosphate for gluconeogenesis in liver.

45. Absence of carnitine would inhibit oxidation of long-chain fatty acids. Depending on severity, may lead to fasting hypoglycemia, which could be life-threatening. Treatment with dietary carnitine.

46. Oxidation of fatty acids in muscle mitochondria produces acetyl-CoA. Metabolism of acetyl-CoA in the TCA cycle requires oxaloacetate for condensation with acetyl-CoA in the citrate synthase reaction. Carbohydrates produce pyruvate, which is converted to oxaloacetate by pyruvate carboxylase, assuring a constant supply of oxaloacetate for acetyl-CoA metabolism.

47. Fatty acid catabolism supports gluconeogenesis and provides energy in most tissues during fasting and starvation. Because of decreased glycolysis in the liver during these conditions, oxaloacetate concentration is low and acetyl-CoA cannot be efficiently metabolized in the TCA cycle. To recover the acetyl-CoA required for continued β-oxidation of fatty acids, the liver converts acetyl-CoA to ketone bodies, exporting them from liver. The CoA is released for continued β-oxidation.

48. A ketogenic diet involves dietary restriction until ketone bodies begin to appear in urine. The presence of urinary ketone bodies signifies active fat metabolism, which will lead to a gradual weight loss.

49. One mole of glucose yields 36–38 moles ATP, or 0.2 mole ATP per gram of glucose. One mole of acetoacetate requires investment of 2 equivalents of ATP in the thiokinase reaction, yielding two moles of acetyl-CoA, each of which yields 24 moles ATP. Thus, the energy yield from acetoacetate is about 52 ATP/mol, or about 0.5 mole ATP per gram of acetoacetate.

50. Review Figures 15.2 and 15.3, discussing the role of the cysteinyl and pantetheinyl sulfhydryl groups, the charging and chain elongation reactions, and the additional enzymatic activities of the fatty acid synthase complex.

51. Acetyl-CoA carboxylase catalyzes the rate limiting step in fatty acid biosynthesis. It is activated by citrate which causes polymerization of inactive protomers into the active polymeric form of the enzyme. It is also inactivated by phosphorylation in response to glucagon, inhibiting lipogenesis during gluconeogenesis.

52. High carbohydrate diets induce a number of glycolytic and lipogenic enzymes which catalyze the conversion of carbohydrates into fatty acids and triglycerides.

53. Triglycerides are delivered to adipose tissue in the form of chylomicrons or VLDL. The triglycerides are hydrolyzed by lipoprotein lipase, the fatty acids are taken up into adipose tissue and esterified to glycerol 3-phosphate, derived from dihydroxyacetone phosphate. Genetic and environmental (diet, activity) factors determine total fat deposition. The hormone leptin, secreted by adipocytes, suppresses food intake by action on the hypothalamus.

54. Mammalian fatty acid desaturases cannot insert double bonds beyond the Δ9 carbon. Linoleic acid has a double bond at $\Delta^{9,12}$ (ω-6) and linolenic acid at the $\Delta^{9,12,15}$ (ω-3 & ω-6) positions. These fatty acids are precursors of prostaglandins.

55. Cholesterol enters the cell by a receptor-mediated pathway. An increase in intracellular cholesterol levels leads to a decrease in receptor number and decreased cholesterol uptake. A decrease in intracellular cholesterol (e.g. when HMG-CoA reductase is inhibited) leads to an increase in receptor number.

56. Cytochrome P450 mono-oxygenase regulates the two enzymes that cleave the cholesterol side chain at C-17 and the aromatase enzyme that converts the A ring of testosterone into the aromatic ring of estradiol with the loss of the C-19 angular methyl group.

57. The enterohepatic circulation allows 98% of bile acids to be reabsorbed from the jejunum, transported via the portal vein and resecreted into the bile duct.

58. In normal subjects about 50% of cholesterol is synthesized de novo. In certain groups of subjects there is abnormal cholesterol synthesis and metabolism that can lead to a high serum cholesterol despite dietary restriction.

59. The vast majority of cholesterol in plasma is bound to hydrophilic protein molecules.

60. Acetyl-CoA accumulation in the mitochondrion, derived from either carbohydrate or fat metabolism, inhibits pyruvate dehydrogenase and stimulates pyruvate carboxylase, providing oxaloacetate for TCA cycle activity.

61. Pyruvate dehydrogenase is inhibited by acetyl-CoA and NADH, both allosterically and by activation of pyruvate dehydrogenase kinase, which inhibits the enzyme; this limits carbohydrate utilization during periods of gluconeogenesis. Mitochondrial dehydrogenase activities are dependent on levels of NAD^+, which depends on NADH utilization to regenerate ATP; this links TCA cycle activity to energy requirements of the cell. Isocitrate dehydrogenase is especially sensitive to ATP and NADH; its inhibition during energy-rich conditions shuttles citrate to the cytoplasm for lipid biosynthesis.

62. Review data in Figure 13.1. Aerobic metabolism of glucose yields about 20 times as much ATP as glycolysis.

63. Review Figures 13.5 and 13.6.

64. Review Malonate Block box in Chapter 13.

65. The yeast convert to more efficient oxidative metabolism of glucose, requiring less glucose and therefore evolving less CO_2.

66. Confirm increased adjusted calcium on at least two occasions. Measure PTH 1–84 and if >3 pmol/L then the cause is hyperparathyroidism. Measure urea creatinine and electrolytes to exclude renal disease and urinary calcium excretion to exclude familial hypocalciuric hypocalcemia. If renal function is normal and urinary calcium elevated, diagnosis is primary hyperparathyroidism. If PTH 1–84 <3 pmol/L then malignancy must be excluded by a combination of history, physical examination, X-rays, CT scan, and magnetic resonance imaging where required. PTH-P can be measured; if >2.6 pmol/L highly suggestive of solid tumor. Myeloma screen should be performed (serum and urine electrophoresis for monoclonal gammopathy). Thyroid function tests, vitamin D, growth hormone, angioconverting enzymes and lithium measurement in serum would all be required when rare causes are suspected.

67. As ionized calcium decreases, this stimulates the chief cells of the parathyroid gland to produce PTH (1–84). The PTH circulates in blood and acts on receptors in the kidney promoting calcium reabsorption and phosphate excretion. It also stimulates the renal conversion of 25-hydroxy cholecalciferol (vitamin D) to 1,25-dihydroxy cholecalciferol which promotes calcium absorption from the gut. PTH acts on osteoblasts/osteoclasts in bone stimulating osteoclast bone resorption which releases calcium and phosphate from the bone matrix. All of these effects act in combination over the short (kidney reabsorption) and longer term (gut absorption, bone resorption) to restore calcium to normal.

68. During the bone remodeling, cycle resorption and formation are 'coupled' so that the amount of old bone removed by osteoclasts is equaled by the amount of new bone formed by the osteoblasts. This is achieved by hormones and cytokines released by the two cell types which regulate the cellular activity. Calcium balance is maintained. In osteoporosis osteoclast activity is increased more than osteoblast with the result that: (a) more bone surfaces are resorbed; (b) deeper 'pits' are seen in bone; (c) less filling in with new bone occurs. The osteoclast and osteoblast are now 'uncoupled' and with the passage of time a decrease is observed in the total amount of bone present throughout the skeleton.

69. Galactose is phosphorylated by a specific kinase to give galactose-1-P which is then converted to UDP-galactose by Gal-1-P:uridyltransferase (the enzyme missing in severe cases of galctosemia). This UDP-galactose is epimerized to UDP-glucose which is then converted to glucose-1-P, then to glucose-6-P and then to fructose-6-P. Fructose is also phosphorylated in liver by a specific kinase to give fructose-1-P which can be cleaved by a specific liver aldolase (aldolase B) to give dihydroxyacetone-phosphose and free glyceraldehyde. The glyceraldehyde can be phosphorylated to give glyceraldehyde-3-P which can enter glycolysis. Fructose utilization is not regulated by factors (ATP, AMP levels, etc.) that control the activity of PFK.

70. N-linked oligosaccharides may be important in helping protein to assume its proper conformation in the endoplasmic reticulum, or these oligosaccharides may increase the stability of the protein to heat or other denaturants. Specific N-linked oligosaccharides with mannose-6-P residues as part of their structure are involved in targeting hydrolytic enzymes to the lysosome. Specific oligosaccharide structures are also involved in chemical recognition reactions that allow certain bacteria and viruses to recognize and bind to host target cells. In addition, many cell:cell interactions that occur during development involve recognition of N-linked oligosaccharides.

71. N-linked oligosaccharides are assembled on a lipid carrier whereas O-linked oligosaccharides are not. For the N-linked oligosaccharides, the individual sugars, GlcNAc, mannose, and glucose, are added sequentially to the lipid carrier, dolichol-P, in the endoplasmic reticulum by a series of glycosyltransferases. The final product is a 14 sugar oligosaccharide-PP-dolichol (i.e. $Glc_3Man_9GlcNAc_2$-PP-dolichol). This intact N-linked oligosaccharide is then transferred to specific asparagine residues on the protein. Further trimming of the protein-bound oligosaccharide, to give a variety of different oligosaccharide chains, occurs in the ER and Golgi apparatus. On the other hand, O-linked oligosaccharides are synthesized in the Golgi apparatus by the transfer of GalNAc directly to serine residues of the protein and then sequential transfer to other sugars (GlcNAc, galactose, silaic acid) to GalNAc without the participation of a lipid carrier.

72. Sugars are activated by converting them to the nucleoside diphosphate sugars (such as UDP-glucose, GDP-mannose, etc.). Polymerization, or glycoside bond formation, is an anabolic reaction and requires an input of energy, since the product is more complex than the starting material. Thus, a high energy phosphate is utilized to make the activated form of the sugar, i.e.

$$UTP + glucose\text{-}1\text{-}P \rightarrow UDP\text{-}glucose + PPi.$$

73. I-cell disease is an inborn error of metabolism characterized by inability of afflicted individuals to degrade (turnover) macromolecules such as proteoglycans, glycolipids and glycoproteins. This defect results from the inability of these individuals to attach the proper targeting signal to their lysosomal proteins (which are synthesized in the ER and must have a mannose-6-P added to the N-linked oligosaccharides) in order to target these proteins to the lysosomes. Individuals with I-cell disease are missing the GlcNAc-1-P transferase that adds GlcNAc-1-P to high-mannose oligosaccharides to give GlcNAc-1-P mannose oligosaccharides. The GlcNAc is then removed to expose the mannose-6-P residues (possibly another form of I-cell disease will be found where people are missing the GlcNAc trimming enzyme). The mannose-6-P residues are recognized by Golgi receptors that target those proteins to the lysosomes.

74. N-linked oligosaccharides are initially synthesized in the endoplasmic reticulum and then modified in the Golgi, as the protein is transported through the various Golgi cisternae. O-linked oligosaccharides are probably mostly synthesized in the Golgi although some of the early reactions such as the xylosyltransferase (for proteoglycans) and the Gal-NAc transferase may be in the ER.

75. Phosphatidic acid is a precursor for phospholipids and for triglycerides. It is used to make DAG as well as CDP-DAG.

76. PE and PC can be made by condensation of CDP-choline or ethanolamine with DAG, or PC can be made from PE by methylation with SAM. PE can also be made by decarboxylation of PS. PS can be made from PC or PE by exchange of the headgroup (i.e., S for C or S for E).

77. Dipalmitoylphosphatidylcholine (DPPC) is a surfactant that facilitates opening of alveoli during inspiration and prevents collapse of the lungs.

78. Inositol triphosphate (IP_3) and DAG are two signaling molecules that come from PI degradation.

79. Because glycolipids can have many different sugars (and linkages) in their structure and therefore contain much more information that can be used as recognition signals.

80. Glycosphingolipidoses are a group of inborn errors where individuals are missing one of the essential enzymes in their lysosomes that are involved in degradation and turnover of glycosphingolipids.

81. Glycolipids are antigens on the surfaces of red blood cells and are responsible for the ABO blood group types. People with A blood type have a certain glycolipid structure that causes formation of antibodies against red cells from persons with type B or AB blood.

82. Review role of repeating tri-peptide, glycine, hydrogen bonding, disulfide bonds, and quarter-staggered array of collagen molecules (Figures 27.1 and 27.2).

83. Nonhelical segments interrupt fibril associations, promoting formation of nonfibrillar, network-type structures.

84. Consider three-dimensional structure, amino acid composition, post-translational modifications and crosslink structures.

85. Describe fibronectin, laminin, and nidogen, their domain structures and interactions with other components of ECM, and the role of RGD sequences in integrin binding.

86. Consider composition, linkage to protein, repeating disaccharide structure, size, and branching of saccharide chains, and polyanionic character.

87. Long, polyanionic chains form extended structure, imparting strength and compressibility to the ECM, and provide a matrix for interaction with other matrix components and cells.

88. 'Direct' bilirubin is an alternative name for conjugated bilirubin, whilst 'indirect' bilirubin refers to the unconjugated fraction of bilirubin. In patients with hyperbilirubinemia, measurement of both the direct and indirect proportions of bilirubin may help to differentiate between pre-hepatic causes, where the serum bilirubin is predominately unconjugated or indirect, and hepatic/post-hepatic causes, when the serum bilirubin is mainly conjugated or direct.

89. Patients with clinically significant disease of the hepatic parenchyma are unable to detoxify nitrogenous substances, since the functional capacity of the hepatocyte urea cycle is impaired. Amino acids and other amines arising from the gut may escape normal hepatic metabolism, and thereby gain access to the systemic circulation. Certain amines may act as neurotransmitters in the brain and alter cognitive function. Low protein diets reduce the nitrogenous load to be metabolized by the liver.

90. The liver is responsible for metabolizing most drugs, and in general the metabolic transformations increase their water-solubility and thereby their rates of excretion in urine or bile. Diseases of the hepatic parenchyma are likely to impair drug metabolism non-specifically, and increase the half-life of the drug. This in turn may lead to a greater, or more prolonged, therapeutic effect in patients with liver disease. For those drugs which are subject to biliary excretion, cholestatic disease will impair the excretion of drug metabolites, which may in turn give rise to pharmacologic effects in their own right. Drug prescriptions for patients with liver disease should be carefully reviewed before any drug is administered.

91. The two essential questions to be answered in any jaundiced patient are first the general cause of the jaundice (pre-hepatic, hepatic or post-hepatic), and secondly the specific disease process. Biochemical tests to delineate the general cause of jaundice.
Serum direct/indirect bilirubin: Pre-hepatic causes of jaundice are generally associated with a rise in the serum concentration of unconjugated (indirect) bilirubin, whilst hepatic and post-hepatic causes lead mainly to a rise in conjugated (direct) bilirubin and to a lesser extent unconjugated bilirubin.
Serum transaminases (AST/ALT): Hepatic causes of jaundice lead to a rise in AST and ALT.

Serum alkaline phosphatase (ALP) and γ-glutamyl transferase (GGT): Post-hepatic (obstructive/cholestatic) causes of jaundice lead to a rise in ALP/ GGT.
Biochemical tests may identify the specific disease process. In general, however, such tests may be helpful only in hepatocellular disease.
α_1-antitrypsin deficiency: Low serum concentration and phenotyping.
Ceruloplasmin: Low serum concentration (Wilson's disease).
Iron, iron-binding capacity, and ferritin: An increased ratio of iron to iron-binding capacity and/or an increased ferritin are good screening tests for hemochromatosis.
Drugs: following an acetaminophen overdose, the plasma acetaminophen concentration predicts those patients likely to suffer significant liver damage. Screening for alcohol abuse is difficult and patients do not always admit to their drinking habits. In some circumstances a serum ethanol level may indicate whether a patient is truly abstinent.

92. Neonatal jaundice which occurs between the second and tenth day of life is common and is usually of no concern unless the degree of hyperbilirubinemia is sufficiently severe to require treatment. Jaundice in the first day of life, or which occurs after 10 days, is always abnormal. Early jaundice may be caused by hemolysis, and late jaundice by inborn errors of metabolism of structural defects in the biliary tree (biliary atresia).

93. See Figures 29.2, 29.3, 29.5, and 29.6 regarding phosphoribosyltransferases.

94. See Chapter 29, suicide inhibition of thymidylate synthase.

95. See Chapter 29. Substrate channeling is important in complex metabolic pathways, especially in lipid metabolism when substrates are not soluble in the aqueous phase. There is some evidence for substrate channeling in glycolysis.

96. See Chapter 29, deficiency of HGPRTase, accumulation of PRPP, leading to excessive purine biosynthesis and uric acid production.

97. Sequence element that might help to identify genes in this 450 kb sequence would be promoter and enhancer consensus sequences such as the basal promoter sequences (TATA box; TATAAT and TGTTGACA) located 5' to the start of genes. Once these areas have been located it will be possible to search the sequences downstream for protein synthesis start and stop codons and poly A addition sequences.

98. The rho protein is involved in transcription termination. It has an ATP-dependent helicase activity. This activity is required because the rho protein must travel along the newly synthesized RNA, chasing the RNA polymerase. When the rho protein catches up with the RNA polymerase it displaces it from the DNA template terminating transcription.

99. Since your goal would be to inhibit bacterial protein synthesis and have no effect on eukaryotic cells so you could use it to fight infections, the most likely candidates would be those enzymes, factors, or structures that are different between the two types of cells. For example, since bacteria typically use a formylated methionine to initiate protein synthesis while eukaryotic cells do not formylmethionine synthase might be a good target for an antibacterial drug. Another likely target would be the bacterial ribosome. Even though the ribosome in both cell types perform similar functions, it is possible to target bacterial ribosomes because their constituents are different from eukaryotic cells.

100. The most likely target of the drug would be the elongation factors responsible for bringing the newly charged tRNA molecules to the protein synthetic machinery. Specific targets of the drug could be either the elongation factors which bind to the tRNA molecules or the factors that allow these molecules to be recharged with GTP.

101. The key features of a transcription unit are the gene template and the mechanism for converting this message into a peptide gene product. This machinery comprises RNA polymerase, RNA Pol II, and other proteins that allow for the correct alignment of the polymerase in relation to the start point of the gene. These are associated factors such as promoters and enhancers that confer tissue and cell phase specificity to the transcription process and determine the efficiency of the process.

102. Key features in the design of this gene would include: a tissue specific promoter to ensure expression in hair follicles, a sex-specific response element (perhaps via estrogen or androgen response elements) that would allow for male pattern baldness to occur, another time-sensitive promoter to allow graying of the hair with age, and even an enhancer that promotes red hair growth in response to bad tempers.

103. There are numerous ways to alter gene transcription – See Table 33.1.

104. Yes. Genomic imprinting is a mechanism whereby the effect of a gene or one allele of a gene can be altered depending on the sex of the parent donating the gene. This means that the same gene or mutant allele can affect offspring differently depending on which parent donated the mutant gene. Examples of this include neonatal myotonic dystrophy (only when the mutant is donated from the mother) and Huntington's disease (where cases inherited from affected fathers have symptoms and signs at an earlier age, including childhood cases).

105. PCR amplification allows for rapid, high volume amplification of potentially very small amounts of template DNA. In addition, it can be used to amplify poor quality DNA template and DNA from other species that may share common ancestral genes. On the down side, the amplification may be inaccurate and amplification relies on knowledge of the nucleotide sequence of the neighboring DNA. In contrast, cell-based cloning is relatively slow and labor intensive. It requires the use of *in vitro* systems and the efficiency of transformation of the replicating cells is poor. However, cell-based cloning can provide large yields of pure target DNA with no sequence errors introduced. In addition, the size of the target DNA is not limited as is the case with PCR.

106. If the sequence of the gene is known then a PCR amplification reaction for each exon could be designed. Ideally the region of primer hybridization would be in the flanking intronic sequences and the resulting PCR products of different sizes. In cases where exons are of equal sizes, an attempt to design primers which allow amplification of a different sized product for each exon based on the flanking intronic sequence should be used. Such PCR products could either be sequenced directly or if of small enough size subjected to methods such as SSCP or DGGE. Alternatively, RNA could be extracted from white blood cells and a reverse transcriptase reaction performed. The resulting cDNA could then be amplified by PCR and then sequenced directly.

107. The ideal PCR reaction would contain a pure template and primers that hybridized only to the regions flanking the target DNA. The polymerase enzyme would accurately and repeatedly transcribe the target DNA to provide an end-product, which consisted of large amounts of target DNA faithfully copied without any sequence errors. In addition, the reaction conditions would be constant throughout the numerous cycles and each subsequent step in the cycle would occur instantaneously. In reality, Taq I introduces a high number of sequence errors in the course of a standard PCR and the template and primers are often far from ideal. The need to change temperatures from 95°C for denaturation to 45°C for annealing and then to 72°C for extension means that each step requires time for heating and cooling which alters the efficiency of each subsequent step in the cycle.

108. Two methods are routinely used for prenatal diagnosis:
Amniocentesis – sampling of amniotic fluid at 16–18 weeks' gestation and culturing the fetally derived amniocytes. Culture of these cells takes 2–3 weeks but often gives rise to potentially large amounts of DNA for analysis.
Chorionic villous sampling (CVS) – sampling of developing chorionic villi at 9–11 weeks' gestation. Sampled tissue is then used to prepare DNA. This method produces DNA for analysis quickly, but in small amounts.
Methods that require small amounts of DNA such as PCR are therefore suited to CVS as results can be obtained very quickly. Examples of this include detection of single gene disorders such as cystic fibrosis or sickle cell disease. However, if the method requires a large amount of DNA, e.g. a Southern blot-based method, then CVS is not practical and amniocentesis is preferred. The drawback of the CVS method is the detection of mutations at 16–20 or more weeks' gestation rather than 9–12 by amniocentesis.

109. There are myriad reasons for PCR failure (and numerous books have been written to explain it!). However, simple things such as incorrect primer design, poor template preparation, incorrect timing and temperature settings for the reaction cycles, poor reaction mixture preparation, and sheer bad luck are among the most common reasons for PCR failure.

110. Essential features for microsatellite paternity testing include:
Accurate documentation and sample collection from tested parties.
Choosing microsatellites which display a large number of alleles.
Choosing microsatellites which have alleles with equal frequencies, i.e. there is no excessive bias toward one allele thus reducing its discriminatory power.
Choosing microsatellites which are easily typed and not prone to typing errors which would invalidate their usefulness.
Using a large enough battery of microsatellite markers to ensure the probability of individuals possessing similar genotypes by chance is sufficiently low.

111. GH is secreted in bursts with greatest activity during the night. The GH concentration at the peak of a burst of secretion may be 100-fold greater than the basal level. Therefore, single GH results are of no diagnostic value. Dynamic tests of GH secretory reserve are required.

112. Autoantibodies are produced which bind to the TSH receptor on the surface of the thyroid cell. However, binding by the autoantibody does not trigger the intracellular sequence of events evoked by binding of TSH. Thus, the autoantibody and TSH compete for available receptor binding sites. As the autoimmune condition progresses, more and more receptor sites are occupied by autoantibody and hypothyroidism results.

113. (a) Prolactin is under inhibitory control from hypothalamic dopamine. All other pituitary hormones are under predominantly stimulatory control from the hypothalamus. (b) Prolactin is not a trophic hormone – in other words its action does not rely on stimulating the release of another hormone (c) There is no known prolactin deficiency syndrome in normal adults

114. Steroid 21-hydroxylase stimulates the conversion of 17-hydroxyprogesterone into deoxycorticosterone in the biosynthetic pathway to cortisol. If the enzyme is deficient there is a build up of 17-hydroxyprogesterone which is converted by side chain cleavage into androgens. This effect is exaggerated because the lack of cortisol feedback results in increased ACTH secretion from the pituitary which causes even more 17-hydroxyprogesterone to be synthesized.

115. FSH is a two chain polypeptide of molecular weight 28 kDa. As such it is big enough to contain many epitopes (antigen sites) and it is easy to obtain antibodies that will bind to two different epitopes on the same FSH molecule. Estradiol is a small molecule, a steroid hormone, which will only fit into one antibody binding site at any one time.

116. Plasma binding proteins provide a subtle control mechanism for the delivery of the hormone to its target cell. The bound hormone acts as a reservoir and there is sufficient excess binding capacity to prevent uncontrolled surges of hormone delivery to the target cell. The free (unbound) hormone is the biologically active form; this is in equilibrium with the bound hormone. Although plasma binding proteins most commonly exist for small molecules (e.g. thyroxine, cortisol) they are also found for polypeptide hormones (e.g. growth hormone).

Abbreviations

A	adenine	CD	cluster designation: classification system for cell surface molecules
ACE	angiotensin-converting enzyme		
acetyl-CoA	acetyl-coenzyme A	CDGS	carbohydrate-deficient glycoprotein syndromes
ACh	acetylcholine		
ACTase	aspartate carbamoyl transferase	CDK	cyclin-dependent kinase
ACTH	adrenocorticotropic hormone	CDKI	cyclin-dependent kinase inhibitor
ADC	AIDS–dementia complex	CDP	cytidine diphosphate
ADH	alcohol dehydrogenase	CFTR	cystic fibrosis transmembrane conductance regulator
ADH	antidiuretic hormone (also known as AVP)		
ADP	adenosine diphosphate	cGMP	cyclic GMP
AFP	α-fetoprotein	CITP	carboxy-terminal procollagen extension peptide
AGE	advanced glycation end-product		
AHF	antihemophilic factor	CML	chronic myeloid leukemia
AICAR	5-aminoimidazole-4-carboxamide ribonucleotide	CMP	cytidine monophosphate
		CNS	central nervous system
AIDS	acquired immunodeficiency syndrome	COAD	chronic obstructive airways disease (synonym: COPD)
AIR	5-aminoimidazole ribonucleotide		
ALDH	aldehyde dehydrogenase	COMT	catecholamine-O-methyl transferase
ALP	alkaline phosphatase	COPD	chronic obstructive pulmonary disease (synonym: COAD)
ALT	alanine aminotransferase		
AML	acute myeloblastic leukemia	CoQ_{10}	coenzyme Q_{10} (ubiquinone)
AMP	adenosine monophosphate	COX-1	cyclooxygenase-1
APC	adenomatous polyposis coli (gene)	CPK	creatine phosphokinase
APO-1	'death domain'-receptor Fas	CPS I, II	carbamoyl phosphate synthetase I, II
apoB	apolipoprotein B	CPT I, II	carnitine palmitoyl transferase I, II
APRT	adenosine phosphoribosyl transferase	CREB	cAMP-responsive-element-binding protein
APTT	activated partial thromboplastin time	CRGP	calcitonin-related gene peptide
ARDS	Acute Respiratory Distress Syndrome	CRH	corticotropin-releasing hormone
AST	aspartate aminotransferase	CRP	C-reactive protein
ATF	activation transcription factor	CSF	cerebrospinal fluid
ATM	ataxia telangiectasia-mutated gene	CT	calcitonin
ATP	adenosine triphosphate	CTP	cytidine triphosphate
AVP	arginine-vasopressin (same as antidiuretic hormone)	CVS	chorionic villous sampling
		DAG	diacyl-glycerol
AZT	3′-azido-3′-deoxythymidine	DCC	'delete in colon carcinoma' gene
2,3-BPG	2,3-bisphosphoglycerate	DEAE	diethylaminoethyl
Bcl-2	B cell lymphoma protein 2	DGGE	denaturant-gradient gel electrophoresis
bp	base pair	DHAP	dihydroxyacetone phosphate
BUN	blood urea nitrogen equivalent of (but not the same as) blood urea	DIC	disseminated intravascular coagulation
		DIPF	diisopropylphosphofluoride
bw	body weight	DNA	deoxyribonucleic acid
C	cytosine	DNP	2,4-dinitrophenol
CA	carbonic anhydrase	Dol-P	dolichol phosphate
CAD	caspase-dependent endonuclease	Dol-PP-GlcNAc	dolichol pyrophosphate-acetylglucosamine
CAIR	carboxyaminoimidazole ribonucleotide		
cAMP	cyclic AMP	DOPA	dihydroxyphenylalanine

DPPC	dipalmitoylphosphatidylcholine	GDP-L-Fuc	guanosine diphosphate-L-fucose
EBV	Epstein–Barr virus	GDP-Man	guanosine diphosphate-mannose
ECF	extracellular fluid	GFAP	glial fibrillary acid protein
ECM	extracellular matrix	γGT	γ-glutamyl transferase
EDRF	endothelium-derived relaxing factor (NO)	GH	growth hormone
EDTA	ethylenediaminetetraacetic acid	GHRH	growth hormone-releasing hormone
EF-1, 2	elongation factor-1, -2	GIP	glucose-dependent insulinotropic peptide
EF2	eukaryotic elongation factor	GIT	gastrointestinal tract
EGF	epidermal growth factor	GK	glucokinase
eIF-3	eukaryotic cell initiation factor(-3)	Glc	glucose
ELK	transcription factor	Glc-1-P	glucose-1-phosphate
ER	endoplasmic reticulum	Glc-6-P	glucose-6-phosphate
ERK	extracellular-regulated kinase	Glc-6-Pase	glucose-6-phosphatase
ESR	erythrocyte sedimentation rate	GlcN-6-P	glucosamine-6-phosphate
F-ATPase	coupling-factor-type ATPase	GlcNAc	N-acetylglucosamine
FACIT	fibril-associated collagen with interrupted triple helices	GlcNAc-1P	N-acetylglucosamine-1-phosphate
		GlcNAc-6-P	N-acetylglucosamine-6-phosphate
FAD	flavin adenine dinucleotide	GlcNH$_2$	glucosamine
FADD	a 'death domain' accessory protein	GlcUA	D-glucuronic acid
FADH$_2$	reduced flavin adenine dinucleotide	GLP-1	glucagon-like peptide-1
FAICAR	5-formylaminoimidazole-4-carboxamide ribonucleotide	GLUT	glucose transporter (GLUT-1–GLUT-5)
		GM1	monosialoganglioside 1
FAP	familial adenomatous polyposis	GMP	guanosine monophosphate
Fas	apoptosis signaling molecule: a 'death domain' accessory protein (CD95)	GnRH	gonadotropin-releasing hormone
		GP1b-IXa (etc)	glycoprotein receptor 1b-IXa (etc)
FBPase	fructose bisphosphatase		
FCγR	group of immunoglobulin receptors	GRE	glucocorticoid response element
FDP	fibrin degradation product	GSH	reduced glutathione
FGAR	formylglycinamide ribonucleotide	GSSG	oxidized glutathione
FGF	fibroblast growth factor	GTP	guanosine triphosphate
FHH	familial hypocalciuric hypercalcemia	GTPase	guanosine triphosphatase
FMN	flavin mononucleotide	5-HIAA	5-hydroxyindoleacetic acid
FMNH$_2$	reduced flavin mononucleotide	5-HT	5-hydroxytryptamine
FRAXA	fragile X syndrome	Hb	hemoglobin
Fru-1,6-BP	fructose-1,6 bisphosphate	HbA$_{1c}$	glycated hemoglobin
Fru-2,6-BP	fructose-2,6 bisphosphate	HbF	fetal hemoglobin
Fru-2,6-BPase	fructose-2,6 bisphosphatase	HCM	hypercalcemia associated with malignancy
		Hct	hematocrit
Fru-6-P	fructose-6-phosphate	HDL	high-density lipoprotein
FSF	fibrin-stabilizing factor	HGF-R	hepatocyte growth factor receptor
FSH	follicle-stimulating hormone	HGPRT	hypoxanthine-guanine phosphoribosyl transferase
G	guanine		
G3PDH	glyceraldehyde-3-phosphate dehydrogenase	HIV	human immunodeficiency virus
GABA	γ-amino butyric acid	HLA	human leukocyte antigen (system)
GAG	glycosaminoglycan	HLH	helix–loop–helix (motif)
Gal	galactose	HMG	hydroxymethylglutaryl
Gal-1-P	galactose-1-phosphate	HMWK	high-molecular-weight kininogen
GalNAc	N-acetylgalactosamine	HNPCC	hereditary nonpolyposis colorectal cancer
GalNH$_2$	galactosamine	hnRNA	heteronuclear ribonucleic acid
GAP	guanosine triphosphatase activating protein	HPLC	high-pressure liquid chromatography
GAR	glycinamide ribonucleotide	HPT	hyperparathyroidism
GDH	glutamate dehydrogenase	HRT	hormone replacement therapy
GDP	guanosine diphosphate	HTGL	hepatic triglyceride lipase
GDP-D-Man	guanosine diphosphate-D-mannose	HTH	helix–turn–helix (motif)

ICAM-1	intracellular cell adhesion molecule-1		MCV	mean corpuscular volume
ICF	intracellular fluid		MEK	mitogen-activated protein kinase kinase
IDDM	insulin-dependent diabetes mellitus		MEN IIA	multiple endocrine neoplasia type IIA
IDL	intermediate-density lipoprotein		met-tRNA	methionyl-tRNA
IdUA	L-iduronic acid		MGUS	monoclonal gammopathy of uncertain significance
IFN(-γ)	interferon(-γ)		MHC	major histocompatibility complex
Ig	immunoglobulin (etc)		mRNA	messenger ribonucleic acid
IGF-I	insulin-like growth factor-I (etc)		MRP	multidrug resistance-associated protein
IL	interleukin (IL-1–IL29)		MS	mass spectrometry
IMP	inosine monophosphate		MSH	melanocyte stimulating hormone
Inr	initiator (nucleotide sequence of a gene)		MSUD	maple syrup urine disease
IP_1 I-1-P_1, I-4-P_1 (etc)	inositol monophosphate		MyoD	muscle-cell-specific transporter factor
IP_2, I-1, 3-P_2, I-1, 4-P_2	inositol bisphosphate		Na^+/K^+–ATPase	sodium–potassium ATPase
			NABQI	N-acetyl benzoquinoneimine
IP_3 I-1,4, 5-P_3	inositol trisphosphate		NAC	N-acetylcysteine
			NAD^+	nicotinamide adenine dinucleotide (oxidized)
IP_4 I-1,3,4, 5-P_4	inositol tetraphosphate		NADH	nicotinamide adenine dinucleotide (reduced)
			$NADP^+$	nicotinamide adenine dinucleotide phosphate (oxidized)
IRE	iron response element		NADPH	nicotinamide adenine dinucleotide phosphate (reduced)
IRF-BP	IRE-binding protein			
IRMA	immunoradiometric assay		NANA	N-acetyl neuraminic acid (sialic acid)
ITAM	immunoreceptor tyrosine activation motif		NF	nuclear factor
ITIM	immunoreceptor tyrosine inhibition motif		NF-II	type II neurofibromatosis
JAK	Janus kinase		NGF	nerve growth factor
JNK	Jun N-terminal kinase		NIDDM	noninsulin-dependent diabetes mellitus
K	equilibrium constant		NMDA	N-methyl-D-aspartate
kb	kilobase		NO	nitric oxide
kbp	kilobase pair(s)		NPY	neuropeptide Y
KCCT	kaolin–cephalin clotting time		NSAID	nonsteroidal anti-inflammatory drug
KIP2	cell cycle regulatory molecule		nt	nucleotide (as measure of size/length of a nucleic acid)
K_m	Michaelis constant			
LACI	lipoprotein-associated coagulation inhibitor		$1,25(OH)_2D_3$	1,25-dihydroxy vitamin D_3
LCAT	lecithin: cholesterol acyltransferase		OGTT	oral glucose tolerance test
LDH	lactate dehydrogenase		8-oxo-Gua	8-oxo-2′-deoxyguanosine
LDL	low-density lipoprotein		OxS	oxidative stress
LH	luteinizing hormone		P-ATPase	phosphorylation-type ATPase
LPL	lipoprotein lipase		3-PG	3-phosphoglycerate
LPS	lipopolysaccharide		p38RK	p38-reactivating kinase
LRP LDL	receptor-related protein		Pa	Pascal
M-CSF-R	macrophage colony-stimulating factor receptor		PA	phosphatidic acid
			PAF	platelet activating factor
Malonyl-CoA	malonyl-coenzyme A		PAGE	polyacrylamide gel electrophoresis
Man	mannose		PAI-1	plasminogen activator inhibitor type 1
Man-1-P	mannose-1-phosphate		PAPS	phosphoadenosine phosphosulfate
Man-6-P	mannose-6-phosphate		PC	phosphatidyl choline
MAO	monoamine oxidase		PC	pyruvate carboxylase
MAPK	mitogen-activated protein kinase (a superfamily of signal-transducing kinases)		PCP	phencyclidine
			PCR	polymerase chain reaction
Mb	myoglobin		PDE	phosphodiesterase
MCHC	mean corpuscular hemoglobin concentration		PDGF	platelet-derived growth factor
MCP-1	monocyte chemoattractant protein-1		PDH	pyruvate dehydrogenase

PDK	phosphatidylinositol trisphosphate-dependent kinase	SAPK	stress-activated protein kinase
PE	phosphatidyl ethanolamine	SCIDS	severe combined immunodeficiency syndrome
PEP	phosphoenolpyruvic acid	scuPA	single-chain urinary-type plasminogen activator
PEPCK	phosphoenolpyruvate carboxykinase		
PF3	platelet factor 3	SDS	sodium dodecyl sulfate
PFK-1 (-2)	phosphofructokinase-1 (-2)	SDS-PAGE	sodium dodecyl sulfate-polyacrylamide gel electrophoresis
PGG_2	prostaglandin G_2 (etc)		
PGK	phosphoglycerate kinase	SGLT	Na^+-coupled glucose symporter
PGM	phosphoglucomutase	SEK	SAPK homologue of MEK
PHHI	persistent hyperinsulinemic hypoglycemia of infancy	SER	smooth endoplasmic reticulum
		ser-P	serine phosphate
PHP	pseudohypoparathyroidism	SH (figs only)	steroid hormone
Pi	inorganic phosphate	SH2	Src-homology region-2
PI-3-K	phosphoinositide-3-kinase	SIADH	syndrome of inappropriate antidiuretic hormone secretion
PICP	amino-terminal procollagen extension peptide		
		snRNA	small nuclear RNA
PIP_2/PIP_3	phosphatidylinositol bisphosphate/trisphosphate	SPCA	serum prothrombin conversion accelerator
		Src	a protein tyrosine kinase
PK	pyruvate kinase	SRE	steroid response element
PKA/PKC	protein kinase A/C	SRP	signal recognition particle
PKU	phenylketonuria	SSCP	single-strand conformational polymorphism
PLA/PLC	phospholipase A/C	SSRI	selective serotonin reuptake inhibitor
PMA	phorbol myristic acetate	STAT	signal transducer and activator of transcription
PNS	peripheral nervous system		
PPi	inorganic pyrophosphate	SUR^-	sulfonylurea receptor
PRL	prolactin	T	thymine
PrP	prion protein	T tubule	transverse tubule
PRPP	5-phosphoribosyl-α-pyrophosphate	T_3	tri-iodothyronine
PS	phosphatidyl serine	T_4	thyroxine
PTA	plasma thromboplastin antecedent	TAG	triacylglycerol (triglyceride)
PTH	parathyroid hormone	TAP	transporters associated with antigen presentation
PTHrP	parathyroid hormone-related protein		
PTK	protein tyrosine kinase	TBG	thyroid-binding globulin
PTPase	phosphotyrosine phosphatase	TCA	tricarboxylic acid cycle
Py	pyrimidine base (in a nucleotide sequence)	TF	transcription factor (with qualifier)
		TFPI	tissue factor pathway inhibitor
R	receptor (with qualifier, not alone)	TG	triacylglycerol (triglyceride)
RAIDD	a 'death domain' accessory protein	TGF(-β)	transforming growth factor(-β)
Rb	retinoblastoma protein	T_{max}	renal transport maximum
RBC	red blood cell		
RDS	respiratory distress syndrome	TNF	tumor necrosis factor
RER	rough endoplasmic reticulum	TNF-R	tumor necrosis factor receptor
RIP	a 'death domain' accessory protein	tPA	tissue-type plasminogen activator
RKK	p38RK homologue of MEK	TRADD	a 'death domain' accessory protein
RNA	ribonucleic acid	TRAFS	a 'death domain' accessory protein
RNAPol II	RNA polymerase II	TRH	thyrotropin-releasing hormone
RNR	ribonucleotide reductase	TSH	thyroid-stimulating hormone (thyrotropin)
RNS	reactive nitrogen species		
ROS	reactive oxygen species	TTP	thymidine triphosphate
S	Svedberg	TXA_2	thromboxane A_2
SACAIR	5-aminoimidazole-4-(N-succinylocarboxamide) ribonucleotide	U	uridine
		UCP	uncoupling protein
		UDP	uridine diphosphate
SAM	S-adenosyl methionine	UDP-Gal	UDP-galactose
SAP1	transcription factor	UDP-GalNAc	UDP-N-acetylgalactosamine

UDP-Glc	UDP-glucose	VIP	vasoactive intestinal peptide
UDP-GlcNAc	UDP-N-acetylglucosamine	VLDL	very-low-density lipoprotein
UDP-GlcUA	UDP glucuronic acid	vWF	von Willebrand factor
UMP	uridine monophosphate	WAF1	cell cycle regulator
uPA	urinary-type plasminogen activator	X-SCID	X-linked severe combined immunodeficiency
UV	ultraviolet	XMP	xanthine monophosphate
VCAM-1	vascular cell adhesion molecule-1	XO	xanthine oxidase
VDCC	voltage-dependent calcium channel	ZP3	zona pellucida 3 glycoprotein

Index

A

A23187, 83
Aβ, 82
ABCA1, 218
ABCG5, 218
ABCG85, 218
abdominal discomfort, 125, 155
abdominal succussion splash, 343
Abl, 585, 595–6
Abl proto-oncogene, 595
ablation, 252
ABO blood-group antigens, 384
ABO blood-group system, 384
abortion, 84
abrin, 371
absorption
   of carbohydrates, 116–20
   of lipids, 120–3
   of nutrients, 113
   of proteins, 123–5
absorption spectra, ultraviolet, 9, 20
absorptive (postprandial) state, 279–82
abstinence, 407–8
acceptor stem, 439
acetaldehyde, 59, 148, 406
acetaminophen (paracetamol)
   hepatotoxicity of, 406–7
   metabolism of, 407
   overdose, 71
acetate, 170, 406
acetic acid, 59, 81, 105
acetoacetate, 195, 333
acetoacetic acid, 195
acetoacetyl-CoA thiolase, 210
acetone, 195
N-acetyl benzoquinoneimine
   (NABQI), 406
acetyl coenzyme A *see* acetyl-CoA
N-acetyl cysteine (NAC), 406
acetyl-CoA, 3, 170–2, 180, 183
   activation of, 183
   and biosynthesis of cholesterol, 210
   carboxylation of, 199–200
   condensation of, 180–1
   from fatty acids, 193–4
   from pyruvate, 177
   metabolic sources of, 177
   oxidation of, 175
   and PDC activity, 178
   product of catabolic pathways, 176
   removal of excess, 195
   sources of, 177
   and TCA cycle, 186
acetyl-CoA carboxylase, 199–200, 203
N-acetyl-neuraminic acid, 366
acetylcholine (ACh), 62, 564–5, 579–80
   naming agonists and antagonists, 564
acetylcholinesterase, 62, 563, 565, 579
   inhibitors, 580–1
acetyldihydrolipoamide, 178
N-acetylgalactosamine (GalNAc), 359
N-acetylglucosamine (GlcNAc), 359–60
N-acetylglutamate, 252, 257
N-acetylneuraminic acid, 361
acetylsalicylic acid (aspirin), 59, 66, 68, 75, 254, 555, 597

Achilles tendon, 235
α₁-acid glycoprotein, 34
acid–base balance, control of, 333–44
acid–base disorders, 337, 341–4
   classification of, 335
   clinical causes of, 343
   compensation in, 334
   and plasma potassium concentration, 342
   respiratory and metabolic compensation, 342
acidemia, 335
   methylmalonic, 257
   propionic, 257
acidosis, 181, 257, 268, 335, 343–4
   lactic, 181, 344, 407
   metabolic, 115, 195, 288, 341, 343–4
   respiratory, 341, 343
   in lung disease, 338, 343
acids, conjugate, 11
aciduria, dicarboxylic, 194
acini, pancreatic, 120
acne, facial, 536
aconitase, 181–2
   cytosolic, 182
aconitase reaction
   isomerization specificity during, 182
   stereochemistry of, 182
   cis-aconitate, 182
acquired (toxic) methemoglobinemia, 44
acrodermatitis enteropathica, 140
acrolein, 504
acromegaly, 353
   GH excess and, 538
actin, 87, 261, 263
   isoforms of, 264
   polymerization, 264
   stress fibers, reorganization of, 584
action potentials, 570–1
   generation of, 571
activated partial thromboplastin time (APTT), 71
activation transcription factor (ATF), 548
actomyosin complex, 267
acute fatty liver of pregnancy *see* AFLP syndrome
acute mountain sickness (AMS), 42
acute phase response, 23, 32–4, 401
acute respiratory distress syndrome (ARDS), 81, 378, 499
acute tubular necrosis, 328
acyclovir, 61
acyl phosphate, 146, 170
acyl–arsenate bond, 148
acyl-carrier protein (ACP), 200–1
acyl-CoA:acylcholesterol transferase (SOAT; ACAT), 230
acyl-CoA, 121
acyl-CoA synthase, 121
N-acylsphingosine, 380
Addison's disease, 530–1
adenine, 95, 97, 413, 416
   bonding, 426, 441
   nucleotides in RNA, 437
adenine deoxyribonucleotide, 421
adenine dinucleotide (FADH₂), 94
adenine phosphoribosyl transferase (APRT), 416

adenoids, 510
adenoma, 329, 593
   parathyroid gland, 353
adenosine, 417, 419
adenosine deaminase, 417, 419
   deficiency, 419
adenosine diphosphate (ADP), 67, 99, 160, 183
   and active transport, 85–6
   availability, 105–6
   cytoplasmic, 98
   inhibition, 108
   phosphorylation, 148–9
   production of, 95, 185, 165
   ratio with ATP, 110
adenosine monophosphate (AMP), 161, 250, 414
   production of, 95, 149, 165
adenosine monophosphate deaminase, 417
adenosine triphosphate (ATP), 2–3, 55, 143–5, 160, 165, 170
   and active transport, 85–6
   and arsenate, 148
   balance, allosteric control of, 149
   biosynthesis driven by, 96
   copper-transporting P-type (ATP7B), 29
   coupling, 95–6
   energy conservation by coupling with, 95–6
   high levels of, 183
   hydrolysis, 451
      products of, 95
   and magnesium, 97
   metabolic function, 97
   and muscle contraction, 261
   pumping, 124
   ratio with ADP, 110
   structure of, 95
   synthesis of, 93, 98–106, 108–10, 147–8, 175, 414–16
      mitochondrial from coenzymes, 96–7
   transmitter functions of, 580
   utilization, 185
   yield reduction, 150
adenosine triphosphate synthase *see* ATPase
adenosine 5′-triphosphate, 413
S-adenosyl methionine, 229
adenosylcobalamin, 136
S-adenosylmethionine (SAM), 377
adenovirus, 591
adenylate cyclase, 161, 276–8, 532, 536, 539
adenylate kinase, 165, 416
adenylate kinase reaction, 149
adenylosuccinate, 414
adenylosuccinate lyase, 414
adenylosuccinate synthetase, 414
adenylyl cyclase, 545, 547
   activated by G-protein, 547
adequate intake (AI), 299–300
adhesion molecules, 511
adipocytes, 205
adipokines, 205
adiponectin, 205
adipose tissue, 77, 84, 166–7
   biosynthesis of fatty acids in, 199–208
   brown, 106
   as endocrine organ, 204–5
   fatty acids released from, 168

   fatty acids stored in, 199–208
   glucagon activated lipolysis in, 282
   hormonally active, 205
   loss of, 168
   normal amounts of, 273
   stress-induced insulin resistance in, 285–6
adrenal cortex, 220, 529
   and steroid hormones, 219
   zones of, 219
adrenal failure, 530
adrenal gland, cortex of, 541
adrenal insufficiency, primary, 531
adrenal medulla, 160
adrenaline *see* epinephrine
adrenergic receptors, 163, 543
adrenergic transmission, 565
adrenocorticotropic hormone (ACTH), 220, 526, 529, 581
adrenoleukodystrophy, 88
adrenoreceptors, 577
Adrucil, 421
advanced glycoxidation end-products (AGE), 288–90, 501, 603–5
   structure of, 604
advanced lipoxidation end-products (ALE), 500, 603–5
   structure of, 604
AFLP syndrome, in mothers of children born with LCHAD, 196
African swine fever virus, 591
agarose, 18
aggrecan, 396
   structure of, 397
aggressiveness, 417
aging, 106, 599–608
   biomarkers of, 604
   chemical theories of, 602
   and chemistry, 602
   of circulatory system, 605
   of complex systems, 599–600
   decline of biochemical and physiological systems during, 600
   error–catastrophe theory of, 601
   free radical theory of (FRTA), 603–5
   genetic models of, 607–8
   interventions to delay, 606
   mathematical models of, 600
   mitochondrial theories of, 605
   of muscle, 606
   organ system theories of, 603
   theories of, 601–5
agonists, dopaminergic, side effects of, 252
agouti-related protein (AgRP), 305
AICAR transformylase, 414
AIDS, 261
   dementia complex, 433
AIR carboxylase, 414
AIR synthetase, 414
airway disease, 88
alamethicin, 83
alanine, 9, 11–12, 85, 161, 168, 170
   from pyruvate, 177
   and inter-organ flow of C and N, 246
   N transport by, 250
   source of pyruvate, 177
   as substrate for gluconeogenesis, 273–4

supply of acetyl-CoA from, 185
transport of amino groups by, 248–9
β-alanine, 421
alanine aminotransferase, 170, 177
alanine transaminase, 170
albinism, 258
albumin, 18, 26, 28, 129
  bile acids bound to, 217
  and drug availability, 28
  human, 28
  as nutritional marker, 306
  and serum calcium concentration, 355
  serum concentration and Ca, 348
  synthesis of, 32, 401
  testosterone binding, 533
  urinary, excretion testing, 296
Alcobon, 421
alcohol, 93
  excess intake and pancreatitis, 121
  intolerance, symptoms of, 407–8
  and liver disease, 12, 203, 406–8
  metabolism of, 168
  oxidation to ketone, 184
alcohol dehydrogenase, 57, 59, 406
alcoholic steatosis, 408
alcoholism, 59
  lipid abnormalities in, 203
  Mg deficiency in, 304
  symptoms of beri-beri in, 180
  thiamin deficiency in, 133, 180
aldehyde dehydrogenase (ALDH), 59, 406
aldol condensation, 391
aldolases, 146, 152, 364
aldose receptor, 152
aldose reductase, 291
aldose–ketose interconversion, 145
aldosterone, 218, 220, 323
  control of renal water and sodium, 330
  disorders of secretion, 329
  regulation of sodium reabsorption by, 327–8
  stimulation of, 327
  synthesis of, 219
alkalemia, 335, 355
alkaline phosphatase (ALP), 409–10
alkalosis, 335, 341, 344
  metabolic, 344
    caused by vomiting, 343
  mixed metabolic and respiratory, 341
  respiratory, 344
    cause of, 337
alkaptonuria, 258
allantoin, 422
alleles
  HLA, 516–17
  preferential activation of, 468–9
allergy, to bee venom, 509
allopurinol, 418
alloster effectors, 2, 40–1, 110
alloxanthine, 418
allysine, 390–1
alopecia, 140
Alu sequence, 428
aluminium, 127
alveoli, 338
Alzheimer's disease, 23, 82, 227, 580, 601
  amyloid in, 455
  neuronal plaque, 500
  role for oxidative stress, 607
Amadori rearrangement, 290
Amanita phalloides, 440
α-amanitin, 439–40
Ames, B, 435
Ames test for mutagens, 435
amidation, 403
amide bond, 13
amidophosphoribosyl transferase, 414–15
amines, biogenic, 574
amino acid analyzer, 22

amino acids, 3, 7–24, 36, 123–4, 168
  accumulation of, 323
  acidic, 9–10
  activation, 450
  active transport of, 124
  aliphatic, 9
  α-amino group, 10, 12–13
  ε-amino group, 10, 15
  aromatic, 9, 125
    catabolism of, 256
  basic, 10
  biosynthesis of, 245–60
  by genetic code, 8
  C-terminal, 13
  α-carbon, 7
  catabolism, 402–3
  classification, 7–8, 10
  cyclic, 10
  deamination, 249
  degradation of, 245–60
  during starvation, 175
  essential, 245, 257, 303
  free, 125
  from body proteins, 245–7
  from diet, 245–7
  fuel, 273
  glucogenic, 170, 253–5
  hydrophilicity, 10
  hydrophobic, 125
  increased demand for, 302
  ionization state of, 10
  ketogenic, 253–4
  metabolic relationships of, 246
  metabolism, 135
    carbohydrate and lipid interfaces with, 253
    of carbon skeletons, 247, 253–5
    and central metabolic pathways, 254
    inherited diseases, 256–9
    screening for defects in newborns, 253
  N-terminal, 13
  as neurotransmitters, 573–4
  neutral polar, 9
  nonessential, 245
    origins of, 257
  nonprotein, 8
  polarity, 10
  as precursors of signaling molecules, 259
  residues of, 13, 79
  structure of, 8
  sulfur-containing, 10
  titration of, 12
  uptake, 124
  urinary, 323
α-amino acids, 7, 100
γ-amino butyric acid (GABA), 248, 574
amino groups (—NH₂), 7, 10, 12
amino sugars, synthesis of, 366
aminoaciduria, 8, 84, 323
aminoacyl-tRNA synthetases, 449
5-aminoimidazole ribonucleotide (AIR), 414
5-aminoimidazole-4-carboxamide ribonucleotide (AICAR), 414
5-aminoimidazole-4-(N-succinylocarboxamide) ribonucleotide (SACAIR), 414
5-aminoimidazole-4-(N-succinylocarboxamide) ribonucleotide synthetase, 414
β-aminoisobutyrate, 421
aminopeptidases, 123, 125
m-aminophenylboronic acid, 292
aminopterin, 421
ammonia, 247
  and brain damage, 403
  encephalopathy, 251
  high blood concentrations of, 251
  metabolic balance, 250
  toxicity, 251, 402
  and urea cycle, 402–3

ammonium, 245
  sulfate ((NH₄)₂SO₄), 17
    fractionation, 17
amniotic fluid, 81
  lecithin:sphingomyelin ratio in, 378
amphetamines, 575
  stimulatory effects of, 576
amphipathic compounds, 79
amphotericin B, 83
amplimers, 481
amputations, lower limb, 289
amylase, 115–16
  increased activity, 121
  pancreatic, 120
amyloid, 455
amyloidosis, 563
amylopectin, 117, 157
amylose, 117, 157
amyotrophic lateral sclerosis, 23
amytal, 108
anabolic pathway, 274
  suppression of, 285
anabolic steroids, 533
anabolism, 3
analbuminemia, 28
analgesia, opiate, 353
anaphylactic response, 377
anaphylactic shock, 509
anaphylatoxin activity, 507
anaphylaxis, 509
anaplerotic reactions, 175, 186
  catalyzed by pyruvate carboxylase, 186
Ancotil, 421
androgen-binding protein, 532
androgens, 218–20, 531
  deficiency, 534
  excess, 535
  hypersecretion of, 536
androstane ring, 218
anemia, 32, 42, 47, 125, 150, 384
  and ATP synthesis, 155
  caused by Cu deficiency, 141
  characterizing orotic aciduria, 419
  Cu deficiency in, 402
  hemolytic, 131, 323, 380
    caused by Glc-6-P dehydrogenase deficiency, 155
  hypochromic, 140–1
  iron deficiency, 48, 99
  macrocytic, 136
  megaloblastic, 136–7
  pernicious, 137
  prolactin amelioration of, 539
  shortness of breath and tiredness caused by, 339
  sickle cell, 448
    RFLP in, 487
  sideroblastic, caused by pyroxidine deficiency, 135
  and vitamin C deficiency, 138
anesthetics, 79
  local, 91
angina, 66, 577
  pectoris, 236, 239
  and plaque growth, 240
  stable, 239
  unstable, 270
angiokeratoma, 383
angiotensin, 13, 57
angiotensin converting enzyme (ACE), 57, 326–7
angiotensin II, 220, 327
angiotensinogen, 57, 326
angular stomatitis, 133
aniline dyes, 44
anion exchange, 18–20
anion gap, 316
ankyrin, 83
anomers, 117, 153
anorexia nervosa, 309, 531
Antabuse®, 59
anti-inflammatory drugs, 555
anti-insulin hormones, metabolic effects of, 276

antibiotics, 136, 441
  induction of ion permeability by, 83
  polyene, 83
  and protein synthesis, 452–3
  targets of, 453
antibodies, 30, 518
  effector functions of, 519
  function of, 518
  structure of, 518
  to phospholipids, 84
anticancer agents, 136
anticardiolipin antibody, 84
anticoagulants, 25
  oral, 71
  long-term, 69
  patient self-monitoring, 69
anticoagulation, effect of heparin, 396
anticodon loop, 438
antidepressants, 575
  tricyclic, 575
antidiuretic hormone (ADH) *see* vasopressin
antifolates, 421
antigens, 30–2
  elimination of, 514–16
  human leukocyte (HLA), 516–17
  Lewis blood group, 385
  P blood group, 385
  reaction with, 514–16
  recognition, molecules involved in, 511–13
  response to, 514–16
antihistamines, 509, 580
antimycin A, 108–9
  inhibition by, 108–9
antioncogenes, 595
antioxidant protection, 151, 242
antioxidant response elements (ARE), 504
antioxidant systems, 499
antioxidants
  β-carotene, 129, 242
  defenses, 3, 501–5
    in RBCs, 503
  lipid-based, 504
  supplements and aging, 606
  vitamin C, 242, 503
  vitamin E, 242, 504
antiphospholipid antibody syndrome, 84
α₂-antiplasmin, 75
antiplatelet drugs, 68–9
  action of, 68
antiporters, 83, 86
antiretroviral chemotherapeutic agents, action of, 434
antithrombin III (AT), 396
antithrombins, 72–4
antitrypsin, alpha-1 (AA1T), 32, 34, 409
anxiety, 44
aortic aneurysm, 34
APC, 597
aplasia, 68
apnea, 171
APO-1, 592
APOB, 468–9
apoB48, 229, 468
apoB100, 468
apoenzyme, 54
apolipoprotein B48, 123
apolipoproteins, 203, 227–9
apoprotein B (apoB), 226, 468
apoprotein C (apoC), 226
apoprotein E
  (apoE), 227, 300
  genetic mutation in, 227
apoproteins, 129, 227–9
  function of, 229
apoptosis, 102, 583, 587, 590–3
  caspases in, 590–1
  galectin induced, 372
  regulation of, 592
appetite, 305
  loss of, 133

AQP1, 328
AQP2, 328
aquaporin A (AQPOP), 328
aquaporin-2, 82, 328–9
aquaporin water channel, 328
arachidonate, 59
arachidonic acid, 67, 203, 302, 554–5, 597
  metabolites, 509
  precursor of eicosanoids, 555
arachnodactyly, 393
areflexia, 559
arginine, 10, 13, 15, 22, 53, 250, 417
  in histones, 429
  residues, 125
  supplementation, 252
L-arginine, 8
arginine-vasopressin (AVP; ADH), 354
argininosuccinate, 250
argininosuccinate synthetase, 250
argininosuccinic acid synthetase deficiency, 419
aromatase, 220, 535
aromatic amino acid carboxylase, 578
  deficiency, 579
arrythmias, 303
1-arsenato-3-phosphoglycerate, 148
arsenic, 148
arteries
  blocking of, 236
  narrowing, 236
  pulmonary, 338
  wall structure, 236
arteriole, afferent, 319
arteriole, efferent, 319
arthritis, 538
  gouty, 417
  and obesity, 206
  OxS, 499
  rheumatoid, 417, 555
ascites, 399
ascorbate, 365, 503
  aqueous-phase antioxidant, 503
ascorbic acid, 109, 138, 140, 258
  see also vitamin C
asialotransferrin, 560–1
asparagine, 9, 15, 21, 85
aspartate, 10, 21, 170, 250, 417
  from TCA cycle, 175
  residues, 13
D-aspartate, 603–4
aspartate aminotransferase, 100–1, 135, 170
aspartate transcarbamoylase (ATCase), 60, 417–18
aspartic acid, 9, 15, 247
  from TCA cycle, 183
aspirin see acetylsalicylic acid
asterixis, 29
asthma, 118, 337, 549, 577
astrocytes, 227, 560, 562–3
ataxia, 133, 179, 601
atherogenesis, 236–40
  inflammation and, 239
  inflammatory phenomena and, 236
  lipid entry into arterial wall, 239
  process of, 237
  role of cytokines in, 238
  role of growth factors in, 238
atherosclerosis, 3, 138, 225, 236, 601
  acid lipase treatment, 383
  development of, 236–8
  low grade inflammatory reaction in, 288
  OxS, 499
  plaques, 500
  relationship with obesity and diabetes, 293
  risk factors for, 194
  risk reduction, 241–2
atherosclerotic plaques, 239–40
  growth and rupture of, 239–40
Atkins, R, 310–11
  high fat/protein diet, 310

ATM gene, 587
atorvastatin, 225
ATPase, 98–9, 103, 105, 120
  binding-change mechanism, 105
  complex, 103–6
  coupling factor (F-ATPase), 85, 103
  F-type, 86
  H⁺-ATPase, 85
  H⁺/K⁺, 90
  inhibitors of, 109
  ion pumps, 85–7
  P-type, 86
  phosphorylation of, 110
  role of Na⁺/K⁺ in glucose uptake, 88–9
  V-type, 86
atractyloside, 110
atrial fibrillation, 69, 132
atrial natriuretic peptide (ANP), 330
atropine, 580
  sulfate, 62
autoactivation, 124
autocatalysis, 124
autoimmune disease, 521
autoimmune thyroiditis, 521
autoimmunity, 521
autonomic nervous system, 579
  transmitters in, 570
autoradiography, 475
autosomal dyskeratosis congenital, 605
avidin, 135
axon hillock, 564
axonal transport, differing speeds of, 562
azide, 102, 109
azido-TTP, 433
azido-2′,3′-dideoxythymidine, 433
AZT, 433
  therapy for HIV infection, 433

B
bacteria, 16, 83, 101, 418, 420–1, 482, 518
  anaerobic, 2, 148, 565
  antibiotic resistant, 58
  binding sites for, 385
  genetic code of, 448
  Gram-negative, 519
  insulin gene copies, 483
  nitrogen fixing, 419
  parasitic, 385
  protein synthesis inhibition, 453
  recombinant DNA, 480
  surface structures of, 373
  symbiotic, 385
  synthesis of vitamin B₁₂ by, 136
  toxins of G-proteins, 545
bacterial artificial chromosomes (BACs), 482
bacterial infection, 32
bacteriophages, 482
  lambda (λ), 482
bacteriorodopsin, 82
Bad, 591
Bak, 591
baldness, frontal, 490
barbiturates, 28, 108, 574
β-barrel structure, 17
basal metabolic rate (BMR), 93, 106, 304
bases, conjugate, 11
basophils, 32
Bax, 591
Bcl-2, 591–3, 596
Bcl-xₗ, 591
Bcl-xₛ, 591
Bcr, 595–6
Becker muscular dystrophy, 265
bee venom, allergy to, 509
beef heart mitochondrial ATPase, 16
Bence-Jones protein, 32, 323, 563
bendrofluazide, 326, 330
Benedict assay, 153
benzoate, 252
benzodiazepines, 574
benzopyrene, 435

benzothiazepine, 91
beri-beri, 133
  thiamin deficiency in, 180
Bernard–Soulier syndrome, 67
Berthelot reaction, 248
betaine, 254
biantennary chains, 361
bicarbonate buffer, 333–5
  components of, 336
bicarbonate generation, 341
bicarbonate reabsorption, 340
biguanides, 275
bile, 29, 86, 121
  salts, 121
bile acids, 209, 217–18, 404
  biosynthesis of, 217
  chemistry of, 123
  in digestion, 115
  of fat, 217
  fecal loss, 217
  formation of, 138
  metabolism of, 404–5
  recirculation of, 217–18
  secondary, in intestine, 217
  structure of, 123, 216
bile canaliculi, 217
bile ducts, 120, 217, 399
bile salts, 79, 150
  inadequate secretion, 356
biliary system, 399, 403–4
bilirubin, 25, 155, 217, 323–4, 411–12
  metabolism of, 403–5
biliverdin, 403
binding-change mechanism, 105
Bio–Gel P series, 18
biochemistry
  human, 1–2
  flowchart of, 2
  overview of, 4
bioenergetics, 2, 93–111
biomembranes see membranes
biosynthesis, driven by ATP, 96
biotin, 127, 135, 170, 177, 193
  binding of, 178
  deficiency, 135
biotin carboxylase, 199
bisphosphates, 354
  in HCM management, 354
  and osteoporosis prevention, 356
1,3-bisphosphoglycerate (1,3-BPG), 143, 146–7, 170
2,3-bisphosphoglycerate (2,3-BPG), 41–2, 143, 155
  binding to deoxygenated hemoglobin, 43
  degradation of, 150
  synthesis of, 150
bisphosphonates, treatment of Paget's disease by, 356
black urine disease, 258
blast cells, 511
bleeding disorders
  excess, causes of, 65
  platelet related, 67–8
  and vitamin K, 132
blindness, 107, 110, 384
  cause of, 129, 289
  and oxygen concentration, 499
bloating, 125
blood
  acid–base balance, 13
  control of, 333–44
  cells, 25–34
  clotting, 26, 60
  coagulation, 1–2, 66
  inhibitors, sites of action, 73
  count (full), reference values, 610
  formed elements of, 25–6
  gases
    measurement of, 335–6
    reference values for, 337, 609
  glucose, 2, 85, 88
  concentration, 149
  and gluconeogenesis, 185

hepatic, pathways of glycogenesis, 158–9
  low, causing stress response, 168
  measurement of, 153–4
  reducing sugar assays, 153
  requirement for, 157
  sources of, 158
occult, peroxidase detection of, 503
plasma, 25
plasma proteins, 25–34
pressure
  control of, 326–8
  diastolic, 330
  genotype-related, 301
  high, 576
  systolic, 330
serum, 25
sinusoids, 399
transfusion, 384
urea nitrogen, measurement of, 248
blood–brain barrier, 42, 85, 559–60
  and leptin, 205
blood–CSF barrier, 560
blood-group substances, 385
blood vessels, 510–11
  occlusions of, 63
  role of collagen in, 66
  wall, 65–6
    adventitia, 65
    endothelium, 65–6
    intima, 65
    media, 65
    nitric oxide generation in, 66
    normal structure of, 65
    prostacyclin generation in, 66
Bloom's syndrome, 601
BNP propeptides, diagnostic utility of, 330
body fluids
  composition of, 317
  electrolyte content of, 317
  loss of, 317
body mass index (BMI), 206
  and nutritional status, 306
body weight, and BMI, 306
Bohr effect, 41–2, 47
bonds
  anhydride, 94
  high-energy, 95
  phosphate anhydride, 96
  thioester, 94
bone
  and calcium circulation, 347–8
  disorders of, 352–6
  endosteal surface, 346
  fragile, 389
  matrix of, 14
  metabolism, 345–58
  mineral, 138
  mineral density reduction, and vitamin supplementation, 139
  overgrowth of, 538
  pain in, 129
  remodeling, 345
    cycle, 346
  resorption, calcitonin inhibition of, 351–2
  types of, 345
bone disease, metabolic, 356
bone marrow, 25–6, 29, 175, 510
  megaloblastic, 136
  transplantation, 419, 586
bone matrix, 345–6
  components of, 345
bone sialoprotein, 346–7
bongkrekic acid, 110
Bordetella pertussis, 545
boronic acid affinity chromatography, 292
Borrelia, 416
bottlebrushes, 396
botulinus toxin, 565
botulism, 567
bovine serum albumin, 9

bowel
biotin synthesis in, 135
small, 125, 128
bowel disorders, inflammatory, 34
Bowman's capsule, 319
Bowman's space, 321
bradykinin, 579
brain, 29, 86
congenital malformations of, 179
cortex, 305
damage, and ammonia, 257, 403
fuel priority during stress, 284–5
and peripheral nerve, 559–60
regional fluids in, 560
brain natriuretic peptide (BNP), 330
brain parenchyma of CNS, 560
brain pathology, markers for, 561
BRCA1 cancer gene, 492
BRCA2 cancer gene, 492
breast cancer, 492
breath
acetone smell to, 288
shortness of, 327, 331, 338
brittle-bone disease, 389
Brody myopathy, 86
bromodeoxyuridine (BrdU), 592
bronchi, 336
bronchioles, 336, 338
bronchitis, winter, 338
browning of proteins, 602
Brownlee, M, 291
bruising
abdominal, 531
easy, 138
severe, 72
brush-border membrane, 117–18, 120–1, 124
buffer concentrations, 1
buffer systems, 333–6
buffering, intracellular, 335
buffers, 12
bicarbonate, 333–5
intracellular
phosphate, 336
potassium exchange, 336
protein, 336
main human, 334
bulimia nervosa, 309
α-bungarotoxin, 91, 565
Burkitt's lymphoma, 596
buspirone, 578
butter, 194
sec-butyl groups, 9
iso-butyl groups, 9

C
C-peptide, 276
C-reactive protein (CRP), 32–4, 236, 507
c-*Src* proto-oncogene, 595
C282Y, 409
CAD, 418–19, 422
metabolic channeling by, 418
cadmium, 127, 141
renal toxic effects of, 141
caffeine, 164, 563, 580
calcidiol, 130, 221
calciol, 129
calcitonin, 346–7, 467
in HCM management, 354
inhibition of bone resorption, 351–2
and osteoporosis prevention, 356
salmon and eel, 352
calcitonin-related gene peptide (CRGP), 467
calcitriol, 130, 221, 319, 347
calcium, 303
absorption, 352
adjusted, calculation of, 348
balance, 352
Ca²⁺ transport and mobilization, 87–8
in coagulation, 25
complexed, 347–8
deficiency, 130
excretion, 352

fluxes, 355
in bone, 345
homeostasis
factors influencing, 348–52
hormones influencing, 347, 357
hormonal control of circulation, 347–8
ionized (Ca²⁺), 347–8, 549
metabolism, 345–58
disorders of, 352–6
metastatic deposition, 131
mobilization, 550
and osteoporosis prevention, 356
protein-bound, 347–8
reference values, 609
requirement for muscle contraction, 267
storage in bone, 347
calcium-activated neutral protease, 288
calcium–calmodulin systems, 536
calcium channel blockers, 91
calcium trigger, 265
calmodulin, 164, 549
structure and function of, 550
Ca²⁺-calmodulin-activated protein, 163
Ca²⁺-calmodulin-dependent protein kinase, 164
calnexin, 369
calorie restriction
and delay of carcinogenesis, 608
and longevity, 607–8
calorimetry, 93
measurement of energy expenditure by, 304
calpain-10, 288
calreticulin, 369
calsequestrin, 549
cAMP–PKA signaling cassette, 548–9
cAMP-responsive-element-binding protein (CREB), 548
Campylobacter jejuni, 559
canaliculi, 345
cancer, 3, 93, 106, 138, 261, 583–98
associated with α-fetoprotein, 402
breast, 492
hereditary, 492
and HRT, 356
protein truncation testing in, 492
classification, 594
colon, 434, 593, 597
colorectal, 312, 421, 593
defined, 594
and DNA mutations, 594
factors involved in cell proliferation, 595
gastric, 421
genetic component of, 431
increased frequency in progerias, 601
influence of lifestyle and diet on, 312
inherited syndromes, 596
liver, and AFP, 402
lymphoreticular, 587
ovarian, 492
pancreatic, 412
and obstructive liver disease, 412
prostate, 312
uterine, 421
and vitamin supplementation, 139
see also carcinoma(s); tumors
Candida albicans, 517
canola oil, 303
capillaries, 65
capillary wall, permeability of, 315
captopril, 57
carbamination, 42
carbamoyl aspartate, 417
carbamoyl phosphate, 247, 417
synthesis, 249–50, 252
carbamoyl phosphate synthetase, 252, 257, 417–18

carbohydrate-deficient glycoprotein syndromes (GDGSs), 371
carbohydrate–lectin interactions, 373
carbohydrates, 2–3, 93, 301–2
blood-group substances, 385
complex, 301, 359–74
conversion to fat, 175
dietary, structure of, 117
digestion and absorption, 116–20, 125
in food, 113
metabolism, 100, 140
in liver, 399–401
refined, 301
storage and synthesis, in liver and muscle, 157–73
carbon, inter-organ flow of, 246
carbon–carbon (C–C) bonds, 14, 77
carbon dioxide (CO₂), 1, 3, 35, 41, 80, 93
daily flux, 333
elimination of, 148, 170
generation of, 98, 144, 151
handling of, 339–40
metabolic, 175
partial pressure (pCO₂), 334, 336–9
in respiration, 337
removal, 25
carbon monoxide (CO), 102, 110, 499
inhibition by, 109
poisoning, 37
carbonic acid (H₂CO₃), 42
carbonic anhydrase, 42, 90, 123
carbonyl group, introduction of, 184
carbonyls, 603
carboxy–biotin intermediate, 178
carboxy-fluoresceindiacetate succinimidyl ester (CFDA SE), 592
carboxyaminoimidazole ribonucleotide (CAIR), 414
carboxyhemoglobin, 37
carboxyl groups (—COOH), 7, 12, 121
α-carboxyl groups, 12–13
β-carboxyl groups, 10
γ-carboxyl groups, 10, 15
carboxyl terminus, 13
carboxylation, 127, 135
carboxylic acid, 9, 11, 146
carboxymethylcellulose, 18
carboxymethylcysteine, 22
carboxymethyllysine, 603
carboxypeptidases, 123–4, 247
carcinogenesis, delayed by calorie restriction, 608
carcinogens and DNA mutation, 181
carcinoid syndrome, 579
carcinoma *in situ*, 594
carcinomas, 129, 594
commonest forms, 594
malignant cervical, 594
see also cancer; tumors
cardiac arrhythmias, 83, 304
cardiac death, 83
cardiac disease, 44
cardiac failure
diuretic treatment for, 326
and renin–angiotensin system, 327
cardiac myocytes, 261
cardiac regurgitation, 393
cardiac weakness, 180
cardiolipin, 78–9, 375
cardiomyopathies, 191, 605
iron overload increase risk of, 497
selenium-responsive, 141
cardiorespiratory arrest, 341
cardiovascular disease, 135, 225
and HRT, 356
links to obesity, glucose intolerance, and diabetes, 292
and metabolic syndrome, 293
risk of, 235, 240–3, 536
and vitamin supplementation, 139
cardiovascular risk, 235, 240–3, 536
assessment of, 240–3

management of, 241
non-lipid marker of, 229
cardiovascular system, 236
carnitine, 257
deficiencies in metabolism, 191
carnitine palmitoyl transferase-I (CPT-I), 189
carnitine shuttle, 189–90
carnitine supplementation, 191, 193
carnosine, Cu chelation, 502
carotene, 504
β-carotene, 128, 239
dioxygenase, 128
carotenoids, conversion of, 129
carrier proteins, 524
cartilage, 14, 394, 538
caspase 8, 592
caspases, 590
in apoptosis, 590–1
overexpression of, 591–2
castanospermine, 369
catabolic pathways, 176, 274
catabolism, 3, 135
after trauma, 286
of catecholamines, 577
increased, 285
catalase (CAT), 52, 100, 102, 502–3
catalysis, rotary, 103–5
cataracts, 47, 107, 289, 364, 601
congenital, 328
diabetic, 291
inherited, 490
catecholamine-O-methyl transferase (COMT), 577
catecholamines, 160, 284, 574–9
catabolism of, 577
multiple receptors for, 578
β-catenin, 597
cathepsins, 346
cation exchange, 18–20
caveolae, 82
caveolins, 82
CD markers, 511, 518
CD95, 592
CDK inhibitors (CDKIs), 589
CDP-choline pathway, 378
CDP-DAG, formation of, 379
CDP-ethanolamine, 376
celecoxib, 555
celiac disease, 356
cell cycle, 430–5, 583–4
analysis of progression, 592–3
and cancer, 591
growth factor regulation of, 590
phases of, 583–4
regulation of, 589
stages of, 431
subversion of, 596
cell death, 102
cell differentiation, 583–98
cell growth, 583–98
cell membranes, 1
cholesterol in, 216
cell proliferation, regulation of, 584–5
cell signaling
mechanisms of, 542
protein tyrosine kinase (PTK) in, 585
systems, 3
cell volume, 318
cell–cell communication, 85
carbohydrate dependent, 373
cells
CNS, 561
complex ecosystem of, 1
CSF circulating, 561
of the nervous system, 560–3
reticuloendothelial, 560
transformed, 583
cellulose acetate, 20
central nervous system (CNS), 84
cells of, 561
ceruloplasmin deficiency, 402
defects in, 215
delivery of vitamin B₁₂, 138
iron in, 561

norepinephrine neurons in, 576
serotoninergic nerves in, 578
centrifugation, 17
cephalosporin, 58
ceramide, 380
cerebronic acids, 381
cerebrosides, 381
cerebrosidoses, 381, 384
cerebrospinal fluid (CSF), 56, 85, 100
analysis of, 579
circulating cells, 560–1
leak, 560
oligoclonal bands in, 563
reference values, 610
rostral–caudal gradient, 579
sources of, 560
ceruloplasmin, 29, 86, 141
deficiency, 402
plasma ferroxidase activity of, 30
cervical carcinoma, malignant, 594
cervix, uterine, 594
channelopathies, 565
chaotropic agents, 16
chaperones, 23, 369–70, 455
Charcot–Marie–Tooth disease, 85
charge–charge repulsion, 148
chemokines, 509
chemotaxis, 507
chemotherapy, 578
applications of ROS, 498
resistance to, 87
side effect, 421
chenodeoxycholic acid, 404
chest pain, in heart attack, 235
child, macrosomic, of diabetic
mother, 168
Chinese Restaurant Syndrome, 248
Chlamydia, 416
chloride, 303
chloroform, 81
p-chloromecuribenzoate, 146
cholecalciferol, 129, 220–1, 348
see also vitamin D$_3$
cholecystokinin, 120–1, 124, 217,
278
cholera, 385
toxin, 385, 545
choleragen, 545
cholestanol, 218
cholestatic disease, 410
cholesterol, 78–9, 82–3, 120, 150,
175
absorption of, 121
biosynthesis, 190, 209–23
circadian rhythm of, 215
regulation of, 212–17
biosynthetic defect, 215
catabolism in liver, 404–5
in cell membranes, 216
delivery to liver, 215
essential component of cells,
225–6
excretion, 218
via feces, 218
factors influencing regulation, 213
free concentration, 214
free and esterified, 209–10
HDL as acceptor of, 215
homeostasis, 218
intracellular concentration of, 214,
226
lack of metabolization, 218
levels, interpretation of, 242
and membrane fluidity, 216
planar ring structure of, 209
as precursor, 225
of steroid hormones, 218–19
removal, 233
reverse transport, 233–4
secretion from liver, 217
sterol ring of, 209
structure of, 209–10
synthesis, control of, 232–3
transport of, 225
uptake, control of, 232–3
cholesterol acyltransferase (ACAT;
SOAT), 210

cholesterol efflux regulatory protein
(CERP), 233
cholesterol ester transfer protein
(CETP), 230
cholesterol esterase, 529
cholesterol-lecithin acyltransferase,
210
cholesteryl esterase, 120
cholesteryl esters, 120, 215
cholestyramine, lowering of plasma
cholesterol by, 218
cholic acid, 121, 123, 404
choline, 62, 78, 377
source of ACh, 579
synthesis, 135
choline acetyl transferase, 579
cholinergic transmission, 564–5
chondrocytes, proliferation of, 538
chondroitin sulfates, 394
chondroitin-6-sulfate, 395
chromatin, 429
condensed, 466
chromatography
affinity, 20
glycated hemoglobin
measurement by, 292
gradient, 20
high performance liquid (HPLC),
20, 22, 133, 421, 579
chromium, 139
chromogenic agents, 22
chromogens, 153
chromophores, 153
chromosomes, packaging of, 430
chronic myelogeneous leukemia
(CML), 594
chronic obstructive airways disease
(COAD), 343
chronic uridine therapy, 419
Chvostek's sign, 355
chylomicrons, 123, 209, 213, 225,
227
fat transport by, 231
chymotrypsin, 52, 59, 124–5, 246
substrate binding sites of, 53
chymotrypsinogen, 60
cimetidine, 91, 581
circulation
peripheral, 166
portal, 165
circulatory system, aging of, 605
cirrhosis, 29, 86, 168
and alcohol excess, 406–7
and Cu excess, 141
and Se excess, 141
citrate, 25, 170, 199
accumulation, 183
achiral, 182
Ca complex with, 347
conversion to α-ketoglutarate,
184
formation in TCA cycle, 181
isomerization of, 182
citrate lyase, 203
citrate synthase, 181
citric acid, 176
in TCA cycle, 181
citric acid cycle, 3, 175
see also tricarboxylic acid (TCA)
cycle
citroyl-CoA, 181
citrulline, 8, 85, 250, 252
classical activation pathways, 518–19
clathrin, 214, 563
clinical laboratory, function of, 27
clonidine, 577
clopidogrel, 68, 555
Clostridium botulinum, 567
clozapine, 578
CNS *see* central nervous system
co-lipase, 121
coagulation, 69–74
pathways in, 71
coagulation factors, 64, 69, 74
activation of, 70
coagulation inhibitors, properties of,
74

coagulation tests, reference values,
610
coated pits, 214
cobalamin *see* vitamin B$_{12}$
cobalt, 136
cocaine, 575
codeine, 408
codon–anticodon base pairing
possibilities, 450
wobble hypothesis of, 450
codons, 447–50
coeliac disease, 125
coenzymes, 1, 3
A (CoA), 122, 135, 183
esters, 183
and PDC activity, 178
B vitamins as, 133
nucleotide, 98
and PDC activity, 178
Q$_{10}$, 98, 101–2
rare deficiency of, 100
redox, 96
concentrations in cell, 151
structure of, 97
reduced, 96–8
and ATP synthesis, 96–7, 175
roles of, 54
vitamins as, 127
cofactors, 1, 54, 183
metal, 138
collagenases, 240, 346
type IV, 595
collagens, 14, 67, 138, 360,
387–90
age-related chemical changes in,
604
basement membrane, 389
biosynthesis and processing of,
390
in bone matrix, 345
classification and distribution of,
388
crosslink formation, 391
and Cu, 141
fibril-associated with interrupted
triple helices (FACITs), 389
fibrillar, 345, 388
glycosylation of, 359–60
multiple triple helices with
interruptions, 389
nonfibrillar, 389
pigment deposition on, 259
role in blood vessels, 66
of skin, 603
amino acid oxidation products
in, 603
slow turn over, 501
structure of, 388
triple-helix, 387
synthesis and modification of,
389–90
types of, 387–9
collodion membrane, 17
colon
bile acids reabsorption, 217
cancer and FAP, 597
cathartics for, 90
color blindness, 431
colorectal cancer, 593
mutations underlying development
of, 593
colostrum, 31
coma, 253, 286
caused by pyroxidine deficiency,
135
hypoglycemic, 2, 157
common bile duct, 218
complement system, 507–8
activation of, 518–19
cascade, 507–8
complete blood count (CBC), 48
complex I (NADH-Q reductase or
NADH dehydrogenase), 98–100,
102, 110
inhibition of, 108
phosphorylation/dephosphorylation
of, 110

complex II (succinate-Q reductase or
succinate dehydrogenase),
99–100, 184
complex III (QH$_2$-cytochrome *c*
reductase or ubiquinone
cytochrome *c* reductase), 98–102,
110
inhibition of, 108–9
complex IV (cytochrome *c* oxidase or
cytochrome oxidase), 98–100,
102, 104, 110–11
inhibition of, 109
phosphorylation of, 110
complex V (ATP synthase or F$_0$F$_1$-ATP
synthase), 99, 103–5
computed tomography imaging
(CTI), 121, 576
concanavalin A, 371
concerted model, 61
confusion, mental, 531
congenital adrenal hyperplasia, 213,
220, 536
conjugase, 135
connexin, 82, 85
Conn's syndrome, 329
consensus elements, 461
constipation, 133
contraceptive pill, oral, 135
convulsions, 286, 574
caused by pyroxidine deficiency,
135
Coomassie Blue, 20–1
copper, 54, 86, 127, 139–41, 498
albumin binding, 502
in complex IV, 102
defective transport of, 86
deposition in liver, 409
excess and cirrhosis, 141
and oxygenase enzymes, 140
transport of, 29
copro-oxidase, 403
coproporphyria, hereditary, 403
coproporphyrinogen III, 403
coprostanol, 218
CoQ$_{10}$, 101
Cori cycle, 170, 246, 282–3, 401
cornea, 14, 86, 398
softening of, 129
in Tangier disease, 233
coronary heart disease, and obesity,
206
corpus luteum, 535
corticoliberin (CRH), 305
corticosteroids, 66, 219–20, 509,
581
corticotrophin releasing hormone
(CRH), 529
cortisol, 160, 218, 524, 541
biosynthesis of, 529–30
diabetogenic effect, 530
excess, 557
influence on gluconeogenesis, 530
reference values, 610
secretion, disorders of, 530–1
synthesis, 219
cortisol-binding globulins (CBG), 524
cortisone, 530, 555
cosmids, 482
costal cartilage, age changes in, 602
counter–current exchange and
multiplication, 322
coupling factor, 103
covalent modification, regulation by,
110
cramps, stimulated by hypocalcemia,
355
creatine phosphate (creatine-P), 268
synthesis and degradation of, 268
creatine phosphokinase, 168
creatinine, 8, 245, 269
assay of, 269
clearance, 324
serum levels of, 325, 328
p-cresol, 106
Creutzfeldt–Jacob disease, 23
Crick, F, 425
Crigler–Najjar syndrome, 412

cristae, mitochondrial, 96
Crohn's disease, 129, 137, 356
crossover point, 108
crystallins, slow turn over, 501
CSF see cerebrospinal fluid
CTP synthesis, 419
CTP synthetase, 419
Cushing's syndrome, 196, 531, 536, 557
cyanide, 102, 109–10
  conversion to thiocyanate, 110
cyanogen bromide, 22
cyanosis, 44, 47
cyclic adenosine monophosphate (cAMP), 347, 546–7
  β-adrenergic receptors coupled to, 546–7
  metabolism of, 547
cyclic 3'5'-adenosine monophosphate, 110, 161, 163–4
cyclic guanosine monophosphate (cGMP), 580
cyclic guanosine-3',5'-monophosphate, 66
cyclin complexes, 589
cyclin-dependent kinases (CDKs), 430, 589
cyclins, 589
cyclo-oxygenase, 66, 597
cycloartenol, 211
cycloheximide, 453
cyclooxygenase, 59
CYP enzymes, 219–20
CYP2C19, 408
CYP2D6, 408
cystathionine, 229, 254
cystathionine β-synthase, 254
cystatin C concentration, and renal function, 324–5
cysteamine, 84
cysteic acid, 22
cysteine, 10, 12, 16, 21–2, 52, 59, 229
  residues, 90, 100, 102, 422
cystic fibrosis, 88, 488
  and pancreatic insufficiency, 118
  transmembrane conductance regulator (CFTR), 88
cystine, 10, 21–2
  accumulation in lysosomes, 84
cystinosis, 84
cystinuria, 259
cytidine, 377, 420
cytidine deaminase, 420
cytidine diphosphate (CDP), 376
cytidine triphosphate (CTP), 376, 417
cytochrome a, 102, 104
cytochrome a3, 102, 104
cytochrome b, 101–2
cytochrome c, 101–2, 104, 108–9, 111, 593
  oxidase, 499
cytochrome c1, 101–2
cytochrome oxidase, 102, 109, 140
  deficiency in aging, 606
cytochrome P450, 405–6
  control of steroidogenesis, 219
cytochromes, 29, 98–100, 102
  and iron, 99, 139
  variation in heme structures, 103
cytoglobin, 43
cytokines, 66, 285, 508–9, 584, 586
  anti-inflammatory, 509
  autocrine action, 508
  characteristics, 508
  classification, 508–9
  immunostimulatory, 509
  osteoclast regulation by, 346
  paracrine action, 508
  pleiotropy, 508
  pro-inflammatory, 205, 236, 240, 509
  receptor signaling, 586–8
  redundancy, 508
cytomegalovirus (CMV), 61
cytoplasmic tubulovesicles, 90

cytoplasmic vesicles, 86
cytosine, 413, 420
  bonding, 441
    in DNA, 426
  methylated, 438
  nucleotides in RNA, 437
cytosine deaminase, 420–1
cytoskeleton, 83
cytosol, 98, 100, 109, 138, 150, 164
  and urea cycle, 250–2
cytosolic enzymes, 143
cytosolic retinal-binding protein (CRBP), 129

D
dansyl chloride, 22
dantrolene, 268
dATP, 419
ddc, 433
de novo pathway, 417–19
deafness, 85
  due to osteosclerosis, 389
death, 107, 110, 253
  rate of, human, 600
debrisoquine, 408
  polymorphism, 406
decarboxylation, 378
decay accelerating factor, 380
deep brain stimulation, 252
deep vein thrombosis (DVT), 74, 132, 254
dehydratase, removal of water by, 247
dehydration, 84, 288, 308, 344, 483
  and fluid intake, 329
  from polyuria, 354
  serum protein increase, 348
dehydroascorbate, 503
dehydroascorbate reductase, 503–4
dehydroascorbic acid, 138
dehydroascorbyl radical, 503
7-dehydrocholesterol, 129, 348
dehydrolysinonorleucine, 391
delusions, 574
dementia, 135, 227, 601
  AIDS-related, 574
denaturants, 16
deoxy-TMP, 421
deoxyadenosine, 419
5'-deoxyadenosylcobalamin, 136, 138
deoxycholic acids, 217, 404
8-oxo-2'-deoxyguanosine, 435
deoxyhemoglobin, 150
deoxynucleotides, formation of, 421–2
deoxyribonucleic acid (DNA), 3, 7, 20, 44, 143, 425–36
  alternate forms of, 426–7
  amplification and cloning, 479–85
    cell-based, 479–81, 483
      restriction fragment length polymorphisms (RFLPs), 486–7
    enzyme-based, 479, 481–5, 487–90
    PCR, 479, 481–5, 487–90
    vector systems for, 482
  analysis, 23, 46
    specific methods for, 485–92
  annealing properties of, 473
  B-, A-, and Z-forms of, 428
  banking, 428
  binding motifs, 463
  compaction into chromosomes, 429–30
  cutting sites, 477
  damage
    nature of, 433
    repair of, 432–5
    to mtDNA in aging, 605
  deamination, 433
  defects in repair, 601
  depurination, 433
  detection of variation in, 490–2
    denaturant-gradient gel electrophoresis, 491–2

    single-strand conformational polymorphism (SSCP), 490–1
  duplex, 427–9
  excision repair, 433
    and folic acid, 136
  labeling of probes, 475–6
  'melting' of double strands in DGGE, 491–2
  melting temperature (Tm), 475
  mismatch repair, 434
  mitochondrial, 428–9
    damage to, 606
  monitoring for damage, 589
  movement through agarose, 479
  mutant, 488, 493
  nick translation, 476
  oxidative damage to, 435
  paternity testing, 427
  polymerase complexes, 431
  polymerases, biochemistry of, 429
  prokaryotic, 432
  recognition sites, 477
  recombinant technology, 473–95
  repair activity and longevity, 601
  replication
    eukaryotic, 432
    separation/copying of strands, 430–2
    site, 431–2
  restriction enzyme digestion, 478
  satellite, 428
  separate strands, 427–9
  sequencing, 492–4
    chain termination (Sanger), 492
    dideoxynucleotides, 494
  Southern blotting, 479
  steroid response element (SRE), 464
  storage, 476–9
  strand breaks, 433–4
  structure of, 425–30
  synthesis, 150–1, 432, 584
  TATA sequence, 428, 441
  template, 481
  tests, 473
  three-dimensional, 426
  transcription, process of, 440–2
  viral, 61
  Watson and Crick model of, 425–7
  Watson–Crick pairing, 466
Z-deoxyribonucleic acid, 427
deoxyribonucleoside phosphates (dNTPs), 475, 481
deoxyribose, 425
deoxyuridine triphosphate diphosphohydrolase, 421
deoxyuridylate (dUMP), 421
depolarization, 571
depression, 133
  amine theory of, 575
  caused by biotin deficiency, 135
  caused by pyroxidine deficiency, 135
  as disease of amine neurotransmitters, 575
  relieved by serotonin, 579
  and Se excess, 141
dermatan sulfate, 394
dermatitis, 129, 135
  caused by biotin deficiency, 135
  pellagra-like, 85
  scaly, 133
desaturase system, 203
desensitization, 161
desmopressin, 67
desmosine, 391–2
developmental delay, 85
dexamethasone, 531
dextrans, 18
diabetes, 2–3, 93, 106, 118, 186, 490, 601, 603
  blood glucose monitoring in, 154
  classification of, 286
  complications of, 288–91
    polyol pathway, 291
  diagnosis of, 149

  false impression of, 153
  and glucose net synthesis, 183
  and impaired renal function, 323
  inflammatory reaction in, 288–9
  iron overload increases risk of, 497
  and kidney disease, 296
    tests for, 296
  laboratory diagnosis, 294
  linkage trait studies, 489
  links to obesity, glucose intolerance, and cardiovascular disease, 292
  maturity onset diabetes of the young (MOBY), 287–8, 401
  and metabolic syndrome, 293
  metabolism in, 288
  and negative N balance, 253
  OxS, 499
  polygenic, 288
  portable pump treatment, 275
  relationship with obesity and atherosclerosis, 293
  toxicity of excess glucose, 288–9
  treatment of, 293
    compliance, 295
  type 1, 2, 199, 275, 286–7
  type 2, 34, 206, 235, 275, 286–8, 308
    β-cell dysfunction in, 106
    genetic component of, 431
    IGF-I therapy in, 538
    low grade inflammatory reaction in, 288
  urine glucose test for, 295
  vascular complications in, 288–9
  worldwide increase in, 286
diabetes insipidus, 325
  nephrogenic, 82, 328
  and vasopressin deficiency, 325
diabetes mellitus, 46–7, 286–93, 312
  diagnosis of, 287
  dyslipidemias in, 235
  management linked to nutrition, 312
  metabolism in, 289
diabetic ketoacidosis, 289, 343
  affect on potassium balance, 290
  development of, 290
  presentation of, 288
diabetic nephropathy, 289, 296
diabetic neuropathy, 289, 291
diabetic patients, hyperglycemic, 170
diabetic peripheral vascular disease, 289
diabetic retinopathy, 289
diacylglycerol (DAG), 122, 164–5, 377, 379, 550–3, 585
  biosynthesis of, 375–6
dialysis, 17, 19
  Cu loss during, 141
  Zn loss during, 140
4',6'-diamidino-phenylindole-2HCl (DAPI), 592
diarrhea, 90, 125, 129, 364, 579
  acute, 559
  and fluid balance, 115
  and fluid loss, 320
  and fungal poisoning, 440
  intermittent, 563
  and Mg deficiency, 303
  and niacin deficiency, 135
  occasional, 529
  osmotic, 385
  severe, 320, 545
  traveler's, 545
  and Zn deficiency, 140
diaspirin cross-linked human Hb, 38
trans-dicarboxylic acid, 184
dicarboxylic aciduria, 194
dicoumarin, 132
dideoxynucleotides, in DNA sequencing, 494
2',3'-dideoxy-3'-thiacytidine, 433
diet
  balanced, 309
  butter–margarine debate, 194

and cardiovascular prevention, 312
and coronary disease prevention, 311
  food guide pyramid, 310
  in health and disease, 309–11
  high-fat, 186
  ketogenic, 85
  low-carbohydrate/high-fat controversies, 310–11
  low-cholesterol, 312
  low-fat, 312
  role of, 2
dietary history, 309
dietary polymers, digestion of, 116
dietary reference intakes (DRI), 299–300
dietary reference values (DRVs), 300
diethylaminoethyl (DEAE) cellulose, 18
diffusion
  through phospholipid bilayer, 80–2
  transport kinetics of, 83
digestion, 113–20
  of carbohydrates, 116–20
  of dietary lipids, 122
  of dietary polymers, 116
  emulsification of fat before, 120
  gastric, loss of, 115
  general principles of, 115
  of lipids, 120–3
  mechanical and anatomical basis of, 113
  of polysaccharides, 116
  of proteins, 123–5
digoxin, 91
dihydrobiopterin, 258
dihydrofolate, 421–2
dihydrofolate reductase, 421
dihydrofolic acid, 135
dihydrolipoamide dehydrogenase, 178
dihydrolipoyl dehydrogenase (E₃) deficiency, 181
dihydrolipoyl transacetylase, 178
dihydroorotase, 418
dihydroorotate dehydrogenase, 417
dihydroorotic acid, 417
dihydropteridine reductase (DHPR), 580
dihydropyridine (DHP), 91
dihydrotestosterone, 523, 532–3
dihydrothymine, 421
dihydrouracil, 421
dihydrouracil dehydrogenase, 421
dihydrouridine, 438
dihydroxyacetone phosphate (DHAP), 99–100, 146, 168, 170, 376
1α,25-dihydroxycholecalciferol (1,25(OH)₂D₃), 130, 221, 319, 347, 350
  Ca and P absorption increased by, 351
dihydroxyphenylalanine (DOPA), 258
L-dihydroxyphenylalanine (DOPA), 580
L-dihydroxyphenylalanine (L-DOPA), 252
diiodothyronine, 104
diisopropylfluorophosphate, 59
diltiazem, 91
dimethylallyl pyrophosphate, 211
dimethylbenzimidazole ring, 136
2,4-dinitrophenol (DNP), 106–7, 109
  induction of weight loss by, 107
  poisoning by, 107
diolepoxides, 435
dipalmitoylphosphatidylcholine (DPPC), 338, 378
dipeptidases, 123, 125
dipeptides, 123
  digestion, 125
  structure of, 13
diphosphatidylglycerol (DPG), 79, 375, 379
dipyridamole, 68, 254, 555

disaccharides, 116
  cleavage of, 117
  inducibility of, 118
dissociation constant (Kₐ), 11
  negative logarithm of (pKₐ), 10–12, 106, 148
disulfide bonds, 10, 15–16
disulfide bridge, 32
disulfiram, 59, 408
dithiothreitol, 10
diuresis, 82
  magnesium deficiency in, 304
diuretic phase, 328
diuretics, 576
  loop, 326
  thiazide, 326
  for treatment of cardiac failure, 326
  for treatment of edema, 326
  for treatment of hypertension, 326
dizziness, 44
  postural, 563
DNA see deoxyribonucleic acid
dominant mutant phenotype, 583
dopa carboxylase, 578
  deficiency, 579
dopamine, 539, 577–8
  catabolism, 578
  deficiency, 565
  disorders of metabolism, 579
  inhibitor of prolactin, 539
  in nigrostriatal tract, 577
  synthesis cofactor, 580
dorsal root ganglia, 560
double vision, 129, 581
drugs
  addictive, 564
  antiarrhythmic, 91
  antibiotic, 136
  anticancer, 136, 421
  antidepressant, 564, 575, 578
  antidiabetic, 233
  antidopaminergic, 539
  anti-emetic, 578
  antihypertensive, 330, 575
  antimalarial, 155
  antiplatelet, 68–9, 555
    action of, 68
  antipsychotic, 578
  antithrombotic, 63, 72, 132
  antitubercular, 135
  bisphosphate, 389
  cardiotonic, 549
  cytotoxic, 594
  diuretic, 326
  hepatotoxicity of, 406
  hypolipidemic, 190
  idiosyncratic toxicity, 406
  inhibition of transporters by, 91
  insulin stimulating, 275
  lipid lowering, 235
  metabolism of, 405–8
    role of cytochrome P450, 406
    and pancreatitis, 121
  statins, 211, 225
  sulfa, 155
  thrombolytic, 75
dual energy X-ray absorptiometry (DEXA), 306, 357
Dubin–Johnson syndrome, 88, 412
Duchenne muscular dystrophy, 265, 467, 490
duodenum, 113, 116, 120–1, 124, 217–18
  acid damage to, 91
  lining of, 123
dwarfism, 601
dynorphins, 581
dyslipidemias, 227, 234–5
  in diabetes mellitus, 235
  most important genetic forms of, 228
  phenotypic classification of, 228
  WHO classification of, 227
dysphagia, 567
dysplasia, 594
dystrophin, 265, 467

E
E-cadherin, 595
Eadie–Hofstee plot, 56–8
eating, 3
echocardiography, in Marfan's syndrome, 254
EcoRI, 477
ectopic ACTH syndrome, 531
edema, 27, 131, 377
  ankle, 327
  bilateral pitting, 308
  cerebral, 252, 257, 286, 401
  CNS, 253
  diuretic treatment for, 326
  in kwashiorkor, 308
  and protein loss, 319
  pulmonary, 499
  and water distribution, 318
Edman degradation, 21–2
Edman's reagent, 22
edrophonium, 565
effectors
  allosteric, 2, 40–1, 110
  intracellular, 546
Efudex, 421
Ehlers–Danlos syndrome, 14, 66
eicosanoids, 555–7
  synthesis of, 203, 556
eicosapentaenoic acid, 203
elastase, 52, 59, 124–5, 246
  substrate binding sites of, 53
elastin, 141, 390–1, 502
  multichain crosslink in, 392
elderly, folate deficiency in, 136
electrochemical gradients, 86
electroimmunodiffusion, 521
electrolytes
  balance and water, 315–32
  in digestion, 115
  imbalance, 385
  reference values, 610
  serum, 307
  status assessment, 331
electron transfer (redox) reactions, 97, 175
electrons, 96
  mitochondrial transport of, 97–102
  shuttles, 100
  transfer of, 101
    from NADH to mitochondria, 100
  transport system, inhibitors of, 106–9
electrophoresis, 479
  denaturant-gradient gel, 491–2
  pulse-field gel, 480
electroporation, 481
electrospray ionization mass spectrometry (ESI MS), 13, 421
embolism, 63
emphysema, 341
enantiomers, 7–8, 82
encephalomyopathy, mitochondrial, 110
encephalopathies, 100, 110, 605
  ammonia in, 251, 403
endocarditis, 307
endocrine disorders, 490
  in female, 535–6
endocrine processes, 524
endocrine tests, reference values, 610
endocrinology, 3
  biochemical, 523–40
endocytosis, 138
endogenous glucose production, 401
endometrium, 535
endonucleases, restriction, 480
endopeptidases, 123, 125
endoplasmic reticulum, 1, 16, 102, 121, 123
  assembly/processing of oligosaccharides, 366–8
  collagen synthesis in, 389–90
  and glycoproteins, 359
  LDL receptor synthesis, 214

  protein modification, 456
  protein synthesis on, 456
endoproteases, 22
endoribonucleases, 443
β-endorphin, 581
endosaccharidases, 117
endosomes, 86
endothelium
  arterial, 236
    control of vasodilation, 236
    inhibition of clotting, 236
  dysfunction of, 236–8
endothelium-derived relaxing factor (EDRF), 65–6, 236, 499
endrophonium, 581
energy
  conservation by coupling with ATP, 95–6
  expenditure during activity, 304
  free, 94
  homeostasis, 304–5
    regulation of, 305
  oxidation as source of, 93–4
  requirements by age and sex, 304
  storage forms of, 246
  transduction of, 96–7
    pathways, 98
enhancers, 460–1
enkephalins, 581
enol–phosphate bond, 170
enolase, 149
  inhibition by fluoride, 149
enolpyruvate, 148
entero-hepatic circulation, 121
Enterobacter cloacae, 373
enterochromaffin cells, 579
enterocytes, 116–17, 121–3, 125, 247, 403
  chylomicron particles in, 280
  fatty acid entering, 231
  triaglycerol resynthesis, 231
  use of glutamine by, 113
enterohepatic circulation, 209, 217–18
enteropeptidase, 116, 124
  duodenal, 124
  intestinal, 60
enterotoxin, 545
enzymatic assays, 153–4
enzymatic reactions, 51–4
  factors affecting, 51–2
  pH effect, 52
  reaction profile, 52
  temperature effect, 51–2
enzyme-linked immunosorbent assay (ELISA), 270, 524–5
enzyme replacement therapy, 383
enzyme–substrate complex, 55
enzymes, 1, 51–62
  activity, definition of, 52–4
  affecting TCA cycle, 185
  allosteric, 60
    regulation of, schematic representation, 61
  antioxidant, 141
  aromatase, 220
  classification of, 54
  CYP, 219–20
  cytosolic, 143, 168
  defects in, 396
  digestive, 115–16
    proteolytic activation of, 60
  erythrocyte, 135
  expression changes on food intake, 203
  function and micronutrient status, 127
  gluconeogenic, 181
  glycogen branching, 158
  glycogenic, 158
  glycogenolytic, 158
  glycolytic, 170
  hepatic, low substrate specificity of, 405
  heterotropic regulation, 60–1
  homotropic regulation, 60–1

human genes for, 54
induction and repression by glucagon, 276
induction and repression by insulin, 276
inhibition of, 57–9
  by drugs and poisons, 59
  by statins, 211
  competitive, 58
  noncompetitive, 59
  transition-state, 58
isoforms of, 100
isosteric, 60
isozymes, 52
kinase, 96
kinetics of, 55–7
leakage into blood, 270
lipogenic, control of, 199–200
lyase/desmolase, 220
lysosomal, 346, 370
malic, 186, 203
measurement of activity in clinical samples, 56
mitochondrial, 168
nomenclature of, 53–4
oxidase, 102
pancreatic, 121
peroxisomal, 87
phosphorylation/dephosphorylation, 170
polymerase, 481
protein digesting, 120
rate-limiting, 210–11
  allosteric regulation of, 60–2
regulation of activity, 59–62
regulatory role of phosphorylation, 280
restriction, 477, 480
  cutting frequency, 478
signaling, 542
specificity of, 52
stereospecificity of, 182
suicide substrate, 58
sulfhydryl, 59
thrombolytic, 498
and transfer proteins, 229–30
of urea cycle, 251
used for clinical diagnosis, 52
eosinophilic degranulation, 31
epidermis, Malpighian layer, 221
epidermolysis bullosa, 392
epilepsy, 580
  high frequency, 257
epimerases, 152
epinephrine (adrenaline), 67, 74, 138, 160, 509, 565
  effects in liver, 278
  hormonal activity of, 523
  ligand, 543
  mobilization of hepatic glycogen, 163–4
  as neurotransmitter, 576–7
  regulation of lipid metabolism, 197
epithelial cells, intestinal, 124
epithelialization, defective, 129
epitopes, 30
Epivir, 433
Epstein–Barr virus, 591
ergocalciferol, 129, 348
ergosterol, 83, 129, 348
error–catastrophe theory of aging, 601
erythroblasts, 25
erythrocyte transketolase, 133
erythrocytes, 25–6, 35, 37, 42, 48, 85, 143–4
  and CO$_2$ transport, 339–40
  count, 47
  distorted morphology, 45
  function of pentose phosphate pathway in, 153
  glucose transport into, 88
  hemolysis of, 29
  metallothioneine levels and Zn status, 140
  regulation of glycolysis in, 148–50

erythropoetin, 319
erythropoiesis, 25
  defective, 140
erythropoietin, 1, 25, 42, 483
  recombinant, preparation of, 480–1
erythrose-4-phosphate, 152
Escherichia coli, 440, 476, 545
  Klenow fragment, 476
  uropathogenic strains, 385
esophagus, 113
estimated average requirement (EAR), 299–300, 304
estradiol, 220, 532
  FSH promotion of, 535
  and GH secretion, 537
  reduced secretion, 536
  synthesis, 535
1,3,5(10)-estratriene nucleus, 220
estrogens, 219–20, 352
  and bone mass, 356
  deficiency, 536
ethanol, 80, 148
  use in methanol poisoning, 57
ethanolamine, 78, 377
ethylene glycol, 57
ethylenediamine tetraacetic acid (EDTA), 25
N-ethylmaleimide, 146
eucaryotic cells, primary transporters in, 87
eunuchoidism, 534
Evans' Blue, 559
excitotoxicity, 574
exercise
  and mitochondrial biogenesis, 96
  prolonged, 160, 164
  regular, benefits of, 267
exocrine pancreatic insufficiency, 88
exocytosis, 123, 546
exons, 439, 443–4, 462, 492
exopeptidases, 123
exoribonucleases, 443
expansive adaptation, 301
extracellular matrix (ECM), 387–98
  changes associated with disease, 387
  collagens in, 387
  macromolecular network of, 387
  noncollagenous proteins in, 390–3
extracellular regulated kinase (ERK), 587
eye coordination, loss of, 133
ezetimibe, 218

F
Fabry's disease, 383–4
factor EF-1α, recycling of, 453
factor VIII deficiency, congenital, 72
FAD, 98–100, 183
  and PDC activity, 178
  prosthetic groups, 99–100
  reduction to FADH$_2$, 184
FADH$_2$, 96–100, 105, 108, 110, 175, 189
  in TCA cycle, 181
failure to thrive, 84, 118
familial adenomatous polyposis (FAP), 597
familial combined hyperlipidemia, 228, 235
familial dysbetalipoproteinemia, 228, 235
familial dyslipidemia, 227
familial hemiplegic migraine type 2, 86
familial hypercholesterolemia, 228, 234–5, 431
familial hypocalciuric hypercalcemia (FHH), 356
familial intrahepatic cholestasis, 86
familial lipid disorder, 243
familial periodic paralysis, 565
familial persistent hyperinsulinemic hypoglycemia of infancy (PHHI), 88

Fanconi syndrome, 341
farnesyl pyrophosphate, 211
  biosynthesis of, 212
  structure of, 211
Fas, 592
Fas-associated death domain protein (FADD), 592
fasciculi, 262
fast-feed cycle, 226
  tests and, 296
fasting, 3
  avoidance of, 191, 193
  excess acetyl-CoA in, 195
  fat metabolism during, 185
  gluconeogenesis in, 194–5
  glucose turnover during, 274
  loss of muscle mass in, 245
  and negative N balance, 253
  overnight (postabsorptive), 282–3, 401
  phosphorylation in, 185
  plasma glucose in, 280, 294
  possible length of, 273
  prolonged, 282, 284
fatigue, 327
fats, 2, 302–3
  catabolism, 157
  deposits, 131
  digestion of, 217
  emulsification of, 120
  metabolism, 186
    bile acids in, 404
  monounsaturated, 302–3
  polyunsaturated, 302–3
  redistribution in Cushing's disease, 196
  saturated, 302
  stores, total body, regulation of, 204–7
  transport and storage, in response to feeding, 207
  unsaturated, 302
fatty acid synthase, 200–1, 203
  reactions catalyzed by, 202
  structure of, 201
fatty acids, 28, 79, 96, 98, 120–1, 150, 175
  absorption, 123
  activation of, 121–3, 189–90
    by fatty acyl-CoA synthetase, 190
  alternative oxidation pathways, 193–4
  biosynthesis of, 177, 199–208
  branched-chain, catabolism, 193
  catabolism of, 189
  desaturation of, 203, 205
  elongation of chains in, 202–3, 205
  entering enterocytes, 121
  essential, 203
  free, 120, 176
  homeostasis, 171
  hydrophobic, 28
  long-chain, 273
    transport of, 191
  medium chain, impaired oxidation of, 193
  metabolic fuel, 273
  metabolism of, 190
  naturally occurring, 78
  nonesterified (NEFA), 120
  odd-chain
    metabolism of, 193
    and TCA cycle, 193
  omega3, 303
  omega6, 303
  oxidation of, 110, 170, 184, 190–4
  β-oxidation of, 189, 192
    alternative pathways in, 194
  place of activation, 189
  plasma concentrations of, 196
  polyunsaturated (PUFA), 500
  release from adipose, 170
  storage of, 199–208
    in adipose tissue, 186

synthesis of, 199–202
  transport of, 189–90, 203–4, 225
  unsaturated, FADH2 yield from, 193
fatty acyl-CoA dehydrogenase, 99–100, 193
fatty streaks, 239
fava beans, 155
fecal urobilin, 404
fecal urobilinogen, 403
feces
  calcium excretion in, 352
  nitrogen loss by, 123
fed state, and fatty acid synthesis, 203
feed–fast cycle, 3
feed-forward regulation, 150
feeding
  frequent, 193
  high carbohydrate, 191
Fehling assay, 153
fentanyl, 46
Fenton reaction, 500
fermentation, 148
ferricytochrome c, 102
ferrihemoglobin, 503
ferritin, 29, 140, 402
  synthesis by CNS, 561
ferrocytochrome c, 102
ferrohemoglobin, 503
fetal yolk sac, 510
α-fetoprotein, associated with liver cancer, 402
fever, 286
fiber, 113, 301
fibrates, 190, 233, 241
fibric acid, 233, 241
fibrin, 25, 60, 63–4, 72
  D-dimer, 74
  degradation products (FDP), 65
  lysis of, 65
fibrinogen, 25, 32, 60, 63–4, 67, 71–2
  deficiency, 67
fibrinolysis, 60, 74–5
fibrinolytic system, 63, 65, 75
  fibrin limitation by, 74
  properties of components, 75
fibroblasts, 601
fibronectin, 346, 391–3
  isoforms, 393
  role of, 391
  structural map of, 393
fibrosis, 406
  pulmonary, 499
fibula, 389
fight or flight response, 164, 576
fingers, spidery, 254
first messengers, 542, 563
flavin adenine dinucleotide (FAD), 3, 94, 96, 133
  reduced (FADH$_2$), 97
flavin mononucleotide (FMN), 96–8, 100, 133
  prosthetic groups, 99–100
  reduced (FMNH$_2$), 96–7
flavoproteins, 98, 100, 102, 247
  FAD containing, 99–100, 184
  FADH$_2$ containing, 108
  FMN containing, 99–100
  mitochondrial, 101
flippase, 79–80
  aminophospholipid, 86
flotation ultracentrifugation, 226
Flucytosine, 421
fluid mosaic model, 82
fluids
  extracellular (ECF), 315–19, 345
  intake and dehydration, 329
  interstitial, 315
  intracellular (ICF), 315–19
  loss and diarrhea, 320
  movement, 318
  regional, within brain, 560
  see also body fluid
fluorescent dyes, 592
fluoride, inhibition of enolase, 149

fluoroacetate, toxicity of, 181
fluoroacetyl-CoA, 181
fluorocitrate, 181
fluorocytosine (FC), 420–1
5-fluorocytosine (FC), 419
fluorodeoxyuridylate (FdUMP), 421
fluorogenic agents, 22
fluorophosphates, 59
    organic, poisoning by, 62
fluorouracil (FU), 420–1
5-fluorouracil (FU), 419
fluorouridine, 421
fluoxetine, 575
Fluracil, 421
flushing attacks, 579
foam cells, 239, 383
folates, 127, 135, 422
    deficiency, 229
folic acid, 135, 229
    analogs, 421
    deficiency, 136
    and DNA synthesis, 136
    polyglutamate forms, 135
    sources of, 136
    supplementation, 139
follicle-stimulating hormone (FSH),
    220, 526, 532
    action on ovary, 535
    action on testes, 532–3
    variation in level with age, 534
follicular maturation, 535
follicular rupture, LH stimulation of,
    535
food
    energy content of, 93
    energy value of, 94
    lubrication and homogenization
        of, 115
    macromolecules in, 113
food guide pyramid, US Department
    of Agriculture, 309–10
food intake, regulation of, 305
Food and Nutrition Board, IOM, 300
food poisoning, 440
foot ulcers, 289
formaldehyde, 57, 422
formate, 57
formic acid, 81
N-formyl methionine (fmet), 451
5-formylaminoimidazole-4-
    carboxamide ribonucleotide
    (FAICAR), 414
formylglycinamide ribonucleotide
    (FGAR), 414
formylglycinamidine ribonucleotide
    (FGAM), 414
formylglycinamidine ribonucleotide
    synthetase, 414
N10-formyltetrahydrofolate, 135
Fos, 587
fragile X sites, 490
Franklin, R, 425
Friedewald formula, 231
fructokinase, 364
fructose, 116, 118, 120, 291, 363–5
    conversion to glucose, 172
    intolerance, hereditary, 365
    metabolism of, 364
fructose-1,6-biphosphate, 144–6,
    364
fructose-1,6-bisphosphatase, 170
fructose-2,6-bisphosphatase, 171
fructose-1,6-bisphosphatase,
    deficiency, 171
fructose-2,6-bisphosphate, 171
    regulation of gluconeogenesis by,
        279
    regulation of glycolysis by, 279
fructose-1-phosphate, 364
fructose-6-phosphate, 145, 150–2,
    362, 365–6
frusemide, 326
fucose, 360–1
fuel
    during fasting, illness or injury, 273
    metabolic, utilization and storage
        of, 274

metabolism, 273–97
    assessment of, 294–6
    storage types, 273
    supply, brain priority for, 284–5
fuel–organ interactions, 273–4
fuel transport pathway, 233–5
fumarase, 184
fumarate, 99, 183–4, 250
fungi, 83, 418, 420–1
Fyn, 55

G
G-cells, 123
G-proteins, 160–1, 164, 542–6
    bacterial toxins of, 545
    heterotrimeric, 546
    and metabotropic receptors, 573
    as molecular switches, 546
    monomeric (Ras-like), 546
    properties of, 546
    signaling mechanism of, 545
gait
    unsteady, 587
    unusual, 257
    waddling, 265, 357
galactokinase deficiency, 364
galactorrhea, 539
galactose, 116, 118, 120, 363
    conversion to glucose, 172
    interconversion, 363
D-galactose, 82
galactose-1-phosphate, 172, 363
galactose-1-phosphate uridyl
    transferase deficiency, 364
galactosemia, 363–5
galactosyl-β1,4-glucose, 365
galectins, 372
gall bladder, 121, 217, 399
    action in digestion, 115
    disease, and obesity, 206
gall stones, 121, 217
    cholesterol in, 209
gammopathy monoclonal, 33
ganciclovir, 61
gangliosides, 381
    degradation (turnover), 383
    formation, 382
    receptor for cholera toxin, 385
    structure and nomenclature of,
        381–2
gangliosidoses, 381, 384
gas chromatography–mass
    spectrometry (GCMS), 213
gas exchange, in lungs, 338–9
gastrectomy, 286
gastric acid, 90
gastric adenocarcinoma, 91
gastric banding, 308, 311
gastric folds, 116
gastric juice, acidification of, 89–91
gastric mucosa, 124
    secretion in, 115
gastric parietal cells, acid secretion
    from, 90
gastric stretch, 305
gastric ulcers, 123, 339
gastrin, 90, 123
gastrointestinal bleeding, and Se
    excess, 141
gastrointestinal tract
    and calcium circulation, 347–8
    function of, 113–26
Gatorade, 365
Gaucher's disease, 383
    enzyme replacement therapy, 383
gel electrophoresis, two-dimensional,
    21
gel filtration, 18
    chromatography, 18–19
gel permeation chromatography, 18
gelatinases, 240
genes
    for ABC transporters, 88
    antiproliferative, 583
    ataxia telangiectasia-mutated ATM,
        587
Bcl-2, 591

Bcl-xL, 591
Bcl-xs, 591
biallelic, 468–9
    restricted expression of, 469
consensus elements, 461
definition of, 462
detection of deletions in, 490
enhancers, 461
expression of, 467–71
    basic mechanisms of, 459–64
    control of, 459–71
    efficiency and specificity of,
        460–1
    processes, 459
    regulation of, 460, 462
        by DNA methylation, 466
fibrillin, 16
    preferential allelic activation,
        468–9
    proliferative, 583
    promoters, 460–1
        access, 465–6
        alternative, 467
        elements of, 461
    regulation, alternative approaches
        to, 465–7
    replacement therapy, 419
    response elements, 461
    superfamilies, 464
    for susceptibility to diabetes, 288
    tissue-specific expression, 467
    transcription, 459
        factors, 461–4
        initiation, 462–3
        requirements for, 459–60
genetic anticipation, molecular basis
    of, 491
genetic code, 447–9
    mutation of, 448
genetic diseases
    modes of inheritance, 431
    X-linked, 431
genetics
    Mendelian, 431
    and nutrition, 299–301
genitalia, ambiguous, 213, 215, 218,
    530–1
genome, 3, 23
    human, 428
        enzyme genes in, 54
    mitochondrial, 429
genomic imprinting, 467
    caused by DNA methylation, 467
genomics
    of liver disease, 408–9
    nutritional, 299–300
ghrelin, appetite stimulant, 305
Gibbs equation, 94
Gibbs free energy (deltaG), 94
gigantism, and GH excess, 538
Gilbert's disease, 409
Gilbert's syndrome, 411
Glanzmann's thrombasthenia, 67
glaucoma, 580
glial cells, 574
glial fibrillary acid protein (GFAP),
    562
glibenclamide, 88
globins, 29, 36–43
    recently identified vertebrate, 43
globosides, 381
globotriaosylceramide, 383
globulins, synthesis of, 401
glomerular basement membrane
    (GBM), 389
glomerular filtrate, 321
glomerular filtration barrier, 321
glomerular filtration rate (GFR), 324
glomerular injury, 84
glomerulonephritis, 344
glomerulus, 320–1
glossitis, 133, 135
glucagon, 160, 164, 167, 170–1
    cascade amplification system, 162
    control of plasma glucose levels,
        274
    declining blood concentration, 163

emergency injections of, 294
hormonal response to, 163
lipolysis activation in adipose
    tissue, 282
metabolic effects of, 276, 278
method of action, 160–3
regulation of lipid metabolism,
    197
release inhibition, 279–82
secretion of, 120
glucagon-like peptide-1 (GLP-1), 278
glucocerebrosidase, 383
glucocorticoids, 66, 219, 319, 529
    regulation of gene transcription,
        464
glucokinase, 55, 96, 158, 170, 203,
    279
    properties of, 55
gluconeogenesis, 135, 148, 157–8,
    167–72, 177
    and blood glucose concentration,
        185
    from amino acids, 170
    from glycerol, 170
    from lactate, 168–70
    influence of cortisol, 530
    limiting of, 193
    in liver, 273–4, 401
    mobilization of lipids during,
        195–7
    pathway of, 169
    regulation of, 170–2
glucose, 2–3, 55, 116–18, 120, 124,
    158
    anaerobic metabolism of, 100,
        143–56
    blood, 85
    bodily stores of, 158
    conversion from fructose, 172
    conversion from galactose, 172
    conversion to lactate, 144, 170,
        184
    defective transport of, 85
    endogenous production, 276
    energy yield, 191
    from TCA cycle, 183
    and GH secretion, 537
    glycolytic yield, 184
    in the gut, 113
    homeostasis, 273–97
        hormonal control of, 274
    infusion of, 168
    insulin-dependent transport, 276
    interconversion, 363
    intolerance
        diagnosis of, 287
        links to obesity, diabetes, and
            cardiovascular disease, 292
    laevo (L-glucose), 82
    as metabolic fuel, 273
    metabolism, 96
    modification of proteins by, 290
    Na+/K+-ATPase role in uptake, 88–9
    net synthesis of, 183
    oxidation, energetics of, 184
    as precursor, 362–3
    protein modification by, 290
    radioactive, 88
    reduction, 291
    reference values, 610
    renal reabsorption of, 89
    stimulation of insulin, 278
    supply of acetyl-CoA from, 185
    synthesis of, 175
    toxicity in diabetes, 289–91
    transport from intestine to blood,
        90
    transport into erythrocytes, 88
    urine, test for diabetes, 295
    utilization in RBC, 144
glucose–alanine cycle, 282–3
glucose-dependent insulinotropic
    peptide (GIP), 278
glucose–lactate cycle, 283
glucose meters, for blood glucose
    measurement, 154
glucose oxidase, 153–4

glucose peroxidase, 153–4
glucose-6-phosphatase, 159, 170
glucose-1-phosphate (Glc-1-P),
  158–9, 161
glucose-6-phosphate (Glc-6-P), 55,
  96, 161, 172, 362
  hydrolysis of, 94
  synthesis of, 144, 158–9
glucose-6-phosphate dehydrogenase,
  203
  deficiency, 431
    and anemia, 155
glucose-6-phosphate hydrogenase,
  151
glucosidase, 159
exo-1,6-glucosidase, 160
α-glucosidases, 116–17
glucosuria, 84, 295
glucuronic acid, 404
  formation, 365
(UDP)-glucuronyl transferase, 403
glutamate, 10, 15, 21, 52, 100, 170,
  448
  excitatory CNS transmitter, 573–4
  and excitotoxicity, 574
  recycling, 574
  residues, 13
  synthesis of GABA from, 574
  and TCA cycle, 175, 186
glutamate decarboxylase, 574
glutamate dehydrogenase (GDH),
  170
  reaction, 247
glutamate-oxaloacetate
  transaminase, 100
glutamic acid, 9, 15, 248
  relationship to glutamate, 249
  relationship to glutamine, 249
  relationship to α-ketoglutarate,
    249
  residues, 131–2
glutaminase, 574
glutamine, 9, 15, 21, 85, 113, 170
  high concentrations of, 252
  N transport by, 250
  transport of amino groups by,
    248–9
glutamine synthetase, 501
γ-glutamyl, 12
γ-glutamyl-cysteinylglycine, 153
L-γ-glutamyl-L-cysteinylglycine
  (GSSG), 12
glutamyl hydrolase, 135
γ-glutamyl transpeptidase (GGP),
  410
glutaraldehyde-polymerized bovine
  Hb, 38
glutaredoxin, 501
glutaryl-CoA, 255
S-glutathiolation, 501
glutathione, 12, 505
  antioxidant activities of, 153
  reduced (GSH), 503
  structure of, 13, 153
glutathione peroxidase (GPx), 141,
  153, 259, 502–3, 606
glutathione reductase, 133, 153
S-glutathionylation, 501
  of proteins, 501
gluten-induced enteropathy, 125
gluten sensitivity, 125
glycated hemoglobin, 295
glycemia, control of, 295
glycemic control, in diabetes care,
  293
glyceraldehyde, 117
glyceraldehyde-3-phosphate, 146–7,
  150–2, 167, 605
glyceraldehyde-3-phosphate
  dehydrogenase (GAPDH), 146–7,
  149
  mechanism of reaction, 147
glycerol, 77, 121, 157, 168, 176,
  379
  esters, 273
  formation from DAG, 379
  release from adipose, 170

as substrate for gluconeogenesis,
  273–4
glycerol kinase, 122, 170
glycerol phosphate, 122
glycerol-3-phosphate (glycerol-3-P),
  99–100, 121, 167–8, 282, 375–6
glycerol-3-phosphate dehydrogenase,
  99–100
glycerol-3-phosphate-Q reductase, 99
glycerol phosphate shuttle, 99–101,
  184
glyceryl trioleate, 77
glyceryl tristearate, 77
glycerophospholipids, 77, 375–9
  see also phospholipids
glyceryl trinitrate, 236
glycinamide ribonucleotide (GAR),
  414
glycinamide ribonucleotide
  synthetase, 414
glycinamide ribonucleotide
  transformylase, 414
glycine, 7–10, 14, 53, 422
  amide linkages, 217
  conjugated, 404
  as neurotransmitter, 574
  synthesis, 135
glycochenodeoxycholic acids, 217
glycocholic acids, 217
glycoconjugates, 117
glycogen, 2–3, 55, 117, 158–9, 164
  bodily stores of, 158
  cascade amplification system, 162
  depletion, 167
  hepatic, 158
    mobilization by epinephrine,
      163–4
  levels in muscle, 269–70
  storage, 166
    diseases of, 163–4, 279
  structure of, 157–8
  synthesis, 3, 167
glycogen phosphorylase, 159, 161,
  166
  reaction, 135
glycogen synthase, 158–9, 161, 166
  maximal inhibition of, 163
glycogenesis, 157–9, 161, 163
  pathways of, 159
    blood glucose in liver, 158–9
  regulation of, 165–7
glycogenin, 157
glycogenolysis, 157–8, 161, 163,
  282
  activation in liver, 165
  hepatic, hormonal regulation of,
    160
  hormonal control of, 160
  in muscle, 164–5
  pathways of, 159
  in liver, 159–60
glycolipids, 3, 78, 80, 159, 381
  classification of, 381
  elongation of, 382
glycolysis, 2–3, 110, 121, 143–50,
  171, 184
  aerobic, 143
  anaerobic, 143–4, 168, 184
  in yeast, 148
  of carbohydrate, 176
  inhibitors of, 149
  investment stage, 144–6
  regulation in erythrocytes, 148–50
  splitting stage, 144, 146
  yield stage, 144, 146–8
glycolytic pathway, 42, 96
glycophorin, 83
glycophospholipids, 380
glycoproteins, 3, 9, 80, 138, 159,
  359–74
  AIDS virus envelope, 369
  deficiencies in synthesis, 371
  N- and O-glycosidic linkages, 361,
    370
  histamine-rich (HRG), 75
  hormones, structures of, 532
  oligosaccharide chains of, 369–72

permeability (P), 87
  receptors, 67
  structures and linkages, 359–61
  ZP3, 371
glycosaminoglycans (GAGs), 74, 394
  lysosomal degradation of, 396
glycose, 122
glycosidases, inhibitors of, 369
glycosides
  cardiac, 91
  poisonous, 318
glycosphingolipids, 381
  ABO blood-group antigens, 384
glycosyl, 116
glycosyl transferases, 158, 367, 381
  inhibitors of, 367
N-glycosylases, 433
glycosylation, 16, 389
glycosylphosphatidylinositol
  anchoring defects, 380
  membrane anchors, 380
glyoxalase, 504
  pathway, 505
goitre, 529
Golgi apparatus, 1, 16, 214, 232,
  367, 455
  collagen synthesis in, 390
  ganglioside production in, 381
  glycoprotein modification, 369
  and glycoproteins, 359
  and insulin secretion, 275
  oligosaccharide synthesis in, 395
  protein modification, 456
  VLDL processing, 204
Gompertz equations, 600
Gompertz plots, 600
Gompertz–Makeham equation, 600
gonadotropin
  chorionic (HCG), 532
  influence of testosterone, 533
gonadotropin-releasing hormone
  (GnRH), 531
Goodpasture's syndrome (GP), 389
gout, 418
  allopurine treatment of, 417
GPIb-IX deficiency, 67
GPIIb-IIIa deficiency, 67
gradient chromatography, 20
gradients
  ATP-synthetic proton, 102–5
  electrochemical, 98, 103
  pH, 103
  proton, 111
graft-versus-host disease (GVHD),
  419
gramicidin A, 83
granulosa cells, 220
granzymes, 516
Graves' disease, 529
Grb2, 585–6
growth factor-mediated cell rescue,
  592
growth factors, 584–8
  insulin-like, 347
  platelet-derived, 347
  regulation of cell cycle, 590
growth hormone (GH), 352–3, 483,
  536–7
  axis, 536–8
  biochemical actions of, 537–8
  clinical disorders of, 538
    deficiency, 538
    excess, 538
  control of secretion, 537
  hypersecretion, 557
  resistance, 538
growth hormone-releasing hormone
  (GHRH), 536
growth retardation, 140
GTPase see guanosine triphosphatase
guanidine hydrochloride, 15
guanidinium ion, 10
guanine, 10, 413, 416–17
  bonding, 441
  in DNA, 426
  nucleotides in RNA, 437
guanine deaminase, 417

guanine deoxyribonucleotide, 421
guanosine, 417
guanosine diphosphate (GDP), 160
guanosine diphosphate-mannose
  (GDP-Man), 362, 365
guanosine monophosphate (GMP),
  414
guanosine monophosphate
  synthetase, 414
guanosine triphosphatase (GTPase),
  167
guanosine triphosphatase-activating
  protein (GAP), 585–6
guanosine triphosphate (GTP), 160,
  175, 276, 362, 580
  equilibrated with ATP, 184
  formation from GDP, 184
  hydrolysis, 451
  synthesis of, 414–16
guanylate cyclase, 66
guanylate kinase, 416
Guillain–Barré syndrome, 559
gums, swollen and bleeding, 135
gynecomastia, 534

H
H substance, 384
H63D, 409
Haber–Weiss reaction, 500
*Hae*III, 477
haemochromatosis, hereditary, 408
hair
  hypopigmented, 86
  loss, 129, 140
  premature graying of, 601
Haldane effect, 339
hallucinations, caused by biotin
  deficiency, 135
Halobacterium halobium, 82
haloperidol, 578
halothane, anesthesia, 268
haptoglobin, 29, 34
Hartnup disease, 85, 124
Hashimoto's thyroiditis, 528
Haversian systems, 346
Hayflick, L, 599
Hayflick limit, 599, 605
headache, 110, 129, 248, 383, 576
  severe, 576
  sinus, 452
healing, impairment by zinc
  deficiency, 140
heart attack, 63, 96, 225, 235
  and insulin resistance, 294
heart contractility, and potassium,
  325–6
heart disease
  increased risk of, 34
  ischemic, 577
heart failure, congestive, 91
heart valve protheses, 69
Heinz bodies, 155
Helicobacter pylori, eradication of,
  91
helix, 39
α-helix, 14–15, 23, 36, 79
helix-loop-helix (HLH) motif, 463
helix-turn-helix (HTH) motif, 463
HELLP syndrome, in mothers of
  children born with LCHAD, 196
hemagglutination reaction, 371
hematocrit (HCT), 47, 99
  low, 155
hematopoiesis, deficient, 380
hematuria, 155
heme, 25, 29, 35, 96, 102, 175
  A, 102
  C, 102
  degradation to bilirubin, 405
  Fe–porphyrin prosthetic group, 35
  from TCA cycle, 183
  iron, 102
  porphyrin structure of, 136
  structure of, 36
    prosthetic group, 35–6
  synthesis, 135, 403
    pathway of, 404

heme–hemopexin complex, 29
hemianopia, 110
hemiparesis, 110
hemoglobin (Hb), 16, 25, 35–6, 42, 100, 102
  A (HbA$_{1c}$), 323
    interpretation of, 296
    measurement of, 295
    and treatment compliance, 295
  allosteric effectors of, 41
  artificial, 38
  chromatography of, 46
  and CO, 109–10
  concentration, 99
  and cyanide, 109–10
  deoxygenated–oxygenated transition, 39–40
  effect of CO$_2$, 41
  effect of temperature, 41
  electrophoresis of, 46
  and Fe, 99, 139
  ferric, 44
  ferrous, 44
  fetal, 45
  free, 29
  glycated, 295
    and glycemic control, 295–6
    measurement of, 292
    reference values, 610
  interactions with NO, 44–5
  interactions with O$_2$, 38
  and kidney failure, 38
  model of, 39
  mutant, 47
  normal variants, 45
  O$_2$ binding by, 41
  O$_2$ saturation curves, 38
  O$_2$ transport by, 37–8, 497
  quaternary structure of, 38
  separation of variants and mutants, 46
  sickle cell molecule (HbS), 45
  sticky patch, 47
  T- and R-states, 39–42, 45, 47, 61–2
hemoglobin-based oxygen carriers (HBOC), 37–8, 497
hemoglobin–haptoglobin complex, 29
hemoglobinopathies, 46–8
  classification and examples of, 48
hemolysis, 29, 47
hemolysis, elevated, liver enzymes and low platelets see HELLP syndrome
hemopexin, 29
hemophilia, 63, 431
  classical, 72
Hemopur®, 38
hemorrhage
  subarachnoid, 85
  subcutaneous, 138
hemorrhagic disease of newborn, 132
hemorrhagic shock, 38
hemosiderin, 29, 140
hemostasis, 63–76
  overview of mechanisms, 64
hemostatic plugs, lysis of, 75
Henderson–Hasselbalch equation, 10–12, 334–6, 341, 343
heparan sulfate, 394–5
  degradation of, 396
heparin, 74, 394–5
  anticoagulation effect of, 396
  half-life of, 396
hepatic damage, 191
hepatic encephalopathy, 399
hepatic failure, 407, 410
hepatic function, 400
hepatic steatosis, 407
hepatic vein, 399
hepatitis, 410
  alcoholic, 406
hepatocellular carcinoma, 12
hepatocellular disease, 410

hepatocrinin, 217
hepatocytes, 55, 190, 397, 399, 403–4
  plasma membrane, 161
  redox potential, 407
hepatomegaly, 364, 383
hepatosplenomegaly, 129
hepatotoxicity
  caused by niacin, 135
  and vitamin supplementation, 139
hereditary fructose intolerance, 153, 365
hereditary hyperammonemia, 252
hereditary nonpolyposis colon cancer, 434
hereditary nonpolyposis colorectal cancer (HNPCC), 593
herpes simplex virus (HSV), 61
herpes virus Saimiri, 591
heterodimers, 39
heterotropic effect, 60
hexanoylcarnitine, 190
hexokinase, 15, 55, 144–6, 148–50, 203
  metabolism of fructose, 364
  properties of, 55
hexose monophosphate pathway, 133
hexose monophosphate shunt, 150
high density lipoprotein (HDL) levels, interpretation of, 242
high endothelial venule (HEV), 511
high-altitude cerebral edema (HACE), 42
Hill coefficient, 38–9, 47, 61
hippocampus, 574
hirsutism, 218, 531, 536
  mild, 536
hirudin, 72
Hirudo medicinalis, 72
histamine, 90–1, 123, 509, 579–80
  receptors, 123
histidine, 10, 15, 37, 39, 52, 85
  Cu complex, 86
histoglobin, 43
histone acetyl transferases, 466
histone deacetylases, 466
histones, 429, 465–6
  acetylation–deacetylation, 466
HIV, 433, 509
  infection, 494
    AZT therapy for, 433
  and nucleotide salvage, 416
HMG-CoA see 3-hydroxy-3-methylglutaryl CoA
holoenzymes, 54
homeostasis
  calcium, hormones influencing, 347, 352
  cellular, 583
homocysteine, 16, 136–8, 229
  in heart disease and stroke, 255
  toxicity, 229
homocystinuria, 137, 229, 254–5
  lens dislocation in, 16
homogentisic acid, 258
homoglucan, 157
homotropic effect, 60
homovanillic acid (HVA), 578–9
hormone replacement therapy (HRT), 356–7, 536
hormones, 3, 523–5
  action, 524–5
    general features of, 171
    adrenocorticotropic hormone (ACTH), 529
  anti-insulin, 274, 284
  assay, 524
  autocrine, 523
  chemical derivation, 524
  circulation, 524–5
  control features of, 523
  corticosteroid, 555
  corticotropin releasing (CRH), 529
  counter-regulatory, 274

dopamine, 539
  endocrine, 523
  feedback regulation, 524
  follicle-stimulating (FSH), 532
    action on testes, 532–3
  glycoprotein, structures of, 532
  gonadotropin-releasing (GnRH), 531
  growth, 536–7
    biochemical actions of, 537–8
    clinical disorders of, 538
    control of secretion, 537
    resistance, 538
  growth axis, 536–8
  growth hormone-releasing (GHRH), 536
  hypothalamo–pituitary regulatory system, 525–6
  hypothalamo–pituitary–adrenal axis, 529–31
  hypothalamo–pituitary–gonadal axis, 531–6
  hypothalamo–pituitary–thyroid axis, 526–9
  immunoassay, 525
  inactivation, 524–5
  luteinizing (LH), 532
    action on testes, 532–3
  measurement, 525
  organs secreting, 523
  paracrine, 523
  pituitary, 525–6
  polypeptide, 584
  pregnancy-related, 539
  prolactin axis, 539
  rates of clearance, 524
  receptors, 541–2
  reverse tri-iodothyronine (rT$_3$), 527–8
  secretion during menstrual cycle, 535
  somatostatin, 120, 536
  steroid, 464, 535, 541
    actions in females, 535
    biosynthesis, 530
    precursor, 464
    secretion disorders in females, 535–6
  testosterone, 533–5
  tetra-iodothyronine, 527
  thyroid, 106, 527–8
    biochemical actions of, 528
  thyroid stimulating (TSH), 526–7
    plasma concentrations, 527
  thyrotropin, 526–7
    releasing (TRH), 526
  thyroxine (T$_4$), 527–8
    transport of, 524
  tri-iodothyronine (T$_3$), 527–8
  types of, 523
  vasopressin, 67, 529
  see also under individual hormone names
human β-adrenergic receptor, 544
human albumin, 28
  molecular model, 28
human carbonic anhydrase I, 13
human genome project, 300, 470
human herpes virus-8 (HHV-8), 433, 591
human immunodeficiency virus see HIV
human leukocyte antigens (HLA), 516–17
  alleles, 516–17
  molecules, 513
human papilloma virus, 594
human serum immunoglobulins, 17
humoral components, 507
humoral specific immune response, 518–19
hunger, 305
  feelings of, 278
Huntington's chorea, 574
Huntington's disease, 455, 489
  molecular diagnosis of, 491

Hutchinson–Gilford syndrome, 601, 603
hyaluronic acid, 394
hybridization, molecular
  DNA, 473–9, 485–7
    base composition effect, 474
    factors affecting, 474
    heteroduplex formation, 474
    nucleic acid probes, 474
    principles of, 473–5
    probe–template, 474
    reaction conditions effect, 474
    restriction fragment length polymorphisms (RFLPs), 486–7
    strand length effect, 474
  dot–blot, 486–7
  of in situ tissue, 477
  microarrays, 478
  probes, labeling, 475–6
  Southern, 427
  transformation, 481
hybridoma cells, 525
hydrochloric acid (HCL), 21, 90
hydrocortisone, 531
hydrogen, 41, 52
  blockers, 91
  bonds, 15
  ion concentration see pH
  ion gradient, 2
hydrogen peroxide (H$_2$O$_2$), 52, 153, 422, 499, 502, 606
  sites of production, 190
hydrolases, 53, 159
hydrolysis, 21–2
  in digestion, 115
  of Glc-6-P, 94
  thermodynamics of, 95
hydroperoxides, dietary, 503
5-hydroperoxyeicosatetraenoic acid (5-HPETE), 557
hydrophobic bonds, 52
hydrophobic interactions, 15
hydrophobicity, 20–1
hydropyrimidine hydratase, 421
hydroquinone, 133
hydrostatic pressure, 318
α-hydroxy acid, 184
L-3-hydroxy-acyl-CoA dehydrogenase, long chain deficiency (LCHAD), 196
hydroxyallysine, 390
hydroxyapatite, 345
  in bone matrix, 345
hydroxybutyrate, 333
3-hydroxybutyrate, 255
β-hydroxybutyrate, 195
β-hydroxybutyrate dehydrogenase, 195
α-hydroxybutyric acid, 343
25-hydroxycholecalciferol (25(OH)D$_3$), 130, 221, 350, 353
hydroxycobalamin, 136, 138
hydroxyethyl group, 178
hydroxyethyl-thiamine pyrophosphate (HETPP), 178
5-hydroxyindoleacetic acid (5-HIAA), 579
hydroxyl groups, 121
hydroxyl radicals, 500–1
  damage to biomolecules, 502
7α-hydroxylase, 214
1α-hydroxylase, stimulation and inhibition of, 350
hydroxylases, 389
hydroxylysine, 360, 389
4-hydroxy-3-methoxymandelic acid, 577
hydroxymethylbilane synthase, 403
3-hydroxy-3-methylglutaryl CoA reductase, 210–11, 214
  activity regulation, 215
  inhibitors, 211
  rate-limiting enzyme, 211
3-hydroxy-3-methylglutaryl CoA synthase, 210
hydroxymethylglutaryl (HMG) CoA, 195

3-hydroxy-3-methylglutaryl-CoA, 210–11, 225, 255
hydroxynonenal (HNE), 500, 504
17-hydroxyprogesterone, 218, 531
hydroxyprolines, 14, 346, 352, 356, 387, 389
5-hydroxytryptamine *see* serotonin
5-hydroxytryptophan, 578, 580
hyperaldosteronism, 329
hyperaminoaciduria, 85
hyperammonemia, 191, 193, 253, 257, 403
hyperbilirubinemia, 410–12
hypercalcemia, 32, 131, 352–4
    associated with malignancy (HCM), 350, 353–4
        major mechanisms of, 354
    causes of, 353
    investigation of, 353–4
    symptoms and signs, 352
    tests for nonparathyroid causes, 353
    thyrotoxic, 353
hypercalciuria, 131
hypercapnia, 338
hypercatabolism, due to injury, 286
hypercholesterolemia, 234–5, 239, 405
hypercortisolism, 531
hyperglycemia, 55, 121, 274, 294
    fasting, 288
    glycation endproducts in, 289
    reduction of, 275
hyperglycemic nonketotic coma, 295
hyperhomocysteinemia, 135, 229
hyperinsulinemia, 168, 267, 536
hyperkalemia, 268, 275, 303, 307, 325, 342
    and renal failure, 325
hyperkalemic periodic paralysis, 565
hyperlipidemia, 227, 234, 267, 603
    acid lipase treatment, 383
hypernatremia, 317, 331
hyperoxia, toxicity of, 499
hyperparathyroidism (HPT), 352, 354–6, 557
    bones, stones, and abdominal groans, 353
    and hypercalcemia, 352–3
    primary, 353
    secondary, 355
hyperphagia, 205
hyperphenylalaninemias, 258
hyperphosphatemia, 355
hyperplasia
    congenital adrenal, 213, 220, 536
    prostatic, 539
hyperpolarization, 571
hyperprolactinemia, 539
hypersensitivity, and platelet activating factor, 377
hypertension, 47, 57, 66, 267, 531
    arterial, 294, 330
    diuretic treatment for, 326
    endocrine causes of, 329
    genetic component of, 431
    and low levels of NO, 236
    and metabolic syndrome, 293
    neurotransmitter as cause of, 576
    and obesity, 206
    and risk of myocardial infarction, 330
    and risk of stroke, 330
hypertensive crisis, 576
hyperthermia, malignant, 268
hyperthyroidism, 528–9
hypertriglyceridemia, 235, 242, 294, 312
hyperuricemia, 422
hyperventilation, 42, 44, 171, 344
    cause of respiratory alkalosis, 337
hypoalbuminemia, 27–8
hypocalcemia, 121, 304, 355–6
    causes of, 355
    familial, 356
    in neonates, 354
    postnatal, 354

hypochlorous acid, 499, 505
hypochromia, 48
hypoglycemia, 85, 157, 163, 171, 278–9, 294, 308
    after alcohol, 168, 278, 407
    after fasting, 163, 278
    in alcoholics, 407
    causes of, 281
    in child of diabetic mother, 168
    in child of malnourished mother, 164
    diabetic complication, 288
    and endocrine syndromes, 278
    and GH therapy, 537–8
    hypoketotic, 191, 193
    severe, medical emergency, 294
hypoglycorrhachia, 85
hypogonadism, 534
hypokalemia, 275, 289, 303, 325, 342, 344
hypomagnesemia, 304
hyponatremia, 286, 317, 331, 530
hypoparathyroidism, 354–6
    magnesium in, 355
hypophagia, 205
hypophosphatemia, 354
hypopituitarism, 538–9
hypotension, 218, 328–9, 343, 377
hypothalamic arcuate nucleus, 305
hypothalamic failure, 530
hypothalamo–pituitary–adrenal axis, 529–31
hypothalamo–pituitary–gonadal axis, 531–6
hypothalamo–pituitary regulatory system, 525–6
hypothalamo–pituitary–thyroid axis, 526–9
hypothalamus, 305, 531, 537, 539, 580
    disorders of, 534–6
    dopamine deficiency, 539
    nuclei of, 328
hypothermia, 308
hypothyroidism, 133, 528
hypotonia, 559
hypovolemia, 320
hypoxanthine, 416–18
hypoxanthine-guanine phosphoribosyl transferase (HG-PRT), 416–17
hypoxemia, 44
hypoxia, 291, 295, 338, 341, 343–4
    chronic, 42
hypoxic drive, 338
hysterectomy, 356

I
I-cell disease, 371
ibuprofen, 555, 607
sIg, 511
IgA, 30–1, 517–18
IgD, 30–2, 518
IgE, 30, 32, 377, 509, 518
IgG, 30–1, 517–19, 521, 563
    and pregnancy, 31
IgM, 30–1, 517–19, 521
ileum, 113, 121, 579
    surgical removal of, 137
    terminal, 137
imidazole ring, 10
imidazolium ion, 10
imine, 390
α-imino acid, 7
immune deficiencies, 587
immune response, 507–22
    the complement system, 507–8
    human leukocyte antigen (HLA) system, 516–17
    humoral specific, 518–19
    inflammatory mediators in, 507–9
    integrated cellular, 515
        cellular and molecular elements of, 519–21
    major histocompatibility complex (MHC), 516–17
        class I and II structure, 517

    expression patterns, 517
    restricted simulation, 517
    nonspecific, 507–9
    specific, 509–10
    summary of, 520
immune system, 3, 507
immunity
    antiparasitic, 32
    cellular and humoral specific, 510
immunoassay, 521, 525
immunocompetence, 138
immunocompromisation, 517
immunodeficiency disease, caused by biotin deficiency, 135
immunofluorescence, 521
immunogens, 30
immunoglobulins, 18, 26, 30–2
    antibody recognition (Fab₂) region, 30
    further constant (Fc) region, 30
    heavy (H) chains, 30
    light (L) chains, 30
    monoclonal, 32
    paraprotein band, 32
    sIg, 511
    structure of, 30–1
    surface (sIg), 511
    V region, 3
    variable gene recombination events, 513
    see also individual entries under Ig
immunologic dysfunction, 521
immunology, regional, 561
immunoparesis, 32
immunoradiometric assays (IMRAs), 348
inborn errors of metabolism, 256–7
indigestion, 125
indomethacin, 59
infections
    chronic, immune response to, 514
    parvovirus, 385
    urinary tract, 385
infertility, 536, 587
    male, 88
inflammation, 372, 507
    cell–cell interaction in, 373
    cells involved in, 508
inflammatory mediators, 507
inflammatory reaction, 377
influenza virus, 373
inheritance, Mendelian, 467
inhibin, 532–3
inhibition, allosteric, 186
inhibitor-1, 161, 163
inhibitors
    COX-1, side effects of, 557
    monoamine oxidase (MAOI), 252
initiator, 460
injury, metabolism during, 285
inosine, 417
inosine monophosphate (IMP), 413–14
    precursor of AMP and GMP, 416
inosine monophosphate dehydrogenase, 414
inosine monophosphate synthase, 414
inositol, 379
inositol trisphosphate, 164–5
inositol 1,4,5-trisphosphate (IP₃), 550, 585
    degradation of, 552
insecticide, poisoning by, 62
insulin, 1, 55, 166, 170–1, 273–97, 305, 584
    cellular response to, 167
    control of action, 233
    control of plasma glucose levels, 274
    human recombinant, 483
        preparation of, 480–1
    inhibition by, 196
    mechanisms of action, 167
    metabolic effects of, 276–7
    molecule, 277
    release stimulation, 279–82

    resistance, 267, 291–2, 536
        and heart attack, 294
        sites of, 292
        stress induced, 285–6
        treatment of, 292
    secretion of, 84, 88, 106, 120, 275
        stimulated by glucose, 278
    signaling, 275–6
    stimulation of ovaries, 536
    stimulation of pyruvate dehydrogenase, 185–6
    structure of, 277
    synthesis, 275
    treatment of diabetes with, 275
insulin-like growth factor (IGF), 535, 538
    binding proteins (IGFBPs), 538
insulinoma, 279
integrins, 595
interferons (IFNs), 240, 508
interleukin-1, 285
interleukins (ILs), 509, 584
    common γ-chain deficiency, 586
intermittent claudication, 239
    and atherosclerosis, 236
interphase, of cell cycle, 583–4
intestinal mucosa, 125
    in Tangier disease, 233
intestine, 2, 113, 124
    bile acids in, 217
    epithelial cells of, 124
    secretions, volume and pH of, 114–15
    small, 121, 139–40
        folic acid absorption in, 135
    sugar recovery in, 88–9
intima, 65
intracellular buffers, 335
    phosphate, 336
    potassium exchange, 336
    protein, 336
intrinsic factors (IFs), 123, 137–8
    B₁₂ complex, 138
introns, 439, 443–4, 462, 492
    self-splicing, 445
    splicing of mRNA, 467–8
iodoacetate, 22
iodoacetamide, 146
iodothyronine-5-deiodinase, 141
ion pumps, 85–7
ion-exchange chromatography, 18–20
ionomycin, 83
ionophores, 82
    bactericidal effects of, 83
    transport mechanism of, 82
ions, 2
    ammonium, 245
    calcium, 549, 565–6, 584
    changes in membrane flow, 570–2
    channels, 84, 565–6, 572–3
    cobalt, 136
    cupric, 153
    cuprous, 153
    dipolar, 12
    ferric, 29
    gradients, 86
    hydride, 96
    hydrogen, 25, 41, 85, 123, 321
        changes in concentration, 333
        daily flux, 333
        excretion, 342
        excretion of, 340–1
    magnesium, 97
    metal, 29
    permeability, 83
    in plasma and intracellular fluid, 316
    potassium, 89–90
    sodium, 89, 317
iron, 36, 54, 139–40, 498
    absorption of, 138
    binding, 29
    binding and transport of, 30
    bodily storage, 139
    chelation of, 25

in the CNS, 561
deficiency, 29, 468
dietary requirement for, 99
dietary sources of, 140
heme, 99
inorganic, 99
oxidation of, 30, 35
protoporphyrin IX, 102
status and mRNA translation, 470
iron–globulin complex, 29
iron–porphyrin prosthetic group, 35
iron-response element IRE-BP, 182
iron–sulfur complexes, 99–100
in redox reactions, 100
iron–transferrin complex, 29
irritability, 252
caused by pyroxidine deficiency, 135
ischemia, 270, 498
ischemia-perfusion injury, 500
islets of Langerhans, 120, 166, 274, 276, 287
isobutylmethylxanthine, 549
isocitrate
chiral, 182
isomerization of, 182
isocitrate dehydrogenase, 110, 182–3, 186
isocratic chromatography, 20
isodesmosine, 391
isoelectric focusing (IEF), 20–1, 23
isoelectric point (pI), 12, 18, 20
isoleucine, 9, 85, 210
accumulation of, 323
catabolism of, 178
isomaltase, 116
isomerases, 54, 145, 152, 362–3
triose phosphate, 146
isomers, 7
chiral, 7
dextro (D), 7
laevo (L), 7
optically active, 7
isoniazid, 135
isoprene, 102, 131
units, 211
isovaleryl-CoA, 255
isozymes, 52, 54–5, 100
desiometric patterns of LDH, 53
selenium containing, 50
tissue specificity of LDH, 54
itching, in liver disease, 404

J
JAK–STAT system, 205
Janus kinases (JAKs), 585, 587–8
jaundice, 29, 133, 364, 399, 403, 410–12
causes of, 409–10
differential diagnosis of, 409
genetic causes of, 411–12
intrahepatic, 411
neonatal, 410
obstructive, 412
posthepatic, 411
prehepatic (hemolytic), 410
of sclera, 155
jejunum, 113, 118
bile acids reabsorption, 217
Jun, 587
Jun N-terminal kinase (JNK), 587
juxtaglomerular apparatus, 320

K
Kallmann's syndrome, 534–5
kaolin–cephalin clotting time (KCCT), 71
Kaposi's sarcoma, 433
k chains, 32
keratan sulfate, 395
keratomalacia, 129
kernicterus, 28, 410–11
Keshan disease, 141
keto acids, 182, 247
α-keto acids, 100, 183
α-ketoacid dehydrogenases, 178, 181

ketoacidosis
affect on potassium balance, 290
diabetic, 275, 422
development of, 290
presentation of, 288
3-ketoacyl synthase, 200
ketogenesis
and glucose net synthesis, 183
in liver, 191, 194–7
pathways from acetyl-CoA, 195
α-ketoglutarate, 100, 170, 191, 247, 421
decarboxylation of, 183
increase in beri-beri, 180
α-ketoglutarate dehydrogenase, 110, 178, 182–3
deficiency, 181
2-ketoisocaproate, 255
ketone bodies, 85, 186, 282, 323
catabolism in peripheral tissues, 196
metabolism of, 196
plasma concentrations of, 196
ketone bodies, in urine, and weight-loss programs, 195
ketones, 184
in urine, and diabetes, 295
ketonuria, 257, 483
in diabetes, 295
and weight loss programs, 195
ketorolac, 46
ketose, donor, 152
Keto-Stix, 195
kidneys, 3, 25, 57, 86, 319–25, 397
and acid–base balance control, 333–44
bicarbonate handling in, 340–1
blood filtration by, 89
and calcium circulation, 347–8
carnitine synthesis in, 191
collecting ducts of, 328–9
Cu accumulation in, 29
damage to, 107
disease, diabetic, 296
distal tubule, 328–9
failure of, 289
function of, 315–32
glomerular filtrate, 321
glomerular filtration
barrier, 321
rate, 324
glomeruli, 320–1
handling of water and sodium by, 330
metabolism and transport
functions of, 320
nephrons, 319
reabsorption and excretion of
water, 329
renal clearance, 324
stones, 131, 259, 353
tubular cells, 320
tubules, 124
water reabsorption, 328–9
kinase reactions, 170
kinases, 110, 163
kinetic assays, for blood glucose
measurement, 154
kininogen, 69
high-molecular-weight (HMWK), 75
Klenow fragment, 476
Klinefelter's syndrome, 534
Koshland, Nèmethy and Filmer
(multistate) model, 62
Krebs cycle, 3, 175, 199
see also tricarboxylic acid (TCA)
cycle
Krebs, HA, 176, 183
kringles, 228
Kupffer cells, 399
kwashiorkor, 308

L
labile toxin, 545
α-lactalbumin, 365
β-lactam ring, 58

lactase, 118
deficiency, 125
lactate, 41, 113, 148, 157, 163, 168
accumulation, 110
CSF, 85, 100
cycle, 170
during starvation, 175
excretion, 172
from pyruvate, 177
measurement of, 177
oxidization by NAD$^+$, 177
as substrate for gluconeogenesis, 273–4
supply of acetyl-CoA from, 185
lactate dehydrogenase (LDH), 148, 170, 177
isozymes, densitometric patterns
of, 53
lactation, 136
lactic acid, 143, 333
accumulation and death, 177
in blood, 168
excess, 168
lactic acidosis, 110, 177
lacticacidemia, 168, 268
lactobacilli, 148
lactose, 3, 116–17, 363
biosynthesis of, 365
intolerance, 125
lactose synthase, 365
Lambert–Eaton (myasthenic)
syndrome, 565, 567
lamin gene, 601
laminins, 393, 595
Langerhans cells, 511
lanosterol, 211–12
lard, 77
large bowel, 113
Laron dwarfism, 538
Laron syndrome, 538
lathyrism, 392
Lathyrus odoratus, ingestion of, 392
laxatives, 90
lead
inhibition of heme pathway, 403
salts, 59
lecithin, 81, 376
lecithin:cholesterol acyltransferase
(LCAT), 230
lectin-blotting assays, 372
lectin–carbohydrate interactions, 373
lectins, 371–2
functions of, 371–2
mistletoe, 371
peanut, 371
toxicity, 371
leflunomide, 417
Leigh's disease, 181
lens dislocation, 16, 254, 393
lens protein, age changes in, 602
leptin, 205, 305, 309
Lesch–Nyhan syndrome, 417, 431
lethargy, 252
leucine, 9, 85, 210
accumulation of, 323
catabolism of, 178, 255
zipper, 463
leukemia, 69
B cell, disruption of apoptotic
machinery in, 591
in progerias, 595
leukocyte adhesion deficiency disease
(LAD), 365
leukocytes, 25–6, 138, 323
count, 42
reduction, 141
leukocytosis, 286
leukotrienes, 509, 555, 557
Lewis blood-group antigens, 385
Leydig cells, 220, 532
lidocaine, 46, 91
lifestyle change, and plasma lipid
profile, 242
ligands, 20, 26–7, 67
gating by, 84
of transport proteins, 28

ligases, 54
ligation, 541
lignoceric acids, 381
limbic system, 574
α-limit dextrin, 116–17
Lineweaver–Burk equation, 82
Lineweaver–Burk plot, 56–8
linoleic acid, 203, 302, 375
linolenic acid, 375
lipases, 115, 120–1
gastric, 120
lingual, 115
pancreatic, 121
salivary, 120
lipation, 16
lipid peroxides, 153, 605
lipid pool, 239
lipid rafts, 79, 82
lipids, 1, 3, 77, 93, 225–43
amphipathicity, 375
biosynthesis, 150
complex, 375–86
developmental importance of, 302
digestion and absorption of, 120–3
disorders
monogenic, 235
testing for, 226
emulsion, 120–1
essential, 303
in food, 113
levels, interpretation of, 242
measurements, diagnostic, 231
membrane, structure and
properties of, 77–8
metabolism of, 133
mobilization during work and
gluconeogenesis, 195–7
oxidative metabolism of, 189–98
peroxidation pathway, 501
polarity, 375
polyisoprenoid, 193
properties of, 375
reference values, 611
regulation of metabolism, 197
saponifiability, 375
solubility, 375
storage diseases, 384
synthesis, methyl and sulfate
donors in, 378
lipoamide, 178
disulfide form, 178
and PDC activity, 178
structure, 179
lipoate, 183
lipofuscin, 605
lipogenesis, 3, 135, 171
of citrate, 183
and obesity, 199
promotion by insulin, 276
lipoic acid, in PDC, 179
lipolysis, 168, 176, 189, 528
glucagon activated, in adipose
tissue, 282
high rate of, 295
regulation of, 197
suppression by insulin, 276
lipoprotein (a), structure of, 228
lipoprotein lipase, 204
lipoproteins, 131, 225–43
apoproteins in, 227–9
classes of, 227
dynamic system of, 225
electrophoretic mobility of, 227
functions of, 229
high-density (HDL), 215
levels, interpretation of, 242
low density (LDL)
receptors, 214, 230, 362
uptake in cells, 231–2
measurement of, 230–1
metabolism, 231–4
control of, 233
integrated view of, 233–4
pathways of, 232
plasma, size and density, 226–7
receptors, 230

structure and function of, 226–30
structure of, 227
very low density (VLDL), 203–4, 209, 213, 225, 276
transport by, 231
liposome-encapsulated Hb, 38
liposomes, 78–9
lipoxygenases, 557
lips, enlarged, 538
lithium, 353
heparinate, 25
lithocholic acid, 217, 404
liver, 2–3, 12, 28–9, 86, 121, 175
action in digestion, 113, 115
activation of glycogenolysis in, 165
biochemical tests of function, 409–10
biosynthesis of fatty acids in, 199–208
cancer, 402
carbohydrate metabolism by, 399–401
carbohydrate storage and synthesis in, 157–73
carnitine synthesis in, 191
ceruloplasmin deficiency, 402
cirrhotic, 407
classification of disorders, 410–12
CRP synthesis, 32
damage, 107
disease, 71, 132
and alcohol, 406–8
α1-antitrypsin deficiency, 402
clinical features of, 400
genomics of, 408–9
reduced serum proteins in, 348
symptoms of, 399
embryonic, 510
extract, 21
function tests, reference values, 611
gluconeogenesis in, 273–4
ketogenesis in, 191, 194–7
lobules, 399
metabolism of lipids in, 189–98
obstructive disease, due to pancreatic cancer, 412
parenchymal cells, 217
pathways of glycogenolysis in, 159–61
protein metabolism, 401–3
protein synthesis, 26
source of vitamin B12, 136
special function, 399–412
storage of fatty acids in, 199–208
stress-induced insulin resistance in, 285–6
structure of, 399–400
TFPI synthesis in, 74
use of NADPH, 150
vitamin A storage in, 127
local anesthetics, 46
locoism, 369
locus ceruleus, 252
long-term potentiation, 574
longevity
and calorie restriction, 606–7
and DNA repair activity, 601
loop of Henle, 319, 321, 326, 343
Looser's zones, 138
lower reference nutrient intake (LRNI), 300
lungs, 3
and acid–base balance control, 333–44
cancer, and vitamin supplementation, 139
CO2 diffusion, 339
disease
α1-antitrypsin deficiency, 402
obstructive, 177
respiratory acidosis in, 338
dysfunction, 88
gas exchange in, 336–40
structure, 336
ventilation and perfusion, 338–9

luteinizing hormone (LH), 220, 523, 526, 532
action on ovary, 535
action on testes, 532–3
variation in level with age, 534
lyases, 53
lymph, 561
nodes, 510
lymphatics, 510–11
lymphocytes, 509, 511, 561
and adhesion molecules, 511
antigen-specific receptors, 511
B cells, 30–1, 419, 510–11, 518
antigen receptor, 512–13
clonal selection in, 514
CD4 T cells, 515, 561
circulation, 511
cytotoxic T (Tc) cells, 516
NK cells, 515
T cells, 30, 237–8, 419, 510–11, 514–18
antigen receptor (TCR), 512–13
T helper (Th) cells, 515
lymphocytic thyroiditis, 528
lymphoid tissues, 510–11
mucosa-associated (MALT), 510
primary, 510
secondary, 510–11
lymphoma, 593
malignant, 54
lymphopoiesis, 591
lymphoreticular cancer, 587
lysine, 10, 13, 15, 22, 53, 191
ε-carbon, 10
in histones, 429
no transamination of, 253
residues, 102, 125, 179, 389
lysosomal pathway, for GM1, 383
lysosomal storage diseases, 383
lysosomes, 1, 16, 86, 370, 563
cystine accumulation in, 84
ganglioside degradation in, 381
and glycoproteins, 359
and hydrolysis, 370
proteoglycan degradation in, 395
lysyl endopeptidase, 22
lysyl oxidase, 141, 390
inhibition of, 392
lytic lesions, 563

M
McArdle's disease, 163, 279
McCune–Albright syndrome, 557
macrocytosis, 408
macrophage colony-stimulating factor (MCSF), 346
macrophages, 561, 590
macula densa, 320
macular corneal dystrophy, 398
mad cow disease, 23
magnesium, 303
and metabolism of ATP, 97
prosthetic, 127
sulfate, 37
magnetic resonance scanning, 576
Maillard products, 604
Maillard reaction, 290
major histocompatibility complex (MHC), 287, 511, 516–17
genetic organization of, 516
malabsorption, 71, 125
fat, 132
intestinal, 118
Mg, 303
vitamin D, 356
malaria, resistance to, 47
malate, 100, 108, 168, 170
from pyruvate, 186
laevo (L-malate), 184
shuttle, 201, 204
carbon unit recruitment by, 201
malate–aspartate shuttle, 100–1, 184
malate dehydrogenase, 184
cytosolic, 170
in TCA cycle, 183
malate–oxaloacetate equilibrium, 186
malic enzyme, 203

malignancy, and hypercalcemia, 352–3
malignant hyperthermia, 268
malnutrition, 121, 307–8
complicated, 308
due to disease, 307, 385
inappropriate treatment, 308
and multiple nutrient deficiencies, 127
protein energy (PEM), 307
protein–calorie effects, 307
protein–calorie, types of, 308
kwashiorkor, 308
marasmus, 308
reduced serum proteins in, 348
refeeding syndrome, 308
uncomplicated, classification of, 308
malonate block, 183
malondialdehyde (MDA), 500
malonic semialdehyde, 421
malonyl transacylase, 200
malonyl-CoA, 190, 200–2
synthesis from acetyl-CoA, 199–200
Malpighian layer, 221
maltose, 116–17
maltotriose, 116–17
manaquinones, 131
manganese, 54, 139, 141, 498
prosthetic, 127
mania, 575
mannitol, 326
mannose, 360–2
interconversion, 363
D-mannose, 82
mannose binding ligand (MBL) pathway, 519
mannose-1-phosphate, 362
mannose-6-phosphate, 362
maple syrup urine disease (MSUD), 259
marasmus, 308
Marfan's syndrome, 16, 254, 393
margarine, 194
marrow neoplasia, 68
mass spectrometry, 13, 16, 22–3
mast cells, 32, 398
mastication, 113, 116
matrix assisted laser desorption ionization time-of-flight mass spectrometry (MALDI-TOF MS), 13–14
maturity onset diabetes of the young (MOBY), 287–8
mediastinum, 510
medium-chain fatty acyl-CoA dehydrogenase (MCAD) deficiency, 193
meiosis, 431, 490
melanin, 258
melanocyte-stimulating hormones, (MSH), 581
melanocytes, 258
MELAS (myopathy, encephalopathy, lactic acidosis, and stroke-like episodes), 110
membranes, 77–92
biological, 1–2
composition of, 78–80
contraluminal, 124
current structural model of, 79
diffusion across, 81
extraction and analysis of phospholipids, 81
fluid mosaic model of, 80
lipids in, 77–8
mitochondrial, 2, 77–8
movement of solutes across, 81
nitrocellulose, 476
organelle, phospholipid composition of, 79
patches, 82
permeability of, 83
pre/postsynaptic, 572
recycling in synaptic transmission, 563

structure and metabolic role of, 80
transport mediated by proteins, 82
transport systems of, 81
saturability and specificity, 82
transport of water through, 328
meninges, 560
meningitis, 560
bacterial, 85
Menkes disease, 86
menopause, 536
and bone loss, 356
menstrual cycle
hormone secretion during, 535
significance of progesterone level, 535
menstruation, 99, 535
infrequent, 536
irregular, 218, 531, 539
mental confusion, 133
mental retardation, 215, 257, 384, 417, 580
meperidine, 46
β-mercaptoethanol, 20
2-mercaptoethanol (MeSH), 10, 22
mercuric chloride, 88
mercury, 59, 127
meromyosin, 264
mesenchyme, 346
metabolic disorders, 44
metabolic fuels, 273
metabolic pathways, interactions between, 144–5
metabolic syndrome, 34, 235, 293–4
metabolic syndrome (Syndrome X), 267
links obesity, diabetes, hypertension, and cardiovascular disease, 235, 293
metabolism
aerobic, failure of, 181
after meal, 279–82
anaerobic, 110
of glucose, 143–56
basal metabolic rate (BMR), 93
bilirubin, 403–5
calcium and bone, 345–58
carbohydrate, 1–2, 150
in liver, 399–401
cellular, 1
in diabetes mellitus, 289
drugs, 405–8
role of cytochrome P450, 406
during stress and injury, 282–6
equilibrium constants in, 94
in fasting state, 279–82
fuel, 273–97
diabetic disorder of, 286–93
generation of acids, 333
inborn errors of, 256–7
lipid, 150
lipoprotein, 536
oxidative, 1–3, 93–111
inhibitors of, 106–10
postabsorptive (overnight fast), 283
postprandial, 281
potassium, 315–17
protein, in liver, 401–3
purine, 413–17
pyrimidine, 417–21
response to injury, 282–6
sodium, 315–17, 331
water, 315–17
water and electrolyte disorders of, 331
stress affect on, 286
water and sodium interrelated, 330–1
metabolites, 2
key, reference values, 611
toxic, 87
metabolomics, 299–300
metalloenzymes, 127, 497
metalloproteinases, 240
metalloproteins, 36
metallothioneine, 140–1
metanephrines, 576–7

metastases, 579, 594
metformin, 275, 292
methanol, 81
    poisoning, treatment with ethanol, 57
methemalbumin, 29
methemoglobin, 35, 44, 503
methemoglobinemia, 503
    acquired (toxic), 44
methionine, 10, 22, 229
    deficiency, 137
    metabolism, 254
    residues, 500–1
    sentinel function of, 501
    synthesis, 135–6, 138
methionine sulfoxide, 500–1, 603
methotrexate, 136, 421
methyl groups, 9
methyl thioether group, 10
N-methyl-L-aspartate (NMDA), 573
N-methyl-D-aspartate (NMDA), 573
    glutamate receptor, 573
methylation, 136, 378, 466–7
methylcitrate, 257
methylcobalamin, 136, 138
methylene blue, 44, 110
N^5,N^{10}-methylene-tetrahydrofolate, 229, 421–2
methylene-tetrahydrofolate reductase, 229
3-O-methyl-D-glucose, 88
methylglyoxal (MGO), 505, 605
    detoxification of, 504
methylmalonate, 257
methylmalonic acid, 137
methylmalonic aciduria, 137
methylmalonic semialdehyde, 421
methylmalonyl-CoA, 136, 138, 170
methylmalonyl-CoA mutase, deficiency, 257
5-methyltetrahydrofolate (N^5MeTHF), 135–7
5-methyl uracil, 420
methylxanthines, 549, 563
metmyoglobin, 35
mevalonate, 226
mevalonic acid, 210, 211
    biosynthesis of, 210
    in cholesterol synthesis, 210–11
mevastatin, 211
mice, knockout, 292, 346, 435, 555, 605
micelles, 121–2
Michaelis constant (K_m), 56, 401
Michaelis–Menten equation, 55–6, 82, 154
Michaelis–Menten kinetics, 61
Michaelis–Menten plot, 56
microalbuminuria, 296, 323
microangiopathy, 289
microarrays, 478
microcytosis, 48
microencephaly, 215
microglia, 560
micronutrients, 2, 127–42
microsatellite repeats, 488–9
    trinucleotide, 490
microsomal triglyceride transfer protein (MTP), 231
microvilli
    disappearance of, 125
    of intestine, 113
mid-arm circumference, 306
migraine, 578
milrinone, 549
mineralocorticoids, 219, 531
minerals, 2, 127–42, 303–4
minimal change disease, 319
mitochondria, 1–2, 16, 35, 102, 143, 170, 172
    in adipose tissue, 106
    biogenesis and exercise, 96
    and energy transduction, 98
    fatty acid transport to, 189–90
    formation of superoxide by, 500
    genetic code, 448
    intermembrane space (IMS), 98

leaky, 105
location of TCA cycle, 175
membrane potential (MMP), 107
membranes of, 96, 99, 101, 107
β-oxidation of, 190–2
oxidation–reduction in, 93, 176
poisons of, 110
synthesis of ATP by, 96–7
and theory of aging, 605
transfer of electrons from NADH, 100
transport of electrons by, 97–102
uncoupled, 105
and urea cycle, 250–2
mitochondrial myopathies, 100
mitogen-activated protein kinase (MAPK), 422, 586–7
    dual specificity kinase (MEK), 586
    signaling cascades, 587
mitogenesis, 589
mitosis, 430, 583
modeccin, 371
molecular sieving, 18
molybdenum, 141
monensin, 83
monoacylglycerol (MAG), 121–2
2-monoacylglycerol (2-MAG), 121
monoamine oxidase (MAO), 575–7
    inhibitor (MAOI), 252
monoamino acids, 10, 85
monocarboxylic acids, 10, 85
monoclonal gammopathies, 33
    of uncertain significance (MGUS), 32
monocyte chemoattractant protein-1 (MCP-1), 237
monocyte colony stimulating factor (M-CSF), 238
monocytes, 237–8
Monod, Wyman and Changeaux (concerted) model, 61
monoglycerides, 120
monosaccharides, 116–17, 120
    transport systems for, 118–20
monosodium glutamate, 248
    reaction, 248
motility, gastrointestinal, 579
mountain sickness, acute, 42
mouth
    dry, 329
    inflammation of, 133
MstII, 487
mucins
    glycosylation of, 359–60
    salivary, 369
    viscous properties of, 361
mucolipidosis, 371
mucopolysaccharidoses, 395–6
mucosal folds, of intestine, 113
multigenes, 581
multiple endocrine neoplasia type 2A (MEN 2A), 467
multiple myeloma, 32
multiple sclerosis, 562–3
multiplexins, 389
mumps orchitis, 534
muscarine, 564, 580
muscle, 2, 84, 166–7
    aging of, 606
    calcium trigger, 265
    carbohydrate storage and synthesis in, 157–73
    cardiac, 75, 83, 86, 88
        contraction, 91
        Ca^{2+} levels, 110
    circumoral, 355
    contractile unit (sarcomere), 262–3
    contraction, 91, 185, 261–71
        high intensity, 268–9
        long duration, 269
        low intensity, 269
        mechanism of, 266
        short duration, 268–9
        sliding-filament model of, 265–6
    contraction cycle, Ca^{2+} movement in, 89, 185
    contraction filaments, 263

development of, 261–2
energy metabolism, 261–71
energy resources, changes in, 269
excitable tissue, 267
excitation–contraction coupling, 265
exercise, 149
fast-glycolytic fibers, 268
fatigue, 163, 269
glucose utilization, 171
glycogenolysis in, 164–5
long-term performance (stamina), 269–70
mass changes
    with age, 301
    in disease, 168, 261
metabolism
    anaerobic, 268
    and contraction, 268–70
    of lipids in, 189–98
    mitochondria, 100
    non-striated, 87, 262
    oxygen debt, 148
    pain, 141
        caused by biotin deficiency, 135
    proteins, 263–7
        functions, 264
    relaxants, 268
    skeletal, 86
        structural elements, 263
        transverse tubular network, 266
        weakness, 180
    slow-oxidative fibers, 268
    smooth, 66
        and vascular wall structure, 239
    stamina, 269–70
    stress-induced insulin resistance in, 285–6
    striated, 87, 262, 268
    structure, 261–3
        hierarchical, 262
    transporter inhibition in, 91
    uterine, 85
    weakness of, 100, 191, 304, 490, 565, 581
        in scurvy, 138
muscarinic receptors, metabotropic, 580
muscular dystrophy, genetic component of, 431
mutagens, Ames test for, 435
mutant hemoglobin, 47
mutarotase, 153
mutase, 170
mutations
    insertional, 595
    underlying colorectal cancer, 593
myasthenia, 581
myasthenia gravis, 565
Myc, 596
Mycoplasma, 416
myelin sheath, 561–2
myelination, 202
myeloma, 32, 353
    globulin, 563
    multiple, 32, 323
myelomatosis, 32
myeloperoxidase (MPO), 499, 505
myeloproliferative disorders, 557
myoblasts, 261
    smooth muscle, 262
myocardial infarction, 66, 84, 168, 225, 498
    and atherosclerosis, 236
    diabetic risk of, 289
    diagnosis of, 270, 611
    plasma glucose level after, 284
    premature, 235
    serum enzyme changes, 270
    thrombolytic treatment in, 75
    thrombus in, 240
myocytes, cardiac, 261, 605
myofibers, 262, 265, 606
myofibrils, 87–8, 262, 265
    A- and I-bands of, 263
    H-zone, 263

M-lines, 263
Z-lines, 263
myofilament proteins, 262
myogenic pathways, 66
myogenic regulatory factors (MRFs), 261
myoglobin (Mb), 29, 35–6, 100, 102
    insights from knockout mice, 44
    and iron, 99, 139
    model of, 36
    O_2 storage by, 37
    O_2 transport by, 197
    oxygen saturation curves for, 38
myoinositol, 291
myokinase, 165
myopathies, 110, 605
myosin, 87–8, 261, 263–4
    isoforms of, 264
    polymerization, 264
myotonia, 565
myotonic dystrophy (MD), 489–91

N
NAD see nicotinamide adenine dinucleotide
NADH see nicotinamide adenine dinucleotide reduced
NADP see nicotinamide adenine dinucleotide phosphate
nails, abnormal beds of, 141
nasal root, short, 215
nasogastric suction, 344
natural killer (NK) cells, 511
nausea, 121, 129, 133, 248, 440, 531
necrosis, cellular, 590
negative acute phase reactants, 32
neonatal severe hyperparathyroidism (NSHPT), 356
neonates, hypocalcemia in, 354
nephron, 319
nephropathy, diabetic, 289, 296
nephrotic syndrome, 24, 27
    reduced serum proteins in, 348
nerve cells, excess glutamate toxicity, 574
nerve function impaired, 289
nerve gases, 580
nerve–muscle conduction, 581
nervonic acids, 381
nervous system, cells of, 560–3
nervousness, caused by pyroxidine deficiency, 135
neurexins, 468
neurochemistry, 559–66
neurodegenerative diseases, 23, 383
neurogenic pathways, 66
neuroglial structures, 562–3
neuroglobin, 43
neuroglycopenia, 278
neurologic deterioration, progressive, 181
neurological damage, 86
neurological disease, 180
neuromodulators, 569–70
    neuropeptides as, 581
neurons, 561–2
    and axonal transport, 560–1
    brain, 305
    features of, 560
    functional structure of, 562
    ion pumping by, 565
    norepinephrine, in CNS, 576
    serotoninergic, 578
    tuberoinfundibular dopamine, 539
neuropathy, 417
    caused by pyroxidine deficiency, 135
    diabetic, 289, 291
    peripheral, 133
neuropeptide Y (NPY), 305, 570
neuropeptides, 305
    multigene families of, 581
    as neuromodulators, 581
    prolactin-releasing properties, 539
neuropsychiatric problems, 29
neurosarcoidosis, 563

neurotransmission, 570–3
disorders of, 575
neurotransmitters, 569–82
action of, 572
autonomic nervous system, 570
as cause of hypertension, 576
classes of, 573–81
classification of, 569–70
definition of, 569
and ion channel activity, 571
low molecular weight, 570
manipulation of concentration, 573
reference values, 611
regulation of, 573
release of, 571
synaptic activity, 571–2
synthesis of, 575
neutropenia, 141
neutrophils, 517
niacin, 54
deficiency, 85, 135
and $NAD^+/NADP^+$ synthesis, 133–5
nickel, 141
nicotinamide, 85, 94, 97, 133, 180
ring, 182
nicotinamide adenine dinucleotide
(NAD), 110, 133, 146–8, 151, 183
cytosolic ratio, 177
high levels of, 182–3
mitochondrial level, 185
(NAD^+), 3, 96–7, 108, 199, 406
and PDC activity, 178
reduced (NADH), 3, 94, 105, 146–7, 175, 189
consumption, 185
cytosolic ratio, 177
hepatic, 168
mitochondrial, 99
oxidation of, 96–100, 110, 148
in TCA cycle, 181
reduced (NADH) dehydrogenase, 99
reduced (NADH) Q reductase, 99–100
reduction of, 182
nicotinamide adenine dinucleotide
phosphate (NADP)
$(NADP^+)$, 133, 199
reduced (NADPH), 143, 150, 153, 210
synthesis of, 151
nicotine, 564
nicotinic acid, 133
nicotinic receptors, ionotropic, 579
NIDDM1 locus, in type 2 diabetes, 288
Niemann–Pick syndrome, 383
nifedipine, 91
nigericin, 83
night blindness, 129
nigrostriatal tract, dopamine in, 577
ninhydrin, 22
nitric oxide (NO), 8, 44–5, 65, 499, 580
generation in blood vessel wall, 66
signaling by, 542
synthase, 8, 66, 580
vasodilation and, 236
nitrites, 44
nitrocellulose membranes, 17
DNA storage, 476–7
nitrogen, 80
balance, 253, 306
excretion of, 245
incorporation into urea, 247–8
inter-organ flow of, 246
loss in feces, 123
reactive species (RNS), 499–500
and urea cycle, 248
urinary excretion and nitrogen
balance, 306
nitrogen dioxide (NO_2), 500
nitroprusside, 195
nitrotyrosine, 500
nodes of Ranvier, 563
noncompliance, 452

nonheme iron proteins, 100
nonsteroidal anti-inflammatory drugs
(NSAIDs), 46, 59, 555, 607
nontropical sprue, 356
nonvolatile acids, 333
noradrenaline *see* norepinephrine
norepinephrine, 135, 565, 575
neurons in CNS, 576
as neurotransmitter, 576–7
normocalcemia, 348
normoglycemia, 294
maintenance of, 160
northern blots, 477
*Not*I, 477–8
nuclear magnetic resonance (NMR)
spectroscopy, 15, 23
nuclei, 1, 16
nucleic acids, 3
excretion, 418
synthesis, 135–6, 140, 151
nucleoside analogs, as anti-viral
agents, 61
nucleosides, 413
purine, 417
nucleosomes, 426, 429, 465–6
5'-nucleotidase, 418
nucleotide coenzymes, production
of, 93
nucleotide diphosphokinase, 416, 419
nucleotides, 461
biosynthesis and degradation of, 413–23
classification of, 414
de novo metabolism, 422
methylation, 466
mismatch repair, 434
reduced, 97
salvage pathway sources of, 416
sequences, 461
synthesis of purines, 414–16
Watson–Crick base pairs, 427, 466
numbness, 44, 563
stimulated by hypocalcemia, 355
nutrients
calorific value of, 304–5
deficiencies, and malnutrition, 127
essential (limiting), 303
functions of, 302
intake, 299
main classes of, 301–3
plasma concentrations, influenced
by genotype, 300–1
nutrition, 299–313
adequate intake (AI), 299–300
biochemical markers of, 306–7
butter–margarine debate, 194
and chronic disease, 311–12
dietary reference intakes (DRI), 299–300
dietary reference values (DRVs), 300
and disease, 301
enteral, 312
estimated average requirement
(EAR), 299–300, 304
factors determining state of, 300
food guide pyramid, 310
and genetics, 299–301
levels of support for, 312
and life cycle, 301
lower reference nutrient intake
(LRNI), 300
and metabolic adaption, 301
parenteral, 307, 312
recommended daily/dietary
allowances (RDAs), 299–300
reference nutrient intake (RNI), 300
and thermodynamics, 93
tolerable upper intake level (UL), 299–300
nutrition science
definitions, 299–300
recommendations, 299–300
nutritional needs, and emergency
treatment, 306

nutritional status
assessment of, 305–7
and body mass index (BMI), 306
determining factors for, 305
laboratory tests for, 307
plasma proteins as markers of, 306–7
nutritional support, 312
nystatin, 83

O
obesity, 93, 106, 186, 205–6, 308–9, 536
and arthritis, 308
and associated diseases, 308–9
central, 531
clinical, 206
and coronary disease, 308
and diabetes, 308
gastric banding, 311
genetic component of, 431
genetic predisposition to, 301, 309
as health problem, 308–9
links to glucose intolerance,
diabetes, and cardiovascular
disease, 292
low grade inflammatory reaction
in, 288
and metabolic syndrome, 293
multiple problems of, 308
relationship with diabetes and
atherosclerosis, 292–3
obstructive jaundice, 71
octanoylcarnitine, 190
Okazaki fragments, 432
oleic acid, 28, 203, 302–3, 375
oligodendrocytes, 559–63
oligomenorrhea, 536
oligomycin, 109
oligonucleotides
allele-specific (ASOs), 486
and dot–blot hybridization, 486–8
primer design in PCR, 485
oligopeptides, 123
digestion, 125
oligosaccharidase, 116
oligosaccharides, 116–17, 120
biosynthesis of, 366–9
high-mannose, 360, 362, 368, 370
N-linked, 360–2, 366–9
O-linked, 362, 369
structure of, 360–1
oliguria, 328
olive oil, 77
omeprazole, 90–1
oncogenes, 583, 595–6
collaboration, 596
dominant mutation, 596
Ras, 593
oncotic pressure, 318, 321
ondansetron, 578
oocyte release, 535
opioid analgesic, 46
opsin, 129
opsonization, 507
optic chiasm, 539
oral glucose tolerance test (OGTT), 282, 294
organ–fuel interactions, 273–4
organophosphates, 580
ornithine, 250–1
ornithine transcarbamoylase, 250
ornithine transcarbamoylase
deficiency, 419
orotate, 252
orotate monophosphate (OMP), 418
orotate monophosphate
decarboxylase, 419
orotate phosphoribosyl transferase, 419
orotic acid, 417–19
in blood, 252
in urine, 252, 421
orotic aciduria, 419
orotidylate decarboxylase, 419
ortho-tyrosine, 603

osmolality
regulation of, 318
and volume of ECF and ICF, 317–19
osmotic diuresis, 288
osmotic pressure, 318
osmotic stress, 481
osteoblasts, 345–7
phosphatase secretion by, 345
osteocalcin, 132, 346–7
osteoclasts, 86, 345–6
osteocytes, 345–6
osteocytic lacunae, 345–6
osteogenesis imperfecta, 14, 389
osteoid, 345
osteomalacia, 131, 345, 351, 356–7
and vitamin D deficiency, 130
osteonectin, 345
osteopenia, 389
osteopetrosis, 346
osteopontin, 347
osteoporosis, 86, 138, 346, 356–7, 601
and estrogen deficiency, 536
risk factors and secondary causes, 357
osteoprotegrin (OPG), 346
ouabain, 91, 318
ovalbumin, 59
ovarian failure, 490
ovary
disorders of, 535–6
granulosa cells, 220
and steroid hormones, 219
overflow pathway, 233–4
ovulation, 535
oxalate, 138
oxaloacetate, 100, 170, 247
condensation of, 180–1
cytosolic, 168
from pyruvate, 177–8
recycling of, 184
sources of, 177
oxaloacetic acid, 176
oxidation
of fatty acids, 193–4
fuel, stages of, 93–4
as source of energy, 93–4
oxidation–reduction reactions, 93
oxidative damage, protection
against, 501–5
oxidative deamination, 247
oxidative phosphorylation, 86, 96
efficiency of, 99
mechanisms of, 98
oxidative stress, 499
oxidoreductase reactions, 54, 127
oxidoreductases, 53–4
oxygen, 3, 35, 80
daily flux, 333
in desaturation reactions, 203
excess reactive, 291
hyperbaric therapy, 37
inertness of, 497–8
and life, 497–506
nature of radical damage, 500–1
in P:O ratio, 105–6
partial pressure (pO2), 106, 320, 336–9
in respiration, 337
properties of, 35
reactive species (ROS), 497–8
beneficial effects of, 505
cellular response to, 504
enzymatic defenses against, 502
formation of, 500
generation and release during
phagocytosis, 505
hydroxyl radical, 500–1
iron-mediated enhancement, 497
and oxidative stress, 499
reduction of, 13, 98–9
saturation (SpO2), 40
structure of, 498
tension, 1

and tissue metabolism, 336–8
transport, 35–49
uptake, 106
ADP effect on, 106
by mitochondria, 106
inhibition of, 109
oxysterol, 214
oxytocin, 305, 525

P
P:O ratios, 99
and respiratory control, 105–6
p21, 587
p21 CDKI (WAF1), induction of, 589
p38-reactivating kinase (*p38*RK), 587
*p44*ERK1, 587
*p47*ERK2, 587
p53, 587, 591, 593
cell-cycle regulation by, 597
p53 protein, 589
Paget's disease, 356
pain
abdominal, 121, 531, 579
bone, 129
in lower extremities, 384
shooting, 383
palate, arched and cleft, 215
palmar xanthoma, 235
palmitate
energy yield, 191
β-oxidation of, 192
palmitic acid, 28, 203, 375
palmitoleic acid, 203
palmitoyl-CoA, 199–200
palpitations, 498, 576
pancreas, 60, 113, 117, 120
action in digestion, 115
auto-digestion of, 118
β-cells, 55, 106
autoimmune destruction of, 287
function, 140
glucagon secretion, 547
loss of function, 115
secretion in, 115, 124
secretions from, 246
pancreatic duct, 120
pancreatic juice, 114, 120
pancreatitis, 60, 121, 304
diagnosis of, 611
panic attacks, serotonin in, 579
pantothenic acid, 135, 180
papain proteolysis, 31
Papanicolaou 'Pap smear' test, 594
paracetamol *see* acetaminophen
Paramecium, 448
paranoia, 574
parasympathetic nervous system
(PNS), 113, 579
parathyroid disease, 355
parathyroid hormone (PTH), 346,
348, 483
and hypocalcemia, 355
and osteoporosis prevention, 356
synthesis and major actions, 349
parathyroid-hormone-related protein
(PTHrP), 350
synthesis, structure and
relationships, 350
parathyroidectomy, 356
paresthesia, 383
Parkinson's disease, 23, 252, 574,
577–8, 580, 607
treatment for, 565
paroxysmal nocturnal
hemoglobinuria (PNH), 380
partial pressure gradients, 338
particle agglutination, 521
parvovirus infections, 385
paternity testing, 427
Pauling, L, 138
pellagra, 135
penicillamine, 86, 392
penicillin, 28, 58
Penicillium citrinum, 211
pentachlorophenol, 106
pentose phosphate pathway, 143,
150–1, 158

equilibrium reactions in, 152
function in RBC, 153
interconversion stage of, 151–2
redox stage of, 151
pentose phosphates, 151
pentoses, 117
pepsin, 31, 52, 116, 123–4, 246
pepsinogens, 115, 123–4
peptidases, 120
hydrolysis of proteins, 123
peptide bonds, 13–14
formation, 454
structure of, 13
peptide chains, 7, 13, 16
charge and polarity of, 13
folding of, 15
interactions between, 16
peptides, 3, 20, 23, 124
amino-terminal procollagen
extension, 347
appetite-stimulating, 305
bond cleavage, 125
carboxy-terminal procollagen
extension, 347
hypothalamic, 529
inhibitory, 124
natriuretic, 330
markers of heart failure, 330
as neurotransmitters, 581
and proteins, 12–16
recombinant human, 483
signal, 26
peptidyl-dipeptidase A, 326
peptidyl transferase, 449, 452
perfluorocarbon emulsions, 38
perfusion, 269
perilymph, 560
perineum, 383
periosteocytic space, 345
peripheral nerve, and brain, 559–60
peripheral vascular disease, 225
peristalsis, 113
permeases, 82
peroxidase, detection of occult blood
by, 503
peroxidation, of lipids, 501
peroxisomes, 1, 190, 499, 502
role in fatty acid oxidation, 190
peroxynitrite, 499
pertussis toxin, 545
petechiae, 138
Peyer's patches, 510
pH, 1, 10, 13, 20, 52
alkaline, 121
blood, 168
changes in, 342
and CO$_2$ removal, 336–8
changes in digestion, 115–16
in GI tract, 114–15
gradient, 20, 98, 103, 106
high blood, 335
low plasma, 335
neutral, 94–5, 106
optimal, 86
plasma, 341–3
of stomach, 123–4
phagocytes
lipid-laden, 383
mononuclear, 399
in pus, 148
phagocytosis, 31, 80, 402, 507,
590
pharmacodynamics, 408
pharmacogenomics, 408
pharmacokinetics, 408
pharmacologic agents, 44
phenolphthalein, 90
phenothiazines, 578
phentolamine, 565
phenyl isothiocyanate (PITC), 22
phenylacetate, 252
phenylalanine, 9, 53, 85
accumulation of, 323
degradation of, 258
hydroxylation of, 257
phenylalanine hydroxylase, 257–8

phenylalanine–tyrosine pathway,
defects in, 256–9
phenylalkylamine, 91
phenylketonuria, 257–8
phenyllactate, excessive excretion of,
257
phenylpyruvate, excessive excretion
of, 257
phenylthiocarbamyl (PTC) amino
acid, 22
phenylthiohydantoin (PTH)
derivatives, 22
pheochromocytoma, 329, 353,
576–7
Philadelphia chromosome, 596
phloretin, 88
phosphatase, 110
bone-specific, 347
dephosphorylation of, 185
phosphates, 97–8, 144, 303
calcium complex with, 347
groups, 95
ionized, 348
in P:O ratio, 105–6
reference values, 609
phosphatidic acid, 554
activation of, 379
biosynthesis of, 375–6
formation and conversion, 377
phosphatidic acid phosphohydrolase,
554
phosphatidic pathway, 121
phosphatidylcholine, 80–1, 375–7
breakdown products of, 554
formation of, 378
hydrolysis of, 553–5
phosphatidylethanolamine, 80, 375,
377
hydrolysis of, 553–4
phosphatidylglycerol, 375, 377, 379
formation of, 379
phosphatidylinositol, 78, 375, 377,
379–80
bisphosphate, 164–5
4,5-bisphosphate (PIP$_2$), 549–50,
585
cascade, 585
signaling cycle, 551
3,4,5-trisphosphat (PIP$_3$), 585,
592
phosphatidylinositol kinases, 550
phosphatidylinositol-3,4,5-
triphosphate (PIP$_3$) dependent
kinase, 585
phosphatidylserine, 72, 79–80, 375,
377, 590
phosphaturia, 84, 354
phosphoadenosine phosphosulfate
(PAPS), 395
phosphodiesterases, 161, 167, 549,
563
inhibitors, 164
phosphoenolpyruvate (PEP), 147
phosphoenolpyruvate carboxykinase
(PEPCK), 170, 184
phosphoethanolamine, 376
phosphofructokinase
regulation of gluconeogenesis by,
279
regulation of glycolysis by, 279
phosphofructokinase-1 (PFK-1), 110,
145–6, 150, 165, 170
allosteric regulation of, 149
inhibition of, 183
phosphofructokinase-2, 171
phosphoglucomutase, 158–9, 172
6-phosphogluconate, 151
6-phosphogluconate dehydrogenase,
151, 203
6-phosphogluconic acid, 151
6-phosphogluconic acid lactone, 151
phosphoglucose isomerase, 145
2-phosphoglycerate!, 147–9
3-phosphoglycerate!, 147, 150
phosphoglycerate kinase, 146–8,
150, 170
phosphoglycerate mutase, 147

phosphoglycerides, 375
major, 553
phosphohistidine, 147
phosphoinositide-3-kinase (PI-3-K),
585, 592
phospholipase A$_2$, 115
phospholipase C, 164
phospholipase C-γ, 585
phospholipases, 67, 379, 553–5
sites of action, 379
phospholipids, 32, 67, 72, 77,
120–1, 377
biosynthesis of, 376–9
enzyme regulation by, 80
extraction and analysis of, 81
formation of antibodies to, 84
interconversion pathways, 378
polar head groups, 79
structure of, 78, 375–6
surfactant function of, 378
turnover of, 379
phosphoprotein phosphatases,
167
phosphoribosyl transferase, 417
5-phosphoribosyl-pyrophosphate
(PRPP), 413
5-phosphoribosyl-pyrophosphate
synthetase, 413
phosphoric acid, 77
phosphorus, 148
phosphorylase, 159, 163–5
deficiency, 163
phosphorylase kinase, 161, 163
phosphorylation, 16, 86, 161, 164,
166, 171
enzyme, regulatory role of, 280
multi-step, 275
oxidative, 2, 97, 100, 184
regulation of, 110–11
uncouplers, 106–7
reactions, 144
of serine residues, 185
substrate-level, 146–8, 175, 181,
184
inhibition by arsenate, 148
synthesis of ATP by, 146–8
phosphorylation–dephosphorylation,
104
phosphotyrosine, 585
phosphotyrosine phosphatases
(PTPases), 585
photophobia, 133
photosensitivity, 601
phototherapy, 133, 410
phrenic nerve, 567
o-phthalaldehyde, 22
phylloquinone, 131
phytanic acids, 190, 193–4
α-oxidation of, 194
phytohemagglutinin, 371
pinocytosis, 28, 563
pituitary
disorders, 534
disorders of, 535–6
hormone disorders of, 526
tumor, 534
pituitary failure, 530
pituitary fossa, 539
pituitary gland, 525
adenohypothesis, 525
neurohypothesis, 525
pituitary tumor, 534, 538
pK_a *see* dissociation constant,
negative logarithm of
placenta, 86
transfer of O$_2$, 150
plasma, 1, 25, 56
albumin, 140
enzyme, and myocardial infarction,
270
glucose
after myocardial infarction, 284
concentration during fasting,
280, 294
hormones controlling levels of,
274
measurement, 294

homocysteine concentration, 229
hydrophilic, 28
lactate, high levels of, 295
lipid profile, lifestyle change and, 242
membrane, 87
nucleotidase, activity increase in disease, 422
platelet-poor, 71
potassium concentration, 325–6
proteins, 26–32
    as markers of nutritional state, 306–7
triglycerols, 121
TSH concentrations, 527
plasma cholesterol, and coronary mortality in men, 241
plasmalogens, 379
plasmids, 480–1
    bacterial, use as vectors, 481–2
    target genes in, 482
plasmin, 75
plasminogen, 74–5, 228–9
plasminogen activator
    tissue type (tPA), 64, 74–5
    urinary type (uPA), 74
Plasmodium falciparum, 47
platelet activating factor (PAF), 64
    and hypersensitivity, 377
platelet factor 3 (PF3), 64
platelet-derived growth factor (PDGF), 542, 584
    receptor signaling, 585–6
    responses to, 584
    signaling element scaffold, 585
platelets, 26, 48, 63–4, 66–9
    activating factor (PAF), 66
    activation, 67
    adhesion, 67
    aggregation, 67
    and bleeding disorders, 67–8
    membrane receptors, 67
    pathways of activation, 68
    production of thromboxane A_2, 66
    shape changes in, 67
    thrombin activation of, 72
β-pleated sheet, 14–15, 23, 563
plethora, 531
podocytes, 321
poisoning
    CO, 499
    mushroom, 440
poisons
    DNP, 107
    small molecule, 102
polyacrylamide, 18
polyacrylamide gel electrophoresis (PAGE), 20
polyanions, 32
polycystic ovary syndrome (PCOS), 536
polycythemia, 42
polydactyly, 215
polydypsia, 288
polyisoprenoids, biosynthesis of, 190
polymerase chain reaction (PCR), 479, 481–5, 487–90
    advantages and disadvantages of, 485
    amplification refractory mutation system (ARMS), 488
    annealing, 483
    applications of, 487
    assay of restriction site polymorphisms, 487
    denaturation, 483
    detection of microsatellite repeats, 488–9
    elongation, 483
    mutation detection, 488
    oligonucleotide primer design in, 485
    real-time, 494
    reverse transcriptase, 493
polymerases
    heat stable, 483–4

Pfu, 484
Taq, 484
polymeric gel, 20
polyol pathway, 288, 291
    and diabetic complications, 291
polyostotic fibrous dysplasia, 557
polypeptides, 20, 123
    α-globin, 47
    β-globin, 45, 47
    induction of antibody response, 125
polypurine, 426
polypyrimidine, 426
polysaccharides, 32, 116, 157
    cleavage of, 117
    digestion of, 116
    hydration of, 116
    hydrolytic cleavage of, 118
polysomes, protein synthesis on, 455
polyubiquitination, 457
polyunsaturates, and plasma cholesterol reduction, 311
polyuria, 84, 288
pores, 84
    and cellular physiology, 85
    endoplasmic reticular, 85
    mitochondrial, 85
    nuclear, 85
porphobilinogen (PBG), 403
porphyrias, 403
    acute intermittent (AIC), 403
    cutanea tarda, 403
    hereditary coproporphyria, 403
    variegate, 403
porphyrins, 35–6, 175
portal vein, 217, 399
porters, 82
postabsorptive (fasting) state, 282
postabsorptive metabolism (overnight fast), 283
postprandial (absorptive) state, 279–82
postprandial metabolism, 281
postreceptors, 285–6
potassium, 303
    balance, 325
        affected by diabetic ketoacidosis, 290
    bodily distribution of, 316
    loss, 115
    metabolism, 315–17
    plasma, concentration, 325–6
pralidoxime, 580
pravastatin, 225
prazosin, 577
prealbumin
    as nutritional marker, 306
    synthesis, 32
pregnancy, 99, 127, 136
    alkalosis in, 344
    biochemical confirmation of, 532
    metabolic adaptation to, 301
    nucleotidase elevation, 422
    premature rupture, 34
pregnane ring, 218
pregnenolone, 220
prekallikrein, 69, 72
premenstrual tension (PMT), 535
preosteoblast, 346
preprocollagen, 389
preproinsulin, 276
prerenal azotemia, 328
Pribnow box, 441
primaquine, 155
primary hyperparathyroidism see hyperparathyroidism
primosome complex, 431
prion diseases, 23
prion protein-cellular form (PrPC), 23
prion protein-scrapie form (PrPSc), 23
prions, 23
pristanic acid, 193
pro-opiomelanocortin (POMC), 529, 581
pro-oxidant systems, 499
pro-urokinase, 74
procarboxypeptidase, 60

procarcinogens, 435
    activation of, 181
procaspases, 591–2
procoagulants, 25
procollagens, 360
prodynorphin, 581
proelastase, 60
proenkephalin A, 581
proenzymes, 60, 120
progerias, 601, 605
progesterone, 356, 535
progressive intrahepatic cholestasis, 88
proinsulin, 276
prokaryotic promoters, 441
prolactin, 539
    axis, 539
    clinical secretion disorders, 539
    inhibited by dopamine, 539
    inhibition of, 539
prolactinoma, 539
proline, 7, 10, 14, 22, 387
    α-carbon, 10
    hydroxylation of, 138
    residues, 389
promoters, 460–2
    access, 465–6
    alternative, 467
    elements of, 461
    enhancers, 460–1
    GC box, 460
    initiator sequence, 460
    TATA box, 460
proopiomelatocortin (POMC), 305
propanolol, 565
propeptides, BNP, diagnostic, 330
propidium iodide (PI), 592
propionyl-CoA, 170, 193
    from fatty acids, 193–4
    metabolism to succinyl-CoA, 193, 255
    in TCA cycle, 193
prostacyclins, 65, 555
    generation in blood vessel wall, 66
prostaglandin synthase, 561
prostaglandins, 59, 68, 509, 535, 555,
    E series PGE_2, 354
    I_2, 65
    pathogenetic role of, 597
    synthesis, 555
prostatic hyperplasia, 539
proteases, 23, 115, 120, 124
    pancreatic, 125
    V8, 22
proteasomes, 457–8
    structure of, 457
protein C, 73–4
protein carbonyls, 603
protein disulfide isomerase, 23
protein glycation, 290
protein kinase A, 161, 163, 167, 171, 422, 547–9
    binding of cAMP, 547–8
    phosphorylation by, 547
    regulation of, 166
protein kinase C, 163–7, 585
    DAG activation of, 550–3
    superfamily, 552
protein kinases, 554–5
protein S, 73–4
protein truncation testing, 492
protein tyrosine kinase (PTK), 585, 587
proteinase inhibitors, 32
proteins, 1–2, 7–24, 302
    abnormal liver concentrations, 402
    acute phase, 46, 401–2
    age-dependent chemical modification of, 603
    aging of, 457
    allosteric, 40–1
    α_1 and α_2, 34
    androgen-binding, 532
    antiapoptotic, 592–3
    binding, 549
    biotin–carboxyl-carrier, 199

bone Gla, 346
    browning of, 602
    c-reactive, 32–4, 236, 401–2
    CAD, 418–19
    carbohydrate-binding, 371–2
    carrier, 82, 212, 524
    catalytic, 51–62
    cell attachment, 346–7
    cellular fate of, 455–6
    chaperone, 23, 369–70, 455
    conformational energy of, 100
    Cu carrying, 141
    cyclin-dependent kinases, 430
    cysteine-rich, 140
    cytochrome P4550, 219
    cytoplasmic, glycosylation of, 359–60
    daily requirements by age, 302
    determination of molecular weight by electrophoresis, 20
    determination of primary structure, 22–3
    determination of purity by electrophoresis, 20
    determination of three-dimensional structure, 23
    dialysis of, 17, 19
    dietary, digestion and absorption of, 246–7
    digestion and absorption of, 123–5
    digestion by enzymes, 120
    dimeric, 16
        structure of, 17
    DNA-binding, 461
    domains of, 15
    endogenous, 123
    folding, 23, 367, 369–70
        disease, 23
    in food, 113
    fractionation by charge, 20
    fractionation by size, 19
    gel filtration chromatography of, 19
    glutathionylation of, 501
    growth-related, 347
    guanosine-binding, 161
    "heat shock", 23
    heme, 29, 100
    hetero-and homotropic binding to, 41
    hydrolyzed by peptidases, 123
    inhibitor, 161
    ionized groups in, 11
    iron-carrier, 468
    iron-sulfur, 182
    kinase A (PKA), cAMP-dependent, 161
    loss and edema, 319
    mammalian globin, 36–43
    membrane anchoring, 83
    metabolism, in liver, 401–3
    metal binding, reference values, 611
    mitochondrial encoded, 429
    modification by glucose, 290
    multidrug resistance-associated (MRP), 87
    multifunctional, 418–19
    multimeric, 16
    muscle, 263–7
    myofilament, 262
    noncollagenous, in ECM, 390–3
    O_2 storage, 37
    O_2 transport, 37–8
    parathyroid-hormone-related (PTHrP), 353
        synthesis, structure, and relationships, 350
    and peptides, 12–16
    pK values of, 11
    plasma, 26–32
    post-translational modifications of, 16
    primary structure of, 12–13
    proteasomal degradation of, 402

purification and characterization of, 16–21
quaternary structure in, 16
secondary structure of, 13–15
separation on the basis of charge, 18–20
signal-transduction, 160
solubility and stability of, 370
SREBP cleavage-activating (SCAP), 215
sterol regulatory element-binding (SREBPs), 215
structural analysis, 21–3
structural elements, 18
sugar–amino acid attachments in, 359
synthesis, 3, 32, 140, 447–58
effect of mutations on, 449
elongation, 452–3
on endoplasmic reticulum, 456
fidelity of translation, 449
initiation of, 451–2
machinery of, 449–51
peptidyl transferase, 452
on polysomes, 455
post-translational modification, 456–7
process of, 451–5
targeting, 455–6
termination, 453–5
TATA-binding, 462
tertiary structure of, 15–16
transfer, 229–30
translation, 447
transport of, 28, 456
trimeric, 16
turnover, 447–58
UMP synthase, 418–19
uncoupling (UPC), 98–9, 106–7
vitamin A transport by, 129
vitamin D-binding, 348
proteinuria, 27, 84, 319, 383
proteoglycans, 3, 345, 347, 394–8
degradation defects, 395–6
distribution, 394
functions of, 396–8
heparan sulphate, 230
structure of, 360, 394–5
synthesis and degradation of, 395–6
proteolysis, 176, 402–3
proteolytic cleavage, 16
proteome, 23
proteomics, 7, 23
prothrombin, 32, 72, 132
time measuring devices, 69
prothrombin-converting complex, 25
prothrombin time (PT), 71, 401
proto-oncogenes, 583
proton pumps, 90
gastric, inhibition of, 91
in stomach, 89–91
protons, 96
and ATP synthesis, 105
channel blocking, 109
controlled leakage of, 98
gradient, 102–5
pumping, 106
pumps, 98
protoporphyrin, 36
IX, 403
protoporphyrinogen III, 403
prourokinase, 75
provitamins, 128
ultraviolet light action on, 129
Prozac, 575
Prusiner, SB, 23
pseudo-Hurler polydystrophy, 371
pseudohypoparathyroidism, 355
pseudouridine, 439
pseudoxanthoma elastica, 88
pterins, 580
pteroyl glutamic acid, 135
puberty
delayed, 534
precocious, 213, 535–6
pulmonary disease, 42, 44

pulmonary thromboembolism, 132
pulse oximetry (pulse-ox), 40
pump ATPase, 85–7
purine monophosphates, 415–16
purines, 136, 413
biosynthetic pathways, 415
bonding in DNA, 426
degradation to uric acid, 416–17
metabolism, 413–17
names and structures of, 414
overproduction, 418
ring, 413
salvage pathway, 416, 419
transmitter functions of, 580
putrescine, 251
pyloric stenosis, 343
pyrexia, 140
pyridinolines, 356
pyridostigmine, 581
pyridoxal, 135
kinase, 135
phosphate, 135, 247, 579
catalytic role of, 247
pyridoxamine, 135
pyridoxine, 135, 247, 254
in amino acid metabolism, 135
supplementation, 139
pyrimidines, 136, 413
analogs, 421
biosynthesis, 252
chemotherapeutic blocking agents, 421
bonding in DNA, 426
degradation of, 420–1
metabolism, 417–21
monophosphates, dephosphorylation of, 420–1
names and structures of, 414
ring, 417
salvage pathways, 419–20
synthesis, 418
triphosphates, synthesis of, 420
pyrophosphatase, 159
pyrophosphate, 159, 354, 421
pyrophosphorylase, 159
pyrrolidine ring, 10
pyruvate, 2–3, 98, 143, 147–8, 163, 170
carboxylation, 178
conversion to metabolites, 177
excretion, 172
from alanine, 185
from glycolysis, 176
from lactate, 185
increase in beri-beri, 180
oxidation, 183
reduction of, 177
pyruvate carboxylase, 168, 170–1, 177–8
pyruvate decarboxylase, 148
pyruvate dehydrogenase, 110, 171, 175–6, 178, 183
complex (PDC), 177–80
deficiency, 179, 181
mechanism of action of, 178
reactions of, 179
regulation of, 185
insulin stimulation of, 185
pyruvate dehydrogenase kinases, 178
control by diet, 186
pyruvate dehydrogenase phosphatase, 178, 185
pyruvate kinase, 147–50, 170–1, 203
deficiency, 155
pyruvic acid, 176

Q
quinone, 258
quinonoid dihydrobiopterin (qBH₂), 580

R
R-proteins, 137–8
racemase, 170
radioimmunoassay (RIA), measure of cAMP by, 557
radioisotopes, 475

radiotherapy, applications of ROS, 498
ranitidine, 91, 581
raphe nuclei, 578
Ras signaling element, in tumors, 585–6, 589, 596
Ras–MAPK cascade, 585
Ras–MAPK pathway, 586
Rb, 597
reagent strips, for blood glucose measurement, 154
real-time PCR, 494
receptor activator for nuclear factor κ β ligand (RANKL), 346
receptor antagonists, 91
receptor interacting protein (RIP), 592
receptor ligation, 542
receptors, 572–3
acetylcholine, 579
adenosine, 580
adrenergic, 543, 546–7, 565, 573
antigen recognition by, 509–10
asialoglycoprotein, 372
calcium-sensing (CaSR), 348, 356
cell-surface, 542
cytokine, 587
dopamine (Dₙ), 578
G-protein, 348
coupled, 543–6
ganglioside, 385
hemopoietic, 587
hormone, 541–2
human β-adrenergic, 544
intracellular, 541–2
ionotropic, 572–3
mechanism of action, 572
lipoprotein, 230
LDL, 226, 229–30, 362
liver X, 214, 217–18, 233
membrane, 275, 541–58
classification of, 543
metabotropic, 573, 578
multiple, 578
muscarinic, 564, 580
nicotinic, 564–5, 579
acetylcholine, 581
NMDA glutamate, 573
nuclear, 220
opioid, 581
oxysterol, 214
PDGF, 585
peptide, 581
peroxisome proliferation activating (PPARS), 233
polypeptide hormone, 542
retinoid X, 215, 233
scavenger, 215, 230
serotonin, 578
SRP docking protein, 455
steroid, 464–5, 541–2
similarities between, 466
TNF, 592
transmembrane glycoprotein, 587
recombinant DNA technology, 473–95
recombinant proteins, 1
recommended daily/dietary allowances (RDAs), 300
recommended nutrient intake (RNI), 300
red blood cell (RBC) see erythrocytes
redox reactions, 144, 150, 175
iron–sulfur complexes in, 100
redox shuttles, 101
reductive adaptation, 301
refeeding syndrome, 308
reference nutrient intake (RNI), 300
Refsum's disease, 194
reinforced concrete, 396–7
renal clearance, 324
renal disease
and malnutrition, 312
tracking of, 248
zinc loss in, 140
renal failure, 38, 422, 578
acute, 84
fall in urine output, 328
high creatinine concentration, 328

high serum urea concentration, 328
and weight loss, 307
renal function
assessment of, 269, 324
impairment by diabetes, 323
testing, 296
renal hypomagnesemia, 83
renal oxalate stones, 138
renal reabsorption and excretion, 329
renal tubular acidoses (RTA), 86, 341
renal tubules, Na reabsorption in, 323
renin, 57, 326, 329
renin–angiotensin system, 326–8
renin-angiotensin, in water and electrolyte disorders, 330–1
renin–angiotensin–aldosterone axis, 330
reperfusion injury, 498
reserpine, 575
resistin, 205
respiration, 2
control of, 337
coupled, 105
pauseless, 288
respiratory acidosis, 341
respiratory alkalosis, 44, 337
respiratory control, 110
respiratory control, and P:O ratios, 105–6
respiratory problems, 338–9
respiratory tract, 336
response elements, 461
restriction endonucleases, 480
restriction enzymes, 477–8, 480
restriction fragment length polymorphisms (RFLPs), 486–7
detection of pathologic mutations by, 487
in sickle-cell anemia, 487
restriction site polymorphisms (RSPs), 487
resuscitation, 341, 344
reticulocytes, 25
high count, 155
reticulocytosis, 155
reticuloendothelial cells, 560
reticuloendothelial system, 28–9
retina, 504
rod cells, 129
retinal, 128–9
11-cis-retinal, 129
retinaldehyde, 128
retinoblastoma gene (Rb), 596–7
retinoblastoma protein (Rb), 589
retinoic acid, 128–9, 541
binding protein (RABP), 129
retinol, 128–9
all-trans-retinol, 129
retinol palmitate, 129
retrolental fibroplasia, 499
Retrovir, 433
reverse aldol reaction, 146
reverse transcriptase PCR, 493
reverse tri-iodothyronine (rT₃), 527–8
rhabdomyolysis, 323
rhinorrhea, 560
rhodopsin, 129, 566
ribitol, 133
riboflavin, 54, 97, 100, 127, 135, 180
deficiency, 133
and oxidoreductases, 133
riboflavin phosphate, 97
ribonucleic acid (RNA), 3, 143, 150–1, 437–45
editing at post-transcriptional level, 468–9
general classes of, 437
hairpin loop, 438
heteronuclear, 442
labeling of probes, 475–6
messenger (mRNA), 437, 447, 449
base pairing possibilities, 450
eukaryotic, 439, 443

interaction with tRNA, 450
prokaryotic, 439
regulation of translation, 470
splicing of, 443, 467–8
structure of, 439
untranslated regions, 451
molecular anatomy of, 437–9
molecules, 51
polymerases, 439–40
post-transcriptional processing,
442–5
pre-mRNA, 463
primary messenger, 463
probes, 477
processing, 443
ribosomal (rRNA), 437–8
formation of ribosome, 438
processing, 443
self-splicing, 444
splicing, 444
transcription
elongation, 441, 451
initiation, 440–1, 451
process of, 440–2
termination, 441–2, 451
transfer (tRNA), 259, 437, 447,
449
amino acid attachment, 450
interaction with mRNA, 450
molecular cloverleaf, 438
processing of, 443
structure of, 438
ribonucleic acid polymerase II
(RNAPol II), 460
ribonucleoprotein, signal recognition
particle, 455
ribonucleotide reductase, 421
feedback control, 422
riboprobes, 477
ribose, 95, 97
ribose-5-phosphate, 151–2, 413
ribose phosphate
pyrophosphokinase, 413
ribosomes, 447
A and P binding sites, 449
mRNA binding by, 451
and protein synthesis, 451
ribosyl-5'-phosphate, 418
ribozymes, 51, 444, 452
ribulose-5-phosphate, 151–2
ricin, 453
toxicity, 371
rickets, 351, 358
and vitamin D deficiency, 130
rifampicin, 441
rifamycin, 441
rigor mortis, 264
RIP-associated ICE-like protease with
a death domain (RAIDD), 592
RNA *see* ribonucleic acid
rosuvastatin, 225
rotenone, 108
Rotor's syndrome, 412
Rous sarcoma virus, 595
ryanodine, 91

S
salbutamol, 118, 337, 577
salicylates, 28
saline, 81, 88
saliva, 114
salivary glands, 117
action in digestion, 115
secretion in, 115
Salmonella typhimurium, 435
salt bridges, 15
salting-out, 17
Sanger, F, 492
sarcolemma, 265
sarcomas, 594
sarcomere, 262–3
structure, 263
sarcopenia, 267, 606
sarcoplasm, 265
sarcoplasmic reticulum (SR), 88, 91,
265
satiety centre, 305

scavenger receptor pathway, 215
Schiff base, 249, 290
adducts, 407
crosslinks, 390
intermediates, 391
schizophrenia, 578
Schwann cells, 559, 563
scrapie, 23
scrotum, 383
scurvy, 14, 66, 138, 389
second messengers, 542, 546–57,
563
lipid, 553
fatty-acid side chains of, 554
secondary hyperparathyroidism *see*
hyperparathyroidism
γ-secretase, 82
secretin, 120
secretions, exocrine, 115
secretory granules, 16, 86
sedoheptulose-3-phosphate, 152
seizures, 85, 100, 110, 179
stimulated by hypocalcemia, 355
selectins, 237
selective estrogen receptor
modulators (SERMs), 356
selenium, 139, 141, 153, 259
in cancer prevention, 312
cellular occurrence of, 141
deficiency, 141
sources of, 141
selenocysteine, 141, 153, 259
selenomethionine, 141
selenoproteins, 141
self-mutilation, 417
sella turcica, 525
semiquinone, 606
senescence, replicative, 599
sensory systems, signal transduction,
542
Sephadex series, 18
Sepharose series, 18
septicemia, 308
sequential (multistate) model, 62
serine, 9, 15, 21, 58, 78, 85, 161,
166, 377
degradation, 422
residues, 163, 167
synthesis, 135
serine dehydratase, 247
serine proteases, 52, 60, 246
catalytic mechanism of, 59
catalytic triad of, 59
substrate binding sites of, 53
serotonin, 65, 135, 575, 578–9
disorders of metabolism, 579
multiple receptors for, 578
synthesis cofactor, 580
serotoninergic nerves, in CNS, 578
serpins, 402
Sertoli cells, 532
serum, 25, 56
alkaline phosphatase, 130
aspartate aminotransferase, 168
creatinine concentration and
clearance, 324
enzyme and myocardial infarction,
270
normal, 33
proteins, reference values, 609
retinal-binding protein (SRBP),
129
sodium, concentration in fluid and
electrolyte disorders, 331
urea, measurement of, 324
severe combined immunodeficiency
syndromes (SCIDS), 419
sex chromosomes, 468–9
sex hormone-binding globulin
(SHBG), 533
sex hormones, 541
sex steroid secretion, in females,
535–6
sexual development, retardation of,
140
Shc, 585
Shine–Dalgarno sequence, 451

shock, 42, 344
anaphylactic, 377
short stature, GH deficiency and,
538
short-term memory loss, 133
sialic acid, 360–1, 365–6
lack of, 560
synthesis of, 366
sickle cell disease, 45–7
sickle cell vaso-occlusive crises,
analgesic treatment of, 46
sickle-cell anemia, RFLP in, 487
side chains (—R), 7
slg immunoglobulin, 511
signal transducers, 542
and activators of transcription
(STATS), 587–8
mutant, 595–6
signal transduction, 541–58
receptor coupling to, 542–6
role of PTK in, 585
signaling
cascades, 275, 548, 587
mechanisms, receptor-
independent, 542
pathways, cytokine receptor
recruitment of, 588
receptor-coupled, 542–3
silly putty, 396–7
silver staining, 20
simvastatin, 225
single-strand conformational
polymorphism (SSCP), 490–1
sinusoids, 399
sitosterolemia, 88, 217
skin, 504
blistering of, 392
integrity and healing, 140
lesions, 140
pigmentation, 587
light, 257
rash, 384
thinning of, 389, 601
xanthomas, 235
sleeping sickness, 380
smell, impairment by zinc deficiency,
140
Smith–Lemli–Opitz syndrome, 215
smoking, oxidative damage caused
by, 435
smooth muscle cells (SMCs), 262
sodium, 303
absorption in gut, 120
bodily distribution of, 316
channel defects, 565
glucose transporter, 2, 89
loss, 115
metabolism, 330–1
pump regulation by, 318–19
reabsorption
regulation of, 327–8
in renal tubules, 323
transport in kidney, 320
sodium bicarbonate (NaHCO₃), 125
sodium dodecylsulfate (SDS), 20
sodium dodecylsulfate-
polyacrylamide gel electrophoresis
(SDS-PAGE), 20–1, 23
sodium fluoride, 149
sodium hydroxide (NaOH), 12
sodium urate, 418
sodium–potassium pump, 317–19
somatostatin, 120, 536
and GH secretion, 537
sorbitol, 291, 319
sorbitol dehydrogenase, 291
Southern blots/blotting, 476–9, 486,
491
Southern, E, 477
Southern hybridization, 427
soybean oil, 303
spasticity, 417
specific serotonin reuptake inhibitors
(SSRIs), 575
spectrin, 83
spectrophotometry, 9
speech, loss of, 255

spermatogenesis, 140
influence of FSH and LH on,
532–3
influence of testosterone on, 533
spermine, 251
sphingolipidoses, 384
sphingolipids, 78, 82, 379–85
synthesis, 202
sphingomyelin, 78–81, 380–1, 383
degradation defects, 383
in Niemann-Pick syndrome, 383
sphingomyelinase, 383
sphingosine, 135, 379–81
structure and biosynthesis, 379–81
spironolactone, 326
spleen, 25, 29, 510
red and white pulp areas, 510
in Tangier disease, 233
splenic tenderness, 155
splenomegaly, 68
and Se excess, 141
spongiform encephalopathy, 23
squalene, 212
biosynthesis, 213
cyclization of, 211
ring formation by, 211
Src, 585, 595
Src kinases, 587
SRY, 469
starch, 117
digestion of, 116
Stargardt disease, 88
starvation
associated with illness and trauma,
301
excess acetyl-CoA in, 195
gluconeogenesis in, 194–5
and glucose net synthesis, 183
Mg deficiency in, 303
and negative N balance, 253
phosphorylation in, 185
prolonged, 282
statins, 215, 225, 241
stature
short, 389, 538
tall, 393
stearic acid, 28, 203, 375
steatorrhea, 121
steatosis, 203, 406, 408
stem cells, 419
stercobilin, 404
stercobilinogen, 403
stereochemistry, 7
sternum, 563
steroid hormones, 150, 218–20
action and elimination of, 220
biosynthesis, 219
excretion of, 220
as nuclear receptors, 220
precursors of, 218
structure and nomenclature of,
219
steroid 21-hydroxylase deficiency,
218
steroid receptors, 464–5
gene family, 464
organization of molecule, 465
similarities between, 466
steroid-thyroid-retinoic acid, 464
steroidogenesis, 138
steroids
adrenal, 213, 352
biosynthesis of, 209–23
excess ovarian secretion, 536
gonadal, 352
measurement of, 213
urinary, separation of, 222
sterol regulatory element-binding
proteins (SREBPs), 215, 232
cleavage-activating protein (SCAP),
215, 232
sterol–polyene complex, 83
sterols, 28, 129
stimulation tests, 127
stomach, 113
acid damage to, 91
digestive functions of, 123

lining, 123
lumen, 114, 123
protein digestion in, 123–4
proton pump in, 89–91
stool, 118
fat content of, 121
pale and bulky, 125
pale-colored, 411–12
water content of, 114
Streptococcus pneumoniae, 236
streptokinase, 5, 75
stress
acute and chronic types, 160
affect on metabolism, 286
fuel priority during, 284–5
metabolism during, 285
oxidative, 604
response, 278, 282–4
and laboratory tests, 286
stress-activated protein kinase (SAPK), 587
stridor, 509
stroke, 34, 63, 69, 84, 110, 225, 236, 574
acute, 329
and atherosclerosis, 236
and HRT, 356
ischemic, 255
and obesity, 206
thrombus in, 240
stromyelysin, 240
strychnine, 574
subacute combined degeneration of the cord, 136
subarachnoid space, 560
substance P, 581
substantia nigra, 252
succinate, 99, 108, 183
succinate dehydrogenase, 99, 184
succinate thiokinase, 183
succinate-Q reductase, 99
succinyl-CoA, 170, 180–1, 183, 193, 196
from methylmalonyl-CoA, 136, 138
from TCA cycle, 175
removal of, 186
succinyl-CoA synthetase, 183–4
sucrase–isomaltase complex, 116
sucrose, 116–17
sugars, 9
dietary, interconversion and activation of, 362–5
metabolism of, 133
nucleotide
interconversion, 363
metabolism of, 365–6
suicide substrate, 181
sulfatides, 381
sulfhydryl, 149
buffer, 153
residues, 146–7
sulfite oxidase deficiency, 16
sulfonamides, 28
sulfonylurea, 88, 275
sulfur, methionine as source of, 256
sumatriptan, 578
superoxide dismutase (SOD), 140–1, 499, 502–3, 606
Cu,Zn-superoxide dismutase, 16–17
superoxide, formation by mitochondria, 500
superoxide radicals, 101
surgery
bowel, 344
magnesium deficiency in, 304
survival, human, 600
swainsonine, 369
swallowing difficulties, 581
sweat, chloride ions in, 88
sweating, 248, 278, 576
excessive, 538
problems of, 317
symporters, 86
and amino acid uptake, 124
Na⁺-dependent, 124
Synacthen, 530–1

synapse, types of, 563–4
synaptic space (cleft), 572–3, 575, 579, 581
synaptic transmission, 563–6
in vision, 566
syndrome of inappropriate antidiuretic hormone secretion (SIADH), 325
Syndrome X, 267
synthases, 54
synthetases, 54
systemic lupus erythematosus (SLE), 84, 521
OxS, 499

T
tachycardia, 286, 320, 327–9, 343, 529
tachykinins, 581
tachypnea, 257, 286
Tangier disease, 88, 215, 233
Tanner Stage 3 breast development, 557
taste, impairment by Zn deficiency, 140
TATA box, 441, 462
TATA-binding protein (TBP), 462
taurine, 319, 404
amide linkages, 217
taurochenodeoxycholic acids, 217
taurocholic acids, 217
Tay–Sachs disease, 384
teeth, transparent and discolored, 389
telangiectasia, 587, 601
telomerase, 605
telomeres, 430, 605
telopeptides, 346, 356
tendon xanthomas, 235, 243
tendons, 14
lipid deposits on, 235
weak, 389
teratogenicity
and vitamin A, 129
and vitamin supplementation, 139
testes, 532
disorders of, 534
Leydig cells, 220, 532
Sertoli cells, 532
and steroid hormones, 219
testosterone secretion by, 533
testosterone, 218, 352, 523, 532
biochemical actions in males, 533
clinical disorders in males, 534–5
mechanism of action, 534
metabolism, 140
tetany, stimulated by hypocalcemia, 355
tetra-antennary chains, 361
tetra-iodothyronine, 527
tetracycline, 452
tetrahydrobiopterin (BH₄), 258, 578–80
tetrahydrobiopterin cofactor, 258
tetrahydrofolate, 135, 421–2
trap, 137
Tetrahymena, 448
tetrapyrrole ring, 36, 102
tetrodotoxin, 91
β-thalassemia, 45
theophylline, 164, 549
therapy, chronic uridine, 419
thermogenesis, 106, 528
thermogenin (UCP1), 106
thiamin, 178, 181
and calorific intake, 133
and carboxylation, 133
deficiency, 133, 308
thiamin pyrophosphate, 133
thiamine, 135
treatment for PDC deficiency, 179
thiamine pyrophosphate, 183
and PDC activity, 178
structure, 179
thiazolidinediones, 1, 233, 275, 292
thienopyridines, 555
thioester bond, 183

thioesters, 147, 183
thiohemiacetal, 147
thiokinase, 190
thiol reagent, 20
thiolase, 192
thioredoxin, 422, 501
thioredoxin reductase, 422
thiosulfate, 110
three-point attachment, 182
threonine, 9, 15, 21, 85, 161, 166
polarity/hydrophobicity, 37
residues, 163, 167
threonine dehydratase, 247
thrombin, 25, 60, 63, 67, 72–4
in blood clotting cascade, 396
role in hemostasis, 72
thrombin–thrombomodulin complex, 74
thrombocytes (platelets), 26
thrombocytopenia, 67, 84
thrombocytosis, 131
thromboembolic disease, and HRT, 356
thromboembolism, venous, 74
thrombomodulin, 74
thromboplastin, 25
thrombosis, 63–76, 240
acute coronary, 69
arterial, 63, 68
risk of, 132
venous, 63, 380
thrombospondin, 346
thromboxane, 68, 555
A₂ (TXA₂), 64–5
production by platelets, 66
thromboxane synthase, 66
thrombus, 67
thymidine, 419–20
thymidine kinase (TK), 61, 419
thymidine monophosphate (TMP), 421
thymidine triphosphate (TTP), 417
thymidylate synthase, 421–2
thymine, 136, 413
bonding, 441
in DNA, 426
thymine dimer, 434
thymine triphosphate analog, 433
thymus, 25, 510
thyreoliberin (TRH), 305
thyroglobulin, iodination of, 527–8
thyroid
carcinoma, 467
disease, 106, 355, 528–9
function, clinical disorders of, 528–9
function tests, reference values, 610
gland, 527
hormone, 104, 106
and bone resorption, 352
regulation by, 111
stimulating hormone (TSH), 353, 526–7
thyroid-binding globulin (TBG), 524
thyrotoxicity, 528
thyrotoxicosis, 557
thyrotropin, 526–7
thyrotropin releasing hormone (TRH), 523, 526
thyroxine, 353, 524, 541
deiodination of, 141
(T₄), 527–8
tibia, 389
ticlopicline, 555
ticlopidine, 68
tingling, stimulated by hypocalcemia, 355
tissue factor pathway inhibitor (TPFI), 73–4
α-tocopherol, 131, 239
tocopherols, 131, 503–4
tocotrienol, 504
tolerable upper intake level (UL), 299–300
tolbutamide, 88

tongue
enlarged, 538
inflammation of, 133
tonsils, 510
in Tangier disease, 233
torticollis, 566
toxins, plant and mould, 110
trace elements, 2, 139–41
toxicity of, 127
trace metals, 127, 304
reference values, 611
trachea, 336
tranquilizers, 79
trans-acting factors, 462
see also transcription factors
trans-fatty acids, 194
transacetylase, 179
transaldolase, 152
transaminases, 409
transamination, 247
transcobalamins, 137–8
transcription, 437
factors, 461–4, 541–2, 548, 584, 589, 595
NKκB, 288–9
of RNA, 440–2
unit, 462
transferases, 53, 133
Golgi, 369
transferrin, 28–30, 140, 371, 402
lacking sialic acid, 371, 560
as nutritional marker, 306
synthesis, 32
transformation, 481
transforming growth factor (TGF), 509, 542
transforming growth factor-β (TGF-β), 589
transglutaminase, 72
transglycosylase, 158–9
transient ischemic attacks, 239
transketolase, 152
translation, 447
translocases, 82, 96
ADP–ATP, 98
inhibitors of, 109–10
ATP–ADP, 86
in inner mitochondrial membrane (TIM complexes), 96, 98
in outer mitochondrial membrane (TOM complexes), 96, 98
phosphate, 98
translocation, 454
transmethylglutaconate shunt, 211
transmissible spongiform encephalopathies, 23
transphosphorylation, 584
transplants, immune response to, 514
transport, 77–92
active, 85–7
antiport (countertransport) mechanism, 87
by channels and pores, 84–5
of carbohydrates, 118
of Ca²⁺ in muscle, 87–8
(cotransport) symport mechanism, 87
defective glucose, 85
in digestion, 115
facilitated secondary active, 87
kinetics of diffusion, 83
processes, types of, 80–91
systems, examples of, 87–9
uniport (monoport) mechanism, 87
transporters, 82
ATP-binding cassette (ABC), 87
and diseases, 88
glucose (uniporters), 83–4
classification of, 84
GLUT-1, 82–3, 85, 88, 90, 144, 149, 401
GLUT-2, 83–4, 88–90, 120, 158–9, 278, 401
GLUT-4, 84, 167, 172, 261, 276, 282, 401
GLUT-5, 83, 90, 120

membrane, 124
for monosaccharides, 118–20
primary active, 87
sodium glucose, 89, 118
transthyretin
as nutritional marker, 306
synthesis, 32
transverse (T) tubules, 87
tranylcypromine, 576
trauma, 96, 344, 574
multiple, 286
trehalose, 117
trembling, 278
tremor, 577
tri-antennary chains, 361
tri-iodothyronine (T_3), 215, 353, 527–8
triacylglycerol (TAG), 77, 120–3, 176
synthesis of, 121–3, 203–4, 206
transport of, 225
tricarboxylic acid cycle (TCA cycle), 3, 99, 110, 170, 175–87, 189
amphibolic nature of, 176
biosyntheses linked to, 175–6
deficiencies in pyruvate metabolism in, 181
energy production, 175, 184
enzymes and reactions of, 180–4
interconversion of fuels and metabolites in, 175
limitation of activity, 282
location of, 175
metabolic defects in, 175
regulation of, 184–6
and urea cycle, 247–8, 250
trichloroacetic acid, 88
triglycerides, 77, 120, 168
hydrolysis, 189
levels, interpretation of, 242
storage, 166
in adipose, 158, 186
transport of, 231
trimethoprim, 136, 421
trinitrotoluene (TNT), 107
trinucleotide repeats, 490
triolein, 77
triose, 117
triose phosphates, 170
tripeptide glutathione (GSH), cysteine containing, 150–1
tripeptides, 13, 123, 125
trisaccharides, 116
tristearin, 77
tropocollagen, 14
tropoelastin, 391
tropomyosin, 265–7
troponins, 265–7
cardiac, measurement of, 270
Trousseau's sign, 355
Trypanosoma brucei, 380
trypanosomes, variable surface antigens of, 380
trypsin, 22, 52, 59–60, 124–5, 246
substrate binding sites of, 53
trypsinogen, 60
tryptophan, 9, 15, 21, 37, 85, 255
conversion to serotonin, 578–9
synthesis of niacin from, 133
tryptophan hydroxylase, 578, 580
tuberculosis, 514
tumor necrosis factor (TNF), 285, 509, 592
receptor, 592
receptor associated death domain protein (TRADD), 592
tumor suppressor genes, 593, 595–6
deleted in colon carcinoma (DCC), 593
tumors
adrenal, 329, 467, 536
benign, 594
carcinoid, 53
catecholamine-secreting, 329
flushing attacks caused by, 579
hypothalamic, 538
immune response to, 514

laryngeal, 355
malignant, 594
occult, 531
ovarian, 536
pancreatic, 538
pharyngeal, 355
pituitary, 531, 534, 538–9
prolactin-secreting, 539
PTHrP in, 354
secondary (metastases), 594
steroid producing, 213
tunicamycin, 367, 370
turgor
poor, 329
reduced, 343
Turner's syndrome, 536
two-dimensional electrophoresis, 23
Tylenol, 607
type V disease, 279
tyramine, 576
tyrosinase, 258
tyrosine, 9, 15, 37, 85, 166
degradation, 138
hydroxylation, 258
residues, 157, 167
tyrosine hydroxylase, 578, 580
deficiency, 579
tyrosine kinase, 167, 538, 584

U
ubiquinone, 98–102, 108, 606
cytochrome c reductase, 101
electron transport system, 417
ubiquitin, 402, 457
carrier protein (E2), 457
role of, 457
ulceration, scarring from, 343
ulcers, 66
bacterial-induced, 91
duodenal, 91
foot, 289
gastric, 91, 123
peptic, 91
ultracentrifugation, 226
ultrafiltration, 17
ultrasound imaging, 121
ultraviolet (UV) radiation, 348
uncouplers, 106
proton transport by, 107
uncoupling proteins (UPC), 106–7
uniporters, 83–4
unsteadiness, 133
uracil, 413, 419–20
nucleotides in RNA, 437
uracil deoxyribonucleotide, 421
uracil phosphoribosyl transferase (UPRTase), 419
urea, 15, 52, 80
excreted in urine, 170, 245
incorporation of N, 247–8
reference values, 610
serum levels of, 325, 328
synthesis, 251–2
urea cycle, 170, 183, 247
and ammonia, 402–3
carbamoyl phosphate in, 417
and central metabolism, 249–53
enzymes of, 251
in mitochondria and cytosol, 250–2
regulation of, 252–3
sources of N, 248
and TCA cycle, 250
X-linked defects in, 253
urease, 52, 248
β-ureidoisobutyrate, 421
β-ureidopropionase, 421
β-ureidopropionate, 421
uremia, 312
uric acid, 245, 417
accumulation of, 418
from human purines, 416–17
oxidation, 422
serum measurement, 422
toxicity, 418
uricase, 422

uridine, 420
residues, 442
uridine diphosphate (UDP), 403
glucuronyl transferase, 411
uridine diphosphate galactose (UDP-Gal), 362
uridine diphosphate glucose (UDP-Glc), 158, 362, 365
uridine diphosphate glucose pyrophosphorylase, 158–9
uridine monophosphate (UMP), 417
uridine monophosphate kinase, 419
uridine monophosphate synthase, 418–19
channeling by, 418
uridine phosphorylase, 420
uridylate, 421
urinalysis
disease diagnosis, 323
dry tests, 324
urinary tract infections, 385
urine, 8, 321–4, 576
analysis and disease diagnosis, 323
Bence-Jones proteins, 32
calcium excretion, 352
catecholamines, 353
dark, 155, 411–12
dilution, assessment, 269
dry testing, 324
glucose, test for diabetes, 295
increased passage of, 125
ketone bodies, 195
ketones, 295
maple syrup odor, 259
nitrogen excretion and balance, 306
orotic acid in, 419, 421
steroid hormones, excretion of, 220
steroid metabolites, excretion of, 213
vitamins, excretion of, 133
urobilin, 411–12
urobilinogen, 323–4, 411
urokinase, 74–5
uroporphyrinogen III, 403
urticaria, 509
US Preventive Services Taskforce (2003), 139
uterus, 356

V
vaccination, and specific immune response, 519
valine, 9, 47, 53, 85, 391, 448
accumulation of, 323
catabolism of, 178
valinomycin, 83
vanadium, 141
vanillylmandelic acid, 576–7
varicella-zoster virus (VZV), 61
vascular endothelial growth factor (VEGF), 205
vascular tone, control of, 326–8
vascular wall, 398
vasoactive intestinal peptide (VIP), 278, 581
vasoconstriction, 66, 236, 238
angiotensin II-induced, 327
serotonin induced, 579
vasodilation, 66, 236, 238, 500
caused by dopamine, 578
caused by NO, 236
vasodilators, 65
vasopressin, 67, 286, 319, 525
control of renal water and sodium, 330
control of water reabsorption by, 328–9
increase in permeability by, 329
increase in response to stress, 529
secretion, disorders of, 325
and water control, 321
in water and electrolyte disorders, 330–1
vegetarianism, nutrient deficiencies in, 302

vegetative behaviors, serotonin implicated in, 579
veins, pulmonary, 338
venom
puffer fish, 91
snake, 91, 555, 565
venous stasis, 348
verapamil, 91
vertigo, 383
Vibrio cholerae, 385, 545
villi, intestinal, 113
viral genes, 595–6
viruses, 591
vision
blurred, 567
double, 129, 581
mechanism of, 566
vitamin A, 128–9, 220
antioxidant, 503–4
deficiency, 129
protective role, 129
sources of, 129
storage in liver, 129
structure, metabolism, and function, 128
supplementation, 139
toxicity of, 129, 353
vitamin B-complex, 133–5
action as coenzymes, 133
deficiency, 133
lack of storage capacity, 133
structure, sources, and deficiency diseases of, 134
vitamin B_1 see thiamin
vitamin B_2 see riboflavin
vitamin B_3 see niacin
vitamin B_6 see pyridoxine
vitamin B_{12}, 136–8, 193
deficiency, 137
digestion, absorption, and transport, 137
and folate, 136–7
and heme structure, 136
need for supplements, 137–9
structure, 136
transport proteins, 138
vitamin C, 138, 239, 503
antioxidant, 503–4
aqueous-phase, 503
role of, 138
deficiency, 66, 138, 389
lability of, 138
as reducing agent, 138
sources of, 138
structure and synthesis of, 139
supplementation, 139
vitamin D, 129–31, 220–1, 348, 541
abnormal metabolism of, 355–6
active metabolite of, 350
deficiency, 130–1
causes of, 35–6
maternal, 354
main storage form of, 350
metabolism, 351
and osteoporosis prevention, 356
sources of, 130
structure, function, and metabolism, 130
supplements, 131, 139
synthesis, 348
toxicity, 131, 354
vitamin D_2, 129, 348, 353
vitamin D_3, 129, 220–1, 348, 353
formation and hydroxylation of, 221
vitamin E, 131, 239
antioxidant, 503–4
function of, 131
in cancer prevention, 312
deficiency, 131
sources of, 131
structure of, 131
supplementation, 139
vitamin K, 131–3
and blood coagulation, 131–2
and carboxylation of glutamate, 132

deficiency, 71, 132
and hydroquinone, 133
inhibitors, 132
sources of, 132
structure and nomenclature, 132
vitamins, 2, 127–42, 304
as coenzymes, 127
dietary supplementation of, 139
fat-soluble, 127–33
storage, 128
hormone-like action, 128
reference values for, 612
sources of, 139
toxicity, 128
water-soluble, 127, 133–9
voltage, changes in, 571
vomiting, 121, 129, 252, 354, 483, 531
during therapy, 578
and fluid balance, 115
Mg deficiency in, 303
profuse, 343
severe, 567
von Gierke's disease, 279
von Willebrand disease, 67
von Willebrand factor (vWF), 64, 66–7

W
waist-to-hip ratio, 306
Waldenström's macroglobulinemia, 32
warfarin, 28, 69, 71, 74, 132
water, 1, 3, 13, 93, 98, 144, 148, 303–4
balance, 319
bodily distribution of, 316
body, compartments, 315–17
deficit, 329
and electrolyte balance, 315–32
elimination of, 13
in GI tract, 114
ICF–ECF redistribution, 318
insensible loss, 286, 319
metabolism, 315–17, 330–1
result of excess, 330
status assessment, 331
water–lipid interface, 121
Watson, JD, 425
Watson–Crick base pairs, 429
weakness in limbs, 567
weight loss, 483
and renal failure, 307
weight reduction, 309–10
Werner's syndrome, 601, 603

Wernicke–Korsakoff psychosis, 133
Wernicke–Korsakoff syndrome, 308
western blot analysis, 265
western blots, 477
wheat gluten antibodies, 125
wheat protein sensitivity, 125
white cells, 48
whooping cough, 545
Wilson's disease, 29, 86, 141, 402, 409
Wolffian ducts, 533
Women's Health Initiative (WHI), 356
Wuthrich, K, 23

X
X chromosome, inactivation, 469
X-linked severe combined immunodeficiency (X-SCID), 586
X-ray crystallography, 15, 21, 23
xanthelasma, and lipid disorder, 243
xanthine, 417–18
xanthine monophosphate (XMP), 414
xanthine oxidase (XO), 417–18
xanthomas, 235, 243
xanthosine, 417
xenobiotics, 87
xeroderma pigmentosum, 425
genetic component of, 431

xylose, formation of, 365
xylulose-5-phosphate, 152

Y
yeasts, 16, 83, 432, 482, 587
anaerobic glycolysis in, 148
artificial chromosomes (YACs), 482
insulin gene copies, 483
origin recognition complex (ORC), 432
receptor pathways in, 546

Z
Zellweger syndrome, 88, 190, 194
Zidovudine, 433
zinc, 139–40
absorption, 140
deficiency, 140
oral treatment with, 86
prosthetic, 127
zinc finger, 220, 463, 465
region, 464–5
zwitterion, 10, 12
zymogens, 60, 124
as cause of hemophilia, 60
digestive, 115–16